D1558041

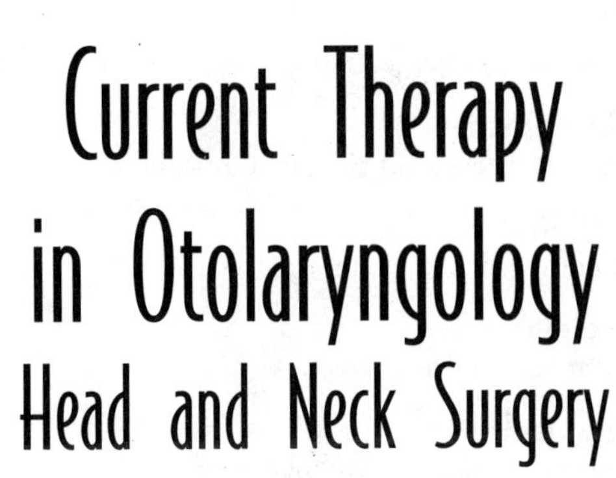

Current Therapy in Otolaryngology Head and Neck Surgery

CURRENT THERAPY SERIES

Bardin:
Current Therapy in Endocrinology and Metabolism

Bayless:
Current Therapy in Gastroenterology and Liver Disease

Brain, Carbone:
Current Therapy in Hematology–Oncology

Callaham:
Current Practice of Emergency Medicine

Cameron:
Current Surgical Therapy

Ernst, Stanley:
Current Therapy in Vascular Surgery

Fazio:
Current Therapy in Colon and Rectal Surgery

Garcia, Mastroianni, Amelar, Dubin:
Current Therapy of Infertility

Gates:
Current Therapy in Otolaryngology—Head and Neck Surgery

Glassock:
Current Therapy in Nephrology and Hypertension

Grillo, Austen, Wilkens, Mathisen, Vlahakes:
Current Therapy in Cardiothoracic Surgery

Johnson, Griffin:
Current Therapy in Neurologic Disease

Kassirer, Greene:
Current Therapy in Adult Medicine

Lichtenstein, Fauci:
Current Therapy in Allergy, Immunology, and Rheumatology

Parrillo:
Current Therapy in Critical Care Medicine

Schlossberg:
Current Therapy of Infectious Disease

Torg, Shephard:
Current Therapy in Sports Medicine

Trunkey, Lewis:
Current Therapy of Trauma

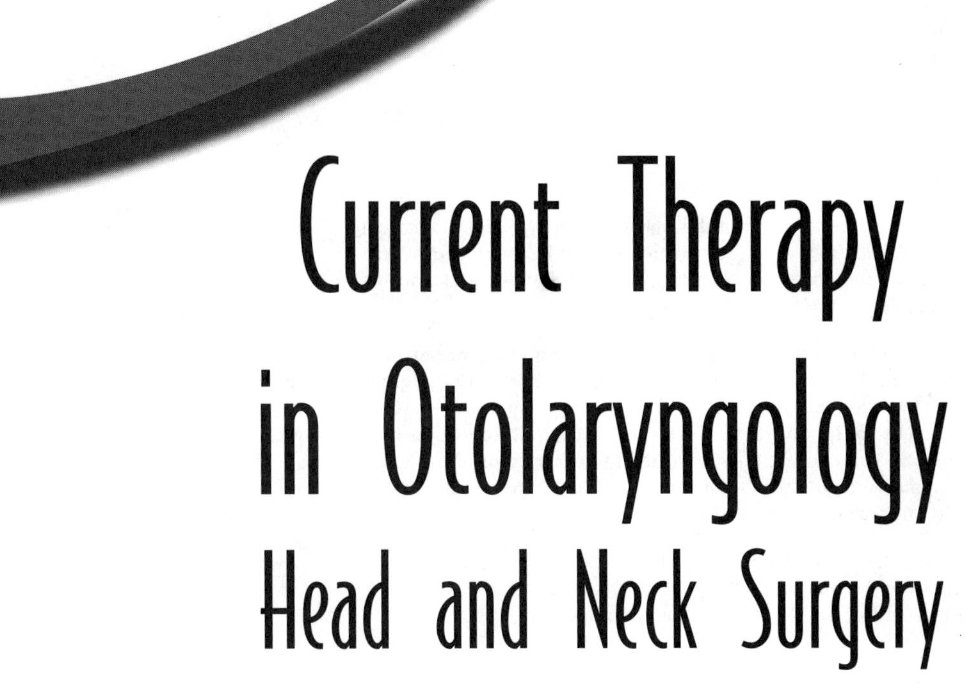

Current Therapy in Otolaryngology Head and Neck Surgery

SIXTH EDITION

Edited by

George A. Gates, M.D., F.A.C.S.

Professor of Otolaryngology—Head and Neck Surgery
Director, Virginia Merrill Bloedel Hearing Research Center
University of Washington
Seattle, Washington

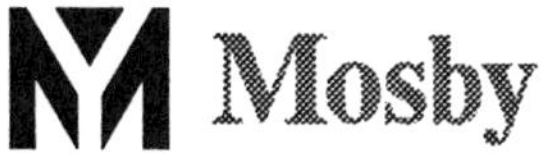

St. Louis Baltimore Boston Carlsbad Chicago Minneapolis New York Philadelphia Portland
London Milan Sydney Tokyo Toronto

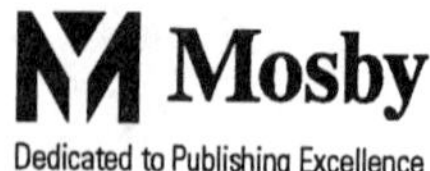

Dedicated to Publishing Excellence

A Times Mirror Company

Senior Managing Editor: Lynne Gery
Editorial Assistant: Amanda Starr
Production Manager: Chris Baumle
Production Editor: Anthony Trioli
Manufacturing Supervisor: William A. Winneberger, Jr.
Design Manager: Carolyn O'Brien

Sixth Edition

Printed in the United States of America
Composition by Maryland Composition Company, Inc.
Printing/binding by Maple-Vail Book Manufacturing Group

Mosby–Year Book, Inc.
11830 Westline Industrial Drive
St. Louis, MO 63146

ISBN: 0-8151-3560-2

99 00 01 02 03 / 9 8 7 6 5 4 3 2 1

Contributors

George L. Adams, M.D., F.A.C.S.
Professor and Head, Department of Otolaryngology, University of Minnesota Medical School, Minneapolis, Minnesota

Malignant Tumors of the Parotid Gland

Kedar K. Adour, M.D.
Senior Consultant and Director of Research, Department of Head and Neck Surgery, and Chairman, Cranial Nerve Research Clinic, Kaiser Permanente Medical Center, Oakland, California

Idiopathic Facial Paralysis

James C. Alex, M.D.
Assistant Professor, Section of Otolaryngology, and Director, Division of Facial Plastic and Reconstructive Surgery, Yale University School of Medicine, New Haven, Connecticut

Permanent Facial Paralysis

Ronald G. Amedee, M.D., F.A.C.S.
Professor, Department of Otolaryngology—Head and Neck Surgery, Tulane University School of Medicine; Staff Surgeon, Tulane University Hospital and Clinic, New Orleans, Louisiana

Wegener's Granulomatosis

W. Douglas Appling, M.D., F.A.C.S.
Clinical Assistant Professor, Department of Otorhinolaryngology and Communicative Sciences, Baylor College of Medicine, Houston, Texas

Zygomatic Fracture

Moises A. Arriaga, M.D.
Adjunct Associate Professor of Surgery, Otorhinolaryngology and Neurosurgery, and Director, Hearing and Balance Center, Allegheny University of the Health Sciences; Associate Clinical Professor of Otolaryngology, University of Pittsburgh School of Medicine, Pittsburgh, Pennsylvania

Traumatic Facial Paralysis

Byron J. Bailey, M.D., F.A.C.S.
Wiess Professor and Chairman, Department of Otolaryngology, University of Texas Medical Branch, Galveston, Texas

Glottic Carcinoma

Shan R. Baker, M.D.
Professor of Otolaryngology and Chief, Division of Facial Plastic Surgery, University of Michigan Medical School, Ann Arbor, Michigan

Cancer of the Lip

Robert W. Bastian, M.D.
Associate Professor of Otolaryngology, Loyola University of Chicago Stritch School of Medicine, Maywood, Illinois

Vocal Problems of Singers

Olga Bedoya, M.D.
Research Assistant, Department of Otolaryngology—Head and Neck Surgery, Northwestern University Medical School, Chicago, Illinois

Cholesteatoma

Joel M. Bernstein, M.D.
Clinical Associate Professor of Otolaryngology and Pediatrics, State University of New York at Buffalo School of Medicine and Biomedical Science, Buffalo, New York

Otitis Media

F. Owen Black, M.D., F.A.C.S.
Director, Neurotology Research, Legacy Holladay Park Medical Center, Portland, Oregon

Perilymphatic Fistula

Elizabeth Blair, M.D., MAJ., MC, USA
Assistant Professor, Department of Surgery, Uniformed Services University of the Health Sciences, Bethesda, Maryland; Chief of Head and Neck Surgery, Otolaryngology Service, Walter Reed Army Medical Center, Washington, D.C.

Thyroid Nodule

Charles D. Bluestone, M.D.
Eberly Professor of Pediatric Otolaryngology, University of Pittsburgh School of Medicine; Director of Pediatric Otolaryngology, Children's Hospital of Pittsburgh, Pittsburgh, Pennsylvania

Perilymphatic Fistula in Children

Charles M. Bower, M.D.
Associate Professor, Department of Otolaryngology—Head and Neck Surgery, University of Arkansas for Medical Sciences, Little Rock, Arkansas
Invasive Fungal Rhinosinusitis

Linda Brodsky, M.D.
Professor of Otolaryngology and Pediatrics, State University of New York at Buffalo School of Medicine and Biomedical Sciences; Director, Pediatric Otolaryngology, Children's Hospital of Buffalo, Buffalo, New York
Tonsil and Adenoid Disorders

Daniel E. Bruegger, M.D.
Assistant Professor, Department of Otolaryngology, University of Kansas School of Medicine, Kansas City, Kansas; Section Chief, Division of Otolaryngology, Children's Mercy Hospital, Kansas City, Missouri
Hyperparathyroidism

Lawrence P. Burgess, M.D., F.A.C.S., LTC., MC, USA
Clinical Professor of Surgery, Uniformed Services University of the Health Sciences, Bethesda, Maryland; Chief of Surgery, Tripler Army Medical Center, Tripler, Hawaii
Large Facial Wounds

Thomas C. Calcaterra, M.D.
Professor of Surgery, Division of Head and Neck Surgery, UCLA School of Medicine, Los Angeles, California
Inverting Papilloma

Karen H. Calhoun, M.D., F.A.C.S.
Professor and Vice Chair, Department of Otolaryngology, University of Texas Medical Branch, Galveston, Texas
Skin Cancer

Stephen P. Cass, M.D., M.P.H.
Associate Professor of Otolaryngology, University of Pittsburgh School of Medicine, Pittsburgh, Pennsylvania
Hemifacial Spasm

Yew-Meng Chan, M.D.
Senior Registrar, Department of Otolaryngology, Singapore General Hospital, Singapore
Cerebrospinal Fluid Otorrhea

W. Gregory Chernoff, B.Sc., M.D., F.R.C.S.C.
Clinical Assistant Professor, Department of Otolaryngology, Indiana University School of Medicine; Private Practice, Chernoff Plastic Surgery and Laser Center, Laser Skin Care Salons International, Inc., Indianapolis, Indiana
The Wrinkled Face

Martin J. Citardi, M.D.
Assistant Professor, St. Louis University School of Medicine, St. Louis, Missouri
Refractory Posterior Epistaxis

William D. Clark, M.D., D.D.S.
Associate Clinical Professor of Otolaryngology, The University of Texas Health Science Center at San Antonio, San Antonio; Chairman, Department of Otolaryngology, Wilford Hall Medical Center, Lackland Air Force Base, Texas
Mandibular Fracture

Lanny Garth Close, M.D., F.A.C.S.
Howard W. Smith Professor and Chairman, Department of Otolaryngology—Head and Neck Surgery, Columbia University College of Physicians and Surgeons; Director, Department of Otolaryngology—Head and Neck Surgery, Columbia Presbyterian Medical Center, New York, New York
Frontal Sinus Fracture

Wayne B. Colin, D.M.D., M.D.
Assistant Professor, Department of Otolaryngology—Head and Neck Surgery, University of Tennessee, Memphis, College of Medicine, Memphis, Tennessee
Pharyngoesophageal Reconstruction

Jacquelynne P. Corey, M.D., F.A.C.S., F.A.A.O.A.
Associate Professor, Department of Otolaryngology—Head and Neck Surgery, University of Chicago Pritzker School of Medicine, Chicago, Illinois
Allergic Fungal Sinusitis

Robin T. Cotton, M.D.
Professor, Department of Otolaryngology and Maxillofacial Surgery, University of Cincinnati College of Medicine; Director, Department of Otolaryngology and Maxillofacial Surgery, Children's Hospital Medical Center, Cincinnati, Ohio
Subglottic Stenosis in Children

Beverly J. Cowart, Ph.D.
Adjunct Assistant Professor, Department of Otolaryngology—Head and Neck Surgery, Jefferson Medical College of Thomas Jefferson University, Philadelphia, Pennsylvania
Anosmia

Charles W. Cummings, M.D.
Professor and Director, Department of Otolaryngology—Head and Neck Surgery, The Johns Hopkins University School of Medicine, Baltimore, Maryland
Carcinoma of the Tongue Base

Judith M. Czaja, M.D.
Head and Neck Fellow, Department of Otolaryngology—Head and Neck Surgery, University of Cincinnati College of Medicine, Cincinnati, Ohio
Tracheal Neoplasms

Bruce J. Davidson, M.D., F.A.C.S.
Assistant Professor, Department of Otolaryngology—Head and Neck Surgery, Georgetown University School of Medicine; Chief of Surgical Services, Section of Otolaryngology, V.A. Medical Center, Washington, D.C.
Cervical Metastasis

Steven H. Dayan, M.D.
Chief Resident, Department of Otolaryngology—Head and Neck Surgery, University of Illinois College of Medicine, Chicago, Illinois
Revision Rhinoplasty

Paul C. Drago; M.D.
Central Carolina Ear, Nose, and Throat Center, Rock Hill, South Carolina
The Crooked Nose

Larry G. Duckert, M.D.
Professor, Department of Otolaryngology—Head and Neck Surgery, University of Washington School of Medicine; Attending Physician, University of Washington Medical Center, Seattle, Washington
Acoustic Neuroma

James A. Duncavage, M.D., F.A.C.S.
Associate Professor and Vice Chairman of Otolaryngology, Vanderbilt University School of Medicine; Attending Physician, V.A. Medical Center and Vanderbilt Medical Clinic, Nashville, Tennessee
Nasal Polyposis

James N. Endicott, M.D.
Professor and Director, Division of Otolaryngology, University of South Florida College of Medicine; Program Leader, Head and Neck Oncology Program, H. Lee Moffitt Cancer Center and Research Institute, Tampa, Florida
Deep Neck Infection

Jay B. Farrior, M.D.
Clinical Associate Professor, University of South Florida College of Medicine, Tampa, Florida
External Otitis

Jose N. Fayad, M.D.
Clinical Fellow, House Ear Institute, Los Angeles, California
Frontal Sinus Fracture

Ugo Fisch, M.D.
Professor and Head, Department of Otorhinolaryngology, University Hospital, Zurich, Switzerland
The Internal Carotid Artery in Skull Base Surgery

James W. Forsen, Jr., M.D.
Instructor, Pediatric Otolaryngology, Washington University School of Medicine, St. Louis, Missouri
Caustic Ingestion

John L. Frodel, Jr., M.D.
Associate Professor and Director, Division of Facial Plastic Surgery, Department of Otolaryngology—Head and Neck Surgery, The Johns Hopkins University School of Medicine, Baltimore, Maryland
Microtia: Reconstructive Methods
Midface Fracture

Gerry F. Funk, M.D.
Associate Professor, Department of Otolaryngology—Head and Neck Surgery, University of Iowa College of Medicine; Attending Physician, University of Iowa Hospitals and Clinics, Iowa City, Iowa
Pharyngocutaneous Fistula

Neal D. Futran, M.D., D.M.D.
Assistant Professor, Department of Otolaryngology—Head and Neck Surgery, University of Washington School of Medicine; Attending Surgeon, Harborview Medical Center and V.A. Medical Center, Seattle, Washington
Mandibular Defect

Bruce J. Gantz, M.D., F.A.C.S.
Professor and Head, Department of Otolaryngology—Head and Neck Surgery, University of Iowa College of Medicine, Iowa City, Iowa
Meniere's Disease: Medical Therapy

George A. Gates, M.D., F.A.C.S.
Professor of Otolaryngology—Head and Neck Surgery; Director, Virginia Merrill Bloedel Hearing Research Center, University of Washington, Seattle, Washington
Acoustic Neuroma

Paul W. Gidley, M.D.
Assistant Professor, Department of Otolaryngology, University of Texas Medical School at Houston, Houston, Texas
Meniere's Disease: Medical Therapy

Richard E. Gliklich, M.D.
Assistant Professor, Harvard Medical School; Attending Physician, Division of Facial Plastic and Reconstructive Surgery, Department of Otolaryngology, Massachusetts Eye and Ear Infirmary, Boston, Massachusetts
Proptosis

Jack L. Gluckman, M.D.
Professor and Chairman, Department of Otolaryngology—Head and Neck Surgery, University of Cincinnati College of Medicine, Cincinnati, Ohio
Tracheal Neoplasms

Helmuth Goepfert, M.D.
Professor and Chairman, Department of Head and Neck Surgery, University of Texas M.D. Anderson Cancer Center; Adjunct Professor, Department of Otolaryngology, Baylor College of Medicine, Houston, Texas
Thyroid Nodule

John D. Goldenberg, M.D.
Head and Neck Oncology and Microvascular Surgery Fellow, University of Pennsylvania School of Medicine, Philadelphia, Pennsylvania
Malnutrition from Cancer

Iain L. Grant, M.D.
Senior Research Associate, Department of Otolaryngology, Ohio State University College of Medicine, Columbus, Ohio
Otosclerosis

John H. Greinwald, Jr., M.D., Cdr., MC, USNR
Assistant Clinical Professor, Department of Otolaryngology—Head and Neck Surgery, Eastern Virginia Medical School, Norfolk, Virginia, and Uniformed Services University of the Health Sciences, Bethesda, Maryland; Pediatric Otolaryngology Fellow, University of Iowa Hospitals and Clinics, Iowa City, Iowa
Hereditary Hearing Impairment

Carla DeLassus Gress, Sc.D., CCC-SLP
Assistant Clinical Professor, Department of Otolaryngology, University of California, San Francisco School of Medicine, San Francisco, California
Postlaryngectomy Aphonia

Kenneth M. Grundfast, M.D., F.A.C.S., F.A.A.P.
Professor of Otolaryngology and Pediatrics, Georgetown University School of Medicine, Washington, D.C.
Progressive Sensorineural Hearing Loss

Robert Guida, M.D., F.A.C.S.
Director, Facial Plastic and Reconstructive Surgery, Department of Otolaryngology, Cornell University Medical Center, New York, New York
Saddle Nose Deformity

A. Julianna Gulya, M.D.
Professor, Department of Otolaryngology—Head and Neck Surgery, Georgetown University School of Medicine, Washington, D.C.; Chief, Clinical Trials Branch, National Institute on Deafness and Other Communicative Disorders, National Institutes of Health, Rockville, Maryland
Sensorineural Hearing Loss: Rehabilitation

Joseph Haddad, Jr., M.D., F.A.C.S.
Associate Professor and Vice Chairman, Department of Otolaryngology—Head and Neck Surgery, Columbia University College of Physicians and Surgeons; Director, Pediatric Otolaryngology—Head and Neck Surgery, Babies Hospital, New York, New York
Velopharyngeal Insufficiency

Ronald C. Hamaker, M.D.
Private Practice, Head and Neck Surgery Associates, Indianapolis, Indiana
Malignant Melanoma

Cecil W. Hart, M.D.
Professor of Otolaryngology—Head and Neck Surgery, Loyola University of Chicago Stritch School of Medicine, Maywood, Illinois
Vertigo

George T. Hashisaki, M.D.
Assistant Professor, Division of Otology/Neurotology, Department of Otolaryngology—Head and Neck Surgery, University of Virginia School of Medicine, Charlottesville, Virginia
Congenital Aural Atresia

Bruce H. Haughey, M.B., Ch.B., M.S., F.R.A.C.S., F.A.C.S.
Associate Professor and Director, Division of Head and Neck Surgical Oncology, Department of Otolaryngology, Washington University School of Medicine, St. Louis, Missouri
Pharyngoesophageal Reconstruction

Fred S. Herzon, M.D.
Professor of Surgery and Chief, Division of Otolaryngology, University of New Mexico Health Sciences Center, Albuquerque, New Mexico
Peritonsillar Abscess

Barry E. Hirsch, M.D., F.A.C.S.
Associate Professor, Department of Otolaryngology, University of Pittsburgh School of Medicine, Pittsburgh, Pennsylvania
Cancer of the Temporal Bone

Henry T. Hoffman, M.D.
Associate Professor, Department of Otolaryngology, University of Iowa College of Medicine, Iowa City, Iowa
Laryngeal Paralysis

Lauren D. Holinger, M.D.
Professor, Department of Otolaryngology, Northwestern University Medical School; Head, Pediatric Otolaryngology, The Children's Memorial Hospital, Chicago, Illinois
Foreign Bodies of the Airway and Esophagus

Larry A. Hoover, M.D.
Professor and Chairman, Department of Otolaryngology—Head and Neck Surgery, University of Kansas School of Medicine, Kansas City, Kansas
Hyperparathyroidism

John R. Houck, Jr., M.D., F.A.C.S.
Associate Professor, Department of Otorhinolaryngology, The University of Oklahoma Health Sciences Center, Oklahoma City, Oklahoma
Floor of the Mouth Cancer

Gordon B. Hughes, M.D.
Director of Education, Otology and Neurotology; Otolaryngology and Communicative Disorders, Cleveland Clinic Foundation, Cleveland, Ohio
Sudden Hearing Loss

Richard M. Irving, M.D., F.R.C.S.
Clinical Instructor of Otolaryngology, University of California, San Francisco, School of Medicine, San Francisco, California
Facial Nerve Tumors

Mark A. Jabor, M.D.
Chief Resident, Department of Otolaryngology—Head and Neck Surgery, Tulane University School of Medicine, New Orleans, Louisiana
Wegener's Granulomatosis

Robert K. Jackler, M.D.
Professor of Otolaryngology and Neurological Surgery, University of California, San Francisco, School of Medicine, San Francisco, California
Facial Nerve Tumors

C. Gary Jackson, M.D., F.A.C.S.
Clinical Professor, Department of Surgery, Otology and Neurotology, University of North Carolina at Chapel Hill School of Medicine, Chapel Hill, North Carolina; Department of Otolaryngology, Vanderbilt University School of Medicine, Nashville, Tennessee; and Department of Otolaryngology—Head and Neck Surgery, Georgetown University School of Medicine, Washington, D.C.; President, The EAR Foundation and The Otology Group, Nashville, Tennessee; Board of Governors, American Academy of Otolaryngology—Head and Neck Surgery
The Chronic Draining Ear

Pawel J. Jastreboff, Ph.D., Sc.D.
Professor of Surgery and Physiology, University of Maryland School of Medicine, Baltimore, Maryland; Visiting Professor, University College, London, United Kingdom, and Yale University School of Medicine, New Haven, Connecticut; Director, University of Maryland Tinnitus and Hyperacusis Center, Baltimore, Maryland
Tinnitus

Calvin M. Johnson, Jr., M.D.
Director, Hedgewood Surgical Center, New Orleans, Louisiana
The Aging Face

Jonas T. Johnson, M.D.
Professor, Departments of Otolaryngology and Radiation Oncology, Vice Chairman, Department of Otolaryngology, and Director, Division of Head and Neck Oncology and Immunology, University of Pittsburgh School of Medicine, Pittsburgh, Pennsylvania
Obstructive Sleep Apnea

Robert W. Jyung, M.D.
Assistant Professor, Department of Otorhinolaryngology and Broncho-esophagology, and Director, Otology, Neurotology, and Skull Base Surgery, Temple University School of Medicine, Philadelphia, Pennsylvania
Glomus Tumors

Frank M. Kamer, M.D.
Private Practice, Lasky Clinic, Beverly Hills, California
Baggy Eyelids

Donald B. Kamerer, M.D., F.A.C.S.
Professor and Director, Division of Otology, Department of Otolaryngology, University of Pittsburgh School of Medicine, Pittsburgh, Pennsylvania
Cancer of the Temporal Bone

Michael J. Kaplan, M.D.
Associate Professor, Departments of Otolaryngology—Head and Neck Surgery and Neurological Surgery, University of California, San Francisco, School of Medicine, San Francisco, California
Benign Parotid Tumors

Jack M. Kartush, M.D.
Clinical Professor, Department of Otolaryngology, Wayne State University School of Medicine, Detroit; Director, Department of Otology/Neurotology, Providence Hospital, Southfield; President, Michigan Ear Institute, Farmington Hills, Michigan
Meniere's Disease: Surgical Therapy

William M. Keane, M.D.
Professor and Chair, Department of Otolaryngology, Jefferson Medical College of Thomas Jefferson University, Philadelphia, Pennsylvania
Tumors of the Parapharyngeal Space

David C. Kelsall, M.D.
Associate Clinical Professor, Department of Otolaryngology, University of Colorado Health Sciences Center; Private Practice, Otology/Neurotology, Denver Ear Associates, Denver, Colorado
Ossicular Problems in Chronic Otitis Media

Theda C. Kontis, M.D., F.A.C.S.
Instructor, The Johns Hopkins Medical Institutions, Baltimore, Maryland
The Difficult Nasal Tip

Charles F. Koopmann, Jr., M.D., M.H.S.A.
Professor and Associate Chair, Department of Otolaryngology—Head and Neck Surgery, University of Michigan Medical School; Attending Physician, University Hospital and C.S. Mott Children's Hospital, Ann Arbor, and Chelsea Community Hospital, Chelsea, Michigan
Congenital Neck Masses

Frederick A. Kuhn, M.D., F.A.C.S.
Director, Georgia Rhinology and Sinus Center, Savannah, Georgia
Refractory Posterior Epistaxis

Paul R. Lambert, M.D.
Professor and Vice Chairman, Department of Otolaryngology—Head and Neck Surgery; Director, Division of Otology/Neurotology, Department of Otolaryngology—Head and Neck Surgery, University of Virginia School of Medicine, Charlottesville, Virginia
Congenital Aural Atresia

Micheal J. Larouere, M.D.
Clinical Assistant Professor, Department of Otolaryngology, Wayne State University School of Medicine, Detroit; Attending Neurotologist, Michigan Ear Institute, Farmington Hills, Michigan
Meniere's Disease: Surgical Therapy

Wayne F. Larrabee, Jr., M.D.
Clinical Professor, Department of Otolaryngology—Head and Neck Surgery, University of Washington School of Medicine; Attending Physician, Facial Plastic Surgery, Swedish Hospital Medical Center, Seattle, Washington

Chin Disproportion

William Lawson, M.D., D.D.S.
Professor, Department of Otolaryngology—Head and Neck Surgery, Mount Sinai School of Medicine of the City University of New York, New York

Oroantral Fistula

Donald A. Leopold, M.D.
Associate Professor, The Johns Hopkins University School of Medicine, Baltimore, Maryland

Chronic Nasal Obstruction

Paul A. Levine, M.D.
Professor and Chair, Department of Otolaryngology, and Director of Head and Neck Surgical Oncology, University of Virginia Medical School, Charlottesville, Virginia

Esthesioneuroblastoma

William H. Lindsey, M.D.
Assistant Professor, Department of Otolaryngology—Head and Neck Surgery, University of Virginia School of Medicine, Charlottesville, Virginia

Submucous Cleft Palate

William H. Lippy, M.D.
Clinical Assistant Professor, Department of Otolaryngology, Ohio State University College of Medicine, Columbus, Ohio, and Eastern Virginia Medical School, Norfolk, Virginia; Clinical Professor, Northeastern Ohio University College of Medicine, Rootstown, Ohio; Instructor, American Academy of Otolaryngology—Head and Neck Surgery, Alexandria, Virginia; Chief of Otology, St. Joseph Health Center, Warren, Ohio

Otosclerosis

Louis D. Lowry, M.D.
Professor and Vice Chairman, Department of Otolaryngology—Head and Neck Surgery, Jefferson Medical College of Thomas Jefferson University, Philadelphia, Pennsylvania

Anosmia

Carol J. MacArthur, M.D., F.A.C.S., F.A.A.P.
Assistant Clinical Professor, Department of Otolaryngology—Head and Neck Surgery, University of California, Irvine, College of Medicine, Orange, California

Vasoproliferative Tumors in Children

Scott C. Manning, M.D.
Associate Professor, Department of Otolaryngology—Head and Neck Surgery, University of Washington School of Medicine; Chief, Pediatric Otolaryngology—Head and Neck Surgery, Children's Hospital and Medical Center, Seattle, Washington

Orbital Cellulitis and Abscess

Douglas E. Mattox, M.D.
Professor and Head, Department of Otolaryngology—Head and Neck Surgery, University of Maryland School of Medicine, Baltimore, Maryland

Cerebrospinal Fluid Otorrhea

Marc R. Mayberg, M.D.
Professor and Chief of Clinical Services, Department of Neurological Surgery, University of Washington School of Medicine, Seattle, Washington

Acoustic Neuroma

Thomas V. McCaffrey, M.D., Ph.D.
Professor, Mayo Medical School; Consultant, Department of Otorhinolaryngology, Mayo Clinic, Rochester, Minnesota

Carotid Body Tumors

Timothy M. McCulloch, M.D.
Associate Professor, Department of Otolaryngology—Head and Neck Surgery, The University of Iowa College of Medicine, Iowa City, Iowa

Laryngeal Paralysis

Michael J. McKenna, M.D.
Assistant Professor, Department of Otology and Laryngology, Harvard Medical School; Associate Surgeon in Otolaryngology, Massachusetts Eye and Ear Infirmary, Boston, Massachusetts

Glomus Tumors

Jesus E. Medina, M.D.
Professor and Chairman, Department of Otorhinolaryngology, The University of Oklahoma Health Sciences Center, Oklahoma City, Oklahoma

Floor of the Mouth Cancer

Ralph B. Metson, M.D.
Associate Clinical Professor, Department of Otology and Laryngology, Harvard Medical School; Surgeon in Otolaryngology, Massachusetts Eye and Ear Infirmary, Boston, Massachusetts
Lacrimal Obstruction

Alan G. Micco, M.D.
Assistant Professor of Otolaryngology— Head and Neck Surgery, Northwestern University Medical School, Chicago, Illinois
Cholesteatoma

Kris. S. Moe, M.D.
Oberarzt, Otolaryngology—Head and Neck Surgery, University of Zurich Hospital, Zurich, Switzerland
The Internal Carotid Artery in Skull Base Surgery

Aage R. Moller, Ph.D.
Professor, University of Texas at Dallas, Dallas, Texas
Hemifacial Spasm

Gary F. Moore, M.D.
Associate Professor and Vice Chairman, Department of Otolaryngology—Head and Neck Surgery, University of Nebraska College of Medicine, Omaha, Nebraska
Cerebrospinal Fluid Rhinorrhea

Susan H. Morgan, M.Ed.
Instructor, Department of Otolaryngology—Head and Neck Surgery, and Director of Audiology, Georgetown University School of Medicine; Washington, D.C.
Sensorineural Hearing Loss: Rehabilitation

Harlan R. Muntz, M.D.
Associate Professor, Department of Otolaryngology—Head and Neck Surgery, Washington University School of Medicine and St. Louis Children's Hospital, St. Louis, Missouri
Choanal Atresia

Craig S. Murakami, M.D.
Associate Professor, Department of Otolaryngology—Head and Neck Surgery, University of Washington School of Medicine, Seattle, Washington
Saddle Nose Deformity

John J. Murray, M.D., Ph.D.
Associate Professor of Medicine and Pharmacology, Vanderbilt University School of Medicine; Chief Operating Officer, Vanderbilt Asthma, Sinus, and Allergy Program; Attending Physician, Nashville V.A. Hospital, Nashville, Tennessee
Nasal Polyposis

Charles M. Myer III, M.D.
Professor, Department of Otolaryngology and Maxillofacial Surgery, University of Cincinnati College of Medicine and Children's Hospital Medical Center, Cincinnati, Ohio
Head and Neck Neoplasms in Children

Eugene N. Myers, MD
Professor and Chairman, Department of Otolaryngology, University of Pittsburgh School of Medicine; Chairman, Department of Otolaryngology, University of Pittsburgh Medical Center, Pittsburgh, Pennsylvania
Cancer of the Anterior Tongue

Jeffrey N. Myers, M.D., Ph.D.
Assistant Professor and Assistant Surgeon, Department of Head and Neck Surgery, University of Texas M.D. Anderson Cancer Center, Houston, Texas
Cancer of the Anterior Tongue

Robert M. Naclerio, M.D.
Professor and Chief of Otolaryngology—Head and Neck Surgery, University of Chicago Pritzker School of Medicine, Chicago, Illinois
Vasomotor Rhinitis

Joseph B. Nadol, Jr., M.D.
Walter Augustus LeCompte Professor, Department of Otology and Laryngology, Harvard Medical School; Chief of Otolaryngology, Massachusetts Eye and Ear Infirmary, Boston, Massachusetts
Glomus Tumors

Vincent P. Nalbone, M.D.
Private Practice, Las Vegas, Nevada
Allergic Fungal Sinusitis

Quoc A. Nguyen, M.D.
Assistant Clinical Professor, Department of Otolaryngology, University of California, Irvine, College of Medicine, Orange, California
Chronic Nasal Obstruction

Richard D. Nichols, M.D.
Chair Emeritus, Department of Otolaryngology—Head and Neck Surgery, Henry Ford Health System, Detroit, Michigan
Non-Neoplastic Disease of the Salivary Glands

John K. Niparko, M.D.
Associate Professor, Department of Otolaryngology—Head and Neck Surgery, and Director of Otology/Neurotology, The Johns Hopkins University School of Medicine, Baltimore, Maryland
Microtia: Reconstructive Methods

Gary J. Nishioka, M.D., D.M.D.
Clinical Faculty, University of Washington School of Medicine; Attending Physician, Swedish Hospital Medical Center, Seattle, Washington
Chin Disproportion

Fred D. Owens, M.D., M.B.A.
President, Dallas Foundation of Otology, Dallas, Texas
The Draining Mastoid Cavity

Ira D. Papel, M.D., F.A.C.S.
Assistant Professor, The Johns Hopkins Medical Institutions, Baltimore, Maryland
The Difficult Nasal Tip

Norman J. Pastorek, M.D.
Clinical Professor, Department of Otolaryngology, and Clinical Director, Division of Facial Plastic Surgery, New York Hospital-Cornell Medical Center, New York, New York
The Large Nose

Susan C. Pesznecker, R.N.
Neurotology Clinical Research Coordinator, Legacy Holladay Park Medical Center, Portland, Oregon
Perilymphatic Fistula

Eric F. Pinczower, M.D.
Assistant Professor, University of Washington School of Medicine; Attending Physician, University of Washington Medical Center and Harborview Medical Center, Seattle, Washington
Snoring

Anna Maria Pou, M.D.
Assistant Professor, Department of Otolaryngology, University of Texas Medical Branch, Galveston, Texas
Malignant Melanoma

Steven D. Rauch, M.D.
Assistant Professor of Otolaryngology, Harvard Medical School; Surgeon in Otolaryngology, Massachusetts Eye and Ear Infirmary, Boston, Massachusetts
Sensorineural Hearing Loss: Medical Therapy

Allyson M. Ray, M.D.
Clinical Instructor and Fellow, Department of Otolaryngology—Head and Neck Surgery, The Johns Hopkins University School of Medicine, Baltimore, Maryland
Microtia: Reconstructive Methods
Midface Fracture

Anthony J. Reino, M.D., M.Sc., F.A.C.S.
Assistant Clinical Professor, Mount Sinai School of Medicine at the City University of New York, New York; Associate Director and Staff Physician, Section of Otolaryngology, Bronx V.A. Medical Center, Bronx; Assistant Attending Physician, Mount Sinai Medical Center, and St. Luke's Roosevelt Hospital, New York; Attending Physician, Sound Shore Medical Center, New Rochelle, New York
Oroantral Fistula

Dale H. Rice, M.D.
Tiber/Alpert Professor and Chair, Department of Otolaryngology—Head and Neck Surgery, University of Southern California School of Medicine, Los Angeles, California
Angiofibroma

Mark A. Richardson, M.D.
Professor and Deputy Director, Department of Otolaryngology—Head and Neck Surgery, The Johns Hopkins University School of Medicine, Baltimore, Maryland
Drooling

William J. Richtsmeier, M.D., Ph.D.
Professor and Chief, Division of Otolaryngology—Head and Neck Surgery, Department of Surgery, Duke University School of Medicine, Durham, North Carolina
Acute Sinusitis

Franklin M. Rizer, M.D.
Clinical Assistant Professor, Department of Otolaryngology, Ohio State University College of Medicine, Columbus, Ohio; Assistant Clinical Professor, Medical College of Hampton Roads, Norfolk, Virginia, and Northeastern Ohio University College of Medicine, Rootstown, Ohio; Instructor, American Academy of Otolaryngology—Head and Neck Surgery, Alexandria, Virginia
Otosclerosis

Jay K. Roberts, M.D.
Clinical Assistant Professor, University of Rochester School of Medicine and Dentistry, Rochester, New York
Injuries of the Pinna

Thomas Romo III, M.D., F.A.C.S.
Director of Facial Plastic and Reconstructive Surgery, The New York Eye and Ear Infirmary; Chief of Facial Plastic and Reconstructive Surgery, Lenox Hill Hospital, New York, New York
Protruding Ears
Nasal Septal Perforation

Richard M. Rosenfeld, M.D., M.P.H., F.A.A.P.
Associate Professor of Otolaryngology, State University of New York Health Science Center at Brooklyn; Director, Division of Pediatric Otolaryngology, University Hospital of Brooklyn and Long Island College Hospital, Brooklyn, New York
Sinusitis in Children

Philip W. Rouadi, M.D.
Fellow, Allergy and Rhinology, University of Chicago Pritzker School of Medicine, Chicago, Illinois
Vasomotor Rhinitis

Robert Thayer Sataloff, M.D., D.M.A.
Professor of Otolaryngology—Head and Neck Surgery, Jefferson Medical College of Thomas Jefferson University; Adjunct Professor, Otorhinolaryngology—Head and Neck Surgery, University of Pennsylvania School of Medicine, Philadelphia, Pennsylvania, and Department of Otolaryngology—Head and Neck Surgery, Georgetown University School of Medicine, Washington, D.C.; Chairman, Department of Otolaryngology, Allegheny University Hospitals, Graduate, Philadelphia, Pennsylvania
Contact Ulcers and Granulomas of the Larynx

Steven D. Schaefer, M.D., F.A.C.S.
Professor and Chair, Department of Otolaryngology, New York Medical College, Valhalla; Chair, Department of Otolaryngology, New York Eye and Ear Infirmary and Affiliated Hospitals, New York, New York
Acute Laryngeal Trauma

Gary L. Schechter, M.D.
Professor and Chairman, Department of Otolaryngology—Head and Neck Surgery, Eastern Virginia Medical School, Norfolk, Virginia
Dysphagia

Stephan Schmid, M.D.
Associate Professor, Department of Otorhinolaryngology—Head and Neck Surgery, University of Zurich, Zurich, Switzerland
The Internal Carotid Artery in Skull Base Surgery

David E. Schuller, M.D.
Professor and Chair, Department of Otolaryngology; Director, Arthur G. James Cancer Hospital and Research Institute, and Co-Director, Comprehensive Cancer Center, Ohio State University Medical Center, Columbus, Ohio
Far-Advanced Head and Neck Cancer

Arnold G. Schuring, M.D.
Clinical Assistant Professor, Department of Otolaryngology, Ohio State University College of Medicine, Columbus, Ohio; Assistant Clinical Professor, Eastern Virginia Medical School, Norfolk; Instructor, American Academy of Otolaryngology—Head and Neck Surgery, Alexandria, Virginia
Otosclerosis

Robert W. Seibert, M.D.
Professor, Department of Otolaryngology-Head and Neck Surgery, University of Arkansas for Medical Sciences; Chief, Pediatric Otolaryngology, Arkansas Children's Hospital, Little Rock, Arkansas
Invasive Fungal Rhinosinusitis

Craig W. Senders, M.D., F.A.C.S.
Associate Professor, Department of Otolaryngology, University of California, Davis, School of Medicine, Sacramento, California
Unilateral Cleft Lip and Palate

Roy B. Sessions, M.D., F.A.C.S.
Professor and Chairman, Department of Otolaryngology—Head and Neck Surgery, Georgetown University School of Medicine, Washington, D.C.

Cervical Metastasis

Reuben C. Setliff III, M.D.
Private Practice, Setliff Clinic, Sioux Falls, South Dakota

Chronic Ethmoid Sinusitis

Pramod K. Sharma, M.D.
Head and Neck Oncologic Surgery Fellow, Department of Otolaryngology, Ohio State University Medical Center, Columbus, Ohio

Far-Advanced Head and Neck Cancer

Kathleen C.Y. Sie, M.D.
Assistant Professor, Department of Otolaryngology—Head and Neck Surgery, University of Washington School of Medicine; Attending Physician, Pediatric Otolaryngology—Head and Neck Surgery, Children's Hospital and Medical Center, Seattle, Washington

Acute Mastoiditis

Eric J. Simko, M.D.
Clinical Assistant Professor, Department of Surgery, Uniformed Services University of the Health Sciences, Bethesda, Maryland, and Departments of Otolaryngology—Head and Neck Surgery, Eastern Virginia Medical School, Norfolk, Virginia, and University of Texas Medical School at San Antonio, San Antonio; Staff Otolaryngologist, Wilford Hall Medical Center, Lackland Air Force Base, Texas

Mandibular Fracture

Mark I. Singer, M.D., F.A.C.S.
Professor and Vice-Chair, Department of Otolaryngology; Chief, Division of Head and Neck Surgery, University of California, San Francisco, School of Medicine, San Francisco, California

Postlaryngectomy Aphonia

Howard W. Smith, M.D., D.M.D., F.A.C.S.
Clinical Professor of Otolaryngology—Head and Neck Surgery, Columbia University College of Physicians and Surgeons, New York, New York

Velopharyngeal Insufficiency

Richard J.H. Smith, M.D.
Professor and Vice-Chairman, Department of Otolaryngology—Head and Neck Surgery, University of Iowa College of Medicine; Head, Division of Pediatric Otolaryngology, and Director, Molecular Otolaryngology Laboratory, Departments of Otolaryngology—Head and Neck Surgery and Genetics, University of Iowa Hospitals and Clinics, Iowa City, Iowa

Hereditary Hearing Impairment

Robert A. Sofferman, M.D.
Professor and Chairman, Division of Otolaryngology, University of Vermont College of Medicine, Burlington, Vermont

Traumatic Optic Neuropathy

Brendan Curran Stack, Jr., M.D.
Assistant Professor, Department of Otolaryngology, St. Louis University School of Medicine, St. Louis, Missouri

Supraglottic Carcinoma

Sarah A. Stackpole, M.D.
Residency Coordinator, Department of Otolaryngology, Manhattan Eye, Ear, and Throat Hospital; Staff, Department of Otolaryngology, Lenox Hill Hospital, New York, New York

Protruding Ears

J. Gregory Staffel, M.D., F.A.C.S.
Associate Professor, Department of Otolaryngology, University of Texas Health Science Center at San Antonio, San Antonio, Texas

Nasal Fracture

David W. Stepnick, M.D., F.A.C.S.
Associate Professor of Otolaryngology—Head and Neck Surgery, Case Western Reserve University School of Medicine; Director, Residency Training Program, Otolaryngology—Head and Neck Surgery, University Hospitals of Cleveland, Cleveland, Ohio

Facial Scars and Keloids

Michael G. Stewart, M.D., M.P.H., F.A.C.S.
Assistant Professor, Bobby R. Alford Department of Otolaryngology and Communicative Sciences, Baylor College of Medicine; Deputy Chief of Otolaryngology, Ben Taub General Hospital, and Attending Otolaryngologist, The Methodist Hospital, Houston, Texas

Zygomatic Fracture

Sylvan E. Stool, M.D.
Professor, Department of Otolaryngology, University of Colorado School of Medicine; Attending Physician, Department of Pediatric Otolaryngology, The Children's Hospital, Denver, Colorado
Inflammatory Laryngeal Disease in Children

John R. Stram, M.D.
Assistant Professor, Department of Otolaryngology, Boston University School of Medicine, Boston, Massachusetts
Allergic Rhinitis

Marshall Strome, M.D., M.S., F.A.C.S.
Professor, Department of Otolaryngology, The Cleveland Clinic Foundation Health Sciences Center of the Ohio State University; Chairman, Department of Otolaryngology and Communicative Disorders, Cleveland Clinic Foundation, Cleveland, Ohio
Aspiration

Chester L. Strunk, M.D.
Clinical Assistant Professor, University of Texas Medical Branch, Galveston, Texas
Necrotizing Otitis Externa

Fred J. Stucker, M.D., F.A.C.S.
Professor and Chair, Department of Otolaryngology—Head and Neck Surgery, Louisiana State University School of Medicine, Shreveport, Louisiana
The Crooked Nose

Charles A. Syms III, M.D., F.A.C.S.
Assistant Professor of Surgery, Uniformed Services University of the Health Sciences, Bethesda, Maryland; Clinical Assistant Professor of Otolaryngology, University of Texas Health Science Center at San Antonio, San Antonio, Texas
Progressive Sensorineural Hearing Loss

Luke K.S. Tan, M.D., F.R.C.S.
Head and Neck Surgery Fellow, Department of Otolaryngology, University of Texas Medical Branch, Galveston, Texas; Staff, Department of Otolaryngology, National University of Singapore, Singapore
Skin Cancer

M. Eugene Tardy, Jr., M.D., F.A.C.S.
Professor of Clinical Otolaryngology, and Director, Division of Facial Plastic Surgery, University of Illinois College of Medicine, Chicago, Illinois
Revision Rhinoplasty

Paul H. Toffel, M.D., F.A.C.S.
Clinical Professor, Department of Otolaryngology—Head and Neck Surgery, University of Southern California School of Medicine, Los Angeles; Chief, Department of Otolaryngology—Head and Neck Surgery, Daniel Freeman Memorial Hospital, Inglewood, California
Nasal Septal Perforation

Dean M. Toriumi, M.D.
Associate Professor, Division of Facial Plastic and Reconstructive Surgery, Department of Otolaryngology—Head and Neck Surgery, University of Illinois College of Medicine, Chicago, Illinois
Permanent Facial Paralysis

Jenny A. Van Duyne, M.D.
Fellow, Facial Plastic and Reconstructive Surgery, Department of Otolaryngology—Head and Neck Surgery, University of Toronto Faculty of Medicine, Toronto, Ontario, Canada
Nasal Polyposis

Luis Victoria, M.D.
Department of Otolaryngology—Head and Neck Surgery, The University of Iowa College of Medicine, Iowa City, Iowa
Laryngeal Paralysis

Randal S. Weber, M.D.
Gabriel Tucker Professor and Vice-Chair, Department of Otorhinolaryngology—Head and Neck Surgery, and Director, Center for Head and Neck Cancer, University of Pennsylvania Health System, Philadelphia, Pennsylvania
Submandibular Gland Tumors

William Ignace Wei, M.S., F.R.C.S.E., D.L.O., F.A.C.S.
Professor of Otorhinolaryngology, University of Hong Kong; Chief of Service, Department of Otorhinolaryngology, Queen Mary Hospital, Hong Kong
Carcinoma of the Nasopharynx

Edward C. Weisberger, M.D.
Professor, Department of Otolaryngology—Head and Neck Surgery, Indiana University School of Medicine, Indianapolis, Indiana

Cancer of the Hard Palate

Barry L. Wenig, M.D., M.P.H.
Professor and Director, Division of Head and Neck Surgery, University of Illinois College of Medicine at Chicago; Chief, Department of Otolaryngology, West Side V.A. Medical Center, Chicago, Illinois

Malnutrition from Cancer

Ernest A. Weymuller, Jr., M.D.
Professor and Chairman, Department of Otolaryngology—Head and Neck Surgery, University of Washington School of Medicine, Seattle, Washington

Supraglottic Carcinoma

Brian J. Wiatrak, M.D., F.A.A.P., F.A.C.S.
Associate Professor of Surgery and Pediatrics, University of Alabama School of Medicine; Chief, Pediatric Otolaryngology, Children's Hospital, Birmingham, Alabama

Respiratory Papillomatosis

Richard J. Wiet, M.D., F.A.C.S.
Clinical Professor of Otolaryngology and Neurosurgery, and Chief, Section of Neurotology and Skull Base Surgery, Northwestern University Medical School; Professor and Head, Department of Otolaryngology, Evanston Hospital, Evanston-Northwestern Health Care, Chicago, Illinois

Cholesteatoma

Mark C. Witte, M.D.
Chief Resident, Department of Otorhinolaryngology, Mayo Clinic, Rochester, Minnesota

Carotid Body Tumors

Gayle E. Woodson, M.D.
Professor, Department of Otolaryngology—Head and Neck Surgery, University of Tennessee, Memphis, College of Medicine; Director, Voice Disorder Clinic, University of Tennessee, Memphis, Medical Group, Memphis, Tennessee

Spasmodic Dysphonia

Audie L. Woolley, M.D.
Assistant Professor of Surgery and Pediatrics, Division of Otolaryngology—Head and Neck Surgery, University of Alabama School of Medicine, Birmingham, Alabama

Pediatric Tracheotomy and Long-Term Management

Mark J. Yanta, M.D.
Attending Physician, Northside Hospital, Atlanta, and North Fulton Regional Hospital, Roswell, Georgia

The Aging Face

Anthony J. Yonkers, M.D.
Professor and Chairman, Department of Otolaryngology—Head and Neck Surgery, University of Nebraska College of Medicine, Omaha, Nebraska

Cerebrospinal Fluid Rhinorrhea

Ross I.S. Zbar, M.D.
Resident, Department of Plastic Surgery, University of Texas Southwestern Medical Center at Dallas, Dallas, Texas; Former Resident, Department of Otolaryngology—Head and Neck Surgery, University of Iowa Hospitals and Clinics, Iowa City, Iowa

Pharyngocutaneous Fistula

Preface

This, the sixth edition of *Current Therapy in Otolaryngology—Head and Neck Surgery,* follows the same format as its predecessors. It is dedicated entirely to the treatment of most of the clinical problems in otolaryngology—head and neck surgery that the average practitioner is likely to encounter. This is not a surgical encyclopedia, rather it focuses on clinical problems that are important because of morbidity, controversy about management, or simply because they are challenging to treat. By comparing one's own management approach to the approaches used by experts in the field, one can hopefully find areas for refinement that will be useful. *Current Therapy in Otolaryngology—Head and Neck Surgery* is also of value for the resident-in-training who needs succinct summaries of the principles of treatment and pertinent "do's and don'ts" that often influence successful outcomes.

Unlike most texts, discussions of basic information such as anatomy, pathology, etiology, and physiology are omitted or minimized (except where essential for therapeutic decision making), not because they are unimportant, but because the average reader is assumed to be well grounded in the basics or because such information is readily available. Diagnostic procedures are also omitted or de-emphasized for the same reasons. As a result, the authors are free to concentrate on the finer points of clinical decision making and to emphasize the technical maneuvers that have been successful in their experience.

This text is intended for the practicing otolaryngologist, but upper level residents will also find much of interest herein. Those unfamiliar with basic clinical therapeutics should exercise caution in applying the material directly to patient care, as the authors may have omitted basic material in order to address more subtle points. There is a trade off between conciseness and readability on the one hand and compendial ponderosity on the other that has encouraged the former approach. The intent of the volume is to provide a consultation with an expert on how he/she solves a specific clinical problem.

Clearly, the emphasis in this book is upon surgical therapy and technique, as this is the mainstay in our field. It must be noted that this is not a surgical primer nor a "how to" manual; surgical technique must be learned in the operating room under the guidance and supervision of a qualified mentor. It would be inappropriate to adopt an author's approach as one's own without consideration of the technical requirements and a realistic assessment of one's own level of experience, skill, and training.

Although the topics covered in this edition are similar to previous ones, each chapter is a new work. Some topics have been updated from the earliest edition, which was published 15 years ago. Indeed, the original intent of the series was to have each author review and update his/her work every decade; however, the number of new techniques being used currently and the fact that some operations evolve slowly, if at all, has led to an expansion of the author list. The authors have been chosen because of their published expertise in their respective clinical areas and their mature, well-considered positions on controversial issues. My appreciation goes to them and to the publisher for their time and effort. I am certain the readers will agree with this sentiment as well.

My personal thanks go to my secretary Leslie Sullivan, who provided capable assistance, and to my loving wife Mary, whose care and support have enriched my life beyond compare.

George A. Gates, M.D., F.A.C.S.

Contents

THE HEAD AND NECK

GENERAL AND PEDIATRIC OTOLARYNGOLOGY

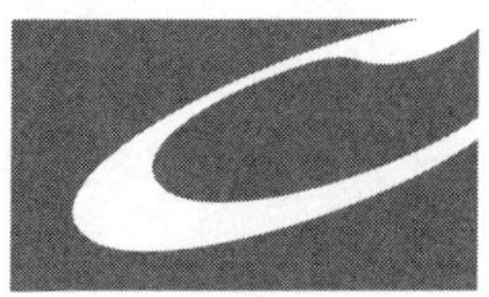

THE EAR AND TEMPORAL BONE

EXTERNAL OTITIS

The method of
Jay B. Farrior

External otitis is a ubiquitous problem that affects approximately 10 percent of the population in the United States annually. The spectrum of the disease ranges from a mild dermatitis of the external auditory canal to extensive osteomyelitis of the skull base. It is necessary to be familiar with the various forms of external otitis. Incorrect diagnosis or treatment may be frustrating for both the physician and the patient. With osteomyelitis, delayed diagnosis or inadequate treatment could lead to severe neurologic and medical complications or death.

■ ACUTE EXTERNAL OTITIS

Acute bacterial external otitis, or swimmer's ear, is often associated with water exposure and most commonly occurs during the summer months. Frequently, there is a history of mild trauma to the ear canal a few days before the onset of symptoms. Common causes of trauma are scratching, hearing aids, and the use of cotton-tipped swabs by the patient. Iatrogenic causes are aggressive cleaning of the external ear canal or the use of high-pressure irrigations. Once the trauma and moisture have disrupted the normal protective layer of epithelium, the acute infective process may become self-perpetuating; the meatus is closed by edema, with desquamation and exudate formation serving as a bacterial culture medium.

Patients commonly complain of pain and exquisite tenderness on manipulation of the pinna. Often, the meatus of the ear canal is narrowed. The external ear canal is commonly filled with moist desquamated debris. Careful cleaning of the ear canal and the use of antibiotic ear drops will cure most cases of acute external otitis.

Acute external otitis is commonly caused by *Staphylococcus aureus* or *Pseudomonas aeruginosa.* Bacterial cultures are not obtained unless there is granulation tissue, profuse drainage, of if the patient is diabetic or immunocompromised and is not responding to treatment within 7 to 10 days. Obtaining material for culture is facilitated by moistening the end of the cotton applicator with the liquid-holding medium before swabbing the external ear canal.

Cleaning of an acutely inflamed ear should be done under direct visualization. A narrowed meatus may be gently dilated with sequentially larger speculums to facilitate visualization. A small, cotton-tipped, wire applicator dipped in benzalkonium chloride (Zephiran) or 3 percent hydrogen peroxide is used to remove moist debris. Larger particulate matter can be gently removed with a smooth ear curet. Gentle suction is used to remove pus and moist debris. In children, a small cotton ball soaked in benzalkonium chloride is placed in the ear canal to reduce noise of the suction. Suction is applied to the cotton ball to avoid trauma to the skin of the canal. Once the cotton ball is saturated, it is removed and replaced with a clean cotton ball. This procedure is repeated until the ear canal is clean. Irrigation is not used in an acutely inflamed ear with a narrowed meatus.

Once the ear canal is clean, a strip of one-quarter inch gauze soaked in antibiotic ear drops is inserted as a wick. In children or in individuals who have a severely swollen external ear canal, an expandable sponge wick, such as a Pope Otowick, is inserted. The wick helps to deliver the antibiotics to the site of infection. It is maintained for 3 to 7 days, depending on the severity of the infection. At that time, the ear canal is cleaned, and the wick is either removed or changed, depending on the patient's progress. Without a wick, a narrow meatus may prevent the antibiotic drops from reaching the deeper portions of the external canal.

The patient is instructed to saturate the wick with antibiotic drops three to four times a day. With adequate treatment, symptoms should begin to improve in 2 to 3 days. Treatment is continued for 5 to 7 days. The patient is reexamined 10 to 14 days after treatment to confirm that the ear canal is fully healed.

The most popular ear drop preparation for external otitis is a suspension of neomycin, polymyxin B sulfate or colistin, and hydrocortisone (Cortisporin; Coly-Mycin S). This combination of aminoglycosides is specifically directed toward the treatment of *Pseudomonas* and other gram-negative organisms. Ophthalmologic solutions—gentamicin (Garamycin), tobramycin sulfate, and ciprofloxacin (Cipro)—may be used as single agents in those individuals who have a contact allergy to neomycin. Acetic acid solutions (VōSoL, VōSoL HC, and Domeboro solution) acidify the external ear canal, creating an environment that is less favorable for the growth of *Pseudomonas* organisms. These solutions may be effective in the early management or prevention of external otitis, but are not as effective as aminoglycosides in more severe cases.

A frequently overlooked aspect in the management of acute external otitis is pain relief. Ibuprofen or acetaminophen with codeine may be required. With adequate treatment, analgesics should not be needed for more than a few days. Deep pain or prolonged requirement for analgesic therapy is an indication for further investigation.

■ PREVENTION OF BACTERIAL EXTERNAL OTITIS

Acute external otitis commonly occurs as a complication of cerumen removal by either the patient or the physician. After cleaning, a strip of one-quarter inch gauze, soaked in antibiotic ear drops or acetic acid ear drops, is placed in the ear canal to be removed by the patient the following day.

Patients who either wear hearing aids or are frequently exposed to water have a greater risk of developing external otitis, particularly during the hot, humid summer months. Irrigation of the external ear canal with a solution of acetic acid and alcohol after bathing or swimming will help prevent external otitis by acidifying and drying the external ear canal.

Boric acid alcohol solution is prepared in two strengths: one contains 70 percent isopropyl alcohol, and the other has 91 percent anhydrous isopropyl alcohol. An irrigation solution of 70 percent acid alcohol is prepared by mixing 500 cc (1 pt) of alcohol plus 2 tbsp of boric acid powder, or 2 oz of white vinegar. The 91 percent solution is prepared from 120 cc (4 oz) of 91 percent isopropyl alcohol plus 1 tsp of boric acid powder.

The patient is instructed to gently rinse the ear with 1 oz of 70 percent boric acid alcohol using a bulb syringe. After removing the 70 percent alcohol from the ear, the ear can be filled with 91 percent alcohol, which is then drained. The patient is instructed to dry the ear with a blow-type hair dryer for 3 to 5 minutes to remove any additional moisture from the ear. The alcohol solutions help to dry the ear and restore the normal acid environment of the external ear canal.

Do not use alcohol irrigation if there is a perforated or monomeric eardrum. Stop irrigation if pain should occur.

Patients who wear hearing aids or other occlusive devices are asked to irrigate their ears with 8 to 16 oz of warm water and hydrogen peroxide to remove ceruminous debris. This is followed by the acid and alcohol irrigations and hair dryer. Commercially available acetic acid solutions may also be used after irrigation to help prevent infections as well. Acetic acid solutions should not be used for at least 2 weeks after the acute infection has subsided. They are also not to be used if there is a question of whether a perforated tympanic membrane exists.

■ DERMATITIS

A history of dermatologic reaction or contact allergy should be sought in a patient who has chronic or recurrent external otitis.

Dermatologic problems are a common cause of chronic or recurrent external otitis. External otitis may be a manifestation of dandruff, seborrhea, or psoriasis. It may also be the result of a contact allergy to soaps, shampoos, hair coloring agents, sprays, jewelry, or hearing aid molds. Frequently, the patient will complain of pruritus, weeping, and excessive desquamation or crusting in the ear. On examination, crusting or scaling around the meatus may be noted. These patients may develop a sensitivity to neomycin-containing solutions.

Dermatitis frequently predisposes the patient to acute external otitis. Once the secondary infection has been controlled, the dermatologic disorder can be treated with steroid creams or solutions. The fluoridated synthetic steroids such as betamethasone valerate (Valisone) and fluocinonide (Lidex) may be used for brief periods to manage severe dermatologic reactions. These solutions should not be used on a continuous basis because of atrophy of the epithelium. Hydrocortisone cream or solution (1 percent) is preferred for the management of chronic dermatologic disorders. These preparations are available over the counter. The patient is instructed to apply them directly to the meatus of the ear canal as needed to control the itching.

Keeping the ear canal clean and dry will reduce the pruritus and likelihood of a secondary infection. Periodic irrigations of the ear canal using hydrogen peroxide and solutions of acid and alcohol after bathing or swimming are helpful in the management of chronic dermatologic external otitis. In patients who have severe dermatitis, salicylic acid solutions or ointments may be helpful. Salicylic acid preparations help to dry the ear and reduce desquamation without causing the atrophic changes associated with the long-term use of fluorinated steroids. Recently, salicylic acid preparations have become available over the counter for the control of dandruff and seborrhea.

■ FUNGAL EXTERNAL OTITIS

Fungal infections are commonly associated with chronic external otitis, particularly if the mucous membrane of the middle ear is exposed. *Aspergillus nigrans* and *Candida* species are common pathogens associated with chronic external otitis. The initial management of fungal external otitis requires careful cleaning of the external auditory canal to remove all squamous debris. An antifungal cream such as ketoconazole (Nizoral) or clotrimazole (Lotrimin) is applied directly to the external ear canal. The patient is instructed to continue applying the cream for 10 to 14 days.

If there is a perforation of the tympanic membrane, the antifungal cream or solution is applied to saturated gauze, which is then placed in the external auditory canal.

Boric acid and alcohol irrigations and the use of a hair dryer will help prevent the recurrence of fungal external otitis.

Fungal external otitis can occasionally progress to osteomyelitis of the skull base as well as to intracranial abscess formation. This is a particular problem in the patient who is immunocompromised. In patients who have fungal external otitis and increasing symptoms of persistent pain, evaluation for deep bone involvement is necessary. For invasive *Aspergillus* infections, intravenous amphotericin B (Fungizone) is required.

■ CHRONIC EXTERNAL OTITIS

Chronic external otitis patients frequently have thickened and stenotic external auditory canals. In severe cases, there may be loss of landmarks of the tympanic membrane, atresia of the ear canal, and shortening of the external auditory canal.

Because of stenosis, the management of chronic external otitis is more difficult. After debris is carefully cleaned from the ear canal, the acute infection is treated as previously described.

Management of the stenotic ear canal may require prolonged packing for 4 to 6 weeks. An expandable sponge wick is placed into the canal. The pack is saturated with an antibiotic ear drop alternating with a fluoridated steroid drop such as betamethasone valerate, four times a day for 7 to 10 days. The pack is removed, the ear canal is cleaned, and then it is repacked as tightly as possible with expandable sponges. The ear canal is repacked every 10 to 14 days until the external ear has dilated to its normal size. Frequently, this may require 4 to 6 weeks. Prolonged follow-up and occasional repacking of the ear canal may be necessary to prevent stenosis. Once the infective process has been controlled, boric acid and alcohol irrigations and the use of a hair dryer should help keep the ear canal clean, which will prevent recurrent infections.

In severe cases, the fibrous stenosis or atresia of the external ear canal will require surgical correction. The scar is dissected out of the ear canal without disturbing the fibrous layer of the tympanic membrane. A plane of cleavage can generally be established at the layer of the fibrous drum, fibrous annulus, or over the short process of the malleus. Frequently, there is an acute anterior tympanomeatal angle, which requires a canaloplasty to enlarge and straighten the bony external ear canal. The ear canal and lateral surface of the tympanic membrane are then resurfaced with a thin split-thickness skin graft. The ear canal is packed with Gelfoam and cellulose sponge wrapped in nonadherent gauze for 2 weeks. It is then repacked at 2 week intervals until fully healed.

■ OSTEOMYELITIS OF THE SKULL BASE

In patients for whom symptoms persist or progress while they receive adequate therapy, the physician must consider contributing factors such as diabetes or immunocompromise. If deep pain or granulation tissue is present, the patient may have osteomyelitis (malignant external otitis) or malignancy. Cultures as well as biopsy of the granulation tissue are indicated to differentiate between an infective or malignant process. In patients in whom osteomyelitis is suspected, a detailed computed tomographic scan of the temporal bone to determine the extent of bone erosion and invasion is necessary. In addition, limited gallium and technetium scans of the head and neck region will help determine the extent of inflammation and bone involvement.

If the infection is limited and it is early in the course of the disease process, Cipro, 750 mg twice a day, in conjunction with either rifampin (Rifadin) or metronidazole (Flagyl), can be used with local treatment to control the infection. Clinical response to Cipro and local treatment should be seen within a 2 week period.

If the patient is not responding to Cipro or if on radiographic evaluation there is extensive involvement of the temporal bone and/or cranial nerve paralysis, then intravenous antibiotics should be instituted. The initial treatment is directed toward *Pseudomonas* osteomyelitis of the skull base and consists of 6 to 8 weeks of intravenous antibiotics. The initial aminoglycoside treatment is ticarcillin disodium (Ticar), 1 g every 6 hours. Therapeutic blood levels of aminoglycosides as well as renal function and cochlear reserves are monitored on a regular basis. Tobramycin is maintained in a therapeutic range of between 3 and 10 μg per milliliter peak levels, with toxic levels being greater than 10 μg per milliliter and trough levels being greater than 2 μg per milliliter. The addition of clindamycin phosphate (Cleocin Phosphate), 300 to 600 mg intravenously every 6 hours, has also been used. Cleocin Phosphate becomes concentrated in bone and is an effective agent against anaerobic bacteria that may be associated with deep-seated osteomyelitis.

Intravenous therapy is done through a home-health agency. Treatment is continued until the ear canal is fully healed and the patient is free of all symptoms for 2 to 3 weeks. After discontinuing the intravenous antibiotics, if there is concern about incomplete healing, then additional treatment with Cipro, Rifadin, and Cleocin Phosphate may be continued for an additional 1 to 3 months.

Hyperbaric oxygen has recently been reported by Davis and co-workers to be a useful adjunct in the management of osteomyelitis of the skull base. It has been helpful in providing more rapid resolution of the infection, as well as healing following surgery. In most cases, the deep pain associated with osteomyelitis of the temporal bone resolves within a few days following the initiation of treatment. Exacerbation or recurrence of symptoms suggest extension of the disease process, which may require further evaluation and a change in the course of treatment.

Planned surgical debridement is indicated in patients who have persistent or progressive symptoms while receiving medical therapy or who have failed a previous course of medical therapy. The removal of osteomyelitic bone may facilitate antibiotic therapy and reduce hospitalization. Extensive surgical resection or radical mastoidectomy that was once described for this disease is seldom indicated.

Osteomyelitis is initially limited to the floor of the external ear canal and involves the facial nerve at the stylomastoid foramen. With advanced disease, osteomyelitis may extend through the mastoid tip and petrous apex along the skull base, but seldom involves the labyrinth. Occasionally, it may extend superiorly along the anterior canal wall and into the zygoma. The extent of surgical debridement should be determined by the disease process, which may be suggested by preoperative bone and technetium scans as well as radiographic evaluation.

■ DISCUSSION

External otitis is a common disorder whose spectrum ranges from acute bacterial external otitis to aggressive osteomyelitis of the skull base. The otolaryngologist should be familiar with both the multiple aspects of this disease and its diagnosis and management. Medical treatment should be combined with judicious use of surgery, when needed. Most cases of external otitis can be managed by careful cleaning. Acute external otitis can be managed by careful cleaning of the ear canal and local antibiotic packs. Prevention of acute external otitis must be considered during ear cleaning and in patients who are either frequently exposed to water or use occlusive devices. Chronic external otitis requires evaluation of the cause of infection as well as contributing factors, such as dermatologic disorders and immunocompromise, in order to prevent recurrent infection. Osteomyelitis of the skull base has become primarily a medical disorder; this condition requires combined use of antibiotic and aminoglycoside therapy. The advent of the increased availability of hyperbaric oxygen has been shown to be a useful adjunct in the management of osteomyelitis of the skull base. However, planned surgical debridement of the diseased bone should be considered in patients who do not respond to medical treatment within a reasonable period of time. Planned surgical debridement may reduce the duration of intravenous antibiotic therapy.

Suggested Reading

Davis JO, Gates GA, Lerner C, et al. Adjuvant hyperbaric oxygen in malignant external otitis. Otolaryngol Head Neck Surg 1992; 118:89-93.

CONGENITAL AURAL ATRESIA

The method of
George T. Hashisaki
Paul R. Lambert

Congenital aural atresia is an uncommon otologic condition. Optimal management addresses issues of hearing loss, cosmesis, aural rehabilitation, and patient or parent concerns. We present an approach to this condition that will arm the otolaryngologist and the parents with information necessary to make reasonable decisions.

■ EMBRYOLOGY

The anatomic changes and variations seen in congenital aural atresia can be understood within the context of arrested embryologic development of the external ear canal. During normal embryologic development, a fascinating sequence of programmed events results in a patent ear canal. The first pharyngeal pouch, first branchial arch, and first branchial groove interact and develop into the middle ear structures, tympanic membrane, and external ear canal. These developments occur after formation of the otic capsule and inner ear structures. The inner ear develops from the otic placode, beginning in the third to fourth weeks of gestation. The inner ear is structurally complete by Week 8, although maturation continues until full gestation. The external canal has its origin in the first branchial groove. The groove and the first pharyngeal pouch meet each other, and the site of contact becomes the tympanic membrane. A solid core of epithelial cells fills the groove from the level of the tympanic membrane out to the surface. In the middle trimester, the epithelial core undergoes programmed cell death, and recanalization of the external ear canal occurs. Recanalization progresses from a medial to lateral direction.

The tympanic portion of the temporal bone forms at the level of the rudimentary tympanic membrane. It surrounds the first pharyngeal groove and the subsequent epithelial cord. As recanalization occurs, the bony portion of the ear canal forms from the tympanic bone.

Congenital aural atresia results from the failure of the recanalization sequence. Because this is a second trimester event, inner ear development is complete. Middle ear structures have formed, but full maturation has not occurred. Ossicles are present, but arrested growth can leave them at various stages of formation. The stapes is often misshapen, but usually mobile. The incus and malleus are commonly fused. Other branchial arch derivatives are affected as well. The facial nerve may have variations in its constituent fibers, anatomic course, or both.

■ EVALUATION

Most cases of major congenital ear malformations are evident at birth because of microtia or other craniofacial anomalies. Patients who have a normal or only slightly deformed pinna and a stenotic ear canal may escape diagnosis for years. When initially evaluating an infant or young child who has congenital aural atresia, the two principle objectives are (1) to assess the overall hearing status and need for immediate amplification, and (2) to formulate a treatment plan in conjunction with a comprehensive medical team (e.g., plastic surgery, genetics, and pediatrics).

Tests of hearing function are performed early. For unilateral cases, standard testing of the contralateral ear can include auditory brain stem response audiometry (ABR) and/or otoacoustic emissions (OAE) testing. Behavioral audiometry can begin at 6 to 9 months of age. For bilateral atresia, bone conduction ABR is performed at an early age.

Radiologic evaluation consists of a high-resolution noncontrast temporal bone computed tomographic (CT) scan. Questions arise as to the indications for CT scans, optimal timing of the scan, and scanning techniques.

CT of the temporal bone is necessary in all patients being considered for surgery. For patients who have ear canal stenosis, CT scans are also recommended to assess for possible cholesteatoma formation. Cholesteatoma formation is uncommon, but otorrhea, fistula drainage, mastoid tenderness, or clinical signs of mastoiditis are indications of that possibility; CT scanning is indicated to evaluate the temporal bone.

CT scans are typically obtained near the time of planned surgery, around age 4 to 6 years. Radiographic studies on infants are usually not recommended because the information gained is usually not applicable to immediate rehabilitative plans. If concerns of cholesteatoma formation arise at a young age, scans are performed then. Almost all patients who have cholesteatomas are older than 3 years, which is another reason to delay the CT evaluation until the patient is beyond that age.

Both axial and coronal views are important. Axial projections (parallel to the line from the infraorbital rim to the external meatus) delineate well the head of the malleus and body of the incus, the incudostapedial joint, and the round window. Coronal projections (parallel to the ramus of the mandible) show the stapes, oval window, and vestibule. Both projections are necessary to follow the course of the facial nerve.

■ MEDICAL THERAPY

Unilateral Atresia

No immediate medical intervention is necessary in the infant or young child who has unilateral atresia if hearing levels are normal in the contralateral ear. The parents can be reassured that speech, language, and intellectual development will proceed normally. For school, preferential seating is advised.

A hearing aid is not recommended, for reasons of poor compliance with wearing the aid and a small benefit to overall audition. Adults are more likely to use a hearing aid to improve communication skills in social and workplace settings. A bone conduction hearing aid is necessary for complete ear canal atresia. An air conduction hearing aid may be fitted to a stenotic ear canal.

Bilateral Atresia

Early amplification using a bone conduction hearing aid is of paramount importance. To foster speech and language acquisition, fitting the infant with a hearing aid early in life is critical. Audiologic and medical evaluations can be completed within the first few months of life, and placement of a hearing aid can proceed quickly.

■ SURGICAL THERAPY

Unilateral and Bilateral Atresia

The hearing loss associated with bilateral atresia carries significant speech and language consequences. Most otologic surgeons would consider surgical repair of one ear an appropriate pursuit. Repair of the second atretic ear, as well as repair of a unilateral aural atresia, is a matter of some controversy.

The issue is not simply the unilateral conductive hearing loss. Most otologic surgeons would explore the middle ear of a child who has a large conductive hearing loss due to other causes. Concerns with atresia repair surgery are the degree and predictability of hearing improvement, potential lifetime care of a mastoid cavity, and risk of facial nerve injury. These concerns have prompted many surgeons to recommend delaying surgery for unilateral atresia or the second ear in bilateral cases until adulthood, when the patient can participate in the decision-making process.

To address these concerns, consider the following. An improvement in the speech hearing threshold to 25 dB or better eliminates the handicap of a unilateral hearing loss. As a surgical result, this degree of hearing improvement is not possible in all atresia patients, but can be achieved in approximately two-thirds of carefully selected patients. A mastoid cavity is avoided if the anterior surgical approach is used, reducing the need for frequent cavity cleaning. Risk of injury to the facial nerve is minimized by understanding the abnormal development and anatomy of this structure and by employing intraoperative facial nerve monitoring. We and others believe that the benefits of binaural hearing and the possibility of achieving that goal are sufficiently great to offer corrective surgery to carefully selected children who have unilateral atresia.

Patients who have bilateral atresia present less of a surgical dilemma. The goal in these cases is to restore sufficient hearing to supplant the bone conduction hearing device. The *better* ear (as determined by CT evaluation) is selected for the initial surgical procedure, which is a departure from standard otologic protocol. Most surgeons recommend operating as the child approaches school age and, depending on the hearing result, operating on the second ear within the next several years. Although the selection criteria are not as stringent as in unilateral atresia cases, careful patient screening is essential for satisfactory results.

Selection Criteria

Following atresia repair, most patients have a residual conductive deficit of at least 10 dB. Therefore, preoperative sensorineural hearing function should be normal to achieve binaural hearing in unilateral cases or to obviate the need for a hearing aid in bilateral cases. Normal or near-normal sensorineural function in the contralateral ear is also important to avoid operating on the ear with better sensorineural function.

Although audiometric criteria can be defined quantitatively, the art of patient selection centers on the CT evaluation of the middle ear. Hypoplasia of the middle ear space, ranging from mild to severe, occurs in most cases of congenital atresia. Ossicular development can be expected to correlate directly with middle ear size. The risk of surgical complications will be minimized, and the chances for a successful hearing result are increased if the middle ear and mastoid spaces are at least two-thirds of the normal size, and if all three ossicles can be identified. Presence of the oval and round windows and a normal or near-normal course of the facial nerve further define the ideal surgical candidate. A CT-based grading system that quantifies the developmental status of the ear has been shown to predict postoperative hearing results. In unilateral cases, only the ideal candidates are selected; in bilateral cases, minimum criteria are a middle ear space of at least one-half normal size and the presence of an ossicular mass. Only about 60 percent of patients who have aural atresia are deemed to be surgical candidates.

Timing of Surgery

If elected, surgery can be performed as early as age 5 or 6 years. By this time, accurate audiometric tests have been obtained, pneumatization of the temporal bone is well advanced, and most children are able to cooperate with postoperative care. This timing also permits any microtia repair to be well under way.

For microtia patients requiring major external ear reconstruction, it is reasonable for the plastic surgeon to operate first. This ensures a surgical field without scars or compromised blood supply, which optimizes survival of the implanted auricular framework. The overall cosmetic result should also be better by not restricting the auricular reconstruction to a specific site. The plastic surgeon can place the auricular framework at a position to his or her satisfaction. Later, during the atresia repair, the reconstructed auricle may be repositioned with appropriate undermining to align the meatus and external canal.

Cholesteatoma

Patients who have cholesteatoma should undergo surgery to eradicate the disease process and, if possible, improve hearing. Patients who have stenosis of the external canal are at risk for cholesteatoma formation and should also be considered for surgery. Cole and Jahrsdoerfer reviewed 50 patients (54 ears) having an average canal diameter of 4 mm or less and found that 50 percent of them developed a cholesteatoma. The patient's age and canal size were important variables in predicting disease. No cholesteatomas were found in patients younger than age 3 years, and bone erosion and middle ear involvement from a canal cholesteatoma were not encountered in patients younger than age 12 years. The preponderance of cholesteatomas developed in ear canals that were 2 mm or less in diameter.

Patients who have stenosis severe enough to prevent adequate cleaning of the canal and examination of the tympanic membrane should have a CT scan by age 4 or 5 years. Assuming that a cholesteatoma is not found, several options are available. If the CT findings are favorable with regard to hearing improvement, canal and middle ear surgery can be considered. Canaloplasty alone is offered to patients who have unfavorable middle ear findings. If the parents are uncomfortable with surgery, a CT scan should be obtained every few years to assess for cholesteatoma development. Periodic CT scans are not necessary in patients who have a completely atretic ear canal, given the rarity of cholesteatoma formation in that setting.

■ SURGICAL TECHNIQUE

There are two basic surgical approaches for repair of aural atresia: the mastoid approach and the anterior approach. In the mastoid approach, the sinodural angle is first identified and followed to the antrum. The facial recess is opened, and the incudostapedial joint is separated. The atretic bone is then removed. In the anterior approach, exposure of the mastoid air cells is limited. Drilling is confined to an area defined by the temporomandibular joint anteriorly, the middle cranial fossa aura superiorly, and the mastoid air cells posteriorly. An advantage of the anterior approach is that a large mastoid cavity is avoided. There is also less surgical manipulation in the area of the mastoid segment of the facial nerve. The more cylindrical contours of the new canal with limited mastoid exposure facilitate placement of the split-thickness skin graft. We prefer the anterior approach.

Incision

A postauricular incision is used to expose the mastoid bone. The soft tissues are elevated anteriorly until a surface depression in the mastoid is encountered. In most major malformations, this depression is the temporomandibular joint, although occasionally a stenotic bony ear canal is found. Dissection within this area may be necessary to differentiate between the two, but the manipulation should be limited because the facial nerve frequently exits the skull into the glenoid fossa.

Canal Drilling

In most atresia cases, a tympanic bone is not identified. Occasionally, it is present and demarcated from the surrounding cortex. This bone serves as a pathway to direct the drilling for the external canal. When a tympanic bone is not identified, there is sufficient space between the glenoid fossa anteriorly and the mastoid air cells posteriorly to drill the external canal. Ideally, drilling is confined to the area just lateral to the middle ear space, using the middle cranial fossa dura as the superior landmark and the glenoid fossa–temporomandibular joint as the anterior landmark. The posterior wall of the glenoid fossa should be thinned to maximize anterior exposure and limit mastoid air cell exposure. As the middle cranial fossa dura plate is followed medially, the epitympanum will be the first portion of the middle ear space identified. The fused head of the malleus and body of the incus are identified next.

This superior pathway has the advantage of protecting the facial nerve because that structure always lies medial to the ossicular mass in the epitympanum. Drilling in a posteroinferior direction brings the dissection closer to the facial nerve. Because of the possible acute anterior and lateral course of the facial nerve at the second genu, the nerve is very vulnerable to injury.

Middle Ear Surgery

The atretic bone lateral to the fused malleus-incus complex is removed circumferentially around the ossicular mass. Visualization of the stapes is often difficult. The stapes may be obscured because of the contracted middle ear cavity, the malformed lateral ossicular mass, or the overlying facial nerve. Usually, enough of the stapes can be seen to assess its mobility and the integrity of the incudostapedial joint. A normal oval window and stapes footplate are anticipated, but the stapes may be fixed in up to 5 percent of patients.

The ossicular chain is maintained in position. In most cases, the ossicular chain, although deformed, is mobile, and hearing results may be better when the chain is left undisturbed.

Tympanic Membrane Grafting

A temporalis fascia graft is placed over the ossicular mass. Because of malleus deformities, it is difficult to anchor the graft medial to the malleus. Absence of a tympanic membrane remnant or annulus further predisposes to graft lateralization. An anterior sulcus can be drilled in the anterior canal wall to stabilize the graft. A second technique to prevent lateralization involves placing a temporary Silastic button at the medial terminus of the exterior canal. The button is placed lateral to the skin graft that overlaps the temporalis fascia.

Meatoplasty

A meatus is created in the reconstructed auricle. A circular meatal opening approximately twice the normal size is made. The alignment of the meatus and the bony external canal is assessed. The reconstructed auricle may require repositioning. Careful undermining of the auricle may be necessary. Because the auricular reconstruction may have caused scarring and tethering of the extratemporal facial nerve, it is vulnerable to injury during the undermining dissection.

Skin Grafting

A thin split-thickness skin graft, 0.008 to 0.010 inch thick, is harvested from the upper thigh or medial upper arm. The thinness of the graft facilitates its placement as the lining of the canal. At the level of the tympanic membrane graft, multiple small wedges are excised from the medial edge of the skin graft to allow coverage and eversion of the skin graft edges. The skin graft may be stabilized with thin gauze impregnated with antibiotic ointment or with three to four sponge ear wicks seated in the ear canal. After the bony canal has been packed, the auricle is returned to its anatomic position. Working through the meatus, the lateral edge of the skin graft is unfolded to line the meatus and sutured in place. Gauze or sponge ear wick packing is placed in the meatus.

Postoperative Care

Approximately 7 to 10 days postoperatively, all the ear canal packing is removed, as well as the Silastic button, if used. Complete survival of the split-thickness skin graft is anticipated at this time. If any granulation tissue is seen, antibiotic-impregnated Gelfoam is placed into the ear canal, and the patient is instructed to keep this moist for 7 to 10 days.

■ HEARING RESULTS

It is difficult to compare hearing results from various series because of differences in selection criteria, reporting hearing results, and length of follow-up. In general, a postoperative hearing level of 30 dB or better can be achieved in approximately 50 percent to 75 percent of major congenital aural atresia patients. A hearing level of 20 dB or better is possible in 15 percent to 50 percent. A recent review of 45 consecutive patients from 1985 to 1996 with a minimum follow-up of 1 year showed hearing levels of 20 dB in 38 percent and 30 dB in 67 percent.

Complications

Given that near-normal hearing is not universally achieved even in carefully selected patients, the surgical complications must be compared carefully with the merits of atresia surgery. The two potential serious complications are sensorineural hearing loss and facial nerve paralysis. Other complications include canal stenosis, chronic infection, and recurrent conductive hearing loss.

Labyrinthine Injury

The anterior surgical approach limits exposure of mastoid air cells, minimizing potential injury to the horizontal semicircular canal. High-frequency sensorineural hearing loss has been noted in some patients postoperatively. Because the ossicular mass is connected to the atretic bone, energy from drilling will be transmitted to the inner ear in all atresia cases. This energy transfer will be limited by the fixation of the ossicles. Direct manipulation of the ossicular chain by instruments or the drill may cause greater damage. Care in dissecting around or manipulating the ossicular chain is particularly important in the anterior approach because the incudostapedial joint is not disarticulated.

Facial Nerve Injury

The abnormal development of the temporal bone in aural atresia places the facial nerve at increased vulnerability. Understanding the anomalies of the facial nerve likely to be encountered and the use of intraoperative facial nerve monitoring enables the surgeon to proceed with confidence. Temporary facial paralysis has occurred rarely. This complication has usually resulted from transposition of the facial nerve to gain access to the oval window. Jahrsdoerfer and Lambert reported a 0.7 percent incidence of facial paresis or paralysis in a series of over 1,000 patients.

Canal Stenosis

Some narrowing of the new external auditory canal develops in as many as 25 percent of patients, particularly in the soft-tissue segment or at the meatus. If a large meatus has been created, this narrowing is of little consequence. Occasionally, a significant stenosis occurs, trapping squamous epithelium and causing infection. Attempts to dilate the canal with soft or hard stents are usually ineffective, and a secondary meatoplasty with skin grafting is necessary.

Chronic Infection

Normal migration of keratin debris is lacking in the skin-grafted ear canal. Protective secretions from sebaceous and apocrine glands are also absent. As a consequence, the incidence of canal infections is higher than in the normal ear. The cylindrical contour of the canal and absence of a mastoid cavity achieved with the anterior surgical approach minimize debris accumulation. A widely patent meatus and soft-tissue canal are important for aeration and cleaning. Most patients are not restricted regarding water activities.

Conductive Hearing Loss

Persistent or recurrent conductive hearing loss is the most common negative outcome in aural atresia surgery. The causes of persistent conductive hearing loss are varied and include inadequate mobilization of the ossicular mass from the atretic bone, and unrecognized incudostapedial joint discontinuity, or a fixed stapes footplate. Wide exposure of the ossicular mass at surgery is necessary to assure ossicular chain mobility and to facilitate assessment of ossicular chain integrity. Recurrence of a conductive hearing loss after an initial satisfactory improvement in air conduction thresholds is usually secondary to refixation of the ossicular chain or tympanic membrane lateralization.

■ DISCUSSION

The objective in congenital aural atresia surgery is to create a functional pathway by which sound can reach the cochlear fluids. This surgery presents a true challenge to the otologic surgeon. A thorough knowledge of the anatomic variations that can occur with abnormal development of the temporal bone is essential. Hearing results that are consistently excellent cannot yet be achieved in atresia surgery. But with adherence to strict selection criterion and further refinements in surgical technique, this goal is realistic.

Suggested Reading

Bellucci RJ. Congenital aural malformations: Diagnosis and treatment. Otolaryngol Clin North Am 1988; 14:95.

Cole RR, Jahrsdoerfer RA. The risk of cholesteatoma in congenital aural stenosis. Laryngoscope 1990; 100:576.

Jafek BW, Nager GT, Strife J, et al. Congenital aural atresia: An analysis of 311 cases. Trans Am Acad Ophthalmol Otolaryngol 1975; 80:588.

Jahrsdoerfer RA. Congenital atresia of the ear. Laryngoscope 1978; 88 (Suppl 13):1.

Jahrsdoerfer RA. Embryology of the facial nerve. Am J Otol 1988; 9:423.

Jahrsdoerfer RA, Yeakley JW, Aguilar EA, et al. Grading system for the selection of patients with congenital aural atresia. Am J Otolaryngol 1992; 13:6.

Lambert PR. Major congenital ear malformations: Surgical management and results. Ann Otol Rhinol Laryngol 1988; 97:641.

Molony TB, De la Crus A. Surgical approaches to congenital atresia of the external auditory canal. Otolaryngol Head Neck Surg 1990; 103: 991.

Schuknecht HG. Congenital aural atresia. Laryngoscope 1989; 99:908.

NECROTIZING OTITIS EXTERNA

The method of

Chester L. Strunk

Necrotizing otitis externa (NOE), formerly known as malignant otitis externa, is a life-threatening infection of the external auditory canal and skull base, usually found in elderly diabetic (80 percent) or other immunocompromised patients, such as those who have acquired immunodeficiency syndrome. One of the reasons diabetics may be more susceptible to NOE is that the pH of their cerumen has been found to be higher and therefore more hospitable for growth of bacteria, such as *Pseudomonas aeruginosa,* the most common bacterium isolated in skull base osteomyelitis (SBO). *P. aeruginosa* colonizes the ear canal when a warm, moist environment is present, such as after swimming or aural irrigation. *Pseudomonas* is resistant to most antibiotics because of its capacity for selective vasculitis, thereby limiting the blood supply and the penetration of antibiotics to infected tissue. NOE initially involves the cartilaginous and bony aspect of the external canal before spreading through Santorini's fissures in the cartilaginous floor to the skull base, parotid, and soft tissues of the neck. Treatment has evolved over the past 30 years from extensive surgical removal of all infected material and adjuvant antibiotic therapy to minimal debridement of the ear canal and prolonged antibiotic therapy.

■ DIAGNOSIS

Successful management of NOE requires early detection and treatment. Severe otalgia in an elderly diabetic accompanied by granulation tissue in the floor of the external canal near the bony-cartilaginous junction should raise suspicion of NOE. A culture should be obtained and sensitivities to all anti-pseudomonal antibiotics should be obtained. A biopsy of the granulation tissue is performed to exclude carcinoma, which may mimic NOE. SBO must be excluded if there is cranial nerve involvement (VII, IX, X, or XI).

Routine laboratory tests should include renal function studies, complete blood count, fasting glucose, and erythrocyte sedimentation rate (ESR). Renal function is monitored in case nephrotoxic antibiotics are needed. The white blood cell count is usually normal. If the fasting glucose is normal, then a 5 hour glucose tolerance test should be obtained. The ESR, although nonspecific, is a valuable test to follow up on the response to antibiotics.

Radiologic tests are needed to confirm the diagnosis of SBO and follow the progression and resolution of the disease process. Computed tomographic (CT) scan should be obtained to define the location and extent of disease. CT is of no use in monitoring resolution of disease, because remineralization is required for the bony changes to return to normal. Remineralization may never occur with resolution of SBO. Magnetic resonance imaging has not proved useful in the diagnosis or management of SBO. If the CT finding is negative, but the index of suspicion remains, then a technetium phosphate radionucleotide scan (bone scan) should be obtained. A positive bone scan is indicative of increased osteogenic activity, whether it be bone destruction or bone repair. A bone scan finding will be positive when there is absence of bone destruction on the CT. A bone scan is not helpful in determining resolution, because the finding may remain positive for 9 months after infection. Gallium-67 citrate is absorbed by macrophages and reticular endothelial cells and is a sensitive indicator of soft-tissue infection. Gallium uptake quickly returns to normal after infection has cleared. Gallium scans are useful in determining the end point of antimicrobial therapy. They are obtained every 3 weeks until normal, at which point antibiotics are discontinued provided clinical stages of infection have also resolved.

■ THERAPY

Treatment is best understood in the context of the following staging system, as recommended by Kinney: stage I—disease confined to the external auditory canal and/or facial nerve paralysis; stage II—osteitis of the skull base and/or multiple cranial nerve involvement; stage III—meninges or brain involvement.

The successful management of diabetics who have NOE includes careful control of their glucose levels and close monitoring of renal function. Antimicrobial therapy remains the mainstay of treatment for SBO. Topical antibiotic therapy is controversial because it alters the flora, rendering future cultures for resistant strains useless. Once the diagnosis of SBO is confirmed, the patient is hospitalized, and an infectious disease consult is obtained. Two-drug therapy is recommended to prevent emergence of resistant bacteria. A frequently suggested intravenous regimen includes aztreonam plus clindamycin. Daily debridement of granulation tissue and removal of sequestered bone of the external auditory canal is recommended. Tympanoplasty with mastoidectomy may become necessary in stage II disease, but more extensive surgery only exposes previously uninfected skull base to *P. aeruginosa.* Home intravenous antibiotic therapy is started once the following clinical signs and symptoms have begun to resolve: (1) resolution of otalgia, (2) decrease in drainage, (3) falling ESR, and (4) reduction in granulation tissue. An alternative oral route using a quinolone such as ciprofloxacin, ofloxacin, or levofloxacin plus rifampin to reduce the emergence of resistant *Pseudomonas* strains has been used. When taking an oral quinolone, the patient should be instructed not to take an antacid preparation containing calcium or magnesium salts, because doing so reduces absorption of the quinolone. An alternative intravenous regimen of ceftazidime plus metronidazole can be equally efficacious. The use of an aminoglycoside with ticarcillin was formerly the treatment of choice, but the possible nephrotoxicity and ototoxicity (aminoglycosides) and penicillin rashes (ticarcillin) makes this a less desirable combination.

Stage I disease responds to 6 weeks of combination antipseudomonal antibiotic therapy and limited debridement. Stage II disease is treated until pain resolves, wound culture findings become negative for *P. aeruginosa,* and the gallium scan returns to normal. Stage III disease was uniformly fatal until hyperbaric oxygen (HBO) therapy was added to the treatment regimen. HBO improves the oxidative killing of aerobic bacteria by phagocytes. Adjuvant HBO therapy should be considered in patients who have advanced SBO (stages II and III) and in recurrent cases. Patients who fail a round of antibiotics and HBO should undergo reculture and be treated for another 6 weeks with antibiotics guided by sensitivities and HBO.

Suggested Reading

Barza M. Use of quinolones for treatment of ear and eye infections. Eur J Clin Microbiol Infect Dis 1991; 10:296-303.

Davis JC, Gates GA, Lerner C, et al. Adjuvant hyperbaric oxygen in malignant external otitis. Arch Otolaryngol Head Neck Surg 1992; 118:89-93.

Gips S, Front A, Meyer SW, et al. Quantitative bone and 67Ga scintigraphy in the differentiation of necrotizing external otitis from severe external otitis. Arch Laryngol Head Neck Surg 1991; 117:623-626.

Slattery WH, Brackmann DE. Skull base osteomyelitis. Otolaryngol Clin North Am 1996; 795-806.

OTITIS MEDIA

The method of
Joel M. Bernstein

Otitis media (OM), the most common illness for which children visit a physician, is an all-encompassing term used to describe an inflammatory process in the middle ear space. However, the disease really begins in the nasopharynx and extends into the eustachian tube and then into the middle ear mucosa. Otitis media may be divided into various categories, including acute otitis media, recurrent acute otitis media, otitis media with effusion, chronic otitis media with effusion, and chronic suppurative otitis media. However, these categories probably represent various stages along a continuum of severity. This chapter addresses the management of three parts of this spectrum, namely, acute otitis media (AOM), recurrent acute otitis media (RAOM), and otitis media with effusion (OME).

With frightening changes in the capacity of the three most common bacterial organisms that cause OM to alter their resistance to antibiotics, it is urgent that clinicians alter and even curtail some medical treatment(s) without subjecting individual patients to undue risk. Although this chapter addresses medical and surgical management, immunology and molecular biology of the inflammatory response will ultimately be the areas upon which clinical otolaryngologists must focus if they are to eradicate or control infectious diseases of the upper respiratory tract, including OM.

PATHOGENESIS

Nasopharyngeal colonization with three major bacterial pathogens—*Streptococcus pneumoniae,* nontypable *Haemophilus influenzae* (NTHI), and *Moraxella catarrhalis*—is the major risk factor for OM. Among the 84 serotypes of *S. pneumoniae,* types 3, 4, 6B, 7, 14, 15, 19F, and 23F are most frequently isolated from the nasopharynx. NTHI may be recovered from the airways of as great as 80 percent of normal children. When colonization with *S. pneumoniae,* NTHI, and *M. catarrhalis* occurs early in life, AOM coincidentally occurs early. For example, among Australian aboriginal infants, who are at high risk for developing OM, colonization with all three pathogens reaches 100 percent by age 4 months. In contrast, low-risk populations in the same community are rarely colonized in the first 9 months of life. Therefore, one of the most important new concepts in the treatment of OM is the prevention of colonization of bacterial pathogens. Preventing bacterial adhesion to the glycoprotein conjugates of mucus or on the surface of nasopharyngeal epithelial cells is one of the strategies for the prevention of OM. Unfortunately, in the United States, most physicians only think of antibiotic therapy as the method of treating this disease. As a result, there has been a dangerous increase in the resistance of *S. pneumoniae* to penicillin. At the Buffalo Children's Hospital, total resistance of *S. pneumoniae* to penicillin from 1994 to 1996 increased from 6 percent to 12 percent, as noted in Table 1. It is therefore critical that otolaryngologists lead the way in evolving new strategies for the prevention and treatment of OM. This chapter is devoted to some of the new concepts in controlling OM.

ACUTE OTITIS MEDIA

The management of AOM depends on the age of the patient and the severity of the disease. Before the introduction of antibiotics, treatment of AOM was primarily directed toward the relief of pain with medication or myringotomy. Today in the United States, as well as in most developed nations, antibiotics are administered to the majority of children early in the course of disease. In 1995, more than 245 million prescriptions for antibiotics were written in the United States for patients who had AOM. The goals of early treatment are presumed to be hastened clinical improvement, eradication of the etiologic event, prevention of recurrence, shortened duration of middle ear effusion, and prevention of complications. The Netherlands stands alone among advanced nations in withholding early antibiotic intervention. Arguments against antibiotic therapy include a high rate of spontaneous resolution, expense of antibiotics, side effects of antibiotics, induction of drug allergy, impairment of the immune response to the etiologic agent, and, most important, the development of antibiotic resistance.

Spontaneous resolution of AOM without therapy is common. In studies conducted with placebo groups, rapid relief

Table 1. Penicillin Minimal Inhibitory Concentration (MIC) Results on *Streptococcus pneumoniae* Isolates from Patients at Buffalo Children's Hospital, 1994–1996*

YEAR	NO. OF ISOLATES TESTED/ TOTAL ISOLATES	PERCENT PENICILLIN SUSCEPTIBLE	PERCENT PENICILLIN INTERMEDIATE	PERCENT PENICILLIN RESISTANT
1994	110/155	86	9	5
1995	97/128	79	13	6
1996	103/138	76	12	12

All isolates from any site that were penicillin resistant by Kirby-Bauer disc diffusion and all isolates from nonpermissive sites (i.e., blood, cerebrospinal fluid) were tested, even if they were penicillin susceptible.

of pain and fever within 3 days of diagnosis was observed in 60 percent to 92 percent of untreated children. In addition, disappearance of all symptoms within 7 to 10 days occurred in 68 percent to 87 percent. Resolution of middle ear effusion occurred within 30 days of disease onset in 48 percent to 65 percent of children, whereas 20 percent to 28 percent of children experience recurrence of acute symptoms. Severe complications occurred at an extremely low rate of less than 0.5 percent in the absence of treatment.

Insight into the process of spontaneous resolution of AOM has come from the studies pioneered by Howie and co-workers, who introduced the concept of the "in vivo sensitivity test" as a way to measure the effectiveness of antibiotics in eradicating bacteria from the middle ear space. As originally described, tympanocenteses were performed before treatment and 2 to 7 days after starting treatment. One author recently summarized results from 11 studies that employed the same dual tympanocenteses approach (Klein, 1993). Placebo groups included in the studies demonstrated the spontaneous disappearance of bacteria in 11 percent of *S. pneumoniae* and 48 percent of NTHI AOM cases. Although placebo groups were not available for *M. catarrhalis* infections, treatment with antibiotics that were ineffective according to in vitro testing demonstrated a spontaneous eradication rate of 79 percent. Because 25 percent of middle ear effusions yield no pathogen upon culture, they are presumed to represent viral infections that will improve without therapy. When the frequency of each bacterial pathogen is multiplied by the corresponding spontaneous resolution rate, the cumulative result represents the proportion of episodes of AOM that may not require treatment to improve. This crude calculation estimates that 50 percent of all patients who have AOM will experience resolution of infection. The other 50 percent of patients may benefit from antibiotic therapy. The basis for spontaneous cure is probably related to restoration of eustachian tube function, drainage of the effusion, and the host-defense response.

Based on this relatively high incidence of spontaneous resolution of AOM, the following recommendations are made for the otolaryngologist as well as for the pediatrician. Children younger than 2 years old probably should always be treated with an appropriate antibiotic. Although millions of dollars have been devoted to the efficacy of various antibiotics, amoxicillin (Augmentin) is still the drug of choice, because most studies do not support the concept that second-generation cephalosporins are any better than amoxicillin in the treatment of AOM. Although there is cross-reactivity between penicillin and the cephalosporins, allergic reactions in my experience are rare, and I would recommend cefuroxime axetil as the drug of choice in patients who are allergic to penicillin. However, in children older than 2 years, I would recommend the philosophy of the Dutch physicians and would closely observe patients for 48 to 72 hours. They should be treated with pain medication, a nasal decongestant such as 0.25 percent or 0.50 percent Neo-Synephrine nasal drops, and followed up in the office in 2 to 3 days. If the child continues to be symptomatic, the antibiotics just mentioned should be given. Surgical intervention should be considered in the following circumstances: AOM in children younger than 6 months old; when an organism may be present that is not the customary bacteria found in AOM; a child who has an impending complication, such as swelling behind the ear or facial nerve weakness; a child who is very ill and experiencing toxicity; or a child with AOM who is still symptomatic after one or two antibiotics have failed.

If a child over the age of 2 years appears to be improving within 48 to 72 hours, I would then recommend follow-up in 2 to 3 weeks, and the parent should be advised to call the physician if any clinical symptoms such as temperature elevation or pain recur. At that point, medical therapy must be instituted. With this method of practice, approximately 80 percent to 90 percent of children will recover from AOM without the use of antibiotics.

It has been demonstrated that there is no significant difference in the following two important outcome results involving AOM and antibiotics. The use of antibiotics does not alter the recurrence rate of AOM and the eventual resolution of fluid in the middle ear. Pain is the major problem about which parents are concerned. Finally, the development of meningitis associated with AOM is most likely related to invasion of the organism from the nasopharynx rather than from the middle ear. Therefore, the presence of AOM per se is not a reason for either medical or surgical intervention to prevent meningitis, because by the time the patient develops AOM, meningeal disease is probably already present. Obviously, aggressive treatment for meningitis must be instituted immediately.

The duration of antibiotic therapy in the United States has empirically been at least 10 days. The reason for this duration has never been completely justified. What now seems reasonable is to individualize the duration of treatment based on various risk factors: the child's age (older children fare better than younger); the season of the year (in summertime most episodes resolve readily); the severity of the episode (mild episodes usually are not problematic); the child's previous history of OM (a relatively otitis-free past bodes well); and the child's response to current treatment (prompt, symptomatic improvement usually foretells continuation of a benign course). In many instances in which those factors, on balance, suggest a favorable near-term outcome, limiting the duration of antimicrobial treatment to 3 to 5 days appears to be a prudent modification of current practice.

One final potential complication of the use of oral antibiotics is the increased duration of carriage of NTHI. This phenomenon was demonstrated in our clinical studies recently. The use of amoxicillin and/or amoxicillin-clavulanate prolonged nasopharyngeal colonization with potential middle ear pathogens and may thus predispose children to recurrent infections.

■ RECURRENT ACUTE OTITIS MEDIA

This disease entity, characterized by recurrent episodes of AOM with either persistent effusion or complete clearance between events, is one of the most difficult problems to eradicate. It is characteristic of the so-called otitis-prone condition and is associated with such variables as immunologic deficiency, possible food allergy, and genetic predisposition, particularly regarding the ability of the child to produce either specific nasopharyngeal secretory immunoglobulin A or specific systemic immunoglobulin G.

Inasmuch as the otolaryngologist usually sees children

with recurrent AOM fairly late in their course, that is, these children have been treated with multiple antibiotics, it is often necessary to select a more aggressive approach in their therapeutic management. These children often are young—between 1 and 3 years of age—and adenoidectomy, although considered by many pediatricians to be too aggressive a therapy, may actually be the best treatment. There is overwhelming molecular biologic evidence that the bacteria that colonize the middle ear and cause inflammation are always present in the nasopharynx at the time of acute or recurrent AOM. Therefore, the disease always begins in the nasopharynx; the philosophy of adenoidectomy is to remove the bulk of bacterial antigenic load that is present in the nasopharynx. Thus, the adenoidectomy is not being performed because of hypertrophy or obstruction, but because the nasopharynx is the source of the bacteria that infect the middle ear. Just as adenoidectomy between ages 4 and 8 years has been shown to significantly improve middle ear status, the effect of adenoidectomy in younger children, although not yet tested in a large study, nevertheless is a clinically useful procedure. Most likely this procedure will be shown to be as effective in younger children as it has in older children in the published studies previously referred to. Even the most knowledgeable pediatricians who have studied OM are now backing away from prophylactic antibiotics because of the serious trend of emerging resistant bacteria, particularly *S. pneumoniae.*

I therefore would advise adenoidectomy as the treatment of choice in children who are otitis-prone, have recurrent AOM, and persistently fail medical therapy. It should also be emphasized that tonsillectomy has never been proved to be of any benefit in the treatment of either AOM, recurrent AOM, or OME.

OTITIS MEDIA WITH EFFUSION

OME is the disease entity in which pediatricians, general physicians, and otolaryngologists must refrain from indiscriminate and unnecessary use of antibiotic therapy. OME is defined as an inflammatory condition of the middle ear in which there is an accumulation of serous or mucoid fluid in the absence of clinical symptoms such as pain and fever. OME may or may not be associated with a significant hearing loss, and there is no hard evidence to correlate the effect of intermittent or even long-term hearing loss with speech or language development later in life. It is important to emphasize that there is a very high incidence of complete recovery from OME without any therapy. By and large, OME is a benign disorder in which probably 90 percent of patients recover spontaneously within 3 to 6 months. OME is virtually never treated with antibiotics in most European countries, but it is frequently treated with antibiotics in the United States. It is unfortunate that the guidelines for OME that have recently been published suggest that antibiotics are an option for this disease. The other option is watchful waiting, which is not only safer but also just as successful based on epidemiologic studies. Even the most astute general physicians have written on this subject and have suggested that OME in young children is "a disease in search of a treatment." Indications for surgical treatment are listed in Table 2.

Table 2. Summary of Management of Otitis Media in an Era of Increasing Bacterial Resistance to Antibiotics

ENTITY	AGE	MANAGEMENT
AOM	Neonate–2 yr	Amoxicillin, cefuroxime axetil, and amoxicillin-clavulanate 3–5 days; tympanocenteses in selected cases
	>2 yr	No therapy for 48–72 hr, but medical therapy as mentioned previously if clinical symptoms persist after this time
RAOM	Neonate–2 yr >2 yr	Same as for AOM, but if effusion or recurrent OM persist, then adenoidectomy and bilateral tympanostomy with tubes
OME	All ages	Watchful waiting for at least 3–6 months; tympanostomy with tubes if hearing loss >20 dB in speech frequencies after 4–6 months; adenoidectomy if these treatments fail

AOM, acute otitis media; RAOM, recurrent acute otitis media; OME, otitis media with effusion.

DISCUSSION

The emergence of multidrug–resistant strains of *S. pneumoniae* and the increasing incidence of β-lactamase–producing strains of *H. influenzae* prompt re-examination of the impact that resistant strains have on the treatment of AOM as well as the spectra of recurrent OM and OME. In response to emerging drug resistance, some experts have suggested that mild to moderate cases of AOM may not need antimicrobial therapy. The use of prophylactic antibiotics for the treatment of recurrent OM must be significantly curtailed or abolished. Finally, the management of OME should *not* include antibiotic therapy. It may be that some of the literature in the 1970s and 1980s overemphasized the presence of bacteria in the middle ear in OME. Based on recent studies from our laboratory, long-standing middle ear fluid is usually sterile and will not respond to antibiotic therapy. The medical and surgical management of these three common childhood problems involving the middle ear are summarized in Table 2. These suggestions may be radically different from what is found in most textbooks of pediatrics and even otolaryngology. But, as we approach the 21st century, it is mandatory that we seek other strategies of management for OM.

Suggested Reading

Bernstein JM. Otitis media with effusion: To treat or not to treat? J Respir Dis 1995; 16:88-99.

Froom J, Culpepper L, Grob P, et al. Diagnosis and antibiotic treatment of acute otitis media: Report from international primary care network. Br Med J 1990; 300:582-586.

Klein JO. Microbiologic efficacy of antibacterial drugs for acute otitis media. Pediat Infect Dis 1993; 12:973-976.

Paradise JL. Managing otitis media: A time for change. Pediatrics 1995; 96:712-714.

ACUTE MASTOIDITIS

The method of
Kathleen C.Y. Sie

Acute mastoiditis is usually a complication of acute otitis media (AOM). The mastoid air cells communicate with the middle ear space through the aditus. Inflammation of the middle ear mucosa causes obstruction of the aditus and secondary changes in the mastoid air cells. One of the reasons to treat acute otitis media with antibiotics is to prevent complications such as mastoiditis. With the widespread use of oral antibiotics in the management of acute otitis media, the incidence of acute mastoiditis has fallen dramatically. However, the likelihood of complications associated with acute mastoiditis remains quite high.

PRESENTATION AND CLINICAL PICTURE

Acute mastoiditis is characterized by postauricular pain, erythema, and tenderness. The patient may or may not have a history of acute otitis media.

Edema of the posterior superior canal skin and proptosis of the pinna may be noted. On otoscopy, the tympanic membrane (TM) is usually intact and shows signs of AOM. On occasion, the TM may have ruptured, with partial drainage of the middle ear space. Rarely, the TM will appear normal, presumably associated with a blocked aditus causing mastoiditis. Signs of systemic illness, such as fever and malaise, may be present. Acute mastoiditis should be differentiated from chronic mastoiditis; the latter is usually associated with chronic otorrhea, chronic TM perforation, and possibly aural polyp.

There is a spectrum of disease, depending on the severity of infection and underlying host factors. The earliest infections may have a presentation of postauricular erythema. Primary care providers often treat this early infection on an outpatient basis, with close follow-up. The early stages of infection may go unrecognized, and patients more often come to otolaryngologists with significant postauricular inflammation, pain, tenderness, erythema, and systemic signs of illness.

Finally, complete physical examination should be performed on all patients who have acute mastoiditis to rule out associated complications (Table 1). The most common complication of acute mastoiditis is subperiosteal abscess. Careful palpation of the mastoid cortex should be performed. Patients without signs of complications on initial presentation should be carefully monitored while being treated.

Table 1. Complications of Acute Mastoiditis

INTRATEMPORAL	INTRACRANIAL
Acute coalescent mastoiditis with subperiosteal abscess	Hydrocephalus
Hearing loss	Meningitis
Tympanic membrane perforation	Encephalitis
Facial nerve palsy	Intracranial abcess (epidural, subdural)
Labyrinthitis	Sigmoid sinus thrombosis

DIAGNOSIS

Presence of the aforementioned clinical findings defines the diagnosis of acute mastoiditis. Computed tomographic (CT) scan of the temporal bones may be used to support the diagnosis, but mastoid opacification is common in patients who have acute otitis media, especially in children. Radiologic evidence of mastoid opacification in the absence of clinical signs of mastoiditis is not clinically significant. In general, temporal bone CT scan is reserved to confirm or diagnose complications of mastoiditis, for example, subperiosteal abscess and intracranial infection. Imaging studies may also be useful in patients who do not respond appropriately to medical therapy to rule out other diseases that may affect the mastoid. If there is suspicion of an intracranial complication, a head CT scan with contrast must also be ordered (Fig. 1).

DIFFERENTIAL DIAGNOSIS

Patients who do not respond to medical therapy should be reassessed. Other diagnoses should be considered (Table 2). Biopsy of the involved mucosa is required for definitive diagnosis.

THERAPY

Medical

Acute mastoiditis is usually caused by the same organisms that cause acute otitis media, *Streptococcus pneumoniae*, β-hemolytic streptococcus, *Staphylococcus aureus*, and *Haemophilus influenzae*. Empiric treatment should be directed at these organisms. Tympanocentesis for culture of the middle ear contents should be performed to identify pathogenic organisms and direct antibiotic management. Empiric intravenous antibiotic management should be initiated pending cultures. Antibiotic choices include ticarcillin/clavulanate and ceftriaxone with or without metronidazole (or imipenem). Acute mastoiditis related to chronic otitis media with effusion should be treated with aztreonam plus clindamycin (or ticarcillin/clavulanate, imipenem plus gentamicin, or ceftazidime plus nafcillin plus metronidazole). The duration of antibiotic therapy for treatment of acute mastoiditis is controversial and probably depends on the severity of infection at the time of presentation. In general, intravenous antibiotics should be given until the soft-tissue infection of the postauricular region and external auditory canal is re-

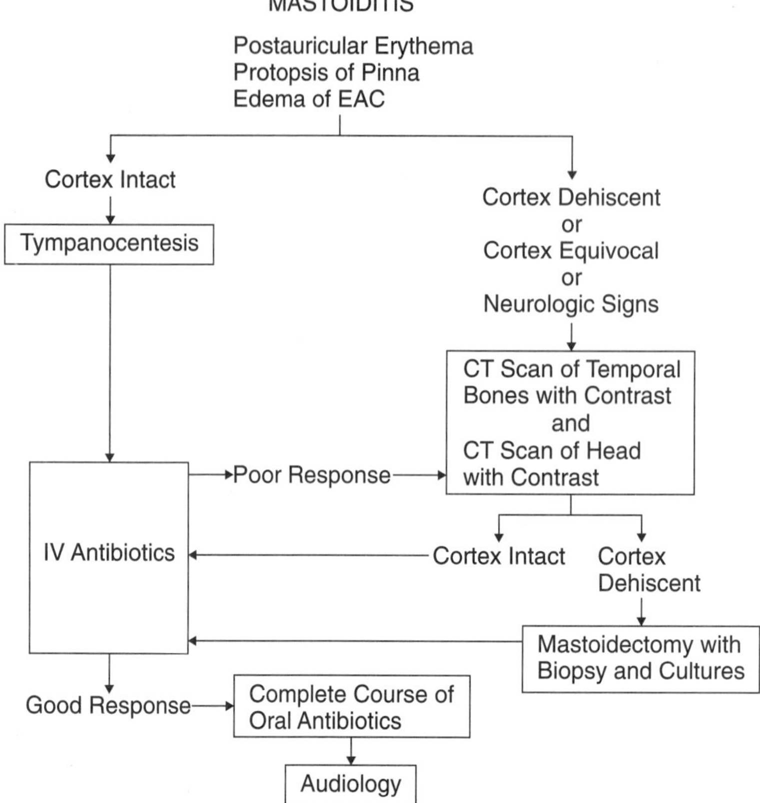

Figure 1.
Algorithm for the treatment of mastoiditis. EAC, external auditory canal.

Table 2. Differential Diagnosis of Acute Mastoiditis

CHILDREN	ADULTS
Rhabdomyosarcoma	Fulminant otitis externa
Histiocytosis X	Histiocytosis X
Leukemia	Metastatic disease
Kawasaki's syndrome	

solved. This usually ranges from 3 to 7 days. I recommend completion of a 3 to 4 week course of oral antibiotic therapy on an outpatient basis.

Patients being treated for mastoiditis require continuous vigilance. If signs of progression of infection or development of complications arise, CT scan of the temporal bones with contrast should be obtained. Wide myringotomy with biopsy of the middle ear mucosa should be considered if there is no significant clinical response 48 hours after instituting antibiotic therapy and the mastoid cortex remains intact by physical examination and CT scan. Patients refractory to culture-directed medical management may require simple mastoidectomy. Tissue sample should be taken for culture and pathology at the time of surgery.

Surgical

Patients who develop significant complications of acute mastoiditis, specifically subperiosteal abscess or intracranial complications, should undergo simple (or cortical) mastoidectomy. A tympanostomy tube may be placed at the same time. The procedure is performed under general anesthesia, with the patient breathing spontaneously, so that facial nerve function can be monitored. I prefer a postauricular approach for mastoidectomy. In children younger than 3 to 4 years of age, the inferior limit of the incision should be positioned over the palpable portion of the mastoid cortex to avoid inadvertent injury to the facial nerve. Intraoperative facial nerve monitoring should be considered for patients who have craniofacial disorders, young patients (i.e., younger than 4 years), and those who have facial nerve palsy.

Cortical mastoidectomy is performed in the standard fashion. Samples of any fluid, or pus, and mucosa should be sent for culture and pathology, respectively. Ideally, mastoidectomy results in communication between the mastoid and middle ear spaces through the aditus. However, some patients will require posterior tympanotomy through a facial recess approach to accomplish free communication between these two spaces. An irrigation catheter, using a 16 or 14 gauge angiocatheter, may be placed into the mastoid cavity through the postauricular wound. The angiocatheter is capped with a heparin lock port. Ototopical drops containing steroids can be instilled through the irrigation catheter in an effort to treat edema of the middle ear and mastoid mucosa. The tympanostomy tube allows egress of the drops. The catheter is usually removed 1 to 3 days postoperatively.

Audiologic testing should be performed in all patients. Any patient who has vestibular symptoms should have a hearing test to rule out cochlear involvement. In the absence of vestibular involvement, audiologic testing should be performed after resolution of the infection. In children, the testing should be repeated until they are able to give reliable, ear-specific responses.

■ DISCUSSION

Acute mastoiditis remains a significant clinical disease, despite widespread use of antibiotics in the management of AOM. In fact, the frequent use of broad-spectrum antibiotics for treatment of AOM has raised the potential for infections with antibiotic-resistant organisms. It is important for clinicians to understand the pathogenesis, differential diagnosis, propensity for associated complications, and management issues in patients who have acute mastoiditis. Neurosurgical consultation may be required for patients with intracranial complications. The diagnosis and monitoring of these patients remains a clinical art. CT scanning should be reserved for patients who have an equivocal examination, poor response to directed therapy, and those who are surgical candidates.

Suggested Reading

Gliklich RE, Eavey RD, Iannuzzi RA, Camacho AE. A contemporary analysis of acute mastoiditis. Arch Otolaryngol Head Neck Surg 1996; 122:135-139.

THE CHRONIC DRAINING EAR

The method of

C. Gary Jackson

Due to the proximity of the middle ear and mastoid air cell system to the vital anatomy of the temporal bone and its intracranial relationships, the presence of chronic infection imparts unique challenges. Once chronicity has been established, the management of this condition is in large part surgical and necessarily pre-emptive.

The traditional outcome objectives for the management of the chronic draining ear are as relevant today as they were 50 years ago. In order of priority, these objectives are (1) to achieve a clean, healed, dry ear; (2) to obtain an air-containing middle ear space; and (3) to rehabilitate hearing. The chronically infected ear is a hostile environment that often confounds the realization of these optimal outcome objectives. This chapter presents my evolved methods for maximizing success in this difficult area.

■ PREOPERATIVE STRATEGY

The patient who is initially seen with active discharge through the tympanic membrane (TM) perforation without cholesteatoma undergoes a thorough otolaryngologic exam to assess the problem as well as any ear, nose, and throat (ENT) disorder that might predispose to this disease or contribute to management failure. Such entities might include nasosinal disease, sinusitis, nasal airway disorders, palatal abnormalities, or nasal allergy. It is important to emphasize the need to evaluate these ears otomicroscopically. Under the microscope debris should be evacuated to permit a thorough evaluation of the disorder. Pure-tone and speech audiometry is assessed. The status of the opposite ear is often important to ipsilateral management decision making.

There are no clinically applicable tests of eustachian tube (ET) function. ET patency, otherwise not germane to the pathophysiology at hand, is assessable (e.g., by Valsalva's or Toynbee maneuver), but adds little to the treatment decision tree. ET testing is not performed.

■ CONTROL OF CONTRIBUTING FACTORS

Contributing factors are those conditions which, when they exist, tend to confound disease resolution or predispose to treatment failure. In a recent national poll of otologists, nasal allergy and adenoidectomy were regarded as factors predisposing to treatment failure. To this, I add nasosinal disease.

In the pediatric patient who has significant adenoidal hypertrophy, the surgical plan is pre-empted to manage this problem which, by consensus, is significant to the outcome of ear surgery. Adenoidectomy and tympanoplasty are not performed at the same time. I have believed it illogical to do so. The patient is referred to an otolaryngologic colleague for surgery. Tympanoplasty is scheduled 4 to 6 weeks later. The same logic applies to *acute* nasosinal disease.

■ PREPARATION FOR SURGERY

Every effort is made to control otorrhea preoperatively. I have found it unnecessary to rigidly mandate that an ear be dry at the time of surgery, even though this is our preference. My primary treatment regimen to control preoperative otorrhea and prepare an ear for surgery is topical. Ear toilet is critical. If the patient resides locally, he or she will be seen frequently for otomicroscopic cleansing of the ear. This is, however, unusual in my practice. Patients are instructed to cleanse the ear by lavage with 1.5 percent acetic acid solution three times daily. Immediately after irrigation, an antibiotic-steroid topical suspension is employed. Water precautions are urged, and surgery is scheduled. This interim in my practice is usually 2 to 4 weeks. Surgery is performed at the prescribed time whether the ear is dry or not. Expensive, labor-intensive intravenous antibiotics are avoided.

A word on intravenous antibiotics. I find them palliative. As a curative therapy, my experience has been that specific intravenous antibiotics are effective in the short term. I reserve this protocol for those patients without cholesteatoma who are otherwise not candidates for the consensus treatment of choice, surgery.

■ RADIOLOGY

Preoperative radiologic studies are not routinely done. Plain mastoid x-ray studies have been abandoned. Magnetic resonance imaging (MRI) has little use in diagnosing chronic ear disease at this time. This will surely change in the future. Currently, MRI is employed very selectively to (1) better image the facial nerve in a complicated ear; (2) define and qualify brain herniation; and (3) better define intracranial complication. In all other cases, a high-resolution temporal bone scan and computed tomography (CT) scan and head CT with contrast are done. Although not done routinely, CT is called for in an only-hearing ear and in the presence of adult long-standing disease commonly heralded by multiple failed surgical revisions. The contrasted head study scouts for intracranial complication which, in this antibiotic era, might exist in a clinically silent stage.

■ PATIENT INFORMATION

All surgical details, more common potential risks and complications, as well as *reasonable* expectations are presented to the patient in person as well as by professionally prepared audiovisual material employing models and diagrams. Receipt of this education and understanding of possible complications of surgery is acknowledged by the patient's signature on printed material that outlines the content of the educational material. Informed consent is an important objective, as is documentation of a legitimate attempt to accomplish it.

■ BASIC TECHNICAL CONCEPTS

The success of any surgical protocol is based on the competent execution of each one of its fundamentals. Every procedure can be distilled down to its elemental components, the completion of which virtually warrants the desired outcome. Often disregarded under the microscope, these basic principles are essential to success.

Infection Control

Surgical preparation takes place in the operating room. One inch of hair is shaved around the ear. Adhesive barrier drapes are employed to avoid bacterial contamination of the surgical field. The ear is prepped with povidone-iodine (Betadine) scrub and paint. Betadine is placed into the ear canal, which is evacuated when the surgeon is first seated.

The secret to pollution is dilution. Copious irrigation is consciously employed throughout the procedure to keep the field clear and reduce colony counts.

In general, antibiotic prophylaxis is not used. The protective umbrella of prophylactic antibiotics does not exist. There is no substitute for careful aseptic technique. The intent to reduce colony counts by antibiotics is, at best, contentious. When clean fields become contaminated by the complex microbiology of the chronic ear, antimicrobial prophylaxis is important. When the dura or labyrinth is violated, when the host is compromised, or when breaks in technique are overt, antimicrobial prophylaxis is indicated. Clearly, prophylactic antibiotics are no insurance of better results. The downside risks of allergic reaction and a false sense of security do not justify the routine application of these agents.

Exposure

Adequate visualization is essential to success, particularly in microsurgery. Nearly 100 percent of my surgery for chronic ear problems, for this reason, is done postauricularly. Transcanal routes are technically restrictive and promote failure. From the postauricular approach, the visualization of the anterior sulcus for accurate graft placement is unsurpassed. In general, I disavow minimally invasive formats (e.g., paper patches, fat "push-throughs").

For prominent anterior external auditory canal (EAC) bulges, a Wright-Guilford window shade flap can be elevated from medial to lateral; the bone is drilled back for visualization; and the flap is rolled back down without risk to the graft or EAC stenosis.

When mastoidectomy is done, it should be complete. Atticotomy, antrostomy, and similar procedures have limited utility. I have, for all practical purposes, abandoned them.

Hemostasis

All the exposure available will not help graft placement under blood. Hemostasis, particularly in microsurgery, is fundamental.

Before the incision is made and after prepping, the postauricular incision site is injected with 2 percent lidocaine (Xylocaine) and 1:100,000 epinephrine (Adrenalin) in a commercially prepared dental carpule. This vehicle avoids loose solution, the identity of which can later be confusing, on the operating table. The surgeon's first task is to evacuate the povidone-iodine from the EAC and then inject the canal using the same anesthetic-hemostatic solution. In this way, hemostasis can be achieved at the critical incision lines.

During the procedure, bleeding can be bothersome in and around granulation tissue. Gelfoam soaked in 1:1,000 epinephrine can be applied, and attention can then be directed elsewhere. Ten minutes or so later, removal of the Gelfoam usually reveals adequate hemostasis to proceed. Frequent irrigation is also useful.

Bipolar electrocautery in chronic ear surgery is very useful. Hemostasis on the facial nerve sheath, the dura, sigmoid sinus, delicate EAC flaps, and other areas is easily achieved. Adopted from our neurosurgery, this tool is invaluable in cases where unipolar cautery is clearly dangerous.

Grafting Techniques

For the surgeon who occasionally works on the ear, undersurface techniques offer higher take rates and fewer complications. Lateral graft placement requires higher levels of proficiency for success—a fact readily acknowledged by those who endorse it.

I prefer "fool's fascia," which is the superficial areolar layer that overlays the temporal fascia. More malleable, it does require some technical facility, which the new surgeon might find daunting. Tragal perichondrium, temporal fascia, temporal periosteum, and vein are all good alternatives. We have disavowed the use of homograft.

Mastoidectomy

The issue of employing mastoidectomy in chronic otitis media with cholesteatoma is clear and uncomplicated. The question of whether to use mastoidectomy in chronic otitis media without cholesteatoma is more clouded. There are no data that establish guidelines for using mastoidectomy in this circumstance.

The guidelines I use to decide whether to perform a mastoidectomy in the chronic draining ear acknowledge that graft failure is usually due to infection in the middle ear (which we control nicely and consistently at surgery) or infection in the mastoid. In certain circumstances when mastoid infection is suspected (e.g., recent otorrhea, multiple failed previous operations, poorly aerated ears), I am more inclined to "just do it." Mastoidectomy takes me 8 to 12 minutes and involves very minimal morbidity, so I am more inclined to perform the procedure than not to do it.

Mastoidectomy nomenclature is confusing. Here I am speaking of a simple (complete) mastoidectomy. Modified radical, "Bondy," and radical mastoidectomies are highly specific protocols rigidly confined to precise indications that are not addressed here.

Staging

Under managed care, staged reconstruction is a precarious strategy. Generally, I do more and more primary reconstructions. Clearly, hearing results are better in the staged ear when the changing anatomic relationships of healing are stable. There are still, however, some very legitimate reasons to stage an ear: (1) extensive granulation or skin on the stapes or footplate not otherwise amenable to laser therapy; (2) extensive mucosal disease; (3) cases in which stapedectomy is required; and (4) extensive disease. I still perform staged reconstruction, and I seek informed consent preoperatively in those patients who have less optimal, more diseased ears.

Surgical Technique

All patients undergo surgery with general anesthesia in the supine position and prepared as already described. The EAC injection should clearly demonstrate the vascular strip area between the tympanomastoid suture and tympanosquamous suture.

Vascular strip incisions are then made, and ear canal skin flaps are then outlined (Fig. 1). A postauricular incision is executed 1 cm behind the postauricular crease. A temporal areolar graft is harvested. Soft tissue overlying the mastoid portion of the temporal bone is incised and elevated, the vascular strip being extracted from the ear canal in the process (Fig. 2). Removal of any bulges or excrescences of the ear canal is done at this time.

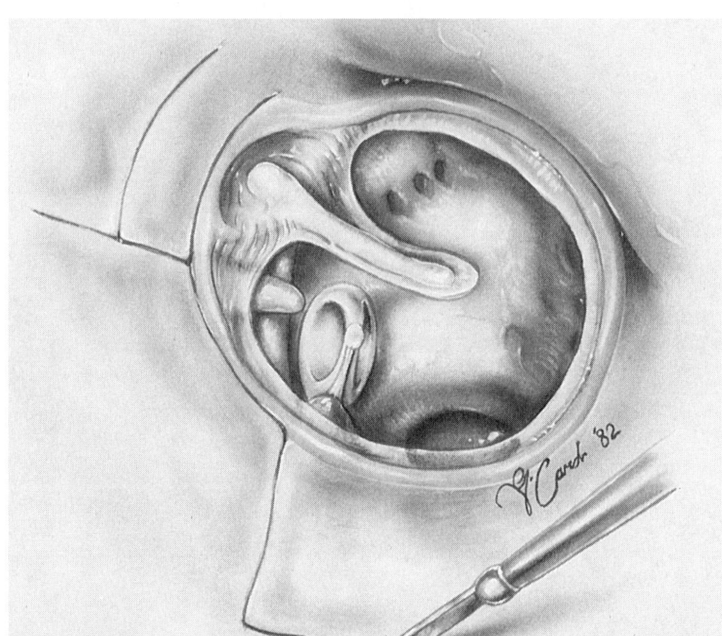

Figure 1.
At the tympanomastoid suture and tympanosquamous suture, vascular strip incisions are made. An inferiorly based flap and a smaller anterior flap are outlined. *(From Glassock ME, Jackson CG, Nissen AJ, Schwaber MK. Postauricular undersurface tympanic membrane grafting: A follow-up report. Laryngoscope 1982;92:718–727.)*

The margins of the tympanic membrane perforation and any diseased tympanic membrane are excised. Perforation size is irrelevant to outcome success. The EAC flaps are then rotated, and the middle ear is inspected. Any ossicular or mucosal disarray is acknowledged and dealt with presently. When indicated, a complete mastoidectomy is performed next. The field is kept well irrigated and clear of bone dust.

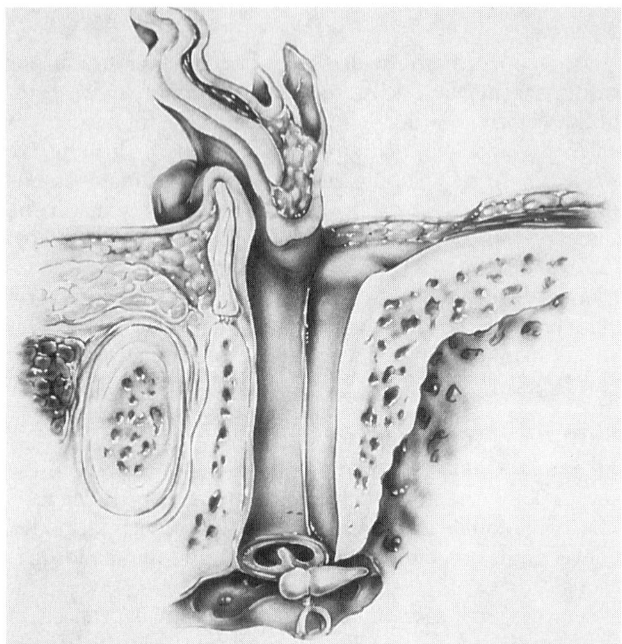

Figure 2.
The postauricular approach affords excellent exposure of the difficult anterior sulcus region. *(From Glassock ME, Jackson CG, Nissen AJ, Schwaber MK. Postauricular undersurface tympanic membrane grafting: A follow-up report. Laryngoscope 1982;92:718–727.)*

In preparation for grafting, the middle ear is filled with Gelfoam that is moistened and pressed (by hand). No antibiotic drops are used. The Gelfoam is hydrated in Tissusol, which serves as a graft bed. Critical areas are medial to lateral transition zones and at the eustachian tube. The graft slit is then placed medial to the malleus handle. The graft is then placed medial to the tympanic membrane and back up the posterior EAC wall. The EAC flaps are then re-rotated (Fig. 3). The vascular strip is returned to its original position, and the EAC is filled with Polysporin ointment. No packing is used. The postauricular incision is closed in two layers with 3–0 and 4–0 Vicryl sutures. The skin closure is subcuticular. A bubble dressing is placed, and the procedure is then terminated.

The dressing is removed in the late afternoon after morning surgery. The patient is discharged on the same day with postauricular bandage in place and EAC cotton to catch the ointment drainage, because the ointment liquefies at body temperature. Written instructions are given to patients, along with a follow-up appointment 3 weeks later. Water should be excluded from the ear, and trauma should be avoided. Air travel to and from the clinic is not discouraged. Clinical course dictates subsequent follow-up, which is liberally infrequent. Expectation of success from my procedures is 95 percent. Complications are minor.

■ SPECIAL CONSIDERATIONS

The difficult chronic ear (some in the field may argue that *all* chronic ears are difficult!) is a special otologic circumstance that consistently challenges our management efforts. These patients exhibit a social and professional incapacity; undergo multiple operations; and are medically dependent and water intolerant. The ear is an unrelenting imposition to the patient and otologist alike. The costs of multiple operations, intravenous antibiotics, drop therapy, and office vis-

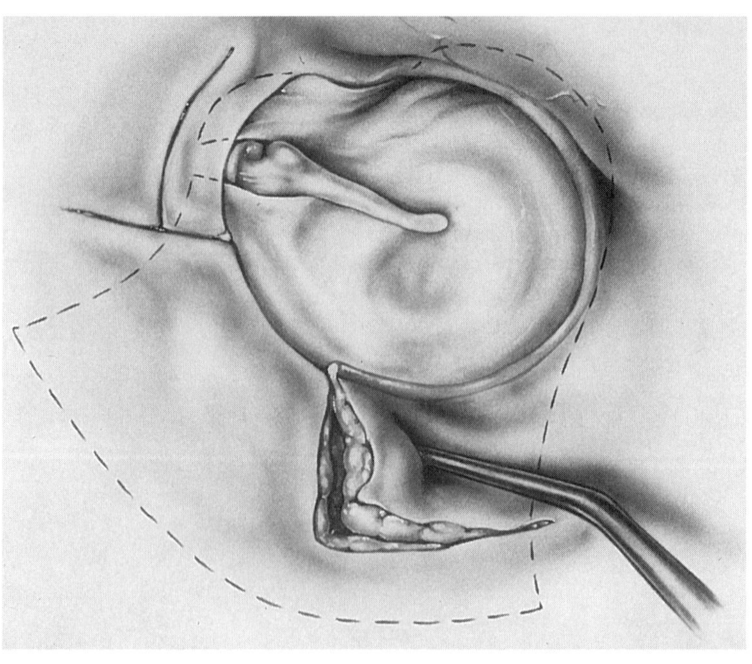

Figure 3.
The underlay graft has been placed medial to the annulus. The graft slit is tucked under the malleus and manubrium. External auditory canal flaps are re-rotated. Ointment will "pack" the EAC. *(From Glassock ME, Jackson CG, Nissen AJ, Schwaber MK. Postauricular undersurface tympanic membrane grafting: A follow-up report. Laryngoscope 1982;92:718–727.)*

its, when coupled with time and money lost to the economy due to the aforementioned incapacities, constitute a socioeconomic problem of significant proportion.

The problem cavity is the aftermath of multiple attempts at surgical correction and is characterized by (1) a small meatus; (2) dependent tip in which debris accumulates; (3) a high facial ridge and/or incomplete levels of EAC wall removal; (4) noisome otorrhea; (5) polyps, granulation tissue, retained cholesteatoma; and (6) water intolerance.

The solution to this problem is always surgical. Objectives include infection control, freedom from future surgery, and hearing rehabilitation. The technique highlights a canal wall-down format and the establishment of a wide meatoplasty. Technical details are provided in the Suggested Reading list. This approach is consistently applied to disease in an only-hearing ear.

Of 541 patients fitting this description in our practice, we were able to achieve infection control and freedom from future surgery in 91 percent. These are our most difficult ear cases: 67 percent exhibited intraoperative complication of disease (e.g., fistula, exposed facial nerve, dural dehiscence). Of 15 patients who had only-hearing ears, none lost hearing, with the majority exhibiting no change in hearing ability after operation.

Suggested Reading

Jackson CG. Antimicrobial prophylaxis in ear surgery. Laryngoscope 1988; 98:1116-1123.

Jackson CG, Glasscock ME, Widick MH. Chronic ear disease: Surgical decisions and techniques. In: Highlights of the AAO–HNS instruction courses—1994 edition. St. Louis: Mosby–Year Book, 1994.

Jackson CG, Pappas DG Jr, Manolidis S, et al. Brain herniation into the middle ear and mastoid: Concepts in diagnosis and surgical management. Am J Otol 1997; 18:198-205.

Jackson CG, Schall DG, Glasscock ME, et al. A surgical solution for the difficult chronic ear. Am J Otol 1996; 17:7-14.

CHOLESTEATOMA

The method of
Richard J. Wiet
by
Richard J. Wiet
Alan G. Micco
Olga Bedoya

The management of aural cholesteatoma is both old and new. We have come to appreciate the collective wisdom of both authors of *Surgery of the Ear,* Fourth edition. The reader who analyzes the discussions of mastoid surgery carefully will note the clash of opinions between George Shambaugh, Jr., and Michael Glasscock. These authors diverge on management issues related to canal wall-up versus canal wall-down. Having the unique privilege of being trained and influenced by both experts (and now seasoned by time), we would argue toward a synthesis of eclectic thought. This chapter first defines terms, then classifies the types of cholesteatoma, and finally discusses the controversies in management influenced by the current health care system.

There are two basic forms of cholesteatoma: congenital and acquired. Congenital cholesteatoma is precisely defined. Authors from Northwestern University have defined congenital cholesteatoma as an epidermoid mass occurring in the middle ear behind an intact tympanic membrane. There is absence of suppuration, with no evidence of a perforation. Congenital cholesteatomas originate during embryonic development when small remnants of ectoderm are trapped within the temporal bone. In Michaels's review of temporal bones, he noted that squamous cells rest in the anterior superior lateral wall of the tympanic cavity from 10 to 33 weeks of gestation. He further noted that this formation was not present after 33 weeks. According to Schuknecht, congenital cholesteatomas may occur in five sites: (1) the petrous apex, (2) the cerebellopontine angle, (3) the mastoid, (4) the middle ear, and (5) the external auditory canal. Each location will have certain presenting signs and symptoms. Generally speaking, the diagnosis of congenital middle ear cholesteatoma is made in childhood; in contrast, acquired cholesteatomas are often diagnosed in later life—the second to the fourth decades. Our focus in this chapter is limited to acquired cholesteatoma of the middle ear and mastoid. Treatment of congenital cholesteatoma is determined by both location clinically and computed tomography (CT). It generally bears a better prognosis than does acquired cholesteatoma.

The acquired cholesteatoma is subdivided between primary and secondary. Both are related to dysfunction of the eustachian tube. This definition, as Shambaugh states, has implications for management. Primary acquired cholesteatoma occurs in the attic at the level of Shrapnell's membrane. It often appears to be a perforation in the pars flaccida, but on closer examination under the otomicroscope there is often a retraction pocket (Fig. 1). A retraction pocket may give rise to a cholesteatoma via invasive activity. There are both anatomic and physiologic reasons for its development. The anatomic reasons relate to lack of support due to the fact

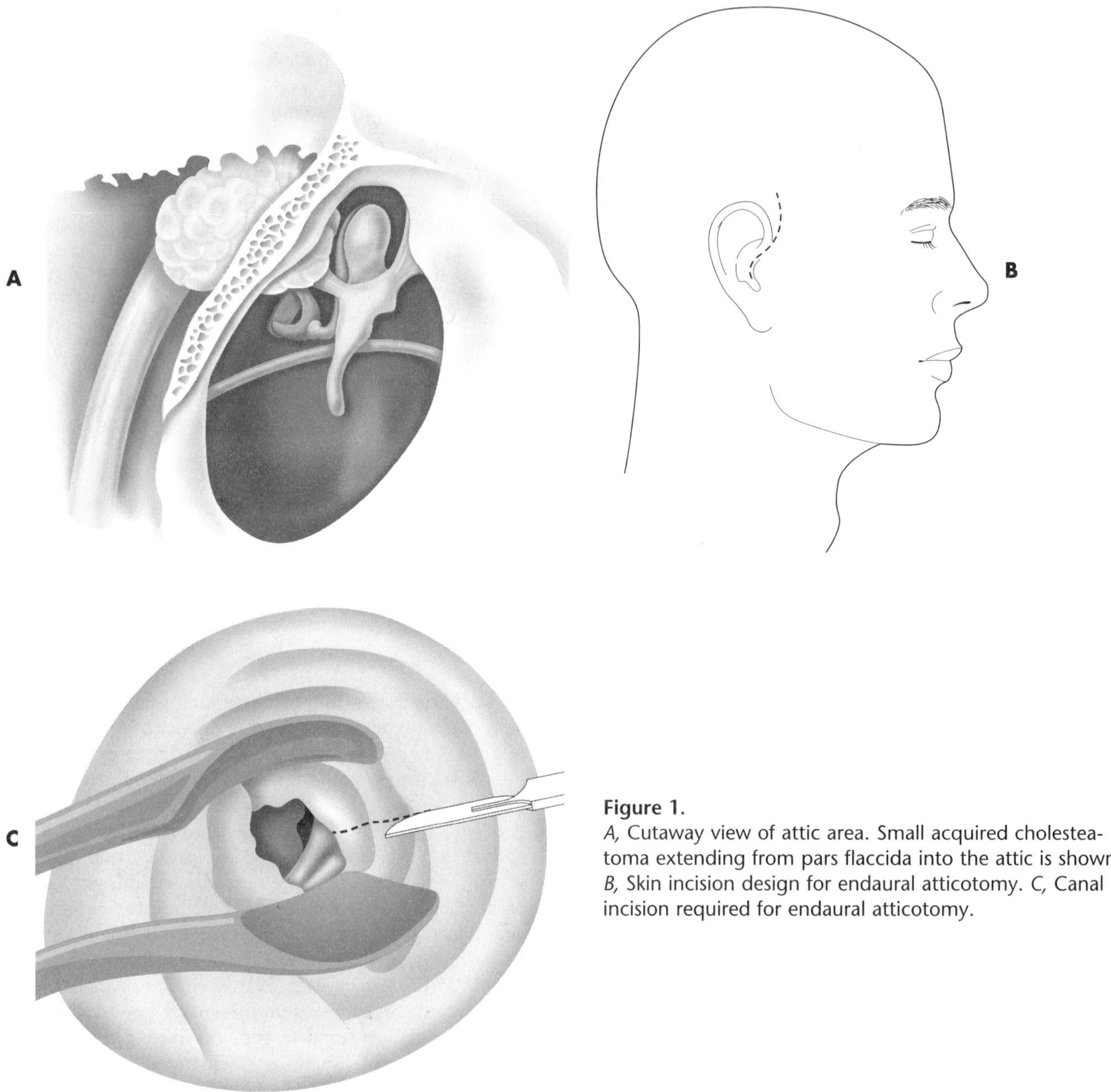

Figure 1.
A, Cutaway view of attic area. Small acquired cholesteatoma extending from pars flaccida into the attic is shown. *B,* Skin incision design for endaural atticotomy. *C,* Canal incision required for endaural atticotomy.

that dense fibers are not found in the middle ear. Chronic eustachian tube obstruction causes high negative pressure in the middle ear, with the eventual collapse or retraction of the tympanic membrane. The progressive collection of squamous debris associated with enzymatic change leads to cholesteatoma. There are two other theories of origin, however: the metaplastic theory and the migration theory.

The secondary acquired cholesteatoma is associated with tympanic membrane perforations and chronic middle ear infection. The concept of squamous migration through an existing perforation is well accepted. Squamous metaplasia of the middle ear mucosa is also a recognized cause of cholesteatoma. Another less common cause is iatrogenic implantation during ear surgery for repair of the tympanic membrane cholesteatoma. In most patients who have cholesteatoma (primary and secondary), at least one ossicle is involved; most commonly, it is the incus. The scutum or upper part of the tympanic ring is eroded in 42 percent of patients.

The management of cholesteatoma is better understood when one studies how cholesteatomas develop related to the ossicular structure. Proctor, and more recently Palva, have clarified these issues. Cholesteatomas tend to follow a pattern of origin in a single space and spread to other compartments by particular routes. The most common sites of origin of primary acquired cholesteatoma in order of frequency are the posterior epitympanum, the posterior mesotympanum, and the anterior epitympanum. If a growing cholesteatoma is medial or lateral to the incus body, *hearing preservation* techniques through atticotomy or endaural approaches are possible (Figs. 1, *B* and *C*). The position of the cholesteatoma is generally determined with coronal midcochlear CT examination. This scan illustrates eligibility for the endaural approach. The posterior epitympanic cholesteatoma occurs in Prussak's space (Fig. 2) and penetrates posteriorly to the superior incudal space lateral to the body of the incus, with progression to the aditus and the antrum. Anterior mesotympanic cholesteatomas pursue a more inferior route, descending to the pouch of Von Troeltch; these cholesteatomas are more prone to involve the stapes and proceed relentlessly toward the sinus tympani and the facial recess (Fig. 3). Our current management of these cholesteatomas involves a facial recess approach. The anterior epitympanic isolated cholesteatoma is infrequent. It is also one of the most challenging management problems. These cholesteatomas generally follow the course of the saccus anticus and also may involve the facial nerve at the level of the geniculate ganglion.

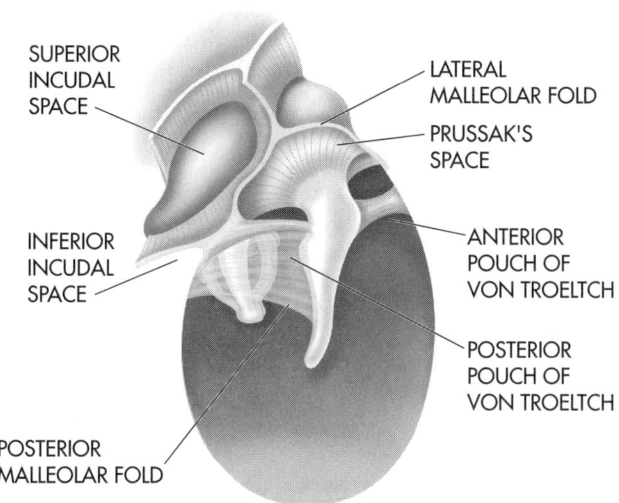

Figure 2.
Diagram of middle ear folds and ligaments that define the routes of cholesteatoma penetration.

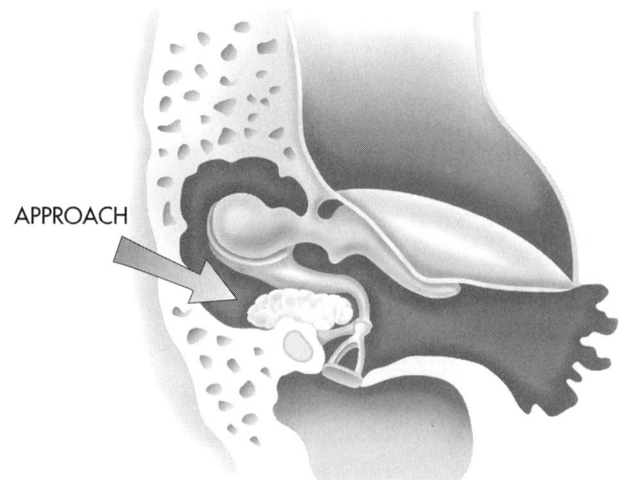

Figure 3.
Diagram of approach through the facial recess to access cholesteatomas medial to the incus and involving the stapes.

■ OFFICE EXAMINATION

After the appropriate history and physical examination, an otomicroscopic examination is performed. The clinician looks for obvious pearl white masses in the middle ear or evidence of posterior superior tympanic membrane retraction and/or perforation. Tuning fork examinations are done to evaluate and confirm a conductive hearing loss. In acquired cholesteatomas, examination of the head and neck should be done to rule out chronic nasal problems such as rhinitis and nasopharyngeal disease. Evidence of submucous cleft palate should also be sought. These conditions predispose to chronic eustachian tube dysfunction, which may limit the success of the procedure. Indeed, Bellucci has classified rates of success in a four-step process. Based on the position of the cholesteatoma and the amount of destruction it has caused, one can decide whether or not conservative surgery can be applied.

Results of the audiogram are carefully assessed, with particular attention to the amount of cochlear reserve, masking, the amount of air–bone gap, and interaural difference between the speech reception thresholds (SRTs). A far more conservative approach in planning surgery is taken for patients who have an only-hearing ear versus surgery planned in patients who have binaural hearing. When appropriate, a tympanic membrane patch is placed over the perforation to evaluate a gain in air conduction, with the implication that the ossicular chain is intact when air conduction improves. CT evaluation of the middle ear and mastoid is frequently obtained to evaluate whether or not conservative surgery can be applied. Conservative surgery is defined as attempting to preserve structure, either ossicular structure or canal wall structure, depending on the pneumatization of the mastoid and the position of the cholesteatoma.

In preoperative discussion with the patient, not only are the risks and benefits of surgery discussed, but also the alternatives of management for dry, inactive disease are mentioned. The possibility of diminished hearing postsurgery is reviewed in the event that the patient is *hearing through the cholesteatoma* or the incus needs removal. Staging is discussed, with the emphasis on operating for disease the first time and for hearing and/or residual lesion the second time. The patient is given information on aural cleansing, the need for antibiotics before surgery, and the possibility of staging is reiterated.

In our review of 97 mastoid cholesteatomas, there was a trend to favor two-stage surgery for intact canal wall mastoidectomy. One-stage procedures were followed with serial office examinations. The residual disease rate for single-stage, intact canal wall procedures was 20 percent compared with a residual rate of 5 percent for the two-stage procedure. However, the difference was not statistically significant due to the small sample size.

■ MANAGEMENT

Hearing Conservation: Intact Chain, Favorable Cholesteatoma

Unfortunately, surgical training in the *endaural* approach as well as the *atticotomy* approach in the United States is diminishing. Both are approaches for treating limited disease in the most common cholesteatomas, which often lend themselves to one-stage surgery.

We use the Lempert incision with the Shambaugh modifications. Adequate mastoid exposure is developed by aiming toward the short process of the incus in drilling. The lateral surface of the temporal bone is saucerized, and a copious suction-irrigation technique is used. The final area of bone removal near the scutum is performed with curets. Often, the cholesteatoma can be removed with laser or Harrison knives. A possible contraindication to the endaural approach is a low-lying temporal lobe seen on coronal CT. The cholesteatoma is removed under direct visualization, and the tympanic membrane is repaired with an underlay technique.

Hearing conservation can also be achieved with the intact wall tympanomastoidectomy. A one-stage procedure for cholesteatoma is possible only under the most ideal circumstances. In this method, a postauricular incision is made. The canal wall is preserved by drilling toward the antrum, with caution not to disrupt the incus. Once it is determined that the incus is eroded and involved, it is removed. Disease is removed from the antral areas as well as the epitympanum. Through the bony canal, disease involving the middle ear can be removed. If the disease in the mesotympanum is extensive, the facial recess can be opened to provide increased exposure to that area. This allows for disease removal from around the stapes as well as the sinus tympani. When using only an intact canal wall technique, a residual and/or recurrent cholesteatoma rate of as high as 36 percent has been reported.

Canal Wall-Down Surgery: Ossicular Chain Not Intact

We follow Sheehy's tenets that the wall should not be removed in an only-hearing ear, in a very contracted mastoid, in a mastoid with a labyrinthine fistula, or in situations in which canal wall erosion is present due to disease. Each patient must be individually assessed preoperatively and intraoperatively for decision making. Canal wall-down procedures are clearly superior in reducing the incidence of residual disease.

Meaningful data regarding residual disease comparing intact canal wall-down mastoidectomy are obtained only from long-term follow-up. It is interesting that Cody and McDonald compared residual and recurrent disease in open cavity versus intact canal wall procedures at 4 and 10 year intervals. Open cavity failure rates increased from 6 percent to 7 percent, whereas intact canal wall failure rates increased from 35 percent to 45 percent. In contrast, Smyth reported an intact canal wall residual rate of 14 percent, whereas the wall-down rate was 1 percent in 13 years of follow-up.

■ EFFECTS OF MANAGED CARE

The changes in managed care in the United States have influenced a trend toward cost containment. Our group has adapted to these changes in the following way. Most of our mastoid surgery is now done on an outpatient basis (overnight stay). This 24 hour time frame is sufficient to manage most patients. When possible, we try to perform one-stage surgery. We follow up patients with CT scans when hearing is sufficient at 6 and 12 months postoperatively, and then annually. Austin has shown data for single-stage surgery, with a total recidivism rate (residual and recurrent disease) of 4 percent for a canal wall-down procedure and 3 percent for intact canal wall procedure. He argues that, by omitting staged procedures in the intact canal wall patient, the surgeon risks undetected disease, but overall performs fewer procedures, which may be more cost effective. Further, Tos and Lau suggest that a clinical examination could replace staging or surgery, because most residual cholesteatoma would occur in the mesotympanum or attic.

Endoscopy as proposed by Silverstein and Poe may have advantages in assessing the presence of cholesteatoma. Using a 1.7 mm 30 degree and 0 degree scope, the clinician can view the middle ear through the perforation and determine cholesteatoma presence or absence. This can at times save costs of scans and/or mastoid surgery. Additionally, ingrowth of squamous epithelium can be noted.

We reserve axial and coronal CT scans for revision cases, endaural surgery planning, and situations in which we may suspect an intratemporal complication. CT is also invaluable in determining the selection of a specific operating technique. This is especially true when one is dealing with a small contracted mastoid.

Suggested Reading

Bellucci R. Selection and cases and classification of tympanology. Otolaryngol Clin North Am 1989; 22:911.

Bluestone CD, Sheehy JL, Jackler RK, Glasscock ME III. Cholesteatoma. Otolaryngol Clin North Am 1989; 22:5.

Deguine C. Staging in cholesteatoma surgery. Ear Nose Throat 1993; 72: 197-200.

Gantz BJ, Ragheb SM, McCabe BF. Hearing results after cholesteatoma surgery: The Iowa experience. Laryngoscope 1987; 97:1254-1263.

Glasscock ME III, Johnson GD, Poe DS. Surgical management of cholesteatoma in an only hearing ear. Otolaryngol Head Neck Surg 1990; 102:246-250.

Michaels L. An epidermoid formation in the developing middle ear, possible source of cholesteatoma. J Otolaryngol 1986; 15:169.

Palva T, Ramsay H, Bohling T. Prussak's space revisited. Am J Otol 1996; 17:512-520.

Proctor B. Surgical anatomy of the ear and temporal bone. New York: Thieme, 1989.

Roden D, Honrubia V, Wiet RJ. Outcome of residual cholesteatoma and hearing in mastoid surgery. J Otolaryngol 1996; 25:178-181.

Rosenberg S, et al. Use of endoscopes for chronic ear surgery in children. Arch Otolaryngol Head Neck Surg 1995; 121:870-872.

Sade J. Treatment of cholesteatoma. Am J Otol 1987; 8:524-533.

Schuknecht HF. Congenital cholesteatoma. In: Pathology of the ear. 2nd ed. Cambridge: Harvard University Press, 1993:161.

Sheehy JL. Cholesteatoma surgery: Canal wall down procedures. Ann Otol Rhinol Laryngol 1988; 97:30-35.

Wiet RJ, Harvey SA, Bauer GP. Management of complications of chronic otitis media. In: Brackmann DE, ed. Otologic surgery. Philadelphia: WB Saunders, 1994:258.

THE DRAINING MASTOID CAVITY

The method of
Fred D. Owens

The purpose of surgery in a chronic draining mastoid cavity is resolution of disease. Hearing improvement is of secondary importance. A draining mastoid cavity that is unresponsive to medical treatment in a compliant patient is an indication of failure of the previous surgery. This failure may be a result of recurrent cholesteatoma, mucosal disease, suppuration in residual mastoid air cells, or failure to exteriorize the disease. Residual cholesteatoma may occur in as high as 30 percent of mastoidectomies with the posterior wall-up and as high as 12 percent with either modified radical or radical mastoidectomies. Mucosal disease frequently emanates from a diseased eustachian tube. Suppuration in mastoid air cells may result from residual disease in the mastoid air cells that may occur in the tip, along the facial ridge, in the zygomatic cells inferior to the tegmen mastoideum, the cells lateral to the sigmoid sinus, along the posterior fossa dura plate, in the cells of the labyrinth, or in the sinodural angle. Failure to exteriorize diseased air cells or to provide an adequate meatus frequently results in a draining mastoid cavity. Other reasons for a mastoid cavity to drain are trauma from self-cleaning of the ear and excessive exposure to water. Allergy, diabetes, and other general health problems also frequently contribute to drainage in a mastoid cavity.

The medical mastoid cavity may frequently be treated successfully in the office. If medical therapy should fail, revision surgery may be necessary.

■ OFFICE TREATMENT

Treatment in the office may include the following:

- Thorough microscopic cleaning of the cavity
- Antibiotic powder
- Silver nitrate application
- Phenol applications for granulations
- Fluorouracil (Efudex) cream for granulations
- Steroid cream
- Docusate sodium (Colace) drops
- Oral antibiotics

Many cavities become active because the patient does not return for routine cavity care. All cavities have their own individual characteristics that require interval cleaning. Most good cavities can be successfully cared for at 6 month intervals. Some may, however, go for a year. No cavity should go for more than 1 year between cleaning. If crusts are encountered in the treatment of the mastoid cavity, they may be softened by using Colace drops. This stool softener is very effective in softening crusts and decreasing the pain in removing these crusts. Frequently, cleaning of the cavity is all that is necessary to restore the cavity to a normal dry state. A variety of treatments can be used for the cavity that has granulation. In most of the cavities, the granulation can be cleaned by using silver nitrate followed by betamethasone valerate (Valisone) steroid cream. The most important step in the treatment of such a cavity is follow-up. This interval, of course, depends on the condition of each draining cavity. In many instances, an interval of one or two treatments per week may be necessary to restore the cavity to a dry, normal state.

If granulations are severe and resistant to treatment, applications of phenol or Efudex may be necessary. The phenol to be applied is an 88 percent solution, which is very effective in removing granulation and can be used in the cavity once per week. The phenol is best applied using a phenol applicator, which was designed by Lloyd Storrs, M.D., and sold by Smith and Nephew Inc. The use of Efudex on granulation tissue was described by Mansfield Smith, M.D. The Efudex can be applied weekly to granulation tissue. Both the phenol and Efudex should be used sparingly because either may perforate the tympanic membrane. Either of these treatments is frequently successful in treating resistant granulations.

There are also two types of powder that are used. One is CSF powder, which is a mixture of chloramphenicol (Chloromycetin), sulfadiazine, and Fungizone. The powder is mixed from the following ingredients: four 250 mg capsules of Chloromycetin, ten 100 mg tablets of Fungizone, and two 500 mg tablets of sulfadiazine. The powder is placed in an insufflator and used each time the mastoid cavity is cleaned and treated for granulations. Frequently, the patient will have some reaction to this powder, which is probably due to an allergy to the sulfadiazine. The second powder, and the one that is more often used, was described by Steve Landers, M.D., and is a mixture of ciprofloxacin (Cipro) and fluconazole (Diflucan). The following prescription is made up and placed in capsules to be put in insufflators and used after cleaning draining mastoid cavities: ten 500 mg capsules of Cipro and two 500 mg tablets of Diflucan. I find this powder much less reactive, and it is used quite frequently for granulations.

Valisone cream is frequently placed in these cavities before insufflation of powder. This tends to hold the powder in position and prevent crusting. This cream is a 0.1 percent concentration.

Some otologists do not choose to use the dry treatment method of these cavities and instead use drops. Drops frequently used are neomycin, polymyxin B sulfates, and hydrocortisone (Cortisporin Otic Suspension), hydrocortisone and acetic acid (VōSoL HC), and aluminum acetate (Domeboro solution).

In our practice, cultures are seldom performed on ears with draining mastoid cavities, and oral antibiotics are infrequently used. If, however, topical treatment fails, systemic treatment may be necessary and useful. The typical organisms encountered in chronic draining cavities are both aerobes and anaerobes. The most common aerobic organisms include *Pseudomonas aeruginosa, Proteus* sp., *Klebsiella pneumoniae, Staphylococcus aureus,* and *Escherichia coli.* Anaerobic organisms isolated may include *Bacteroides* sp. and gram-positive cocci. Antibiotics usually fail because of suppuration in the mastoid air cells, which have such a minimal blood supply available.

Of utmost importance is the prevention of any water getting into the draining cavity. This is best accomplished by placing cotton saturated with petroleum jelly in the ear during bathing or washing of the hair. Following the bathing or washing of the hair, the cotton and petroleum jelly are removed, and the ear is held back with one hand and gently dried with a hair dryer. If the ear is not kept free of water, it will be very difficult to obtain a dry cavity under any circumstances.

■ SURGICAL THERAPY

Revision Mastoidectomy

If medical therapy fails, revision surgery is often necessary. The most common cause of a chronic draining mastoid cavity following a modified radical or radical mastoidectomy is diseased cells that have not been removed. More often than not, these diseased cells are in a facial ridge that has not been lowered. This facial ridge needs to be lowered to the level of the facial nerve after identification of the nerve just inferior to the second genu. The facial nerve should not be exposed, but the bone over the facial nerve should be thinned sufficiently to identify the nerve. Once identified, the level of the facial nerve should be followed inferiorly as the facial ridge is lowered to the level of the inferior portion of the bony external auditory canal. If the cells in the mastoid tip are diseased, the tip can be completely amputated down to the level of the digastric ridge. This will also help in the obliteration of the cavity at the termination of the procedure.

The cells in the zygomatic ridge are frequently the cause of chronic drainage. These cells can be removed all the way to the level of the anterior limit of the bony external auditory canal. The cells lateral and posterior to the sigmoid sinus are easily removed by skeletonizing the sigmoid sinus in its lateral and posterior limits. The mastoid emissary vein can be protected while these cells are removed. The cells along the posterior fossa dura plate can be removed down to the level of the skeletonized posterior fossa plate. The cells inferior to the tegmen mastoideum must also be removed. The cells of the labyrinth cannot all be removed, but certainly the majority of cells lateral to the labyrinth can be removed. Frequently, diseased cells going down the sinodural angle can be removed by drilling posterior and medial to the posterior and superior semicircular canals. If one is to attain a dry cavity in these cases, it is most important to remove as many of the diseased cells as possible.

Obliteration

Once as many of the diseased cells as possible are removed and/or exteriorized, the mastoid cavity can be obliterated. The majority of the skin in the cavity is frequently normal. Inasmuch as it is possible, the skin is preserved and used in reconstruction of the cavity. The temporalis muscle is often used to obliterate the mastoid cavity. In some instances in which there is no skin in the cavity, a split-thickness skin graft may be used. In other instances, the temporalis fascia can be used. However, in most cases, the temporalis fascia has been previously harvested during the primary surgery. The skin incision in a revision of a modified or radical mastoidectomy is usually made through the original incision used in the primary surgery. The incision is usually postauricular. The incision through the musculoperiosteum is made just superior to the linea temporalis, just posterior to the posterior limit of the mastoid cavity, and then inferiorly over the mastoid tip and anteriorly back to the auricle. The skin and underlying soft tissue are carefully dissected away from the sigmoid sinus, posterior fossa dura, and tegmen mastoideum in a posterior-to-anterior direction. The skin and/or the tissue filling the cavity are dissected off the facial ridge and the drum remnant, if one is present, and retracted laterally and anteriorly to expose the middle ear. All mucosal disease possible is removed from the middle ear.

After all the suppurative mastoid air cells, mucosal disease, and cholesteatoma (if present) are removed, the cavity can be obliterated. If obliteration is anticipated in the initial planning of the surgery, a large inferiorly based musculoperiosteal flap can be developed. This can extend superiorly as far as necessary to provide adequate tissue for obliteration. If grafting of the tympanic membrane is necessary, the temporalis fascia is placed medial to the drum remnant and over the facial ridge medial to the obliteration flap. The obliterated flap is then placed in the mastoid cavity, and the salvaged skin is placed lateral to the musculoperiosteal flap and temporalis fascia. Other methods of cavity obliteration include bone plate, bone fragments, and autologous fat. If the external os is not of adequate size, a meatoplasty should be performed. The external canal and cavity is packed with cotton oxidized cellulose (Oxycel) and the incisions are closed in layers.

■ POSTOPERATIVE CARE

Packing is removed after 1 month. Any postoperative granulations are treated with either of the office treatments previously indicated. Complications of cavity obliteration include cholesteatoma covered by the flap, necrosis of the flap, failure of epithelialization over the flap, and abscess formation medial to the flap. Therefore, meticulous removal of all disease is essential if obliteration of the cavity is to be performed. Complications that may occur in the revision of a radical mastoidectomy or modified radical mastoidectomy include infection of the soft tissue and cartilage, bleeding from the sigmoid sinus, violation of the dura with subsequent cerebrospinal fluid drainage, facial nerve injury, and loss of hearing and balance due to injury to the semicircular canals. These complications differ very little from those involved in primary radical mastoidectomies or modified radical mastoidectomies.

DISCUSSION

Control of mucosal disease, exenteration of all possible suppurative mastoid air cells, and exteriorization of disease, including an adequate meatoplasty, are necessary for success when surgery is required for resolution of a draining mastoid cavity. Reconstruction of the ossicular chain can often be accomplished in the same procedure.

Meticulous microscopic cleaning of the cavity at appropriate intervals is essential to maintaining a dry cavity once this condition has been attained. The patient should be informed and the fact should be stressed that the goal of office or surgical management is to render the disease inactive and maintain that state of inactivity. Furthermore, the natural history of this chronic disease is to become active. The otologist and the patient must work in concert to prevent the return to an active draining mastoid cavity state.

Suggested Reading

Beales PH. Complications following obliterative mastoid operations. Arch Otolaryngol 1969; 89:223-224.

Jackson GC, Glasscock ME III, Nissen AJ, et al. Open mastoid procedures: Contemporary indications and surgical technique. Laryngoscope 1985; 95:1037-1043.

Nadol JB. Causes of failure of mastoidectomy for chronic otitis media. Laryngoscope 1985; 95:410-413.

Palva T. Operative technique in mastoid obliteration. Acta Otolaryngol 1973; 75:289-290.

Pillsbury HC III, Carrasco VN. Revision mastoidectomy. Arch Otolaryngol Head Neck Surg 1990; 116:1019-1022.

Schuknecht H, Bocca E. Guilford F, Rambo T. Panel on surgical approach, cavity management, and postoperative care in ear surgery. Arch Otolaryngol 1963; 78:142-150.

Shea MC Jr, Gardner G Jr. Mastoid obliteration using homograft bone. Arch Otolaryngol 1970; 92:358-364.

Sheehy JL, Brackmann DE, Graham MG. Cholesteatoma surgery: Residual and recurrent disease (a review of 1,024 cases). Ann Otol 1977; 86: 451-462.

OSSICULAR PROBLEMS IN CHRONIC OTITIS MEDIA

The method of
David C. Kelsall

Ossicular reconstruction is an integral part of the management of chronic otitis media. It is often a challenging endeavor, and frequently requires some degree of creativity and artistry. Successful outcomes depend on the surgical techniques used, but also on the severity of disease, status of the residual ossicular chain, and underlying eustachian tube function. The overall surgical treatment usually includes some type of mastoidectomy, tympanic membrane repair, and ossiculoplasty, often with a staged approach. Although it is difficult to isolate this procedure from other components of surgical treatment, I focus only on techniques of ossicular reconstruction.

The original techniques of tympanoplasty included little attempt at reconstruction of the ossicular chain. Over the next decade, early polyethylene prostheses were used only to be replaced by cartilage techniques, and then by incus interposition. The sculpted incus interposition gave uniformly good results, but concerns were raised regarding bony fixation and the possibility of harboring residual cholesteatoma. In addition, difficulties made the development of artificial prostheses prudent and necessary. Currently, there is a wide array of artificial prostheses, and the novice is often overwhelmed by the choices available.

Like most procedures in otology, there are many successful, proven techniques. Rarely is there only one right way to do things. Wise otologic surgeons will review the techniques available at the time, and perfect for themselves the procedures that make the most sense. Ossiculoplasty techniques and prostheses are in a stage of transition, and in the future, different techniques or prostheses may give better results.

PROSTHETIC MATERIAL AND DESIGN

In evaluating a substance as an optimal prosthetic material, there are numerous qualities to consider. The foremost is biocompatibility. A biocompatible material is not likely to extrude and causes a minimal amount of tissue reaction. The material should be stable initially and over time, easy to insert, and the best at sound transmission to ensure maximal hearing improvement. In addition, there should be a low risk of infection, minimal time required for preparation, easy storage requirements, acceptable cost, and, ideally, no need for tissue interposition grafting. The prosthesis should also be acceptable to most surgical situations.

Autografts have had a historical place in the story of ossicular reconstruction and continue to be of prime importance in locations where synthetic materials are not readily available. Fashioning and positioning an autologous incus requires time and skill to minimize the risk of bony fixation and ensure stability. The remnant of incus often is too small to be of use, and the risk of harboring microscopic disease is very real.

Homografts are a tempting alternative to ossicular reconstruction, but they require complex storage and preparation, and they possibly transmit infectious disease. Although this risk is no doubt quite low, and safeguards could be taken to further reduce this risk, patients and surgeons are acutely aware of the possibility of disease transmission and, in my opinion, this limits the potential use of homografts.

Synthetic materials are generally readily available, easy to store, require minimal time to prepare, and are free of infectious disease–causing agents. Their cost is offset by ease of use, and therefore less patient time in the operating room. There are numerous synthetic materials used in commercially available prostheses. These include metals, plastics, glass, ceramics, hydroxyapatite ceramics, polymaleinate ionomer, composites, and semibiologic materials. No one prosthesis currently solves all of the problems inherent to ossiculoplasty, but many of these newer materials are quite promising.

The two most commonly used materials for ossicular reconstruction prostheses are Plastipore and hydroxyapatite. Plastipore, introduced in 1978, is a high-density polyethylene sponge. This substance is very easy to work with and easily trimmable with a knife or scissors in the operating room. Its major drawback is a high incidence of extrusion, unless it is used with cartilage interposition.

Hydroxyapatite seems, at this time, to be superior to other materials readily available. Hydroxyapatite is a dense calcium phosphate ceramic. It has high biocompatibility and the capacity to form bonds with living bone. There is general consensus that bone-to-bone grafting gives the best long-term results. Hydroxyapatite is available in either a dense or porous state. The dense form appears to conduct vibratory energy quite well.

The prostheses I find most useful are composites of Plastipore and hydroxyapatite. The hydroxyapatite head can be hooked under the malleus, which allows excellent stability and bone-to-bone bonding. The hydroxyapatite head also allows use directly against the tympanic membrane. The Plastipore shaft allows precise trimming for length and shape, but does not directly contact the tympanic membrane, so there is no need for interposition grafting. This line of prosthesis is manufactured by Smith and Nephew Inc., Memphis, Tennessee, and was developed by R.A. Goldenberg, M.D.

With an absent incus, the choice of prosthesis design depends on two variables. The condition of the malleus will determine whether the prosthesis can be anchored on its undersurface or if the prosthesis will need to go to the tympanic membrane directly. The condition of the stapes superstructure will determine what length of prosthesis is needed. The four designs available are an incus replacement, incus-stapes replacement, partial ossicular replacement prosthesis (PORP), and total ossicular replacement prosthesis (TORP).

■ PATIENT SELECTION

The indication for ossicular reconstruction is to improve or maintain sound conduction to a functional cochlea. This can include cases of chronic otitis media or traumatic hearing loss where ossicular continuity has been lost, as well as cases of ossicular fixation. Surgeons should discuss other therapeutic options, such as hearing aid amplification, with the patient when applicable. These reconstructive techniques are best used when the middle ear is healthy and free of mucosal disease and cholesteatoma. Contraindications include severe eustachian tube dysfunction, unrepaired tympanic membrane perforation, severe tympanic membrane atelectasis, and prior extrusions of this type of prosthesis.

In canal wall-up tympanomastoidectomy for cholesteatoma, and in cases of active mucosal disease, the ossicular reconstruction is performed as a staged procedure 4 to 6 months following the primary surgery. The reconstruction is performed during the primary procedure in cases of chronic otitis media without mucosal or squamous disease, traumatic ossicular discontinuity, ossicular fixation, and in most canal wall-down mastoidectomy procedures.

■ SURGICAL TECHNIQUE

Incus Prosthesis

This prosthesis is used when the malleus is present, mobile, and in a favorable position relative to the stapes, and when the stapes superstructure is present and the footplate is mobile. The prosthesis consists of a hydroxyapatite head, with a hook for placement under the long process of the malleus and a hollow Plastipore shaft. The placement under the shaft of the malleus provides stability to the prosthesis, but probably offers no significantly better sound transmission than a stapes to tympanic membrane reconstruction.

The distance between the stapes capitulum and undersurface of the malleus is measured to aid in approximation of the prosthesis length. It is very important that the length of the prosthesis be adjusted to allow slight tension on the hook of the prosthesis when it is in position under the long process of the malleus. The Plastipore shaft of the prosthesis is trimmed with a scalpel or small scissors to the appropriate length. Notches are then cut anteriorly and posteriorly in the hollow Plastipore shaft. The anterior notch is for the anterior crus of the stapes, and the posterior notch is for the stapedial tendon. These notches result in a very stable arrangement when the prosthesis is appropriately positioned. The notches do cause the prosthesis to sit slightly more medial on the stapes superstructure, so this needs to be considered when judging the overall length.

The prosthesis is first placed on the capitulum of the stapes with the hook pointed inferiorly. With gentle lateral elevation of the malleus handle, the hook of the prosthesis is rotated under the malleus handle. As the prosthesis is rotated, the notches are engaged, and the prosthesis settles into a very stable, "locked" position. The hook of the prosthesis should be positioned as far down on the handle of the malleus as possible, because placement under the short process does not seem to be as favorable for hearing improvement. The position of the prosthesis can be checked by visualizing the stapes capitulum through the cannulated hydroxyapatite head. Once the prosthesis is in position, the round window reflex can be assessed, and for patients who have undergone general anesthesia, subjective hearing improvement can be judged. The middle ear is then packed with pledgets of Gelfoam, and the tympanic membrane is repositioned anatomically.

Incus-Stapes Prosthesis

This prosthesis is used when there is a mobile malleus and stapes footplate, but no useful stapes superstructure. It consists of a hydroxyapatite head that also has a hook for placement under the malleus handle. The Plastipore shaft is longer than the incus prosthesis, not cannulated, narrower in diameter, and wire-reinforced.

The distance between the malleus handle and stapes footplate is measured, and the prosthesis is trimmed to allow slight tension on the hook when in position. The wire shaft can also be bent slightly if needed for a more favorable alignment. The shaft of the prosthesis is then centered in the midportion of the stapes footplate. The wire in the shaft of the prosthesis will embed slightly in the stapes footplate to prevent slippage. There is also a specifically designed hydroxyapatite footplate shoe that can be placed on the end of the prosthesis shaft to aid in centering the prosthesis in the oval window niche. Gentle lateral elevation of the malleus is then performed, and the hook of the prosthesis is rotated under the long process of the malleus. Care must be taken to ensure that there is not too much tension, and therefore, too much depression of the oval window. Round window reflex and subjective hearing improvement can then be assessed, and the middle ear is packed with Gelfoam pledgets.

This prosthesis can also be used in cases in which the stapes footplate is immobile. The implantation of this prosthesis is always performed, however, as a staged procedure. At the first stage, stapedectomy is performed and a tissue graft is placed over the oval window. At the second stage, 3 to 6 months later, the prosthesis is placed from oval window graft to malleus. To perform this procedure as one stage is unwise because of the risk of displacement of the prosthesis shaft into the vestibule.

Partial Ossicular Replacement Prosthesis (PORP)

This prosthesis is used in cases where there is absence of the malleus and incus, but presence of a stapes superstructure and mobile footplate. The prosthesis consists of a hydroxyapatite, rounded, egg-shaped head, and a cannulated shaft of Plastipore

The technique is similar to the placement of the incus prosthesis. The distance is measured from capitulum to tympanic membrane. The shaft of the prosthesis is then trimmed to the appropriate length. The cut can be angled to assist with the appropriate orientation of the prosthesis head to the tympanic membrane, in order to maximize surface contact. Notches are cut in the Plastipore shaft to accept the anterior stapes crus and the stapedial tendon. The prosthesis is then placed on the capitulum of the stapes and rotated until the notches engage the anterior crus and stapedial tendon.

The tympanic membrane or previously reconstructed tympanic membrane graft is then repositioned, and the position of the prosthesis is checked. There should be enough length of the prosthesis to slightly "tent-up" the surface of the tympanic membrane. In some cases, a cartilage interposition graft is placed over the head of the prosthesis. The cartilage is obtained from either the tragus or the pinnae. It is trimmed so that it just covers the head of the prosthesis, and is thin and flexible. The cartilage is placed to support the tympanic membrane (TM) or graft and to prevent extrusion. It is placed in cases of TM atelectasis or atrophy, severe eustachian tube dysfunction, and when there has been previous prosthesis extrusion or failure. It also assists with preventing formation of retraction pockets in the posterior TM and pars flaccida.

Total Ossicular Replacement Prosthesis (TORP)

This prosthesis is used when there is absence of the malleus, incus, and stapes superstructure. It can also be used in cases of absent stapes footplate as part of a staged procedure. TORP consists of a rounded, egg-shaped head composed of hypoxyapatite and a solid, wire-reinforced shaft of Plastipore.

The distance between the footplate and tympanic membrane (or TM graft) is measured, and the shaft is trimmed to the appropriate length. The shaft is then placed in the oval window and centered on the footplate. The wire end of the prosthesis will assist with stability in relation to the footplate. A footplate shoe can be used to assist with centering of the prosthesis in the oval window niche. The head is then placed under the TM surface, and the prosthesis is angled to ensure maximum contact with the tympanic membrane. Packing of the middle ear is very important in this situation because the prosthesis is not as stable as the three prostheses already discussed. Cartilage interposition grafts can be used when risk factors for extrusion exist (as discussed previously).

Additional Procedures

Tympanostomy is rarely performed at the time of ossiculoplasty. Patients are followed up, however, with frequent microscopic examination. If middle ear effusion develops and persists, or if there is evidence of tympanic membrane retraction, then tympanostomy with PE tube placement is performed, usually as an office procedure.

In patients who have severe eustachian tube dysfunction, a mastoidectomy is often performed for the "reservoir" effect. Opening the mastoid air cells, epitympanum, and facial recess allows excellent communication between the middle ear and mastoid; there is less chance for future development of chronic negative pressure and serous otitis media, and therefore, less chance of prosthesis extrusion. Allergy evaluation should also be performed in symptomatic patients, and allergies should be aggressively treated before attempts at ossicular reconstruction occur.

■ SURGICAL RESULTS

Hearing Results

I have used the techniques previously described for the past 2 years. Hearing results have been comparable to the results reported by other surgeons using this or similar prosthetic materials and designs. Overall, for all prosthetic designs, the mean air–bone gap at 1 year has been approximately 20 dB, with approximately 50 percent of patients achieving closure of the air–bone gap to less than or equal to 20 dB. The incus prosthesis gives the best overall results, as expected with both the malleus and stapes superstructure present. The worst results are with TORP, also as expected with the absence of the malleus, incus, and stapes superstructure. As I gain more experience with this implant system, I will be able to produce more detailed reporting of results. The long-term success rate of these prostheses has not yet been determined.

Complications

Extrusions of these prostheses certainly do occur, and initially the extrusion rate was higher than expected. As more experience is gained with this system and the use of a cartilage cap in patients who have risk factors for extrusion, the extrusion rate has sharply declined. Other complications include displacement of the prosthesis, fixation to the bony canal wall posteriorly, granulation tissue over the hydroxyapatite head (without eventual extrusion), and lateralization of the tympanic membrane so that contact with the prosthesis head is lost.

■ DISCUSSION

The composite system of hydroxyapatite-Plastipore prostheses has proved to be effective for successful ossicular reconstruction. They are highly biocompatible, stable over time, and easy to store, prepare, and insert. They have a low risk of infection, no risk of disease transmission, acceptable cost, and, in most cases, there is no need for tissue interposition grafting. The four designs are adaptable to most surgical situations. The hearing results appear to be favorable, and complication rates are relatively low with appropriate surgical techniques.

Ossicular reconstruction techniques and materials have been evolving over many years, and the evolution is far from complete. The future will undoubtedly bring new materials, new techniques, and new claims of success. Additional research is needed to define the optimal prosthetic design to maximize sound transmission and minimize complications. Success of ossicular reconstruction will undoubtedly also be increased with improved treatment of eustachian tube dysfunction, cholesteatoma control, and techniques to minimize fibrosis.

Suggested Reading

Goldenberg RA. Ossiculoplasty with composite prostheses. Otolaryngol Clin North Am 1994; 27:727-745.

Goode RL, Nishihara S. Experimental models of ossiculoplasty. Otolaryngol Clin North Am 1994; 27:663-675.

Monsell EM. Results and outcomes in ossiculoplasty. Otolaryngol Clin North Am 1994; 27:835-840.

Treace HT. Biomaterials in ossiculoplasty and history of development of prostheses for ossiculoplasty. Otolaryngol Clin North Am 1994; 27: 655-662.

Wehrs RE. Hydroxyapatite implants for otologic surgery. Otolaryngol Clin North Am 1995; 28:273-286.

OTOSCLEROSIS

The method of
William H. Lippy
by
William H. Lippy
Iain L. Grant
Franklin M. Rizer
Arnold G. Schuring

Unique to human beings, otosclerosis is a disease of the endochondral bone of the otic capsule. Excessive bony overgrowth of the annular ligament results in a conductive and occasionally a sensorineural hearing loss. The etiology is genetic, although viral factors have been implicated. Inheritance is autosomal dominant with variable penetrance. Recent evidence links the disease to abnormalities in the type 1 collagen gene COL 1A1. Otosclerosis occurs far more commonly in persons of European origin than in Africans or Indians.

■ PATHOLOGY

The active stage of otosclerosis is noted for the basophilic appearance seen in hematoxylin and eosin staining known as the "Blue Mantles of Manasse." Immature bone with a higher content of ground substance is laid down. Clinically, disease foci are soft and bleed easily. Rarely, they may be seen as "Schwarze's sign," a flamingo-colored blush on the promontory.

Subsequently, the process enters the sclerotic phase where remodeling results in denser, more mature bone. This process is similar to new bone formation elsewhere in the body and occurs at certain defined sites within the temporal bone; the anterior oval window (fissula ante fenestrum) is the most commonly involved site, with the round window less frequently involved. The focus then becomes quiescent.

Histologic otosclerosis occurs 10 times more commonly than clinical disease and appears to be decreasing as a result of increased water fluoridation. In 85 percent of patients, the process is bilateral, with the presentation peaking in the third decade. Pregnancy has been suspected of accelerating the hearing loss.

It is common that the process results in fixation of the annular ligament and footplate, with a resultant conductive hearing loss. Once present, fixation tends to progress rapidly. Foci not directly involving the labyrinth or oval window may remain asymptomatic. Otosclerosis may also initially involve a sensorineural loss. Rarely, otosclerosis may cause postural imbalance or vertigo.

Conductive hearing loss behind a normal and intact eardrum should raise otosclerosis high on the list of differential diagnoses. More subtle clues include a positive family history, bilateral hearing loss, absence of stapedial reflexes, female gender, a negative finding from the Rinne test, a finding from Weber's test that lateralizes logically, and a paucity of cerumen. These features help strengthen the diagnosis; however, the ultimate confirmation is surgical.

We present in the following pages a safe surgical technique that in this practice alone has been used in more than 14,000 stapedectomies. It requires little special instrumentation and is appropriate for the occasional operator. Most important, it has withstood the test of time.

■ PATIENT SELECTION

The patient should have two appropriately masked audiograms that confirm adequate bone thresholds and an air–bone gap in excess of 15 dB. The conductive loss must be confirmed with a reversed 512 Hz tuning fork, or at least a plus-minus test, and a Weber's test that lateralizes to the appropriate ear.

Surgery should generally be performed on the poorer hearing ear. When hearing levels are similar and one ear has been previously operated on, the unoperated ear should be operated on rather than revising the already operated ear. When the ears are equal, a right-handed surgeon should select the left ear, especially in a large-chested patient with a short neck. Speech discrimination should be appropriate to the hearing loss. In a pure conductive loss, discrimination should reach 100 percent with a very loud stimulus. The patient should be in reasonable health.

Advanced age is not a contraindication to surgery. Stapedectomy in very young children (younger than 5 years old) is contraindicated until it is demonstrated that they are not prone to otitis media. The benefits of surgery for both children and the elderly have been demonstrated.

Stapedectomy can be beneficial in patients who have far-advanced otosclerosis. These patients have a severe or profound mixed loss. Surgery may raise their thresholds into the aidable range, when previously a hearing aid could not be worn. Typically, these patients have excellent speech production and air conduction no better than 95 dB, with bony thresholds in excess of 60 to 75 dB (the limit of the audiometer). The conductive element may be detectable with the 512 Hz tuning fork applied to the teeth when it is not heard on the mastoid. The upper central incisors and the alveolar ridge given an 11 dB gain over applying the fork to the mastoid. The examiner must be sure that the fork is heard and not felt by the patient.

Most patients who will benefit from a stapedectomy will also benefit from a hearing aid. This alternative must be offered to the patient. Successful surgery, however, is associated with better fidelity of sound and none of the ongoing problems of hearing aid management.

All patients who have otosclerosis and a sensorineural hearing loss are treated with a minimum course (2 years) of sodium fluoride, as Florical, two tablets twice daily. Supplemental vitamin D and Florical act to prevent further hearing loss. For patients with a progressive sensorineural hearing loss or only one hearing ear this can be a lifelong regimen.

■ CONTRAINDICATIONS

Active middle or external ear disease is an absolute contraindication to surgery. Surgery should be delayed for active upper respiratory tract infection. Any tympanic membrane perforation should be repaired months before stapedectomy. Meniere's syndrome is a potential problem. A dilated saccule may sit immediately beneath the footplate and be damaged upon entry into the vestibule, with resultant sensorineural loss. Surgery in patients who have poor discrimination scores who are not severely hard of hearing should be avoided.

Occupation does not constitute a contraindication. The senior author has performed this procedure for six active fighter pilots and several ballerinas.

Before any operation, the patient should be advised of the potential benefits, significant risks, and alternatives to surgery.

■ SURGICAL TECHNIQUE

Before surgery, the clinic nurse counsels each patient on what to expect, which assists in calming an anxious patient. Patients are reminded to indicate if they experience any vertigo during the procedure. It is our preference to perform all surgery under local anesthesia with sedation. Aside from less nausea and a shorter hospital stay, benefits of this anesthetic regimen are most apparent in revision surgery, where it is critical not to injure the saccule. Manipulating adhesions from the underside of the footplate will produce vertigo, which the patient can communicate to the surgeon, thus preventing a potentially disastrous complication. Because 30 percent of the senior author's practice is in revision stapedectomy, local anesthesia is used routinely.

The patient is premedicated with midazolam 1 hour preoperatively. On arrival in the operating room, an air threshold audiogram is performed (described later). The ear and ipsilateral forearm are prepped with povidone-iodine solution. As large a vein graft as possible is harvested from the ipsilateral arm, placed in saline solution, slit open, and pressed.

Intravenous sedation with propofol is temporarily increased to provide amnesia and sedation for the ear canal injections. A four-quadrant injection of 4.0 cc lidocaine 2 percent mixed with 0.5 cc 1 : 1,000 epinephrine is completed. Excess iodine from the prep solution is irrigated from the ear.

An easily insertable speculum is introduced into the ear canal and rotated so as to dilate the external cavity, bringing the short process of the malleus into view. The size of the speculum is gradually increased. Patient position is critical and should be adjusted so that the short process can be easily seen with the majority of the drum before proceeding. A further injection is made into the vascular strip until a very slight hydrodissection of the flap occurs.

A sickle knife is used to make external canal incisions in the 12 and 6 o'clock positions; these incisions are joined approximately 6 mm lateral to the drum with a round knife. Several interrupted passes with the knife are made so as to take the incision through the periosteum and prevent tissue tags tethering the flap. During these stages, it is possible to gradually increase the size of the speculum. The speculum is then fixed using a speculum holder. The holder is always used because it assists with hemostasis, helps to secure the patient's head, provides a firm base against which to curet, and allows both hands free to work. The canal elevator is passed firmly along the bone to elevate a tympanomeatal flap down to the annulus. Every effort is made to avoid tearing the flap. The middle ear is entered in the posterior superior quadrant, and a blunt instrument is used to dissect the annulus and identify the chorda tympani if it is not encased in the bone. An annulus elevator is inserted, and the annulus is freed from the sulcus. The chorda is dissected free from its fold of mucosa and then followed anteriorly as it becomes medial to the malleus. The chorda is regularly moistened during the procedure.

A Gelfoam pledget saturated with the original anesthetic solution is placed in the middle ear. This serves to anesthetize the mucosa and also to collect bone chips created by curettage. Malleus and incus mobility are checked by vision and palpation. This is always done with the same instrument to maintain a standard reference. The malleus must be visualized from the underside of the eardrum, pushing the eardrum aside with a 20 gauge suction needle in one hand and palpating with a strong blunt instrument in the other hand. This is done to exclude other forms of ossicular pathology, such as malleus or incus fixation. Curettage must always be done in a direction away from the incus to avoid its dislocation. Enough bone is removed to be able to view the course of the horizontal facial nerve, the oval window, and the origin of the stapes tendon. A rotatory motion is used, and curettage is commenced slightly lateral to the scutum to create a furrow. This area of bone is thinned, and this thinning subsequently allows easier removal of the annular margin and reduces the possibility of injury to the incus. Once the curettage is finished, only a 26 gauge suction needle is used in the middle ear.

An assessment is made of the oval window region; any dehiscence over the seventh nerve is noted, and stapes fixation is checked. Subtle fixation may be detected by palpating the footplate while observing the annular ligament for change in color or width. After the diagnosis of otosclerosis has been confirmed, a sharp needle is used to perforate the footplate at the junction of the posterior and middle thirds. In small footplates, this control hole would be made more anterior, because more of the footplate should be removed. The control hole facilitates later footplate removal, minimizes hydraulic injury to the cochlea, and allows early detection of the rare perilymphatic gusher.

The incudostapedial joint is divided in a motion that pushes against the pull of the stapedius tendon. The tendon is divided close to its origin with Bellucci scissors. A Storz No. 3 chisel is positioned inferior to the chorda onto the capitulum of the stapes. A sharp thrust toward the promontory down fractures the superstructure free of the footplate. Mucosa is removed from the footplate and the promontory to control the bleeding during subsequent footplate removal. At this stage, the areas anterior to the footplate and over the facial nerve are avoided to lessen bleeding from any vascular otosclerotic foci.

Approximately the posterior one-third to one-half of the footplate is removed. The smaller the footplate area, the greater the proportion of the footplate that should be removed. Care is taken not to suction perilymph from the vestibule. Small fragments of bone falling into perilymph are left untouched. After the footplate is removed, further mucus is removed from the facial nerve and the area anterior to the footplate. This further secures bleeding and provides for purchase of the vein graft.

The vein graft that has been cut to a square approximately 4 x 4 mm by the scrub nurse is placed adventitia side down over the fenestra. The graft is draped up over the facial nerve and inferiorly onto the promontory. It is crucial that the graft generously overlaps the vestibule, because this creates a trampoline-like self-centering action for the prosthesis, and any gap may predispose to a later perilymphatic fistula.

A dimple is made in the center of the graft to aid prosthesis placement (Fig. 1). This dimple is very important in facilitating prosthesis placement; thus, it must be deep enough to indicate the position of the open vestibule and

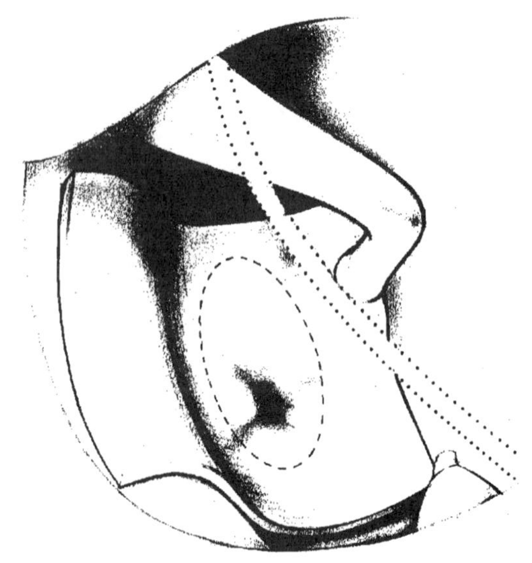

Figure 1.
Dimple in vein graft for placement of prosthesis.

allow for placement of the prosthesis. It should not extend into the vestibule, but it should indicate the correct position for the prosthesis.

The microscope is positioned to allow a good view of both the incus and the footplate. This is best accomplished by pulling the head of the microscope toward the surgeon and then refocusing. A 4 mm Robinson prosthesis is placed in the dimple of the graft and rested against the incus (Fig. 2).

Irrespective of the side, an incus hook is taken in the left hand and a strut guide in the right hand. The hook is placed anterior to and beneath the incus, but no attempt is made to pull it laterally. The strut guide engages the prosthesis and is used to manipulate it beneath the incus (Fig. 3). As the prosthesis approaches the lenticular process, the hook is used to steady and minutely lift the incus. Once underneath the lenticular process, the incus hook is released, and the prosthesis tends to snap onto the lenticular process (Fig. 4).

The bucket handle is flipped over the long process, and the mechanical action of the prosthesis is checked. If it is difficult to fit the bucket handle, it should be left alone. The bucket handle should not be forced onto the incus, because too tight a fit prevents the prosthesis from centering. The tympanic membrane is replaced, and the blood is removed from its surface. An intraoperative air threshold audiogram is obtained by the technique described next. We expect this to be within 15 dB of the preoperative bony threshold. If it is not, the eardrum is lifted, and a cause is sought for the failure to improve. Gelfoam and then a cotton ball saturated with bacitracin ointment are placed in the external canal, and the patient is returned to the recovery room.

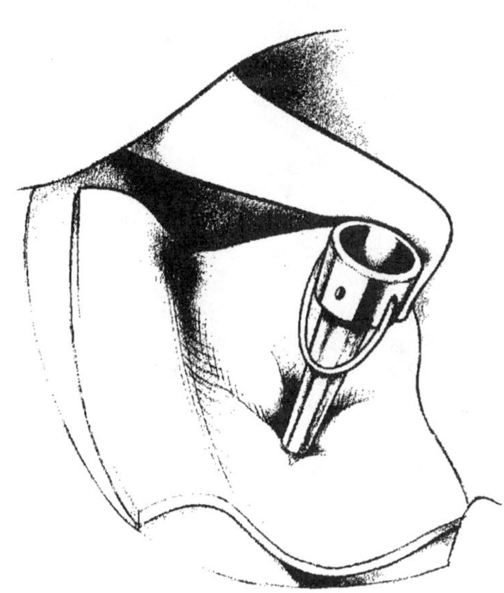

Figure 2.
Placement of Robinson prosthesis against incus.

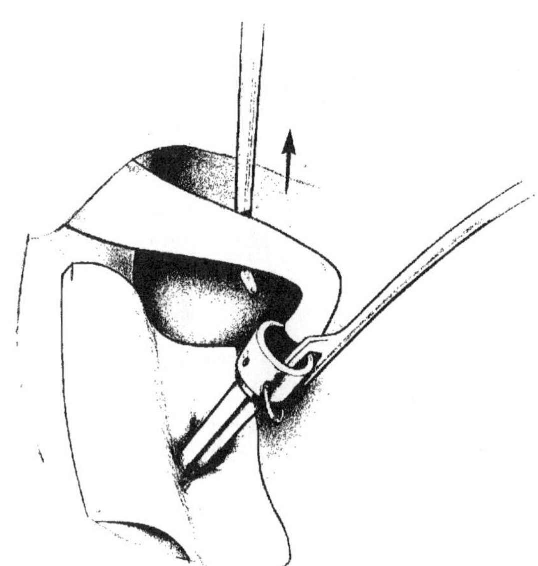

Figure 3.
Two-handed technique for placing prosthesis under incus.

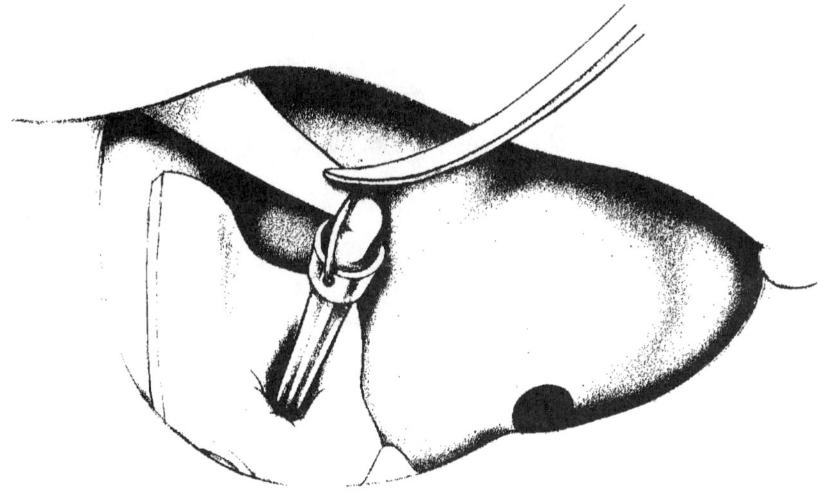

Figure 4.
Palpating prosthesis in place.

■ POSTOPERATIVE CARE

Patients are cautioned not to blow their nose and to sneeze with their mouth open in the 3 week postoperative period. Some patients experience mild dizziness that will resolve within hours of surgery, If symptomatic, dizziness may be controlled with ondansetron or droperidol. The majority of patients go home within 24 hours of surgery; many return home on the same day.

■ RESULTS

This is a safe technique of stapes surgery and requires no special equipment. In the senior author's series of 12,241 stapedectomies, there was 96 percent closure to within 10 dB and a 0.7 percent sensorineural loss rate. There is an 80 percent overclosure rate.

Intraoperative Problems

Tympanic Membrane Perforation and Flap Tears

Most torn flaps heal with simple reapposition of the edges. Any significant tissue defect or injury to the tympanic membrane can be repaired in an underlay fashion, with a vein graft placed adventitia side up under the perforation. A generous graft should always be taken from the arm in case a repair is required.

Chorda Tympani

It is often preferable to section a stretched chorda to prevent prolonged taste disturbance. In the majority (>98 percent) of cases, adequate surgical access can be gained without sacrificing the chorda. When operating on a second ear, every effort should be made to preserve the chorda if it was damaged in the opposite ear. If the original first ear was operated elsewhere, you must assume it was damaged. If the chorda tympani nerve is stretched or cut on both sides, there may be a permanent dry taste disturbance, but what is more important, a permanent dry mouth may result.

Ossicular Dislocation

The incus may be inadvertently injured during curettage. If only subluxation has occurred, a rigid stapes prosthesis may assist in fixing the incus in position. As the joint capsule heals and undergoes fibrosis, surprisingly good hearing may result. A more severe injury may require revision or management with a different ossicular solution.

Malleus Fixation

Reduced malleus mobility on pneumatic otoscopy may provide a preoperative clue to this diagnosis. If this situation is suspected, the malleus can be palpated in the office. Phenol is placed on the umbo for anesthesia, and a rigid instrument is used to touch the manubrium under microscopic control. At surgery, once the middle ear is entered, the malleus should always be palpated under direct vision. An assessment is made of the fixation: slight, moderate, or total.

The operation should continue until an assessment of footplate mobility can be made. If otosclerosis coexists, a stapedectomy is indicated. In cases in which malleus fixation is slight or moderate, the result will be as if there were no fixation. If the malleus is totally fixed, a large amount of footplate should be removed in case a second or revision procedure involving a TORP is necessary. In 45 of our patients who had both stapes and complete malleus fixation, 70 percent improved to within 10 dB and 84 percent to within 20 dB of the preoperative bone conduction level when they were treated with stapedectomy alone. Those patients who fail to improve may require a secondary procedure with another ossicular solution.

Incus Necrosis

This condition is often evident preoperatively if it is secondary to retraction, or it may be noted during revision stapedectomy when the lenticular process is eroded or missing. A Lippy Modified Robinson prosthesis (Fig. 5) that is 4.5 mm or longer in length, depending on the extent of necrosis, is used. Incus necrosis is most likely to occur when the tympanic membrane is atrophic. In these cases, the eardrum should be thickened by using a tissue graft on the underside.

Facial Nerve Anomalies

The facial nerve is frequently dehiscent and yet rarely presents a problem. When overhanging with some footplate visible, a 26 gauge suction needle is used to gently push the nerve aside. This may allow enough access to the footplate for the operation to proceed. If the footplate is not visible, a Hough hoe is used to protect and retract the facial nerve, and a microdrill may be used to drill off the promontory and open the inferior margin of the oval window. Place the drill on the footplate and gently sweep up several times. There will be no damage to the hearing or the nerve. Remove whatever footplate you can and blindly perforate the rest. A prosthesis and vein graft can then be applied. Even though the prosthesis indents the facial nerve, there will no damage or paralysis. This solution requires a two-handed technique

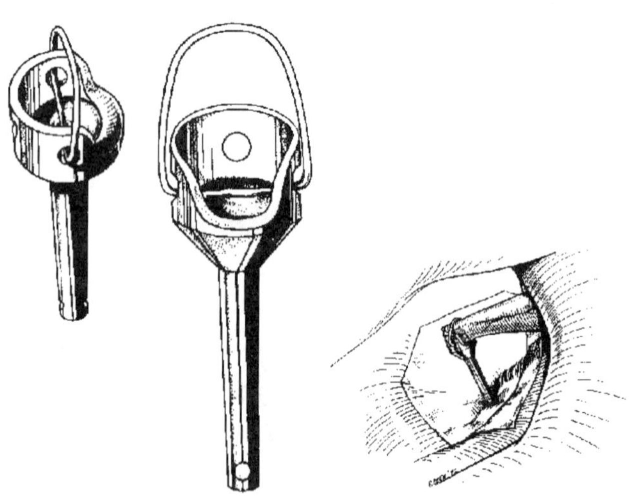

Figure 5.
Lippy modification of Robinson prosthesis for absent lenticular process.

and a great deal of dexterity. It is unwise to attempt this technique without experience.

Obliterative Otosclerosis

This extensive form of otosclerosis is dramatically less common than it was in the 1960s. The footplate is considered to be obliterated when the margins cannot be seen or removed. Occasionally, the footplate is partially or totally obliterated with only the top of the superstructure visible. A 0.7 mm diamond bur should be used to saucerize the footplate region, drilling gently and slowly. Irrigation should be used to minimize heat transfer. The bone should be removed on a broad front, avoiding a small opening into the vestibule. The vestibule should be blue-lined, with the final layer of bone removed with a needle and pick. On occasion, the superior margin of the promontory may need to be drilled. A slightly longer prosthesis may be required. If the bone is well saucerized, prosthesis action should be near normal. Results, however, are not as good as a routine stapedectomy (80 percent success).

Floating Footplate

The footplate may inadvertently mobilize when it is manipulated. Regardless of whether it is solid (white) or diffuse (blue), a vein graft should be placed over the floating footplate and a 4 mm prosthesis is inserted. Long-term success rates with this technique are 97 percent with a blue footplate. If this occurs with a white footplate, hearing success is only 52 percent. Unsuccessful cases can be safely revised. Should the footplate mobilize again during revision, no future surgery should be advised. In a series of 8,000 stapedectomies, there were no cases of sensorineural hearing loss in 147 cases of floating footplates treated in this fashion. An inadvertently mobilized footplate treated in this manner becomes a fortuitous event, not a disaster.

Intraoperative Audiometry

Immediately before surgery, a portable audiometer is used by the circulating nurse to measure an air threshold at 500 or 1,000 Hz wherever the air–bone gap is greater. The single TDH 39 headphone is then placed in a sterile drape so that it can be handled in the sterile field. The drape attenuates the tone by 5 dB at 500 Hz and 2 dB at 1,000 Hz. At the completion of surgery, all blood is cleaned from the middle ear, and an air threshold is measured in a descending manner. No masking is used. Despite a flaccid tympanic membrane and blood in the perilymph, if the surgery has been successful, hearing should be within 15 dB of the preoperative bone threshold; frequently, it is within 5 dB. If it fails to reach this level (15 dB), the prosthesis should be reinspected, and any abnormality should be corrected. Intraoperative audiometry gives the surgeon instant and accurate feedback on the success of the procedure and defines the end point of surgery. It is particularly useful in revision surgery where the hearing can be measured in several different prosthesis positions and the optimum location ascertained. With an accurate knowledge of the outcome, the surgeon can counsel the patient and relatives with confidence at the end of the operation.

Laser Stapedectomy

Many surgeons make the laser a routine part of their stapedectomy technique. Crural division and sectioning of the stapedius tendon can be easily accomplished. If the footplate is thin, it allows a no-touch stapedectomy technique with consequently less risk of a floating footplate. If the footplate is thick, extensive char may need to be removed with rasps, which negates this advantage. In the ear filled with dense adhesions, the laser is advantageous, allowing trauma-free and bloodless division of adhesions. A laser, in the senior author's opinion, is not essential for stapes surgery, but it may have some advantages in revision surgery.

Revision Stapedectomy

Revision surgery may be considered in the situation of conductive loss, sensorineural loss, or vertigo. A careful decision as to whether a revision procedure is in the patient's best interests should be based on the history and audiogram. The original operative note may also be useful. The experience of the original surgeon is often indicative of the likelihood of a reversible problem being found. In careful revision surgery, the risk of further loss is no higher than in an original procedure. However, the success rates are lower.

Conductive Loss

A history of hearing improvement at surgery with later deterioration is a good indicator that revision may be successful. Stapedectomy in which the anterior footplate has been removed and reconstructed with stapes crura (anterior crurotomy technique) has a high rate of successful revision.

Wire prostheses are often associated with incus necrosis and can be easily revised. In occasional cases, the prosthesis may be too short, and the patient will sense vibrations with distorted hearing. Replacing a wire or the same 4 mm Robinson prosthesis over a second vein graft usually retrieves the hearing. Valsalva's maneuver may momentarily restore hearing. This indicates a prosthesis out of an optimal position.

Sensorineural Hearing Loss

In patients who have a delayed sensorineural hearing loss after stapedectomy, revision is only indicated for trauma or vertigo. If a tissue seal was placed, the surgeon should be reluctant to undertake a revision. If no tissue graft was used, 50 percent of sensorineural loss will be fistulas and should be revised.

Vertigo

Tullio's phenomenon (vertigo with loud noise) or a positive fistula test finding is suggestive of a prosthesis impinging on the saccule. At revision, a shorter prosthesis should be used.

The Tissue Seal

When performing revision, it is our belief that the tissue seal of the oval window must not be breached. Occasionally, if the first prosthesis cannot be removed because manipulation causes the patient to be dizzy, a second prosthesis (a Bailey) can be placed alongside the original, and the position can be checked audiometrically. Undoubtedly, this may deprive some patients of an improvement in hearing, but results in fewer patients suffering a sensorineural loss and being made worse as a result of further surgery.

Suggested Reading

Lippy WH. Special problems in otosclerosis. In: Brackmann DE, Shelton C, Arriaga MA, eds. Otologic surgery. Philadelphia: WB Saunders, 1994.

Lippy WH, Schuring AG. Prosthesis for the problem incus in stapedectomy. Arch Otolaryngol 1974; 100:237-239.

Lippy WH, Schuring AG. Treatment of the inadvertently mobilized foot plate. Arch Otolaryngol 1973; 98:80-81.

Lippy WH, Schuring AG. Solving ossicular problems in stapedectomy. Laryngoscope 1983; 93:1147-1150.

Lippy WH, Schuring AG, Ziv M. Stapedectomy for otosclerosis with malleus fixation. Arch Otolaryngol 1978; 104:388-389.

HEREDITARY HEARING IMPAIRMENT

The method of
Richard J.H. Smith
by
John H. Greinwald, Jr.
Richard J.H. Smith

Hereditary hearing impairment (HHI) is an important and probably underdiagnosed disorder in children and adults. It is estimated to affect one in 2,000 newborns and, if delayed onset and progressive forms of HHI are included, this condition affects a substantially higher number of persons in the United States. In more than half the children who have severe to profound hearing impairment, a genetic etiology can be found. The recent explosion of molecular biology has given clinicians a wealth of information concerning the pathophysiology and diagnosis of HHI. Coupled with developments in cochlear implant and hearing aid technology, the otolaryngologist can now offer persons who have hearing impairment the option of integrating more fully into the hearing world. These advances have brought HHI into the forefront when the otolaryngologist evaluates, diagnoses, and treats patients who have hearing impairment, and will require for the future increasingly more knowledge in the fields of genetics, genetic counseling, and gene therapy.

Hearing loss can be defined in a number of ways. The terms *syndromic* and *nonsyndromic* are most commonly used, reflecting the presence or absence, respectively, of coinherited abnormalities. Nonsyndromic hearing loss (NHL) accounts for the majority of cases of HHI (approximately 75 percent). Typically monogenic, it is a highly heterogeneous disorder, with some estimates of the number of genetic loci exceeding 100. Other descriptors applied to HHI include progressive or nonprogressive, and congenital or delayed onset. Quantitating the degree of hearing loss by audiometry is important in terms of diagnosis and treatment options.

Characterization by inheritance pattern is determined by examining the family pedigree. Affectation status will be consistent with autosomal recessive (AR) inheritance in approximately 75 percent of patients, autosomal dominant (AD) inheritance in approximately 20 to 25 percent of patients, and X-linked inheritance in the remaining 1 to 2 percent. Maternal inheritance through mitochondrial DNA also has been implicated in forms of HHI associated with skeletal muscle disorders and in nonsyndromic hearing loss associated with increased susceptibility of the inner ear to aminoglycoside ototoxicity. The diagnostic challenge for the otolaryngologist is that most infants and children with HHI have NSHL inherited in an autosomal recessive manner.

The views expressed in this chapter are those of the author and do not reflect the official policy or position of the Department of the Navy, Department of Defense, or the U.S. Government.

■ PATTERNS OF INHERITANCE

Recessive Inheritance

The ability to distinguish modes of inheritance is made during the patient interview as a pedigree is developed for the family. Autosomal recessive hearing loss (ARHL) is characterized by a *horizontal* pattern on the pedigree (Fig. 1). Because the phenotypic expression requires a mutation in both

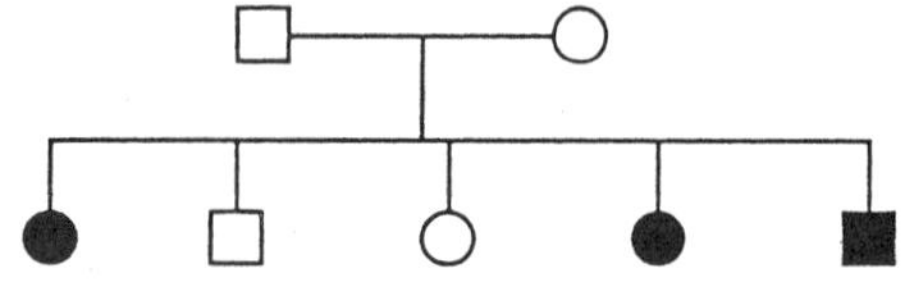

Figure 1.
Pedigree of a typical family with autosomal recessive hearing loss. Note that the parents are not affected. □, unaffected male; ■, affected male; ○ unaffected females; ● affected females.

copies of a given gene, the parents are heterozygous (carriers) and unaffected. Recessive disorders are usually monogenic (involve only one gene), and progeny have a 25 percent chance of being affected. In most families, there will be no history of hearing impairment, although an exception to this rule is when the coefficient of inbreeding is high. Examples include consanguineous marriages and population isolates in which multiple generations may be affected. The paucity of affected persons in nonconsanguineous unions makes differentiating nonsyndromic ARHL from spontaneous mutations and nongenetic or acquired types of hearing impairment difficult. Many so-called idiopathic cases of hearing impairment may be examples of recessive inheritance.

Syndromic and nonsyndromic ARHL usually cause severe to profound hearing impairment that starts in the pre- to perilingual stages of language development (Table 1). Two exceptions are DFNB8, which has been mapped to chromosome 21q22 in a Pakistani kindred, and Usher's syndrome type III, which is found in Finland. Both of these disorders are associated with a postlingual, slowly progressive sensorineural hearing loss (SNHL).

In many syndromic forms of ARHL, the hearing impairment is recognized before other associated abnormalities; the progressive pigmentary retinopathy of Usher's syndrome, the goiter of Pendred syndrome, and the conduction defects of Jervell and Lange-Nielsen (JLN) syndrome may remain undiagnosed for many years. The diagnostic dilemma of testing for these disorders thus becomes an important issue.

Dominant Inheritance

Autosomal dominant hearing loss (ADHL) is easier to identify than is ARHL due to the *vertical* pattern of transmission from one generation to the next (Fig. 2). Because phenotypic expression requires only one copy of the disease gene, no true carrier state exists, and the risk of transmission from one affected parent to progeny is 50 percent. However, disease phenotype can differ considerably from one individual to the next due to variance in gene penetrance and expressivity. Penetrance can be thought of as an "all or none phenomenon" and refers to the presence of any clinical evidence of gene expression. In contrast, expressivity as a measure of the extent the phenotype is clinically evident. For example, Waardenburg's syndrome type 1 is greater than 95 percent penetrant (most patients have at least one clinical manifestation), but this syndrome has a highly variable expression pattern (great variability in the number of findings in af-

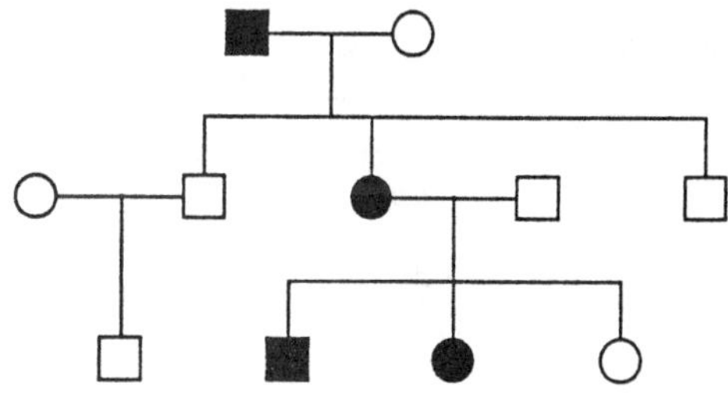

Figure 2.
Pedigree of a typical family with autosomal dominant hearing loss. Note the multiple affected family members; transmission can be either maternal or paternal. □, unaffected male, ■, affected male; ○ unaffected females; ● affected females.

Table 1. Autosomal Recessive Forms of Hereditary Hearing Impairment

LOCUS	LOCATION	GENE	ONSET	FREQUENCY	TYPE‡
DFNB1	13q12	Unknown	Prelingual	All	Stable (profound)
DFNB2	11q13.5	MYOSIN VII	Pre- and postlingual	All	Stable (profound)
DFNB3	17p11.2–q12	Unknown	Prelingual	All	Stable (profound)
DFNB4	7q31	Unknown	Prelingual	All	Stable (profound)
DFNB5	14q12	Unknown	Prelingual	All	Stable (profound)
DFNB6	3p14–21	Unknown	Prelingual	All	Stable (profound)
DFNB7*	9q13–21	Unknown	Prelingual	All	Stable (profound)
DFNB8	21q22	Unknown	Postlingual	All	Stable (profound)
DFNB9	2p22–23	Unknown	Prelingual	All	Progressive (profound)
DFNB10	21q22.3	Unknown	Prelingual	All	Stable (profound)
DFNB12	10q21–22	Unknown	Prelingual	All	Stable (profound)
DFNB15	3q21–25 19p13	Unknown	Prelingual	All	Stable (profound)
Usher's†					
Type 1a	14q	Unknown	Prelingual	All	Stable (profound)
Type 1b	11q13	MYOSIN VII	Prelingual	All	Stable (profound)
Type 1c	11p13	Unknown	Prelingual	All	Stable (profound)
Type 1d	10q	Unknown	Prelingual	All	Stable (profound)
Type 2a	1q41	Unknown	Prelingual	All	Stable (moderate to severe)
Type 3	3q21–25	Unknown	Pre- and postlingual	All	Progressive (moderate to severe)
Pendred	7q31	Unknown	Prelingual	All	Stable (profound)
Jervell and Lange-Nielsen	11p15.5	KVLQT1	Prelingual	All	Stable (profound)

* DFNB11 maps to the same region as DFNB7.
† Usher's syndrome type 1 consists of sensorineural hearing loss (SNHL), normal vestibular function, and PPR.
‡ Degree of SNHL.
DFNB, nonsyndromic autosomal recessive hearing loss.

fected persons). An added consideration is the spontaneous mutation rate. In some diseases, such as neurofibromatosis type 1, spontaneous mutations are common, and although the inheritance pattern is known to be AD, the disease gene will not be traceable to earlier generations if the affected person is expressing a new mutation.

Genetic linkage analysis has shown that nonsyndromic ADHL is a heterogeneous disorder; 13 loci have been identified, and more than 60 are estimated to exist. With the exception of DFNA3 and DFNA8, all of the localized genes cause postlingual, progressive hearing impairment that ranges from moderate to profound in intensity (Table 2). Variable expressivity is common, and even within families, affected persons can have different degrees of hearing loss.

With nearly all types of syndromic ADHL, the associated anomalies can be recognized at birth and should prompt auditory testing to establish whether a significant degree of hearing impairment exists. Waardenburg's, Treacher Collins, and branchio-oto-renal syndromes are relatively common and can be diagnosed by physical examination. Rarer syndromes, such as Alport's, Crouzon, and Stickler, also have an easily recognized phenotype.

X-Linked Inheritance

X-linked hearing impairment is uncommon, although several X-linked disorders should be considered in persons who have HHI (Table 3). The important feature to recognize in this type of inheritance is that *only males are affected* (Fig. 3).

Table 2. Autosomal Dominant Forms of Hereditary Hearing Impairment

LOCUS	LOCATION	GENE	ONSET	FREQUENCY	TYPE*
DFNA1	5q31	Unknown	Postlingual	Low	Progressive
DFNA2	1p32	Unknown	Postlingual	High	Progressive
DFNA3	13q12	Unknown	Prelingual	High	Stable (moderate)
DFNA4	19q13	Unknown	Postlingual	Mid/All	Progressive
DFNA5	7p15	Unknown	Postlingual	High	Progressive
DFNA6	4p16.3	Unknown	Postlingual	Low	Progressive
DFNA7	1q21–23	Unknown	Postlingual	High	Progressive
DFNA8	11q	Unknown	Prelingual	Mid/All	Stable (moderate to severe)
DFNA9	14q12–13	Unknown	Postlingual	High	Progressive
DFNA10	6q22–23	Unknown	Postlingual	Mid/All	Progressive
DFNA11	11q13.5	Unknown	Postlingual	Mid/All	Progressive
DFNA12	11q14–22	Unknown	Postlingual	Mid/All	Progressive
DFNA13	6p21	Unknown	Postlingual	Mid/All	Progressive
Waardenburg's					
Type 1	2q35	PAX3	Postlingual	High/All	Progressive
Type 2	3p12–14	MITF†	Postlingual	High/All	Progressive
Type 3*	2q35	PAX3	Postlingual	High/All	Progressive
Branchio-oto-renal	8q12–13	Unknown	Postlingual	Mid/High	Progressive (mild to profound)
Treacher Collins	5q32–33.1	TREACLE	Prelingual	All	Stable (mild to severe)
Stickler	6p21–22	COL11A2	Postlingual	High/All	Progressive (mild to severe)
	12q12–13.2	COL2A1	Postlingual	High/All	
Alport's	2q	COL4A3/4	Postlingual	High/All	Progressive
Neurofibromatosis					
Type 2	22q12.1	SCH	Postlingual	High/All	Progressive

* Usually a mixed hearing loss with a predominantly conductive component.
† Degree of sensorineural hearing loss unless otherwise specified.
DFNA, nonsyndromic autosomal dominant hearing loss.

Table 3. X-Linked Forms of Hereditary Hearing Impairment

LOCUS	LOCATION	GENE	ONSET	FREQUENCY	TYPE*
DFN1	Xq22	Unknown	Postlingual	All	Progressive
DFN2	Xq22	Unknown	Prelingual	All	Stable (profound)
DFN3	Xq21.1	POU3F4	Prelingual	All	Stable (moderate)†
DFN4	Xp21.2	Unknown	Prelingual	All	Stable (profound)
DFN6	Xp22	Unknown	Postlingual	High	Progressive
Otopalatal-digital	Xq28	Unknown	Postlingual	All	Conductive
Alport's	Xq22	COL4A5	Postlingual	High/All	Progressive

* Degree of sensorineural hearing loss otherwise specified.
† Mixed hearing loss.
DFN, X-linked hearing loss. Reanalysis of the DFN1 kindred has demonstrated additional features making this a syndromal type of hearing loss.

Male-to-male transmission does not occur. Affected males have no affected progeny, although all female progeny are carriers. Males born to carrier females have a 50 percent chance of being affected, whereas female progeny have a 50 percent chance of being carriers.

X-linked nonsyndromic hearing loss has a variable presentation that can include a mixed type of hearing impairment (DFN3). The conductive component in DFN3 is caused by stapes fixation that mimics otosclerosis. Stapedectomy should be avoided because the risks of a perilymphatic gusher and a subsequent "dead" ear are high. X-linked SNHL includes Alport's syndrome (SNHL and glomerulonephritis) and oto-palato-digital syndrome.

Mitochondrial Inheritance

Mitochondria have their own circular DNA that encodes 13 enzymes necessary for oxidative phosphorylation (i.e., Krebs cycle), 22 transfer RNAs, and 2 ribosomal RNAs. Because all mitochondrial DNA (mtDNA) is derived from the oocyte (the spermatocyte sheds its non-nuclear DNA), inheritance is unique. It follows *only the maternal line,* with affected females producing affected male and female progeny, and affected males producing no affected descendants at all (Fig. 4).

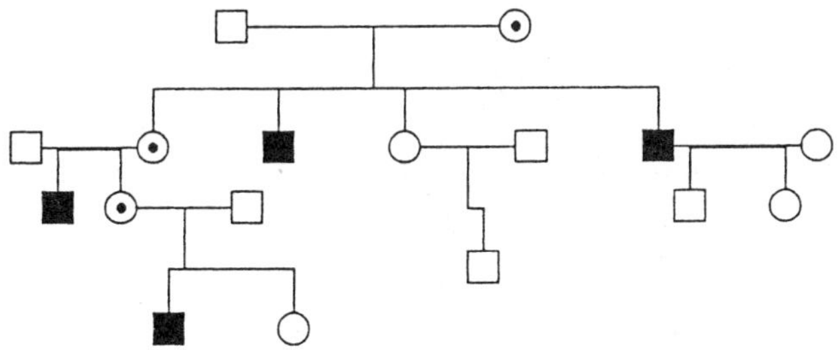

Figure 3.
Pedigree of a typical family with X-linked recessive hearing loss. Note that only males are affected with transmission through a carrier female. Males cannot transmit the disease. □, unaffected male; ■, affected male; ○ unaffected females; ● affected females; ⊙, carrier female.

Mutations in mtDNA produce a wide range of clinical signs and symptoms, especially in tissues with a high metabolic demand. Although the myopathies are biochemically and genetically heterogeneous, they share the common histologic diagnostic criteria of ragged red fibers in muscle stained by Gomori's trichrome method. Important diseases associated with mtDNA syndromic hearing loss include Kearns-Sayre syndrome; myoclonic epilepsy and ragged red fibers; and mitochondrial encephalopathy, lactic acidosis, and strokelike episodes. Two mutations in mtDNA have been identified that produce nonsyndromic hearing loss (Table 4). One of these mutations, an A-to-G transversion in nucleotide 1555 of the 12rRNA gene, is associated with a genetic predisposition to aminoglycoside-induced ototoxicity.

Multifactorial Inheritance

Many inherited disorders cannot be attributed to a single mutation, and the interaction of numerous genes is posited to play an important role in disease pathogenesis. Gene-to-gene interactions are said to occur when the combined effect of two or more genes on a phenotype is not predictable as the sum of their separate parts. This synergism or interaction deviation is known as *epistasis.* It is probably important in presbycusis, and may reflect the impact of both genetic and environmental factors on the auditory system over a lifetime.

■ PATIENT EVALUATION

A genetic etiology should be considered in any person who has hearing impairment. Historical information is the paramount tool that the otolaryngologist has to make this diagnosis, which can be affirmed by several findings. Most important is the occurrence of a similar type of impairment in other family members, particularly if age of onset and severity of hearing loss are similar. It is important to inquire about parental consanguinity and ethnic origins. A negative family history on the initial interview should not be accepted at face value, and the patient or parents should be encouraged to complete a medical health pedigree by contacting several other family members.

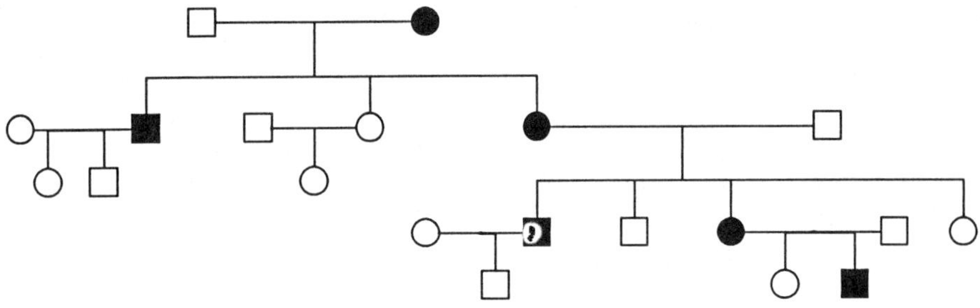

Figure 4.
Pedigree of a typical family with mitochondrial inherited hearing loss. Note that only female transmission occurs. Although males can be affected, they cannot transmit the disease. This is because all of the mitochondrial DNA of an offspring comes from the mother. Incomplete penetrance of the mutation accounts for not all offspring having the disease phenotype. □, unaffected male; ■, affected male; ○ unaffected females; ● affected females.

Table 4. Mitochondrial Forms of Hereditary Hearing Impairment

GENE	MUTATION POSITION	ONSET	FREQUENCY	TYPE
MELAS	3243,3271	Postlingual	High/All	Progressive
MERRF	8344,8356	Postlingual	All	Progressive
12S rRNA	A1555G	Postlingual	All	Progressive
tRNA-Ser(UCN)	T7445C	Postlingual	High	Progressive

Although physical evaluation may uncover craniofacial abnormalities consistent with a recognized syndrome, the possibility of nonpenetrance and variable expressivity must be considered and explored by directed questioning. For example, questions focused on premature graying, heterochromia iridis, and dystopia canthorum should be a routine part of the history if Waardenburg's syndrome is considered in the differential diagnosis.

Physical examination should be complemented by appropriate consultations and a limited and directed laboratory and radiologic evaluation. The life-altering impact of progressive pigmentary retinopathy and vestibular dysfunction (Usher's syndrome), cardiac dysrhythmias (JLN syndrome), renal abnormalities (branchio-oto-renal syndrome), or cafe-au-lait spots (neurofibromatosis) should be ascertained. Audiometry may reveal a conductive hearing loss (DFN3, otosclerosis, branchio-oto-renal syndrome) or a midfrequency deficit ("cookie-bite" audiogram), which can be associated with postlingual, progressive ADHL. Unfortunately, audiometry is not a reliable indicator of the type of inheritance pattern, and a single examination provides little prognostic information about the possibility of further progression.

Genetic counseling should be provided to ensure that families understand the scope and consequences of the information presented to them. Hearing impairment involves cultural and linguistic differences that have ethical and social implications. Genetic counselors trained to address these subjects can assist family members by exploring the options and implications, including psychological, that arise when HHI is diagnosed. Information should be provided in a nondirected manner with the focus on autonomy.

Neonates and Infants

Despite technologic advances in hearing screening through the use of otoacoustic emissions and recommendations to implement routine screening for all neonates and infants, age at detection of congenital hearing impairment remains greater than 24 months. Etiology is equally divided among hereditary and acquired causes, making it imperative to rule out nongenetic possibilities. Most common among these are infectious etiologies and "risk factors" typically seen in very sick babies.

If HHI seems likely, an extended family pedigree should be constructed to establish the inheritance pattern. The typical pattern of hearing impairment in this age group is a severe to profound, nonprogressive loss, although in the interpretation of the audiometric brain stem response the clinician must recognize that low-frequency (<1,000 Hz) hearing is not accurately measured.

Of congenital types of HHI, nonsyndromic ARHL represents the predominant etiology and is the most difficult to diagnose. Nonsyndromic ADHL is uncommon, although DFNA3 and DFNA8 must be considered. X-linked types of hearing loss include DFN2, DFN3, and DFN4. Usher's syndrome is the most common type of congenital syndromic ARHL. It belongs to a heterogeneous group of disorders characterized by the eventual development of progressive pigmentary retinopathy. In Usher's syndrome type 1, vestibular dysfunction is present and is manifest by the delayed attainment of motor milestones. Affected infants are slow to sit and walk. An ophthalmologist can often detect the associated retinal pathology by electroretinography at 4 to 6 years of age, before the onset of visual difficulty.

Routine laboratory tests and radiographic evaluations in neonates and infants should be discouraged, because the probability of finding a positive result argues against this practice. It is a more cost-effective approach to direct testing based on historical information and diagnostic possibilities. This approach requires the clinician to have an excellent understanding of all of the common types of syndromic hearing loss and know the general features of the various types of nonsyndromic hearing loss. For example, a history of sudden infant death syndrome or fainting episodes in siblings of an infant who has severe to profound SNHL should prompt electrocardiography to explore the diagnostic possibility of JLN syndrome. Branchio-oto-renal syndrome should be considered in a child who has hearing impairment and preauricular pits or a branchial cleft sinus, especially if these features are present in family members of the older generations, and abdominal ultrasonography should then be ordered to assess renal anatomy. Although computed tomography (CT) or magnetic resonance imaging (MRI) can confirm the presence of inner ear malformations (i.e., Mondini's dysplasia), we do not routinely order these studies unless X-linked nonsyndromic hearing loss is being considered (i.e., DFN3), or if there is fluctuating hearing impairment, vestibular dysfunction, or recurrent meningitis.

The emotional impact of the diagnosis of HHI on the parents must be acknowledged, and appropriate counseling should be extended to the family. Time must be available to explain inheritance patterns and types of HHI in infants in terms that the family can understand. The sense of guilt or failure that parents often feel also must be addressed. If the clinician does not feel competent to deal with these issues, appropriate genetic counseling must be offered to the family.

Children and Adolescents

This age group is a lesser diagnostic challenge than are neonates and infants, because the auditory history is more precise and most prelingual severe to profound forms of hearing impairment can be excluded. Many of the disorders are AD, so the pedigree can be very informative. However, mild to moderate degrees of hearing impairment can pass unnoticed, and unless audiometric testing of the parents is performed, some types of ADHL will be unrecognized.

The important diagnostic issue is the possibility of progression of the hearing impairment. Careful documentation on repeat audiograms is required. The enlarged vestibular aqueduct syndrome will usually occur in this age group and is known to occur as an AR form of HHI. CT scanning or MRI can confirm this diagnostic impression. These tests are also indicated if neurofibromatosis type 2 is suspected or in cases of the presence of conductive hearing loss consistent with either X-linked inheritance (i.e., DFN3) or branchio-oto-renal syndrome.

The types of SNHL often diagnosed during this time period include Waardenburg's, branchio-oto-renal, Treacher Collins, and Usher's syndromes. The first three should be recognized on physical examination, and the last by ophthalmoscopy. Routine laboratory analysis is again not required.

Adults

Hearing difficulty in this age group is extremely common. It is estimated that 50 percent of octogenarians have significant problems with daily communication. The impairment usually takes the form of a progressive SNHL or mixed loss, undoubtedly reflecting the synergistic impact of a lifetime of environmental and genetic factors.

The most common type of HHI that is diagnosed is some form of nonsyndromic ADHL. Although most types appear in the second to third decades and slowly progress to a severe to profound loss over the ensuing years, DFNA10, DFNA11, and DFNA13 can occur with a mid- to high-frequency loss in the late 40s or early 50s. The loss caused by DFNA4 seems to be potentiated by noise exposure. Although in most instances the high frequencies are initially affected, an exception is DFNA1, which primarily causes a low-frequency hearing loss.

DFN3 is characterized by a mixed hearing loss, in which the conductive component is caused by stapes fixation. The hearing loss usually occurs in a manner similar to otosclerosis (ages 20 to 30 years), except that sensorineural impairment may contribute significantly to the overall hearing loss. The critical feature of this disease can be seen on CT of the temporal bones. There is a widened lateral internal auditory canal that creates an abnormal communication with the inner ear at the lamina cribosa, which predisposes the patient to increased perilymphatic pressure and subsequent perilymphatic gushers if the vestibule is opened. These gushers have been reported to result in a high rate of subsequent severe to profound SNHL. Because this condition is X-linked, a careful history should be performed to uncover a family history of males who have had complications during otosclerosis surgery or a high rate of "cochlear" involvement with the otosclerosis.

Adults who have rapidly progressive SNHL should be evaluated for retrocochlear pathology to exclude the possibility of an acoustic neuroma. One form of syndromic ADHL, neurofibromatosis type 2, has the highest spontaneous mutation rate of any form of HHI and can occur in persons who do not have a family history of the disease.

■ THERAPY

Initial Treatment Plan

For a medical team to be well trained in the care of persons who have HHI, there must be sufficient depth of expertise to deal with a chronic problem that has far-reaching emotional, social, ethical, and educational ramifications. In addition to the otolaryngologist, integral to this team are the primary care physician, speech pathologist, audiologist, educator, psychologist, geneticist, genetic counselor, and representative from the hearing-impaired community. Generally, the otolaryngologist plays the pivotal role in initiating and coordinating appropriate treatment and habilitation.

One of the most difficult tasks is to inform a family of a genetic hearing loss, particularly if the loss is severe to profound and affects a child. A feeling of significant parental guilt is not uncommon, especially if neither parent is similarly affected. Thorough and compassionate counseling is imperative, thus acknowledging the emotional and psychological impact that the diagnosis of HHI can cause. Issues that must be covered include habilitation and treatment options; prognosis (i.e., stable versus progressive); pattern of inheritance; and risk of recurrence. The amount of information is too much to comprehend on a single visit, and in general it is a better policy to plan several return visits over the ensuing 2 to 4 weeks. This approach allows families to take a proactive role in the workup and affords more opportunities to review the diagnosis and its implications.

An aggressive broad-based treatment regimen appropriately tailored for patient age, functional ability, and degree of hearing impairment is the cornerstone of a strong habilitation program. Educational options include home or public schooling, special classes or focused day schools for the hearing-impaired, and residential schools. When a child is diagnosed with severe to profound hearing impairment, the first important decision is whether to educate the child partially or wholly in the hearing community ("mainstreaming") or to send the child to a school for the deaf. Total communication is an amalgamation of all potential forms of hearing amplification, supplemented by lipreading and American sign language, in an effort to maximize avenues for communication.

Each option has its relative merits that can be the subject of intense and emotional debate. For the infant who has severe to profound hearing loss, the otolaryngologist must fully and impartially educate the parents, a process that can be facilitated by meetings with other families who have affected children, public educators, and representatives of the hearing-impaired community. For the postlingually deafened child or adult, the best treatment is usually a total communication program.

Although the otolaryngologist must be impartial in counseling families, it is also important to dispel false statements or claims. For example, many leaders in the hearing-impaired community believe it is counterproductive to have a severely hearing-impaired child outside the "deaf culture" and that cochlear implants should not be offered as a habilitation option. However, medical technology has made rapid advances that have enabled many patients to integrate into the hearing world. Significant benefit from cochlear implantation has been shown in postlingually deafened children (deafness after age 4 years) and adults. Older congenitally hearing-impaired persons achieve less dramatic open set speech testing scores after implantation. However, significant benefits, such as better compliance to a total communication program, improved behavior and attentiveness, and perception of an environmental sound can be seen.*

Usher's syndrome patients possess a special need to maximize their auditory input, due to their dual sensory impairment. Children with Usher's syndrome have gained benefit from implantation, achieving significant gains in speech production and auditory perception before visual loss.

By establishing the inheritance pattern, the broader implications of HHI can be covered, including the risk of additional affected offspring. Ideally, as many family members as possible should be informed of the findings. This practice not only ensures that accurate firsthand information is provided to family members, but also allows the otolaryngologist to evaluate the family's support system.

A difficult counseling situation arises when only one family member is affected, but the suspicion of HHI is high. The empiric risk of other affected offspring when the firstborn is diagnosed with "idiopathic" SNHL is estimated to be 10 percent to 16 percent. With subsequent nonaffected offspring, the likelihood of a genetic etiology is diminished. In contrast, a hearing-impaired couple face more than a fivefold greater risk of further affected offspring if their firstborn is hearing impaired.

Amplification

Close ties with an experienced team of audiologists is essential to gain the maximum benefit from hearing aids. For a child, a team of professionals accustomed to working with pediatric patients is particularly important, because children present unique challenges to fit with hearing aids. The infant and young child are often not able to verbalize their preferences, and with adolescents, developmental and emotional issues can make compliance marginal. If the loss is progressive, frequent adjustments and even changes in the hearing aids may be necessary to maximize potential benefits. An adequate trial of hearing aids, complemented with aggressive speech therapy and lipreading, may require up to 2 years to adequately determine the benefit of these interventions. For many persons, amplification may provide only gross auditory cues, which are nevertheless helpful as part of a total communication program.

Cochlear implantation offers an alternative form of amplification to persons who have HHI. The criteria for implantation are identical to those for persons who have acquired forms of hearing loss. Patients should have a stable severe to profound hearing impairment and gain no benefit from hearing aids. In adults, the latter criterion has now been amended to include any hearing loss with no greater than 60 dB hearing with maximum amplification. An older person can be expected to find an implant more beneficial if the loss is postlingual (i.e., ADHL) as opposed to prelingual (i.e., congenital ARHL). The maintenance of linguistic skills is an important goal of all forms of amplification and speech therapy.

* Prelingually deafened children undergoing early implantation (<4 years) are now achieving high speech recognition and experience language development that is near their normal-hearing peers.

THE FUTURE OF HEREDITARY HEARING LOSS

Hearing Loss Genes

Numerous genes that cause HHI have been discovered by linkage analysis in affected families in many laboratories around the world. The human genome contains approximately 3 billion nucleic acid-base pairs, and most of these genes have been localized to regions of only a few million base pairs. This step is a necessary precursor to gene cloning and mutation analysis.

Several genes that cause syndromic hearing loss have now been cloned. Waardenburg's syndrome type 1 is caused by mutations in PAX3, a gene that encodes a transcription factor essential for regulation of cell migration during embryogenesis. Inappropriate migration of neural crest–derived melanocytes to the intermediate layer of the stria vascularis of the cochlea results in hearing impairment. The human microphthalmia (MITF) gene is associated with Waardenburg's syndrome type 2. The functional elements of the encoded protein include a DNA-binding region and dimerization motifs. Mutations in a series of collagen genes have been identified in Alport's syndrome, Stickler syndrome, and osteogenesis imperfecta. Investigators have discovered the sequence and mutations for the TREACLE gene of Treacher Collins syndrome, although its function is not known.

Progress with nonsyndromic hearing loss has not been as rapid, because only two genes have been cloned. The gene that causes DFN3 was identified by studying small deletions in affected families and is known as POU3F4. It encodes a POU-domain–containing transcription factor that is expressed in the fetal brain, kidney, and inner ear. Amino acid substitutions or protein truncation has been demonstrated in affected patients. The second nonsyndromic gene is myosin VIIA. Unconventional myosins are important intracellular molecules that generate intracellular mechanical forces. Myosin VIIA causes DFNB2, in addition to Usher's syndrome type 1B, which illustrates how different mutations in a single gene can result in two distinct phenotypes.

Many types of ARHL are hypothesized to reflect lack of expression of the wild-type (normal) protein, which implies the presence of mutations in each of the two copies of the relevant gene (or in the only copy if the disease is X-linked). Findings in USH1B are consistent with this hypothesis, as missense mutations in both alleles of the myosin VIIA gene have been demonstrated in affected persons and result in premature termination of mRNA translation.

The pathophysiology underlying ADHL is not as clear and may involve many different mechanisms. Simple haploinsufficiency (only one working copy of the gene) may result in a disease phenotype (i.e., hearing impairment and the other stigmata of Waardenburg's syndrome) as a result of a dosage effect. However, if the mutation results in inappropriate gene expression, a dominant negative can be produced as the mutant gene product over-rides the control mechanisms that normally exist to regulate gene function. Dominant negative effects may be associated with the mutations in the MITF gene.

Other possible mechanisms of action that can result in an AD phenotype include increased protein activity (i.e., loss of repressor function); altered components of a larger structural protein (i.e., weak link in the chain); and toxic protein alterations. A single inherited mutant allele also may unmask acquired mutations that develop in the wild-type allele. For example, the neurofibromatosis type 2 gene (SCH) acts as a recessive tumor suppressor gene. If a spontaneous mutation develops in the other allele, a neurofibroma develops.

Gene Replacement

The rapid explosion of knowledge on molecular genetics will change the way the otolaryngologist diagnoses and treats HHI. It will be possible to screen a small sample of DNA from a person in whom HHI is suspected, and by analyzing this DNA, determine the type of genetic defect involved. As knowledge of the types of genetic defects expands and their mechanism of action becomes clarified at the molecular level, some forms of hearing impairment will become amenable to medical treatment. For example, alleles that result in incomplete mRNA translation by using cryptic splice sites to reveal premature stop codons may be correctable using intranuclear-directed antisense nucleotide technology. It also may be possible to deliver normal copies of the malfunctioning gene to the inner ear using select viral vectors.

Suggested Reading

Andreoli SP, Deaton M. Alport's syndrome. Ear Nose Throat J 1992; 71: 508-511.

Brookhouser PE. Diseases of the inner ear and sensorineural hearing loss. In: Bluestone CD, Stool, SE, Kenna MA, eds. Pediatric otolaryngology. Philadelphia: WB Saunders, 1996:649.

Brookhouser PE. Hereditary hearing loss. In: Gates GA, ed. Current therapy in otolaryngology—head and neck surgery. St. Louis: Mosby–Year Book, 1990:44.

Grundfast KM. Hearing loss. In: Bluestone CD, Stool, SE, Kenna MA, eds. Pediatric otolaryngology. Philadelphia: WB Saunders, 1996:249.

Grundfast KM, Lalwani AK. Practical approach to diagnosis and management of hereditary hearing impairment (HHI). Ear Nose Throat J 1992; 10:479-493.

Hereditary hearing loss. Home page-http://dnalab-www.uia.ac.be/dnalab/hhh.html, sponsored by the Universities of Iowa and Antwerp (Belgium).

Joint commission on infant hearing 1994 position statement. Otolaryngol Head Neck Surg 1995; 113:191-196.

Lalwani AK, Mhatre AN, San Augustin TB, et al. Genotype-phenotype correlations in type 1 Waardenburg syndrome. Laryngoscope 1996; 106:895-902.

Online mendelian inheritance in man. Internet resource-http://www3.ncbi.nlm. gov/omim/

Reardon W, Harding AF. Mitochondrial genetics and deafness. J Audiol Med 1995; 4:40-51.

Smith RJ, Berlin CI, Hejmancik JF, et al. Clinical diagnosis of Usher syndrome. Am J Med Genet 1994; 50:32-38.

Steel KP, Brown SD. Genes and deafness. Trends Genetics 1994; 10:428-435.

Van Camp G, Willems P, Smith RJ. Non-syndromic hearing loss: Unparalleled heterogeneity. Am J Hum Genet (in press).

SUDDEN HEARING LOSS

The method of

Gordon B. Hughes

Sudden hearing loss (SHL) often is defined as 30 dB or more of sensorineural hearing loss over at least three contiguous audiometric frequencies occurring within 3 days or less. Of course, many patients perceive small degrees of loss. Slower loss over more than 3 days usually is described as "rapidly progressive" as opposed to "immediate."

SHL accounts for approximately 1 percent of all cases of sensorineural hearing loss; approximately 4,000 new cases of SHL occur annually in the United States, and 15,000 new cases occur worldwide. Infectious, traumatic, neoplastic, immunologic, toxic, circulatory, neurologic, metabolic, and other disorders can produce SHL (Table 1). The most popular theories of etiology are viral and circulatory causes. Cytomegalovirus, mumps, and rubeola have been identified in the inner ears of patients who have SHL, which provides the strongest evidence for a viral etiology. Circulatory disorders have reportedly been associated with SHL. Smoking may be a contributing factor, but apparently hyperlipidemia and aberrations of hemostasis are not. Although circulatory impairment of the cochlea would seem to be an obvious cause of SHL, definitive proof is lacking. A careful history indicates the likely cause of SHL in only 10 to 15 percent of patients. When no cause can be identified, SHL is deemed to be "idiopathic."

■ EVALUATION

The first priority is to discover potentially treatable causes of sensorineural hearing loss, especially ototoxicity that can be profound and permanent if medication is continued. Is

Table 1. Partial List of Causes of Sudden Sensorineural Hearing Loss

INFECTIOUS	**TOXIC**
Meningococcal meningitis	Snake bite
Herpesvirus (simplex, zoster, and varicella)	Ototoxicity
Mumps	**CIRCULATORY**
AIDS	Vascular disease/alteration of microcirculation
Mononucleosis	Vascular disease associated with mitochondriopathy
Lassa fever	Vertebrobasilar insufficiency
Mycoplasma	Red blood cell deformability
Cryptococcal meningitis	Sickle cell disease
Toxoplasmosis	Anomalous carotid artery
Syphilis	Cardiopulmonary bypass
Cytomegalovirus	**NEUROLOGIC**
Rubeola	Multiple sclerosis
Rubella	Focal pontine ischemia
TRAUMATIC	**METABOLIC**
Perilymphatic fistula	Thyrotoxic hypokalemia
Inner ear decompression sickness	Disturbances of iron metabolism
Temporal bone fracture	Diabetes mellitus
Inner ear concussion	Renal failure/dialysis
Otologic surgery	**OTHER**
Operative complications of nonotologic surgery	Meniere's disease
NEOPLASTIC	Pseudopsychosis
Acoustic neuroma	Neurosarcoidosis
Leukemia	Cyclosporine-treated renal transplantation
Myeloma	Dental surgery
Metastasis to internal auditory canal	Hyperostosis cranialis interna
Meningeal carcinomatosis	Genetic predisposition
IMMUNOLOGIC	Stress
Primary immune inner ear disease	
Temporal arteritis	
Wegener's granulomatosis	
Cogan's syndrome	
Polyarteritis nodosa	
Delayed contralateral endolymphatic hydrops	

AIDS, acquired immunodeficiency syndrome.
From Hughes GB, et al. Sudden sensorineural hearing loss. Otolaryngol Clin North Am 1996; 29:393–405.

the patient taking any medication? Does the patient have other medical problems that might predispose to SHL?

The exact circumstance and characteristic of the onset of hearing loss should be determined. Was the loss instantaneous or progressive over several days? The patient may recall the exact event or may awaken with hearing loss. Perilymphatic fistula can be considered only if SHL is closely associated with a well-defined event of trauma, exertion, or barotrauma. Is there vertigo, imbalance, tinnitus, and aural pressure, which suggest Meniere's disease or syndrome?

Because SHL often occurs in healthy patients, the general physical examination results are usually normal. Routine otoscopy should be performed in every patient; sometimes a simple plug of wax can create sudden conductive loss. Many SHL patients who experience dizziness should also have neurotologic examination including cranial nerves, cerebellar function, and spontaneous nystagmus using Fresnel lenses to determine if SHL is part of a more generalized neurologic disorder. Fistula testing can be performed in patients who are suspected of having this condition (gentle positive pressure in the ear canal may elicit subjective dizziness or objective nystagmus). Systemic disorders can be evaluated as indicated clinically. The physician should be alert for diabetes, syphilis, Lyme disease, acquired immunodeficiency syndrome, as well as renal, cardiovascular, immunologic, metabolic, and other systemic diseases that can produce SHL.

Table 2 lists some of the various laboratory tests that can be obtained, depending on clinical circumstances. Audiometry should be obtained to document the type and severity of loss. Electronystagmography usually is not helpful unless aminoglycoside ototoxicity is suspected; these agents are preferentially vestibulotoxic, so bilateral caloric weakness (canal paresis) is expected.

Unless hearing quickly returns to normal or its previous level, I routinely obtain magnetic resonance imaging with gadolinium enhancement for detecting possible acoustic neuroma (vestibular schwannoma), even though these tumors are rare. Enhanced computed tomography is not as sensitive for detecting tumor but will provide bone detail if trauma or developmental anomaly is suspected.

When SHL is bilateral and rapidly progressive or occurs in an only-hearing ear, or when systemic immune disease is present, immune-mediated inner ear disease must be sus-

Table 2. Diagnostic Tests Indicated Clinically for Sudden Hearing Loss

INDICATIONS	TEST(S)
All patients	Basic audiometry
Acoustic neuroma or skull base lesion	MRI or CT with contrast
Immune inner ear disease	Western blot immunoassay
	LTT
	Antigen-specific serologic tests
Syphilis	FTA-ABS
	MHA-TP
Other bacterial infections	Lyme disease titer
	Cultures as indicated clinically
Virus	Acute and convalescent titers
	HIV testing as indicated
Various indications	BAEP
	ENG
	ECoG
	Perilymphatic fistula "tests"
	CBC, blood chemistries, metabolic studies

MRI, magnetic resonance imaging; CT, computed tomography; LTT, lymphocyte transformation test; FTA-ABS, fluorescent treponemal antibody absorption; MHA-TP, microhemagglutination assay-*Treponema pallidum*; HIV, human immunodeficiency virus; BAEP, brain stem auditory evoked potentials; ENG, electronystagmography; ECoG, electrocochleography; CBC, complete blood count.

From Hughes GB, et al. Sudden sensorineural hearing loss. Otolaryngol Clin North Am 1996; 29:393–405.

Table 3. Procedure for Collecting and Mailing Serum Specimen for Western Blot Immunoassay

Frozen serum may be shipped overnight express to:
Clinical Immunology Laboratory
c/o Jose San Martin, M.D.
Massachusetts General Hospital
32 Fruit Street, Bullfinch 4, Room 442
Boston, MA 02114
Tel: 617-726-3743
Costs of labor and supplies are $150. Samples from outside Massachusetts must be accompanied by a check payable to the Massachusetts Eye and Ear Institute.
Results usually are available within 2 weeks.

pected. Serum can be sent to the Massachusetts Eye and Ear Institute for Western blot immunoassay (Table 3). An alternative is to purchase the test through Otoimmune Diagnostics, a division of IMMCO Diagnostics, Inc., Buffalo, New York (800-537-TEST). This test is probably more sensitive than the lymphocyte transformation test (LTT), and serum is preserved and transported more easily than whole, fresh blood. Moreover, the Western blot test result will remain positive even if steroid treatment has been started. In a patient who has suspected immune-mediated inner ear disease, a positive result should be considered a true-positive, and steroid treatment should be offered. If there is no contraindication, I prescribe prednisone, 1 mg per kilogram per day for 1 month, followed by a tapering dose and maintenance therapy as needed for an additional 3 to 6 months, or until normal hearing has been recovered. If antigen-specific testing cannot be obtained, antigen-nonspecific tests (antinuclear antibody, rheumatoid factor, complement studies, and so on) and acute phase reactants (erythrocyte sedimentation rate, C-reactive protein) may support a presumptive clinical diagnosis.

Syphilis is a well-known, treatable cause of bilateral, rapidly progressive hearing loss that can be sudden; however, the relatively low prevalence of the disease limits the predictive value of a positive fluorescent treponemal antibody absorption (FTA-ABS) or microhemagglutination assay-*Treponema pallidum* (MHA-TP) test. The clinician should decide first whether clinical circumstances warrant testing, and then be prepared to treat positive results as true-positives, administering antibiotics and cortisone to the patient. In nonallergic patients, I prescribe benzathine penicillin, 2.4 million units IM on each of 3 weeks, then every other week for a total of 3 months, and prednisone, 1 mg per kilogram per day for 30 days, if tolerated, followed by slow tapering and a low maintenance dose.

Again, disease prevalence greatly influences test predictive value. Syphilis and immune inner ear disease are more prevalent in patients who have bilateral symptoms. Therefore, patients who have *bilateral* hearing loss are more likely to have a true-positive immune or syphilis test; those who have *unilateral* hearing loss are more likely to have a false-positive Western blot or MHA-TP. In my practice, therefore, most patients who have bilateral hearing loss undergo MRI, Western blot (or LTT), and MHA-TP (or FTA-ABS), whereas most patients who have unilateral hearing loss undergo only MRI. Other tests are ordered as clinically indicated.

■ THERAPY

When a cause of SHL can be identified, treatment is specific, but may or may not be helpful: stop ototoxic medication, recompress inner ear decompression sickness, treat perilymphatic fistula, administer famciclovir for herpesvirus and antibiotics for bacterial infection, and correct metabolic imbalance. When a cause cannot be found, treatment of idiopathic SHL is much more controversial.

Although many treatment regimens have been proposed for idiopathic SHL (Table 4), prospective, controlled trials have not yet confirmed significant benefit from treatment with any medication compared with spontaneous recovery, because patients are not necessarily treated at comparable stages of disease. Approximately two-thirds of patients improve without treatment of any kind, usually within the first 2 weeks. The prognosis for recovery from idiopathic SHL is best when patients are seen early, begin recovery within 2 weeks, and have mild loss, an upward sloping audiogram, and no vertigo. The prognosis is worse when patients fail to begin recovery within 2 weeks, have severe loss, a downward sloping audiogram, and vertigo. In 15 percent of patients, hearing loss progresses. Thus, even prospective studies are prone to interpretive error unless patient groups are matched exactly.

Prospective, controlled studies have not confirmed any benefit from infusions of dextran 40 and/or pentoxifylline, nor from procaine and low molecular weight dextran, compared with spontaneous recovery. Even a "shotgun" regimen

Table 4. Partial List of Treatment(s) for Sudden Sensorineural Hearing Loss

ANTI-INFLAMMATORY/IMMUNOLOGIC AGENTS
Cortisone
Prostaglandin
DIURETICS
Hydrochlorothiazide-triamterene
Lasix
ANTIVIRAL AGENTS
Acyclovir
VASODILATORS
Carbogen (5 percent carbon dioxide, 95 percent oxygen)
Papaverine
Buphenine (nylidrin)
Natfidrofuryl (nafronyl)
Thymoxamine
Prostacyclin
Nicotinic acid
Pentoxifylline
VOLUME EXPANDERS/HEMODILUTION AGENTS
Hydroxyethyl starch
Low molecular weight dextran
DEFIBRINOGENATION AGENTS
Batroxobin
CALCIUM ANTAGONISTS
Nifedipine
OTHER TREATMENTS
Amidotrizoate
Acupuncture
Iron
Vitamins
Procaine

From Hughes et al. Sudden sensorineural hearing loss. Otolaryngol Clin North Am 1996; 29:393–405.

of dextran, histamine, Hypaque (diatrizonate meglumine), diuretic, steroid, vasodilator, and carbogen (5 percent carbon dioxide, 95 percent oxygen) inhalation failed to have measurable benefit in a prospective, controlled clinical trial.

Despite these studies, I still believe that three treatment modalities are justifiable and should be used in selected patients: corticosteroid, low-salt diet and diuretic, and carbogen. The specific action of corticosteroids is unknown, but they may help infectious, inflammatory, and immune-mediated conditions. Despite disappointing results of early steroid studies that used lower doses and/or short treatment duration, and despite the lack of a prospective, randomized controlled study of high-dose, long-term (30 days) corticosteroids, abundant clinical experience now supports the use of prednisone, 1 mg per kilogram per day for 1 month in patients who have immune-mediated or syphilitic SHL, and for at least 10 days in patients who have idiopathic SHL. If the exact cause is unknown, I prefer to treat idiopathic SHL with prednisone, 1 mg per kilogram per day if hearing loss is *unilateral,* following the same reasoning as previously described in ordering laboratory tests.

Low-salt diet and diuretic therapy is a well-accepted treatment for Meniere's disease and syndrome. SHL can be associated with hydrops, a nonspecific response to injury. I frequently prescribe a low-salt diet and diuretic therapy to patients who have SHL because it may help and is convenient and inexpensive. The low-salt diet averages 2 to 4 g of sodium per day. Patients are asked to avoid salty food, not to add table salt to the food when prepared, and not to add salt to the food when served. Hydrochlorothiazide 25 mg combined with triamterene (Dyazide, Maxzide) is selected for diuretic therapy because it is potassium sparing. One tablet per day with fruit juice will not deplete potassium if the patient is taking a prostaglandin inhibitor (nonsteroidal anti-inflammatory agent), because it can cause severe renal failure.

Carbogen increases perilymphatic oxygen and may provide better SHL recovery compared with traditional intravenous vasodilators. Unfortunately, carbogen usually is administered in the hospital, and insurance companies still consider it experimental and will not pay for hospitalization. Although oral outpatient steroid and diuretic therapy are readily accepted by most patients, inpatient carbogen treatment is more controversial and requires informed patient consent. There is no guarantee of benefit, and the patient may have to pay the entire hospital bill. Therefore, I offer carbogen for 10 minutes, six times daily, over 3 days to a relatively small group of patients: those who have SHL in an only-hearing ear or better-hearing ear, those who are professional musicians, and any others who are highly motivated to do anything that might help.

■ DISCUSSION

The treatment physician's primary responsibilities are to: (1) diagnose treatable underlying disease, particularly ototoxicity; (2) discuss risks, benefits, and alternatives of treatment with the patient; (3) treat aggressively or not at all; (4) rehabilitate with hearing aid or other assistive device those patients whose hearing does not improve; and (5) follow up adequately all patients for possible delayed symptoms and contralateral ear disease.

Suggested Reading

Fisch U. Management of sudden deafness. Otolaryngol Head Neck Surg 1983; 91:3-8.

Hughes GB, Freedman MA, Haberkanp TJ, Guay ME. Sudden sensorineural hearing loss. Otolaryngol Clin North Am 1996; 29:393-405.

Kronenberg J, Almagor M, Bendet E, Kushnir D. Vasoactive therapy versus placebo in the treatment of sudden hearing loss: A double-blind clinical study. Laryngoscope 1992; 102:65-66.

Probst R, Tschopp K, Kellerhals B, et al. A randomized, double-blind, placebo-controlled study of dextran/phenoxifylline medication in acute acoustic trauma and sudden hearing loss. Acta Otolaryngol 1992; 112: 435-443.

Wilkins SA Jr, Mattox DE, Lyles A. Evaluation of a "shotgun" regimen for sudden hearing loss. Otolaryngol Head Neck Surg 1987; 97:474-480.

Wilson WR. The relationship of the herpesvirus family to sudden hearing loss: A prospective clinical study and literature review. Laryngoscope 1986; 96:870-887.

PROGRESSIVE SENSORINEURAL HEARING LOSS

The method of
Kenneth M. Grundfast
Charles A. Syms III

Current therapy for progressive sensorineural hearing loss (P-SNHL) remains perplexing and controversial. Although attempts have been made in recent years to gain better understanding of the involved biologic mechanisms so that rational approaches to therapy might be offered, in fact, the causes of P-SNHL remain obscure and mysterious. Accordingly, audiologists and otologic surgeons who share responsibility for case management remain frustrated when confronted with patients who have P-SNHL. Unfortunately, for most patients, there simply is no medical or surgical treatment that can be depended on to cure P-SNHL.

Not only is the management of P-SNHL fraught with frustration because of lack of any generally accepted cure, but also definition of the disorder and clinical diagnosis are problematic. Some of the uncertainties inherent in diagnosis and management of P-SNHL are summarized as follows:

- What are the criteria for diagnosis of *progressive* sensorineural hearing loss?
- How can *progressive* sensorineural hearing loss be differentiated from *fluctuating* sensorineural hearing loss (F-SNHL)?
- If a patient who has newly diagnosed hearing loss that is thought to be progressive actually has a hearing loss that eventually is seen to fluctuate, how can any incremental improvement that occurs after treatment is provided be attributed to the treatment rather than to the improvement that is known to occur repeatedly when a hearing loss fluctuates?
- Is *rapidity* of progression of hearing loss a significant factor in determining what type of therapy might be warranted?
- Is the goal of therapy for P-SNHL *improvement* in hearing or *stabilization* of hearing at a certain threshold level? If the goal is stabilization, then how is stabilization defined?

■ DEFINITION

To treat progressive sensorineural hearing loss, we must have a way of determining specifically when a patient has this disorder. That is, there is a need to distinguish between fluctuating hearing loss that does not appreciably "progress," becoming worse over time, and the hearing loss that fluctuates within relatively short periods but also progresses and becomes appreciably worse over longer periods.

Recently, the American Academy of Otolaryngology–Head and Neck Surgery (AAO–HNS) has revised the definition of fluctuating and stable hearing for patients who have Meniere's disease. The AAO–HNS now suggests that a *significant* change in hearing be defined as follows:

- Change of 10 dB or greater in the four pure-tone average (PTA) at frequencies of 500 Hz, 1 KHz, 2 KHz, and 3 KHz, or
- Change in the word recognition score (speech discrimination) of 15 percentage points or more.

Although this definition helps in providing quantifiable parameters that are used to measure magnitude of change, the definition does not include a time factor that might be used to quantify rate of change in hearing. Therefore, although the AAO–HNS definition can be used to determine when a hearing loss is to be considered significant, it cannot be used to determine whether a hearing loss is sudden, fluctuating, or progressive.

Sudden Hearing Loss

This condition is defined as a significant change in hearing (as defined by the AAO–HNS) occurring in an individual who has not had prior history of change in hearing.

Fluctuating Sensorineural Hearing Loss

This condition represents a significant change in hearing (as defined by the AAO–HNS) occurring in an individual who has had prior history of significant change in hearing followed by significant improvement in hearing in the affected ear. Significant improvement in hearing is defined using the AAO–HNS definition of change.

Progressive Sensorineural Hearing Loss

This condition is defined as a significant change in hearing (as defined by the AAO–HNS) occurring in an individual who has had prior history of decrement change in hearing without any evidence of improvement in hearing since the time that the hearing loss was initially detected and measured with audiologic assessment.

Fluctuating and Progressive Sensorineural Hearing Loss (F-P-SNHL)

This condition is defined as a hearing loss that both fluctuates within short periods of time *and* progresses (worsens) over a longer period of time. That is, a significant change in hearing (as defined by the AAO–HNS), occurring over more than 6 months' time, in an individual who has had prior history of decrement change in hearing with some evidence of improvement in hearing occurring sporadically since the time that the hearing loss was initially detected and measured with audiologic assessment.

Rate of Change in Hearing

With the aforementioned definitions in mind, the other parameter that needs to be considered in management of the patient who has P-SNHL is the rate of change in hearing. Hearing loss that is *rapidly* progressive most likely has an underlying cause that is different from a hearing loss that is *slowly* progressive. For example, a rapidly progressive sensorineural hearing loss could be caused by autoimmune inner ear disease or syphilis, whereas a slowly progressive sensorineural hearing loss is more likely to be diagnosed as presbycusis, which is believed to be caused by the loss of inner hair cells that occurs with aging.

■ EVALUATION

History

In taking the medical history from a patient who has P-SNHL, an attempt should be made to elicit specific information about the following:

- Time of onset: When was the hearing loss first noticed?
- Involved ear: Is the hearing loss in both ears, or only in one ear?
- Associated symptoms: Is there tinnitus, aural fullness or pressure, dizziness, vertigo, headache, or visual disturbance?
- Family history: Are there other family members who have had similar hearing loss? Have any family members been diagnosed with otosclerosis, acoustic tumor, or neurofibromatosis?
- Medical history: Was there any event or trauma before the onset of the hearing loss that might be causally related, such as blunt head injury, barotrauma, or noise exposure? Is there a history of autoimmune disorder, thyroid disease, exposure to ototoxic medications, or irradiation to the head?

Examination

On examination, look specifically for clues that could help determine the cause of the hearing loss, such as:

- Pigmentary abnormalities that might be consistent with a diagnosis of Waardenburg's syndrome: two eyes of different color, an iris that contains pie-shaped segments of blue and brown, white forelock, and depigmented or hypopigmented areas of skin.
- Funduscopic abnormalities, such as pigmented spicules that might suggest retinitis pigmentosa and a possible diagnosis of Usher's syndrome.
- Thyromegaly.
- Positional vertigo, nystagmus, or both, which might be consistent with a diagnosis of perilymphatic fistula.
- Neurologic assessment, including tests of cerebellar function, cranial nerve function, Romberg's test, and gait testing.

Audiologic Assessment

Complete audiologic assessment is essential. Having serial audiologic testing at the same facility using the same test equipment helps to minimize variability that can confuse the issue of whether hearing is changing over time. The initial audiologic assessment should include (1) pure-tone audiography, (2) pure-tone average, (3) speech reception threshold, (4) speech discrimination score, and (5) tympanography.

Subsequent hearing assessments should include a similar test battery, but tympanography need not be repeated if the initial findings were normal and there is no evidence on examination of an abnormal middle ear condition.

Timing of follow-up visits and repeat audiologic assessment is important in making a diagnosis and developing an approach to case management. When there is a history to suggest fluctuating or progressive SNHL, the patient should be instructed to return for repeat hearing testing once every 3 months for at least 1 year and should be encouraged to come in for a hearing test on an urgent basis at any time that there is a perception of significant change in hearing. In this way, fluctuations in hearing can be documented and considered in further attempts to uncover a cause for the hearing loss.

Saeki and Kitahara have presented an innovative way of graphically representing cumulative results of serial audiograms. They present the three-dimensional audiogram, which displays duration of the hearing loss on the x-axis, frequency on the y-axis, and hearing threshold level on the z-axis.

Imaging Studies

Once serial tests have demonstrated progression of hearing loss, the decision needs to be made whether to request an imaging study. The best imaging study in adult patients is magnetic resonance imaging (MRI), with gadolinium used to detect either the presence of an acoustic tumor (cochlear or vestibular schwannona) or the enhancement of the cochlea, which is believed to be due to inflammatory or infectious disorders, perhaps viral infection of the cochlea. When multiple sclerosis is suspected, imaging of the entire brain may help detect the sclerotic plaques that can be diagnostic. The best imaging study in children is the computed tomographic (CT) scan, which is used to look for congenital abnormalities. These are, in order of frequency of occurrence, (1) enlarged vestibular aqueduct, (2) incomplete cochlear partition (Mondini's deformity), and (3) bulbous internal auditory canal, described by Phelps as associated with the hereditary disorder known as X-linked mixed hearing loss with stapes gusher.

Laboratory Studies

Since the cause of P-SNHL is usually obscure, there has been a tendency by many clinicians to order a battery of hematologic and blood chemistries in the hope of uncovering an abnormal result that will lead to diagnosis of a disorder that is not yet apparent. However, after taking the history, carefully examining the patient, and analyzing results of an imaging study, the likelihood is not high that a discrete diagnosis will be made on the basis of detecting elevated serum glucose, cholesterol, triglycerides, or glucose levels; elevated erythrocyte sedimentation rate; electrolyte abnormalities; or abnormal thyroid function. The laboratory tests most likely to be helpful in diagnosis are the Western blot assay for autoimmune inner ear disease (AIED), and serologic tests for syphilis. The Western blot assay for detection of antibodies to the 68 kD antigen associated with AIED is not a test that can be done in any laboratory. To do this test, send 5 to 100 cc of serum (red top tube on ice) to any of the laboratories listed next:

IMMCO Diagnostics
60 Pineview Drive
Buffalo, NY 14228
Tel # 800-537-TEST

Harvard Medical School
The Massachusetts Eye and Ear Infirmary
The Coolidge Clinical Laboratory
Antibody to Inner Ear Immunoassay
243 Charles Street
Boston, MA 02114-3096
Tel # 617-573-3654

The Cleveland Clinic Foundation
9500 Euclid Avenue
Cleveland, OH 44195
Tel # 800-628-6816
216-44-5755

In evaluation of children who have F-P-SNHL, the question often arises about how to use laboratory tests to detect the viral disorders that might cause hearing loss Many textbooks recommend that infants and children with SNHL have the TORCH (toxoplasmosis, rubella, cytomegalovirus, herpes) assay done in an attempt to uncover the cause of hearing loss. However, interpretation of the assay titers in a child who does not currently have acute or subacute infection is so difficult as to render the testing of little diagnostic value in most cases. In general, if an infant or child has F-P-SNHL caused by a serious viral infection, there will be other manifestations of the infection, such as congenital cataract or neurologic sequelae that are more helpful than is an elevated serologic titer in leading to the proper diagnosis.

■ DIAGNOSTIC POSSIBILITIES AND TREATMENT RECOMMENDATIONS

An algorithm for the diagnosis and management of progressive hearing loss is given in Figure 1.

Idiopathic

In most cases of progressive hearing loss, no specific cause can be detected and confirmed with reasonable assurance. This has created a problem in case management. Patients who have P-SNHL are frightened that they may have further hearing loss and become deaf. Similarly, parents of children who have P-SNHL are frightened that their child may become deaf. Patients and parents want an explanation of what is causing the loss of hearing, and all caring physicians naturally want to help in allaying the fears of patients and parents. However, if diagnostic studies have failed to reveal a discrete diagnosis, predictions about probability of further loss of hearing mostly are conjectural and can be misleading. Sometimes, empathy and compassion on the part of the clinician rather than a tentative or circuitous explanation of cause are more appreciated and lead to better patient rapport in the future. Unfortunately, physicians have little understanding of what causes P-SNHL in most cases, and until we have a better understanding of the biologic mechanisms involved, we probably can serve our patients best by simply being honest and letting the patients or parents know when we cannot explain why hearing is deteriorating.

When P-SNHL is believed to be idiopathic, a short course of high-dose steroids is recommended, with repeat hearing test within 2 weeks following cessation of steroid. The recommended dose is prednisone, 1 mg per kilogram daily, to a maximum of 60 mg per day, and tapered over 14 days.

Hereditary

The U-shape or "cookie-bite" audiogram is supposedly suggestive of hereditary hearing impairment. Recent studies, however, have raised questions about the extent to which configuration of the audiogram correlates with hereditary cause of the hearing loss.

A common hereditary disorder causing progressive SNHL is autosomal dominant, nonsyndromic, delayed-onset, progressive sensorineural hearing loss. Typically, the hearing loss begins in the second decade of life and the rapidity of progression of the hearing loss is variable, but progression to severe or profound SNHL in the fourth decade is not uncommon. Because the disorder is autosomal dominant, a key to diagnosis is the family history of affected parents, grandparents, or siblings.

There are many different types of nonsyndromic autosomal recessive P-SNHL, and there are probably many different genes that can cause them. Diagnosis depends on learning that siblings or cousins of the patient have progressive hearing loss, but parents and grandparents would not be expected to be affected.

X-linked mixed hearing loss with stapes gusher occurs in males. The hearing loss can occur after relatively minor head trauma. Phelps has described the characteristic bulbous shape of the lateral aspect of the internal auditory canal associated with this hereditary disorder.

At present, there is no treatment for the hereditary causes of SNHL. In the future, as understanding increases of the molecular mechanisms involved, gene therapy may become available to prevent these types of hearing loss or ameliorate the effects of aberrant gene expression.

Enlarged Vestibular Aqueduct Syndrome

The most common radiographic abnormality found in children who have F-P-SNHL is the enlarged vestibular aqueduct. Typically, children with this disorder have hearing that periodically becomes worse, often reaches a plateau, and then worsens again at a later time. Findings on CT scan are diagnostic. Although this condition is not usually known to be a hereditary disorder, there have been cases of multiple family members affected with enlarged vestibular aqueduct syndrome (EVAS), so there may be a genetic predisposition for this disorder.

There have been reports that a short course of high-dose steroids may help hearing return to a previous level. Endolymphatic sac shunt surgery is not helpful and can be associated with worse hearing following surgery. There have been reports suggesting that patients who have EVAS are prone to developing perilymphatic fistula, and one of the reports suggests middle ear exploration in patients who have EVAS to look for and repair perilymphatic fistula. We are skeptical of the validity of these reports and would not advise exploration of the middle ear simply on the basis of radiographic

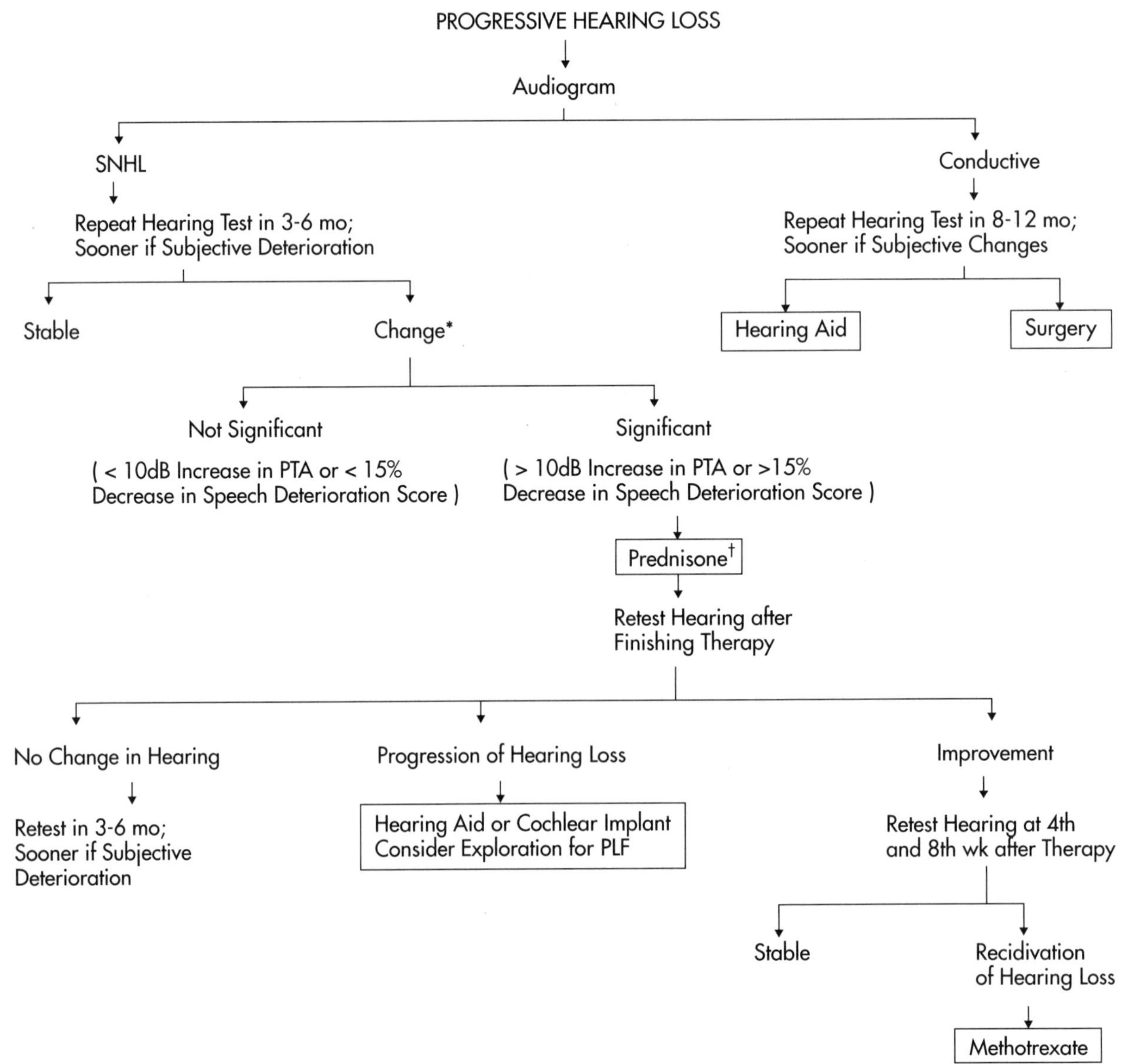

Figure 1.
Algorithm for the diagnosis and management of progressive hearing loss. SNHL, sensorineural hearing loss; PLF, perilymphatic fistula; FTA, fluorescent treponemal antibody.
* Obtain otometabolic screening (complete blood cell count, erythrocyte sedimentation rate, urinalysis, FTA-ABS or MHA-TP, thyroid function tests, cholesterol and triglycerides, antinuclear antibody, rheumatoid factor, and other tests, if indicated) and consider high-resolution computed tomography of the temporal bone or high-resolution spin echo magnetic resonance imaging if available.
† A trial of 10 to 14 days of prednisone (7 to 10 days of 30 mg twice daily, with a rapid taper) is considered in all patients, but strongly encouraged in patients who have large or rapidly progressive losses and patients who have laboratory evidence of autoimmune disease. All patients should have their hearing retested 14 days after starting therapy.

finding of EVAS without signs and symptoms to suggest a perilymphatic fistula. Also, there have been reports that surgical compression of the endolymphatic sac may ameliorate the hearing loss.

Incomplete Cochlear Partition (Mondini's Deformity)

Patients with Mondini's deformity do have F-P-SNHL. Low-sodium diet is advisable, and a short course of high-dose steroids may be helpful at times when the hearing becomes worse.

Autoimmune Inner Ear Disease

Autoimmune inner ear disease is perhaps the single most treatable cause of F-P-SNHL. Initial treatment is prednisone, 1 mg per kilogram daily, to a maximum dose of 60 mg daily. In some patients, the hearing promptly begins to worsen when the prednisone is withdrawn. In such patients, long-term low-dose methotrexate can be given to adults in a dose of 7.5 to 15 mg per week for at least 8 weeks. For children and adolescents who have AIED and for women of childbearing age, methotrexate can be given, but the side effects and potential adverse results of long-term administration of methotrexate must be considered before initiating therapy. The most common side effects of prolonged administration of methotrexate are elevation of liver enzymes, nausea, vomiting, diarrhea, stomatitis, thrombocytopenia, and dermatologic conditions. If methotrexate is not successful in maintaining a patient's hearing threshold or cannot be tolerated because of side effects, cyclophosphamide can be given in a dose of 2 to 5 mg per kilogram for a 3 month trial.

Perilymphatic Fistula

Certainly, perilymphatic fistula (PLF) can cause sudden hearing loss. In some patients, PLF can also cause F-P-SNHL. When a patient with F-P-SNHL has a history of antecedent barotrauma, symptoms of dysequilibrium, a positive fistula test, and reproducible nystagmus with subjective vertigo elicited during positional testing, a diagnosis of PLF must be considered. Inspection of the middle ear with a tiny endoscope to look for evidence of a fistula is recommended if PLF is suspected, and surgical middle ear exploration with PLF repair is indicated either if middle ear endoscopy detects leak of perilymph or if middle ear endoscopy cannot be done and there is high suspicion of PLF. This having been said, PLF does *not* have to be suspected in every case of F-P-SNHL without apparent cause. Raising the possibility of PLF as a possible cause of F-P-SNHL when there really are no findings typical of PLF is not intellectually honest and may be misleading to patients and parents. We must all remind ourselves that patients and parents who face the prospect of losing their hearing are frightened individuals who will grasp at any hope of preventing further hearing loss. Recommending middle ear exploration "to see if there might be a fistula" because the procedure "can't hurt" is not an optimal approach to patient management and will not help those of us involved with care of these patients to find the valid scientific explanations that eventually will be found.

Delayed Effect of Ionizing Radiation

Patients who have had ionizing radiation to the head and neck for treatment of malignancy can develop sensorineural hearing loss months to years after completion of the radiotherapy. Histologic studies in chinchillas reveal that radiation to the temporal bone can cause delayed loss of sensory and supporting cells in the organ of Corti. Although there is no specific treatment known to be helpful in restoring hearing in cases of P-SNHL suspected to be caused by prior radiotherapy, recognizing the relationship between the hearing loss and the radiotherapy may help to explain why the hearing loss has occurred. A short course of high-dose steroids can be tried, but there have been no reports or studies suggesting that steroid administration has therapeutic value.

Bacterial Meningitis

The hearing deficit resulting from bacterial meningitis may not be entirely apparent within weeks or months after the meningitis is recognized and treated. Hearing threshold may worsen years after the meningitis has been treated and the patient has recovered. Some children who have severe hearing impairment that has been attributed to bacterial meningitis and remained stable for many years may, upon reaching puberty, have progressive further loss of hearing resulting in profound hearing loss or even an anacoustic ear. Therefore, when an adolescent who is severely hearing impaired as a result of bacterial meningitis complains that his or her hearing aid is no longer functioning properly, retest the hearing thresholds in each ear and look for evidence of delayed progression of a hearing loss that had remained stable for many years.

SENSORINEURAL HEARING LOSS: MEDICAL THERAPY

The method of
Steven D. Rauch

Medical management of sensorineural hearing loss? Implicit in this concept is the notion that sensorineural hearing loss (SNHL) is reversible. Although every medical student learns the simple dogma that SNHL is irrevocable, in fact, there are several examples of reversible SNHL. These include the temporary threshold shift of acoustic trauma, salicylate or loop diuretic ototoxicity, some cases of idiopathic sudden sensorineural hearing loss, Meniere's disease, immune-mediated inner ear disease, and perhaps others. It is fascinating to speculate on the possible underlying pathophysiologic mechanisms that might explain reversibility. Inner ear ion homeostasis and endocochlear potential, cochlear and hair cell micromechanics, neurotransmitters and their receptors, and signal transmission along neurons are all critical to normal audition and are all conceivable sites of reversible dysfunction.

Reversible causes of SNHL are not the most common conditions encountered by the clinical otologist, but they are of disproportionate significance by virtue of the opportunity they provide for study of basic aspects of inner ear physiology and pathophysiology. Discussion of these basic physiologic mechanisms is beyond the scope of this chapter. I review two specific types of reversible SNHL: idiopathic sudden SNHL and idiopathic, progressive, bilateral SNHL (a.k.a. immune-mediated SNHL; a.k.a. "autoimmune" SNHL). Although these two entities share a clinical feature of reversibility by treatment with corticosteroids, they seem to share little else.

IDIOPATHIC SUDDEN SENSORINEURAL HEARING LOSS

Clinical Presentation

Idiopathic sudden sensorineural hearing loss (ISSNHL) has a reported incidence of five to 20 per 100,000 population per year. ISSNHL was first described in 1944 by De Kleyn and attributed to a brain stem abnormality and possible vitamin deficiency. There are currently two widely held etiologic theories: vaso-occlusive and viral. Histopathologic study of temporal bones from patients who have ISSNHL demonstrates degeneration of the hair cells and supporting cells of the organ of Corti, the tecorial membrane, and, to a lesser degree, the stria vascularis and spiral ganglion. These findings are virtually identical to those seen in cases of known viral cochleitis, such as measles, mumps, rubella, or herpes infection. In contrast, known cases of vaso-occlusive disease are virtually always associated with fibrosis and ossification of the cochlea, findings absent from the ISSNHL temporal bones reported by Schuknecht and Donovan. However, vascular insult is still an appealing explanation in those patients with known systemic microangiopathy and hyperviscosity or hypercoagulability states. Autoimmune inner ear injury and inner ear membrane rupture have also been invoked as possible explanations, but these etiologic hypotheses are less plausible for a variety of reasons.

ISSNHL is defined as the appearance of unilateral SNHL in less than 48 to 72 hours that cannot be attributed to other known causes of sudden hearing loss, such as acoustic neuroma, multiple sclerosis, Meniere's disease, perilymphatic fistula, systemic autoimmune disease, syphilis, and neoplasm metastatic to the temporal bone. It is a diagnosis of exclusion. Diagnostic workup consists of a careful history and appropriate serologic and imaging studies to make such determination. It is noteworthy that there have been no reports of confirmed simultaneous ISSNHL. All such cases of bilateral hearing loss have eventually been determined to be functional, immune-mediated, retrocochlear, or paraneoplastic. Immune-mediated hearing loss affects both ears but is rarely (if ever) simultaneous and sudden.

The natural history of ISSNHL was studied prospectively by Mattox and Simmons. Subsequent prospective study by Wilson and co-workers and retrospective study by Fetterman and co-workers have generally corroborated earlier reports. Nearly two-thirds of all patients who have ISSNHL will recover to normal or near-normal hearing levels without treatment. Detailed analysis reveals several predictors of outcome. Those who recover spontaneously tend to do so within the first 2 weeks after onset of hearing loss. Thus, patients who are initially seen more than 2 weeks after symptom onset with persistent hearing loss have a worse prognosis. Younger patients have a greater likelihood of spontaneous recovery, as do those patients who have no associated vestibular symptoms and those who have milder hearing loss. Wilson and co-workers noted that all patients who had less than 40 dB of hearing loss confined to the mid-frequencies made full recovery, whereas no patients who had greater than 90 dB of hearing loss recovered. Patients who had between 40 and 90 dB had an approximately 38 percent spontaneous recovery rate.

Therapy

ISSNHL is a medical emergency in which prompt diagnosis and treatment is essential if outcome is to be optimized. Unfortunately, many patients who have this condition experience considerable delay in diagnosis. They perceive a blocked ear, consult their primary care physician, and receive weeks of therapy with decongestants, antihistamines, and antibiotics before eventually seeking otolaryngologic and audiometric assessment. Spontaneous recovery is likely in those who have mild hearing loss and unlikely in those who have profound loss. In those who have moderate loss, there is a window of opportunity for treatment with systemic steroids. This time window is probably 2 weeks long and may possibly last up to 4 weeks. Use of vasodilators and volume expanders, although popular in the past, has generally fallen out of favor in recent years. New antiviral drugs are beginning to have application for ISSNHL, but controlled trials have not yet been conducted. It is in the best interests of patients and otolaryngologists to help make primary care physicians more aware of this clinical entity in order to facilitate rapid diagnosis and appropriate treatment.

Treatment of ISSNHL has changed over the years as different proposed etiologies have fallen in and out of favor. Volume expanders and vasodilators were popular in the 1970s and early 1980s, but these agents have gradually seen less use as evidence has mounted in favor of the viral etiology. Fisch did conduct a prospective, randomized study comparing carbogen (95 percent oxygen and 5 percent carbon dioxide mixture) inhalation to intravenous administration of papaverine and low molecular weight dextran. Although no difference was observed between groups at the end of the 5 day treatment period, those patients in the carbogen inhalation group had better hearing at 1 year follow-up. Fisch concluded that carbogen was not a cure for ISSNHL but was safe and perhaps improved the rate of spontaneous recovery.

The cornerstone of therapy for ISSNHL is systemic steroids. The prospective, randomized, double-blind study of Wilson and associates remains the best demonstration of the efficacy of steroids in treating this disorder. As stated previously, patients who were initially seen early in the course of their illness with hearing loss of less than 40 dB all recovered; those patients who had more than 90 dB of hearing loss never recovered; and those patients who had dB losses between 40 and 90 had a spontaneous recovery rate of 38 percent. The researchers showed that administration of a tapering course of methylprednisolone or dexamethasone increased the recovery rate in this moderate hearing loss group to 78 percent. A subsequent smaller study by Moskowitz and coworkers confirmed this finding, noting hearing recovery in 89 percent of steroid-treated subjects compared with 49 percent of controls. Both studies began administration of steroids within a few days of onset of hearing loss. As stated previously, there appears to be a window of opportunity for steroid administration that is certainly 2 weeks long and may reach up to 4 weeks. It is unlikely that a benefit of steroid use would be seen thereafter.

In recent years, systemic antiviral agents have become available. Their use in treating ISSNHL has not been studied thoroughly; no controlled trials of their use in this condition have been reported. Nonetheless, these agents are beginning to be used on an anecdotal basis by many practitioners. The pharmacology of the antiviral drugs (such as acyclovir and ganciclovir) requires that they be used before or immediately after onset of symptoms in order to have demonstrable benefit. Because the temporal relationship of viral insult to onset of hearing loss has not been defined, and most patients do not visit the otolaryngologist within the first 72 hours after onset, use of these drugs is of questionable merit.

■ IMMUNE-MEDIATED INNER EAR DISEASE

In 1979, McCabe described 18 patients who had idiopathic, rapidly progressive, bilateral sensorineural hearing loss who regained hearing after administration of corticosteroids. He theorized about an autoimmune etiology based on the patient's response to immunosuppressive drugs. The next decade saw proliferation of a host of clinical reports, diagnostic tests, and treatment protocols for this entity, few of which have subsequently been validated. The next significant step toward understanding this disorder came in 1990, when Harris and Sharp reported circulating antibodies against inner ear antigens detected by use of a Western blot technique. Four years later, Moscicki and co-workers presented the clinical correlation of idiopathic, progressive, bilateral sensorineural hearing loss (IPBSNHL) with circulating antibodies against a 68 kD protein antigen present in bovine inner ear and renal extracts. They demonstrated that the presence of these antibodies correlated with both activity of disease and steroid responsiveness. Using different experimental approaches, Billings and associates and Block and associates both identified the 68 kD protein antigen as heat shock protein 70 (Hsp 70) in 1995. Whether Hsp 70 within the inner ear is the target of these antibodies or simply has a shared epitope with the actual target antigen is unknown. This uncertainty notwithstanding, it is reasonable to refer to these antibodies as anti-Hsp 70 antibodies, because it is immunoreactivity with Hsp 70 that is the basis for their detection in the Western blot assay. This assay for circulating anti-Hsp 70 antibodies remains the only diagnostic study with proven prognostic significance for IPBSNHL.

Although the Western blot assay for detecting circulating antibodies reactive with Hsp 70 has prognostic significance, its diagnostic value is unproved. The assay has not been widely applied to other inner ear disorders nor to other autoimmune disorders in order to characterize its sensitivity and specificity. Therefore, IPBSNHL remains a clinical diagnosis based on historical and audiometric criteria. Likewise, there has been no certain confirmation that IPBSNHL is actually an autoimmune disorder. Such confirmation must meet the three criteria of Witebsky's postulates: (1) identification of antibodies or activated T cells reactive with a "self" protein; (2) identification of a characteristic immune-induced "lesion"; and (3) reproduction of this lesion by introduction of the specific antibodies or activated T cells into a naive host. Until these criteria are met, it is more accurate to refer to this entity by its clinical description (i.e., IPBSNHL) or acknowledge the undefined role of the immune system and call the condition "immune-mediated inner ear disease."

Clinical Presentation

The hallmark of the condition originally described by McCabe was the presence of rapidly progressive sensorineural hearing loss: too fast to be age-related degeneration and too slow to be sudden sensorineural hearing loss. This remains the most salient distinguishing feature of the disorder. Moscicki and co-workers articulated a precise clinical description of IPBSNHL that enabled them to minimize heterogeneity in their study population and, ultimately, correlate this clinical presentation with results of Western blot assays. Specifically, they defined IPBSNHL as a bilateral sensorineural hearing loss of equal to or greater than 30 dB at any frequency *and* evidence of progression in at least one ear on two serial audiograms that are performed equal to or less than 3 months apart; progression here is defined as a threshold shift of equal to or greater than 15 dB at one frequency, 10 dB at two or more consecutive frequencies, or a significant change in discrimination score. A single episode of threshold shift occurring in less than 72 hours and then stabilizing was classified as sudden sensorineural hearing loss and excluded. Fluctuating hearing loss, however, qualified if there was also progression according to the just described criteria. This is still the most explicit description of IPBSNHL in the literature. Analogous to the diagnostic situation with Meniere's disease, in the absence of a "gold standard" diagnostic test, adherence to these diagnostic criteria permits comparison of observations and results between different studies.

In the paper by Moscicki and associates, demographic features, test results, and treatment outcome were reported for 72 patients who had IPBSNHL. Recently, I reviewed the records of 66 new patients who were evaluated at the Massachusetts Eye and Ear Infirmary for possible immune-mediated inner ear disease. Five patients who had a diagnosis of Cogan's syndrome, an autoimmune vasculitis characterized by SNHL, vertigo, and interstitial keratitis of the eyes, were excluded, which left 61 cases for analysis. Results are tabulated in Tables 1 and 2. IPBSNHL diagnostic criteria were the same as for Moscicki's study. Demographic features and trends in the correlation of Western blot assay with steroid response in the present group of patients are essentially the same as those of Moscicki's original cohort.

Approximately half of IPBSNHL patients also experience vestibular symptoms (Table 1). These can include dysequilibrium, motion intolerance, positional vertigo, and episodic whirling vertigo of the Meniere's type. Approximately 20 percent of IPBSNHL patients have a combination of fluctuating and progressive sensorineural hearing loss and episodic vertigo that meets strict American Academy of Otolaryngology–Head and Neck Surgery diagnostic criteria for Meniere's disease. Rauch and co-workers and Gottschlich and co-workers have reported that approximately one-third of classic Meniere's disease patients have a Western blot assay positive for anti-Hsp 70 antibodies. This overlap between IPBSNHL and Meniere's disease suggests that a subset of patients falling into both diagnostic categories may share a common pathophysiologic mechanism.

IPBSNHL can occur in combination with other systemic autoimmune diseases. Nearly 15 percent of IPBSNHL patients have another autoimmune diagnosis (Table 1). These diagnoses include multiple sclerosis, inflammatory bowel disease (ulcerative colitis and Crohn's disease), systemic lupus erythematosus, rheumatoid arthritis, and ankylosing spondylitis. Although not definitely autoimmune, several other IPBSNHL patients included in the Table 1 data had diabetes or thyroid dysfunction. There are reports of certain human leukocyte antigen subtypes that correlate with immune-mediated inner ear disease. This suggests the possibility of a genetic predisposition to autoimmune disease that may include IPBSNHL as well as other systemic disorders.

Diagnosis

As previously noted, the salient feature of IPBSNHL is audiometric evidence of progression over days to months. Serial audiometry performed at an interval equal to or less than 3 months is necessary to confirm the diagnosis. When in doubt, monthly audiograms for several months can be helpful. The pattern of hearing loss is highly variable. As yet, no one has described a characteristic pattern of hearing loss. The loss may be high tone, low tone, up- or downsloping, or predominantly affecting discrimination rather than threshold. Exclusion of retrocochlear disease such as multiple sclerosis or acoustic neuroma is mandatory and can be accomplished by evoked response audiometry and/or gadolinium-enhanced magnetic resonance imaging.

Routine serologic tests in possible IPBSNHL patients include complete blood count with differential white blood count, erythrocyte sedimentation rate, rheumatoid factor, antinuclear antibody (ANA), C3 and C4 complement levels, and Raji cell assay for circulating immune complexes. Serologic workup is aimed at detecting evidence of systemic immunologic dysfunction; none of these tests has been shown to correlate with the diagnosis of IPBSNHL.

Western blot assay for anti-Hsp 70 antibodies is a useful adjunct in diagnosis and management of IPBSNHL. As previously noted, the sensitivity and specificity of this test has not been validated, and it should not be used as the absolute determinant of whether a patient has actual immune-mediated inner ear disease, nor should it be the sole determinant of whether to treat with immunosuppressive drugs. On the other hand, Moscicki and associates have shown that the presence of these antibodies is correlated with both active disease and steroid responsiveness. Review of Western blot results in our most recent 61 cases of IPBSNHL reveals similar findings (Table 2). It may therefore be an aid to clinical decision making in difficult cases. For example, a patient who has either brittle diabetes or peptic ulcer disease may

Table 1. Clinical Features of 61 Patients Evaluated at the Massachusetts Eye and Ear Infirmary for Possible Immune-Mediated Inner Ear Disease

DEMOGRAPHIC CHARACTERISTICS: IPBSNHL	PATIENT NO. (61)
Male-female ratio	32:29
Mean age (range)	47 (4–72)
Vestibular symptoms	30 (49.2%)
Meniere's disease	13 (21.3%)
Unilateral : bilateral	5:8
Other autoimmune diagnosis	9 (14.8%)

IPBSNHL, idiopathic, progressive, bilateral sensorineural hearing loss.

Table 2. Relationship of Western Blot Assay for Anti-Hsp 70 Antibodies and Response to Corticosteroid Therapy in 61 Patients with IPBSNHL

WESTERN BLOT (ANTI-HSP 70)	STEROID RESPONSE +	STEROID RESPONSE −	NO THERAPY
+	14	11	7
−	5	12	8
?	2	2	—

IPBSNHL, idiopathic, progressive, bilateral sensorineural hearing loss; +, antibody present; −, antibody absent; ?, status unknown.

be at considerable risk from treatment with high-dose corticosteroids. Such risk may be more acceptable if one finds a positive Western blot for anti-Hsp 70, indicating as much as a 75 percent chance of steroid response. Conversely, a high-risk patient might forgo therapy if the assay result is negative, which suggests that the chance of response is less than 20 percent.

In addition to the lack of sensitivity and specificity data, the Western blot assay for anti-Hsp 70 antibodies has other shortcomings. It is not a quantitative assay. Because the antigen used is a relatively crude protein extract from bovine renal cells rather than a single purified protein or polypeptide, the exact amount of Hsp 70 is not standardized. The test is therefore reported only as antibodies "present" or "absent." Eventually, an enzyme-linked immunosorbent assay or quantitative Western blot could be developed based on identification of the specific epitope(s) relevant to this disorder. Results would then be reported as antibody titer, as is currently done for ANA and many other routine immunologic studies. Antibody titers could then be measured serially to monitor progress of the treatment or possibly to herald relapse. Despite its limitations, to date the Western blot assay for anti-Hsp 70 antibodies remains the only serologic study with demonstrated prognostic significance for IPBSNHL.

Immunosuppressive Therapy

Corticosteroid therapy for IPBSNHL at the Massachusetts Eye and Ear Infirmary has evolved over the last 15 years based on clinical experience with more than 150 IPBSNHL patients. There have not been any prospective, randomized clinical trials to validate this empiric approach. Initial therapy for adults consists of a therapeutic trial of prednisone, 60 mg daily for 4 weeks. Pediatric patients receive prednisone, 1 mg per kilogram per day for 4 weeks. Although occasionally patients may show a response early in the 4 week period, many do not begin to improve until late in the month; shorter courses of treatment usually result in relapse. Patients' hearing is tested at the initiation of therapy and again at 4 weeks. If the threshold has improved by equal to or greater than 15 dB at one frequency, or 10 dB at two or more consecutive frequencies, or if the discrimination score is significantly improved, patients are considered to be steroid responders. Nonresponders are tapered off their medication in 12 days. Responders continue full-dose therapy until monthly audiograms confirm that they have reached a plateau of recovery. They are then slowly tapered over 8 weeks to a maintenance dose of 10 to 20 mg every other day. This maintenance dose is continued for a variable length of time. Clinical observation suggests that patients who receive a total treatment duration of less than 6 months are at increased risk compared with those treated for 6 months or longer.

Patterns of response to corticosteroid therapy vary. Some patients have improvement in threshold, some in discrimination score only, and some in both areas. Some patients who have fluctuation and progression before therapy show stabilization of their hearing without actual improvement. Historically, these patients have been considered to be nonresponders, but this issue is currently under reassessment. The majority of responders are carried through a slow taper to complete weaning from steroids, and they do well. A subset of IPBSNHL patients relapse while tapering or after discontinuing their medication. In some instances, re-treatment is effective. However, occasionally the hearing loss becomes refractory to corticosteroids. In such cases, alternative immunosuppressive drugs are considered. An occasional patient, especially in the pediatric age group, may show steroid-dependent hearing loss. In other words, they cannot be weaned below a certain level of steroid dosage without experiencing a decline in hearing. Such patients often develop unacceptable side effects from chronic steroid administration. Recently, we have observed benefit from combining prednisone with low-dose (15 mg per week) methotrexate in these steroid-dependent patients. After several weeks of combined therapy, the prednisone can be tapered and discontinued, and the patient is then maintained on methotrexate alone for an additional 2 to 3 months, at which time this second drug is also successfully discontinued.

Corticosteroid therapy has obvious limitations. There are risks of long-term administration that include gastritis and ulcers, fluid retention and weight gain, blood pressure lability, altered blood sugar metabolism and diabetes, mood changes or psychiatric problems, sleep disturbance, accelerated cataract formation, and cushingoid habitus. Ischemic necrosis of bone is a rare complication, more likely to be seen in patients who receive prolonged high-dose steroid administration, although none of our patients have had this problem. We have observed an overall steroid response rate of approximately 60 percent in IPBSNHL patients. Some initial responders become refractory to steroid therapy at the time of subsequent relapse. Despite these limitations, corticosteroid therapy remains the mainstay of IPBSNHL treatment based on the extensive clinical experience with its use.

Alternatives to systemic corticosteroids include methotrexate and cyclophosphamide. We have found low-dose methotrexate to be especially useful as an adjunct in the management of steroid-dependent hearing loss. It is the first-line drug of choice for patients who are unable to take corticosteroids. A low-dose protocol, as is the case for rheumatoid arthritis or psoriasis, is used. Methotrexate is administered by mouth in three doses given at 12 hour intervals once weekly. The initial dose is 7.5 mg per week (three doses of 2.5 mg). If this is tolerated without toxic effects for 2 weeks, the dose is doubled to 15 mg per week. This dose is continued for 6 to 8 weeks as a therapeutic trial. Nonresponders are discontinued; responders are carried on the 15 mg per week dose for 6 months. Potential toxicity includes myelosuppression, gastrointestinal upset, oral ulceration, acute pneumonitis, and hepatic fibrosis. This last complication is insidious and generally seen only when methotrexate is given for more than 1 year. It may be associated with abnormal liver function tests, and early diagnosis is achieved by liver biopsy. Weekly testing that includes complete blood count with differential white count, liver function tests, blood urea nitrogen, creatinine, and urinalysis is recommended to monitor for signs of toxicity.

Cyclophosphamide is a potent cytotoxic agent generally used for cancer chemotherapy. It is somewhat selective for B-cell and monocyte-macrophage function. Although some physicians advocate its use as a first-line drug, the high risk of toxicity makes it a better choice as a salvage drug or treatment of last resort. We have used this drug in a small number of patients at an initial dose of 1 mg per kilogram per day orally for 4 to 6 weeks. When no response is apparent, the dose is doubled to 2 mg per kilogram per day. Responders are treated for 6 to 12 months. Toxicity includes severe myelosuppression, opportunistic infection, hair loss, cystitis, infertility, and increased risk of malignancies. Weekly monitoring of hematologic status is mandatory. Many patients, when confronted with the risks of taking this medication, would rather consider cochlear implantation.

Intratympanic steroid therapy, systemic immunoglobulin G injections, and plasmapheresis are possible treatments with sound theoretic justification. Intratympanic steroid therapy is particularly appealing because it is minimally invasive and enables direct application of the drug to the affected site with a low risk of systemic effects. There are, however, no published series in which these treatments have been systematically applied. Determination of the best role for any of these treatment modalities remains to be established.

■ DISCUSSION

IPBSNHL and idiopathic sudden sensorineural hearing loss are two distinct disorders (Table 3). IPBSNHL is far rarer than is sudden SNHL. IPBSNHL is by definition bilateral, whereas sudden hearing loss is virtually always unilateral. Sudden hearing loss develops in less than or equal to 72 hours. In contrast, IPBSNHL progresses over days to months such that serial audiograms on a monthly basis will show continued decline. Sudden hearing loss is an otologic emergency with a treatment window of perhaps 2 to 4 weeks, during which time a short "burst and taper" of corticosteroids must be administered in order to achieve optimum recovery. IPBSNHL is not urgent. Patients who have progression over 6 to 12 months can still achieve significant recovery with administration of a long course of high-dose corticosteroids or other immunosuppressive drugs. Throughout the otolaryngologic community, there is wide awareness that some cases of sensorineural hearing loss are potentially reversible with corticosteroid treatment. However, there is unfortunately little awareness of the fact that these two entities are quite different in etiology, presentation, workup, and management. Hasty administration of a short tapering course of steroids can delay diagnosis of IPBSNHL and can confuse interpretation of serologic testing.

Table 3. Comparison of Idiopathic, Progressive, Bilateral SNHL (IPBSNHL) and Idiopathic Sudden SNHL (ISSNHL)

IPBSNHL	ISSNHL
Bilateral	Unilateral
Progressive over days to months	≤72 h drop and stabilize
Not urgent	Urgent
Treatment window ± 6 mo	Treatment window ~ 14–30 d
Long, high-dose course of steroids	Short "burst and taper" of steroids

SNHL, sensorineural hearing loss.

The story of IPBSNHL from initial description by McCabe to present therapy routines has been presented here as a simple and direct path. That has not been the actual case. It has been a broad and meandering path with significant contributions by many investigators and numerous interesting and important digressions. The story still has far to go. The clinical description of this disorder is confined to its auditory manifestations. However, as previously noted, approximately 50 percent of IPBSNHL patients have vestibular symptoms. This aspect of the illness has not been well characterized clinically. Just as there are many IPBSNHL patients who have exclusively auditory symptoms, there may well be an equal number who have exclusively vestibular symptoms. Such a presentation has not yet been reported. Until the Western blot assay for anti-Hsp 70 antibodies is systematically applied to a wide range of vestibulopathy patients, this possibility will be unexplored.

Little is understood about the underlying pathophysiology of IPBSNHL. The very fact of reversible sensorineural hearing loss flies in the face of accepted dogma that sensorineural hearing loss is not medically recoverable. It is interesting to consider what pathophysiologic mechanism could disable neural signal transduction and/or transmission in the auditory system yet be reversed months later by anti-inflammatory or immunosuppressive drugs. The solution to this puzzle will come from systematic research into the nature of the humoral and cell-mediated immune response of affected patients. As yet, there is no good animal model of the IPBSNHL phenomenon in which to carry out such research, and human studies progress slowly due to the rarity of the clinical material. This rarity does not diminish the significance of the topic, however. Understanding the mechanism of IPBSNHL will provide a new level of insight into the role of systemic and organ-specific immune reactions in disease of the inner ear. The fact that 20 percent of IPBSNHL patients have a clinical presentation overlapping with Meniere's disease and 33 percent of Meniere's disease patients have evidence of anti-Hsp 70 antibodies as evidence by Western blot assay is strong evidence of a shared pathophysiologic mechanism. Although IPBSNHL is rare, Meniere's disease is not. In the United States alone, there are an estimated 125,000 cases yearly. New ways of understanding Meniere's disease could have great public health benefit.

Diagnosis of IPBSNHL currently relies on clinical factors alone, supplemented by the Western blot assay for anti-Hsp 70 antibodies. As stated earlier, the observation that many IPBSNHL patients carry serum antibodies reactive with Hsp 70 does not prove that Hsp 70 is the actual inner ear target antigen. Alternatively, the antibodies may not be pathogenic at all. They may simply be reactive antibodies, reflecting up-regulation of Hsp 70 synthesis in inner ear cells injured by some unknown mechanism. Despite our poor understanding of IPBSNHL pathophysiology, detection of these marker antibodies remains clinically useful. The utility of the assay will be greatly enhanced by development of a quantitative measure enabling clinicians to follow antibody titers by serial testing. In addition, estimation of sensitivity and specificity of the assay must be made by its broad application to a wide variety of ear diseases and immunologic disorders.

Current therapy for IPBSNHL is based on empiric experience over the last 15 years rather than on a clear understanding of the underlying pathophysiology. In the future, therapeutic protocols must be informed by expanding knowledge of the pathophysiology of the disorder. Large multicenter studies are necessary to carefully evaluate the best use of corticosteroids and other immunosuppressive drugs. Consensus must be achieved on the clinical diagnostic criteria and treatment regimens in order to enable comparison between studies. Even with strict adherence to rigorous methodology, it may take many years to address these questions. For the foreseeable future, IPBSNHL will remain one of the most interesting, important, and challenging problems confronting otologists and otologic researchers.

Acknowledgments
I wish to acknowledge collaboration of Richard A. Moscicki, Jose E. San Martin, Stacey B. Weston, Donald B. Bloch, and Kurt J. Bloch in the research and clinical work described in this chapter.

Suggested Reading

Billings PB, Keithley EM, Harris JP. Evidence linking the 68 kilodalton antigen identified in progressive sensorineural hearing loss patient sera with hear shock protein 70. Ann Otol Rhinol Laryngol 1995; 104:181-188.

Bloch DB, San Martin JE, Rauch SD, et al. Serum antibodies to heat shock protein 70 in sensorineural hearing loss. Arch Otolaryngol 1995; 121:1167-1171.

Byl FM. Sudden hearing loss: Eight years' experience and suggested prognostic table. Laryngoscope 1984; 94:647-661.

Cao M-Y, Thonnard J, Deggouj M, et al. HLA class II-associated genetic susceptibility in idiopathic progressive sensorineural hearing loss. Ann Otol Rhinol Laryngol 1996; 105:628-633.

Cole RR, Jahrsdoerfer RA. Sudden hearing loss: An update. Am J Otol 1988; 9:211-215.

De Kleyn A. Sudden complete or partial loss of function of the octavus system in apparently normal persons. Acta Otolaryngol 1944: 32:463-480.

Fetterman BL, Saunders JE, Luxford WM. Prognosis and treatment of sudden sensorineural hearing loss. Am J Otol 1996; 17:529-536.

Fisch U. Management of sudden deafness. Otolaryngol Head Neck Surg 1983; 91:3-8.

Gottschlich S, Billings PB, Keithley EM, et al. Assessment of serum antibodies in patients with rapidly progressive sensorineural hearing loss and Meniere's disease. Laryngoscope 1996; 105:1347-1352.

Hadden JW, Smith DI. Immunopharmacology: Immunomodulation and immunotherapy. JAMA 1992; 268:2964-2969.

Harris JP, Sharp PA. Inner ear autoantibodies in patients with rapidly progressive sensorineural hearing loss. Laryngoscope 1990; 100:516-524.

Moskowitz D, Lee KJ, Smith HW. Steroid use in idiopathic sudden sensorineural hearing loss. Laryngoscope 1984; 94:664-666.

Mattox DE, Simmons FB. Natural history of sudden sensorineural hearing loss. Ann Otol Rhinol Laryngol 1977; 86:463-480.

McCabe BF. Autoimmune inner ear disease: Therapy. Am J Otol 1989; 10:196-197.

McCabe BF. Autoimmune sensorineural hearing loss. Ann Otol Rhinol Laryngol 1979; 88:585-589.

Moscicki RA, San Martin JE, Quintero CH, et al. Specificity of serum antibodies to a 68 kD inner ear antigen in disease associated with hearing loss and responsivity to corticosteroid therapy. JAMA 1994; 272: 611-616.

Rauch SD. Clinical management of immune-mediated inner ear disease, Ann NY Acad Sci (in press).

Rauch SD, San Martin JE, Bloch KJ. Prevalence of anti-heat shock protein 70 (HSP70) antibodies in Meniere's disease. Research Forum of the Association for Research in Otolaryngology and the American Academy of Otolaryngology–Head and Neck Surgery 1995; New Orleans (abstract).

Schuknecht HF, Donovan ED. The pathology of idiopathic sudden sensorineural hearing loss. Arch Otorhinolaryngol 1986; 243:1-15.

Wilson WR, Byl FM, Laird N. The efficacy of steroids in the treatment of idiopathic sudden hearing loss. Arch Otolaryngol 1980; 106:772-776.

Zizic TM, Marcoux C, Hungerford DS, et al. Corticosteroid therapy associated with ischemic necrosis of bone in systemic lupus erythematosus. Am J Otol 1985; 79:596-604.

SENSORINEURAL HEARING LOSS: REHABILITATION

The method of
Georgetown University Medical Center
by
Susan H. Morgan
A. Julianna Gulya

Nearly 22 million Americans have some degree of hearing impairment. Although the vast majority of those who have hearing loss are adults, most commonly persons older than age 65, it is important to remember that more than 1 million children are also included in this population.

The consequences of hearing loss in the adult, especially the elderly adult, revolve around impaired social interaction, with its repercussions in feelings of isolation, depression, and diminished self-worth. In children, such difficulties are compounded by problems in the acquisition of speech and language and in learning.

Upon delineation of a not otherwise treatable hearing loss, hearing aid evaluation and fitting constitute recommended rehabilitation. Advances in hearing aid design and performance, facilitated by technologic progress, have in turn driven change in the paradigm used in fitting individuals who have hearing loss.

■ HEARING AID CANDIDACY

The first step in determining candidacy for amplification is a complete audiologic evaluation, including otologic acoustic immitance measures, pure-tone threshold testing, and speech audiometry. The type, degree, and slope of the hearing loss are quantitated, and any central auditory disorder is identified. If a hearing impairment, regardless of its degree, is causing a communication handicap for an individual, then that person is a candidate for amplification. With today's hearing device technology, there is virtually no one who cannot be helped by some type of hearing aid or assistive listening device (ALD).

Individuals deriving the most benefit from hearing aids have moderate or severe peripheral hearing losses and require amplification to hear conversational speech; however, even individuals who have mild, high-frequency, or unilateral deficits experience hearing problems, especially in difficult listening environments. Such individuals may not be full-time hearing aid users, but the benefit derived from amplification on a part-time basis should not be underestimated. Generally speaking, individuals who have profound hearing losses benefit the least from hearing aids, due to their poor speech discrimination, and in some cases, these persons may benefit more from cochlear implantation.

Elderly persons often have hearing problems that are characterized by peripheral sensitivity loss combined with a central auditory processing disorder that can be identified by a thorough audiometric evaluation and that complicates the determination of candidacy for amplification. Remote microphone ALD technology that enhances the signal-noise (S-N) ratio may be a better intervention strategy in such cases.

Other factors to consider in the determination of hearing aid candidacy are patient acceptance of the hearing loss and motivation to wear hearing devices. A person who denies the existence of a hearing problem is unlikely to comply with a recommendation to use hearing aids. Some patients do not perceive any hearing problems and come for audiologic evaluation only on prompting by a spouse or other family member; a successful hearing aid fitting can be exceedingly difficult in such situations.

Having determined candidacy for hearing aid use, it must then be determined whether one or two devices should be recommended. As a general rule, we recommend binaural amplification unless there are clear contraindications. With binaural amplification, speech is reported to sound better and is more easily understood in noisy listening circumstances as compared with monaural amplification. With a microphone at each ear, binaural amplification improves sound localization ability and eliminates the head shadow effect, thus enhancing high-frequency amplification and improving speech intelligibility. Moreover, there is evidence that late-onset auditory deprivation can develop with monaural hearing aid use; that is, the unaided ear demonstrates a significant decline in speech discrimination when compared with the aided ear. Subsequent amplification of the previously unaided ear may halt further deterioration.

■ HEARING AID CANDIDACY IN CHILDREN

With the proliferation of universal newborn hearing screening programs, hearing losses are being identified in ever younger infants. Hearing aid fitting and remediation should begin as soon as the hearing loss is identified, regardless of the infant's age. As complete audiometric data are often not available, auditory brain stem response testing is used to fit amplification until behavioral testing can be performed.

■ HEARING AID SELECTION

Our methods for selecting amplification have evolved over recent years, predominantly in response to advances in hearing aid technology. In the past, the initial decision involved the style of the hearing instrument, as determined by the type, degree, and slope of the hearing loss. Severe, profound, and sharply sloping, high-frequency losses nearly uniformly were fitted with behind-the-ear devices. In-the-ear or in-the-canal devices could be fitted for mild or moderate losses without risking acoustic feedback. Patient factors, such as age, manual dexterity, life-style, and personal preference also played a role in the style of aid selected. Once style was determined, electroacoustic characteristics, including gain, output, and frequency response, were selected, often on the basis of one of many widely used prescriptive fitting methods that use pure-tone thresholds or thresholds and loudness comfort levels to select optimal hearing aid characteristics. Ideally, the aid would amplify conversational speech to a level near the patient's most comfortable listening level, but amplification would not exceed a level uncomfortable to the wearer. Decisions regarding circuit options or other features were facilitated by both the limited range of possibilities available and patient awareness of the technical aspects of device selection. In hard-to-fit cases, speech audiometric testing of several devices, often from different manufacturers, was used to determine the "best" device, which was then fitted and dispensed to the patient for a trial of use.

Recent advances in hearing aid technology, such as better amplifiers, improved microphones, digital circuits, and miniaturization, combined with a more knowledgeable hearing-impaired public, have had a substantial impact on the process of hearing aid selection. Patient needs, driven by technology, now form the basis for selecting appropriate amplification. Prescriptive methods still are used to select optimal hearing aid circuitry, but the abundance of options has transformed the once straightforward process into one that is complex at best, and confusing at worst.

To simplify explaining amplification options and assisting the patient in making a hearing aid selection, we use a format in which the devices are categorized into groups, or levels, based on complexity of technology. The various levels are described to the patient, who then selects the level from which a device will be chosen. We find that this format allows for a clear, concise delineation of available options that does not consume an inordinate amount of time.

In our hierarchy, level I devices comprise conventional hearing aids. These basic devices consist of a microphone, an amplifier, and a receiver; they function by converting environmental sounds into electrical signals, which after amplification, are transduced back into an acoustic signal and sent to the ear. Space permitting, external controls may be added to allow adjustment or fine-tuning of the electroacoustic characteristics by the dispenser. The user may have a volume control, telephone coil, or some other control capable of altering the degree or mode of amplification delivered to the ear. Traditional contralateral routing of signals (CROS) and bilateral routing of signals (BiCROS) hearing aids are also considered conventional devices, and they are designed for an individual who has one unaidable ear and a contralateral normal (CROS) ear, or an impaired but aidable (BiCROS) ear. These aids improve perception of sounds on the side of the unaidable ear by eliminating the head shadow effect.

Second-level hearing aids are less complex programmable aids, which differ from conventional devices in that their amplifiers are controlled by digital electronics. Second-level devices typically have a specific set of electroacoustic parameters programmed within a single frequency band and/or channel that can be changed by the dispenser through programming, using either a dedicated programmer or a PC-based computer. If the device has more than one memory program, the patient may also change parameters.

Multiple-channel programmable hearing aids constitute the third level of hearing aids; they tend to be complex and often have multiple memories per programs under user control. The circuitry characteristics of these devices are programmed in two or more frequency bands. In essence, these devices divide the audiogram into multiple frequency regions and adjust the gain, compression, and other factors independently for each region in an attempt to fit target goals more accurately.

The fourth level of hearing instruments are the truly digital devices. Although at the present time there are only two digital devices on the market, there is little doubt that digital technology is the future of hearing aids. Our experience with digital aids is limited to date, but we are confident that the numerous advantages of digital technology will lead to their increased use.

Currently, we prefer to fit our patients with programmable hearing aids rather than conventional devices. Although the initial fitting and follow-up times are usually longer with the programmable devices, patient satisfaction tends to be higher, especially for the experienced user, and the versatility offered by programmable devices has enhanced our ability to provide beneficial amplification to our patients.

There are numerous advantages offered by programmability, such as flexibility in shaping the frequency response to better match the sensitivity loss. Programmability also offers an ability to obtain desirable compression characteristics. Compression reduces the gain of high-intensity input signals so that they are not perceived as being too loud by the hearing aid user, and is routinely incorporated into the hearing aids we fit. One type of compression, referred to as wide dynamic range compression, is of benefit to patients who have mild and moderate losses; this type of compression provides maximum gain for soft signals, for example, speech, and progressively less gain for greater intensity sounds. We no longer routinely recommend linear amplification with peak-clipping output limitation.

Another advantage offered by programmability is the ability to fit devices with more than one program or memory. Multiple memory hearing aids have more than one set of electroacoustic characteristics, controllable by the hearing aid user by means of either a switch located on the aid or a remote control; this feature facilitates communication in different listening environments.

Multimicrophone technology is another feature of programmability that can improve speech understanding in background noise. Typical hearing aid microphones are omnidirectional, picking up all sounds equally well; such microphones work well for hearing speech in quiet environments and listening to music, and for those individuals who need to hear information from behind, for example, teachers and cab drivers. Directional microphones pick up sounds arriving from the front better than those arriving from the back or sides, which results in sounds from the front being amplified normally, while those from other directions are suppressed. Clearly, directional microphones are superior for communication in noisy environments. Advanced technology currently available in one programmable hearing aid allows the user to switch between omnidirectional and directional microphones, which achieves maximum sound quality and speech understanding in different listening environments.

Progressive miniaturization of hearing aids has encouraged individuals who are swayed by cosmetic concerns to seek help for their hearing loss. The most miniaturized device available today is the completely-in-the-canal (CIC) aid. By definition, a CIC hearing aid has a lateral end terminating either adjacent to, or 1 to 2 mm medial to, the opening of the external auditory canal. For maximum acoustic benefit, the medial end of the CIC should terminate within 5 mm of the superior aspect of the tympanic membrane. Because the CICs are barely noticeable, they have high cosmetic appeal, but they also have a number of excellent acoustic features. High-frequency input to the microphone of the CIC aid is enhanced by the resonance characteristics of the pinna and concha. Because there is a reduced residual ear canal volume with the deep-canal fitting of the CICs, less actual gain is required to produce the desired sound pressure level at the tympanic membrane. The deep-canal fitting paradoxically is associated with a diminished occlusion effect, because the CIC extension into the bony canal reduces cartilaginous canal vibration. Other benefits of CIC devices include reduced wind noise and improved use of telephones and/or headsets, because they can be directly placed on the ear without feedback.

■ HEARING AID EVALUATION AND FITTING

Upon receipt of a hearing aid from the manufacturer, a series of electroacoustic measurements are performed according to American National Standards Institute standards (S3.22, 1987) to verify that the device is performing according to specifications. The patient hearing aid evaluation follows, consisting of probe microphone measurements and aided speech understanding at different S-N ratios.

Probe microphone instrumentation, invaluable in hearing aid evaluation for both children and adults, is used to measure acoustic levels in the ear canal, with and without the hearing aid in position. A broad-band signal, such as composite noise, is presented through a loudspeaker. A miniature, self-calibrating microphone with a soft silicone tube extension is inserted near the tympanic membrane, and measurements are made in the ear canal. An electret reference microphone, located near the patient's ear, serves as the standard against which the probe signal is compared. Responses are displayed graphically, using real-time analysis, and a hard copy is printed for the patient's records. The information so gathered is used to verify hearing aid real-ear gain, frequency response, and saturation levels. Adjustments of the electroacoustic parameters of the aid continue until the original goals of the fitting are validated.

Having established the electroacoustic parameters of the hearing aid, unaided and aided speech in noise testing is done. Noisy environments adversely impact hearing aid benefit to the user, a defect commonly cited in rejection of the device. Accordingly, our ability to determine speech discrimination in a variety of listening environments is an important part of our management of communication disorders, and we believe it is important to evaluate the patient's speech discrimination in some type of realistic environment. Of the many methods available, including adaptive tests of S-N ratio, paired comparison techniques, traditional speech audiometry measures, and quality measurements, we use the synthetic sentence identification test, in which nonsense sentences embedded within a story are identified at different message-competition ratios.

■ COUNSELING AND FOLLOW-UP

The most important appointment is the one at which the patient receives the hearing aids, and sufficient time must be allotted to explain adequately the use and care of the device, as well as to answer any questions the patient may have. Family members should participate in the counseling process to learn about the hearing loss and what benefit to expect realistically from the hearing aid. Issues discussed during the counseling session should be documented in the patient record. We give all our patients a folder containing material describing basic instrument care, maintenance, and warranty information, as well as the names and addresses of consumer information and patient support groups. Patients should be informed as to available speech reading and aural rehabilitation classes. Follow-up appointments are scheduled during the instrument 30 day trial period and thereafter as needed.

Self-assessment inventories provide good subjective measures of hearing aid benefit that can validate the fitting, and are now an integral part of many hearing aid dispensing practices. These inventories are relatively simple to administer, and there are computer programs that can assist in scoring.

■ ASSISTIVE DEVICE TECHNOLOGY

Hearing aids alone may not meet the needs of hearing-impaired persons in all listening environments. Background noise and reverberation have deleterious effects on speech understanding that may not be improved with hearing aids. In specific listening situations, ALDs may be helpful, and these devices may be used alone or coupled directly with hearing aids for added versatility. In this section, we consider ALDs in three areas: (1) face-to-face communication; (2) telecommunications; and (3) alerting devices.

The most versatile technology for improving face-to-face communication in noisy environments is the FM (frequency modulation) system. By improving the S-N ratio, FM systems allow the user to understand speech under adverse conditions far better than possible with any of today's hearing aids. In the usual FM system, the speaker wears a lapel microphone that is attached to a transmitter; the signal is sent by FM broadcasting to a receiver unit worn by the listener. A pressure zone microphone is substituted for the lapel model if placement in the center of a table is desired. An FM system may be coupled with hearing aids by either direct audio input or an induction coil; the induction coil provides maximum benefit by allowing the listener to switch between the hearing aid and the FM system.

Hard-wired personal amplifiers are relatively inexpensive devices that work well in enhancing communication. The typical device consists of a headset that plugs into a small microphone and amplifier unit. An extension cord is available to attach the device to televisions or telephones. We use them routinely in counseling hearing-impaired patients who either do not possess hearing aids or whose aids are undergoing repair.

Infrared systems are found in a variety of public facilities, such as theaters, churches, auditoriums, and courtrooms. The infrared device transmits signals by infrared light waves to a receiver unit worn by the listener. Infrared systems provide very good sound quality, and these systems are the preferred ALDs for listening to television.

There are a number of devices and services to assist the hearing-impaired listener with telecommunications. Telephone amplifiers or induction coils are practical options, whereas teletypewriters remain a common mode of communication for the profoundly hearing-impaired individual. Local relay services enable a hearing-impaired person to call another person by telephone, with the conversation translated from text to voice (or vice versa) by the relay operator. Combination voice-text telephones allow direct communication among hearing-impaired persons, thus eliminating the need for relay services. A more recently available telecommunication device is the alpha-numeric cellular pager, which beeps or vibrates to signal message arrival, and then delivers the message in text form.

There are a number of alerting devices available to assist individuals who have severe or profound hearing losses. The sound of a baby's cry, a telephone, a doorbell, an alarm clock, or a smoke detector can be perceived by a hearing-impaired individual through visual (flashing lights) or tactile (vibration) stimuli.

Suggested Reading

Compton CL. Clinical management of assistive technology users: Issues to consider. In: Studebaker GA, Bess FH, Beck LB, eds. The Vanderbilt hearing aid report. Parkton, Md: York Publishing, 1991.

Cox R. Using loudness data for hearing aid selection: The IHAFF approach. Hear J 1995; 48:39-44.

Jerger J, Silman S, Lew HL, Chimel R, Case studies in binaural interference: Converging evidence from behavioral and electrophysiologic measures. JAAA 1993; 4:122-131.

Mueller HG, Hawkins DB, Northern JL, Probe microphone measurements: Hearing aid selection and assessment. San Diego: Singular Publishing Group, 1992.

Sandlin RE, ed. Handbook of hearing aid amplification. Vol. II. Boston: College-Hill Press, 1990.

Stelmachowicz PG. Current issues in pediatric amplification. Hear J 1996; 49:10, 12, 16-20.

CEREBROSPINAL FLUID OTORRHEA

The method of
Douglas E. Mattox
by
Yew-Meng Chan
Douglas E. Mattox

Most cases of cerebrospinal fluid (CSF) otorrhea result from skull base fractures, mastoid and skull base surgery, and mastoid encephaloceles. The incidence of CSF leak after skull base surgery has been reported to be between 6.2 percent and 22 percent. Seventy percent of post-traumatic CSF leaks seal spontaneously.

However, in a small proportion of patients, the CSF leak persists. The main concern in these patients is meningitis. The role of prophylactic antibiotic therapy in CSF leak is still debated. Although antibiotic therapy with the newer generation of CSF–penetrating drugs may have contributed to the decline in the incidence of meningitis and brain abscess associated with CSF leak, there is also a risk of selecting resistant nosocomial bacteria.

Identifying the exact site of the dural and bony defect may be difficult. Fluorescein and metrizamide contrast media and biochemical analysis of beta-2 transferrin have been described. Advanced localization techniques such as flow-sensitive magnetic resonance imaging may also be useful if the leak is brisk enough to detect. The intraoperative use of angled endoscopes sometimes allows precise visualization of exposed air cell tracts that were previously not recognized with the operating microscope.

Repair of a CSF leak once it is identified can be problematic. Small defects can be repaired transmastoid with or without bony support. Larger defects in the tegmen can be repaired through a limited middle fossa approach. Other leaks may require closure of the eustachian tube and obliteration of the mastoid with fat. Newer techniques using ionomeric bone cement also have been described. In all cases, a team approach between the neurosurgeon and the neurotologist is essential so as to offer the patient the best modern therapy available.

■ POSTOPERATIVE CSF LEAK

Intraoperative prevention of CSF leaks should be an overriding consideration in closure of any skull base defect, and several techniques are important to all the approaches listed next.

First, all exposed air cells should be obliterated. The degree of temporal bone pneumatization is highly variable, and well-pneumatized temporal bones require special consideration at closure. Small air cells can be closed with bone wax; larger cells may need a muscle or fat plug. Angled telescopes may be beneficial in identifying air cells that are not seen readily through the operating microscope, especially in the posterior fossa.

Second, dead space between the remaining temporal bone remnants and the dura should be obliterated to reduce the likelihood of a CSF fistula and to support the dura in its normal anatomic position.

Third, the wound should be meticulously closed in layers, including muscle flaps and skin. The skin should be closed in at least two layers, preferably with a running locked skin suture to provide a watertight closure.

Fourth, a snug pressure dressing will serve to keep skin flaps against the skull and reduce the incidence of subcutaneous CSF accumulations.

We do not routinely use wound drainage, preferring to keep the wound sealed. However, a wound hematoma can be disastrous to healing, and a suction drain adjacent to a muscle flap (e.g., temporalis flap) may be important. A lumbar subarachnoid drain or a wound drain to divert CSF pressure can be considered if there is a large defect that is tenuously closed.

Middle Fossa Surgery

The middle fossa approach usually entails opening into the middle ear, as well as mastoid and petrous apex air cells, either for identification of landmarks or for exposure. A free piece of temporalis muscle is used to plug apical air cells and the internal auditory canal. If there is a significant tegmen defect over the middle ear cleft, a fragment of the temporal craniotomy bone flap can be used to support the dura and keep it from prolapsing onto the ossicles, which causes a conductive hearing loss.

There is frequently a significant dead space between the dura and the remaining bone after removal of the middle fossa retractor. This dead space should be obliterated with a temporalis muscle flap. The dura should also be suspended to the edges of the craniotomy with sutures to prevent epidural accumulations of CSF or serum.

After this closure, some accumulation of CSF under the skin flaps is not unusual; however, the path from the internal auditory canal to the mastoid defect is usually so circuitous that these leaks nearly always seal spontaneously.

Jugular Foramen Surgery

The lateral approaches to the skull base tend to have a higher incidence of CSF leak compared to other types of skull base surgical techniques. Rates of CSF leak up to 25 percent have been reported.

In 1988, Fisch reduced the incidence of CSF leak in skull procedures using a subtotal petrosectomy, permanent closure of the eustachian tube, and tympanomastoid obliteration with fat. This technique requires closure of the external auditory canal and eradication of all accessible air cell tracts and mucous membrane in the petrous pyramid.

Other techniques described include muscle flap obliteration of the cavity with temporalis or a superiorly based sternocleidomastoid muscle flap. The sternocleidomastoid muscle is detached at the clavicular end and rotated superiorly to obliterate the tympanomastoid cavity. One note of caution: It is important to ensure that the superior blood supply of the sternocleidomastoid muscle has not been compromised by the surgical approach. Alternatively, a rectus abdominis or latissimus dorsi free flap can be used.

Translabyrinthine Surgery

Cerebrospinal fluid leakage is the most common and life-threatening complication following translabyrinthine acoustic neuroma surgery. The incidence of CSF leakage after translabyrinthine approach varies from 6.2 percent to 21 percent.

I have found that careful muscle packing into the aditus, leaving the incus in place for support and fat obliteration with moderate overfilling of the mastoid cavity, has been adequate in most cases. Others in the field have advocated plugging the eustachian tube with bone wax and a muscle plug as well as obliteration of the middle ear space with fat. If this is done, it must be performed through a facial recess approach, and the tympanic membrane should be left intact. I have preferred to leave the middle ear untouched because it is a valuable window through which to see fluid accumulation if the patient is complaining of postoperative rhinorrhea.

Retrosigmoid Surgery

The usual classes of CSF leak in the posterior fossa approach are inadequate closure of the posterior fossa dura or open air cells in the petrous apex or the retrosigmoid cells. Twenty-two percent of temporal bones have a posteromedial air cell tract extending into the posterior wall of the internal auditory meatus. There is little native soft tissue in this area, which reduces the likelihood of a spontaneous closure of a CSF leak from this site. Clinical findings of clear rhinorrhea with a fluid level in the middle ear at postoperative Days 2 to 5 should alert the physician to this complication.

Intraoperative technique is very important in preventing this complication. All open air cells of the petrous apex around the internal auditory canal must be closed. I have found that identification of all air cells by angled endoscope is useful when the drilled surface of the bone is slightly undercut and cannot be seen directly with the operating microscope. All open cells must be carefully sealed with bone wax. I have used a flat fingernail-shaped piece of bone wax to cover the entire surface of the bone drilled around the internal auditory canal. Care must be taken to prevent the bone wax from compressing the facial and cochlear nerves in the internal auditory canal. The bone wax is further supported by application of muscle graft sutured to the remnant dural edges.

Postoperative persistence of a CSF leak may respond to a trial of continuous lumbar drainage for 5 days. If surgical intervention is needed, a transmastoid approach is recommended, with specific identification of the site of the leak and obliteration with a muscle or fat plug as described for the translabyrinthine approach.

Mastoidectomy for Chronically Infected Ears

Management of cerebrospinal fluid leakage in chronic ear disease presents special problems that are different from the procedures already described. Factors such as the nature of the middle ear disease, size of the dural defect, and the type of mastoidectomy (canal wall-up or wall-down) need to be considered; the worst situation is a large dural defect and cholesteatoma in a canal wall-down mastoidectomy.

A small dural defect can be approached by positioning fascia supported by a cartilage or bone graft placed through the defect from the mastoid. Additional soft tissue can be placed over the defect on the mastoid side.

A larger defect requires a combined middle fossa and mastoid approach. A small temporal craniotomy superior to the defect will allow elevation of the surrounding dural edges, and a temporalis muscle flap is rotated between the dura and the floor of the middle fossa. Sutures placed in small bur holes around the edge of the bony defect can anchor the muscle flap in place. The temporalis flap is usually thick enough that additional bony support is not needed.

In a chronically infected ear with cholesteatoma and CSF leak (and usually an encephalocele), the management of the cholesteatoma matrix in the middle ear and mastoid cannot be overlooked. Cholesteatoma matrix and skin of the external auditory canal may be easily buried or left behind during the repair of the dural defect. Here, the challenge is to have an open cavity and yet repair the CSF leak. Because the tissue used in the repair will be exposed to air and local bacteria, a vascularized flap, usually temporalis muscle, is required. Because the cavity is left open, a split-thickness skin graft is laid over the muscle flap within the mastoid cavity to promote rapid epithelialization and prevent desiccation of the flap. This closure is tenuous at best, and continuous lumbar drainage is mandatory for 5 days to a week.

Persistence of the CSF leak may require an obliteration technique, because the priority is now the prevention of meningitis. If known or suspected cholesteatoma matrix is left behind, follow-up computed tomographic and magnetic resonance imaging scans will help to detect recurrent cholesteatoma. The recurrent cholesteatoma can then be removed by the same or alternative surgical approaches once the subarachnoid space is fully sealed.

■ IDIOPATHIC AND SPONTANEOUS CSF LEAK

There are two types of idiopathic and spontaneous CSF leak. Seventy-two percent of cases are congenital defects of the otic capsule that are usually associated with Mondini's deformity. There usually is severe hearing impairment, and treatment can consist of stapedectomy and packing the vestibule with muscle, or a subtotal petrosectomy with complete obliteration of the tympanomastoid air cell system. If there is residual useful hearing, a specific defect may be identified—for example, a fistula through the footplate of the stapes—and this defect may be repaired with a tissue graft.

Twenty-eight percent of spontaneous CSF leaks are characterized by bony dehiscence of the tegmen tympani, and less commonly of the posterior fossa plate. These defects are most commonly seen in adults. The underlying pathophysiology in these cases includes benign intracranial hypertension, a low-grade inflammation, age-related dural atrophy, arachnoid granulations, and congenital defect in the dura bone. These defects frequently have associated meningoceles or encephaloceles. There are several reports in the literature of multiple sites of leakage on the same or contralateral side.

Spontaneous leaks generally occur at three sites: at the tegmen tympani through the middle fossa dura; through the posterior fossa dura between the labyrinth and the sigmoid sinus; and occasionally at the jugular foramen. Surgical repair is essentially the same as that used for postsurgical defects.

CSF leaks from the posterior fossa and jugular foramen are managed with subtotal petrosectomy. CSF leaks through the middle fossa are approached through a combined transmastoid, middle fossa approach.

After the repair, it may be useful to monitor the patient for signs of benign intracranial hypertension. CSF pressure is usually normal when there is a leak because of the release of pressure, but the pressure may be elevated once the leak is repaired. Sequential leaks at different sites have also been reported; therefore, it is important to continue to follow up these patients because significant time intervals may exist between the leak presentations.

■ ENCEPHALOCELE AND BRAIN HERNIATION

The majority of encephaloceles are related to previous surgery or trauma; however, they can occur from congenital defects or infection. Small defects in the tegmen of the middle ear or mastoid without meningeal or cerebral herniation are found in 20 percent of normal temporal bones. Furthermore, removal of a small amount of tegmen bone is common in mastoid surgery, and encephalocele formation is rare; therefore, bony dehiscence is not sufficient for encephalocele formation. Kuhn and Neely in 1985 hypothesized that dural injury, rather than dural exposure, is necessary for herniation to occur.

In general, the brain tissue within the encephalocele is abnormal, ischemic, and necrotic, and can be excised without significant neurologic sequelae. Hernias with small defects ($<1 \times 1$ cm) are repaired through a transmastoid approach. The encephalocele is resected with bipolar cautery, and the defect is repaired with fascia supported with bone or cartilage.

Medium-sized defects (1 to 2 cm^2) are repaired by combining the transmastoid approach with a minicraniotomy, which allows the placement of a muscle flap or large piece of cartilage for reconstruction. Larger defects are approached through an extended middle fossa approach. This latter technique allows safe treatment of large hernias, hernias located far anteriorly, and/or hernias with active infection.

■ CSF OTORRHEA IN PETROUS TEMPORAL BONE FRACTURES

Post-traumatic CSF leaks can be classified as either closed or open. In a closed leak, the tympanic membrane is intact, and the spinal fluid leaks through the middle ear and out to the nasopharynx through the eustachian tube. It is important in evaluating a patient who has CSF rhinorrhea to exclude the ear as the source of the leak.

In an open leak, the tympanic membrane is perforated, and the external canal may be lacerated. These patients should be examined with sterile instruments to prevent introduction of nosocomial bacteria into the CSF in the ear canal.

CSF leaks occurring from a transverse fracture of the temporal bone are treated with subtotal petrosectomy. This is necessary because a fracture of the otic capsule heals by fibrous union and not by new bone formation. Without surgical correction, the danger of meningitis persists for life even though the CSF leak subsides. The auditory status helps to determine the type of approach employed. If hearing is to be preserved, the middle fossa approach is preferred and should include a multilayer fascia and muscle repair, with special attention to providing structural support to the middle fossa floor. The techniques of repair are the same as previously outlined.

Persistence of CSF leak after temporal bone fracture is a rare event. When it occurs, there will most likely be a large bone–defect, often with brain herniation. Repair is the same as previously described.

Direct trauma to the ossicular chain resulting in stapes luxation or after longitudinal fractures of the pyramid can also cause CSF otorrhea. Such cases are managed by sealing off the oval window with perichondrium through a transmeatal approach.

Suggested Reading

Aristegui M, Falcioni M, Saleh E, et al. Meningoencephalic herniation into the middle ear: A report of 27 cases. Laryngoscope 1995; 105:513-518.

Celikkanat SM, Saleh E, Khashaba A, et al. Cerebrospinal fluid leak after translabyrinthine acoustic neuroma surgery. Otolaryngol Head Neck Surg 1995; 112: 654-658.

Coker NJ, Jenkins HA, Fisch U. Obliteration of the middle ear and mastoid cleft in subtotal petrosectomy: Indications, technique, and results. Ann Otol Rhinol Laryngol 1986; 95:5-11.

Fisch U, Mattox DE. Microsurgery of the skull base. New York: Thieme, 1988.

Fishman AJ, Ronald AH, Roland T, et al. Cerebrospinal fluid drainage in the management of CSF leak following acoustic neuroma surgery. Laryngoscope 1996; 106:1002-1004.

Gacek RR. Arachnoid granulation cerebrospinal fluid otorrhea. Ann Otol Rhinol Laryngol 1990; 99:854-862.

Giddings NA, Brackmann DE. Surgical treatment of difficult cerebrospinal fluid otorhinorrhea. Am J Otol 1994; 15:781-784.

Graham MD. Surgical management of dural and temporal lobe herniation into the radical mastoid cavity. Laryngoscope 1982; 92:329-331.

Kerr AG, Lang J. Pneumatization of the posteromedial air-cell tract. Clin Otolaryngol 1989; 14:425-427.

Kuhn JR, Neely JG. Diagnosis and treatment of iatrogenic cerebrospinal fluid leak and brain herniation during or following mastoidectomy. Laryngoscope 1985; 95:1299-1300.

Myers DL, Sataloff RT. Spinal fluid leakage after skull base surgical procedures. Otolaryngol Clin North Am 1984; 17:601-612.

Ramsden RT, Herdman RCD, Lye RH. Ionomeric bone cement in neuro-otological surgery. J Laryngol Otol 1992; 106:949-953.

Rodgers GK, Luxford WM. Factors affecting the development of cerebrospinal fluid leak and meningitis after translabyrinthine acoustic tumor surgery. Laryngoscope 1993; 102:959-962.

Wetmore SJ, Hermann R, Fisch U. Spontaneous cerebrospinal fluid otorrhea. Am J Otol 1987; 8:96-102.

Wiet RJ, Monsell EM, Hahn YS, O'Connor CA. Brain herniation and space-occupying lesions eroding the tegmen tympani. Laryngoscope 1987; 97:1172-1175.

VERTIGO

The method of
Cecil W. Hart

Patients and doctors tend to use the term *vertigo* differently. In lay usage the word *vertigo* most commonly describes a fear of heights, although it is sometimes used to refer to generalized feelings of giddiness, faintness, confusion, anxiety, or insecurity. The conclusion from this is that when a patient tells us that he or she feels vertiginous or dizzy, we need to consider not only a possible physical abnormality but also a possible emotional disturbance—or both.

Physicians use the term *vertigo* in a somewhat different sense. In medical usage, the sensation of vertigo may best be simply defined as a hallucination of motion. Vertigo is frequently a sensation of rotation (spinning or turning), and this may be one of self-rotation (subjective vertigo) or rotation of the environment (objective vertigo). Sometimes the hallucination of motion is linear, or the patient may experience a tilting sensation. Normally, if a patient feels vertiginous at rest, he or she will also experience the additional symptom of unsteadiness when walking.

Dizziness, on the other hand, is best defined medically as a sensation of the loss of immediate relationship to one's surroundings. By definition, therefore, all vertiginous patients simultaneously feel dizzy.

The sensation of vertigo presupposes a disturbance of function of the vestibular system. This may involve the central vestibular system or any of its three inputs. The labyrinth is a well-recognized site. The visual system is an integral part of the central vestibular system, such that patients may feel vertiginous in response to the flow of certain visual surroundings, for example, walking in supermarket aisles, traffic, crowds, and so forth. Whether the proprioceptive system, for example, the neck, can produce a vertiginous effect has always been somewhat controversial, but it probably can be a factor.

Our knowledge of the physiology of the vestibular system would suggest that a disturbance of a semicircular canal should produce a sensation of rotation (in the plane of that particular canal). Clinical experience, however, reveals that in patients who have gross paroxysmal positioning nystagmus, which is generally accepted to arise from the posterior semicircular canal, the accompanying sensation is not always one of rotation. Also, when one performs a caloric test, deliberately stimulating the horizontal semicircular canal, some patients deny that the resulting sensation is one of rotation. Why this is so is unclear, but the conclusion is very clear, that is, the absence of a sensation of vertigo does *not* exclude disease of the vestibular system.

■ DIAGNOSIS

A distinction needs to be made between an isolated episode of vertigo, for example, vestibular neuronitis, and recurrent episodes, for example, Meniere's syndrome. A single episode of vertigo could be, of course, the first of a series—only time can tell! However, patients who have recurrent vertigo may be distinguished by the fact that they tend to be older and have more in the way of concomitant emotional problems.

Specific treatment depends on the diagnosis. Because there are three types of diagnosis, there are three types of treatment. (1) For an anatomic diagnosis, treat the site (for example, benign paroxysmal positioning vertigo is a disturbance of the inner ear). (2) For a physiologic diagnosis, treat the system (for example, ototoxic drugs may reduce the function of the vestibular system). (3) For an etiologic diagnosis, treat the cause (for example, diabetes mellitus).

Because treatments for diagnoses 1 and 2 are mainly empiric, I only discuss these treatments here.

■ MEDICAL THERAPY

Symptomatic Therapy

Patients who have severe vertigo are frequently seen in the hospital emergency room. Intravenous (IV) treatment offers the most rapid relief of the symptom. Intravenous diazepam is very effective. Five to 20 mg can be given fairly rapidly intravenously (use a large vein in order to minimize the possibility of vein sclerosis). More drug can then be added to the IV bottle and infused slowly. By this means, it is possible to titrate the dosage by observing its effect on the nystagmus, which is also usually present, turning both the nystagmus and the sensation of vertigo on or off by slowing or quickening the IV rate.

For the accompanying nausea and vomiting, intravenous droperidol is very effective. Dosage again should be individualized. Promethazine and prochlorperazine are other useful antiemetics. They can be given intravenously, intramuscularly (IM), orally, or by suppository. The dosage of promethazine is 12.5 to 25 mg, which may be given intravenously, diluted to 25 mg/mL, at a maximum infusion rate of 25 mg per minute. The dosage for prochlorperazine is 5 to 10 mg IV, by slow injection (5 mg per minute), or IM (repeat once in 30 minutes if necessary). Ondansetron, a useful drug for postoperative and chemotherapy-induced vomiting, may also help in this situation. It is available in both intravenous and oral preparations. Intravenously, it may conveniently be given as a single 32 mg dose over 15 minutes. Diphenidol may help both vertigo and vomiting. It is now only given orally and should be administered under close medical supervision (it may cause hallucinations, disorientation, and confusion). The recommended dosage is 25 to 50 mg every 4 hours, as necessary. Finally, IV fluid and electrolyte replacement may be important. An anesthesia consultation may be very helpful for all of the aforementioned.

■ MAINTENANCE THERAPY

Once the acute vestibular symptoms have subsided, the patient can be sent home with oral medication. Vertigo, of either peripheral or central origin, may continue to be treated with vestibular function suppressant drugs. When used after an acute episode, however, such drugs are known to slow the normal rate and completeness of recovery. For this reason, it is usually wise to wean the patient off such drugs as rapidly as the symptoms will allow. Diazepam should only be used on a short-term basis, that is, weeks, to avoid addiction. This drug is especially useful if the patient is also anxious. Dosage levels may be 2, 5, or 10 mg four times per day, depending on the severity of the patient's symptoms. Meclizine and dimenhydrinate are more appropriate for peripheral rather than central vestibular disturbances, and these drugs can be used over the long term. The usual meclizine dosage is 12.5 to 25 mg four times per day. The usual dimenhydrinate dosage is one or two 50 mg tablets every 4 to 6 hours. Promethazine, 25 mg four times per day, and prochlorperazine, by mouth three or four times per day, or by rectal suppository at 25 mg twice a day, are also useful for the control of nausea and vomiting on an outpatient basis.

There has been some interest in the use of drugs to accelerate vestibular compensation, including calcium antagonists, melanotropic peptides, and gangliosides (ginkgo biloba extract). All three of these drugs can be used in humans, and the last two seem to be most promising.

Patients who have recurrent attacks of vertigo may require long-term maintenance treatment with vestibular function suppressant drugs in order to reduce the frequency and severity of recurrent episodes. However, all vestibular function suppressant drugs may lose their effect over time, and it may be necessary to change back and forth from one drug to another. In some patients, especially those who have concomitant fluctuating low-frequency hearing loss, the etiology may be a migraine variant, and prophylactic treatment with a β-adrenergic blocker such as propranolol may be helpful. An appropriate starting dosage might be 40 mg twice a day, and then a gradual increase of the dosage over the course of a few weeks up to 120 to 240 mg daily, or until the symptoms have been controlled.

■ PHYSICAL THERAPY

In order to facilitate compensation, physical therapy is particularly useful following a single severe episode of vertigo, an attack of vestibular neuronitis, or for vertigo following a surgical intervention. The Cooksey-Cawthorne exercises, or some modification of them, are appropriate. These are outlined in the appendix. Balance exercises are also helpful for patients who have chronic dysequilibrium, and even patients who have oscillopsia. However, these exercises are less helpful when the cause lies in the central vestibular system, especially if there is also damage to other supranuclear ocular motor systems that may play a part in the compensatory process, for example, the saccadic, pursuit, and fixation reflex systems. Balance stratagems and a list of assistive devices are also found in the appendix.

The physical therapist is also likely to spend considerable time with the patient and in the process establish a good relationship with him or her. This encourages the patient to share information and accept responsibility for exploring diagnostic and rehabilitative possibilities.

Another common problem for which the physical therapist has much to offer is benign postural vertigo with paroxysmal position nystagmus (BPPV). The two most commonly used physical therapy treatments are some form of liberatory movement (e.g., the Semont maneuver, the Epley maneuver) and the Brandt-Daroff exercises. These therapies have approximately a 95 percent success rate with one treatment, even if the patient may have had the problem for years!

The Epley maneuver usually requires one treatment. Once the diagnosis of the involved side is made, the patient is moved quickly from sitting with legs extended, head turned 45 degrees toward the involved side, into the provoking Hallpike-Dix position (i.e., supine with head rotated and extended off the edge of the plinth toward the involved side). This position is maintained for 2 to 3 minutes. Then the head is slowly rotated toward the other side (while maintaining some neck extension). The patient then rolls from supine onto the side that the head is now turned to and is maintained in this position with the head facing downward for 2 to 3 more minutes. The patient is then assisted back to sitting and is fitted with a soft cervical collar and instructed not to bend over or extend the neck for 48 hours. For 48 hours the patient should sleep semiupright; and for 7 days the patient should not lie on the affected side.

For patients who cannot undergo or are refractory to this treatment, there are the Brandt-Daroff exercises. The patient is seated and moves as fast as tolerated into a side-lying position, with the head turned to the opposite direction (i.e., right side–lying, head turned left). If the patient feels symptoms, he or she waits until they have subsided, adds 30 seconds, and then returns to sitting. If the patient feels no symptoms in the position, he or she waits only 15 seconds until moving into the next position. Once sitting, the patient moves quickly into the opposite side-lying position (i.e., left side–lying, head turned right) for 15 seconds if he or she does not experience symptoms, or for 30 seconds if symptoms occur. This exercise is repeated five to 20 times, depending on patient tolerance, three times per day. The patient can stop once the exercises are performed at this frequency for 2 consecutive days without producing any symptoms.

■ RELAXATION THERAPY

Relaxation training with electromyography biofeedback may be beneficial for patients who have concomitant neck tension, hyperventilation, jaw clenching, or teeth grinding, or when the vertigo is provoked by stress.

Autogenic feedback training, which is a combination of biofeedback and learned control of the autonomic nervous system by means of cognitive imagery, may help patients control their level of arousal and cope with their disorientation. Motion sickness has been shown to be ameliorated by biofeedback training to control skin conductance levels, muscle relaxation, and diaphragmatic breathing, as well as by autogenic feedback training. Such techniques may also be applicable to patients who have vertigo.

Holistic Therapy

The patient is not simply the passive victim of the event. He or she has to adapt his or her life-style to the illness. By doing this, the patient can actually influence the nature and course of the symptoms and disability.

Every patient reacts to the sensation of vertigo in a slightly different way. The presence of a sensation of vertigo makes the patient distressed and handicapped, and recurring episodes of vertigo may increase these disabilities. Vertigo is usually accompanied by other symptoms and signs of autonomic system malfunction, which add insult to injury. All of this induces an emotional response on the part of the patient, further stimulating the autonomic system, which in turn acts upon the vestibular system. This sets up a vicious cycle. If the patient had an anxious disposition to begin with, the whole process may be magnified many times.

The patient cannot proceed to the socially normative and rewarding task of successfully coping with illness until its authenticity has been confirmed by doctors and acknowledged by family, friends, employers, and colleagues. The role of the physician is to facilitate the individual's attempts to adapt by providing the necessary information, training, skills, and support, in addition to providing the necessary medical and sometimes surgical treatment. Patient support groups may also help in this regard.

■ SURGICAL THERAPY

If it proves impossible to control the patient's vertiginous episodes satisfactorily by medical means, various nondestructive surgical treatments have been devised, such as decompression or drainage of the endolymphatic sac or the intratympanic application of steroids. If this is insufficient, some form of surgery to either reduce unilateral vestibular function (e.g., intratympanic application of gentamicin) or destroy function (e.g., vestibular neurectomy) may help.

Acknowledgment
I am grateful to Lyn Fuller, P.T., for her contribution to the physical therapy portion of the chapter. She is not only a knowledgeable individual in the field, but also an excellent practitioner, as many of my patients can attest.

Suggested Reading

Baloh RW, Halmagyi GM, eds. Disorders of the vestibular system. New York: Oxford University Press, 1996.
Blakeley BW, Siegel ME. Feeling dizzy: Understanding and treating dizziness, vertigo, and other balance disorders. New York: Macmillan, 1995.
Brandt T. Vertigo: Its multisensory syndromes. London: Springer Verlag, 1991.
Herdman SJ, ed. Vestibular rehabilitation. Philadelphia: FA Davis, 1994.
Smith PF, Darlington CL. Can vestibular compensation be enhanced by drug treatment? J Vestibul Res 1994; 4:169-179.
Yardley L. Vertigo and dizziness. In: Fitzpatrick R, Newman S, eds. The experience of illness series. London: Routledge, 1994.

APPENDIX

■ COOKSEY-CAWTHORNE BALANCE EXERCISES

Aims

- To relax the muscles of the neck and the shoulder, in order to overcome the protective muscular spasm and the tendency to move "in one piece"
- To train movement of the eyes independently of the head and to enhance the visual fixation reflex system
- To develop proprioceptive and visual mechanisms to compensate for a disturbance in labyrinthine function, for example, the cervico-ocular reflex
- To improve overall muscle coordination
- To practice balancing under everyday conditions, with special attention to developing the use of the eyes and muscle and joint sense
- To practice head movements that cause dizziness, and thus gradually overcome the disability, that is, vestibular habituation
- To become accustomed to moving about naturally in the daylight and in the dark
- To encourage the restoration of self-confidence and easy spontaneous movement

Exercises

1. Seated or in bed
   a. Eye movements: move the eyes slowly at first, then quickly
      1) Up and down
      2) Side to side
      3) Diagonally
      4) Focus on the finger moving from 1 foot to 3 feet away from the face
   b. Head movements: move the head slowly at first, then quickly, with the eyes open
      1) Bending forward and backward
      2) Turning from side to side
      3) Tilting from side to side
      4) Diagonal movements
      5) Repeat with the eyes closed
   c. Coordinate movements of both eyes and the head in the same direction, as in subsections a. and b.
   d. Shoulder shrugging and circling
   e. Bending forward and picking up objects from the ground
2. Standing
   a. Repeat section 1 exercises while standing
   b. Change from a sitting to a standing position, first with the eyes open, and then with the eyes closed
   c. Throw a ball from hand to hand above eye level
   d. Throw a ball from hand to hand under the knees
   e. Change from sitting to standing, turning first to one side and then to the other
3. Moving about
   a. Walk across the room with eyes open, and then with eyes closed
   b. Walk up and down a slope with eyes open, and then with eyes closed
   c. Walk up and down steps with eyes open, and then with eyes closed
   d. Sit up and lie down in bed
   e. Stand up and sit down on a chair
   f. Recover balance when pushed in each direction
   g. Throw and catch a ball
   h. Engage in any game involving stooping or stretching and aiming, such as bowling, volleyball, or shuffleboard

■ BALANCE ADVICE

When Moving from Lying to Standing

When getting up in the morning and on first opening your eyes, focus on something on the ceiling in order to help develop your stability. Next, slowly move to the side of the bed and sit up, again focusing on something before you stand up. Finally, stand up, but be sure to focus on something once more before you start to walk.

When Moving from Sitting to Standing

First, slide to the middle of your chair. Next, place your hands next to your hips on the chair seat. Then, focus on an object straight ahead. Rise slowly with your head and back straight and upright. Stand and perform isometric exercises (contract your muscles without moving) for your trunk muscles before you walk. When you stand, be sure to keep your knees slightly bent.

When Moving from Standing to Sitting

Walk to your chair and turn slowly until the back of your knees touch the chair. Reach back with both hands to hold the chair so that it will not slide. Focus on something straight ahead, then sit down slowly with your head and back straight and upright.

When Starting to Walk

It is important that you feel stable while standing still before walking. When you start to walk, focus on something straight ahead. When you look down, try to use your eyes rather than your head.

Walking or Standing

- Position feet comfortably apart (not too close together)
- Focus on distant objects, using side vision for close objects
- When walking, do not look down, but select a distant point for fixation, using peripheral vision to avoid nearby objects
- Do not use bi- or trifocal glasses, especially when going downstairs
- Avoid dark areas and places, for example, dark restaurants

Bending Over

- When getting up from bending over, look up and away at a distant object

Close-up Work

- When sitting, become aware of the feel of your feet on the floor
- When reading, try to limit the amount of time; if you notice a problem after 5 or 10 minutes, do something else and go back to reading later
- When standing, and before attempting to work, steady your feet apart in a comfortable position

Driving

- Ride in the front seat of the car
- Look out the window at distant earth-fixed objects
- When going around curves, look at a distant object, for example, a tree that is beyond the curve

Airplanes

- The larger the airplane, the better the cabin pressure, so the less possible turbulence effects
- Sit near the front where the turbulence is less
- Sit in a window seat so you can see the horizon

■ GENERAL ADVICE TO PATIENTS WHO HAVE VERTIGO AND BALANCE PROBLEMS

Vertigo and unsteadiness can often be very unpredictable. Depending on the cause, these symptoms may sometimes occur at any time, even after long periods of remission. Therefore, it is important to take proper precautions in order to avoid accidents and mishaps. This is particularly important if you are taking medications, such as (but not limited to) sedatives, antihistamines, antidepressants, and/or pain medication. You should not perform activities that might jeopardize your own or other person's lives. These may include driving a car, operating heavy machinery, or working in precarious situations, for example, on ladders or rooftops. It is important that you: remove sharp or easily breakable objects; try to reduce stress; avoid, as much as possible, caffeine, alcohol, and nicotine; eat a well-balanced diet, avoid excessive salt intake, perform regular exercise, and get plenty of sleep; and seek emotional support from your family, friends, and persons where you work.

■ BALANCE ASSISTIVE DEVICES

- Glasses: the best visual function possible should be achieved; use separate glasses for distance and close-up work
- Good hearing also helps orientation; use hearing aids and other hearing assistive devices, if appropriate
- Cervical collar, if appropriate; in patients who have significant cervical spondylosis, and particularly if head turning increases unsteadiness, use a soft, foam rubber cervical collar, which often limits this motion and improves stability
- Cane(s) for walking; carry a light cane, which is often extremely valuable not only for support, but also to provide additional tactile and proprioceptive orientating information
- Use a walker if appropriate
- Wear substantial lace-up shoes with wide rubber soles and low or flat heels
- Choose carpets with a thin pile; the fewer scatter rugs the better; be sure that they do not slip; use non-skid floor wax
- Leave a light on in different areas of the house, including the bathroom, corridors, and stairways; have a bedside lamp
- Staircases: place colored tape on the first and last steps
- Install handrails wherever appropriate
- Use bath bench, shower chair, and non-slip bath and shower mats
- Use goggles when swimming in order to maintain orientation

PERILYMPHATIC FISTULA IN CHILDREN

The method of
Charles D. Bluestone

I am pleased to be asked to describe my experience in the diagnosis, management, and outcomes of perilymphatic fistula (PLF) in children. In my mind this is one of the few conditions that clinicians were unaware of in the past, but now this condition can be effectively treated. I define PLF as an abnormal communication between the middle ear—mastoid and labyrinth, and it can be *congenital* or *acquired.*

In the past, idiopathic sensorineural hearing loss (SNHL) in children that was progressive or fluctuating, or both, was usually considered to be due to hereditary causes, and nothing but habilitation or rehabilitation was possible—certainly not surgery! Yes, we otolaryngologists were aware that children who had a history of trauma to the temporal bone could develop a fracture of the labyrinth, or subluxation of the stapes, and this could lead to SNHL or vertigo, or both. But even these children were often not managed appropriately if they subsequently developed progressive and/or fluctuating hearing loss or vertigo. In addition, children who complained of dysequilibrium or vertigo—or whose parents described "clumsiness" or "bumping into objects"—for which there was no obvious history of an antecedent event such as trauma, rarely, if ever, had the diagnosis of PLF entertained by their physicians. Children who had progressive and/or fluctuating SNHL or vertigo, or both, which was otherwise unexplained, frequently would go through a battery of tests that only occasionally proved fruitful; and then, if the diagnosis was still uncertain, they would receive a variety of medical treatments usually prescribed for adults with Meniere's disease. More often than not, we clinicians would not offer any medical treatment, but would just throw up our hands and recommend "watchful waiting." I can vividly remember that approximately 30 years ago I evaluated just such a child; this child had progressive SNHL of unknown origin, and I gave this sage advice of watchful waiting only to find out from the mother 6 months later that her son's hearing had deteriorated so much that he was enrolled in a school for the deaf.

In the past, we otolaryngologists (as well as neurosurgeons) were also aware that congenital or acquired defects of the temporal bone might predispose a child to either spontaneous cerebrospinal fluid (CSF) otorrhea or recurrent episodes of meningitis, usually as a complication of acute otitis media and frequently caused by a pneumococcal infection, for which the physicians would surgically explore the ear or intracranial cavity, or both, and correct the defect. Also, we were fully aware that cholesteatoma (or tumor) could invade the labyrinth, primarily the footplate of the stapes, or the lateral semicircular canal. We certainly knew we could enter the inner ear at the time of middle ear surgery. Soon after stapedectomy for otosclerosis was introduced in the late 1950s, some patients developed PLF, especially those who had had the early—and since abandoned—procedure that involved insertion of a polyethylene tube prosthesis and Gelfoam to cover the oval window; perilymph could be seen flowing through the polyethylene tube at the time of exploratory tympanotomy. We were also made aware that scuba divers who had sudden SNHL and vertigo during a dive were found to have PLF and a lateral-facing round window. But the concept that a child might have an occult communication between the middle ear and labyrinth, without an obvious connection to the brain, was not considered until recently.

The management of PLF is one of the most satisfying clinical experiences in my 40 years of medicine. After reading this chapter, I hope you will agree with me, and thus more effectively diagnose and manage *congenital PLF* in children.

■ BACKGROUND

A little over 20 years ago, I had the opportunity to be at the Boston City Hospital—like many great institutions today, it is now unhappily called the Boston Medical Center—and came in contact with Stuart Strong, then Professor and Chairman of Otolaryngology at Boston University, and Gerald Healy, who was just beginning his illustrious academic career. They made me aware that adults who had progressive and/or fluctuating SNHL, with or without vertigo, may have an occult PLF. My first case was an adult male recreational pilot who would become vertiginous when he did certain stunts in the air. Important in his medical history was that as a child he had sustained a blow to his head when he was accidentally hit with a baseball bat during a game. At exploratory tympanotomy, I repaired a PLF of the oval window. However, it was not until I returned to Pittsburgh and the Children's Hospital in 1975 that the "light bulb went on" in my brain that children can also have PLF.

In 1977, Kenneth Grundfast and I published our experience managing six children who had PLF; before that publication, only a few isolated cases involving children had been reported. But at that time, I did not recognize the problem to be caused by a congenital abnormality. After the publication of our report, there was considerable skepticism among otolaryngologists that children did indeed have PLF, which was a carryover from the heated controversy concerning the existence of spontaneous PLF in adults that exists to this day. Even when John Supance and I published our second review of a series of 26 children in 1983, I still did not realize what we were dealing with. This report still did not convince many of my colleagues.

It took the painstaking work of Blas Perez, who was a visiting professor from Spain, and Peter Weber, one of our residents, who reviewed the medical records of the 94 patients we operated on between 1980 and 1989 for suspected PLF, to enlighten me. As I describe in detail later, almost 90 percent of the 60 children who had a PLF visualized at surgery had a *congenital defect* of the middle ear or inner ear (as visualized by computed tomography [CT]), or both.

For the first time, Perez and Weber summarized what each of the dozen surgeons who had operated on these children described in their operative notes; we each had recorded our findings, but no one had put all of the observations together. The most common site was the oval window, and the superstructure of the stapes was frequently abnormal, as was the long process of the incus; in some patients, we also found a lateral-facing round window. We concluded in our 1993 publication that these children had a congenital middle or inner ear defect that predisposed them to PLF. But still most of the otolaryngologic community remained unconvinced.

Then Peter Weber—along with an immunopathologist at our medical school, Robert Kelly—informed me that a routine test used by neurosurgeons, beta-2 transferrin, could detect CSF and perilymphatic fluid, and he suspected that this test might be helpful. The title of our paper published in 1994 describing the study was "Beta-2 Transferrin Confirms Perilymphatic Fistula in Children." For the first time, we had a test to prove that *congenital PLF really exists.* The test was not sensitive, but it certainly was specific; that is, if the test results are positive, the child has a fistula, but if the test results are negative, the possibility that a fistula exists cannot be ruled out. A subsequent study of 43 children published in 1995, in which the beta-2 transferrin test was re-evaluated, confirmed my conclusion about this test's lack of sensitivity. Other investigators have also come to the same conclusion. But the *bottom line* is that congenital PLF is a real entity; it is fact, not fiction. Currently, the test, if its results are positive, can be helpful in deciding whether or not to explore a contralateral ear (see text following).

In the remaining portion of this chapter, I describe how we diagnose and manage *congenital PLF* in infants and children.

■ CLINICAL PRESENTATION

Hearing Loss

I have encountered approximately 150 infants and children with congenital PLF in a little over 20 years, and there have been many different clinical presentations. Typically, however, a child has a history of SNHL that has been slowly *progressive* for years. The patient is brought to the attention of the physician after failing an initial screening hearing test upon entering school, and subsequent tests reveal progression of hearing loss. Although a less common presentation, a similar child may demonstrate *fluctuating* SNHL after an initial audiometric test. Still others have both fluctuation and progression of the hearing loss. There is a negative history for the classic causes of SNHL, such as prematurity, ototoxic drugs, viral infections (e.g., cytomegalovirus), and teratogens. There is an absence of the stigmata of syndromal SNHL, such as Waardenburg's syndrome. Likewise, there is no evidence of eye involvement, for example, cataracts (rubella), myopia (Stickler), or retinal changes (Usher's syndrome).

However, important in the history is the occurrence of *otitis media,* especially if a child develops SNHL (or further loss) during an acute attack; the child is then showing signs of some degree of *labyrinthitis.* Likewise, if a child develops acute suppurative labyrinthitis as a complication of acute otitis media while receiving antibiotics, the clinician should obtain a CT and consider exploration of the ear to rule out PLF. More obviously, if a child developed *meningitis* associated with a past episode of acute otitis media and also developed SNHL, and now has progressive and/or fluctuating loss, PLF must be ruled out; another episode of acute otitis media could be a life-threatening situation.

A child may have a *craniofacial malformation,* which could include a middle or inner ear anomaly; any malformation of the head and neck can be associated with PLF. There is usually no family history of SNHL, but I have seen at least five families in which a sibling or parent has had progressive and/or fluctuating SNHL, and a similar malformation was found at the time of exploratory tympanotomy.

Very important in the history is the association of *vigorous physical activity* with either the onset of SNHL or the progression of the loss. Remember, during growth and development children are always exploring new physical activities. Typical antecedent events are usually related to an activity that increases intracranial pressure—the communication is not just between the middle and inner ears, but also the CSF—such as lifting weights, push-ups, pull-ups, sit-ups, climbing rope, and gymnastics.

Another important antecedent event is *barotrauma.* Scuba diving is an uncommon cause in children, but hearing loss may be associated with the onset of swimming lessons, especially diving. Similarly, the onset may occur on descent in an airplane, frequently when a child has an upper respiratory infection. Also, forceful blowing of the nose or sneezing can result in PLF in an ear that has a congenital middle ear or inner ear defect, albeit rare.

The hearing loss is unilateral in approximately two-thirds of patients and bilateral in one-third. When there is a permanent conductive hearing loss associated with progressive and/or fluctuating SNHL (i.e., *mixed hearing loss),* the child most likely has a malformation of the ossicular chain that causes the conductive component in addition to the PLF. Any child who has a mixed hearing loss should have relatively frequent audiograms, for example, every 3 months for 1 or 2 years, to determine if the sensorineural component is stable. If it is not, we would work up the child and seriously consider exploring the ear for suspected PLF, irrespective of the level of conductive loss. If the clinician is uncertain about the effect of recurrent or chronic middle ear effusion on the decision to explore or not, a myringotomy tube should be inserted, and the child should be re-evaluated when the middle ear is free of effusion. Also, if PLF is suspected and tympanotomy is planned, and a middle ear effusion is also present, a tympanostomy tube should be inserted before the tympanotomy; the exploration can then be carried out later, when the ear is free of effusion.

It is uncommon to find PLF in a child with apparently normal hearing who develops *sudden* SNHL in one or both ears. Such children may have another condition, such as an autoimmune disorder. However, we have encountered a few patients who have had unilateral SNHL, subsequently developed sudden SNHL in the contralateral ear, and PLF was found at surgery in both ears. Also, a child who has PLF may have rapidly progressive SNHL, as opposed to a slowly progressive loss.

Vertigo and Dysequilibrium

The most common cause of vertigo and/or dysequilibrium in infants and children is otitis media or eustachian tube dysfunction. In my experience, the second most common cause is PLF. Many children who have vestibular complaints are either too young to verbalize about their imbalance or they grow older thinking everyone is a little "off balance." Frequently, the parents describe the infant or child as "clumsy." The symptom is most commonly associated with progressive and/or fluctuating SNHL, but may be an isolated complaint. On rare occasion, nystagmus can be elicited, especially during an episode of acute otitis media. The same antecedent events that are associated with progressive and/or fluctuating SNHL can be associated with vestibular involvement.

An area of interest of mine today is the significance of the so-called *large vestibular aqueduct syndrome,* characterized by progressive SNHL, with or without vertigo and/or dysequilibrium, and the possible association of PLF. These patients frequently develop progression of their SNHL or recurrence of vertigo, or both, when a relatively mild trauma to the head occurs. However, when these children (and teenagers) undergo repair of their windows, the outcome is excellent, but another traumatic event may necessitate revision surgery. This clinical picture may be explained by our current concepts about the pathogenesis of PLF.

■ PATHOGENESIS

The pathogenesis of congenital PLF is still under investigation and remains controversial. My current hypothesis is that the middle ear malformations we are identifying at surgery are not the *cause* of PLF, but the *result* of abnormal perilymphatic fluid pressure during the development of the middle and inner ear. There is likely an increase in inner ear fluid pressure due to an enlarged cochlear or vestibular aqueduct, or both, during gestation. Why else would the stapes superstructure, incus, and round window be so abnormal? Also, the stapes is a complicated structure to develop, because the inner ear—and medial footplate—is developed from the otic capsule (i.e., the neuroectoderm), whereas the ossicles—and lateral footplate—develop from the branchial arches: two different anlages. These abnormally large aqueducts between the CSF and the inner ear remain more open after birth and probably do not become less open until adolescence. I have observed that a few of the children who have had a PLF, and have had recurrence of the PLF during childhood, which was secondary to physical activities I had counseled against, also engaged in these same activities when they became teenagers without a recurrence. Thus, I am less restrictive about physical activities with teenagers if they are not prone to recurrence.

■ THE WORKUP

Over the years, I have progressively eliminated almost all the traditional tests that are recommended when a child has SNHL of unknown etiology. When the clinical picture is consistent with the description I have previously described, I obtain the following:

1. All of the prior audiograms to *document* the progressive and/or fluctuating nature of the SNHL.
2. An auditory brain stem response evaluation for site of the lesion, for example, to rule out a retrocochlear lesion, and in infants for documentation of the laterality; type (SNHL or conductive, or both); and degree of hearing loss.
3. A CT scan of the temporal bones to determine if there is any malformation of the middle or inner ear (and to rule out retrocochlear disease).

The CT scan is obtained in order to help confirm the diagnosis, which aids in counseling the parents regarding the likelihood of PLF being the cause. The scan is highly specific but not sensitive; its results are positive in only approximately 20 percent of PLF. The absence of a malformation on the scan does not necessarily rule out exploratory surgery. It just makes me less confident about finding PLF. Also, the scan can help in making decisions about the contralateral ear after surgical exploration of one ear (see next section).

If a child has vertigo or dysequilibrium without SNHL, I also obtain a *vestibular evaluation* to document involvement of the vestibule and laterality, and to rule out other causes of the symptom. If the child has progressive and/or fluctuating SNHL, I forgo the vestibular workup. (After 20 years of searching for a vestibular test that is both sensitive and specific in diagnosing PLF, we have yet to find one!)

If no congenital middle ear defect or PLF is found at surgery, and the beta-2 transferrin test result is negative, we frequently obtain laboratory tests to uncover another cause of SNHL, especially when a child continues to have progressive hearing loss. On occasion, we have diagnosed an autoimmune disorder.

■ WHICH EAR TO EXPLORE?

The selection of the ear to explore is not an easy decision. On the one hand, if a child has preoperative evidence of PLF, such as unilateral progressive and/or fluctuating SNHL, with or without vertigo, and only a malformation of that labyrinth (as visualized on CT scan), the decision is easy. Operate only on that ear, and watch the other one. Also, if a child has bilateral signs and symptoms, and bilateral anomalous inner ears, operate on the ear with the worst hearing first, followed by the contralateral ear a few months later. However, if the hearing in one ear is rapidly deteriorating, despite the fact that this ear is the better-hearing ear, operate on that ear first. If a child has classic evidence of congenital PLF in an only-hearing ear, and the hearing is rapidly deteriorating, operate on that ear, but very carefully!

On the other hand, the selection of the ear to explore when a child has bilaterally symmetric hearing loss is arbitrary. The presence of a unilateral malformation of the inner ear can be helpful. When all else fails, I usually choose the ear with a larger ear canal. Also, the decision can be difficult when vertigo is present. This is when vestibular tests can be helpful. Operate on the ear with the abnormal findings.

Before surgery, we discuss the benefits and risks of the exploration. To date, the only postoperative complication in my patients has been a tympanic membrane perforation, which either was not recognized during the procedure or developed postoperatively; the perforation has always been subsequently repaired successfully.

To the best of my knowledge, we have not had a permanent conductive hearing loss from the surgery, nor have we encountered SNHL as the result of the operative procedure. However, it is important to stress that a child might have progressive SNHL *despite* the surgery, not because of it. These issues are discussed with the parents before the procedure.

■ EXPLORATORY TYMPANOTOMY

The procedure is performed with the patient under general anesthesia. The external auditory canal is infiltrated with local anesthetic and vasoconstrictive agents. An incision is made above the pinna slightly above the hairline to remove a small piece of temporalis muscle for grafting the windows. The traditional transcanal tympanomeatal flap is then elevated to explore the middle ear. (In infants, a modified endaural incision is used, and a large ear speculum, or self-retaining retractor, is inserted.) A thorough search for a malformation of the stapes, incus, round window, and promontory is conducted. Because the anatomy of the stapes superstructure is difficult to visualize, a *90 degree pick* is used to palpate the crura and obturator foramen to determine if an abnormality is present. When found, the stapes may have either a retropositioned or absent anterior crus, or it may be monopod. The long process of the incus is frequently malformed, with an obvious concavity facing anteriorly. The round window niche may be facing laterally (as opposed to the normal window, which faces posteriorly), or it may be grossly abnormal. Also, we have encountered PLF when both windows are *retropositioned;* a rare anomaly involving the promontory may be present. This anomaly appears as a fissure between the oval and round windows, and may have perilymph emanating from it. The finding of one or more of these malformations is evidence that the child most likely has a fistula, even if no obvious leak of perilymph is visualized.

The oval and round windows are inspected for a leak. A leak is most frequently seen in the area of the anterior footplate, but it can occur anywhere in the footplate. On rare occasion, a small hole can be seen in the middle of the footplate, but it is unusual to find a relatively large defect in the anterior portion of the footplate. Because the child is under general anesthesia, a voluntary Valsalva's maneuver is not possible, so we ask the anesthetist to perform a Valsalva on the child, during which time we look for PLF. Small pledgets of Gelfoam are then placed over the stapes footplate and round window, which remains in place for a few minutes; we then ask the anesthetist to repeat Valsalva's maneuver. The pledgets are then sent to the immunopathology laboratory for beta-2 transferrin testing. The area around the stapes footplate and round window niche is then denuded of mucosa for the graft site. Small pieces of muscle, which have been previously diced, are then laid over the stapes footplate and in and around the round window niche. A layer of Gelfoam is then placed over the muscle grafts, and the tympanomeatal flap is replaced. *NOTE:* We patch the oval and round windows irrespective of the operative findings. (Despite the recent suggestion that PLF can be simply identified using an endoscopic procedure, we would never consider this method, because we graft the windows whether we see a PLF or not.)

■ POSTOPERATIVE CARE

If PLF is identified at surgery, the child is kept for bed rest overnight, and the patient and parents are counseled about the type of physical activity permitted in the future to prevent *recurrence* of PLF. In general, we warn against activities that grossly elevate CSF pressure (e.g., weight lifting, push-ups, sit-ups) and activities that rapidly alter middle ear pressure, such as diving in water (especially scuba) and flying in unpressurized cabins of airplanes. We have found that these activities are associated with a recurrence of PLF. If the child and parents are properly counseled, recurrence is uncommon. The patient can still play ball games and ride a bicycle.

■ THE CONTRALATERAL EAR

The decision concerning exploring the contralateral ear is frequently difficult. As previously stated, when both ears are involved and a child has bilateral inner ear malformations, we stage the two ears. When the child has unilateral progressive and/or fluctuating SNHL, with an inner ear malformation limited only to that ear, we watch the other ear. However, in a similar child, in whom the CT scan demonstrates bilateral inner ear malformations, we encourage the parents to have the other, normal-hearing ear explored at a later date; benefits versus risks are thoroughly discussed.

If a child has bilateral SNHL, but the CT scan is bilaterally normal, we recommend surgical exploration of the contralateral ear if we find one or more of the following: a congenital malformation of the middle ear, an obvious leak, or positive beta-2 transferrin test results. Currently, if none of these findings are present, we usually advise watching the opposite ear; if the operative ear maintains stable hearing, but the contralateral, nonoperated ear develops progressive SNHL, we explore the other ear.

■ OUTCOMES

We have reviewed the medical records of 137 children we operated on during the 1980s and found that when PLF was identified at surgery, hearing was stabilized in 83 percent of patients, improved in 10 percent, decreased in 3 percent, and 10 percent of patients did not participate in follow-up. The change in hearing was defined as a speech reception threshold (SRT) equal to or greater than 10 dB. When no fistula was visualized, we had similar outcomes (93 percent stabilization rate). It is as a result of the analysis of these outcomes that we graft the windows irrespective of whether or not we find a fistula.

Of these 137 children, 31 (37 percent) had vestibular complaints (with and without SNHL), and *all* were found to have PLF at surgery. Of 31 patients, 22 (71 percent) had resolution of symptoms, six (19 percent) had no change, one (.03 percent) was worse, and four (.12 percent) children were lost to follow-up.

In this group of children, 9 percent had recurrence of their progressive and/or fluctuating SNHL or vestibular complaints, or both, and PLF was found at re-exploration in approximately half of them. My impression is that the rate of recurrence has probably decreased during the last several years, because we are counseling our children more effectively about avoiding certain physical activities.

Suggested Reading

Bluestone CD. Otologic surgical procedures. In: Bluestone CD, Stool SE, eds. Atlas of pediatric otolaryngology. Philadelphia: WB Saunders, 1994:27.

Grundfast KM, Bluestone CD. Sudden or fluctuating hearing loss or vertigo in children due to perilymph fistula. Ann Otol Rhinol Laryngol 1978; 87:761-771.

Reilly, Weber PC. Perilymphatic fistulas in infants and children. In: Bluestone CD, Stool SE, Kenna MA, eds. Pediatric otolaryngology. 3rd ed. Philadelphia: WB Saunders, 1996: 371.

Supance JS, Bluestone CD. Perilymph fistula in infants and children. Otolaryngol Head Neck Surg 1983; 91:663-671.

Weber PC, Bluestone CD, Kenna MA, Kelly RH. Correlation of beta-2 transferrin and middle ear abnormalities in congenital perilymphatic fistula. Am J Otolaryngol 1995; 16:277-282.

Weber PC, Bluestone CD, Perez B. Surgical outcome of perilymphatic fistula surgery. Annual meeting American Otological, Rhinological, and Laryngological Society, Los Angeles, April 1993 (abstract).

Weber PC, Kelly RH, Bluestone CD, Bassiouny M. Beta-2 transferrin confirms perilymph fistula in children. Otolaryngol Head Neck Surg 1994; 110:381-386.

Weber PC, Perez BA, Bluestone CD. Congenital perilymphatic fistula and associated middle ear abnormalities. Laryngoscope 1993; 103:160-164.

PERILYMPHATIC FISTULA

The method of
F. Owen Black
by
F. Owen Black
Susan C. Pesznecker

A perilymphatic fistula (PLF) is a defect in the otic capsule, oval window (OW), or round window. When present, PLFs disrupt auditory and vestibular function by allowing ambient air or cerebrospinal fluid (CSF) pressure changes to stimulate vestibular or auditory hair cells. PLFs may also permit leakage of perilymphatic fluid from the labyrinthine compartment, and, if persistent, may result in permanent end-organ damage.

Benign paroxysmal positional nystagmus and vertigo (BPPN&V), Meniere's disease (primary or idiopathic endolymphatic hydrops), secondary endolymphatic hydrops (SEH), and PLFs are the four most common peripheral vestibular disorders seen by the tertiary care otologist, particularly in practices associated with a trauma center. PLFs often occur in association with comorbid conditions, particularly secondary post-traumatic endolymphatic hydrops and BPPN&V. As for most other otologic diagnoses, PLFs cannot be confirmed histopathologically in the living patient and consequently, there exists no "gold standard" for clinical diagnosis. Histopathologic confirmation can be established only by postmortem examination. Recently, histopathologic confirmation of PLF has been described in a patient who underwent successful PLF closure antemortem.

■ HISTORY

Patients who have PLF typically appear more chronically ill than most otologic patients and are often disabled by their symptoms. No other otologic diagnosis is associated with as much morbidity, obligatory life-style change, and disability. The most common presenting symptoms of an active PLF are dysequilibrium (postural instability), headache (particularly if provoked or exacerbated by exertion), dizziness, tinnitus, cognitive dysfunction, nausea, vertigo, hearing loss, visual disturbances, and aural fullness, in that order.

The diurnal symptom pattern is distinct: PLF symptoms are usually least intense when the patient first awakens in the morning (or after extended rest periods) and worsen progressively as physical activity increases. By day's end, PLF patients are exhausted and miserable. The only means of reliably improving active PLF symptoms is avoiding activities that increase intracranial, intrathoracic, or intra-abdominal pressure.

PLF symptoms tend to be persistent, insidious, and progressive in nature rather than episodic, although various factors may cause symptoms to exacerbate. The well-defined, spontaneous attacks and contrasting symptom-free periods characteristic of Meniere's disease symptomatically differentiate that disorder from PLF.

Increased intracranial, intrathoracic, and/or intra-abdominal pressure (e.g., Valsalva's maneuver) may alter the pressure gradient between the middle and inner ears (across the fistulous opening). If the pressure differential is sufficient to cause loss of perilymph or to stimulate labyrinthine hair cells, PLF symptoms may result. Activities that exacerbate symptoms include coughing, sneezing, vomiting, straining at stool, lifting, sexual activity, singing, yelling, or any strenuous physical activity. Passive (e.g., barometric fluctuations, high-intensity sound) or active (e.g., airplane flight, traveling over mountain passes) changes in ambient air pressure may also precipitate or exacerbate PLF symptoms. In patients who have patent PLFs, symptom exacerbations have been caused by elevator travel of several floors, altitude change of as little as 400 to 500 feet, and airplane travel (particularly in private aircraft with unpressurized cabins).

Dysequilibrium is reported by approximately 90 percent of patients who have active PLFs and is their most common presenting complaint. Postural instability can be documented by computerized dynamic posturography (CDP), which typically shows falls or abnormally increased sway during sensory conflict conditions (sensory organization tests [SOTs] 3 to 6) in approximately three-fourths of patients who have PLFs.

At least 85 percent of PLF patients complain of headaches, which are similar to the "low-pressure" headaches that accompany a CSF leak. The headache tends to involve the same (ipsilateral) side. With bilateral PLFs, the headache pain may be bilateral, but may be more severe on the side of the most active fistula. PLF headaches tend to be severe, are often pulsatile, and are frequently associated with visual photosensitivity. They may be present on a near-continual basis, waxing and waning according to the severity of symptoms. Unilateral headaches related to PLF are often erroneously attributed to migraine. Because of their chronic nature, they are almost invariably accompanied by secondary cervical muscle contraction pain. PLF headaches resolve immediately following successful closure of the fistula, which is similar to the resolution of postspinal tap headaches after blood patching.

Dizziness is experienced by 83 percent of patients, and tinnitus affects almost 79 percent of patients. Seventy-five percent of patients complain of adult-onset motion sickness that follows the development of the PLFs. Nausea, subjective hearing loss, vertigo, and cognitive dysfunction (short-term memory loss, "word search" problems, concentration difficulties, and so forth) are reported by 74 percent of patients. Sixty-two percent of PLF patients describe aural fullness or pressure, and 45 percent experience hyperacusis, especially to low-frequency (e.g., trucks) or high-intensity (e.g., children squealing or screaming) sounds.

The majority of PLF patients, if seen early, have primarily vestibular symptoms and little or no hearing loss. Objective hearing loss typically occurs later, especially in patients who have mild head trauma, and is an emergent complication of PLFs. Speech reception threshold or three-frequency pure-tone average poorer than 25 dB hearing loss is present in 55 percent of PLF patients.

Assuming that no secondary complications develop, most symptoms resolve with PLF closure, albeit at different rates. Cognitive dysfunction is often the last symptom to resolve. If a comorbid condition has developed, or if damage to the vestibular and/or auditory end organs has occurred, symptoms may persist even with optimal closure.

■ ETIOLOGY

The most common cause of PLFs is head trauma, primarily related to motor vehicle accidents. In the majority of post-traumatic PLFs, the head trauma is mild, without loss of consciousness. Whiplash has also been linked to PLFs. In many surgically documented PLF cases that follow motor vehicle accidents, there is no clear history of direct head trauma. External pressure changes exerting sufficient force to cause rupture of the oval and/or round windows (implosive fistulas) or increased intracranial pressure sufficient to produce an explosive fistula were originally described by Goodhill.

Barotrauma, usually via deep-sea or scuba diving, is a well-documented cause of both implosive and explosive PLFs. From our own experience, other causes include rapid descent in commercial aircraft, explosions in close proximity, violent vomiting, difficult and prolonged childbirth, weight lifting, and heading the ball in soccer.

Perilymphatic fistulas may occur following otologic surgery, as with the classic poststapedectomy PLF, or in association with entry into the bony labyrinth during a mastoid procedure. Erosive PLFs may also complicate chronic temporal bone infections or cholesteatoma.

Congenital PLFs associated with stapes footplate anomalies or defects of the superior canal have been reported. Many patients with suspected congenital PLFs have also shown temporal bone abnormalities on computed tomographic (CT) scan and often have a family history of deafness or dizziness strongly suggestive of PLFs. A few patients have spontaneous PLFs. Some spontaneous PLFs probably result from congenital defects, judging from the stapedial footplate dehiscence observed at operation. Several of our pediatric cochlear implant patients who have had deafness since birth have been found at the time of implantation to have active PLFs, with no other apparent etiology for their hearing loss. Congenital footplate dehiscence often presents as repeated episodes of meningitis.

■ DIAGNOSIS

The clinical diagnostic criterion for PLF is the demonstration of a defect in the oval window or round window or a leak of crystal clear fluid from the depths of the oval or round window upon repeated suctioning. Therefore, the only way to definitively diagnose a PLF is to visualize it directly by performing a diagnostic tympanotomy and using the binocular operating microscope to identify the defect or the leak of perilymph. Endoscopy has recently been advocated for examination of the middle ear space for PLFs. The major limitation of endoscopy is the monocular view, which prevents stereopsis. Stereoscopic depth perception is critical for differentiating the welling up of crystal clear fluid from the perilymphatic space versus the dripping of operative fluids (e.g., local anesthetic residue, serous exudate) into middle ear crevices. Thus, successful identification using monocular endoscopy establishes the diagnosis of PLF, but a negative examination finding does not exclude PLF. Without direct visualization of the middle ear windows, the clinical diagnosis of PLF is presumptive.

Because it is not reasonable to perform diagnostic tympanotomies on all suspected PLF patients, other diagnostic criteria must be used. Presumptive diagnostic criteria for PLFs are constant or persistent symptoms of dysequilibrium, ataxia, vertigo, dizziness, hearing loss, and/or tinnitus, particularly (1) if symptom onset followed head trauma, (2) if symptoms are exacerbated by exertion or physical activity, and/or (3) if symptoms are improved by restricting physical activity or avoiding exertion.

There are no "gold standard" auditory or vestibular function tests for PLF or any other otologic disorder. Our patients undergo standard vestibulo-ocular (VOR) and vestibulospinal function tests, computerized dynamic posturography (CDP), electronystagmography, tests of visual-vestibular interactions, and a CDP fistula test. Our audiometric battery includes air- and bone-conducted pure-tone thresholds, speech intelligibility scores, and screening tympanometry. If ossicular discontinuity is suspected, multiple-frequency tympanometry is performed. If a secondary or post-traumatic endolymphatic hydrops is suspected, electrocochleography (ECoG) may be performed. These tests are essential in establishing an auditory and vestibular baseline and in screening for comorbid conditions before therapeutic intervention.

As many as 50 percent of PLF patients complain of positional vertigo and demonstrate a positional nystagmus. Cawthorne-Hallpike test results are often positive in head trauma patients, which confirms BPV as a comorbid condition. Results of rotation tests and tests of visual-vestibular interaction are almost always normal in PLF patients who have mild head trauma. Conversely, CDP results are abnormal in at least three-fourths of PLF patients. CDP motor coordination tests are normal in patients who have PLF secondary to mild head trauma.

Although objective hearing loss can be documented in approximately half of PLF patients, most PLF patients complain of subjective transient hearing loss, distortion, or fluctuation of hearing. Speech intelligibility scores are usually normal; however, reduced speech intelligibility is often the first clinical test of auditory function to deteriorate in association with PLFs. Single-frequency tympanometry results are virtually always normal, but reduced resonant frequencies demonstrated by multiple-frequency tympanometry are very common in patients who have post-traumatic PLFs. When a reduced middle ear resonant frequency is present, fistula tests must be interpreted with caution. False-negative fistula test rates are very high in this group of PLF patients. Results of ECoG are usually normal in patients who have acute uncomplicated PLFs, but often these results become abnormal with time if SEH develops. Auditory brain stem response is normal in PLF patients who have normal hearing, unless brain stem injury has occurred.

Some PLF patients respond abnormally to external auditory canal pressure changes—a response that is the basis of the fistula test. The typical tympanometric fistula test introduces a sinusoidal pressure stimulus ($\pm$300 to 500 mm H_2O) to the suspect ear using an impedance bridge. Eye movement responses may be observed directly or monitored with electro-oculography or infrared video recordings. The test results are considered positive if nystagmoid eye movements are generated in response to the changing pressure stimulus. The CDP fistula test uses the impedance bridge to introduce pressure stimuli to the external ear canal while the patient is standing on a computerized dynamic moving platform. A positive response occurs when the patient sways or when balance is perturbed in response to external auditory canal pressure changes. In either type of test, a subjectively positive response occurs if the pressure stimulus induces unsolicited complaints of nausea and/or vertigo, or if the patient's PLF symptoms are reproduced by changing external canal pressures.

The CDP fistula test is both sensitive and specific for the presumptive diagnosis of PLF. When combined with history and physical findings, a positive CDP fistula test finding in the suspect ear(s) greatly increases the probability of demonstrating a PLF at surgery. In at least 88 percent of our patients, a positive CDP fistula test response correlated with positive findings of PLF at tympanotomy. Tympanometric fistula tests, with observation for nystagmus, have low rates of sensitivity and specificity, and consequently are rarely of diagnostic assistance.

Vestibular function loss sometimes occurs in patients who have persistent PLFs. Subjects who have a unilateral or bilateral loss of vestibular function show abnormal vestibulo-ocular reflex (VOR) responses to rotation testing (phase advance, reduced time constant, and low or low-normal vestibulo-ocular gain constant), and may also show caloric abnormalities if the low frequencies of vestibular function are involved. In addition, CDP may show a "vestibular deficient" (5 to 6) SOT pattern after PLF repair, particularly if the patient has suffered loss of vestibular hair cell function.

■ TREATMENT CONSIDERATIONS

Aspects of Disease Severity Affecting Outcome

Perilymphatic fistulas may occur in one ear or (in 40 percent of patients) both ears. Head trauma patients are the most likely to have bilateral PLFs. However, because the symptoms in the most symptomatic ear dominate the clinical picture, the inexperienced clinician may assume that there is only unilateral involvement. Bilateral PLFs should be considered in the diagnosis of patients who have complaints of fullness, tinnitus, and subjective or objective hearing loss in both ears. Patients who have bilateral PLFs are generally "sicker" than those who have PLFs in one ear. When considering which ear to explore surgically in a patient suspected of having bilateral PLFs, the surgeon must determine which ear is the most troublesome to the patient. The patient's complaints and the presence or absence of objective hearing loss or other objective findings will assist in making this critical decision. In our experience, most patients who have bilateral PLFs identify the more problematic ear without prompting.

When to Treat

All patients who have clinically suspected PLF should receive immediate treatment. Early diagnosis and treatment improve outcome and quality of life and help to avoid the development or progression of complications. Approximately 80 percent to 85 percent of patients with suspected PLFs respond to conservative treatment (modified bed rest and/or activity restriction). Many PLF patients whose diagnosis and management has been delayed often end up disabled, unemployed, and on public assistance because of irreversible complications, even with successful PLF closure. Many, if not most, of these PLF patients have been misdiagnosed as having mental problems, "cervical vertigo," or other problems as the source of their symptoms, or have been falsely accused of "malingering." It is not uncommon to see a secondary or "reactive" depression in these patients as a result of life-style changes superimposed on disabling vestibular symptoms and compounded by delays in management, particularly as imposed by the current health care system.

Effects of Patient Condition and Age

Although we have not found age to be directly related to any outcome parameter, certain issues may warrant special consideration. We have successfully treated PLF patients of all ages, from infants through the elderly. Successful closure of PLF in an infant or young child requires continuous attention to activity restriction, particularly after surgical closure. Successful closure in toddlers and young children may require a brief interval of mild sedation, in addition to close activity supervision. Elderly patients often have systemic medical conditions that may affect general health, wound healing, or compensation for vestibular deficits or vestibular asymmetry, for example, diabetes mellitus, peripheral vascular or cerebrovascular disease, osteoarthritis, vision deficiencies, poor nutritional status, and peripheral neuropathies. Patients of all ages who have long-term inner ear disease and chronic nausea may develop poor eating habits and consequently may develop nutritional deficiencies. A pretreatment regimen of vitamin and mineral supplements is recommended for these patients.

The condition of the ossicles and temporal bone must be considered. Of particular concern are ossicular discontinuities and/or stapes fractures, which are frequently encountered in head trauma patients, and which will complicate oval window PLF closure. It is often difficult to close an oval window fistula when a stapes footplate fracture is present, although fistula closure should be attempted initially without stapedectomy if the footplate fragments can be placed in normal position. In case of failure to close after an initial attempt, stapedectomy should be performed, and a tissue (preferably vein or fascia) graft should be placed under a stable stapes prosthesis at revision.

Two of the most important socioeconomic factors related to outcome of PLF management regimens (conservative or surgical) are (1) the presence of an adequate support system at home, and (2) a source of interval income. Many, if not most, PLF patients are unable to work during their treatment. Activity levels may be restricted for relatively long periods, making it impossible for PLF patients to participate in activities of daily living, care for children, or work outside the home. Unless these obstacles can be dealt with, even the best medical care may fail. These factors have proved to be so important that our treatment plan includes pretreatment counseling and social service referrals to increase the probability that the proper support network has been established before conservative treatment begins or surgery is performed.

Type of Treatment: The ABCs

Table 1 describes the management of perilymphatic fistula. The primary goal of conservative PLF therapy is to minimize pressure changes across the PLFs. Because most PLF patients respond well to conservative therapy (physical activity restriction and/or bed rest), conservative treatment should be attempted first, unless a progressive, sensorineural hearing loss develops. Several weeks of physical activity restriction and/or bed rest may be required in order to achieve PLF

Table 1. The ABCS of Perilymphatic Fistula Management

A	Activity restriction	Avoid physical exertion and strenous physical activity, e.g., heavy lifting, Valsalva's maneuver, and so forth—any activity associated with increased intracranial pressure Helpful medications: stool softeners, nausea medication Most sensitive tests for change in function: audiometry (pure-tone and speech), CDP
B	Bed rest	Three to 6 weeks best rest with head elevated at 30 to 45 degrees Before beginning bed rest, support system in place to help with housework, child care, errands, and so forth Helpful medications: stool softeners, nausea medication, vitamins, and so forth Audiometric monitoring
C	Carbogen	If hearing loss develops, 24–48 hours strict bed rest, OR carbogen treatment (hospitalization for hourly treatments of 95 percent O_2, 5 percent CO_2, for 24 to 48 hours), in association with bed rest Audiometric monitoring every 1 to 2 days until stable
S	Surgery: Tympanotomy and closure of PLFs	Before surgery, support system must be in place to help with housework, child care, errands, and so forth Surgery under local anesthesia with intravenous sedation (monitored anesthesia care) 1 to 2 day hospitalization Modified bed rest and/or activity restriction after discharge

PLF, perilymphatic fistula; CDP, computerized dynamic posturography.

closure. We have developed an incremental, six-stage system of physical activity, ranging from stage I (complete bed rest with bathroom and meal privileges) to stage VI (near-normal activity with avoidance of certain high-risk activities, such as contact sports, scuba diving, and so forth). This management paradigm is based on well-established principles of wound healing (Table 2).

Vestibular suppressants (e.g., meclizine) and antinausea drugs (e.g., promethazine) may help relieve symptoms of nausea and dizziness in certain patients, especially during the early stages of treatment. Stool softeners are given to all patients on bed rest or following PLF surgery, along with dietary instructions for avoiding constipation.

A secondary goal of PLF treatment, conservative or surgical, is to create a healthy internal environment to allow healing to take place. This means working with the patient to ensure optimal nutritional status, sufficient fluid intake, adequate sleep, and appropriate activity. We often recommend a multiple vitamin and mineral supplement, particularly when nausea limits food intake.

If hearing loss develops or progresses, and particularly if there is a sudden or precipitous loss of hearing, PLF treatment becomes emergent. This includes absolute bed rest and/or carbogen treatment in association with daily audiometric monitoring. Carbogen therapy (5 percent CO_2 and 95 percent O_2) is administered 15 minutes every hour, round-the-clock. If there is no hearing recovery after 48 to 72 hours, surgical exploration is offered to the patient. We have used carbogen successfully in many PLF patients who have sudden or progressive hearing loss. It has resulted in at least temporary improvement in virtually every patient, and in many patients it has stabilized hearing to the point where surgical intervention was not required.

Indications for Surgery

If conservative PLF treatment fails, or if hearing loss persists or worsens despite conservative treatment, tympanotomy should be considered. Because of the clinical variability (high interobserver variability) associated with visual identification of PLFs at tympanotomy, various perilymph "markers" have been evaluated toward the development of a diagnostic "gold standard." Fluorescein, injected intravenously, enters the perilymph and upon properly timed observation will reveal oval and round window perilymph leaks under fluorescent illumination at tympanotomy. Unfortunately, intravenous fluorescein may also enter the middle ear cavity upon disruption of the middle ear mucosa vasculature during surgical exposure, therefore limiting usefulness of this technique as a PLF marker. Beta-2 transferrin is a protein specific to CSF and perilymph. Detection of beta-2 transferrin in the middle ear, if there is certainty of no CSF contamination, confirms the presence of perilymph. But because analysis for beta-2 transferrin cannot be conducted in the operating room, this technique confirms PLF only in retrospect. Negative results do not rule out a PLF using either of these techniques. Concentrations of free amino acids have also been used to test middle ear aspirates and to differentiate between whole blood, serum and plasma, and perilymph. The reported sensitivity and specificity of these techniques are inconsistent, but for the present, they may support diagnosis of PLF if their findings are positive.

Argon laser-assisted PLF repair has been available since the 1980s. Advantages include a less traumatic middle ear dissection and a relatively atraumatic preparation of the graft bed. The laser can also be used to "weld" the graft and microfibrillar collagen stent over the tissue graft into place. Laser dissection combined with cryoprecipitated fibrinogen "glue" (Table 3) to bind the areolar tissue graft has greatly decreased the incidence of PLF surgical recurrence.

Careful attention to technique is critical for successful surgical closure of PLFs. After much experimentation with graft materials, we recommend tiny pledgets of postauricular areolar tissue as the tissue graft of choice. The best results are obtained if the graft tissue is impregnated with autologous cryoprecipitated fibrinogen (Table 3) and placed in layers in the oval and round window niche after laser vaporization or mechanical removal of the surrounding mucoperiosteum. Large, single-piece tissue grafts should be avoided because of the tendency to retract out of the oval or round window niche upon healing. Small, layered, multiple tissue grafts tend to contract into the niche during healing. The layered tissue graft is covered with microfibrillar (bovine) collagen and autologous cryoprecipitate, which provides support to the underlying tissue graft during the fibrous ingrowth phase of wound healing. This technique has greatly decreased the incidence of postoperativc PLF graft failure and has significantly reduced PLF recurrence rates.

We perform surgery on a 24 hour outpatient basis, usually discharging patients the morning following the operation. Before discharge, we obtain a vestibular physical therapy consultation, both to ensure that the patient can ambulate safely and to assist with instructing the patient and family in postoperative physical activity limitations. The postoperative PLF patient leaves the hospital with external canal packing and absorbable subcutaneous sutures in place. Packing removal is accomplished by a family member or friend 1 week postoperatively. During the first 6 weeks following operation, the patient must maintain strict, modified bed rest (stage 1; see Table 2). The typical PLF patient returns for follow-up office visits at 6 weeks, 3 months, 6 months, and 1 year following surgery.

If the patient has bilateral PLFs, and closure of the most symptomatic ear has been successfully accomplished, the unoperated ear usually becomes the more symptomatic ear during the postoperative period, or shortly after the patient resumes physical activity following bed rest. If surgery is to be performed on the second ear, it is important to wait at least 3 months between operations, if possible. In approximately 50 percent of patients, symptoms coming from PLFs in the unoperated ear subside during recovery from the operation on the most symptomatic ear. In the remainder of patients, an active PLF in the unoperated ear results in a "symptom shift" to the unoperated ear.

Risks of Treatment

There are three main risks associated with conservative treatment: (1) worsening of the PLF; (2) physical deconditioning associated with bed rest; and (3) development of, or deterioration in, comorbid conditions. Many PLF patients develop SEH. A secondary hydrops may worsen or may initially appear (become symptomatic) following conservative treatment or surgical PLF repair. Patients who have BPV often worsen as a consequence of bed rest. Canalith repositioning

Table 2. Levels of Activity Restriction

STAGE	I BED REST	II HOUSE REST	III INCREMENTAL ACTIVITY INCREASE	IV PROGRESSIVE ACTIVITY INCREASE	V NEAR-NORMAL ACTIVITY	VI NORMAL ACTIVITY
Activity Level	Strict bed rest with head elevated 30 degrees at all times Up for meals and BRP only (<1.5 hr/day) Do not leave house	Spend time sitting or reclining; head of bed elevated 30 degrees at all times Up and about *inside house* for up to 4 to 6 hrs/day Do not leave house	Up and around house; head of bed gradually lowered as tolerated Short walks outside Short car rides	Up and around, in and out of house at near-normal levels Walking good, no strenuous exercise Rest as needed	Fairly normal days Adequate sleep, and rest periods p.r.n.	Normal days Adequate sleep, and rest periods p.r.n.
PLF Precautions	Strict	Strict	Continue to follow "Gentle" sexual activity okay	Continue to follow as closely as possible	May lift to 25 lbs Avoid altitude change >1,500 ft No airplane travel, scuba, contact sports	May lift to 50 lb No scuba Avoid contact sports if possible Avoid airplane travel for at least 1 yr after PLF closure
Medications	Stool softener b.i.d. Multivitamin Nausea medications p.r.n.	(Same as stage 1)	Multivitamin	Multivitamin	Multivitamin	Multivitamin
Leisure	Simple activities that can be performed while reclining Adequate rest periods between activities Limit visitors	(Same as stage 1)	Trips to library, movies, friend's house, restaurant, and so forth	Simple activities and outings Longer walks, surface swimming, exercise bike Avoid weights, aerobics	Any activity that complies with fistula precautions	Unrestricted within aforementioned guidelines
Chores	None	Simple meal preparation, folding laundry, dusting, hand-washing dishes	Simple chores that meet fistula precautions No bending, straining, heavy lifting	Add more complex chores Avoid bending and heavy lifting	Any chores that meet fistula precautions Stay off ladders or heights (trees, roofs, and so forth)	Unrestricted within aforementioned guidelines
Work	No	No	Discuss with physician Part-time may be considered	Modified return to work Work evaluation may be required if changes needed	Normal schedule	Normal schedule
Driving*	No	No	Discuss with physician Daytime hours only, short distances, no traffic	Daytime hours only; avoid conditions of poor visibility or uncertain road surfaces	Unrestricted if symptom-free Do not drive if actively symptomatic	Unrestricted if symptom-free Do not drive if actively symptomatic
Help Needed	Full-time help needed for housework, child care, and so forth	4 to 6 hours daily help needed for housework, child care, and so forth	Help still needed with young children 1–2 hours help each day for heavier jobs, grocery shopping, and so forth	Varies; may need help only with heavy chores—furniture moving, mopping floors, yard work, and so forth	None	None

* An updated driver's test may be suggested in some cases.
BRP, bathroom privileges.

Table 3. Preparation of Graft Using Cryoprecipitated Fibrinogen Adhesive

Timing	Action
Blood bank, 24 (or more) hours before surgery	Patient's blood is used to prepare sterile autologous cryoprecipitated fibrinogen (CF). Blood bank is kept informed of surgery schedule and thaws CF at the proper time.
Immediately before surgery	CF is transferred, on ice, to the operating room.
In operating room, before grafting	Surgeon harvests graft material, and assistant divides it into two portions of multiple small pledgets. Avitene (microfibrillar bovine collagen) is divided into two portions of multiple small pledgets.
Minutes before grafting (while surgeon obtains exposure)	CF is mixed with 10 percent $CaCl_2$ and used to saturate one portion of graft material and one portion of Avitene. α-amino caproic acid (Amicar 250 mg/dL) is mixed with bovine thrombin and used to saturate the other portion of graft material and the other portion of Avitene.
At time of grafting	Graft material from CF and Amicar portions is applied alternately to the graft site. Avitene from CF and Amicar portions are applied alternately over the tissue graft material. A coagulant forms, buttressing the site. Laser may be used to "weld" the tissue graft and coagulate the Avitene.

From Black FO, Pesznecker SC, Norton TL, et al. Surgical management of perilymph fistulas: A new technique. Arch Otolaryngol Head Neck Surg 1991; 117:641–648; with permission.

procedures are generally contraindicated in PLF patients until successful, permanent PLF closure has been accomplished.

In the hands of a properly trained, experienced otologist, risks of exploratory tympanotomy are minimal. The most serious risk of tympanotomy, for any indication, is complete sensorineural hearing loss. This complication is extremely unusual, but the potential risks must be explained to the patient. Besides hearing loss, other risks involve damage to the chorda tympani nerve, and rarely, the facial nerve itself. Occasionally, a perforated tympanic membrane and/or otitis media complicates tympanotomy.

Vertigo, ataxia, and tinnitus may worsen after tympanotomy for repair of PLFs. None of our patients have experienced a permanent facial palsy following tympanotomy for PLF repair, although transient, local anesthetic-induced facial palsies in patients who have congenitally dehiscent facial nerves have occurred.

Pitfalls

Persistence of vestibular symptoms following PLF repair does not necessarily indicate a failed closure or a recurrent PLF. The most common cause of persistent symptoms is a PLF in the unoperated ear. Another frequent cause of a "poor result" in PLF management is the failure to recognize a comorbid condition in the same or opposite ear. For example, after an apparently successful surgical PLF repair, the patient may begin resuming activity and find that he or she is troubled with positional vertigo. If the preoperative baseline testing showed a positive Cawthorne-Hallpike test result, the clinician can safely attribute the symptoms to a BPV that has decompensated during the inactivity of postoperative bed rest. After the PLF has healed, the physician can institute an appropriate treatment plan. In another instance, preoperative and postoperative VOR testing may show asymmetric responses between the two ears; in this case, the clinician can anticipate the eventual need for vestibular protocol physical therapy. Tinnitus, aural fullness, and "soft" vestibular symptoms may suggest an SEH; in our patients, many postclosure SEHs resolve within 12 to 18 months postoperatively.

Another cause of treatment failure is PLF recurrence. In our experience, it is critical that patients observe strict "fistula precautions" following spontaneous or surgical PLF closure (Table 4). These include avoidance of Valsalva's maneuvers (any activity known to increase intracranial pressure), avoidance of rapid altitude changes greater than 300 to 500 feet (at sea level), and maintaining the head above the level of the heart at all times. These precautions must often be strictly adhered to for 3 to 6 months after surgery, followed by avoidance of activities that produce symptoms for at least 1 year following initiation of conservative management or surgery, in order to maximize achievement of a stable PLF closure. Again, these therapeutic guidelines were developed on the basis of well-established principles of wound healing.

A surprisingly frequent cause of "spontaneous" PLF recurrence is unrecognized obstructive sleep apnea (OSA). Consequently, it is very important to query about the symptoms of OSA before institution of PLF management. If symptoms of OSA are present, the patient should be referred for appropriate sleep studies and treatment before attempting management of PLFs.

Our experience suggests that other types of sleep disturbances, including restless legs syndrome, early wakening, delayed sleep onset, patterns of insomnia, and disturbances in REM sleep, are extremely common in patients who have all types of vestibular disorders, including PLF. Fatigue will complicate management of any vestibular disorder and will interfere with both adaptation and compensation. Patients who have sleep dysfunction may benefit greatly from referral to a sleep disorders program.

Table 4. Abbreviated Perilymphatic Fistula Precautions

AVOID ANY ACTIVITY THAT PRODUCES OR INCREASES SYMPTOMS

For example, avoid the following:
- Strenuous activity, e.g., exercise, housework, yard work, sexual activity.
- Activities associated with Valsalva's maneuver, e.g., lifting over 5 lb, straining (as in having a bowel movement), coughing and sneezing, nose blowing, shouting, singing, bending, squatting, unscrewing tightly sealed jars, throwing objects, and so forth.
- Sharp, jerking motions of the head and neck.
- Significant air pressure changes, including:
  - Airplane travel (for 1 year following successful closure; may not travel if otitis media or upper respiratory infection present).
  - Any travel exceeding 500 ft elevation change from baseline.

Modifications to the daily routine:
- Keep head elevated above 20 to 30 degrees at all times, including while sleeping. *Do not lie flat.*
- When sitting up from bed, roll to one side first and push yourself up slowly with your arms. Do not do a sit-up using abdominal muscles.
- Do not bend over so that your head is below the level of your heart, e.g., when putting on or tying shoes.
- When coughing or sneezing, do so as gently as possible, with mouth held wide open.
- Do not hold your nose and "pop" your ears!
- Do not yell or sing.
- Do not drink from a straw or suction device.
- Do not climb on chairs, ladders, or other heights from which you might lose your balance and fall.

Notify physician if:
- You experience a sudden drop in hearing that persists for longer than an hour.
- You experience a sudden worsening of dizziness symptoms that persists for longer than a few hours.
- You experience the onset of severe nausea and/or vomiting.
- You develop a "cold" or "flu," and over-the-counter medications do not control your symptoms.
- You develop a temperature elevation above 100° F.

The longer the interval between the onset of PLFs and their treatment, the more difficult it will be to secure a lasting closure and the greater the chance of recurrence, even with minimal exertion. For most PLF patients, the investment of time and need to comply rigorously with the treatment plan may seem daunting; much support is needed to assist the PLF patient in seeing the long-term result and its benefits. Without full compliance with the PLF treatment regimen, risk of PLF treatment failure or recurrence increases.

Recognition and Treatment of Complications

We monitor vestibular and auditory function at baseline (before treatment) and, depending on symptoms, at regular intervals (e.g., 6 weeks, 3 months, 6 months, and 1 year) after treatment is initiated. PLF patients are instructed to immediately report hearing loss or any acute change in vestibular symptoms.

The potential of a postoperative otitis or meningitis is reduced by the prophylactic use of a broad-spectrum antibiotic following surgery and by careful instruction regarding aural hygiene and wound care.

Results of PLF Management

We consider PLF treatment to be successful when symptoms are eliminated or brought under control (to a level acceptable to the patient), when the patient is able to tolerate exertion and external pressure changes without exacerbation of symptoms, and when the patient is able to resume normal activities of daily living and/or return to school or work. In our hands, 80 percent or more of PLF patients reach this level of improvement following conservative or surgical treatment. Another 10 percent report symptomatic improvement but are unable to return to activities of daily living. Fewer than 10 percent are "worse" or "unchanged," and the majority of these patients have associated comorbid conditions (BPV, hydrops), bilateral PLFs, or underlying systemic problems that were present before conservative or surgical treatment.

Most PLF patients experience onset or exacerbation of motion sickness. It is interesting that following successful PLF closure, virtually all of the affected patients report resolution or marked improvement of their motion sickness symptoms.

Suggested Reading

Black FO, Lilly DJ, Nashner LM, et al. Quantitative diagnostic test for perilymph fistula. Otolaryngol Head Neck Surg 1987; 96:125-134.

Black FO, Pesznecker SC, Norton TL, et al. Surgical management of perilymph fistulas: A new technique. Arch Otolaryngol Head Neck Surg 1991; 117:641-648.

Cole GG. Validity of spontaneous perilymphatic fistula. Am J Otol 1995; 16:815-819.

Glasscock ME, Hart MJ, Rosdeutscher JD. Traumatic perilymphatic fistula: How long can symptoms persist? Am J Otol 1992; 13:333-338.

Goodhill V. Leaking labyrinthine lesions, deafness, tinnitus, and dizziness. Ann Otol 1981; 90:99-106.

Grimm RG, Hemenway WG, LeBray PR, Black FO. The perilymph fistula syndrome defined in mild head trauma, Acta Otolaryngol 1989 (Suppl) 464:5-40.

Healy GB, Friedman JM, DiTroia J. Ataxia and hearing loss secondary to perilymphatic fistula. Pediatrics 1978; 61:238-241.

Kohut RI, Hinojosa R, Thompson JN, Ryu JH. Idiopathic perilymphatic fistulas. Arch Otolaryngol Head Neck Surg 1995; 121:412-471.

Parell GJ, Becker GD. Inner ear barotrauma in SCUBA divers. Arch Otolaryngol Head Neck Surg 1993; 119:455-457.

Strohm M. Traumatic lesions of the round window membrane and perilymphatic fistulae. Adv Otol Rhinol Laryngol 1986; 35:177-247.

Woodson BT, Fujita S, Mawhinney TD, et al. Perilymphatic fistula: Analysis of free amino acids in middle ear microaspirates. Otolaryngol Head Neck Surg 1991; 104:796-802.

MENIERE'S DISEASE: MEDICAL THERAPY

The method of
Bruce J. Gantz
by
Bruce J. Gantz
Paul W. Gidley

The complaint of "dizziness" can be most confusing and discouraging. Much of the confusion arises from the fact that dizziness is a vague symptom with multiple individual interpretations. It is important that a detailed and focused patient history be obtained. This fact is particularly important for patients who have Meniere's disease, because subjective historical information usually provides more information regarding the diagnosis of the disease than does objective laboratory testing.

■ CLINICAL EVALUATION

Meniere's disease is characterized by episodic vertigo, fluctuating hearing loss, fluctuating tinnitus, and aural fullness. The spells of vertigo are spontaneous episodes of a sense of motion that are unprovoked, intermittent, and, often, prostrating. Nystagmus (horizontal or horizontal rotatory) always accompanies the vertigo. It is not uncommon for the patient to describe a sense of aural pressure, increasing tinnitus, and reduced hearing in one ear before the onset of the vertiginous episode. Rotational vertigo is usually described, but a sense of falling or other movement may occur. Characteristically, the vertigo lasts at least 20 minutes and abates by 24 hours. A 30 second spell of vertigo, or one that lasts for days, is not Meniere's disease. Variations of the intensity of symptoms occur among patients and among spells in a given patient. Nausea is quite common during the vertiginous episode and may be severe enough to induce vomiting. Movement during the attack worsens the symptoms. A typical history includes the fact that during the vertigo the patient does not want to move and cannot ambulate to the bathroom. This feature is helpful in differentiating the intensity of the spell from more vague spells of dysequilibrium or central causes of vertigo. Following the vertigo, patients can usually continue their daily activities without residual symptoms. A rare symptom of drop attacks of Tumarkin have been described. Patients describe spontaneous, unprovoked spells of falling to the ground without loss of consciousness. These rare occurrences are thought to be related to aberrant discharges down the spinal motor neural tracts. Meniere's disease patients do not complain of headaches, dysequilibrium, incontinence, or syncope during their attacks.

The auditory symptoms of Meniere's disease include hearing loss, fluctuating tinnitus, and a sense of aural fullness. These symptoms can fluctuate independent of the vertigo, but usually intensify before the onset of vertigo. Early in the disease, after a spell of vertigo, it is common for hearing to improve, tinnitus to decrease, and aural fullness to resolve. Pure-tone audiograms usually demonstrate low-frequency neurosensory hearing loss when symptoms are present, but normal hearing levels between episodes are not uncommon early in the disease. Flat audiometric curves, as well as high-frequency loss, have also been described. Serial audiograms should be obtained to document the fluctuating hearing patterns. As the disease continues, the entire hearing spectrum can be affected, and permanent hearing loss can occur. Discrimination scores usually parallel the hearing loss. It is suspected that hearing worsens with increasing frequency and intensity of the vertiginous spells, but hearing can continue to deteriorate when the attacks are controlled medically or surgically. Special audiometric testing will demonstrate recruitment. Typically, we do not place a label of Meniere's disease on a patient until the changing hearing pattern is documented. The aural symptoms are usually isolated to one ear, but may become bilateral over time. The rate of bilateral disease has been stated to occur in 5 percent to 50 percent of patients. In our series at the University of Iowa College of Medicine, only 2 percent of patients displayed bilateral symptoms while they were followed up for 15 years.

Two variants of Meniere's disease have been described. Cochlear Meniere's disease is characterized by fluctuating cochlear hearing loss, tinnitus, and aural fullness. Spells of vertigo are absent. Vestibular Meniere's disease similarly consists of typical Meniere's spells of vertigo without aural symptoms. Initially, some patient experience isolated vestibular or aural symptoms, but these symptoms evolve into a classic Meniere's pattern with time. The variants usually respond to medical management. If no alteration of symptoms occurs with treatment, the original diagnosis should be considered suspect.

Detailed present and past medical histories should search for details to identify evidence of stroke, diabetes, hypertension, migraine headaches, epilepsy, or other neurologic diseases. Other peripheral causes of vertigo, such as motion sickness, benign paroxysmal positional vertigo, vestibular neuritis, labyrinthitis, perilymphatic fistula, and cerebellopontine angle tumor, must be differentiated from Meniere's disease.

The physical examination is usually normal in patients who have Meniere's disease; however, a detailed head and neck and neurotologic examination is important to exclude other possible etiologies that might account for the patient's symptoms. The neurotologic examination includes careful scrutiny of the tympanic membrane and middle ear. A pneumatic aural speculum (fistula test) should be used to observe tympanic membrane movement and determine if positive or negative pressure reproduces either vertigo or the patient's symptoms. Visual observation for nystagmus with pressure change during the fistula test suggests an inner ear pathology such as perilymphatic fistula, circumscribed labyrinthitis, or neural syphilis. Rinne and Weber tuning fork tests are used to confirm audiometric findings. A careful cranial nerve check, including a corneal reflex test, is performed along with general neurologic testing that includes gait, quick turning to each side, tandem gait, Romberg's test, finger-to-nose testing, pointing tests, heel-to-shin cerebellar tests, general motor strength, and sensory testing. A Hallpike maneuver with Fresnel lens must be included to rule out positional vertigo. Auscultation of the neck should be done along the course of the carotid arteries from the subclavian artery to the skull base. Bruits of the skull may be present over the mastoid and through the orbital fissures to the eyes and squamous portion of the temporal bone. If pulsatile tinnitus is described, a double-headed stethoscope is used to determine the presence of objective tinnitus, which would be suggestive of a vascular tumor or arteriovenous malformation.

Laboratory testing for the evaluation of the dizzy patient can be quite extensive and expensive. The minimal baseline tests should include an audiogram with pure-tone and speech discrimination tests, acoustic reflex decay, and an electronystagmogram. Imaging studies, such as magnetic resonance imaging with contrast or high-resolution computed tomographic scans, should be obtained only if symptoms warrant evaluation. Venereal Disease Research Laboratory and fluorescent treponemal antibody should be obtained in cases of bilateral symptoms. Other hematologic studies are obtained in selected instances. In our clinic, the electronystagmogram (ENG) is obtained before the detailed history. Caloric tests provide an excellent demonstration of a peripheral vestibular disorder, and they are a reference against which patients can compare their symptoms. If their dizziness is unlike that of the caloric stimulation, it is likely that a peripheral vestibular disorder is not the cause of their symptoms. Many patients with Meniere's disease will have symmetric caloric responses and an otherwise normal ENG. Some patients will have unilateral caloric weakness. Positional test results will be normal, along with no evidence of spontaneous or latent nystagmus.

Several other tests have been described in the literature to help differentiate Meniere's disease from other disorders causing dizziness. For decades, the glycerol dehydrating test was used to determine if hearing improved with rapid diuresis. We currently do not use this test because of unrewarding results. More recently, electrocochleography has been touted as a means of diagnosing Meniere's disease. Various authors report different criteria for a significant summating potential to action potential ratio. However, in a study performed here, the ratio was not significantly different between normal subjects and Meniere's disease patients. Therefore, we do not use electrocochleography to diagnose Meniere's syndrome.

The pathophysiology of Meniere's disease remains obscure. Inflammatory changes within the inner ear have been described, but their etiology is unknown. A characteristic histopathologic pattern in temporal bones from patients who have Meniere's disease demonstrates endolymphatic hydrops with bulging of both Reissner's membrane and otolithic membranes.

■ THERAPY

The medical management of Meniere's disease is based on theoretic pathophysiologic mechanisms that are thought to induce endolymphatic hydrops. The mainstay of the treatment is observing a low-sodium diet (1,500 mg per day for the average-weight patient) and using a thiazide diuretic. We counsel patients on dietary habits and provide a sodium content food guide. A combination thiazide and triamterene medication such as Dyazide has the added benefit of potassium sparing and is prescribed one two times per day. Patients are instructed to increase their intake of potassium-rich foods such as bananas and orange juice. Potassium levels are obtained at the first 3 month follow-up visit. Direct vestibular suppressants such as diazepam (Valium) can be of limited benefit for severe spells of vertigo, but these agents should not be prescribed for daily use because of their highly addictive nature. Other drugs such as nicotinic acid are not used. In a few instances, high-dose steroids have been found to be helpful in patients experiencing repeated spells and significant drops in hearing. In these instances, a 2 week burst of 60 to 80 mg (1 mg per kilogram per day) of prednisone has been of anecdotal benefit. No long-term prospective clinical trial using prednisone for treatment of Meniere's disease has been published. Meclizine (Antivert) is a common drug prescribed for patients who have complaints of dizziness. This medication may be useful in treating motion intolerance, but it should not be used chronically for most peripheral vestibular disorders. Long-term use of meclizine may prevent vestibular compensation and should be eliminated in Meniere's disease patients.

This medical regimen controls the spells of vertigo in more than two-thirds of patients who exhibit symptoms of Meniere's disease, as previously described. Almost all patients who have Meniere's disease experience some alteration and improvement of their symptoms with the medical regimen. If there is absolutely no alteration of symptoms with strict sodium regulation and the use of a thiazide diuretic, the diagnosis of Meniere's disease should be questioned. Other indications that the symptoms may not be due to Meniere's disease include daily spells of vertigo and bilateral aural symptoms on presentation. If the latter symptoms are present, neural syphilis or autoimmune inner ear disease must be excluded.

Failure to control spells of vertigo is considered a medical management failure. The critical defining point of failure of medical management must be individualized. In these cases, a surgical management strategy or chemical ablation procedure is adopted. Surgical options include an endolymphatic shunt, destructive labyrinthectomy, or vestibular nerve section. A review of our experience at the University of Iowa reveals that 84 percent (N = 286) of patients who experienced medical failure for treatment of Meniere's disease had their spells of vertigo controlled with an endolymphatic shunt procedure. Significant hearing loss occurred in 1 percent of patients who underwent the shunt procedure. Failures were controlled with a middle fossa vestibular nerve section. Recently, intratympanic gentamicin injections have gained popularity for managing Meniere's disease medical failures. Early reports have documented up to 40 percent hearing loss with this regimen. Weekly injections may reduce hearing loss. Long-term trials may define the limits of these chemical ablative techniques.

Suggested Reading

Campbell K, Harker L, Abbas P. Interpretation of electrocochleography in Meniere's disease and normal subjects. Ann Otol Rhinol Laryngol 1992; 101:496-500.

MENIERE'S DISEASE: SURGICAL THERAPY

The method of
Jack M. Kartush
by
Micheal J. Larouere
Jack M. Kartush

The treatment of Meniere's disease (MD) unresponsive to medical therapy remains controversial. When serviceable hearing is present, options include endolymphatic sac (ELS) surgery, vestibular neurectomy, and aminoglycoside treatment.

For years, sac surgery was considered the best initial treatment because it is the only nondestructive option. Scores of papers have been published attesting to the safety and efficacy of ELS surgery, although the average reported vertigo control rates varied widely between 60 percent and 80 percent.

Vestibular neurectomy via middle fossa craniectomy was shown to demonstrate superior control of vertigo in the 1980s. Technical difficulties and surgical complications forestalled widespread use of neurectomy until Silverstein and others refocused attention on the generally safer posterior fossa approach.

Nonetheless, due to the greater risks associated with a craniotomy, most otologists continued to offer their patients a choice between sac and neurectomy surgery, particularly early in the course of the disease.

However, a "paradigm shift" in thought occurred in the 1980s after publication of two papers that convinced many casual readers to conclude that ELS surgery was an outdated, ineffective procedure: (1) Thomsen and co-workers, 1981, and (2) Glasscock and co-workers, 1989. (See Suggested Reading at the end of this chapter for a complete listing.)

Although we will publish an in-depth analysis of the literature disputing this conclusion elsewhere, the present discussion focuses on why most otologists continue to offer ELS surgery as a low-risk procedure that controls vertigo for the majority of patients.

■ ABLATIVE THERAPY: THE CLINICIAN'S DILEMMA

Medical therapy, including diet and diuretics, is effective for most patients. For those patients with serviceable hearing who fail medical therapy, surgical options fall within two categories: enhancement versus ablation. The literature clearly shows that surgical and chemical ablation of the vestibular system have a higher vertigo control rate than does ELS surgery. Therefore, is there ever justification for choosing a treatment with a lesser success rate?

Absolutely. Whenever an ideal treatment (low risk–high success) does not exist, patients typically choose low risk–low success options unless the severity of a disease forces them to choose a high risk–high success therapy. Examples abound, such as diet and exercise versus coronary artery bypass surgery. Physicians must keep in mind that low risks and rapid recovery are important factors to patients. Most persons will choose to follow a serial path of increasing risk as long as they "burn no bridges" along the way.

Ablative procedures carry a higher rate of hearing loss and postoperative dysequilibrium compared with sac surgery (Table 1). In addition, any destructive procedure increases a Meniere's patient's risks due to the possibility of contralateral disease. Neither vestibular neurectomy nor transtympanic gentamicin is recommended for patients who present with either bilateral disease or an only-hearing ear. Most studies predict that one-third of Meniere's disease patients will develop contralateral disease. Destructive procedures (and craniotomies) are not as well tolerated in the elderly.

Vestibular Neurectomy

Vestibular nerve section (VNS) cures or significantly controls vertigo in 95 percent of Meniere's disease patients, but it subjects patients to the risks of a craniotomy, that is, death, stroke, seizure, cerebrospinal fluid leak, cranial neuropathies, and meningitis. (The first histologic specimens by which Hallpike and Cairns demonstrated endolymphatic hydrops came from two patients who died following neurectomy.) Middle fossa VNS has largely been abandoned because of greater risks to the cochlear and facial nerves as well as difficulty in reliably sectioning the inferior vestibular nerve. Posterior fossa VNS allows superior exposure, but because the cleavage plane between vestibular and cochlear nerves is anatomically ambiguous at this more proximal level, residual vestibular fibers may remain. Drilling out the porus acusticus improves the ability to attain a more complete neurectomy, but worsens the risk of severe disabling headaches.

Although surgeons focus on the high cure rate of vertigo, patient surveys reveal a significant incidence of postoperative dysequilibrium. More than 62 percent of the patients of Kemink and co-workers complained that their balance was worse after surgery. Postneurectomy imbalance is usually mild, but 26 percent of the patients of McElveen and co-workers complained that their disability was worse after surgery. Dysequilibrium and light-headedness can be disabling, particularly to laborers, pilots, school bus and truck drivers, and others. Furthermore, VNS has the longest period of postoperative recovery before patients can safely return to work and driving.

The risk of profound hearing loss following vestibular neurectomy at experienced centers is small, but the review of Nguyen and co-workers revealed that 38 percent of their 112 patients had a sensorineural hearing loss (SNHL) greater than 10 dB.

Table 1. Results of Treatment of Meniere's Disease with 2 Year Follow-Up

	SAC-VEIN DECOMPRESSION (MICHIGAN EAR INSTITUTE) (%)	VESTIBULAR NEURECTOMY (HOUSE EAR INSTITUTE) (%)	GENTAMICIN (UNIVERSITY OF TORONTO) (%)
VERTIGO CONTROL			
Complete	59	82	83
Substantial	41	11	17
Insignificant	—	6	—
Worse	—	1	—
HEARING			
Improved	59	6	30
Same	23	56	43
Worse	18	38	27
DISABILITY			
None	81	78	86
Mild	14	17	7
Severe	5	5	7
DYSEQUILIBRIUM			
Worse postop	0	11	7

Chemical Ablation

Chemical vestibular ablation has recently generated considerable interest. Gentamicin and streptomycin, however, have been tried in various protocols since Fowler's description nearly 50 years ago, but an unacceptably high incidence of hearing loss and dysequilibrium precluded the routine use of these two drugs.

To reduce the side effects of high-dose intramuscular streptomycin, Graham and associates and Silverstein and co-workers independently suggested lower dose "titration" therapy for bilateral disease. The use of transtympanic aminoglycosides for treating unilateral Meniere's disease seems to be taking a parallel course: beginning with Schuknecht's original description using high-dose streptomycin in 1956, Magnusson and Padoan subsequently suggested low-dose transtympanic gentamicin. The recent protocols are of interest, but enthusiasm should be tempered until further results become available. Streptomycin perfusion of the horizontal semicircular canal was recently touted as the "cure for Meniere's disease," but has since been abandoned due to the high risk of SNHL.

Nedzelski and associates promoted a uniform "shotgun" approach for chemical ablation. Patients are hospitalized, and catheters are sutured to the ear to deliver intratympanic gentamicin via myringotomy. Vertigo control is very high, but 27 percent of patients incurred a significant SNHL. Of greater concern is that 10 percent of patients develop profound deafness immediately after therapy. Complete abolition of caloric responses was observed in half of these researchers' patients. This subset had 100 percent control of vertigo, but they also had a 20 percent chance of profound deafness. In contrast, patients with persistent caloric response were never totally deafened, but vertigo recurred in more than 20 percent. These statistics reveal a significantly higher risk of hearing loss than either sac decompression or neurectomy.

Thus, with chemical ablation, there appears to be a trade-off: high doses improve vertigo control at the risk of increasing SNHL. Low-dose titration protocols currently being investigated will likely incur a higher recurrence rate and a lower control rate. Yet this protocol may still lead to a certain risk of profound hearing loss for those patients with "idiosyncratic" reactions to aminoglycosides. The latter may be due to unpredictable variations in (1) genetic susceptibility to aminoglycosides at a molecular level, (2) round window perfusion, or (3) eustachian tube function (i.e., how much gentamicin stays within the middle ear and for how long).

Although chemical vestibular ablation is clearly promising, it must be acknowledged that it is still an investigational procedure; the ideal drug, dosage, and means of delivery have yet to be determined.

■ ENHANCEMENT SURGERY

Georges Portmann described incision of the ELS in 1926. Sac surgery is the only enhancement procedure in current use. Other attempts at enhancement (e.g., Cody tack and cochleosacculostomy) have been abandoned due to inadequate efficacy and an unacceptably high incidence of hearing loss. The great variance in reported vertigo control rates may be due to a number of factors: (1) completeness of sac-dura-vein decompression, (2) operating at different stages of the disease, and (3) operating on different diseases (i.e., Meniere's disease is a *syndrome* that may have many different causes).

To Shunt or Not to Shunt

In the same year in which Portmann described ELS surgery, George Shambaugh questioned how a small incision could stay open. Portmann replied that he did not know, but "only knew the result," which was the first nonablative control of vertigo. Since that time, many variations of the procedure have been tried, including subarachnoid shunts, mastoid shunts, and simple decompression.

Brackmann has performed more than 500 sac operations. He initially shunted the sac into the subarachnoid space, but now only shunts into the mastoid because he found identical efficacy and fewer complications with the mastoid shunt. With the latter, he reported a 1 percent risk of profound hearing loss and attributes this to opening the sac rather than inadvertent injury to the labyrinth.

Our own experience and that of most of the literature (e.g., Shambaugh as early as 1966) indicates no significant benefit to shunts over wide decompression. Furthermore, by not opening the sac, we have had no case of profound hearing loss.

Sac-Vein Decompression

Anatomic Anomalies in Meniere's Disease

The sigmoid sinus in Meniere's disease patients is typically in an abnormal anterior location within the mastoid. Because of this anatomic anomaly, we often removed the bone from the sigmoid sinus and posterior cranial fossa to assure adequate exposure of the endolymphatic sac. When anatomic constraints occasionally made sac exposure impossible, we found that shrinkage of the sigmoid sinus allowed us total sac exposure and decompression in every case (Fig. 1). This is accomplished using bipolar electrocautery parallel to the sinus surface at very low settings. Only a 15 percent reduction in size is typically needed. Silastic sheeting is usually placed over the exposed dura and sinus to prevent adhesions, which reduces postoperative soft-tissue retraction and pulsatile tinnitus.

Sac-Vein Decompression

From a retrospective review of our earlier sac decompressions, one of us (JK) observed improved benefit when the sigmoid sinus was included in the decompression, particularly when it was anteriorly displaced. Consequently, we altered our surgical technique to include routine decompression of the sigmoid sinus as well as the posterior fossa dura and sac, that is, "sac-vein decompression."

Results

A subsequent prospective study was designed to assess this technique. Gianoli and co-workers reviewed 35 patients who underwent sac-vein decompression and had at least 2 years of follow-up to comply with the 1985 AAO–HNS reported guidelines. Vestibular symptom severity was resolved or mild in 92 percent, and disability severity was mild or none in 95 percent of patients at 2 years after surgery. Vertigo control was complete or substantial in 85 percent and 100 percent of patients at 1 and 2 years postoperatively. Audiologic data showed stable or improved hearing in 86 percent and 85 percent of patients at 1 and 2 years postoperatively. Thus, our ELS results significantly improved using this technique.

ELS surgery has the lowest risk of hearing loss (especially if the sac is not opened) and the greatest chance of hearing stabilization or improvement. As Table 1 shows, our 1997 study of sac-vein decompression demonstrated hearing improvement in 59 percent of patients versus only 6 percent of VNS patients in Nguyen's House Ear Institute study.

Mechanism of ELS Surgery

Although many publications attest to the safety and efficacy of sac surgery, the mechanism of its effect is unknown. Some clinicians have cast a skeptical eye on whether ELS surgery might only be a placebo given the similarity of results with and without shunting. We believe this skepticism *is* warranted. However, our conclusion is not that ELS surgery is a placebo but that (1) there is no significant benefit of shunting over decompression, and (2) there is a nonspecific effect related to the mastoidectomy.

We cannot accept the most simplistic mechanisms of action, that is, "opening the sac allows continuous drainage of perilymph to relieve intralabyrinthine pressure." Like Shambaugh in 1927, we find it difficult to believe that any

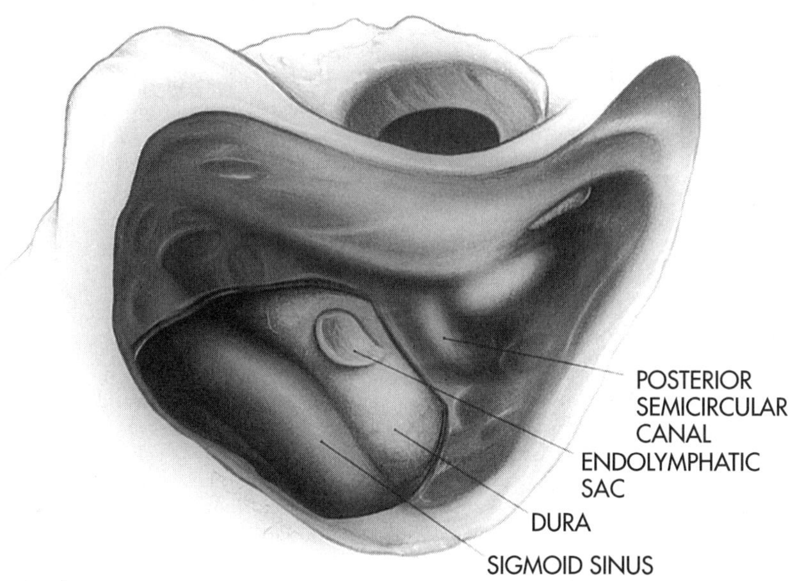

Figure 1.
Wide surgical decompression of sac, dura, and sigmoid sinus.

incision in the sac could remain patent—with or without a shunt. Other possible mechanisms might include simple decompression of the sac (to allow expansion and/or equalized pressure into the mastoid cavity), decompression of the posterior fossa dura or sigmoid sinus, neovascularization of the exposed sac, vibration or noise exposure of the cochlea from the drill, anesthetic or perioperative drugs, and so forth.

Certainly, a portion of the beneficial effects of sac surgery could be due to a placebo effect, but I do not accept that it accounts for the total effect for the following reasons:

- If we select only those patients who fail standard medical therapy, most of the placebo responders have already been filtered out. If these patients later try equivocal therapies, for example, vitamin E, niacin, papaverine, ginkgo, and so forth), they rarely respond. If the average reported success following sac surgery is 70 percent in this subset of medically unresponsive patients, it is hard to invoke the placebo effect.
- Just like VNS, sac surgery has very poor results in non–Meniere's vertigo; thus, why is the effect any different if it is only a placebo?

Even if the effect of sac surgery is part placebo, would it not still be a reasonable option if it can reliably and safely benefit three of four patients when other "placebos" have not?

In "What I Think of Sac Surgery in 1989," Glasscock and associates eloquently explain why they abandoned sac surgery in favor of vestibular nerve section because of the higher rate of *complete* control of vertigo. Despite their conclusion, it is interesting to note their own rather favorable results with sac surgery; they report complete control of vertigo in 65 percent of patients at 3 years. Furthermore, 71 percent of their patients were "very pleased" with the results of their surgery, and 60 percent noted subjective hearing improvement. These favorable results are attributed to placebo effect. We differ with this conclusion, as do the authors of the classic "placebo" study (vide infra).

We also differ with Glassock's opinion that the only criterion for success must be "complete control of vertigo." If vertigo control were the *only* criterion for success, then labyrinthectomy with sacrifice of normal hearing would be considered a "success." As noted, we believe a risk-benefit analysis must be made for each patient, including the risks of dysequilibrium, hearing loss, disability, intracranial complications, and the possible development of Meniere's disease in the contralateral ear.

Effective Treatment or Placebo?

In 1981, Thomsen and co-workers designed a double-blind randomized study to compare ELS mastoid shunt surgery with a placebo. Unfortunately, selecting a mastoidectomy as a placebo was inappropriate because it is far from an "empty" treatment. The study, however, consequently serves as a comparison of endolymphatic shunting versus mastoidectomy.

Not surprisingly, many individuals point to the "Danish sham" study as evidence that shunt surgery is of no value. This conclusion is incorrect for a variety of reasons:

- Reanalysis of these results by Pillsbury and associates identified numerous statistical flaws and in fact concluded that there was a significant benefit to shunting.
- A sham is "something false or empty that is purported to be genuine," as defined by the American Heritage Electronic Dictionary, 1995. By definition, the "placebo cohort" is certainly not a sham. A procedure that includes an anesthetic, perioperative medications, an incision, a mastoidectomy, and removal of bone near the sac and sigmoid sinus is far from empty. Any one or a combination of these parameters might have an unknown effect on the inner ear.
- A placebo is "an inactive substance or preparation used as a control in an experiment to determine the effectiveness of a drug," as defined by the American Heritage Electronic Dictionary, 1995. By definition, the choice of a mastoidectomy as a placebo was clearly inappropriate for this study, as even the original investigators later admitted; 9 years after the Danish study, Bretlau and coworkers state, "To speak of a 'placebo effect' after performing a mastoidectomy is not entirely justifiable."
- The Danish investigators continue to offer their own patients sac surgery as a procedure of "indisputable" efficacy.

■ OUR CLINICAL APPROACH

Patients at the Michigan Ear Institute are counseled regarding the various treatment options, benefits, and risks in order to help them choose their therapy. The patient's age, health, and occupation are all taken into consideration. They are advised of the average duration of surgery, hospitalization, and postoperative recovery (Tables 2 and 3).

Table 2. Summary of Information Presented to Patients Regarding Treatment Options for Meniere's Disease

1. "Sac surgery" is a 1 hour outpatient mastoid operation, with a return to normal activities within a few days. Eighty percent of our patients achieve significant or total control of vertigo. Dysequilibrium and hearing loss secondary to surgery rarely occur. For those patients who do not benefit from this treatment, vestibular neurectomy will be advised.
2. "Vestibular neurectomy" is a 3 hour craniotomy requiring approximately 1 day in the intensive care unit, 4 additional inpatient hospital days, and a 1 month or longer recovery to achieve central compensation. Ninety-five percent of our patients achieve significant or total control of vertigo. Ten percent of patients have persistent dysequilibrium. Five percent of patients may incur a hearing loss.
3. "Chemical vestibular ablation" with aminoglycosides is a promising investigational therapy that can be performed on an outpatient basis via a myringotomy; the ideal drug, dosage, and means of delivery have not yet been determined. Eighty percent of our patients achieve significant or total control of vertigo. Five percent of patients have persistent dysequilibrium. Hearing loss may occur in up to 30 percent of patients, depending on drug dosage and individual sensitivity to the drug.

Table 3. Summary of Risks and Benefits for Various Treatments of Meniere's Disease

RISKS/BENEFITS	SAC SURGERY	NEURECTOMY	GENTAMICIN
Vertigo control	Moderate	High	Moderate-High
Risk of SNHL	Low	Moderate	High
Dysequilibrium risk	Low	Moderate	Low-Moderate
Recovery time	Short	Long	Short
Potential for CNS complications	Low	Moderate	None

SNHL, sensorineural hearing loss; CNS, central nervous system.

Labyrinthectomy

Patients who have profound hearing loss are advised to have a transmastoid labyrinthectomy. Translabyrinthine vestibular neurectomy has a slightly higher success rate, but in order to avoid a craniotomy, it is reserved for the rare patient who has persistent dizziness after labyrinthectomy. For the elderly patient who has poor hearing, topical gentamicin may be a suitable alternative to surgery.

Sac-Vein Decompression

In our experience, sac surgery has its greatest efficacy in treating patients who have early, classic disease, that is, true vertigo, aural fullness, tinnitus, and fluctuating hearing loss. End-stage disease (severe SNHL without fluctuation, lightheadedness rather than true vertigo) and atypical symptoms rarely achieve as much benefit. The reason for this is unknown, but this situation is analogous to vestibular neurectomy; patients who have vestibular neuritis and atypical vestibulopathy achieve a far lower success rate following neurectomy than do classic Meniere's disease patients.

Sac surgery is a reasonable option for patients who have bilateral disease or, occasionally, those with severe symptoms in a better-hearing ear.

Our patients who choose ELS surgery are advised preoperatively that they could eventually require ablative therapy if their vertigo persists. With realistic expectations generated from preoperative counseling, patients rarely begrudge the need for additional treatment should it be necessary.

Vestibular Neurectomy

Vestibular neurectomy is recommended for patients with good hearing and unilateral disease who are willing to accept the higher potential risk of a craniotomy for a higher vertigo control rate.

Transtympanic Aminoglycosides

Topical streptomycin or gentamicin are considered for patients with unilateral disease and serviceable hearing who are willing to accept the risk of hearing loss but not a craniotomy. As noted previously, these patients are advised that this is still an investigational procedure wherein the ideal drug, dosage, and means of delivery have not yet been determined.

Intramuscular Streptomycin

Low-dose intramuscular streptomycin given over a few weeks is a reasonable treatment option for patients who have bilateral active disease. Audiograms and caloric testing are closely followed up to minimize oscillopsia and permanent vestibular hypofunction.

■ FUTURE

None of the current Meniere's disease treatments are ideal. We anticipate that the future may allow improved therapy by a variety of means:

1. New diagnostic tests to identify the exact etiology of each patient's syndrome. This will allow prescription of only the specific treatment suited to the individual patient's underlying disease.
2. Better predictors of each patient's responsiveness (or lack of tolerance to) particular therapies.
    - Refinements in posturography may be able to predict dysequilibrium following ablative surgery.
    - Testing for mutant mitochondrial DNA may detect hypersensitivity to aminoglycoside toxicity, which will alert the otologist that alternative treatment is indicated.
3. An "ideal" topical aminoglycoside therapy will likely obviate the need for vestibular neurectomy.
    - Improved regimens for transtympanic aminoglycosides will be determined following additional empiric trials.
    - Novel delivery systems may be developed (e.g., Cass's intratympanic streptomycin pump).

Suggested Reading

Brackmann D. Emdolymphatic sac–mastoid shunt: Operative techniques. Otolaryngol Head Neck Surg 1991: 2:9-11.

Bretlau P, Thomsen J. Placebo effect in surgery for Meniere's disease: 9 year follow-up. Am J Otol 1989; 10:259.

Cass SP, Kartush JK, Graham MD. Clinical assessment of postural stability following vestibular nerve section. Laryngoscope 1991; 101:1056-1059.

Fischel-Ghodsian N, Prezant T, Bu X, Oztas S. Mitochondrial ribosomal RNA gene mutation in a patient with aminoglycoside ototoxicity. Am J Otolaryngol 1993; 14:399-403.

Fowler EP. Streptomycin treatment of vertigo. Trans Am Acad Ophthalmol Otolaryngol 1948; 52:239-301.

Gianoli G, LaRouere M, Kartush J, Wayman J. Sac-vein decompression for intractable Meniere's: Two year treatment results. Otolaryngol Head Neck Surg 1997 (in press).

Glassscock ME, Jackson CG, Poe D, Johnson G. What I think of sac surgery in 1989. Am J Otol 1989; 10:230.

Graham M, Saraloff R, Kemink J. Titration streptomycin therapy for bilateral Meniere's disease: A preliminary report. Otolaryngol Head Neck Surg 1984; 92:440.

Hallpike C, Cairns H. Observations on pathology of Meniere's syndrome. J Laryngol 1938; 53:625.

Kemink JL, Telian S, El-Kashlan H, et al. Retrolabyrinthine vestibular

nerve section: Efficacy in disorders other than Meniere's disease. Laryngoscope 1991; 101:523-528.
Magnusson M, Padoan S. Delayed onset of ototoxic effects in gentamicin treatment of Meniere's disease: Rationale for extremely low dose therapy. Acta Otolaryngol (Stockholm) 1991; 11:671-676.
McElveen J, Shelton C, Hitselberger E, et al. Retrolabyrinthine vestibular neurectomy: A re-evaluation. Laryngoscope 1988; 98:502-506.
Nedzelski J, Chiong C, Fradet G, et al. Intratympanic gentamicin installation as treatment of unilateral Meniere's disease: Update of an ongoing study. Am J Otol 1993; 14:278-282.
Nguyen C, Brackmann D, Crane R, et al. Retrolabyrinthine vestibular nerve section: Evaluation of technical modification in 143 cases. Am J Otol 1992; 13:328-332.
Paparella MM, Sajjadi H, DaCosat SS, et al. Significance of the lateral sinus and Trautmann's triangle in Meniere's disease. In: Nadol JB Jr, ed. Second International Symposium on Meniere's Disease. Amsterdam: Kugler & Ghedini Publications, 1989:139.
Pillsbury HC, Arenberg I, Ferraro J, Ackley R. Endolymphatic sac surgery: The Danish sham surgery study: An alternative analysis. Otolaryngol Clin North Am 1983; 16:123-127.
Portmann G. Le traitement chiurgical des vertiges par l'ouverture du sac endolymphatique. Presse Med Dec 29, 1926.
Reid C, Eisenberg R, Halmagyi M, Fagan P. The outcome of vestibular nerve section for intractable vertigo: The patient's point of view. Laryngoscope 1996; 106:1553-1556.
Shambaugh G. Surgery of the endolymphatic sac. Arch Otolaryngol 1966; 83:29.
Schuknecht HP. Ablation therapy for the relief of Meniere's disease. Laryngoscope 1956; 66:859.
Shah D, Kartush J. Endolymphatic sac surgery for Meniere's disease. Otolaryngol Clin North Am 1997 (in press).
Silverstein H, et al. Use of streptomycin sulfate in the treatment of Meniere's disease. Otolaryngol Head Neck Surg 1984; 92:229.
Thomsen J, et al. Placebo effect in surgery for Meniere's disease, a double-blind, placebo-controlled study on endolymphatic sac shunt surgery. Arch Otolaryngol 1981; 107:27.

ACOUSTIC NEUROMA

The method of
the University of Washington
by
Larry G. Duckert
Marc R. Mayberg
George A. Gates

The development of more sophisticated imaging techniques has resulted in earlier tumor diagnosis in patients who have intact and serviceable hearing. Although tumor eradication remains the primary focus of surgical treatment, the possibility of hearing preservation (once remote) has become an important determinant of surgical approach. In a recent series, hearing was retained in 75 percent of patients whose tumor size was 2.5 cm and smaller. In this group of patients, 86 percent had hearing that was serviceable and unchanged from preoperative levels. In this chapter, we examine those factors that may predict or influence favorable outcome and reduce patient morbidity.

■ TREATMENT ALTERNATIVES

Surgical resection holds the most promise for tumor removal and hearing preservation. Watchful waiting has been recommended in cases of small intracanalicular tumors, many of which do not demonstrate clinically significant enlargement over time. Unfortunately, it is also the case that as many as 75 percent of patients may lose candidacy for hearing preservation surgery during this observation period due to tumor growth or deterioration of hearing. Stereotactic radiotherapy has been shown to arrest tumor growth while preserving hearing in a limited number of patients, but the long-term results have not yet been determined. To the contrary, hearing pressure after surgery is generally maintained.

Surgery for hearing preservation is performed either by the retrosigmoid (RS, suboccipital) or middle fossa (MF) approach. The latter approach is used by this group for small essentially intracanalicular tumors in patients younger than 65 years. The RS approach, which is more widely employed, is used exclusively for the purpose of tumor removal with hearing conservation or for tumors in excess of 2.5 cm. The translabyrinthine approach is used in the case of tumors smaller than 2.5 cm in either nonserviceable or nonhearing ears.

■ PRETREATMENT SELECTION

Whether hearing conservation in acoustic tumor surgery is even a consideration will depend on a number of factors. These include baseline hearing, demands placed on the patient's hearing, likelihood of success, and relative operative morbidity. Selection criteria based on preoperative hearing have varied among authors. Ideal criteria may be defined as speech reception threshold (SRT) of 30 dB, a speech discrimination score of 70 percent, and tumor size of less than 1.5 cm. Less conservative parameters of pure-tone average equal to or greater than 50 dB, and a speech discrimination score of 50 percent have also been used. The poor correlation between preoperative hearing levels alone and hearing preservation argues in favor of tumor size as the most reliable predictive index. If there exists a statistically significant difference in the complication rate between the hearing conservation (RS and MF) and nonconservation (translabyrinthine) approaches, such factors would have to be weighed in the decision-making process. There is no general consensus of opinion on this issue, and depending on the individual surgeon's experience, complications may be more or less frequently encountered with either approach. A comparison of results between institutions is compromised by different selection criteria, definition of success, and reporting strategies.

With respect to the issues of patient selection and morbidity, this chapter includes a review of our experience with a recently studied series of patients selected for hearing preservation surgery at the University of Washington Medical Center using selection and success criteria based on function. Our complication rate was examined with attention to cerebrospinal fluid (CSF) leak, headache, and tumor recurrence or persistence. We projected that our data would be used to advise patients preoperatively about potential benefit of hearing conservation surgery versus the morbidity associated with the retrosigmoid approach. Moreover, we sought to identify procedural modifications that would positively influence the risk-benefit ratio.

Our series consisted of 22 patients who underwent removal of a vestibular schwannoma via a retrosigmoid approach for hearing preservation. All tumors were unilateral; contralateral hearing was intact with respect to age. Selection criteria included a pure-tone average of 50 dB and speech discrimination score of 50 percent or greater. Our criteria evolved to exclude patients who had tumors in excess of 3 cm.

Tumor size was determined by measuring the maximum diameter of the tumor medial to the porus acusticus. Tumors that were primarily intracanalicular were combined with those in the first group. To be sure, a number of methods have been used for measurement, and the bias imposed by these methods must be taken into consideration if comparison among centers is to be made. We were satisfied that tumor measurements in 0.5 cm increments would be suitable for purposes of internal review and our patient consultation procedures.

The definition of successful surgery and successful hearing preservation varies among surgeons in reported series, again making comparisons difficult. We have agreed that when preoperative hearing is not serviceable, the question of conservation is moot. With this in mind, we accepted the 50-50 selection criteria with respect to the concept of serviceability, and surgery was considered successful when postoperative hearing levels remained within these limits. In patients whose preoperative hearing was borderline, success was defined as hearing preservation to within 10 dB of the preoperative pure-tone average and 10 percent of the preoperative speech discrimination score. Simply stated, for our reporting purposes, a successful outcome was synonymous with preservation of serviceable hearing.

■ RESULTS

Table 1 expresses the results of surgery with respect to our criteria for successful hearing preservation. Tumor size varied, with a greater percentage falling within the 1.1 cm to 2 cm range. The number of patients in each group is small, and for this reason statistical analysis was not undertaken. We readily accept that the potential for hearing preservation is directly related to tumor size; however, this relationship may not immediately be apparent from this patient series. In any event, 73 percent (8 of 11) of the patients who had tumors of 1.5 cm or less of extracanalicular extension retained serviceable hearing. Our success rate was reduced to 65 percent (13 of 20) if the group was expanded to include patients who had tumors of 2.5 cm. Neither of two patients who had tumors larger than 2.5 cm retained any hearing. Overall, only two patients retained hearing that was unserviceable.

Complications were infrequent in this group of patients. Two developed postoperative CSF leaks. One leak sealed spontaneously, but a second patient was returned to the operating room for wound exploration. Operative findings included displacement of the muscle plug from the petrous bone defect. The tissue plug was replaced, with control of the leak and no change in hearing. Three patients suffered postoperative headaches that persisted for more than 3 weeks after surgery. Two responded to nonsteroidal anti-inflammatory agents, but a third required additional physical therapy. Headaches were not problematic after 6 months. The longest patient follow-up is 3 years, and to date there have been no recurrences.

Preservation of Hearing

Strict adherence to any preselection process that mandates one surgical approach over another will certainly deny hearing to some patients postoperatively. The more conservative the indices, the larger will be the number of patients with nonhearing ears. On the one hand, we respect the opinion of some surgeons whose experience dictates that hearing preservation may not be economically sound or even practically attractive. The feasibility of complete tumor removal with hearing preservation has been questioned on histologic grounds. On the other hand, we have remained sensitive to the demands of our patients who may elect to have hearing conserved for individual reasons.

Table 1. Treatment Results of Restrosigmoid Approach to Treat Acoustic Neuroma

TUMOR SIZE (CM)	NO. OF PATIENTS TREATED SUCCESSFULLY/ TOTAL NO. OF PATIENTS TREATED (N = 22)
0.5	3/4
0.6–1.0	1/1
1.1–1.5	4/6
1.6–2.0	4/8
2.1–2.5	1/1
2.6–3.0	0/2

Hearing preservation rates after acoustic neuroma surgery range from 20 percent to 70 percent. Differences in selection criteria and definition of success account in part for the variability. As stated earlier, we imposed selection criteria based on the concept of serviceability. We cannot say based on our experience that the 50-50 rule can be used to identify patients who have a better chance of retaining hearing. These selection criteria established a threshold of serviceability that, if maintained postoperatively, was equated with a successful outcome. These criteria may be forced, but they are not completely arbitrary, because the conservation of useless hearing is not an attractive surgical goal. We do not suggest that retaining serviceable hearing in one ear provides binaural hearing. However, bidirectional hearing may provide certain individuals with a significant advantage, depending on their particular needs. On the rare occasion that hearing is lost in the uninvolved ear, a serviceable ear will become the patient's only hearing ear.

No statistical correlation could be made between tumor size and success given the small numbers in each of our groups. However, we were surprised and gratified to find that in relative terms our success rate did not dramatically decline with tumors larger than 1.5 cm, as has been reported elsewhere. Admittedly, ours is a small series; however, had we imposed stricter selection criteria based on size alone, we would have denied hearing to 5 of 11 patients whose tumors were in excess of 1.5 cm.

Value of Intraoperative Monitoring

Preoperative auditory brainstem response (ABR) data were available in all patients in our series. Intraoperative monitoring of ABR and facial nerve integrity was also employed in all patients. We did not analyze these data relative to the hearing outcome; the prognostic utility of ABR findings in other series is both favorable and unfavorable. Better waveform integrity facilitated monitoring, and in the case of hearing retention, waves I, III, and V remained intact. In a single patient, the waveform amplitude increased after decompression of the porus. Loss of wave V, unless by technical difficulty, was consistently associated with profound hearing loss, as has been reported elsewhere.

Intraoperative facial nerve monitoring was accomplished using electromyogram and constant voltage stimulation during dissection. This procedure facilitated nerve identification, reduced mechanical trauma, and was used to confirm functional integrity at the end of the procedure. The incidence of permanent facial nerve paralysis is known to vary according to tumor size, and the overall incidence is 0 percent to 5 percent in small to medium-sized tumors (<3 cm). Clearly, facial nerve monitoring and improved dissection strategies are responsible for the high incidence of normal or near-normal function postoperatively. In our series, 100 percent of patients had a postoperative facial nerve functional status of House grade I to II.

■ AVOIDING COMPLICATIONS

Surgical Approach and Morbidity

Whether the retrosigmoid approach is associated with more morbidity than the translabyrinthine approach has been the subject of philosophic and scientific debate. In most series, the complication rates are essentially equivalent. At least there appears to be no compelling reason to sacrifice hearing in an effort to reduce patient morbidity.

The choice between the middle fossa or retrosigmoid approach for hearing preservation may be a matter of surgeons' preference, although some series would demonstrate an advantage using the latter approach. More specifically, hearing preservation rate may be higher, whereas the complication rate may be lower. On the other hand, the middle fossa approach may be preferred in cases of tumor occupying the lateral internal auditory canal, because the lateral end of the canal is more difficult to visualize from the posterior route. This being the case, a higher recurrence rate might be anticipated following a retrosigmoid dissection. Experience would indicate, however, that recurrence is uncommon when complete tumor removal is accomplished, regardless of approach. In our series, we consistently used the posterior approach to achieve total tumor removal. In cases in which control of the lateral extension was an issue, endoscopically guided dissection was used. In this way, we were comfortably able to visualize and remove tumor remnants that approached the fundus of the internal auditory canal. Endoscopy is also useful upon completion of tumor removal to verify closure of petrous air cells with bone wax. The longest follow-up in our series has been only 3 years, and to date we have identified no recurrences. We accept the fact that longer follow-up will be necessary to complete our analysis.

Cerebrospinal Fluid Leak

CSF leakage is one of the most common complications following acoustic neuroma surgery. Whether it is more commonly experienced following surgery by the translabyrinthine approach versus the posterior approach has been a source of controversy. In early reports, the overall incidence was reported to be as high as 50 percent; however, refinements of surgical technique have reduced this incidence significantly. More recent series have reported an incidence of from 5 percent to 30 percent. In summary, the data do not suggest that the risk of CSF leakage should exclude the patient from a hearing conservation approach.

Two patients of 22 developed CSF leaks in our series. One patient required surgical exploration for control. In all patients, air cells of the petrous ridge were packed with wax, and the defect was filled with soft tissue glued in position. Despite this technique, CSF leak may occur if the tissue plug is displaced, as occurred in one of our patients. A technique designed to secure the tissue plug has been described, in which the inferior and superior dura flaps are preserved and sutured over the muscle within the petrous defect. Although conceptually attractive, this is a technically challenging procedure. Following the two complications in this series, we modified and simplified the dural flap procedure (Fig. 1). We used a single dural flap that is based superior to the meatus. The flap margin is defined laterally by the endolymphatic sac, superiorly by the superior petrosal sinus, and medially by the lip of the porus acusticus. After elevation, this flap can be rotated and turned down over the seventh and eighth nerve complexes during drilling. Upon completion of the tumor resection, the flap is replaced over the muscle and retained with sutures or buttressed with tissue

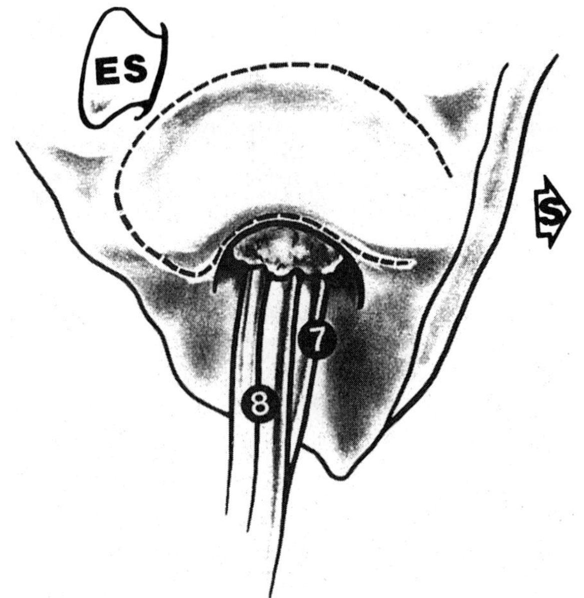

Figure 1.
Posterior surface of left petrous tip and meatus of internal auditory canal, including indwelling seventh and eighth cranial nerves as well as acoustic tumor. Superiorly based dural flap is outlined. ES, endolymphatic sac; S, superior.

glue. If the flap is not allowed to desiccate during the procedure, a tidy edge-to-edge closure is frequently possible.

Several authors have described similar technical modifications to reduce the incidence of CSF leak with minimal effect. Although this technique may alter the outcome of our patients in the future, it awaits further analysis.

Postoperative Headache

It is a popular conception that the posterior approach is associated with a higher incidence of postoperative pain—specifically headache—than the translabyrinthine approach. In some series, the incidence after suboccipital craniotomy has been reported to be in excess of 60 percent, whereas reported pain after labyrinthectomy may be in excess of 50 percent. Concern that the pain was a result of manipulation of the nuchal musculature resulted in modification of the skin incision. Moreover, it became clear that craniectomy without replacement of the bone flap and resultant dural traction promoted postoperative headache. Subsequent modifications of the posterior surgical approach to include replacement of the bone flap have significantly reduced the incidence of postoperative headache, which is currently equivalent to that of the translabyrinthine approach. The reported incidence ranges from 14 percent to 34 percent; however, comparison among series is difficult, because patient assessment parameters vary considerably.

In our series, three patients suffered postoperative headaches that responded to a combination of anti-inflammatory agents or, in the case of one patient, physical therapy. An overview of these patients' cases failed to reveal any apparent contributing factors, because the approach and closure was similar in all instances. We agree that more invasive surgical techniques in general are associated with greater patient morbidity. For this reason, we have modified our retrosigmoid approach to require a conservative amount of bone removal. In most cases, the craniectomy is limited to a defect less than 2 cm x 2 cm, which is meticulously reconstructed.

It is also our practice to remove all bone dust from the posterior fossa before closure. Contamination of the posterior fossa contents can be limited during drilling by strategic placement of sheet Silastic dams that collect the dust. It has been our clinical impression that these efforts help reduce the frequency and severity of postoperative headache, but we concede that an in-depth analysis of the data has yet to be completed. Certainly, the incidence of postoperative headache should not discourage efforts to preserve hearing in acoustic neuroma surgical patients.

■ DISCUSSION

The choices of surgical approach for patients who have residual hearing is limited if function is to be preserved. In our series, hearing was retained in 75 percent of patients who had tumors smaller than 2.5 cm. The definition of successful surgery for hearing conservation varies among surgeons. In our case, when hearing was retained, 86 percent of ears remained serviceable. Patient morbidity associated with the retrosigmoid approach was not significantly greater than the translabyrinthine approach; therefore, the relative advantages and disadvantages of this surgical approach do not invalidate surgery for hearing preservation.

Minimally invasive surgical technique, posterior fossa endoscopy, and meticulous attention to wound closure may reduce the incidence of postoperative complications while the percentage of patients who have useful postoperative hearing continues to improve.

Suggested Reading

Baldwin DL, King TT, Morrison AW. Hearing conservation in acoustic neuroma surgery via the posterior fossa. J Laryngol Otol 1990: 104: 464-467.

Charabi S, Tos M, Thomsen J, Borgesen SE. Suboccipital acoustic neuroma surgery: Results of decentralized neurosurgical tumor removal in Denmark. Acta Otolaryngol (Stockholm) 1992: 112:810-815.

Cohen NL, Hammerschlag P, Berg H, Ransohoff J. Acoustic neuroma surgery: An eclectic approach with emphasis on preservation of hearing. The New York University–Bellevue experience. Ann Otol Rhinol Laryngol 1986; 95:21-27.

Dornhoffer JL, Helms J, Hoehmann DH. Hearing preservation in acoustic tumor surgery: Results and prognostic factors. Laryngoscope 1995: 105:184-187.

Ebersold MJ, Harner SG, Beatty CW, et al. Current results of the retrosigmoid approach to acoustic neurinoma. J Neurosurg 1992; 76:901-909.

Frerebeau P, Benezech J, Uziel A, et al. Hearing preservation after acoustic neurinoma operation. Neurosurgery 1987; 21:197-200.

Gantz BJ, Parnes LS, Harker LA, McCabe BF. Middle cranial fossa acoustic neuroma excision: Results and complications. Ann Otol Rhinol 1986; 95:454-459.

Gardner G, Robertson JH, Hearing preservation in unilateral acoustic neuroma surgery. Ann Otol Rhinol Laryngol 1988; 97:55-66.

Glasscock ME, McKennan KX, Levine SC. Acoustic neuroma surgery: The results of hearing conservation surgery. Laryngoscope 1987; 97: 785-789.

Harner SG, Laws ER Jr, Onofrio BM. Hearing preservation after removal of acoustic neuroma. Laryngoscope 1984; 94:1431-1434.

Jenkins HA. Hearing preservation in acoustic neuroma surgery. Laryngoscope 1992; 102:125-128.

Josey AF, Glasscock ME, Jackson CG. Preservation of hearing in acoustic tumor surgery: Audiologic indicators. Ann Otol Rhinol Laryngol 1988; 97:626-630.

Kemink JL, LaRouere MJ, Kileny PR, et al. Hearing preservation following suboccipital removal of acoustic neuromas. Laryngoscope 1990; 100:597-602.

McKennan KX. Endoscopy of internal auditory canal during hearing conservation acoustic tumor surgery. Am J Otol 1993; 14:259-262.

Nadol JB, Levine R, Ojemann RG, et al. Preservation of hearing in surgical removal of acoustic neuromas of the internal auditory canal and cerebellar pontine angle. Laryngoscope 1987; 97:1287-1294.

Palva T, Troupp H, Jauhiainen T. Hearing preservation in acoustic neuroma surgery. Acta Otolaryngol (Stockholm) 1985; 99:1-7.

Sanna M, Zini C, Mazzoni A, et al. Hearing preservation in acoustic neuroma surgery: Middle fossa versus suboccipital approach. Am J Otol 1987; 8:500-506.

Shelton C, Brackmann D, House WF, Hitselberger WE. Acoustic tumor surgery: Prognostic factors in hearing conservation. Arch Otolaryngol Head Neck Surg 1989; 115:1213-1216.

Silverstein H, McDaniel A, Norrell H, Haberkamp T. Hearing preservation after acoustic neuroma surgery with intraoperative direct eighth cranial nerve monitoring: Part II. Otolaryngol Head Neck Surg 1986; 95:285-291.

Smith MF, Lagger RI. Hearing conservation in acoustic neurilemmoma surgery via the retrosigmoid approach. Otolaryngol Head Neck Surg 1984; 92:168-175.

Wade PJ, House W. Hearing preservation in patients with acoustic neuromas via the middle fossa approach. Otolaryngol Head Neck Surg 1984; 92:184-193.

TINNITUS

The method of
Pawel J. Jastreboff

The diagnosis of "tinnitus" is given when a patient reports hearing a sound that is not related to any external sound in the environment. These reported sounds have enormous variability, with ringing, hissing, buzzing, and cricket sounds being the most common. The perception of tinnitus is pervasive, affecting approximately 17 percent of the general population, and creates a clinically significant problem for approximately 4 percent to 5 percent of the population, that is, approximately 12 million persons in the United States. The impact of tinnitus on the patient's life can vary from mild irritation to total disability and, in some reported cases, suicide. The common scenario is that a patient experiences problems with sleeping and concentration, which in turn affects his or her work, recreational activities, and social interactions. For most patients, their quality of life deteriorates profoundly, and many patients restlessly pursue a "cure" for their tinnitus.

Unfortunately, the most common treatment approach was, and still is, to advise the patient to learn to live with it. Expectations rose when "masking" tinnitus by external sound was introduced in the late 1970s. This approach, however, can only be used on some patients, and it has not been shown to be consistently helpful in clinical practice.

Distressed tinnitus patients frequently exhibit depression and anxiety; consequently many patients are treated with antidepressant and antianxiety medications. Although these drugs may help the patient cope with tinnitus, they have not been shown to affect tinnitus directly. Some of these drugs may actually enhance tinnitus or hyperacusis, in addition to creating personality changes and suppressing the plastic changes within the brain that are needed for therapy.

Various categories of drugs have been tried, and although the initial reports looked promising for some drugs, subsequent controlled studies have failed to prove their effectiveness. Presently, we are unable to recommend any drug specifically to treat tinnitus. This does not rule out the future possibility of developing a drug that would offer significant help. Indeed, a substantial amount of our research is devoted to the search for mechanism-based medications that can suppress the tinnitus source, or suppress tinnitus-related neuronal activity within the nervous system.

At the moment, we are unable to suppress the tinnitus source, and therefore we do not have a cure. However, another method, called tinnitus retraining therapy (TRT), is being used at the University of Maryland Tinnitus & Hyperacusis Center and in a number of centers around the world, with a success rate that represents significant improvement in more than 80 percent of patients.

■ TINNITUS RETRAINING THERAPY

A description of the neurophysiologic model and TRT derived from it is presented in my list of suggested reading. To understand the basis of this approach it is helpful to note several points. First, epidemiologic data show that only approximately one-quarter of persons who have tinnitus are suffering from it, whereas the remaining majority just experience the condition without any problem. Notably, there is no difference in the psychoacoustic characterization of tinnitus between these two populations. Contrary to intuitive prediction, there is no correlation between the severity of tinnitus and its perceived loudness, pitch, or maskability, thus indicating that the auditory system plays only a secondary role in the development of tinnitus annoyance, and that the emotional (limbic) and autonomic nervous systems are the primary players. In other words, the auditory system provides a signal—tinnitus—but the clinical problem is created when this signal, through activation of the limbic and autonomic nervous systems, evokes a strong negative reaction in the brain and consequently throughout the body. Typically, these reactions involve "fight or flight" status, resulting in problems with sleep, inability to pay attention to issues other than tinnitus, a high level of reactiveness, suppression of positive emotions, and disappearance of the "joy of life" (Fig. 1, *A*). A vicious cycle is created which, depending on the psychological structure of the patient, may drive the patient to a high level of anxiety and depression. It is important to realize that these reactions of the limbic and autonomic nervous systems are of a conditioned reflex type, and as such cannot be changed by conscious will; for example, the patient cannot just say, "I am not bothered by tinnitus anymore," and not be bothered anymore.

The second point from the neurophysiologic model is that neurophysiologic and behavioral studies have demonstrated that the brain exhibits a high level of plasticity, and that the brain can habituate any sensory signal, if it does not have a negative association. Therefore, even though there is no effective method for suppressing the source of tinnitus, it should be possible to attenuate the connections between the auditory, limbic, and autonomic nervous systems by interfering with tinnitus-related neuronal activity above the tinnitus source, and thus achieve habituation of tinnitus.

There are two different subtypes of tinnitus habituation: uncoupling the perception of tinnitus from the negative reaction of the brain and the body—habituation of the reactions introduced by tinnitus (Fig. 1, *B*); and blocking (filtering out) the tinnitus-related neuronal activity before it reaches the level of consciousness—habituation of tinnitus perception (Fig. 1, *C*). TRT is aimed at inducing and facilitating both subtypes of habituation. Once the habituation of a *reaction* is achieved, patients are no longer annoyed by tinnitus, and they can disregard the fact that their tinnitus has the same loudness and pitch as before treatment. Once habituation of *perception* is achieved, the percentage of time when the patient is aware of tinnitus decreases radically, typically to the single percentiles. Both types of habituation are usually achieved; patients are much less aware of their tinnitus, and they are not annoyed when they do perceive it. Consequently, tinnitus ceases to have an impact on their life.

The third point from the neurophysiologic model is the prediction that a significant proportion of tinnitus patients should experience hypersensitivity to sound—hyperacusis. Although this postulate was contrary to data presented in the literature at the time, our clinical data later showed that indeed approximately 40 percent of tinnitus patients have hyperacusis, and this finding has been confirmed by centers in the United Kingdom. Linking tinnitus and hyperacusis has enormous theoretic and clinical significance, and plays a crucial role in the clinical implementation of the therapy.

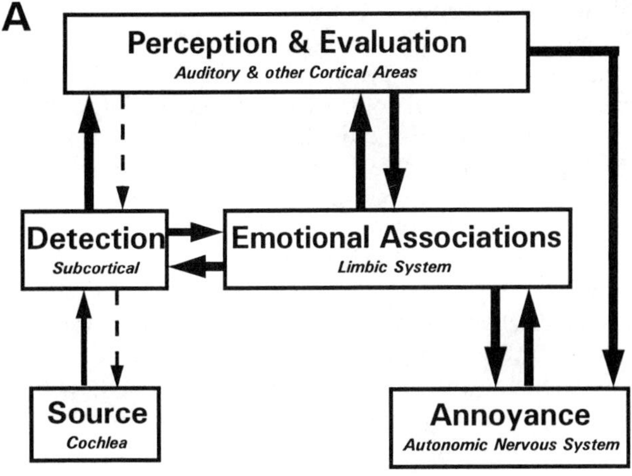

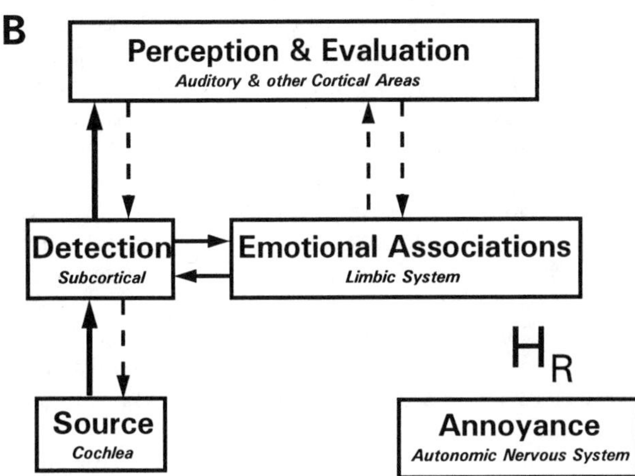

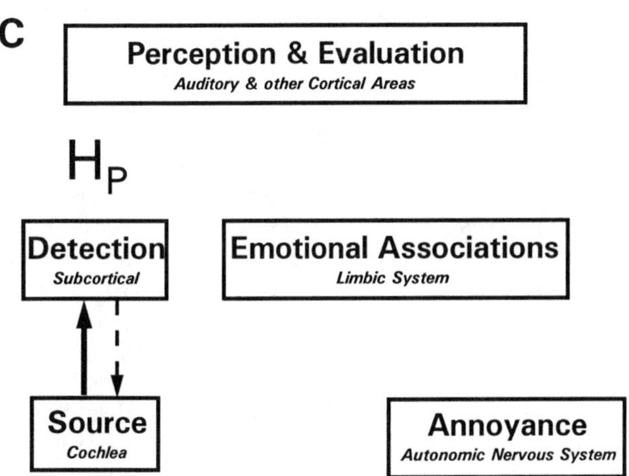

Figure 1.
Block diagram outlining systems involved in clinically relevant tinnitus and changes occurring as a result of tinnitus habituation. Thickness of the arrows indicates the significance of a given connection. *A*, Before treatment; *B*, Habituation of reactions to tinnitus; *C*, Habituation of tinnitus perception.

Clinical Implementation

The approach to therapy consists of a combination of counseling and sound therapy, for which the patient uses low-level sound for several hours a day. Both counseling and the protocol of sound depend on the category in which the patient is placed. In practice the treatment consists of an initial 2 day visit and a number of follow-up appointments that continue for up to 18 to 24 months. The treatment can be divided into the following stages: (1) patient evaluation (includes taking tinnitus and hyperacusis history and audiologic-medical evaluations) and determining the category of treatment; (2) session of retraining counseling; (3) fitting of instruments (noise generators or hearing aids) and/or additional instruction on how to enrich and use environmental sounds; and (4) follow-up visits.

Patient Evaluation

The tinnitus and hyperacusis history is an important part in determining the category of TRT treatment. Consequently, enough time has to be allotted for an interview (approximately 30 minutes), during which the following information is obtained: (1) a characterization of negative associations, patient's fears, and beliefs about their tinnitus; (2) whether hyperacusis is present, and the relative components of hyperacusis and phonophobia; (3) the significance the patient places on the hearing loss; (4) a general psychological profile; and (5) the impact of tinnitus, hyperacusis, and hearing loss on the patient's life.

The audiologic evaluation mainly provides the following information: (1) hearing loss (audiogram); (2) sensitivity to sound (loudness discomfort levels—LDL); and (3) functional integrity of the outer hair cell system (otoacoustic emission distortion product). Results presented in the literature and findings of my colleagues and I show that there is no relationship between the psychoacoustic description of tinnitus, standard audiologic measurements, and the severity of tinnitus and treatment outcome. Therefore, although we perform a number of standard audiologic measurements (matching tinnitus loudness, pitch, maskability, speech discrimination, and acoustic reflexes), these measurements are performed for descriptive purposes, and are presented to the patient during the counseling session to describe the tinnitus, but otherwise have no impact on the treatment.

The main role of the medical evaluation is to ensure that no otologic or health problems are overlooked. Assuring the patient that there is no medical problem related to the tinnitus is a very important factor in the retraining counseling session. If an otologic problem that may be related to the tinnitus is detected, such as Meniere's syndrome, otosclerosis, or acoustic neuroma, then the problem is further assessed and treated as needed, and the potential relationship to tinnitus is discussed in detail with the patient during counseling. Typically, however, the majority of patients exhibit no medical problems related to their tinnitus.

Patients who have clinical depression, whether it is related to tinnitus or not, may need antidepressant therapy. Although we do not prescribe psychotropic medications, if we detect possible clinical depression during the medical evaluation, we advise the patient to contact a psychiatrist for evaluation and treatment. Furthermore, we stress that we will be happy to be in close contact with this specialist to coordinate our efforts while treating the tinnitus.

There is a small population of patients who perceive somatosounds, which can result from blood flow (venous hums, arterial turbulence, arterial venous fistulas, vascular tumors); muscular myoclonus (typically involving the palate); or a patent eustachian tube. These cases are detected through standard otolaryngologic procedures. Some patients can be treated surgically; however, in most cases, the risk of complications outweighs the benefits, particularly because these patients can be treated with TRT to achieve habituation of somatosounds.

Many tinnitus patients take various psychotropic drugs, most commonly antidepressants and benzodiazepines. It is essential to obtain from the patient a list of all medications and doses being taken, as well as medications they have used in the past.

Questionnaires and forms for taking tinnitus history and medical-audiologic evaluations assure consistency of gathered data.

Components of Therapy. The treatment for all patients always consists of two components: counseling and sound therapy. These two components, however, differ for each category.

Counseling. The common element in counseling is explaining to the patient the physiology of the auditory pathways (including, but not limited to, the cochlea); the basic principles of brain function, with focus on the mechanisms of perception, attention, and emotions; the role of the autonomic nervous system; and the mechanisms behind creating and retraining conditioned reflexes, with emphasis on the defensive reflexes aimed at protecting us from danger. Basically, the neurophysiologic model of tinnitus is explained to the patient in simple and understandable terms. All the main points are illustrated with real-life examples, and patients are encouraged to ask questions and interact actively with the presenter. The session lasts at least an hour, and it is usually run by a specially trained audiologist, except when the difficulty of the case requires M.D. or Ph.D. trained personnel to be involved. Proper counseling is imperative for initiating and sustaining the process of tinnitus habituation.

During counseling the issue of psychotropic medications frequently emerges. These medications may improve the patient's ability to cope with tinnitus; however, some of these drugs may actually enhance tinnitus or hyperacusis in addition to creating personality changes, and they can also suppress plastic changes within the brain, thus slowing down the process of TRT. The general approach is to not change the medications in the initial stage of treatment. Only after improvement has been noted do we encourage the patient to gradually wean away from the medications that were taken because of tinnitus. The patient should be made aware that any rapid changes in taking these drugs might affect the tinnitus, hyperacusis, or well-being, and that it is imperative that these changes are done under the close supervision of their physician.

Approximately 20 percent of patients report that their tinnitus can be modified, or that a new sound can be evoked by manipulating the jaw or pressing some parts of the face or skull (indicating the involvement of extralemniscal pathways and multisensory neurons in processing of the tinnitus-related neuronal activity). This issue is discussed during counseling, but mainly it is of research rather than clinical interest. Attempts to treat tinnitus by treating temporomandibular joint disorder have not produced consistent results.

Modification of the general stress level influences tinnitus for many patients. Accordingly, patients are encouraged to decrease their stress level by using any method that works for them (e.g., relaxation techniques, biofeedback).

Sound Therapy. Sound therapy increases the amount of sound the patient is exposed to. Notably, it is not any particular device, but the sound that is important. The use of environmental sounds, enriched by playing low-level music, radio, or television, is always recommended to all tinnitus patients. In the case of hearing loss, these sounds can be amplified by hearing aids, but the basic principle is the same, and it is stressed in our advice to the patient to "avoid silence."

In theory, by extensive use of enriched environmental sounds, it should be possible to implement sound therapy for all patients. In practice, however, it is advantageous to use sound generators, which produce stable, low-level, broad-band noise to provide patients with well-controlled sound for at least 8 hours a day, in addition to the environmental sounds. The generators allow easy and precise control of the amount and timing of sound delivery, and assure a relatively broad frequency range. Moreover, like tinnitus, the perception of the sound generated by them is fixed to the head, so when the patient moves both tinnitus and the sound from the generators remain the same. The stability of sound delivery is particularly important for patients who have hyperacusis, when the amount of sound has to be carefully controlled. Finally, it is easier to put on noise generators, set the level, and forget about them, which helps patients to comply with the protocol. For these reasons, the noise generators are used in most cases.

The specific use of sound depends on the patient's category, with the major difference depending on whether the patient has hyperacusis. If hyperacusis is present, it has to be treated first, with an initial disregard for tinnitus and hearing loss. For hyperacusis patients the sound from noise generators is used to gradually desensitize the auditory system, starting with low-level sound, close to the patient's threshold of hearing. The sound level is then gradually increased, depending on the type of hyperacusis and the speed of the patient's recovery.

For patients who do not have hyperacusis the level of external sound presented will have various effects, depending on its intensity (Fig. 2). For the purpose of habituation the sound level can be anywhere between the threshold of perception and the "mixing point," where the patient perceives that the tinnitus sound and the external sound start to mix or blend together. If there is no hyperacusis, the optimal level is just at or below the "mixing point." The sound from noise generators should never be set at a level that induces annoyance. If this happens, patients are advised to decrease the level to the point where it is neutral, and increase it gradually over a period of weeks until the needed level is reached. Shortening the duration of noise generator use per day is discouraged.

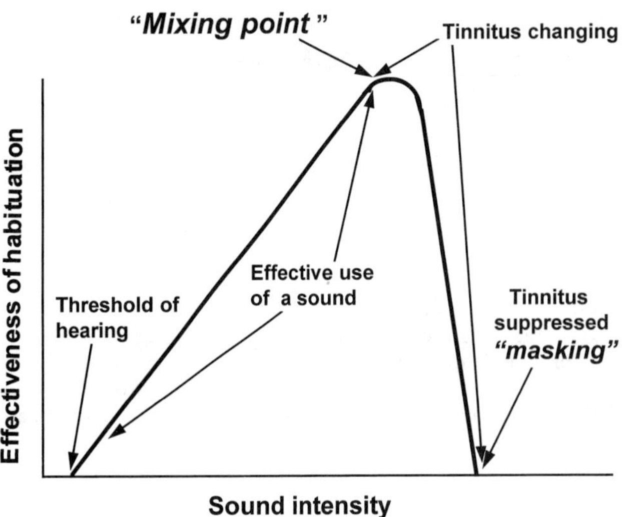

Figure 2.
Dependence of habituation effectiveness on the intensity of the sound used for sound therapy.

Notably, when the perception of tinnitus is suppressed by external sound (typically referred to as "masking"), the habituation of tinnitus cannot occur by definition, because it is impossible to recondition to a stimulus that cannot be detected. Thus, "masking" tinnitus is counterproductive for habituation. The intensity range between "mixing" and "masking" points is commonly referred to in the literature as "partial masking." The effectiveness of habituation decreases rapidly once the intensity of the external sound passes the "mixing point," because retraining occurs on different signals (signal of tinnitus is modified by external sound), and the effectiveness drops to zero once "masking" of tinnitus occurs.

Determining Treatment Category. The following specific factors are used to determine the category of the treatment:

- Hyperacusis (presence and extent of hyperacusis, which is defined as increased sensitivity to sound reflected in the average of LDLs below 100 dB HL)
- Prolonged sound-induced exacerbation (presence of prolonged exacerbation of symptoms following sound exposure persisting into the following day)
- Hearing loss (patient's *subjective* perception of the significance of the hearing loss)
- Impact on life (severity of tinnitus measured in the extent of impact on the patient's life)

The presence and extent of these factors determines the patient's category of treatment (Table 1); however, it is important to recognize that the following five categories offer a general direction only as each patient is treated individually.

Categories of Treatment

Category Zero. Patients who do not have hyperacusis and whose tinnitus has only a low impact on their life are placed

Table 1. Treatment Categories for Tinnitus Patients

CATEGORY	HYPERACUSIS*	SIE	HL	IMPACT†	TREATMENT‡
0	−	−	−	Low	Counseling, environmental sounds
1	−	−	−	High	NG, mixing point
2	−	−	+	High	HA, environmental sounds
3	+	−	NR	High	NG, over threshold
4	+	+	NR	High	NG, threshold, very slow increase

* Hyperacusis: significant hearing level sensitivity to environmental sounds typically associated with loudness discomfort levels below 100 dB.
† Impact: extent of impact of tinnitus on patient's life.
‡ Treatment for each category involves counseling and use of environmental sounds ("avoid silence").
SIE: prolonged sound-induced exacerbation of tinnitus and/or hyperacusis persisting to the following day.
HL: hearing loss has a significant subjective impact on patient's life.
NR, not relevant; NG, noise generators; HA, hearing aids; −, absent; +, present.

in this category. They are more curious than suffering from tinnitus and they "would like to have something done with it." Patients with very recent onset (days, weeks, or a month) of tinnitus can be included in this category, and for this category one session of intensive retraining counseling, including the advice to avoid silence, is usually sufficient to quickly habituate tinnitus. Patients are told that if rapid improvement does not occur within a few weeks, then they should contact the Center again, and then they are treated as patients in category 1.

Category 1. Although annoying tinnitus is present and is the dominant problem, there is no hyperacusis or significant subjective hearing loss. Most patients fall into this category. Although approximately 20 percent to 30 percent of patients experience temporary worsening of their tinnitus after exposure to loud sound, for most the effect disappears within minutes or hours, sleep resets the situation to the pre-exposure level, and high sound levels are needed to induce this phenomenon. This effect is of no clinical relevance, and the treatment can be carried out as for other patients in this category. These patients receive retraining counseling and are fitted with noise generators set to a level close to the mixing point (see Fig. 2).

Patients with somatosounds are treated according to this protocol as well. The retraining procedure acts on the perception of sound and on the reactions of the brain to this signal; thus, it is irrelevant if the sound is real (somatosound) or phantom (tinnitus).

Category 2. Patients in this category are similar to those in category 1; however, they also have hearing loss, which is perceived subjectively as creating significant problems, or they are already using hearing aids. For these patients we use hearing aids to achieve two goals. The primary goal is to provide the patient with amplification of enriched environmental sounds, whereas the secondary goal is to improve the patient's communicating ability and everyday use of sound. It is stressed strongly that the hearing aid is just an amplifier of sound, which the patient has to provide, and will not work on tinnitus if there is no sound around.

Category 3. Category 3 consists of patients who exhibit significant hyperacusis but do not exhibit prolonged sound-induced exacerbation of tinnitus and/or hyperacusis. Approximately 40 percent of tinnitus patients have hyperacusis to various extents, with or without hearing loss. Care is taken not to expose the patient to loud sound, which would be extremely unpleasant for these patients. Accordingly, we do not perform any measurements that would exceed the tolerance levels of these patients.

Hyperacusis is always treated first by a desensitizing procedure using a low level of broad-band noise. Because my chapter is focused on treating tinnitus, the specifics of treating hyperacusis and phonophobia (categories 3 and 4) are not presented here.

Category 4. This category includes patients who exhibit a prolonged sound-induced exacerbation phenomenon. Worsening of their tinnitus and/or hyperacusis lasts for days or weeks, frequently as a result of exposure to moderate or even low-level sound. This is the most difficult category to treat, but it occurs least commonly. Typically, hyperacusis is the dominant problem. These patients usually report that their hyperacusis developed as a direct result of a single exposure to loud sound (e.g., firecrackers, loud concert). Patients in this category have to be treated with extreme care; treatment is prolonged, and the success rate is lower.

Notably, Lyme disease induces hyperacusis of the category 4 type in more than 80 percent of patients, with hyperacusis related to the stage and the extent of Lyme disease. Therefore, it is recommended that patients in this category be tested for Lyme disease and, if necessary, undergo appropriate treatment.

It is of the utmost importance to recognize patients from this category early during the evaluation to avoid the potential problems caused by exposing them to sound that is too loud for them (which can be of a generally moderate level). For example, performing acoustic reflex measurements, or treating them with the protocol used for category 1 patients, may worsen their hyperacusis or tinnitus significantly for an undetermined period of time.

Retraining Counseling Session

In addition to the common elements, for each category there is a different variant of counseling. The session is carried out in an atmosphere of interaction, and explanation is adjusted to the needs and educational and cultural level of the patient.

Fitting Instruments and Teaching How to Enrich and Use Sound Environment

At the moment, the most suitable instrument for TRT is the behind-the-ear Viennatone AMTi (Vienna, Austria), which is used for generating noise. This instrument has a reasonably wide frequency output, and it provides a stable sound level that can be controlled smoothly from below the hearing threshold of a person who has normal hearing. Typically, patients use the Viennatone at a setting close to 2, which provides approximately 60 dB SPL (sound pressure level) of sound. Because most patients experience enhancement of their tinnitus when the ear canal is totally or partially occluded, only behind-the-ear devices are used. The Viennatone provides maximal output up to 90 dB SPL, and therefore there typically is no need for in-the-ear noise generators.

The fitting of hearing aids is subject to the same principle—open, behind-the-ear fitting. During the fitting procedure, it is strongly stressed that the hearing aids are only a tool to amplify sounds that are crucial for the treatment and that the patient has to provide.

Bilateral devices (noise generators or hearing aids) are always recommended to assure a symmetric stimulation of the auditory system, even in patients who have unilateral tinnitus. Both theory and our practice argue against using unilateral devices.

Follow-Up

The follow-up visits are essential for the treatment; without them the success rate would decrease. The visits should be performed after 3 weeks and 6 weeks (preferably more frequently), and after 3, 6, 12, and 18 months. For practical reasons, the first two follow-up visits are replaced by telephone contact for patients coming from far away; telephone contact is encouraged for all patients if they have any further questions or problems. During each visit, the fundamental elements of counseling are repeated to reinforce the initial counseling session and clarify any issues that may have arisen in the meantime. A standard questionnaire is used to assess changes in the patient's tinnitus or hyperacusis and thus determine the progress of treatment. During visits at 6 months and after, the audiogram and LDLs are repeated.

Outcome

The fundamental criterion of improvement is the decrease of the impact of tinnitus and/or hyperacusis on the patient's life. The main parts of the questionnaire are assessed on a point scale (which offers the possibility of both improvement and decline): (1) Is the patient performing activities that were prevented or interfered with previously? (2) Is there a change in the level of annoyance of tinnitus when it is perceived? (3) Is there a change in the percentage of time when the patient is aware of the tinnitus? For a patient to qualify as showing significant improvement, positive changes have to occur in at least two of these general categories, with the extent of change at least 20 percent. Typically, the improvement is much larger, and patients report that their awareness of tinnitus has dropped to percentages of time in the single digits, and there is minor to no annoyance when it is perceived.

Of more than 900 patients treated at the University of Maryland Tinnitus & Hyperacusis Center, I have analyzed 152 consecutive patients who received treatment for at least 6 months. Of this group of 152, 84.9 percent (N = 129) received full treatment involving both counseling and sound therapy facilitated by broad-band noise generators or hearing aids, whereas 15.1 percent (N = 23) received only the initial session of counseling. In the group who had full treatment, 81.4 percent (N = 105) were classified as showing significant improvement, whereas only 17.4 percent (N = 4) showed improvement in the group who had only initial counseling. The difference in treatment outcome between these two groups is highly statistically significant ($P < 0.001$).

Positive and Negative Aspects of TRT

The TRT approach has a number of positive features: (1) because it acts at the level of the brain higher than the tinnitus source, the etiology of tinnitus is irrelevant, and accordingly all patients qualify for the treatment; (2) the treatment requires a limited period of time, after which the patients do not have to follow any special procedures to sustain their improved status; (3) the procedure cannot create harm; (4) it offers a high success rate; and (5) in 6 years of monitoring patients at the University of Maryland, there has only been a handful of patients who have reported relapse, and these cases involved the emergence of a serious medical problem, such as cancer.

On the negative side, the procedure requires a substantial amount of time, especially in the beginning of the treatment; it requires personnel specifically trained for treating tinnitus and hyperacusis patients, and it can take 18 to 24 months to complete. Thus, it is essential to involve properly trained audiologists to assure the financial efficacy of the treatment.

Factors of Concern While Treating Tinnitus and Hyperacusis Patients

Frequently, the first reaction to a patient who has tinnitus, particularly unilateral or dominant on one side, is to recommend a magnetic resonance imaging (MRI) test for detecting acoustic neuroma. Notably, MRI creates a very high level of noise, reaching peaks of 130 dB SPL. For patients who have hyperacusis this noise level may create a significant problem. This issue is of particular importance in patients who exhibit a prolonged sound-induced exacerbation effect. These patients are at high risk for worsened hyperacusis and tinnitus as a result of this test. Indeed, some patients claim that their tinnitus or hyperacusis started or worsened significantly as a result of MRI evaluation. Typically, the MRI testing can be delayed until hyperacusis has improved. If immediate testing is recommended, the patients are made aware of the problem of sound levels during MRI evaluation, and advised to use maximal ear protection with both earplugs and muffs.

Suggested Reading

Jastreboff PJ. Clinical implication of the neurophysiological model of tinnitus. Proceedings of the 5th international tinnitus seminar 1995.

Jastreboff PJ. Phantom auditory perception (tinnitus): mechanisms of generation and perception. Neuroscience Res 1990; 8:221-254.

Jastreboff PJ. Tinnitus as a phantom perception: Theories and clinical implications. In: Vernon J, Møller A, eds. Mechanisms of tinnitus. Boston: Allyn & Bacon, 1995:73.

Jastreboff PJ, Gray WC, Gold SL. Neurophysiological approach to tinnitus patients. Am J Otol 1996; 17:236-240.

Jastreboff PJ, Hazell JWP. A neurophysiological approach to tinnitus: Clinical implications. Br J Audiol 1993; 27:7-17.

IDIOPATHIC FACIAL PARALYSIS

The method of
Kedar K. Adour

Before 1965, acute unilateral facial paralysis—Bell's palsy— was labeled *idiopathic facial paralysis* and was considered to be a diagnosis of exclusion. This most common form of facial paralysis is now known to be caused by the herpes simplex virus (HSV) and can be diagnosed by history and astute observation of presenting signs and symptoms. Any discussion of Bell's palsy must include mention of herpes zoster virus (HZV) facial paralysis (Ramsay Hunt syndrome, or herpes zoster cephalicus), the second most common cause of facial paralysis. Both diseases are herpetic in origin and have a similar history and presenting signs and symptoms. The major difference is degree of severity; herpes zoster facial paralysis has a much graver prognosis. In a general medical clinic setting, these two diagnoses account for 90 percent to 95 percent of all facial paralysis patients seen. In the past, when the disease was considered idiopathic, surgical decompression of the facial nerve was the preferred treatment option. Today, prednisone and acyclovir therapy are recommended to treat both the pathology and the cause of the disease.

■ TYPICAL CASE PRESENTATION

An otherwise healthy 40-year-old woman awakens with pain behind the right ear and numbness of the right side of her face. When she looks in the mirror, she is shocked to see that the right eye does not close, tears run over her right cheek, and the right side of her mouth droops. She immediately calls her health care provider and arranges a same-day appointment or is referred to the emergency department. When she attempts to drink a cup of coffee, liquid drools from the right corner of her mouth, and the coffee has a peculiar taste. When she turns on the radio to hear the morning news, sounds appear louder in the right ear than in the left ear. When seen by the physician, she has partial paralysis of all muscles on the right side of her face. She tells the physician that her face is "numb," and he replies that he can see that the right side of her face is partially paralyzed. She emphasizes that besides being unable to move the right side of her face, that side also feels as though it has been injected with anesthetic, things do not taste right (dysgeusia), and sounds in the right ear and too loud (hyperacusis, dysacusis).

Physical examination shows normal ear findings, no masses in the parotid gland, inflammation of the fungiform papillae of the tongue (right greater than left), and hypesthesia on the right side of the face and behind the right ear.

■ DIAGNOSIS

Accurate medical history and complete physical examination should yield sufficient information to provide the diagnosis of peripheral facial paralysis (Bell's palsy). The clinician should document that all branches of the nerve are affected, no ipsilateral parotid masses are present, the chorda tympani nerve is inflamed (papillitis of the fungiform papillae is present), ear examination results are normal, and no skin blebs or blisters are evident (as in herpes zoster). These points distinguish herpes simplex facial paralysis (Bell's palsy) from non–HSV infection, tumor, trauma, and stroke.

■ EXCLUSION CRITERIA

The diagnosis of HSV (Bell's palsy) or HZV facial paralysis should not be made when:

1. Partial facial paralysis does not resolve in 3 to 6 weeks or is accompanied by either electrical evidence of nerve degeneration or ipsilateral hearing loss.
2. Any facial paralysis is accompanied by evidence of chronic otitis media or history of previous ear surgery.
3. Total facial paralysis is followed by no return of facial motion within 4 months. Even with total loss of nerve excitability, nerve regeneration ensues and results in midfacial contracture with synkinesis in 99 percent of all patients who have Bell's palsy or Ramsay Hunt syndrome. The earliest sign of regeneration is return of the stapedial reflex; the next earliest sign is mouth motion with voluntary forced closures of the eyes (synkinesis).
4. Any facial paralysis with electrical evidence of nerve degeneration resolves without midfacial contracture with synkinesis (facial nerve degeneration with regeneration after HSV or HZV paralysis is followed by midfacial contracture with synkinesis).
5. Facial paralysis progresses during weeks or months (damage to the nerve is complete by Day 14 in Bell's palsy and by Day 21 in Ramsay Hunt syndrome).
6. Recurrent ipsilateral facial paralysis is accompanied by recovery and electrical evidence of nerve degeneration but not by contracture with synkinesis within 4 months.

■ THERAPY

Corticosteroid agents remain the best treatment for inflammatory, virally induced, immune-mediated disease. Because Bell's palsy can progress from a mild, incomplete paresis to a severe, complete paralysis, all patients should be treated with corticosteroid agents. Predicting which patients will experience progression to the severe form of the disease is impossible. If treatment is delayed until severity is determined, irreversible nerve damage may occur. Patients should receive both prednisone and acyclovir (Tables 1 and 2), and treatment should be tailored to degree of disease severity.

Prednisone treats the inflammatory immune response, and acyclovir treats the causative agent, the herpes simplex virus.

For adults, a total daily dose of 1 mg per kilogram of body weight of prednisone is taken in divided doses in the morning and evening. From a practical standpoint, prednisone given in a dose of 30 to 40 mg twice daily is therapeutic and should be taken with food at breakfast and dinner.

Table 1. Recommended Prednisone* Treatment Schedule for Adult Patients with Bell's Palsy

DAY	DOSE TAKEN WITH BREAKFAST (MG)	DOSE TAKEN WITH DINNER (MG)
1	30–40	30–40
2	30–40	30–40
3	30–40	30–40
4	30–40	30–40
5	30–40	30–40
6	25–35	25–35
7	20–30	20–30
8	15–25	15–25
9	10–20	10–20
10	5–15	5–15
11	0–10	0–10

* The cost of generic prednisone is negligible. No advantage can be obtained by giving dexamethasone (Decadron) or methylprednisolone (Medrol).

Table 2. Recommended Acyclovir* Treatment for Adults with Bell's Palsy

DRUG USED	DOSAGE	COST (7 DAY TREATMENT)
Acyclovir (Zovirax)	200–400 mg 5 times daily	$63 ($126)
Famciclovir (Famvir)	500 mg t.i.d.	$143
Valacyclovir (Valtrex)	500 mg t.i.d.	$95

* The newer forms of acyclovir, famciclovir and valacyclovir, are given t.i.d. Famciclovir is a prodrug of penciclovir, which is chemically similar to acyclovir. Valacyclovir is the prodrug of acyclovir. Both are more rapidly and more extensively absorbed than is acyclovir.

The patient should be seen on the fifth or sixth day after onset of paralysis (Table 3). If paralysis is incomplete, prednisone can be tapered during the next 5 days, and acyclovir can be discontinued. If any question about severity or progression arises, the full dose of prednisone and acyclovir should be continued for 7 to 10 days, and the prednisone should then be tapered to zero beginning at Day 10.

No reliable, widely available tests for early identification of HZV infection currently exists. Because HZV carries a considerably poorer prognosis than does HSV, patients infected with HZV require longer follow-up, longer treatment, and greater emotional support.

Until early diagnosis is feasible, all therapeutic decisions must be made on a clinical basis. As in the past, reliance on history and physical examination results is crucial in selecting patients for aggressive treatment. If a patient complains of concomitant severe pain or experiences sensorineural hearing loss, consider the diagnosis to be HZV rather than Bell's palsy (HSV) and treat the patient for 14 to 21 days.

In most managed health care systems, patients are often referred to otolaryngologists after Day 3. If a Bell's palsy patient comes in with incomplete clinical paralysis and no evidence of electrical degeneration between Days 5 and 10, I treat with prednisone alone (30 mg twice daily for 5 days, and then taper). If a Bell's palsy patient comes in with complete clinical paralysis between Days 5 and 7, I treat with prednisone and acyclovir for 7 to 10 days, regardless of the result of electrical tests, because the active disease process for herpes simplex lasts from 8 to 10 days. In herpes zoster, active disease continues until Days 14 to 21, and I therefore treat herpes zoster patients for up to 14 to 21 days after onset of paralysis.

■ PROGNOSIS

Treatment should include providing a prognosis (Table 4), which can be reliably and easily done with maximal stimulation tests (MST) using the Hilger Model 2-R Facial Nerve Stimulator or any similar instrument.

The temporal, orbital, and marginal branches of the facial nerve should be stimulated on the unaffected side, and the results should be recorded separately. The corresponding nerve branch on the affected side should be stimulated at the same setting. Although performing MST is a simple procedure, determining the location of the peripheral branches

Table 3. Recommended Schedule of Medical Office Visits and Treatment for Adults with Bell's Palsy

DAY OF VISIT	TREATMENT	REASONS
1 to 3	Confirm diagnosis, begin medical treatment, perform MST	MST is used on the first visit to ascertain the diagnosis
5 to 7	Ascertain clinical severity, perform MST, encourage eye care, and provide reassurance	To determine continuation of treatment
14 to 21	Ascertain clinical severity, perform MST, encourage eye care, and provide reassurance	To do MST to predict prognosis
30	Encourage eye care and provide emotional support	To provide follow-up care
60	Encourage eye care and provide emotional support	To provide follow-up care
120	Record recovery	To obtain follow-up data

MST, maximal stimulation tests.

Table 4. Prediction of Prognosis in Bell's Palsy Using Maximal Stimulation Tests*

MST FINDINGS	PERCENT OF RECOVERY	TIME (WKS)	CONTRACTURE WITH SYNKINESIS (SEVERITY)
Equal	100	3–6	None
Mild decrease	75–100	4–8	Mild
Moderate decrease	75	6–12	Mild to moderate
Severe decrease	50–75	8–12	Moderate to severe
Complete decrease	<50	12–20	Severe

* Final prediction of prognosis cannot be made until 10 to 14 days after onset of paralysis in Bell's palsy (HSV) and 14 to 21 days in HZV paralysis.
MST, maximal stimulation test.

requires experience. The branch to the frontal muscle is usually found approximately 1 cm lateral to the eye; the branch to the orbicular muscle of the eye is stimulated at the lateral border of the orbit. The location of the branch to the orbicular muscle of the mouth varies the most of all three branches and is usually just anterior to the notch where the facial artery traverses the mandible. The stimulating probe may need to be moved to enable determination of the point of maximal response because the facial nerve can branch in many directions beyond the stylomastoid foramen.

The observer should be placed so as to see both sides of the patient's face simultaneously. The stimulating probe should be applied to the nerve branch at the intensity that produces a just visible muscle twitch. When the first contraction is observed, the area should be explored to find the most sensitive point—that which displays the maximal amount of muscle motion. Current is then increased to 1 to 2 μamp above this threshold to obtain maximal nerve excitability stimulation. Test results are expressed as the difference between facial muscle movement on the affected side of the face and the normal side; results are recorded as equal or decreased movement. In addition, when muscle response to maximal nerve excitability stimulation is decreased, the observer should note whether this decreased response is on the affected side and whether it is minimal, moderate, or severe compared with that of the nonaffected side. These findings equate well with the degree of denervation. No response indicates complete denervation of the nerve branch.

If testing indicates equal muscle response on both sides of the face, the patient can be expected to have complete return of facial function in 3 to 6 weeks without having contracture with synkinesis.

■ OTHER CONSIDERATIONS

Eye Care

Protection of the affected eye is paramount. Encourage the patient to protect the eye from foreign bodies and drying by wearing dark glasses during the day. At the slightest evidence of drying, advise the patient to instill artificial tears and a bland eye ointment at night. Taping the eye closed is not recommended, but early exposure keratitis may require patching or, rarely, tarsorrhaphy.

Electrotherapy

Electrotherapy is of no benefit and may be harmful during the acute or convalescent phase. Experimental research has shown that electrical stimulation of denervated muscle retards ingrowth of neurofibrils to the motor endplates.

Other Tests

Magnetic resonance imaging, computed tomography, and electroneurography are not needed. Besides medical therapy, the greatest benefit to the patient is provided by an understanding doctor who offers emotional support for this psychologically devastating disease.

Acknowledgments
I thank the Medical Editing Department, Kaiser Foundation Research Institute, Oakland, CA, for providing editorial assistance.

Suggested Reading

Adour KK. Acute facial paralysis. In: Rakel RE, ed. Conn's current therapy. Philadelphia: WB Saunders, 1996:906.

Adour KK. Who's afraid of the facial nerve? In: Lucente FE, ed. Highlights of the instructional courses. St. Louis: Mosby–Year Book, 1995: 249.

Adour KK, Ruboyianes JM, Von Doersten PG, et al. Bell's palsy treatment with acyclovir and prednisone compared with prednisone alone: a double-blind, randomized controlled trial. Ann Otol Rhinol Laryngol 1996; 105:371-378.

Austin JR, Peskind SP, Austin SG, Rice DH. Idiopathic facial nerve paralysis: a randomized, double-blind controlled study of placebo versus prednisone. Laryngoscope 1993; 103:1326-1333.

Murakami S, et al. Bell's palsy and herpes simplex virus: identification of viral DNA in endoneural fluid and muscle. Ann Intern Med 1996; 124: 27-30.

FACIAL NERVE TUMORS

The method of
Robert K. Jackler
by
Richard M. Irving
Robert K. Jackler

Tumors account for an estimated 5 percent of patients who are seen with facial paralysis. They are thus rare, but this should not, however, make the physician complacent. Sir Terrence Cawthorne's aphorism "all that palsies is not Bell's" should be kept in mind. The diagnosis of a facial nerve (FN) tumor is frequently delayed or missed. Early diagnosis is important because this influences the eventual outcome for FN function. Prognosis is related to both the size of the tumor and the duration of preoperative paralysis.

Clinical features of FN dysfunction that suggest a tumor include slowly progressive weakness, hyperfunction (full facial spasm or limited twitching), persistence of an acute palsy beyond 3 months, multiple cranial neuropathies, and the presence of persistent pain. Remarkably, only 50 percent of patients who have FN tumors manifest with FN dysfunction. Other patients demonstrate hearing loss (either conductive or sensorineural), tinnitus, or even vestibular complaints.

Primary FN tumors are characteristically slow growing and are almost invariably benign. Schwannomas and hemangiomas represent the vast majority of primary FN tumors (Table 1). Schwannomas were previously believed to be multicentric, but it is more likely that in these cases there is just extensive contiguous involvement of the nerve. These tumors tend to spread longitudinally within the fallopian canal, which results in a smooth, fusiform expansion of its bony wall. Although schwannomas may involve any segment of the nerve, they are predominantly intratemporal, with a predilection for the region of the geniculate ganglion. Although the literature cites an appreciable incidence of FN schwannomas arising within the internal auditory canal (IAC) and cerebellopontine angle (CPA), origination in this location is rare. Most purportedly FN schwannomas in this location are likely to have been vestibular schwannomas that adhered to the adjacent FN.

Hemangiomas are extraneural tumors that are believed to arise from rich capillary plexuses around the geniculate ganglion and in relation to Scarpa's ganglion within the IAC. There are a number of other tumors that can secondarily involve the FN, including vestibular schwannomas, meningiomas, and malignant tumors of the temporal bone. These are not the subject of this chapter, and the therapeutic principles described next cannot necessarily be applied to the management of these other lesions.

■ DIAGNOSIS

Assessment and grading of facial movement, cranial nerve examination, otoscopy, and examination of the parotid region should be done in any case of facial paralysis. However, clinical examination only rarely demonstrates an FN tumor. Intratympanic lesions can occasionally be visualized otoscopically, whereas extracranial lesions can often be palpated in the parotid region. The definitive diagnosis of FN tumor rests with comprehensive imaging of the FN course.

Enhanced magnetic resonance imaging (MRI) is superior to computed tomography (CT) as a screen for FN tumor, because it is capable of visualizing extraosseous lesions in the parotid bed and cerebellopontine angle. It also identifies inflammatory lesions (e.g., Bell's palsy, Lyme disease) that may simulate the presentation of a tumor. For intratemporal lesions, CT is complementary to MRI because it provides essential information concerning fallopian canal erosion, breaches in the osseous labyrinth, and surgical landmarks. To be of optimal value in FN diagnosis, both CT and MRI must be thin section and properly targeted on the FN course from brain stem to terminal branches. Physiologic topologic testing, a mainstay of FN diagnosis in the era before high-resolution imaging, is of little value today.

Hemangiomas demonstrate a characteristic honeycombed or spiculated appearance on CT with flecks of intra-

Table 1. Characteristics of Facial Nerve Tumors

CHARACTERISTIC	SCHWANNOMA	HEMANGIOMA
Location	Intratemporal (most) Extratemporal Intracranial	Geniculate ganglion Distal IAC Petrous apex
Shape	Fusiform multisegment involvement, regular margin	Focal, irregular
Gadolinium enhancement	Homogeneous	Variegated
CT appearance	Smooth fallopian canal expansion	Irregular bone erosion Entrapped bony spicules
Presentation	Weakness > twitch Slow progression typical	Twitch > weakness Acute episodes common
Hearing loss	CHL > SNHL (intratemporal) SNHL > CHL (intracranial)	SNHL > CHL

CT, computed tomographic; IAC, internal auditory canal; CHL, conductive hearing loss; SNHL, sensorineural hearing loss; >, more frequent than.

tumoral bone. The lesion usually has indistinct tumor margins and enlargement of the facial canal. A meticulous approach to imaging is required because it is easy to miss small lesions, especially hemangiomas.

An unsuspected tumor in the vicinity of the FN found incidentally during middle ear or mastoid surgery is best left alone. Biopsy typically results in complete facial paralysis that usually does not recover spontaneously. The most common scenario is a planned stapedectomy, during which tumor erosion of the stapes is found. In this situation, it is advisable to abandon surgery, order appropriate neurotologic and radiologic evaluation, and subsequently review management options with the patient.

■ FUNCTIONAL ASSESSMENT

In addition to appropriate imaging, an audiometric investigation is indicated. The patient needs to be counseled about hearing loss, because the tumor may have eroded the otic capsule, and in some cases preservation of hearing is not compatible with total tumor removal. Electrophysiologic tests can provide useful data concerning the likelihood of success in preserving residual FN fibers. Both electroneurography (ENOG) and electromyography (EMG) are obtained to characterize the functional integrity of the FN.

■ CONSERVATIVE MANAGEMENT

Primary tumors of the FN are benign, slow-growing lesions. These tumors threaten function rather than life, and thus decision making largely considers the long-term functional implications of each management choice. The duration of an individual's predicted life span is highly relevant, particularly for patients who have excellent facial function. In such circumstances, simple observation (yearly MRI) is a wise selection. By contrast, tumors associated with poor facial function are usually managed surgically. Difficult decisions arise in younger patients who have excellent facial function. If they undergo resection, they may sustain a permanent worsening of facial function. Engraftment achieves, at best, a 3/6 result. However, early intervention maximizes the possibility that tumor can be microdissected from the native FN fibers, with preservation of normal or near-normal function. Delaying tumor resection until FN dysfunction has become manifest renders this fortuitous outcome much less likely. In addition, the longer the duration of preoperative FN dysfunction (paresis or paralysis), the less successful FN grafts become. For these reasons, early intervention is usually in the long-term interest of younger patients who have good FN function, although a well-informed patient may elect a treatment delay. Observed patients who have good facial function undergo both yearly MRI scans and ENOG testing. ENOG may detect subclinical deterioration in nerve function and point to the need for intervention. Imaging alone is insufficient, because facial function may often deteriorate even in the presence of a radiographically stable lesion.

■ SURGICAL MANAGEMENT

General Principles

The selection of surgical approach is determined by the site and extent of the tumor as determined by CT and MRI, and the status of hearing in the ipsilateral ear (Table 2). Curative excision is the therapeutic aim. This goal is enhanced by frozen section control of the proximal and distal surgical margins. Neuromonitoring may be useful in cases in which the FN remains electrically stimulable. Comprehensive management of FN tumors requires that the surgeon be able to expose the nerve from the proximal root at the brain stem to the terminal branches distal to the parotid gland. The approaches used may involve extratemporal, intratemporal, and intracranial exposures. A combination of approaches is often required for multisegmental lesions.

Exposure

Parotidectomy. Extracranial tumors are approached by a standard superficial parotidectomy approach. Proximal extension of tumor along the nerve into the stylomastoid foramen necessitates the addition of a transmastoid approach. In this instance, the nerve is found within the mastoid in its vertical portion by following the digastric ridge anteriorly to fascia of the stylomastoid foramen. Removal of the mastoid tip and full exposure of the nerve into the parotid then allows for primary FN grafting onto healthy nerve within the mastoid.

Mastoidectomy. For intratemporal tumors confined to vertical and distal horizontal portions of the FN, the transmastoid approach provides adequate exposure. Following a standard cortical mastoidectomy, the nerve is best identified at the stylomastoid foramen and followed proximally, working from normal nerve toward tumor. Similarly, proximal dissection is also best carried out working from normal nerve to tumor. By extending the posterior access into the epitympanum, a view of the lateral canal and horizontal FN can be obtained. Exposure of the proximal horizontal portion of the nerve is the most difficult part of the procedure; a posterior tympanotomy (facial recess approach) helps in identifying the horizontal FN, but access is still limited by the ossicles. One option is to remove the incus, with or without the malleus head, to gain access and reconstruct the ossicular chain at the end of the procedure. The surgeon who undertakes this type of resection should have consent for, and be prepared to do, a middle fossa exposure in case at surgery the tumor is found to be extensive and proximal frozen section margins are positive.

Tympanotomy. The addition of a standard transcanal tympanotomy to either a transmastoid or middle fossa approach gives access to the horizontal portion of the FN. In such cases, removal of the incus and malleus head is usually required, with reconstruction of the ossicular chain following tumor removal and nerve grafting.

Middle Fossa Approach. The middle fossa (MF) approach is most suitable for tumors of the geniculate ganglion and IAC. This makes it the procedure of choice for the vast majority of hemangiomas. It also has utility, either alone

Table 2. Selection of Surgical Approach for Primary Facial Nerve Tumors

	PREOPERATIVE HEARING	
TUMOR LOCATION	**SERVICEABLE**	**NONSERVICEABLE**
FOCAL LESIONS		
Extracranial	Parotidectomy	Same
Vertical	Transmastoid	Same
Horizontal	Transmastoid and tympanotomy	Same
Geniculate	Middle fossa	Transcochlear
IAC	Middle fossa	Translabyrinthine
CPA	Retrosigmoid	Translabyrinthine
MULTISEGMENT LESIONS		
Extracranial + vertical	Parotidectomy + transmastoid	Same
Vertical + horizontal	Transmastoid + tympanotomy	Same
Horizontal + geniculate	Tympanotomy + middle fossa	Transochlear
Vertical to CPA (<2 cm)	Transmastoid + middle fossa	Transcochlear
IAC + CPA (<2 cm)	Middle fossa	Translabyrinthine
IAC + CPA (>2 cm)	Retrosigmoid	Translabyrinthine
CPA (>2 cm) + IAC + geniculate	Retrosigmoid + middle fossa	Transcochlear

CPA, cerebellopontine angle; IAC, internal auditory canal.

or in combination with other approaches, for a substantial fraction of FN schwannomas. The MF approach may be extended to provide access to the CPA with visualization of the FN root entry zone at the brain stem. The limited posterior fossa access provided precludes approaching tumors with a CPA component exceeding 2 cm in diameter. By opening the roof of the middle ear, this approach affords access to the tympanic (horizontal) segment of the nerve. Greater access is provided to the anterior segment (proximal to the cochleariform process) than to the posterior segment coursing superior to the stapes. Tumors with extension distal to the midtympanic segment are usually addressed with a combination of middle fossa and transmastoid approach. This technique provides access to the entire FN from the brain stem to the stylomastoid foramen without violation of the inner ear.

In the MF approach, the surgeon sits at the head of the table and addresses the temporal fossa from above. The skin incision we prefer is an inferiorly based U-shaped flap positioned above the ear. The advantage of this flap is that the temporalis muscle can be reflected with the skin flap, which maintains the muscle's innervation and blood supply. The skin and muscle flap is reflected inferiorly with skin hooks, and the external auditory canal is identified from above. A craniotomy positioned two-thirds anterior and one-third posterior to the ear canal and measuring approximately 4 cm x 4 cm is fashioned. This is beveled off posteriorly to avoid entry into the mastoid air cell system. The dura is elevated from the bone flap and middle cranial fossa. It is usually necessary to remove a residual rim of bone to lower the craniotomy to the level of the middle fossa floor. Elevation of the dura proceeds from posterior to anterior, with the surgeon first identifying the arcuate eminence created by the superior semicircular canal. Anteriorly, the greater superficial petrosal nerve is encountered. It is the most prominent of several nerve branches that may be present on the temporal floor. When adherent to the dura, it must be liberated sharply. Bleeding is a feature of middle fossa surgery, especially anteriorly from the middle meningeal artery. It can be controlled by a combination of bipolar cautery, hemostatic material, and packing bone wax into the foramen. The dural retraction is maintained by a middle fossa retractor engaged in the crest of the petrous bone.

A tumor of the geniculate is often evident at this stage as a prominence on the temporal floor. The identification of the geniculate ganglion in such cases is by tracing the greater superficial petrosal nerve back to the ganglion and then exposing the tumor and labyrinthine segment. Access to the horizontal portion of the nerve, if required for grafting, is by drilling through the tegmen, exposing the ossicular heads and epitympanum. A tympanotomy can also be simultaneously employed in this instance. Sacrifice of the nerve at the geniculate will require exposure of proximal healthy nerve for grafting, and bone removal will need to be extended over the labyrinthine segments of the nerve, and in some cases opening of the IAC will be required. The geniculate ganglion is immediately adjacent to the basal turn of the cochlea, and tumors at this site can erode the otic capsule. This may not be evident on preoperative imaging, and patients who have tumors at this site should be warned about the possibility of hearing loss. At closure, any defect in the tegmen should be sealed with either a free muscle graft or a bone fragment to prevent brain herniation into the middle ear.

Combined Transmastoid–Middle Fossa Approach. Lesions involving the geniculate ganglion extending into the vertical portion of the FN require simultaneous exposure via the middle fossa and mastoidectomy. An inverted J-shaped supra- and postauricular incision is fashioned. The mastoid and middle fossa exposures employed are exactly as previously described. This approach allows the most extensive intratemporal exposure of the FN from the CPA to the stylomastoid foramen in patients who have serviceable hearing.

Retrosigmoid Approach. Tumors involving the FN in the CPA and proximal IAC with serviceable hearing can be removed by the retrosigmoid (RS) approach. These tumors can be difficult to differentiate from vestibular schwannomas on either clinical or radiographic grounds. In many cases, the diagnosis is made at the time of surgery, when the entire surface of a suspected vestibular schwannoma has a low threshold for CNVII on electrical stimulation. The problem with this approach is poor access to the FN within the lateral IAC. This can be especially limiting when an FN graft is required. We limit use of the RS approach to tumors exceeding 2 cm in diameter in the CPA with involvement of only the lateral two-thirds of the IAC. In patients who have FN tumors with good hearing, a large CPA component, and deep IAC involvement, the approach can be a combined RS-MF approach.

Translabyrinthine Approach. The translabyrinthine operation provides access to the FN from the stylomastoid foramen to the brain stem. Because the semicircular canals are removed during the course of FN exposure, this procedure is suitable only for patients without serviceable hearing. This approach also affords excellent access to the intracranial portion of FN tumors. In cases in which the FN cannot be kept in anatomic continuity, rerouting the convoluted intratemporal course can provide an extra 10 to 15 mm length and may, in the case of small defects, allow for a primary anastomosis.

Transcochlear Approach. The geniculate ganglion and the takeoff of the greater superficial petrosal nerve lie immediately superior to the cochlea. When the ipsilateral ear does not have serviceable hearing, removal of the cochlea substantially facilitates access to the geniculate ganglion. The transcochlear approach is also suitable for accessing a posterior fossa tumor component. When the CSF space is entered, the eustachian tube must be sealed, the meatus sutured closed, and the cavity obliterated with an adipose tissue graft. Such measures are not required for entirely extradural approaches.

■ MANAGEMENT OF THE FACIAL NERVE

Fallopian Canal Decompression

The intratemporal group of tumors cause a higher percentage of facial paralysis than do the parotid or CPA lesions. This is believed to be due to compression of the healthy fibers by the tumor in the nonyielding fallopian canal. In individuals who have mild paralysis, one option to be considered is osseous decompression as opposed to tumor resection. This aims to delay the onset of progressive paralysis die to entrapment neuropathy. Although this concept has considerable theoretic appeal, the efficacy of this management option is unknown.

Preservation of Uninvolved Fibers

The goal of FN tumor surgery is removal of the neoplasm with preservation of the remaining viable FN fibers whenever possible. Preservation of residual fibers is more often achievable with hemangiomas, which arise outside the epineurium, than it is with schwannomas that are intrinsic to the nerve. Nevertheless, maintenance of neural integrity is occasionally possible for schwannomas, especially for small focal lesions. Preoperative paralysis or marked paresis is a notable adverse predictor for residual fiber preservation.

Difficult judgments arise when a tumor has partially destroyed the FN. As a general rule, when greater than 50 percent of the FN fiber bulk has been disrupted, results are better with complete resection and engraftment (achieves at best grade 3/6 function). Experience with split grafts aimed at replacing the missing fraction of nerve has not been favorable. The surgeon must take caution not to misinterpret swelling of the residual epineurium and fiber bundle as possessing more substance than it actually does. It is possible for a 10 percent remnant to swell to a size exceeding 50 percent of the diameter of a normal nerve. Electrophysiologic conductance across the site of tumor resection can provide helpful information about the functional integrity of the remaining fibers.

Nerve Repair

In cases in which nerve integrity cannot be preserved, repair must be undertaken. Simple reapproximation is virtually never possible. Rerouting of the redundant intratemporal course of the FN can sometimes liberate sufficient extra length to accommodate the resected segment and thus permit direct nerve repair. This maneuver has the advantage of achieving repair with a single anastomosis. When the apex of the geniculate ganglion has been destroyed (especially with hemangiomas), rerouting across the base of the geniculate triangle brings together the labyrinthine and posterior tympanic segments. Most other forms of rerouting (e.g., mastoid–meatal) require labyrinthectomy and thus are suitable only for nonhearing ears.

When a direct anastomosis is impossible, the defect should be spanned with a nerve graft. Either the greater auricular or transverse cervical nerves are an excellent size match for the FN. Anastomoses where epineurium is present can be approximated with an interrupted series of 9–0 monofilament sutures (usually 3 to 6 sutures). Proximal to the fundus of the IAC, no epineurium is present, and the nerve is sheathed in a fragile glial layer of little tensile strength. Reapproximation in this segment of the nerve is usually achieved with a single suture placed through the middle of the nerve. Some experts have advocated use of a collagen tube rather than suture (more technically demanding) in this location.

Repair of extracranial lesions that extend beyond the pes anserinus constitutes a special case. Such grafts often need to be branched to meet up with the distal branches of the nerve. In this situation, a sural nerve graft is often superior because of its greater length and better bulk that allows for splitting of fascicles.

■ MANAGEMENT OF LONG-TERM PARALYSIS

A surprising fraction of patients who have FN tumors present with long-standing (>1 year) total facial paralysis. In such cases, the vitality and regeneration capacity of the proximal facial nerve is in doubt. Engraftment following tumor resection might not be successful. Preoperative EMG is helpful in assessing the status of the denervated facial musculature. Electrical silence is ominous. Our general policy is to undertake engraftment only when complete palsy has existed for less than 2 years. With favorable EMG findings (fasciculations, polyphasic potentials), grafting may be attempted even beyond this date. Persistent palsy beyond 5 years nearly always indicates the need for a reanimation strategy not based on the native facial musculature. Options include static and dynamic slings as well as innervated microvascular muscle transfer.

Crossover anastomosis between the hypoglossal and FN (CNXII–CNVII) is indicated in several circumstances. One situation occurs when a large intracranial tumor has rendered the proximal stump at the brain stem useless for grafting purposes. Another situation is a failed FN repair. When no recovery has occurred 1 year following the repair attempt, EMG assessment is undertaken. Unless it is technically well performed, repair is seldom successful. Delay beyond 18 months (combined preoperative and postoperative duration of paralysis) jeopardizes the efficacy of XII–VII due to atrophy of the denervated facial musculature.

Suggested Reading

Dort JC, Fisch U. Facial nerve schwannomas. Skull Base Surgery 1991; 1: 51-56.

Janecka IP, Conley J. Primary neoplasms of the facial nerve. Plast Reconstr Surg 1987; 79:177-185.

O'Donoghue GM, Brackmann DE, House JW, Jackler RK. Neuromas of the facial nerve. Am J Otol 1989; 10:49-54.

Saleh E, Achilli V, Naguib M, et al. Facial nerve neuromas: diagnosis and management. Am J Otol 1995; 16:521-526.

Shelton C, Brackmann DE, Lo WWM, Carberry JN. Intratemporal facial nerve hemangiomas. Otolaryngol Head Neck Surg 1991; 104:116-121.

HEMIFACIAL SPASM

The method of
Aage R. Moller
by
Stephen P. Cass
Aage R. Moller

Hemifacial spasm (HFS) is a rare disorder (incidence of 0.74 per 100,000 in white men and 0.81 per 100,000 in white women) characterized by paroxysmal contractions of the facial muscles on one side of the face. Between attacks, the face is normal with respect to tonus and function. There is no facial weakness except in some patients who have had HFS for many years. The spasm typically involves the muscles around one eye early in the course of the disorder. Over the course of several years, the spasm may progress downward on the face until the entire facial musculature, including the platysma, is involved. In rare cases, the spasm may begin in the lower face. Spasm may occur during sleep, and the frequency of attacks increases during periods of stress. Emotions as well as strong voluntary contractions of facial muscles (especially those around the eyes) can elicit attacks of spasm, Typically, HFS occurs relatively late in life, but occasionally young people are affected. HFS has many similarities to face pain (trigeminal neuralgia), but, unlike trigeminal neuralgia, HFS does not seem to occur more frequently in combination with other diseases such as multiple sclerosis.

The diagnosis of HFS is usually made on the basis of clinical examination. In uncertain cases, electromyography can be used to confirm the diagnosis. In HFS, the affected facial muscles show synchronized activity of many motor units and an abnormally high firing rate (350 discharges per second compared with a normal maximal firing rate of 50 to 70 per second).

There are other disorders that are associated with involuntary contractions of facial muscles, but HFS is usually easily distinguished from such disorders. Postparalytic facial spasm should be distinguished from HFS on the basis of patient history. Blepharospasm is bilateral in contrast to HFS, which is distinctly unilateral. Certain forms of orofacial, oromandibular, or orolingual dystonia, such as Meige's syndrome, may resemble HFS in the beginning of their course. However, these disorders involve the tongue and muscles of mastication in addition to facial muscles, and that characteristic makes it relatively easy to distinguish them from HFS. Trigeminal neuralgia may occasionally be accompanied by facial muscle contractions that may, by superficial observation, resemble HFS. However, simultaneously occurring trigeminal neuralgia and HFS is extremely rare (known as tic convulsive). Facial myokymia, characterized by flickering spasm that resembles crawling of worms, is often the symptom of serious disorders such as brain stem tumors. Probably the most difficult disorder to distinguish from HFS is the common nervous tic involving habitual facial movements.

It is believed that hemifacial spasm is caused by hyperactivity of the facial motonucleus that is brought about by irritation of the facial nerve by a blood vessel. It is known that close contact between blood vessels and the facial nerve is rather common, and it is therefore assumed that some other factors are necessary in addition to a blood vessel being in contact with the facial nerve in order for HFS to develop.

■ THERAPEUTIC ALTERNATIVES

HFS is a benign disorder, and the decision of treatment depends on the extent to which a patient is bothered by the spasm. Persons who have close contact with the public have a high degree of motivation for treatment, whereas people with little such contact may elect to live with the disorder untreated.

There is no known medical treatment that is effective against HFS. Although carbamazepine and baclofen have been suggested as treatments, we have not found these medications to be effective and do not use them to treat HFS.

There are basically three alternative treatments for HFS: microvascular decompression (MVD) of the facial nerve, injection of botulinum toxin into selected facial muscles, and partial selective neurectomy of the facial nerve. MVD of the facial nerve in the cerebellopontine angle is presently in common use and is our preferred approach.

An alternative approach for patients who are unwilling or unable to undergo microvascular decompression is injection of botulinum toxin into the affected facial muscles. Injection of botulinum toxin can also be used to treat blepharospasm and facial synkinesis following facial nerve injury. Botulinum toxin blocks the neuromuscular junction (muscle endplates), and thus the therapeutic goal of reducing the severity of spasm involves a trade-off with induced facial weakness. The amount of botulinum toxin injected and the locations of the injections are crucial factors for obtaining acceptable results; thus, it can be a demanding task to obtain an acceptable balance between facial weakness and relief of spasm. Common side effects of the botulinum toxin injection include mild ptosis of the upper lid; excessive tearing; and lower facial weakness, which produces a lopsided smile. More troublesome side effects such as vertical diplopia, blurred vision, and exposure keratitis can occur after excessive injections or if the injection diffuses beyond the intended target muscle. The incidence of these complications is reported to be 10 percent to 30 percent at the beginning of treatment, but it becomes less frequent following adjustment of the injection site and dose. One disadvantage of treatment with botulinum toxin is that the treatment has to be repeated periodically, usually at 3 to 6 month intervals.

Botulinum toxin blocks the neuromuscular junction (muscle endplates), and although this effect was initially thought to be fully reversible, permanent changes in the form of axonal sprouting and the creation of new motor endplates have recently been shown to occur following botulinum treatment. These changes cause abnormalities in muscle function and a reduction of the effect of future administration of botulinum toxin. Although the incidence of reported systemic complications is low, changes in cardiovascular reflexes have been demonstrated in as many as 80 percent of individuals treated with botulinum toxin.

A third alternative treatment is partial selective neurectomy of the facial nerve. This method consists of selectively sectioning parts of the temporal branch of the facial nerve. It was described by McCabe and used by Fisch, who treated a large number of patients and described the method in detail. In this procedure, control of spasm is obtained in exchange for a certain degree of facial weakness. Naturally, the goal is to limit the weakness while reducing the spasm. With skill and experience, this goal can be obtained in the majority of patients, according to the 1986 study by Dobie and Fisch. We view the results of selective neurectomy as less satisfactory regarding relief of HFS than that of MVD of the facial nerve, and the risk of permanent facial weakness is greater. It should be noted that selective neurectomy may be considered for treatment of blepharospasm for which there is no other suitable surgical treatment available.

Microvascular Decompression

MVD of the facial nerve in the cerebellopontine angle (CPA) is our preferred approach. This operation treats HFS by moving a blood vessel off the facial nerve where it exits the brain stem and placing an implant (shredded Teflon, muscle, or fascia) between the vessel and the nerve. This procedure provides total relief of spasm in a large percentage of patients, but it requires a retromastoid craniectomy, and therefore, it carries certain risks.

The operation was first described by Gardner and Sava in 1962, and later refined by Jannetta and others. The success rate of the operation varies among surgeons; for experienced surgeons, the rate ranges between 80 percent and 90 percent. In a study of 703 patients at the Department of Neurological Surgery at the University of Pittsburgh, the success rate was 84 percent. The recent introduction of intraoperative monitoring of the abnormal muscle response has improved the success rate and decreased the need for reoperation, which carries a higher risk of complications. Surgeons who perform fewer operations are likely to have a lower success rate. Studies of patients over many years reveals that recurrences are very rare.

Patients are selected for microvascular decompression of the facial nerve to relieve HFS based on their history and physical examination. If the diagnosis is uncertain, special electromyographic testing is performed to confirm the diagnosis. Alternative treatments, including the option of no treatment, are reviewed with the patient. The preoperative evaluation includes pure-tone audiometry, air and bone conduction, and baseline brain stem auditory evoked potentials (BAEP). Prior magnetic resonance imaging studies of the brain are reviewed.

The operative procedure is performed under general anesthesia without the use of muscle relaxants so that intraoperative facial nerve monitoring can be performed along with intraoperative monitoring of the BAEP. The patient is placed in a lateral decubitus position with the head secured using Mayfield pins and holder. The head is positioned with the sagittal axis of the head tilted slightly vertex down, and the head is slightly rotated nose down in the axial place. The retromastoid area is shaved and prepped.

An oblique linear skin incision is used that begins approximately 4 cm behind the mastoid tip and angles anteriorly and superiorly for 5 cm. This incision lies within the shaved margin of the natural hair line. Typically, the epidermis is incised with a knife, and cutting cautery is used to divide the dermis and subcutaneous tissues. The subcutaneous dissection is carried first posteriorly and then medially down to the bony cranium. The subcutaneous tissues and deep musculature overlying the retromastoid cranium are elevated forward using a combination of blunt dissection and electrocautery. The mastoid emissary vein is isolated and divided, and the bony foramen of the vein is occluded with bone wax. The dissection is carried inferiorly until the cranium curves medially near the margin of the foramen magnum. Anteriorly, the posterior insertions of the digastric muscle are released, and superiorly, the inferior margin of the temporalis muscle is exposed. Self-retaining retractors are positioned, and hemostasis is secured.

The courses of the sigmoid and transverse sinuses are estimated by examining the surface anatomy of the mastoid and retromastoid cranium. Using a craniotome, dural elevators, and rongeurs, a retromastoid craniotomy approximately 30 mm (inferior–superior) x 30 mm (anterior–posterior) is created. Before opening the dura, hemostasis is checked, and all exposed mastoid air cells are occluded with bone wax. The dura is incised in a curvilinear manner using a No. 15 blade. Once a small dural incision is complete, the dural edge is grasped with a fine-toothed pickup, and Metenzbaum scissors are used to complete the dural incision. It is helpful to apply gentle pressure to the lateral surface of the cerebellum during the dural incisions to prevent possible herniation of the cerebellum through the incision. Neurolon sutures (4–0) are used to retract the anterior dural flap anteriorly.

A 0.5 x 3 mm neurosurgical cottonoid patty with rubber dam (strip of surgical glove cut to the size of the neurosurgical patty) is then placed onto the surface of the cerebellum. A microsurgical suction and bayonet forceps are used to advance the patty until the arachnoid surrounding the CPA cistern is exposed. An arachnoid hook is then used to open the arachnoid and release cerebrospinal fluid (CSF) from the CPA cistern. Once CSF is released, the cerebellum will relax and fall away. posteriorly. Self-retaining brain retractors are seldom necessary.

The structures identified within the posterior fossa include the tentorium; the fifth cranial nerve; the eighth nerve complex, which should be in the middle of the field; the seventh cranial nerve; and cranial nerves IX, X, and XI near the jugular foramen.

Microvascular compression of the facial nerve typically occurs along the pontine segment of the facial nerve by either the vertebral artery, the posterior inferior cerebellar artery, the anterior inferior cerebellar artery, and/or by veins. Veins are coagulated and divided. Arteries are displaced laterally off the brain stem and nerve. Small pieces of shredded Teflon felt are then interposed between the nerve and the vessels. Successful microvascular decompression is enhanced by concurrent monitoring of the abnormal electromyographic response that is characteristic of hemifacial spasm. This response must totally disappear before the operation is concluded. Complications related to hearing loss and facial paralysis are reduced through attention to the occurrence of delays in the BAEP and facial nerve injury potentials.

Once the microvascular decompression is completed, the neurosurgical patty is removed, and the cerebellum is inspected for any bleeding sites using multiple Valsalva's maneuvers. The dura is then closed with a 4–0 Neurolon suture. The craniotomy site is reconstructed using collected bone dust and chips wrapped in Surgicel. Alternatively, methylmethacrylate is used to perform a cranioplasty.

The incision is then closed in three layers, with a deep layer of 2–0 Vicryl reapproximating the musculoperiosteal tissue over the cranium. The deep cutaneous tissues are then closed with 2–0 Vicryl. The skin incision is closed with a running subcuticular 4–0 Vicryl suture, and a light dressing is applied.

Complications

The complications associated with microvascular decompression for HFS are potentially severe but infrequent. The most common complication is partial or total hearing loss, which is sometimes accompanied by severe tinnitus. Barker reported 2.6 percent partial or total losses of hearing over a 20 year period. This number includes operations performed over an extended time period before the introduction of routine intraoperative monitoring of BAEP. The use of intraoperative monitoring of BAEP can reduce the risk of hearing loss to less than 1 percent. Facial palsy, brain stem strokes, and death may also occur rarely as a complication of MVD of the facial nerve. Barker reported a 0.9 percent incidence of permanent severe facial weakness, one operative death (0.1 percent), and two brain stem infarctions (0.3 percent) in a study of 703 patients.

Naturally, the risk of complications is smaller when the operation is performed by surgeons who are experienced in microvascular decompression of the facial nerve; less experienced surgeons are likely to produce more complications. Most of the operations in the study reported by Barker were done by a surgeon who does 300 or more MVD cases per year in an institution with perhaps the greatest amount of experience in the world with that type of operation.

The claim has been made that it is not at all a blood vessel in contact with the facial nerve that causes the symptoms of HFS. This claim is based on the observation that as many as 30 percent to 50 percent of asymptomatic individuals have similar blood vessels in contact with the facial nerve of patients with HFS. The use of MVD as a treatment of HFS has consequently been disputed. However, the high success rate of MVD operations for treating HFS seems to contradict that statement. The controversy can be explained by assuming that the vascular compression is a condition that is *necessary* but not *sufficient* to cause symptoms and that other factors, such as changes in the facial motonucleus, in addition to vascular compression, are needed to cause symptoms. Elimination of one of these *necessary* factors (such as the vascular compression of the facial nerve) totally cures the disease, and that may explain the high success rate of MVD operations for HFS.

■ PROS AND CONS OF TREATMENT

Not all cases of HFS require treatment. HFS is a benign, although annoying disorder, and certain patients may elect to live with the spasms. For patients who feel significantly handicapped, we feel that the microvascular decompression operation is an ideal treatment that is capable of rendering the patient totally free from spasm with no trade-off involving facial weakness. The patient must understand and accept the low but real risk of serious complications related to the intracranial nature of the procedure. The other two alternative treatments, selective neurectomy and treatment with botulinum toxin, can be used effectively to treat HFS, but these procedures have a lower success rate and a higher recurrence rate compared with MVD for HFS. Although the incidence of serious complications associated with selective neurectomy and botulinum toxin injections is very low, the expected sequelae (facial weakness) and inconveniences (recurrences and required frequent re-treatments) inherent to these therapies must be considered.

Suggested Reading

Barker FG, Jannetta PJ, Bissonette DJ, et al. Microvascular decompression for hemifacial spasm. J Neurosurg 1995; 82:201-210.

Digre D, Corbett JJ. Hemifacial spasm: Differential diagnosis, mechanism, and treatment. Adv Neurol 1988; 49:151-176.

Dobie RA, Fisch U. Primary and revision surgery (selective neurectomy) for facial hyperkinesis. Arch Otolaryngol Head Neck Surg 1986; 112: 154-163.

Moller AR. Cranial nerve dysfunction syndromes: Pathophysiology of microvascular compression. In: Barrow DI, ed. Neurosurgical topics book 13, 'Surgery of cranial nerves of the posterior fossa.' Park Ridge, Ill: American Association of Neurological Surgeons, 1993:105.

Møller AR, Lovely TJ. Microvascular decompression of the seventh and eighth cranial nerves. In: Myers EN, ed. Operative otolaryngology. Philadelphia: WB Saunders, 1997:1559.

Sindou M, Keravel Y, Moller AR. Hemifacial spasm: A multidisciplinary approach. Wien: Springer-Verlag (in press).

GLOMUS TUMORS

The method of
Joseph B. Nadol, Jr.
by
Robert W. Jyung
Michael J. McKenna
Joseph B. Nadol, Jr.

Paragangliomas (glomus tumors) of the temporal bone are neoplasms arising from neural crest–derived paraganglia, which were meticulously described by Guild in 1941. The site of origin of these tumors can be predicted by the location and density of these paraganglia (in order of descending frequency): (1) in the adventitia of the jugular bulb, (2) within the inferior tympanic canaliculus, (3) in the mucosa over the promontory, (4) within the nodose ganglion and the vagus nerve trunk, or, rarely, (5) in the fallopian canal itself. Paragangliomas of the temporal bone range in size from small, easily treated tympanic lesions (glomus tympanicum) to extensive jugular foramen lesions (glomus jugulare or glomus vagale) with cranial nerve deficits, great vessel involvement, and intracranial extension. Although many staging systems for paragangliomas have been described, perhaps the most commonly used scheme for conveying tumor data is the Fisch system (Table 1). Staging systems provide a guideline for choosing the surgical approach but cannot substitute for meticulous review of computed tomography (CT) and magnetic resonance imaging (MRI) scans and angiogram images.

DIAGNOSIS AND EVALUATION

Presenting Symptoms

Patients typically have complaints of pulsatile tinnitus, with or without an associated conductive hearing loss, bloody otorrhea, or a mass in the ear canal. Facial paralysis, hoarseness, and dysphagia secondary to cranial nerve palsies are other common presenting complaints. Once a paraganglioma is suspected, careful attention should be paid to any feature of the patient's history that would indicate a secreting tumor (1 percent to 3 percent of tumors), such as episodic flushing, sweating, palpitations, tachycardia, chest pain, headache, or hypertension. These symptoms should prompt a 24 hour urine collection to screen for catecholamine metabolites, including metanephrine and vanillylmandelic acid (VMA). In the event of negative results from urine collection despite clear-cut symptoms of catecholamine excess, direct venous sampling by an interventional radiologist should be considered. A patient who has a symptomatic secreting

Table 1. Fisch Classification of Glomus Tumors

Type	Subtype	Description
Type A		Tumors limited to the middle ear cleft
Type B		Tumors limited to the tympanomastoid area without bone destruction in the infralabyrinthine compartment
Type C		Tumors extending into and destroying bone in the infralabyrinthine and apical compartments
	C1	Tumors destroying the jugular foramen and bulb
	C2	Tumors invading the vertical portion of the carotid canal
	C3	Tumors invading the horizontal portion of the carotid canal
Type D		Tumors with intracranial extension
	D1	Tumors with <2 cm intracranial extension
	D2	Tumors with >2 cm intracranial extension
	D3	Tumors with inoperable intracranial extension

tumor should be referred for antihypertensive treatment with appropriate α- and β-blocking medication.

Family History

Approximately 10 percent of head and neck paragangliomas are familial. It is important to elicit any family history of paragangliomas, because the incidence of multiple, synchronous tumors in familial cases is 30 percent to 40 percent, compared to approximately 10 percent for sporadic cases. The gene for familial paragangliomas is transmitted in an autosomal dominant pattern; therefore, any child of a patient who has familial tumors has a 50 percent chance of inheriting the gene. However, only children who inherit the gene from their fathers have the potential for developing tumors, based on the phenomenon of genomic imprinting.

Physical Examination

Otologic examination may reveal a vascular mass in the middle ear that can be blanched with positive pressure on pneumotoscopy (Brown's sign); alternatively, in some patients, paragangliomas can erode through the tympanic membrane, which results in purulent otorrhea or the presentation of a "polyp" on the ear canal. However, negative results from otoscopy do not rule out a paraganglioma, because jugular and vagal paragangliomas often do not have a middle ear component. When a paraganglioma is visible within the middle ear, differentiating between a tympanic and jugular paraganglioma can be difficult, unless one can visualize the maximum diameter of the tumor above the tympanic annulus. This finding strongly supports the diagnosis of a tympanic paraganglioma.

The remainder of the head and neck examination should be directed toward ruling out other paragangliomas, either ipsilateral or contralateral; this part of the examination may reveal a palpable neck mass or a bruit at the skull base upon auscultation. A detailed cranial nerve examination is important to document all deficits associated with the tumor. Early signs of cranial nerve compromise should prompt the otolaryngologist to counsel the patient that surgery may worsen the pre-existing deficits. Although it has been suggested that pre-existing cranial nerve deficits make the patient's postoperative recovery easier (because some degree of compensation will already have occurred), we have found that often even compromised cranial nerves maintain some low level of function that is lost when these nerves are sacrificed.

Diagnostic Evaluation

Standard evaluation includes air- and bone-conduction audiometry, which will establish a baseline for post-treatment comparison or for serial audiograms if the tumor is observed.

Diagnostic imaging consists of a high-resolution temporal bone CT scan with fine cuts in the axial and coronal planes. An axial CT image of a glomus jugulare tumor demonstrates erosion of the lateral cortical plate of bone at the jugular bulb (Fig. 1); in addition, it provides the bony detail to evaluate tumor relationships to the facial nerve, cochlea, and carotid artery. An MRI scan complements the CT images by demonstrating the typical "salt and pepper" consistency and serpiginous flow voids within the tumor, intracranial and/or intradural extension, presence or absence of flow

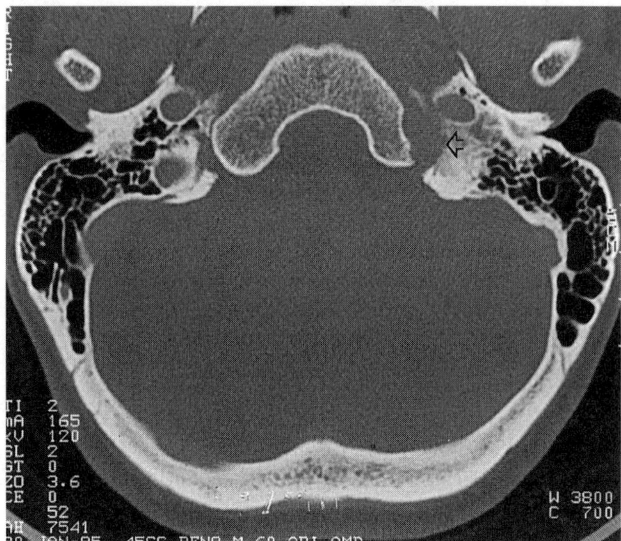

Figure 1.
Erosion of the lateral cortical plate of the jugular bulb (open arrow), indicating a left glomus jugulare tumour.

in the ipsilateral and contralateral sigmoid sinus, as well as the relationship of the tumor to the carotid artery.

If surgical treatment is planned, four-vessel angiography is critical for several reasons: (1) it is the "gold standard" for detection of multicentric tumors; (2) it identifies both extra- and intracranial feeding vessels; (3) it allows embolization for preoperative control of external carotid artery blood supply to glomus jugulare and vagale tumors; (4) it identifies intrasinus and/or intravenous tumor extension; and (5) it provides information regarding adequacy of flow in the contralateral sigmoid sinus and/or internal jugular vein. Documenting flow in the contralateral sigmoid sinus and/or jugular vein is critical for ensuring that tumor resection will not compromise intracranial venous return.

We routinely embolize glomus jugulare and glomus vagale tumors before surgery. Embolization with Gelfoam significantly decreases intraoperative blood loss if surgery is performed within 24 to 48 hours; otherwise, recanalization of feeder vessels will occur. The exception occurs in some familial cases, where a symptomatic patient may have a glomus vagale and a contralateral glomus jugulare. In an effort to ensure preservation of vagus nerve function on the side of the glomus jugulare, resection may be attempted without embolization, thus avoiding the risk of edema secondary to embolization causing nerve compression.

A final imaging modality for glomus tumors is radionuclide imaging with somatostatin analogues such as octreotides. We have used octreotide scans in a few cases in which multicentric or recurrent tumors were suspected, but the ultimate value of these scans has yet to be determined.

When a paraganglioma extensively involves the carotid artery in a patient who has been selected for surgery, test balloon occlusion can be used, followed by assessment of cerebral blood flow with xenon or positron emission tomography (PET) scanning. Test results will determine whether carotid reconstruction would be necessary in the event of carotid artery injury during attempted tumor "peeling" from the adventitia or following planned carotid artery resection. However, in most cases, we do not believe that the typically benign nature of glomus jugulare tumors warrants aggressive measures such as carotid artery resection; a small amount of tumor residual on the carotid artery can be treated with postoperative radiotherapy or followed with serial MRI scans. The avoidance of complications related to carotid artery reconstruction or sacrifice, then, may be worth the trade-off of incomplete tumor removal.

Treatment Options

Our philosophy of treating paragangliomas is based on two main principles: (1) the decision to sacrifice structures during surgery should always be tempered by the fact that most of these tumors are benign; and (2) the morbidity of lower cranial nerve deficits, especially combinations of ipsilateral glossopharyngeal and vagal nerve palsies or ipsilateral vagal and hypoglossal nerve palsies, should be avoided whenever possible.

As a general rule, we encourage surgical removal of tympanic and/or hypotympanic paragangliomas, given the high likelihood of total tumor removal with minimal risks of hearing loss or cranial nerve deficits. For jugular paragangliomas, the decision to use radiotherapy, surgery, or combined therapy should be individualized based on the patient's wishes, the patient's age and coexisting medical conditions, the size of the tumor, and the number of associated cranial nerve deficits. In counseling the patient, it is important to clarify that the goals and risks of the two treatment modalities are different. The object of surgical treatment is total or near-total tumor removal, with the acute risks of new cranial nerve deficits, vascular injury and/or bleeding, and cerebrospinal fluid leak, whereas the goal of radiotherapy is arrest of tumor growth, with the long-term risks of tumor regrowth, late-onset cranial nerve deficits, and osteoradionecrosis of the temporal bone.

We prefer to avoid primary radiotherapy for jugular paragangliomas in young patients given the long-term potential for tumor growth and the increased risk of cranial nerve damage incurred by salvage surgery in an irradiated field. In evaluating patients for surgery, physiologic age is probably more relevant than chronologic age, and therefore an older but healthy patient is still a viable surgical candidate, whereas a younger patient who has significant cardiac or pulmonary problems may be better suited for radiotherapy. Candidates for surgical treatment include (1) patients who have small jugular paragangliomas that can be safely removed without significant risk to cranial nerves, and (2) patients who have larger tumors with established cranial nerve deficits. Patients who have larger tumors but no associated cranial nerve deficits are better treated with radiotherapy, followed by serial MRI scans. Radiation can be delivered over a 4 to 5 week, with the total dose ranging between 40 and 50 Gy. Rarely, a patient who has a larger jugular paraganglioma but no cranial nerve deficits may be reluctant to accept treatment; such a patient can be followed up with serial MRI scans, with the trigger for intervention being significant growth or onset of cranial nerve deficits.

Surgical Approaches

When doubt exists as to whether a jugular foramen lesion is truly a paraganglioma, the surgeon should consider performing a biopsy in the operating room, especially when a component of the tumor is easily accessed. For example, a polypoid mass extruding through the external auditory canal can be sharply transected, followed by canal packing to achieve hemostasis. In some cases, a biopsy may reveal unexpected pathology that could drastically alter treatment planning.

Glomus Tympanicum

For small tympanic paragangliomas (Fisch type A), a simple transcanal tympanotomy may be all that is required (Fig. 2). However, a preferable approach usually is a postauricular tympanotomy accompanied by hypotympanotomy (inferior canaloplasty) to expose the inferior aspect of the promontory and the hypotympanum. The bony canal is exposed as for a standard canaloplasty through the postauricular approach and, after the tympanic membrane is reflected superiorly, the inferior canal wall is lowered, along with the inferior bony annulus. The tumor is then dissected from the promontory under magnification. Direct visualization and bipolar cautery of the feeding vessel to these lesions (inferior tympanic artery) can be easily accomplished with this method. Alternatively, an argon laser with a slightly defocused beam can effectively cauterize the base of the tumor on the promontory. The hypotympanum is packed with Gelfoam, and reconstruction is achieved with a temporalis fascia graft bridging from the undersurface of the tympanic membrane to the inferior canal wall. Split-thickness skin grafts are used to cover the fascia graft as well as any exposed bony canal wall. The external auditory canal is packed with an outer layer of antibiotic ointment–soaked gauze (removed at 1 week) and an inner "rosebud" pack of silk strips around surgical cotton (removed at 2 weeks).

For larger lesions that extend into the mastoid but do not involve the jugular bulb or carotid artery (Fisch type B), the preferred method is a canal wall-up mastoidectomy with an extended facial recess approach. This approach can

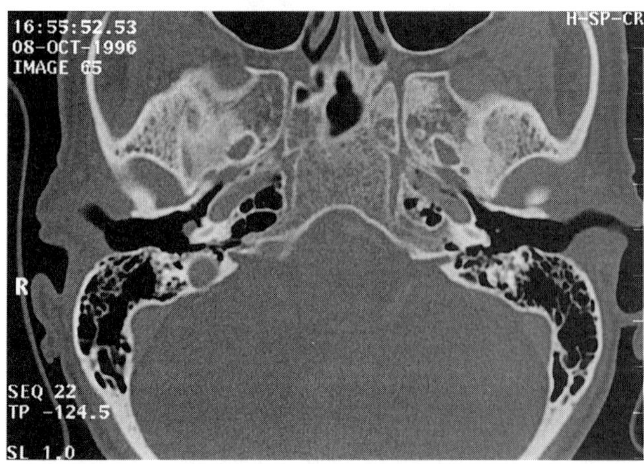

Figure 2.
Right glomus tympanicum, adjacent to the basal turn of the cochlea, in an extensively pneumatized temporal bone.

also be used for tympanic paragangliomas. Exposure is obtained with a postauricular incision, turning the pinna forward after elevating a Korner's canal flap as is done for chronic ear surgery. After a canal wall-up mastoidectomy, the mastoid segment of the facial nerve is identified through thin bone and followed to the stylomastoid foramen, which is skeletonized. Retrofacial air cells can be opened to delineate the superior and inferior limits of the mastoid component of the tumor, and the proximity of the tumor to the jugular bulb is determined. An extended facial recess is created, sacrificing the chorda tympani nerve. The tympanic bone is then thinned, following the contour of the inferior aspect of the bony external auditory canal toward the temporomandibular joint. The fibrous annulus of the tympanic membrane can be turned forward within the preserved bony external auditory canal, and tumor dissection in the middle ear can proceed. The tumor can then be mobilized from multiple routes, anteriorly through the middle ear, inferiorly through the extended facial recess, and posteriorly through the retrofacial air cells. Again, access to the main feeding vessel (inferior tympanic artery) for bipolar cautery is easily obtained with this approach. Ossicular and tympanic membrane reconstruction are performed as for chronic ear surgery.

Glomus Jugulare

For jugular paragangliomas (Fisch type C), a standard infratemporal fossa approach is used, with continuous facial nerve monitoring (Fig. 3). A wide postauricular C-shaped incision is extended down into an upper neck skin crease, staying 2 fingerbreadths inferior to the angle of the mandible to protect the marginal mandibular branch of the facial nerve. The broad anteriorly based skin flap and pinna are then elevated in a plane just superficial to the temporalis fascia and mastoid periosteum up to the external auditory canal. A square flap of periosteum can be elevated and left attached on the undersurface of the soft-tissue flap just posterior to the external auditory canal, which is sharply transected lateral to the bony cartilaginous junction. The skin of the cartilaginous canal is circumferentially elevated and everted through the meatus, where a blind sac closure is performed. The periosteal flap can then be turned forward and sutured to reinforce the closure of the external canal skin. The pinna is now reflected anteriorly to the external canal, with a segment of parotid fascia forming the anterior limit of the field.

A canal wall-down mastoidectomy is performed, with identification of the digastric ridge and skeletonization of the mastoid segment of the facial nerve to the stylomastoid foramen. The sigmoid sinus is identified, leaving a thick layer of bone over it superiorly. Starting in its midportion, all bone is removed from the sinus down to the jugular bulb. This creates a superiorly based "hood" of bone to brace an extraluminal pack of Surgicel, which is used to occlude the sinus. The external auditory canal skin, tympanic membrane, malleus, and incus are removed, and the tympanic bone is drilled away to expose the tumor in the hypotympanum. Diamond burs are used to skeletonize the tympanic segment of the facial nerve; the vertical segment of the carotid artery is likewise identified through thin bone anteroinferior to the promontory. Identification of the carotid artery at this level allows the eustachian tube orifice to be safely enlarged with diamond burs. This facilitates obliteration of the eustachian tube lumen with muscle and bone wax. All remaining bone is removed from the jugular bulb anterior to the facial nerve. The mastoid tip is removed after detaching the sternocleidomastoid muscle (SCM) tendon and then drilling away the bone along the digastric ridge and lateral to the stylomastoid foramen.

A neck dissection is required for identification and control of the internal jugular vein as well as the internal and external carotid arteries. Cranial nerves X, XI, and XII are identified inferiorly, and the digastric muscle is mobilized out of its groove, elevating it from the lateral surface of the internal jugular vein. Facial nerve mobilization begins by picking away the remaining eggshell-thin bone of the fallopian canal in its tympanic and mastoid segments. The extratemporal trunk of the facial nerve need not be dissected into the parotid gland; instead, the periosteum of the stylomastoid foramen is skeletonized with diamond burs without directly exposing the nerve trunk at this level. The entire complex, consisting of the facial nerve, stylomastoid foramen, and digastric muscle is mobilized anteriorly, reflecting the facial nerve at its anterior tympanic segment or at the geniculate ganglion. The digastric muscle can be sutured anteriorly to maintain the facial nerve in a tension-free, transposed position; moist Gelfoam should be draped over the nerve to prevent desiccation.

The jugular bulb is now exposed so that tumor removal can proceed without risk to the facial nerve. In some smaller tumors, a limited mobilization of only the mastoid segment of the facial nerve may be sufficient. All remaining bone and fibrous bands are removed from the lateral aspect of the jugular foramen, exposing the junction between the jugular bulb and the internal jugular vein; the vein is now ligated

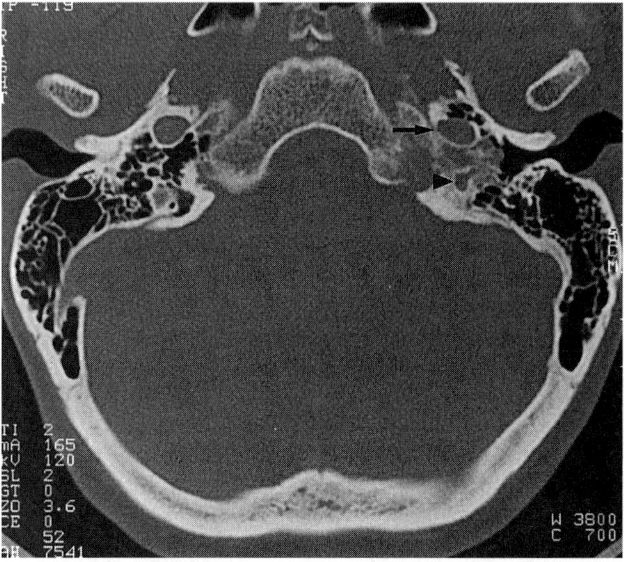

Figure 3.
Left glomus jugulare, in contact with the carotid canal anteriorly (solid arrow) and the fallopian canal posteriorly (arrowhead).

and divided in the neck. The vein should be palpated before dividing it to ensure that any intravenous tumor extension is fully incorporated in the specimen. The superior extents of cranial nerves X, XI, and XII are visualized medial to the proximal stump of the internal jugular vein.

The superior aspect of the tumor is mobilized away from the promontory and carotid artery and is debulked, if necessary. A series of incisions are made in the wall of the jugular bulb around the inferior and posterior borders of the tumor, which usually elicits brisk venous bleeding. Intrasinus tumor extension may require an incision into the lateral wall of the sigmoid sinus as well. Rapid but controlled intraluminal packing of Surgicel is directed toward the lumen of the inferior petrosal sinus, which opens on the medial wall of the jugular bulb. Once the initial bleeding has been controlled, the incision can be extended around the superior tumor border, leaving the tumor and the proximal stump of the jugular vein pedicled on the remaining medial wall of the jugular bulb. This final attachment is divided, while protecting the trunks of the lower cranial nerves.

The facial nerve is left draped in a tension-free position in the anterior mesotympanum. After copious irrigation, the wound is obliterated with abdominal fat, and a small suction drain is placed posteriorly, superficial to the fat graft. Tacking sutures are placed between the lateral aspect of the SCM and the anterior skin flap to obliterate any potential dead space, and the wound is closed in layers.

Intracranial Extension

Tumors with intracranial and/or intradural extension (Fisch type D) are treated in collaboration with a neurosurgeon (Fig. 4). The infratemporal fossa approach previously described is used for exposure. Access to the posterior fossa is obtained by first completely removing bone from the sigmoid sinus and the posterior fossa dura up to the bony labyrinth, and then dividing the sigmoid sinus distal to the junction of the lateral and sigmoid sinuses. This is incorporated into the subsequent dural incisions. The intracranial portion of the tumor is then resected by the neurosurgeon using microdissection and bipolar cautery; a plane often can be developed between the tumor and adjacent cerebellum and brain stem. Whether lower cranial nerves can be dissected free from intracranial tumor is determined at this time.

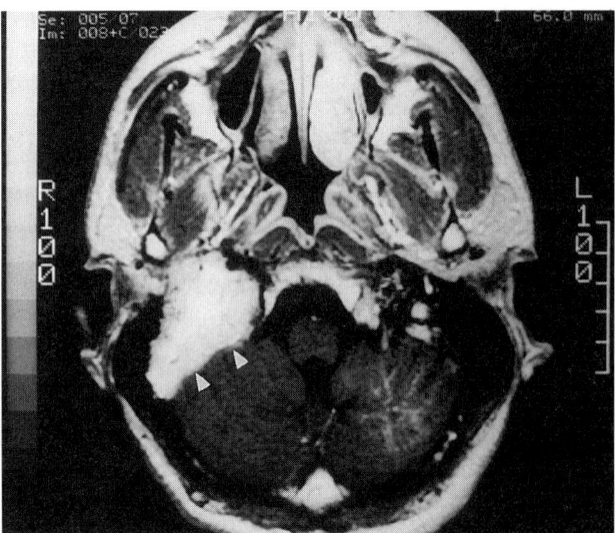

Figure 4.
Right massive glomus jugulare with posterior fossa extension. Note the interface between the tumor and cerebellum (arrowheads).

Care should be exercised to preserve the temporalis muscle and its vascular supply during the exposure and closure of the infratemporal fossa approach. Transposition of this muscle for facial reanimation may be one of the rehabilitation options needed for some patients who have facial nerve paralysis and associated lower cranial nerve deficits.

Postoperative Care

After infratemporal fossa surgery, patients are extubated in the operating room and placed in the intensive care unit for 1 night, with continuous pulse oximeter, electrocardiogram, and arterial line monitoring. In patients who have pre-existing or anticipated swallowing difficulties, a nasogastric tube is left in place postoperatively. The patient's hematocrit should be monitored as it equilibrates, but rarely does it drop sufficiently to warrant transfusion. Most of the postoperative care for glomus jugulare tumors is dictated by the number and severity of cranial nerve deficits.

Care for Facial Nerve Paralysis

Eye protection is the most important element of treatment for a postoperative facial nerve palsy. Initially, passive eye closure may be incomplete secondary to lid edema. However, closure will soon become complete as the edema resolves. Early prevention of corneal exposure is accomplished with artificial tears, lubricating ointment, and taping of the eyelid at night. Oculoplastic consultation is then indicated for either a gold weight implant and/or a lateral tarsorrhaphy. The patient is counseled regarding the prognosis for facial nerve recovery, based on the condition of the nerve at the conclusion of the procedure. A transposed but otherwise intact facial nerve may recover adequate function within 3 to 6 months, at which time the gold weight and tarsorrhaphy can be reversed. A facial nerve that has been cable grafted secondary to tumor involvement will not demonstrate signs of regeneration until 9 to 12 months postoperatively, and the patient's expectations should be guided accordingly. A patient who has a grafted facial nerve should be given realistic goals of regaining full eye closure, facial symmetry at rest, and some motion of the oral commissure; however, the anticipated development of some motor synkinesis should be reinforced as well.

Ultimately, procedures selected to rehabilitate the paralyzed face will depend on which associated cranial nerve deficits exist, if any. Obviously, an associated hypoglossal nerve palsy rules out the option of a hypoglossal-facial anastomosis, but even a vagal nerve palsy with an intact hypoglossal nerve should make the surgeon consider alternatives to this procedure, given the risk of creating a combined ipsilateral vagal and hypoglossal deficit. Masseter and temporalis transposition procedures can be used for facial reanimation when reinnervation is impossible or inadequate.

Care for Lower Cranial Nerve Palsies

Mobility of the vocal cords is determined with a bedside fiberoptic examination of the larynx early in the postoperative period. A speech pathology consultation is obtained whenever a vagus nerve injury is identified, usually prompting a modified barium swallow test. Mild aspiration can be treated with a medialization laryngoplasty with or without a cricopharyngeal myotomy after sufficient recovery from the primary procedure. Percutaneous endoscopic gastrostomy is performed to facilitate tube feeding when significant aspiration is identified on modified barium swallow.

Follow-Up Care

Postoperative radiotherapy can be used to treat residual tumor on or near the carotid artery. Alternatively, serial MRI scans can be used to monitor residual tumor, with radiotherapy reserved until significant tumor growth is documented.

Long-term follow-up (>10 years) is necessary for patients who have these tumors. For tympanic paragangliomas, otoscopic examination is usually sufficient for surveillance. For larger hypotympanic paragangliomas, CT scans improve detection of recurrences by demonstrating further bone erosion. Jugular paragangliomas can be evaluated with a baseline MRI scan obtained soon after surgery or at the time of radiotherapy, followed by repeat scans at 1, 5, and 10 years post-treatment, with earlier re-evaluation prompted by symptoms at any point. Postsurgical recurrences can be treated with either radiotherapy or revision surgery, depending on many of the same factors that dictated the original treatment choice. The status of the facial and lower cranial nerves and the location of the recurrent tumor become the key factors in this situation. Radiotherapy failures often require surgery for salvage, but the decision to operate should be made only after careful review of the previously discussed factors and determination of the approximate rate of tumor growth. We find that decision making in complex cases is facilitated by case presentation in a multidisciplinary tumor board setting.

Suggested Reading

Dutcher PO, Brackmann DE. Glomus tumors of the facial canal: A case report. Arch Otolaryngol Head Neck Surg 1986; 112:986-987.

Farrior JB. Anterior hypotympanic approach for glomus tumor of the infratemporal fossa. Laryngoscope 1984; 94:1016-1020.

Fisch U. Infratemporal fossa approach for glomus tumors of the temporal bone. Ann Otol Rhinol Laryngol 1982; 91:474-479.

Guild SR. A hitherto unrecognized structure, the glomus jugularis in man. Anat Res 1941; 79 (Suppl 2):28.

Megerian CA, McKenna MJ, Nadol JB Jr. Non-paraganglioma jugular foramen lesions masquerading as glomus jugulare tumors. Am J Otol 1995; 16:94-98.

van der May AG, Maaswinkel-Mooy PD, Cornelisse CJ, et al. Genomic imprinting in hereditary glomus tumors: Evidence for new genetic theory. Lancet 1989; 2:1291-1294.

THE INTERNAL CAROTID ARTERY IN SKULL BASE SURGERY

The method of
Ugo Fisch
by
Stephan Schmid
Kris. S. Moe
Ugo Fisch

Management of the internal carotid artery (ICA) in skull base surgery is uniquely challenging. Encasement deep within the temporal bone makes surgical access and vascular control difficult. Interruption of its blood flow can lead to severe neurologic deficits in patients who have poor collateral circulation, and its proximity to numerous critical structures in an anatomically complex area makes any manipulation of the vessel technically difficult and potentially dangerous. This places extremely high demands on the surgeon. To safely and effectively manage these patients requires expertise in the relevant three-dimensional anatomy, neuro-otology, head and neck surgery, oncology, neuroradiology, and neurosurgery. Requisite technical skills include mastery of microsurgery, vascular surgery, and temporal bone dissection.

The pathology encountered in dealing with problems of the ICA can also be unusual and varied, ranging from benign and malignant tumors to iatrogenic and violent trauma. The approaches necessary for eradication of this pathology may require exposure of the entire intratemporal course of the vessel, and it is the development of safe and effective techniques for this exposure that have been a central effort during the last 3 decades at our institution. The result of this work has been the development of the type A, B, and C lateral skull base approaches. The concurrent development of reliable tests of collateral cerebral blood flow (temporary balloon occlusion) with the capability of permanent balloon occlusion of the ICA has also been critical in making excision of advanced disease in this area possible and has greatly advanced this surgical frontier.

PREOPERATIVE EVALUATION

The evaluation of patients whose disease may require manipulation of the ICA begins with a thorough history and physical examination, applying special emphasis on deficits of those cranial nerves and vascular structures that course through the cavernous sinus and temporal bone. These include cranial nerves II through XII, the internal jugular venous system, and the ICA. Based on the differential diagnosis, neuroradiologic imaging studies are then selected and typically include computed tomographic (CT) scans, magnetic resonance imaging (MRI), and selective angiography. High-resolution, contrast-enhanced axial and coronal CT scans and multiplanar MRI are complementary studies and are used together. CT provides information on the bony involvement of a lesion (particularly of a tumor), including its relationship to the carotid, hypoglossal, and facial canals, as well as involvement of the infralabyrinthine compartment and petrous apex. MRI provides optimal definition of tumor size, intradural extension, and the existence of neurovascular or cavernous sinus invasion. A detailed characterization of the tumor by digital subtraction angiography is necessary to demonstrate the feeding arteries, angioarchitecture, venous drainage, and circulation time.

PREOPERATIVE THERAPEUTIC OPTIONS

If, during angiography, it appears that embolization of a vascular tumor would be beneficial (e.g., glomus tumors, meningiomas, and nasopharyngeal angiofibromas), this intervention can be carried out synchronously. This may decrease intraoperative hemorrhage, improve the demarcation of the tumor from the surrounding tissue, and thereby shorten the duration of the operation.

Another procedure that may be undertaken during angiography is awake temporary balloon occlusion (TBC). Because the ICAs together provide 90 percent of the cerebral blood supply, disruption of an ICA without preoperative evaluation of collateral blood flow carries a rate of major neurologic complications of up to 30 percent. When preoperative imaging indicates encasement or invasion of the ICA in the cavernous, petrous, or cervical aspects of the ICA, permanent balloon occlusion (PBO) of the vessel proximal to the ophthalmic artery in the cavernous sinus, and at the carotid foramen, is desirable (Table 1). PBO causes devascularization of the tumor, aids in tumor mobilization and control of hemorrhage, and increases the possibility of complete eradication of disease. In order to perform PBO, the following is required: functional angiography, TBO, and placement of the detachable balloons. TBO is performed in the conscious patient and includes occlusion of the ICA for 15 minutes with careful clinical monitoring to identify any change in neurologic status, blood pressure, or pulse rate. The delay in ipsilateral arterial and venous filling noted on angiography after temporary occlusion is a good indication of whether PBO will be tolerated (Fig. 1).

SURGICAL THERAPY

Approaches

Although there are numerous surgical approaches for treatment of pathology involving the ICA, at our institution the lateral skull base approaches, types A, B, and C, are favored (Fig. 2, *A* and *B*). The goal of these approaches is to preserve, if possible, the integrity of the dura and to reduce the incidence of intracranial complications due to cerebrospinal fluid (CSF) leaks and infections by eliminating the pneumatic space of the middle ear cleft through subtotal petrosectomy.

The *type A approach* exposes the cervical and intrapetrous (vertical and horizontal) segments of the ICA. The typical tumor requiring this exposure is the temporal paraganglioma. A postauricular incision is extended superiorly onto the temporal scalp and inferiorly into the neck. Cranial nerves VII, X, XI, and XII are exposed in the neck along with the ICA and the internal jugular vein. Subtotal petrosectomy is then performed with closure of the eustachian tube and external auditory canal. A permanent anterior transposition of the facial nerve is performed to expose the tumor within the jugular foramen and along the ICA. The middle ear cleft is obliterated with abdominal fat to avoid postoperative meningitis.

The *type B approach* focuses on the horizontal and proximal cavernous segments of the ICA. The most common tumors for which we use this approach are chordomas, chondroid chordomas, and chondrosarcomas of the temporoclival junction. The skin incision is retroauricular, with an anterior extension in the temporal region toward the lateral orbit. The main trunk and frontal branch of the facial nerve are identified in the parotid region. The zygomatic arch is

Table 1. Tumors for Which Permanent Balloon Occlusion (PBO) Was Performed at the University of Zurich, 1983 to 1993

TUMOR TYPE	NO. OF PATIENTS	PBO PREOPERATIVE	PBO INTRAOPERATIVE
BENIGN TUMORS			
Paragangliomas	31	27	4
Neuromas	6	5	1
Others	3	2	1
MALIGNANCIES			
Adenoid cystic carcinomas	4	4	0
Nasopharyngeal carcinomas	2	2	0
Others	6	6	0

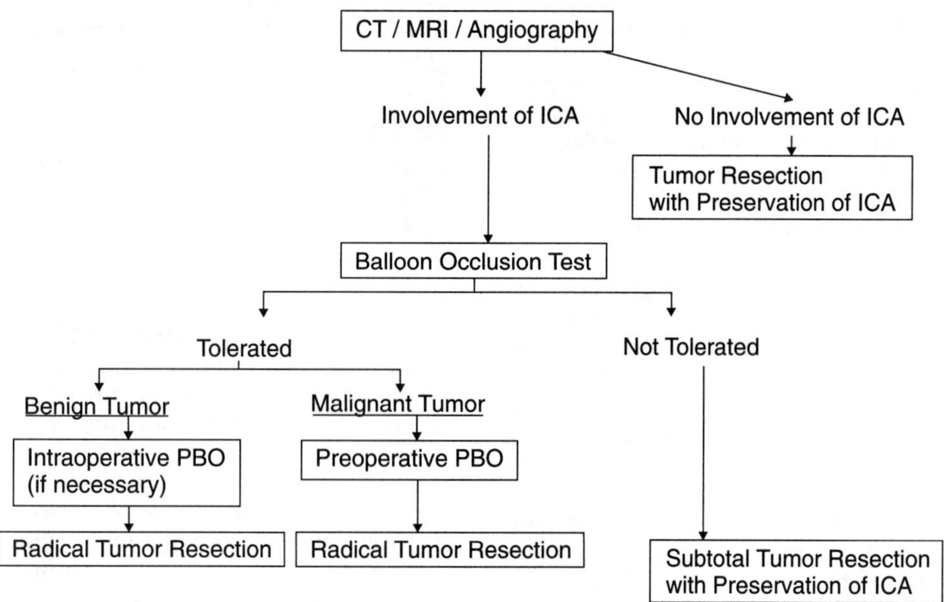

Figure 1.
Preoperative evaluation of skull base tumors with suspected internal carotid artery involvement. PBO, permanent balloon occlusion; ICA, internal carotid artery.

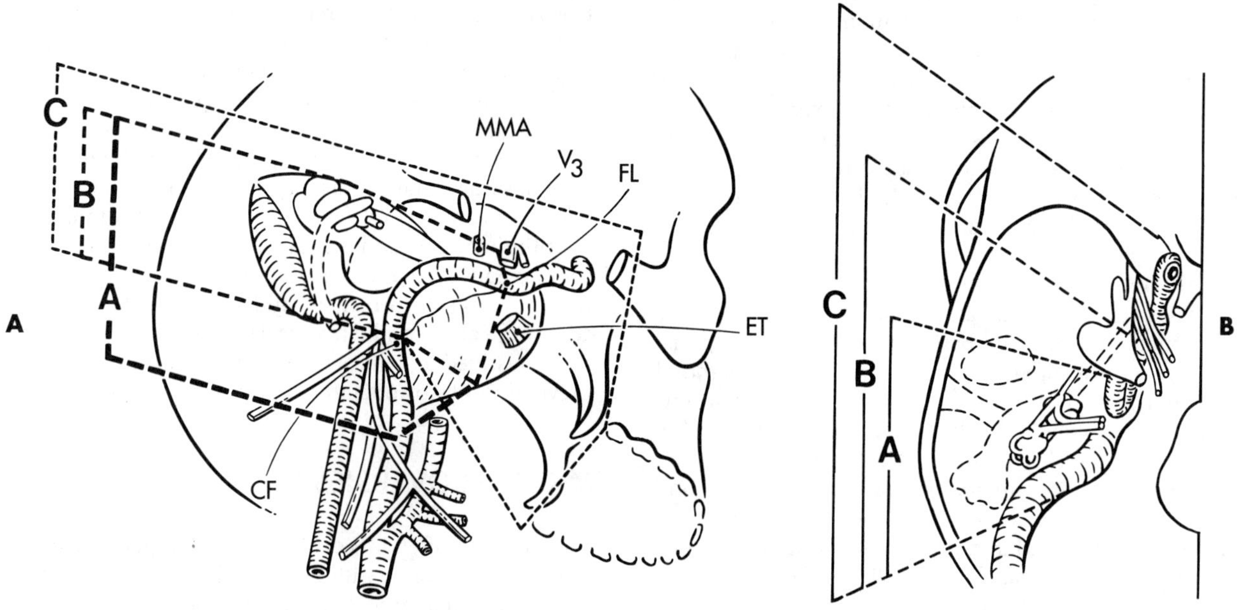

Figure 2.
A, Lateral view of extent of infratemporal fossa skull base approaches, types A, B, and C. *B*, Superior view of extent of infratemporal fossa skull base approaches, types A, B, and C. CF, carotid foramen; ET, eustachian tube; FL, foramen lacerum; V3, mandibular division of trigeminal nerve; MMA, middle meningeal artery.

divided with two osteotomies and reflected inferiorly with the temporalis muscle. A subtotal petrosectomy is performed, and the vertical segment of the ICA is exposed. The identification of the horizontal segment of the ICA requires drilling away the bone that forms the mandibular tubercle. In this way, the foramina spinosum and ovale are exposed, and the horizontal segment of the ICA is identified medial to the proximal cartilaginous eustachian tube. The ICA is usually isolated and preserved; PBO is rarely indicated. Again, the middle ear cleft is obliterated with fat. This technique provides excellent exposure of lesions situated in the petrous apex and clivius.

For lesions involving the anterior infratemporal and pterygopalatine fossae, parasellar region, and nasopharynx, the *type C approach* is used. The most common pathology encountered in this area is the juvenile nasopharyngeal angiofibroma, the persistent nasopharyngeal carcinoma after previous radiotherapy, and the adenoid cystic carcinoma of the peritubal space. The skin incision and initial surgical steps are the same as for the type B approach. Subtotal petrosectomy is performed for better exposure of the tumor and to avoid possible postoperative infectious complications. After transection of the middle meningeal artery and supraorbital nerve (V3), the dissection is continued anteriorly, removing the pterygoid processes with the drill. After identification of the sphenoid sinus, the ICA is exposed along the foramen lacerum toward the cavernous sinus. This may require transection of the infraorbital nerve (V2) and extradural elevation of the temporal lobe. The latter surgical step is performed after exposure of the temporal dura by drilling away a sufficient area of underlying bone. The dural elevation necessary to visualize the lateral wall of the cavernous sinus through the inferior "otologic" approach is minimal. An excellent view of the sixth cranial nerve lateral to the cavernous ICA is achieved in this way, and intracavernous tumor portions can be removed without danger of CSF leaks. Bleeding from the cavernous sinus is stopped by a free muscle graft that is sutured to the surrounding dura and bone.

If the lesion extends to the neck, the cervical ICA can be exposed through a cervicoparotid extension of the primary retroauriculotemporal skin incision. Although benign lesions such as angiofibromas do not typically infiltrate the ICA, malignant lesions tend to invade and necessitate resection of the vessel for tumor control. In these latter instances, PBO is an essential step of the procedure.

Technical Considerations

Regardless of the approach, safe exposure of the intrapetrous ICA through a lateral skull base approach requires special knowledge of otologic microsurgical techniques. Diamond burs should be used with aid of the microscope and continuous irrigation to skeletonize the vessel. The final eggshell of bone covering the skeletonized periosteum of the carotid canal is removed with a microdissector. The exposed carotid periosteum is then separated from the carotid adventitia with a curved clamp and incised using small curved scissors. The artery may be elevated out of its bony canal and retracted with vessel loops (in our experience, gentle handling of the ICA has not induced vascular spasm). Dilated adventitial vessels and the caroticotympanic artery supplying the tumor must be coagulated with fine bipolar forceps. Removal of tumors infiltrating the adventitia of the ICA can weaken the vessel wall. In this case, serious thought should be given to intraoperative PBO. Incomplete tumor removal along the carotid adventitia is the alternative if the central contralateral circulation is insufficient. Avoidance of both CSF leaks around the ICA and ascending infection in the wound is achieved by subtotal petrosectomy, with obliteration and closure of the eustachian tube and external auditory canal. The operative cavity is obliterated with abdominal fat and/or a temporalis muscle flap.

Table 2. Operation Time for Types A, B, and C Surgical Approaches to the ICA

APPROACH	OPERATING TIME: AVERAGE/RANGE
Type A	6 hr 50 min (4:00–9:30)
Type B	6 hr 35 min (5:00–7:00)
Type C	5 hr 30 min (2:30–7:00)

Postoperative Management

A major advantage of the otologic approaches to the lateral skull base is that patients do not require intensive care postoperatively. An intermediate care unit for 2 to 3 days is sufficient. Continuous monitoring of neurologic and cardiovascular status and oxygenation are imperative. Hypotension and hypovolemia must be prevented, and mini-dose heparin is used for thromboembolic prophylaxis. A tracheostomy is rarely required, although intravenous feeding is given for the first 3 to 4 days.

Morbidity and Mortality

The morbidity and mortality of the types A, B, and C infratemporal approaches is minimal. The operating time is not prolonged (Table 2), and the brain is not retracted. In the type A approach where the facial nerve is transposed, grade I or II facial function is retained in 80 percent of patients, and grade III postoperative facial palsy occurs in 20 percent of patients. Swallowing disorders may be encountered after total removal of the pathology through a type A approach, and intraoperative monitoring of the vagus nerve in these cases is essential. With the type C approach, the mandibular (and in some instances the maxillary) branch of the trigeminal nerve is resected. Facial and orodental numbness in the distribution of V and V3 can be expected, but there is a spontaneous recovery of sensation in 50 percent of patients within 1 year. Types A, B, and C approaches will all, in addition, cause conductive hearing loss, but we think that this is justified in light of the superior surgical exposure and prevention of postoperative infection and CSF leak.

■ CONTROVERSIES

The question often arises whether one should attempt total resection of a tumor with extensive involvement of the ICA, either for benign or malignant pathology. The answer to this question has to take into account the chance of cure or long-term tumor control versus the risk of significant morbidity and mortality, as well as the subsequent quality of life that the patient will experience. Our philosophy is that for benign tumors, radical resection of the ICA is performed only in the presence of massive infiltration of the vessel wall in a young patient, when angiography shows that preoperative PBO will be tolerated with minimal risk. Intraoperative PBO for benign tumors is used only in rare emergency situations, for example, danger of rupture of the carotid wall or for distal ICA control. The situation with malignant tumors is easier to define, because the chance of cure or long-term survival is disappointingly small when the ICA is heavily involved with tumor. In the presence of malignant disease, resection of the infiltrated ICA is performed when PBO is well tolerated. It is our policy not to use this procedure for palliation.

The topic of ICA occlusion versus revascularization is also highly debated. When vein grafting is performed, an intracranial access procedure for the distal anastomosis is mandated with increased operative time and morbidity. Additional complications of immediate or delayed graft occlusion or blowout may also be encountered. The only patient group for whom we consider revascularization is the patient who will not tolerate PBO but has limited ICA involvement by a malignant tumor with potential for surgical cure.

Another question is whether unnecessary preoperative ICA occlusion could be avoided by waiting until surgery to perform intraoperative PBO, when the actual extent of the tumor can be visualized, because even with the combination of CT, MRI, and angiography, there is a 30 percent incidence of false-positive prediction of involvement of the ICA by tumor. It is our experience that intraoperative PBO increases the risk of neurologic complications. In a series of 52 patients studied at the University of Zurich, one of 46 (2.2 percent) who received preoperative PBO suffered a lasting neurologic complication, whereas one of six patients (17 percent) who received intraoperative PBO suffered a sustained neurologic deficit. This difference is probably due to impaired hemodynamic situation created by surgery. We have found that the incidence of additional postoperative complications is minimized by performing PBO 1 to 3 weeks before surgery, which allows a better adaptation of the central nervous system to the altered circulation. This delay does not negate the beneficial hemostatic effect of adequate embolization.

■ DISCUSSION

Much progress has been made in our ability to treat disease that involves the ICA at the skull base. Close cooperation with the neuroradiologist who performs CT, MRI, angiography with embolization, and possibly PBO has decreased the surgical morbidity and mortality and improved our ability to achieve total tumor ablation. The use of the "otologic" lateral skull base approaches largely obviates the need for intradural surgery and reduces the operation time, intraoperative blood loss, and postoperative morbidity and mortality. The price is a conductive hearing loss when subtotal petrosectomy is necessary and the (incomplete) loss of facial sensation due to the section of V2 and V3. The challenge for the future remains to balance the potential morbidity and mortality of tumor resection with the chance of cure or long-term survival, and to learn what extent of surgery is actually in the patient's best interest.

Suggested Reading

Andrews J, Valavanis A, Fisch U. Management of the internal carotid artery in surgery of the skull base. Laryngoscope 1989; 99:1224-1229.

Fisch U. Infratemporal fossa approach to tumors of the temporal bone and base of the skull. J Laryngol Otol 1978; 92:949-967.

Fisch U, Mattox D. Microsurgery of the skull base. New York: Thieme, 1988: Ch. 3, 4, 5, and 10.

Pauw BKH, Makek MS, Fisch U, Valavanis A. Preoperative embolization of paragangliomas (glomus tumors) of the head and neck: Histopathologic and clinical features., Skull Base Surgery, Vol. 3, January 1993.

Valavanis A, Fisch U. Balloon occlusion of the internal carotid artery in extensive skull base tumors. Neurological surgery of the ear and skull base. Proceedings of the Sixth International Symposium, Zurich. Amsyterdam: Kugler & Ghedini, 1988:82-86.

Zane RS, Aeschbacher P, Moll C, Fisch U. Carotid occlusion without reconstruction: A safe surgical option in selected patients. Am J Otol 1995; 16:353-359.

THE FACE

FACIAL SCARS AND KELOIDS

The method of
David W. Stepnick

Among darker-skinned persons in much of Africa, in Australian and Tasmanian aborigines, and in many Melanesian and New Guinean groups, the practice of cicatrization or scarification involves intentional mutilation and modification of the skin by incision or burning to create raises scars, or keloids. These scars are usually created in decorative patterns and, in some cases, are for aesthetic effect, whereas in others, the scars indicate status or lineage. Although these cultures utilize this abnormal process of wound healing by intentionally creating wounds that are meant to develop keloids, Western cultures generally regard these scars as undesirable outcomes of tissue trauma. Despite surgeons' best efforts to handle tissue carefully, close wounds with minimal tension, and precisely appose wound edges, scars may hypertrophy or develop into a keloid. Especially in the case of keloids, frustration results from a poor understanding of a *specific* pathogenesis, the variable biologic behavior of these scars, unpredictable outcomes of therapeutic intervention, and frequent recurrences despite "proper" treatment.

■ EPIDEMIOLOGY

The incidence of keloids in darker-skinned races is from 6 percent to 16 percent, which is five to 15 times greater than that in whites. However, keloids have been reported in all races and in patients of any age, including a case of a congenital keloid. Within a racial group, the incidence is higher in individuals with darker pigmentation; keloids have not been reported in albinos. The peak incidence of keloid formation seems to be between the ages of 10 and 30 years. Susceptibility to keloid scarring decreases with age.

■ ETIOLOGY

Trauma to the skin—surgical, accidental, and intentional—is the most well documented etiologic factor leading to the development of keloids and hypertrophic scarring. However, even in persons who have a documented history of keloid formation, this entity is not an invariable outcome of skin injury. The clinician should realize that keloids may also appear with no apparent antecedent history of trauma. Careful examination of earlobe keloids not infrequently reveals a normal epithelialized tract through the ear separate from, but nearby the actual keloid.

Anatomic site appears to be another important etiologic factor. Keloids and hypertrophic scars may occur on virtually any skin surface on the body, but there is a definite predilection for certain areas that are either under increased skin tension or subjected to frequent motion. As with trauma, tension and movement are not *necessary* factors, because earlobe keloids are not subjected to either of these factors.

Frequently, keloids appear during puberty and resolve after menopause, which suggests an endocrinologic role in this disease. One attractive hypothesis is that the metabolism of melanocytic-stimulating hormone (MSH) is disrupted. This theory is based on the observations that keloids usually affect darker-skinner persons; almost never develop in amelanotic areas such as mucosal surfaces, the palms, or the soles; and have a higher incidence in periods of generalized increase in MSH levels, such as puberty and pregnancy.

Familial predisposition for the development of keloids seems to be present in certain individuals; evidence suggests that this *tendency* may be transmitted through simple mendelian inheritance patterns. To date, no clear association with a particular human leukocyte antigen haplotype has been identified.

Other dermatologic disorders, such as acne vulgaris, hidradenitis suppurativa, and pilonidal cysts; infections such as herpes zoster and vaccinia; and connective tissue diseases such as Ehlers-Danlos syndrome and scleroderma may be associated with the development of keloids, especially in areas of the body in anatomic sites predisposed to keloid development. Whether these disorders are truly etiologic factors for the development of these scars remains unclear.

CLINICAL MANIFESTATIONS

The cosmetic deformity that results from the development of a hypertrophic scar or keloid is usually the primary concern of most patients afflicted with this problem. There are wide variations in the appearance of the tumor; some are little more than tiny papules, whereas others are grossly lobulated, pendulous, and extend well beyond the original boundaries of the original inflammation or trauma. Especially in very large keloids, infection may develop. Spontaneous drainage of purulent material may ensue, probably developing as a result of suppurative necrosis resulting from vascular compromise in the center of these lesions. Keloids may also cause significant pain and pruritus, especially in periods of rapid growth.

As previously mentioned, there is documented predilection for the development of hypertrophic scarring and/or keloids in certain areas of the body, such as anterior chest (especially the presternal area), the upper back, shoulders, upper arms, neck, and the earlobes (especially posteriorly). Keloids are rare in areas such as the central third of the face, the palms of the hands and soles of the feet, the eyelids, the genitalia, and the mucous membranes.

Keloids and hypertrophic scars often begin to develop within weeks to a few months after trauma, but can occur many months later. Typically, keloids have a recognizable phase of active growth that eventually stabilizes for a time. Spontaneous regression is rare, in contradistinction to hypertrophic scarring, in which regression is not unusual. Malignant transformation of these entities is poorly documented and, if it occurs at all, is rare.

HISTOPATHOLOGY

A number of early reports indicated that histopathologic differences between keloid and hypertrophic scars were insignificant and that these entities looked, under the light microscope, much the same as a normally healing wound. Over the past several years, reports confirming differences have appeared in the literature. Indeed, histopathologic differences between normal and abnormal scars are hard to detect early in their development. However, as a keloid matures, the presence of abundant mucin and large, thick, brightly eosinophilic bundles of collagen distinguish it from the hypertrophic scar. Keloid scars are more vascular than normal scar tissue, and the collagen fibers lie haphazardly within the dermis, in a less organized manner. Polarized light microscopy and electron microscopy show the collagen structures of keloids to be organized in thicker fibers than that of hypertrophic scars. The extracellular matrix, composed of glycoproteins and water, accounts for the majority of excessive tissue bulk.

The identifying structural subunit of hypertrophic scars appears to be the presence of distinct collagen nodules containing a high density of cells and fine fibrillar collagen; these are absent in keloid and normal scar. These nodules contain α-smooth muscle actin–expressing myofibroblasts, which are also generally absent in keloids. This seems to be correlated with the ability of hypertrophic scars to participate in scar contracture, whereas keloids do not.

PATHOGENESIS

The pathogenesis of keloid development is still very poorly understood. The ratio of collagen deposition to degradation is abnormal, and conflicting results regarding this tissue appear in the literature. It is unclear if there is an overabundant deposition of collagen, decreased collagen degradation, or both. In some studies, collagenase (the enzyme responsible for collagen breakdown) levels are elevated in keloid tissue, whereas in other studies, levels are normal. If the latter situation is characteristic of keloid scars, it is possible that the bioactivity of collagenase may be diminished, which would lead to collagen excess. Collagenase inhibitors, such as α 2-macroglobulin and α 1-antitrypsin, have been found to accumulate in keloid tissue, and their excess could produce similar end results (increased collagen). Abnormal growth regulation of fibroblasts may be another underlying mechanism by which keloids develop. For example, vascular damage may be a possible initiating event through the release of transforming growth factor-β, which stimulates keloid growth.

Increased cellularity and metabolic activity is seen in keloids as compared with normal tissues; yet keloid fibroblasts have the same karyotype, mean population doubling time, confluent density, and cell volume as do their normal counterparts. Some investigators have reported that relative amounts of type III collagen are increased in keloid tissue as compared with normal dermis, whereas other researchers have shown normal amounts of type III collagen, but an increased activity and collagen messenger RNA expression in keloids reflects the roughly 20-fold increase in collagen synthesis seen in immature keloids. A disproportionate increase in type I collagen synthesis leads to its accumulation within the wound. It also appears that the collagen found in keloids is more acid-soluble.

A variety of cytokines and migratory inflammatory cells are present in the wound environment that play an important role in regulation of cellular activity as related to wound healing. The interleukins (IL-1, IL-6, IL-8, IL-10); the growth factors (tumor necrosis factor-alpha [TFN-α] and transforming growth factor-beta [TGF-β]; and humoral- and cell-mediated immunity all potentially could play a role in the development of keloids. TGF-β and IL-1 have attracted a great deal of attention because they specifically increase collagen gene expression in vitro. Identification of the specific pathogenetic mechanisms by which keloids develop remains fertile ground for wound-healing research.

THERAPY

No single form of treatment exists for keloids and hypertrophic scars; numerous techniques have been described over the years. Therapy depends on the size, extent, location, and age of the scar. Argon, CO_2, and ND:Yag lasers; radiotherapy and/or surgical excision; intralesional steroids, hyaluronidase, interferon, adrenocorticotropic hormone or mustine; oral tetrahydroquinone, vitamin E, beta-aminopropionitrile (BAPN)/colchicine or penicillamine/colchicine; intramuscular asiaticoside; intramuscular and/or intraoral madecassol; topical retinoic acid, thiotepa, zinc tape, silicone gel, or silicone sheeting; and pressure devices have all been used to treat these lesions. Many of these modalities must be considered purely experimental; others, such as radiotherapy, have utility in some physicians' hands, but most are unwilling to expose patients to possible deleterious effects of ionizing radiation simply to treat a scar.

Low-Risk Patients

It is important to distinguish between treating a person who is at high risk for developing a keloid or hypertrophic scar based on their race or history of previous scar development, a person who has an established lesion, and a person who has a traumatic facial scar in an undesirable location or orientation who is at low risk for hypertrophic scar development. In the latter group, principles of surgical management involve an understanding of relaxed skin tension lines, facial subunits, scar camouflage, and techniques such as serial excisions, Z-plasty, W-plasty, geometric broken line closures, and dermabrasion. Generally, these techniques are not used in patients who are prone to keloid formation, because most involve lengthening the wound and subsequently increasing the potential size of the keloid.

In the former group (those patients who have a predilection toward hypertrophic scarring without an established lesion), treatment begins with prevention. Every attempt should be made to design incisions such that scars will fall into relaxed skin tension lines, to minimize tension by sufficient undermining, and to do a layered closure using minimally reactive suture material. No attempt is made to infiltrate corticosteroids at the time of the initial operative procedure if the surgery is not for excision and/or revision of a hypertrophic scar or keloid. Some surgeons infiltrate 10 mg per milliliter triamcinolone acetonide adjacent to the wound edges to help prevent development of a keloid scar in high-risk areas in dark-skinned people. Careful observation of such high-risk patients is essential, and office visits every 2 to 3 weeks for a period of 6 to 8 weeks allows early detection of hypertrophy before true keloid formation occurs. If the wound remains flat and soft to the touch, monthly observation for the balance of 3 months and then quarterly visits for the remainder of the first year are planned to help ensure that healing is proceeding uneventfully.

If one determines that a scar is beginning to feel or appear hypertrophic, either 10 mg per milliliter triamcinolone acetonide is infiltrated directly into the scar, or silicone sheeting treatment (discussed next) is instituted, depending on the site of the scar and the perceived likelihood of patient compliance with the latter form of treatment. Once therapy has been initiated, patients are seen every 4 weeks for assessment of response, and if they are treated with triamcinolone, they are seen for additional administration of this drug, as needed. Additional steroid injections are titrated to scar response; high concentrations (40 mg per milliliter of triamcinolone acetonide) are used if there is progression of the disease; additional drug is used if there has been minimal regression or no improvement; and no additional steroid is given if significant improvement is achieved. Patients are seen (and treated) monthly until resolution of the hypertrophy, stabilization of keloid growth, development of unwanted local effects from steroid use (discussed next), or a decision is made to surgically excise a growing lesion. If topical silicone gel sheeting is chosen as the preferred treatment, every attempt is made to continue application of the sheeting for 8 to 12 months.

Established Keloids

Patients who have established keloids are treated in a similar manner, but additional decisions are required in the treatment algorithm (Fig. 1). Although some clinicians do not begin to inject triamcinolone acetonide until *after* an established keloid is surgically excised, I prefer to institute intralesional steroid therapy before deciding to excise the lesion (except in the cases of pedunculated earlobe keloids). First, significant regression is sometimes achieved using intralesional steroids alone, to the extent that surgical excision may not be required. Pretreatment thus may avoid a surgical procedure that is not uniformly successful and prone to recurrences. Second, unless silicone gel sheeting is to be used, patients invariably require postoperative intralesional corticosteroids. It is a useful measure of a patient's compliance to initiate intralesional steroid injections; noncompliance with this treatment following surgical excision predictably results in recurrence of the lesion. Patients to a certain extent grow accustomed and perhaps develop more tolerance to the injections. They tend to develop a sense of the degree of discomfort associated with infiltration of the pharmaceutical into the scar tissue. Finally, there is, at least in theory, reason to have a residual depot of steroid in the tissues at the time of the operative procedure, thereby potentially decreasing the likelihood of recurrence.

Triamcinolone acetonide 40 mg per milliliter is infiltrated directly into the scar tissue; the surgeon should take care not to inject too superficially or into the dermis, to decrease the likelihood of tissue atrophy or hypopigmentation. A 1 cc or 3 cc Luer-Lok syringe is used with a 25 gauge needle. These small syringes develop more hydraulic pressure than do larger ones and facilitate injection into the dense scar tissue. A 25 gauge needle allows relatively easy passage of the emulsion through its hollow bore; larger needles make injection easier, but should only be used if the lesion has been previously anesthetized. Many clinicians inject the triamcinolone acetonide mixed 1:1 with 2 percent lidocaine with 1:100,000 epinephrine to minimize discomfort. Uniform deposition of the drug into the scar is attempted, and the patient is instructed to follow up in 4 weeks. Intralesional infiltration of steroid is again done, and the patient is seen after yet another month. At that time, a decision is made, based on the degree of response to therapy (decreased keloid volume and other symptoms), to either continue treatments until resolution occurs, or to excise the keloid. In the case of earlobe keloids, the decision to operate usually comes much earlier, often at the time of the initial evaluation. This is because these keloids are typically more pedunculated and therefore more easily excised, and because there is minimal tension at the site compared with almost every other head and neck location.

Once the decision is made to excise a keloid, excision is accomplished with removal of as little "normal" surrounding tissue as possible. Some surgeons intentionally leave a very thin margin of mature keloid behind at the edges of the wound, because it is believed that this tissue is metabolically different from surrounding tissue and less prone to scar de-

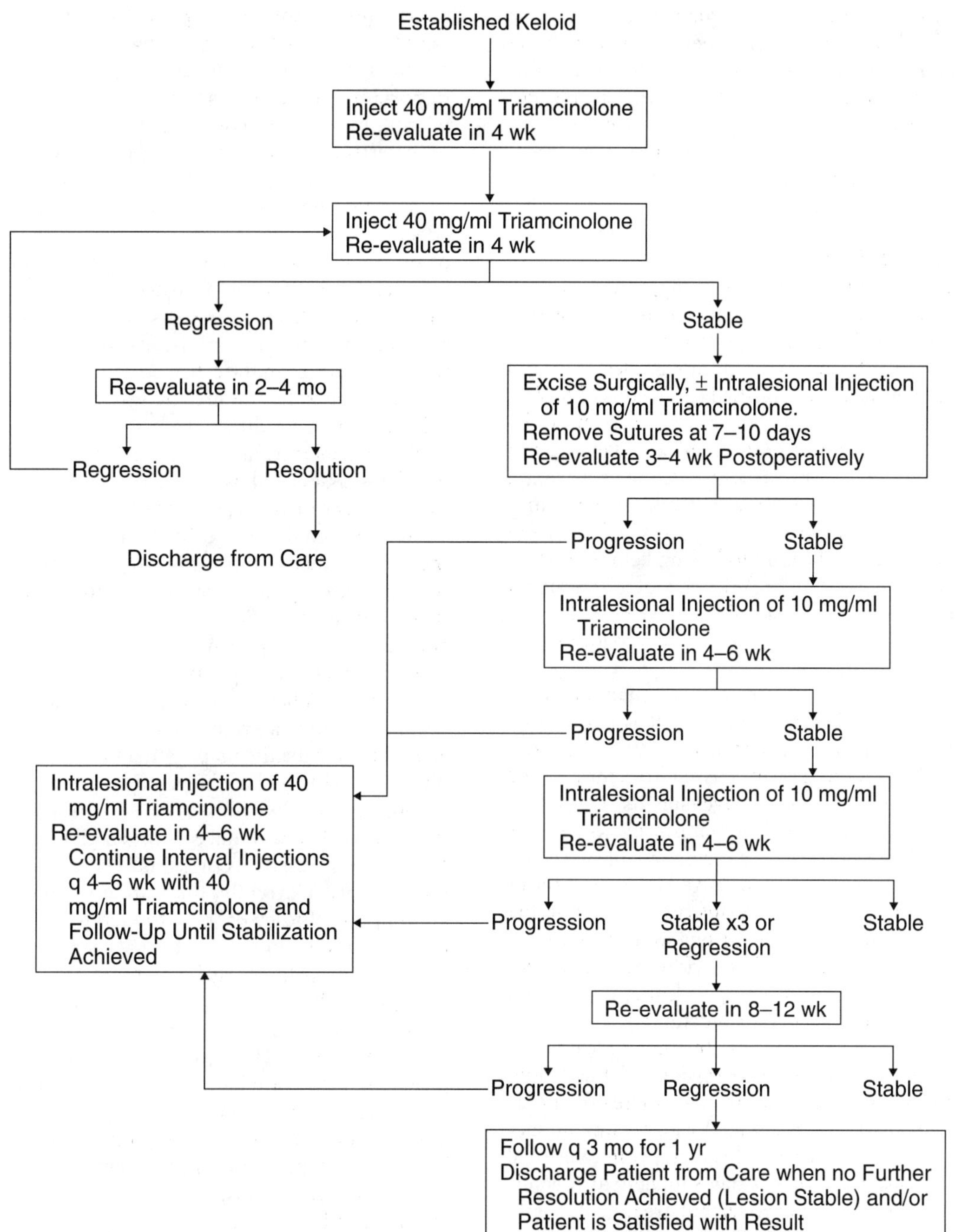

Figure 1.
Treatment algorithm for a patient who has established keloid.

velopment, thus minimizing chances of recurrence. In my hands, however, the wound usually has no palpable induration after excision of the keloid. The wound is undermined sufficiently such that the wound can be closed with little or no tension, although excessive undermining is avoided. Flap reconstruction is not used because of the increased chances of exacerbating the problem. Minimally reactive suture material is chosen to minimize the inflammatory response. Clear polydioxanone suture is often used for the deep layer(s); interrupted or subcuticular monofilament nylon or polypropylene is used for final skin closure. Especially for previously excised lesions, and occasionally for bulky keloids, wound margins are infiltrated with 10 mg per milliliter of triamcinolone acetonide before closure.

Skin sutures are removed at 5 to 7 days, unless steroids have been used, in which case they are left in place approximately 10 days, especially if the strength of the closure was predominantly (although not ideally) in the epidermal layer or if the wound closing tension was higher than desired. Patients are seen on approximately postoperative Day 21 and then every 4 to 6 weeks for approximately 3 months; the wound is closely monitored for evidence of hypertrophy or keloid formation. If this occurs, or empirically for a multiply recurrent lesion, the wound is treated with 40 mg per milliliter of triamcinolone acetonide to circumvent the abnormal healing. Steroid concentration for subsequent injections is chosen based on the degree to which a lesion appears to be developing or regressing.

Silicone Gel Sheeting

Convincing scientific data are accumulating from well-controlled studies showing the efficacy of silicone gel sheeting for the treatment of keloids and hypertrophic scars. Subjective clinical assessment, improvement in scar elasticity, and decrease in scar volume are established end results of topical silicone sheeting treatment. Silicone sheeting appears to be beneficial in the treatment of both established keloids and evolving keloids. Daily treatments with silicone gel sheeting should begin as soon as an itchy red streak develops in a maturing wound. For the past several years, I have been using topical silicone gel sheeting following keloid excision on wounds of the head and neck in lieu of intralesional steroid injections. Intralesional steroids are used supplementally *only if* hypertrophic scar appears to be developing despite the silicone sheeting therapy.

Silicone sheeting is available from several manufacturers and is tailored to the surface of the scar. It is cut so that approximately 1 cm overlaps the perimeter of the scar, and is held in place with skin adhesives purchased from the silicone sheeting manufacturer or with bandage tape. Its action does not appear to be related to the mechanism by which it is secured on the skin, because some patients are able to secure it in place using a scarf or nonadhesive bandage without compromising results. Patients are instructed to wear the sheeting as many hours as possible throughout the day (and night), removing the sheeting only for cleaning and in special social circumstances. The sheeting is cleaned with a mild soap and water and may be reused indefinitely.

A minimum of 8 months of therapy—ideally, 12 months—should be planned. Progression of the keloid should not occur after the first month or so; thereafter, gradual improvement over time is equated with treatment success. If progression occurs despite this therapy, intralesional steroids, as previously described, may supplement the silicone sheeting therapy. With improvement, treatment should continue as described previously. During the interval from 6 to 12 months, the size of the silicone sheet may be reduced to cover only the raised portion of the scar if regression from a true keloid to soft, nonraised scar has been witnessed. Little evidence exists to support the use of silicone sheeting beyond the 12 month period. Silicone sheeting is not painful, as is the injection of steroids, nor is it associated with hypopigmentation or skin atrophy. Its effects can be dramatic when one examines pre- and post-treatment photo documentation. Managed care organizations may look favorably upon this type of therapy, because it potentially substitutes for what may be more costly approaches, that is, surgery or repeated intralesional steroid injections. However, careful monitoring of these lesions is essential, and physician visits must be clinically rather than financially driven.

Leakage of silicone from fluid silicone gel–containing breast implants and its alleged deleterious system effects has raised public awareness regarding medical uses and potential problems with this biomaterial. Especially in this light, it is important that clinicians try to understand the mechanism(s) by which silicone sheeting acts in the management of hypertrophic scars and keloids. It is especially important to know if "leeching" of the silicone into adjacent skin occurs. Fulton explored the possibility that a direct chemical effect of silicone was responsible for the therapeutic effects of silicon gel. Hypertrophic scars treated with Silastic sheeting were compared with adjacent untreated control sites. Biopsies were taken, frozen, and sent for spectrochemical analysis; silica per gram of tissue was reported as the percent total trace metals in the burnt ash of the samples. No significant difference in the groups was found, which provided evidence against a direct chemical effect.

Despite its advantages, there are two not insignificant problems associated with silicone gel sheeting. First, the three-dimensional topography of the head and neck is often so complicated that it is difficult, if not impossible, to apply the sheet so that it uniformly covers the scar. Second, compliance is clearly an issue, in that the effectiveness of the treatment seems to be directly correlated to the willingness and ability of the patient to keep the gel in place (nearly continuously) over a period of 6 to 12 months.

Recently, Allied Biomedical (Paso Robles, Calif.) has begun marketing a product known as Kelocote, a polysiloxane derivative for the management of keloids and hypertrophic scars. This gel has the properties of an "ointment" and is applied much like most pharmaceuticals delivered in this form. It has the advantage of much greater ease of application than silicone sheeting, and there is almost effortless maintenance. Currently, there are no published reports examining the efficacy of this product, but it appears that keloid resolution comparable to that seen with topical steroid preparations, silicone gel sheeting, and pulsed-dye laser therapy, with improvement of erythema, and collagen shrinkage and reorientation parallel to the surface, has been seen in one study. This product may go a long way in solving problems with compliance with the sheeting, due to easier maintenance and conformability; however, it remains largely untested. I have no experience with this product, but believe it may play an important role in the clinician's armamentarium against keloids, assuming that its safety and efficacy can be verified.

Suggested Reading

Ahn ST, Monafo WW, Mustoe TA. Topical silicone gel for the prevention and treatment of hypertrophic scar. Arch Surg 1991; 126:499-504.

DiCesare PE, Chaung DT, Perelman N. Alteration of collagen composition and cross-linking in keloid tissue. Matrix 1990; 10:172-178.

Ehrlich HP, Desmouliers A, Diegelmann RF. Morphological and immunohistochemical differences between keloid and hypertrophic scar. Am J Path 1994; 145:105-113.

Ford T, Widgerow AD. Umbilical keloid: An early start. Ann Plast Surg 1990; 25:214-215.

Fulton JE. Silicon gel sheeting for the prevention and management of evolving hypertrophic and keloid scars. Dermatol Surg 1995; 21:947-951.

Ketchum LD, Cohen I, Masters FW. Hypertrophic scars and keloids: A collective review. Plast Reconstr Surg 1974; 53:140-154.

Koonin AJ. The etiology of keloids: A review of the literature and new hypothesis. S Afr Med J 1964; 38:913.

Lawrence WT. In search of the optimal treatment of keloids: Report of a series and a review of the literature. Ann Plast Surg 1991; 27:164-178.

Murray JC. Scars and keloids. Derm Clin 1993; 11:697-708.

Oluwasanmi JO. Keloids in the African. Clin Plast Surg 1974; 1:179-195.

Omo-Dare P. Genetic studies on keloids. J Natl Med Assoc 1975; 76: 428-432.

Peltonen J, Hsiao LL, Jaakola S, et al. Activation of collagen gene expression in keloids: Co-localization of type I and type VI collagen and transforming growth factor-β mRNA. J Invest Dermatol 1991; 97:240-248.

Stucker FJ, Shaw GY. An approach to management of keloids. Arch Otolaryngol Head Neck Surg 1992; 118:63-67.

Thomas DW, Hopkinson I, Harding KG, Shepherd JP. The pathogenesis of hypertrophic/keloid scarring. Int J Oral Maxillofac Surg 1994; 23: 232-236.

TRAUMATIC FACIAL PARALYSIS

The method of

Moises A. Arriaga

Traumatic facial paralysis is a difficult clinical problem involving a wide range of possible diagnostic tests and interventions. The challenge to the otolaryngologist is to approach this problem in an organized manner to offer the patient appropriately timed, helpful interventions.

I first review diagnostic and decision-making principles, including pertinent findings on history, physical examination, use of electrical testing, use of imaging, and timing of surgery. In the second section on treatment planning, I review specific clinical situations. In the third section on surgical repair of the traumatized facial nerve, I discuss techniques regarding surgical exploration, facial nerve decompression, repair, and grafting techniques.

■ DIAGNOSIS AND DECISION MAKING

Timing is of the essence in assessing facial nerve injury. An accurate observation at the time of initial evaluation documenting any degree of facial function that subsequently deteriorates has important prognostic and management implications. Unfortunately, patients sustaining trauma sufficient to damage the facial nerve often sustain other life-threatening injuries that make facial function a lower priority or simply not assessable given the patient's other injuries. The otolaryngologist usually is consulted 3 to 5 days after severe head trauma as the patient is recovering from major intracranial injuries, and a deficit in facial function is then noted.

The otolaryngologist must be very cautious about examining facial function in a patient following trauma. Head dressings often create upper eyelid edema that gives the illusion of retained facial function in the branches supplying the orbicularis oculi muscle. This can easily mislead the clinician into believing that the patient has maintained some facial nerve function. In addition, young patients who have particularly good muscle tone on the contralateral side can often create facial motion on the ipsilateral side of the injury simply by the pulling effect of the facial muscles on the intact side. General otologic examination techniques are helpful in considering the possible extent of damage to the facial nerve. Specifically, ecchymosis of the mastoid cortex or a visible step-off in the external canal or cerebrospinal fluid otorrhea all suggest a severe temporal bone injury with possible facial nerve damage. In the extratemporal trauma situation, specific note must be made of the function in each branch of the facial nerve. Time is particularly important in these patients, because surgical exploration of the extratemporal facial nerve branches is substantially facilitated by intraoperative electrical stimulation, which can only be done up to approximately 3 days following the injury.

Electrical testing is a very important aspect of decision making in patients who have facial nerve paralysis. The electrical tests include Hilger nerve stimulation (minimal nerve excitability testing [NET]): electroneuronography (ENOG), voluntary motor unit potentials, and spontaneous EMG responses. In the setting of temporal bone trauma or postoperative facial paralysis, the presence of EMG voluntary facial motor unit potentials despite clinically absent motion has important prognostic implications, because the clinician has evidence that the facial nerve has not been transected. After the acute trauma phase (after 3 days), ENOG is used to document the extent of degeneration in comparison to the contralateral side. Specifically, ENOG provides valuable information up to 21 days after the injury. Degeneration to less than 10 percent function in comparison to the contralateral side is considered significant, and this percentage is considered to be the threshold for considering surgical exploration according to the indications described later in this chapter. Hilger NET also provides useful clinical information and is employed in similar indications as ENOG testing. In NET, a 3.5 mA difference between sides for stimulation threshold is considered significant. Hilger NET testing is used to corroborate findings on ENOG as well as a substitute for ENOG in good prognostic situations. Hilger stimulation is usually quicker, easier to perform, and more economical to the patient than is ENOG testing. However, if a significant difference in stimulability is identified, ENOG is employed before making a surgical decision.

Spontaneous EMG activity is tested at 6 months following a major intratemporal facial nerve injury. Fibrillation potentials in the muscle are considered evidence of continuing complete denervation, and polyphasic potentials are considered evidence of regeneration and a good prognostic finding. The 6 month point is selected because this provides adequate time for an intratemporal facial nerve injury to regenerate at the expected 1 mm per day growth rate to the facial periphery.

Temporal bone imaging is critical information in decision making for intratemporal facial nerve injuries. Although these patients often have had computed tomography (CT) scans performed before otolaryngology consultation, the usual head CT algorithm is inadequate to fully evaluate the temporal bone. Ideally, the temporal bone CT should be performed in 1 mm thin cuts in an axial and coronal plane through the temporal bone. (I prefer direct coronal cuts rather than coronal reconstructions for the finest detail of the course of the facial nerve. However, associated injuries, including cervical spine trauma, often limit patient positioning for coronal images.) The full course of the nerve should be evaluated, including the internal auditory canal, labyrinthine portion, geniculate ganglion, tympanic segment, and vertical segment of the nerve. Magnetic resonance imaging has not been helpful for evaluating the status of the facial nerve in the intratemporal or extratemporal course following trauma.

■ TREATMENT PLANNING

The only medical intervention available for post-traumatic facial paralysis is steroid therapy. Prednisone, 30 mg twice a day for 10 days, is recommended in the absence of medical contraindications. The principal therapeutic decision is whether to offer surgical intervention.

Intratemporal Injury

Closed Head Trauma

In my experience, closed head trauma is the most common etiology of traumatic facial paralysis. These patients often have numerous life-threatening injuries and other systemic problems, so clinical decision making is always individualized. There is a strong emphasis by managed care to shift the nonacute management of these patients to rehabilitation facilities. Otolaryngologists often must coordinate serial evaluation of these patients with such facilities. In general, a patient who has partial paralysis, House-Brackmann grades II to V, is managed with observation. Despite radiologic evidence of a temporal bone fracture adjacent to the course of the facial nerve, partial paralysis indicates an anatomically intact and functional facial nerve with a good prognosis without intervention. However, the clinical assessment of minimal function (grade V) must be viewed with circumspection. This is the setting in which contralateral function or nearby muscle groups (innervated by cranial nerves III or V) may mislead the clinician. Accordingly, EMG is helpful for confirming voluntary motor action potentials if there is any doubt of residual function.

Table 1 shows an algorithm for managing complete facial paralysis (grade VI) in the patient who has closed head trauma. Although it is generally assumed that delayed paralysis has a better prognosis than immediate paralysis, reliable information concerning the timing of the facial paralysis is difficult to obtain. In the typical scenario of a closed head trauma patient, the timing of the development of facial paralysis is simply unknown. Both CT imaging and electrical facial nerve testing are used to guide the management of these patients. A positive CT finding would include a temporal bone fracture through the course of the facial nerve with a 1 mm or greater diastasis in that location or an apparent spicule of bone in the facial nerve along its course. Electrical testing includes voluntary EMG in the early course (first 3 days after injury) if there is any question of retained motion, Hilger nerve excitability testing if there is a strong suggestion that the paralysis was delayed in onset or if there is no CT evidence of a significant fracture or spicule along the course of the facial nerve, and ENOG testing in the face of a significant fracture on CT and loss of Hilger excitability. In general, surgical exploration of the course of the facial nerve is advocated in patients who have complete facial paralysis, evidence of a significant diastasis along the course of the facial nerve or spicule along the course of the facial nerve on CT scan, and electrical evidence of degeneration within 3 weeks of their injury. Patients who have temporal bone fractures on CT but without significant findings along the facial nerve and electrical degeneration within the 3 week period are encouraged to await spontaneous recovery for months. However, the possible value of facial nerve exploration is mentioned, because there is some anecdotal evidence to support decompression and facial nerve exploration for patients who experience significant electrical degeneration within 2 to 3 weeks following temporal bone trauma.

Unless there is evidence of a significant facial nerve diastasis on CT scan, patients who have had complete paralysis for more than 3 weeks after their injury are observed for 6 months for spontaneous regeneration (Table 2). Patients who develop any motion during this time period are observed and are not candidates for temporal bone facial nerve surgery. Patients who do not develop spontaneous activity during this time are restudied with EMG for spontaneous

Table 1. Closed Head Trauma Paralysis: 3 Week Decision Algorithm

CT*	ELECTRICAL TESTING†		THERAPY
+	−	→	Observe
+	+	→	Surgery
−	−	→	Observe
−	+	→	Observe‡

* CT+: 1 mm diastasis along course of facial nerve, or spicule in nerve.

† Electrical Testing+: <10 percent residual function on electroneuronography.

‡ Patients are informed that some anecdotal evidence supports facial nerve exploration and decompression. However, I encourage these patients to await the 6 month point.

muscle fibrillation or polyphasic potentials. Patients who demonstrate fibrillations have not experienced reinnervation of their facial musculature, so surgical exploration of the temporal course of the nerve should be considered. Patients who demonstrate polyphasic potentials are undergoing reinnervation of their facial musculature, so they should be managed with additional observation

An unusual presentation of traumatic facial paralysis is bilateral post-traumatic paralysis. In this setting, the paralysis is usually delayed and difficult to diagnose because the patient has symmetric facial function. Electrical testing cannot be used to compare with the contralateral side; thus, the findings on CT are crucial for deciding on surgical intervention.

Penetrating Trauma

The management of patients who have facial paralysis following penetrating trauma to the temporal bone (e,g., missile injuries) is usually more straightforward than that in closed head trauma. The timing of the paralysis is usually well known, and the location of the injury can often be followed in a straightforward manner on radiologic studies. Patients who have CT evidence of penetrating temporal bone trauma to the facial nerve and electrical evidence of degeneration are offered surgery. If the patient's CT scan does not indicate a direct missile injury to the facial nerve, but electrical degeneration reaches less than 10 percent of function, these patients are also offered surgery (unlike the closed head trauma patients), because heat or associated trauma from the missile injury may be responsible for the delayed paralysis (Table 3). Such a direct injury may be amenable to surgical decompression or repair.

Iatrogenic Trauma

Unlike the closed head trauma patient who has associated injuries, the timing of the injury in iatrogenic situations is very specific. The patient is usually recognized to have facial paralysis in the recovery room immediately after surgery. The danger of a tight mastoid dressing misleading the clinician into believing that function remains in the orbicularis oculi branch must not be overlooked. Nonetheless, facial paralysis immediately following ear surgery obviously suggests that the surgical procedure is the cause of the paralysis.

The first step in management of such patients is to realistically consider each of the steps of the procedure and the proximity and involvement of the facial nerve. Reasonable time should be given for dissipation of the effects of local anesthetic agents that may produce reversible paralysis. In addition, if the ear or mastoid cavity was packed with firm material, this should be loosened to give an opportunity for any direct pressure effect on the nerve to dissipate as well. After a number of hours to allow these maneuvers to take effect, consideration should be given to early exploration of the facial nerve. This is another situation in which voluntary EMG may be helpful. Evidence of volitional motor action potentials corroborates an intact nerve that will recover with time. However, neurapraxia sufficient to prohibit facial nerve motion most likely will also prevent adequate conduction for recording of a compound motor action potential.

Immediate postoperative facial paralysis is an emotionally charged situation for the patient as well as the surgeon, The surgeon should seek consultation readily in this situation, and preferably he or she should perform the facial nerve exploration in conjunction with another surgeon who has particular expertise in facial nerve surgery. This provides the additional objectivity of another observer, as well as a surgeon less emotionally involved in the decision-making process regarding a patient who has recently undergone surgery and developed facial paralysis. Because there are potential medicolegal ramifications to this situation, the presence of another surgeon also offers an additional observer to record findings and decision making. Although prompt exploration is indicated, waiting until the next morning for availability of the complete surgical team is preferable to the patient undergoing reoperation the same day with a tired or incomplete surgical team.

Table 2. Closed Head Trauma—Complete Paralysis: 6 Month Decisions

Motion	→	Observe		
No Motion	→	EMG		
		Fibrillations	→	Surgery
		Polyphasic	→	Observe

EMG, electromyography.

Table 3. Management of Patients Who Have Facial Paralysis from Penetrating Trauma

CT*	ELECTRICAL TESTING†		THERAPY
+	−	→	Observe
+	+	→	Surgery
−	−	→	Observe
−	+	→	Surgery

* CT+: 1 mm diastasis along course of facial nerve, or spicule in nerve.

† Electrical Testing+: <10 percent residual function on electroneuronography.

Extratemporal Injury

Penetrating Trauma

Penetrating trauma to the extratemporal course of the facial nerve should be suspected in any patient who has penetrating wounds of the periauricular and face region. Careful systematic examination must be performed of each of the branches of the facial nerve. This situation must be particularly considered in motor vehicle injuries with multiple glass wounds to the face.

A deficit found in any division of the facial nerve requires prompt surgical exploration. The opportunity to stimulate the peripheral branches of the facial nerve will be lost by the third day following injury if the nerve has been severed. Accordingly, it is imperative to explore these branches as soon as possible following the injury. If there is a significant blast injury or other wound with substantial devitalized tissue, then the branches of the nerve should be identified during wound debridement in the early postinjury period, and they should be tagged for subsequent repair.

Iatrogenic Trauma

Surgery of the parotid gland, submandibular gland, and rhytidectomy are all in close proximity to the main trunk or branches of the facial nerve. If the facial nerve branches in proximity to the surgery have been directly identified and visually confirmed to be intact at the conclusion of the procedure, then paralysis in those branches can be expected to recover, and surgical exploration will be of no benefit. For instance, short-term facial paralysis is not uncommon in patients undergoing parotidectomy for chronic infection. Uniformly, this type of paralysis can be expected to improve. In contrast, paralysis of the upper division of the facial nerve following repair of a zygomatic fracture would indicate acute trauma to those branches of the facial nerve. If no effort is made to identify those branches at the time of surgery, they require surgical exploration as soon as possible to permit electrical stimulation of the distal branches.

■ SURGICAL REPAIR OF THE TRAUMATIZED FACIAL NERVE

Intratemporal Injury

Unlike the situation in surgical decompression of idiopathic facial paralysis, radiographic findings guide the surgical exploration and repair of a traumatized facial nerve. The majority of the injuries are in the vicinity of the geniculate ganglion: proximal tympanic segment, geniculate ganglion, or labyrinthine segment. Surgical exploration of the facial nerve following temporal bone trauma is initially performed as a transmastoid approach. Often a canal wall-up mastoidectomy approach with facial recess is adequate for surgical exploration and decompression of the facial nerve from the proximal tympanic segment through the distal vertical segment of the facial nerve. If exploration of the geniculate ganglion or labyrinthine internal auditory canal (IAC) segments is necessary, a middle cranial fossa approach is employed as well. Because temporal lobe retraction is necessary for middle fossa surgery, I limit acute surgical exploration of temporal bone facial nerve trauma to situations with a combination of positive findings on CT scan (diastasis or spicule) and positive findings of significant degeneration on electrical facial nerve testing. If the patient has suffered total sensorineural hearing loss from the trauma, a translabyrinthine approach is preferable to the middle fossa approach to obtain total facial nerve exposure without temporal lobe retraction in an acute head injury scenario.

If the nerve is anatomically intact, it is widely decompressed around the fracture site, and the sheath is opened if hematoma is identified. Bony spicules are removed directly from the facial nerve. A large diastasis in the course of the facial nerve usually requires facial nerve interposition grafting. The greater auricular nerve is an excellent source for this graft. Because the temporal bone course of the facial nerve is an immobile area, interposition grafts can often be placed in the trough of the fallopian canal that are held in place with absorbable hemostatic material. If suture is required, which is usually the case in the labyrinthine or proximal tympanic portions, then two or three 10–0 monofilament sutures are used. The least suture material possible is used to perform this repair. Damage in the perigeniculate region of the nerve often requires middle fossa exposure for complete visualization, In those cases, the tympanic segment may be rerouted directly to the labyrinthine or IAC portion. Suture repair or grafting of the IAC portion of the facial nerve is difficult. Usually only one suture can be placed to approximate the ends of the nerve. This anastomosis is reinforced with absorbable hemostatic material. A fenestrated suction device with holes at the tip and sides is a useful platform for suture repair in the IAC. The nerve is placed on the suction, and the needle is directed through a side hole and the tip hole. In this fashion, the anastomosis is performed on a stable surface.

The most difficult clinical decision is determining how to treat a partial transection injury of the facial nerve. I employ the rule of one-half, that is, if half of the width of the facial nerve has been transected, the remainder of the nerve is probably sufficiently traumatized to require repair with an interposition graft. At this point, the remaining tissue is completely transected, the edges are fastened, and the interposition graft is placed.

If an injury of the sheath is identified with herniation of the nerve fibers through the damaged sheath, a segment of the nerve on either side of the injury is decompressed and the sheath is opened to prevent strangulation of the nerve.

Extratemporal Injury

Extratemporal injuries are dealt with as soon as possible after the trauma. Use of facial nerve stimulation allows identification of the distal segments of the injured nerve if exploration is performed sooner than 3 days after injury. Repair is performed with 8–0 or 10–0 monofilament suture, with the minimal number of sutures necessary for good coaptation. Fascicular repair is not attempted. The sutures are placed through the epineurium for extratemporal injuries.

■ POSTOPERATIVE CARE

The most important priority for any patient who has facial nerve paralysis is adequate care of the eye on the paralyzed side of the face. Aggressive use of ophthalmic drops, ointment, and moisture chambers is necessary. Once an injury is clearly going to be long-standing, the risk of exposure keratitis should prompt early placement of either gold weights or springs for appropriate corneal protection. Occasionally, lower lid procedures are necessary as well. These procedures are best coordinated through an ophthalmology consultation.

Patients are counseled that despite appropriate repair, time is necessary for the nerve fibers to regenerate, and another 6 to 9 month time frame is necessary to await the reinnervation, If no reinnervation is seen by 1 year, nerve substitution procedures can be considered if EMG shows no evidence of reinnervation. On the other hand, if the physician encounters the patient late in the course of recovery, absence of reinnervation by 1 year should prompt surgical exploration of the course of the nerve if this has not been done previously. In most situations, reconstitution of anatomic integrity of the facial nerve provides superior facial function to nerve substitution procedures. Direct or graft repair of the facial nerve permits emotive facial function, which is not obtained with nerve substitution procedures.

Suggested Reading

Brodie HA, Thompson TC. Management of complications from 820 temporal bone fractures. Am J Otol 1997; 18:188-197.

Coker NJ. Management of traumatic injuries to the facial nerve. Otolaryngol Clin North Am 1991; 24:215-227.

Duncan NO, Coker NJ, Jenkins HA, Canalis RF. Gunshot injuries of the temporal bone. Otolaryngol Head Neck Surg 1986; 94:47-55.

Fisch U. Facial paralysis in fractures of the petrous bone. Laryngoscope 1974; 84:2141-2154.

Fisch U. Prognostic value of electrical tests in acute facial paralysis. Am J Otol 1984; 5:494-498.

Jenkins HA, Atar GA. Traumatic facial paralysis. In: Brackmann DE, Shelton C, Arriaga M, eds. Otologic surgery. Philadelphia: WB Saunders, 1994:397.

PERMANENT FACIAL PARALYSIS

The method of
Dean M. Toriumi
by
James C. Alex
Dean M. Toriumi

For patients who have permanent facial paralysis, the cosmetic and functional deficits are both physically and emotionally devastating. Rehabilitation of these patients is a continuing challenge for the otolaryngologist due to the intricate three-dimensional mimetic nature of the 17 paired muscles of facial expression. Although there are several reanimation techniques, each has its limitations. The best reconstruction option is dependent on several considerations, including the individual patient's desires, expectations, and motivation; the cause of facial paralysis; the duration of symptoms; and the status of the facial motor endplates. This information, together with a thorough physical examination, allows the surgeon to propose the optimal strategy for reconstruction.

The goals of reconstruction are both functional and cosmetic. Functionally, the surgeon has to consider the patient's eye closure, speech difficulties, oral competency, and nasal airway patency. Cosmetically, the surgeon must try to reestablish coordinated facial motion on the paralyzed side of the face as well as balance and symmetry between both sides of the face.

■ REANIMATION OF UPPER THIRD OF FACE

Permanent facial paralysis with secondary paralytic lagophthalmos can lead to devastating sequelae, including corneal drying, ulceration, and ocular perforation. Lack of orbicularis function impairs upper and lower lid closure, which causes poor tear film movement and increased tear evaporation. Other contributing problems, such as fifth nerve paralysis and poor Bell's phenomenon, also place the eye at risk for complication. Because 85 percent of lid closure is performed by the upper lid and 15 percent by the lower lid, both lids must be assessed and treated when the eye is rehabilitated.

The Upper Lid

Options for rehabilitating the upper lid include gold weight implants, palpebral wire spring, Silastic-elastic prosthesis, and temporalis or masseter muscle transfer.

Temporalis muscle transfer, a popular method of reanimating the eyelids, can provide complete dynamic eye closure. However, there are several drawbacks to this technique. Often, it creates a slitlike appearance to the palpebral fissure and a visible bulge of the lateral orbital region secondary to muscle bulk. In addition, the temporalis muscle transfer technique, although providing dynamic eyelid closure, interferes with the natural eyelid blink reflex.

An implantable palpebral wire spring is an effective option and has the added advantage of providing closure regardless of position. Initially introduced in 1964 by Morel-Fatio and Lalardie, the procedure has undergone several modifications that have considerably improved the functional and cosmetic result. Despite being the preferred technique of several authors experienced in their use, palpebral springs can be difficult to implant, often need postoperative readjustment, and have been reported to have a significant infection and extrusion rate.

In the past, Silastic-elastic implants have also been used to correct upper lid ptosis. However, these implants tend to stretch over time and lose effectiveness; therefore, they are seldom used today.

Gold Weight Implantation Technique

Our current method for managing paralysis of the upper eyelid is to use gold weight implants. Lid loading with gold weights is (1) successful approximately 90 percent of the time, (2) easy to perform, (3) well tolerated by the patients,

(4) relatively low in complications, and (5) complementary with the blink reflex.

Preoperative evaluation includes complete ocular, neurologic, and otolaryngologic examination. Particular attention is paid to the patient's visual acuity, degree of exposure keratitis, fifth and seventh nerve function, lagophthalmos, degree of Bell's phenomenon, levator function, and eyelid palpebral distances. Photographic documentation of the patient's eyelid function is obtained for all patients.

Thorough analysis is particularly important if gold weight placement is intended, because the lid is not subject to the effects of gravity when the patient is recumbent, and lid closure tends to be incomplete. If, in addition, the patient's Bell's reflex is poor, exposure of the cornea can occur, resulting in exposure keratitis, ulceration, or ocular perforation.

Selection of the proper gold weight implant is determined preoperatively by taping different size weights to the patient's upper lid. Gold implants ranging in weight from 0.6 to 1.6 g are sequentially tested, and the weight that eliminates lagophthalmos without causing excessive ptosis is determined.

Surgery can be performed at the same time as reanimation of the lower two-thirds of the face or in a separate procedure using local anesthesia. With a protective corneal contact lens in place, an incision line is marked out along the superior eyelid crease of the paralyzed eyelid. This line is injected with 2 percent lidocaine with epinephrine and then incised through the skin, anterior lamella layers, and the orbicularis muscle to the tarsal plate, after allowing sufficient time for vasoconstriction. The dissection is carried out to within 1 to 2 mm of the eyelash roots. The gold weight implant is centered in the midpupillary plane. Three 5–0 Prolene sutures are passed through the implant's preformed holes and secured to the anterior tarsus with firm partial-thickness bites. Full-thickness sutures should be avoided. Once the proper position and contour of the implant are achieved, the underlying orbicularis muscle is meticulously sutured together with 6–0 Monocryl sutures. The skin is closed with running 7–0 nylon, and ophthalmic ointment is applied to the suture line. Artificial tears are used for 1 to 2 weeks, and sutures are removed after 7 days. Visual acuity, exposure keratitis, lagophthalmos, levator function, and eyelid palpebral distances are assessed at this initial postoperative visit.

Although lid loading can be an effective, essentially maintenance-free management approach to the paralyzed eyelid, some studies have reported a relatively high complication rate, primarily because of extrusion. The likely mechanism for extrusion is that the delicate, atrophic denervated orbicularis cannot support the long-term weight and bulk of the implant, particularly in the elderly. There are several modifications to our technique that minimize this tendency and decrease the extrusion rate: (1) a modified gold weight implant is used that has a thickness of 1.0 mm, a width of 3.2 mm, and a length that varies according to the weight (a standard implant is 1.0 mm × 5.0 mm × length according to weight). This modified implant distributes the weight more evenly across the lid and gives the lid a more uniform appearance; (2) the implant is secured with nonabsorbable sutures that prohibit movement of the implant and decrease pressure on the adjacent tissues; (3) the smallest weight possible, based on the preoperative examination, is implanted in order to minimize pressure on overlying tissues.

The Lower Lid

Management of the lower lid begins with a close examination of the lid position. In neutral gaze, the lid should be at or just above the limbus. The presence of scleral show or an ectropion should be noted, and a snap test should be performed. The position of the punctum is critical. It should be against the globe and nondisplaced. A lateral traction test of the lower lid (simulating lid tightening) is used to assess the effect on lid apposition to the globe and displacement of the punctum. The traction test also determines if the middle and medial thirds of the lid have adequate support or whether additional procedures such as cartilage grafting may need to be performed. If lateral traction displaces the punctum to an excessive degree or does not provide proper lid support, this may interfere with proper tear flow movement and require an alternative surgical approach.

Treatment methods include lid tightening procedures (lower lid tightening procedures, horizontal eyelid shortening, the Bick procedure, lateral tarsal suspension, and lateral canthopexy); cartilage grafting; and medial canthal ligament imbrication and canthoplasty. The key to selecting the best corrective technique(s) depends on accurate evaluation and diagnosis of lower lid abnormalities.

Eyebrow

After restoration of eyelid function and appearance, additional cosmetic benefit is often achieved with the treatment of any existent unilateral forehead-brow-glabellar complex asymmetries. Two effective corrective procedures are the unilateral midforehead lift and the direct brow lift. The former procedure is typically used in males who have deep transverse midforehead creases. When rhytids are unavailable for scar camouflage, then the direct brow lift is preferred. It should be underscored that when lifting the brow for permanent unilateral facial paralysis, the orbicularis muscle must be suspended to the frontal bone periosteum or the fascia of the frontalis muscle in order to effect permanent ptosis correction.

In our hands, proper rehabilitation of the eye has yielded consistently excellent results, with satisfaction among the patients in the 90 percent range. The more difficult area to reanimate successfully is the lower two-thirds of the face. In this area, methods of correction are technically more involved, and facial symmetry is more difficult to achieve.

■ REANIMATION OF LOWER TWO-THIRDS OF FACE

The treatment modalities for the lower third of the face can be divided according to whether the facial muscles have intact motor endplates and whether dynamic or static reanimation is contemplated. Before discussing treatment modalities, the process and timing of nerve and motor endplate degeneration must be understood.

Neuropathophysiology

The degree of facial nerve and motor endplate degeneration in a patient who has facial paralysis is directly related to the nature of the injury. If the injury is due to pressure on the nerve trunk causing a conduction block (a neurapraxia), then complete recovery will occur. A more severe injury, axonotmesis (a conduction block with wallerian degeneration) will also result in full recovery; however, the recovery time will be longer because the axon must regrow from the site of injury to the motor endplate at a rate close to 1 millimeter per day.

Disruption of the connective tissue elements of the nerve produces varying degrees of nerve injury. The severity of injury depends on whether endoneurium, perineurium, or epineurium is injured (Sunderland classes III to IV). The fewer connective tissue elements intact within the nerve, the less likely the regenerating nerve fibers will find their appropriate motor endplates.

Other factors that adversely affect nerve regeneration include previous radiotherapy to the nerve injury site, diabetes, and advancing age. In addition to providing a framework for understanding a given patient's underlying pathology, the degree of nerve regeneration or degeneration also influences which reanimation procedure(s) would be best suited for the patient.

An important diagnostic tool in the evaluation of facial nerve regeneration or degeneration is electromyography (EMG). The presence of polyphasic or normal voluntary action potentials in a patient who has facial paralysis of greater than 12 months' duration suggests that the motor endplates are intact and reinnervation is present but insufficient to produce facial movement. Fibrillation or denervation potentials indicate that although the motor endplates are intact, they will degenerate over time and be lost. This situation requires that innervation in the form of direct nerve grafting or cross-facial nerve grafting be performed expeditiously. In the case of EMG electrical silence, all the muscles of facial expression have undergone denervation atrophy. Therefore, direct nerve grafts or cross-over grafts are pointless and contraindicated. The only options are a microneurovascular muscle transfer procedure or a temporalis or masseter muscle transfer. The details of these management situations are detailed below.

Functional Motor Endplates, Dynamic Reconstruction

For patients who have intact motor endplates and wish to undergo dynamic rehabilitation, direct facial nerve anastomosis or interposition grafting produces the most desirable effect. When only the distal facial nerve is available, anastomosis to other motor neurons can be performed (hypoglossal, trigeminal, phrenic, accessory, and ansa hypoglossus nerves). Although these techniques provide facial tone, symmetry at rest, and learned voluntary facial movement, they do not restore involuntary, independent mimetic facial expression or allow protective eye closure.

Cross-facial nerve grafting is also used when motor endplates are functional. This technique involves linking the peripheral facial nerve branches on the paralyzed side of the face to a functional facial nerve branch from the opposite side of the face using a nerve graft (sural, lateral femoral cutaneous, superficial radial, antebrachial cutaneous). By connecting facial nerve branches from the functioning side of the face to the nonfunctioning side, both sides of the face are stimulated by the cortical area that corresponds to the facial homunculus. This identical cortical representation permits a more balanced mimetic facial expression to occur.

The difficulty with this procedure is the 9 month regeneration interval necessary for axons to traverse the nerve and reach motor endplates on the paralyzed side of the face. When added to the 12 month observation period before such surgery is typically contemplated, more than 20 months can pass before the motor endplates are restimulated and maintained.

When the EMG indicates polyphasic or normal action potentials, the motor endplates can be assumed to be stable, and this length of time for regeneration poses no problems. The presence of fibrillation potentials indicate that the motor endplates would continue to degenerate as the regenerating axons make their way across the nerve graft. A solution to this problem is an interim hypoglossal nerve transposition graft that can maintain motor endplate viability while the regenerating nerve fibers traverse the cross-facial nerve graft.

Nonfunctional Motor Endplates

When the motor endplates are not viable, rehabilitation options include static procedures (fascial sling, facelift, nasolabial fold incision) and dynamic procedures (free neurovascular muscle transplantation and temporalis or masseter transfer procedures). Static procedures, because they are nearly as involved as muscle transfer techniques, are used primarily in an adjunctive role. The current state-of-the-art method for facial reanimation in a patient who has nonfunctional motor endplates is dynamic reconstruction using free neurovascular muscle transplantation.

Nonfunctional Motor Endplates, Dynamic Reconstruction

Free neurovascular muscle transplantation allows the transfer of innervated vascularized muscle to the face to replace atrophic or fibrotic facial muscles. It is a two-staged procedure that combines an initial cross-facial nerve graft with a subsequent neurovascular free muscle transfer.

The cross-facial nerve graft is performed in the usual fashion with reversal of the donor nerve graft to maximize the number of axons crossing the cross-facial nerve graft from the recipient nerve. During the regenerative phase, Tinel's sign is used to clinically assess the growth of the regenerating nerve axons. Complete migration of the regenerating nerve fibers usually takes roughly 6 months. To ensure the maximal number of axons at the time of free muscle transfer, an additional delay of 3 months is suggested.

Although several different muscles can be used for facial reanimation (most commonly gracilis or serratus anterior), the basic operative approach and techniques are the same. A two-team approach is preferred, with one team preparing the paralyzed side of the face while the other team harvests the neurovascular muscle graft. The free muscle graft is positioned under the zygomaticus major muscle and fixated to the upper lip, oral commissure, and nasolabial groove using 3–0, nonabsorbable sutures. The neurovascular anastomosis is performed next and followed by attachment of the proximal end of the muscle to the zygomatic arch and the temporal region.

It is is difficult to judge the success of this technique

because there is no established grading system that enables the results of staged neurovascular graft procedures to be assessed. However, the preponderance of the literature suggests that facial reanimation with free muscle grafting produces some degree of mimetic function in approximately 65 percent to 70 percent of patients. A major cosmetic disadvantage to this technique is that free neurovascular grafts are bulky, which creates an unnatural skin contour and obvious facial imbalance.

■ TEMPORALIS MUSCLE TRANSPOSITION TECHNIQUE

The most common experience that we encounter in our clinic is the patient who has normal integrity of an intact facial nerve but due to the injury has persistent loss of facial tone symmetry and movement. In this group of patients, we have had success using the temporalis muscle transposition technique, which provides improved facial tone, movement, and balance without interfering with neuronal recovery. It also provides an emotional balm for recovering patients who may suffer as long as 2 years before spontaneous nerve recovery occurs.

The broad fan-shaped temporalis muscle arises from the temporal line and inserts into the coronoid process of the mandible. The muscle is 3 to 5 cm in longest dimension, with a contractile capability of 1 to 5 cm. The muscle thickness is approximately 2 to 3 cm. The trigeminal nerve that traverses the undersurface of the muscle in an arcadian pattern provides innervation in the temporalis muscle. The vascular supply is from the internal maxillary artery and the middle temporal artery.

Preoperative evaluation includes a thorough otolaryngologic and neurologic evaluation. Existing asymmetries, impairment of function, and the patient's smile pattern are assessed and photographically documented. Equally important, the function, strength, and tone of the temporalis muscle is also evaluated to ensure that it is suitable for the required reconstructive task.

Elevation of Temporoparietal Fascial Flap

First, the course of the superficial temporal artery is determined by manual palpation or Doppler probe and marked on the skin surface. The scalp incision we use is similar to that described by Cheney and May. Once marked on the skin, hair is shaved 1 cm on either side of the incision line; the area is injected with 1 percent lidocaine with 1 : 100,000 epinephrine, and the remaining hair is slicked back with bacitracin. After incising the skin to the temporoparietal fascial and dissecting in a subdermal plane, a temporoparietal fascial flap based on the superficial temporal artery is created. Care must be taken to preserve the superficial temporal artery and vein and avoid injuring superficial hair follicles, which can result in hair loss.

Temporalis Muscle Transposition

With the temporoparietal fascial flap protected in a moist sponge, the skin incision is extended inferiorly following the pretragal crease and around the attachment of the lobule in a similar fashion as a facelift. The plane of dissection is immediately subdermal, staying above the superficial musculoaponeurotic system and away from the branches of the facial nerve.

From the zygomatic arch, the dissection is continued anteroinferiorly to the cheek–lip crease (adults) or the oral commissure (children), where skin incisions will be made to gain access to the orbicularis oris. Once the lateral aspect of the orbicularis oris muscle is identified, two fingers are passed through to the zygomatic arch, thus creating a tunnel wide enough to allow passage of the transposed muscle. The middle third of the temporalis muscle is incised and elevated with pericranium on its medial surface, carefully lifted over the zygomatic arch tunnel with preservation of the neurovascular supply, and passed through the tunnel in a superior to inferior direction.

Using three to five 3–0 Prolene sutures, the muscle is fixed to the medial border or the orbicularis oris muscle near the submucous layer of the corner of the mouth. Muscle-to-muscle contact between the temporalis muscle and the orbicularis oris muscle is critical to the final result, as is gross overcorrection and exaggeration of the nasolabial fold at the time of surgery. The amount of overcorrection required depends on each patient's unique smile pattern (as determined preoperatively from the functional side of the face) and with the amount of postoperative muscle relaxation that occurs in each surgeon's experience. The perioral incision is closed using 5–0 nylon horizontal mattress sutures.

We obliterate the donor site defect by transposing the temporoparietal fascial flap into the temporal defect and suturing it to the remaining temporalis muscle using 4-10 PDS sutures. A closed suction drain and a compressive dressing are used for the first 24 hours postoperatively to prevent swelling and hematoma formation.

■ POSTOPERATIVE COURSE

One gram of cefazolin is administered intravenously every 8 hours for 24 hours. After that, cephalexin, 500 mg three times a day for 5 days, is instituted. The suture lines are covered with bacitracin ointment until crusting stops. The results of transposing the temporalis muscle to reanimate the mouth are evident within 3 to 6 weeks after the procedure. This recovery time can be greatly enhanced by patient instruction on how to activate the transposed muscle by voluntary effort. In patients who are motivated to learn the necessary motor-sensory coordination techniques, achievement of mouth symmetry at rest and a balanced voluntary smile is obtainable.

Technically, there are several aspects of the temporalis muscle transposition technique that are important for yielding a beneficial result and deserve highlighting:

1. It is important that the superficial tunnel that conveys the temporalis muscle from the temporal area to the lip–cheek crease or vermilion is made superficial to the superficial musculo aponeurotic system (SMAS). Taking care to create the tunnel in this plane protects functioning facial nerve fibers from injury and allows the temporalis muscle to augment residual facial nerve function in patients.

2. Making the conveying tunnel at least two fingerwidths wide permits the muscle to lie flat in the tunnel with minimal bulging. Using only the middle third of the temporalis muscle also reduces bulging.
3. Placing multiple sutures in the muscle submucous layer at the level of the corner of the mouth is essential in order to initially overcorrect the smile. As the temporalis muscle relaxes and stretches over 3 to 6 weeks, the proper long-term balance and symmetry is obtained.
4. In order to close the donor site defect, a temporoparietal fascial flap is used. To establish adequate contour, it may be necessary to fold this fascial flap upon itself in order to provide the necessary bulk.
5. The middle one-third of the temporalis muscle (2.0 to 2.5 cm) is the optimal choice for reanimation of the midface. The anterior and posterior thirds of the temporalis muscle lack the length, orientation, and contractile properties required for facial nerve reanimation.

■ DISCUSSION

Correcting the functional and cosmetic deficits in patients who have permanent facial paralysis is one of the more challenging and rewarding reconstructive procedures performed by the otolaryngologist. It requires an accurate evaluation of the patient's psychological and neuromuscular status and a comprehensive understanding of the different reanimation procedures and their application. It is the proper marriage of these insights tempered by the surgeon's experience that leads to an optimal reconstructive result.

Suggested Reading

Aviv JE, Urken ML. Management of the paralyzed face with microneurovascular free muscle transfer. Plast Reconstr Surg 1964; 33:446-449.

Cheney ML, McKenna MJ, Megerian CA, Ojemann RG. Early temporalis muscle transposition for the management of facial paralysis. Laryngoscope 1995; 105:993-1000.

Harii K. Refined microvascular free muscle transplantation for reanimation of the paralyzed face. Microsurgery 1988; 9:169-176.

Hoffman WY. Reanimation of the paralyzed face. Otolaryngol Clin North Am 1992; 25:649-666.

Keen MS, Burgoyne JD, Kay SL. Surgical management of the paralyzed eyelid. Ear Nose Throat J 1993; 72:692-701.

Levine RE, Pulec JL. Eyelid reanimation with the palpebral spring after facial nerve graft surgery. An interdisciplinary approach. Ear Nose Throat J 1993; 72:686-691.

Mackinnon SE, Dellon AL. Technical considerations of the latissimus dorsi muscle flap: A segmentally innervated muscle for facial reanimation. Microsurgery 1988; 9:36-45.

May M. Gold weight and wire spring implants as alternatives to tarsorrhaphy. Arch Otolaryngol Head Neck Surg 1987; 113:656-660.

May M. Paralyzed eyelids reanimated with closed eyelid spring. Laryngoscope 1988; 48:382-385.

May M, Drucker C. Temporalis muscle for facial reanimation. Arch Otolaryngol Head Neck Surg 1993; 119:378-384.

Morel-Fatio C, Lalardie JP. Palliative surgical treatment of facial paralysis: The palpebral spring. Ann Clin Plast Esthet 1962; 7:275.

O'Brien BM, Pederson MC, Khanzanchi RK, et al. Results of management of facial palsy with microvascular free muscle transfer. Plast Reconstr Surg 1990; 86:12-22.

Pickford MA, Scamp T, Harrison DH. Morbidity after gold weight insertion into the upper eyelid in facial palsy. Br J Plast Surg 1992; 45:460-464.

Terzis JK. Pectoralis minor: A unique muscle for the correction of facial palsy. Plast Reconstr Surg 1989; 83:767-776.

Townsend DJ. Eyelid reanimation for the treatment of paralytic lagophthalmos: Historical perspectives and current applications of the gold weight implant. Ophthalmic Plast Reconstr Surg 1992; 8:196-201.

INJURIES OF THE PINNA

The method of
Jay K. Roberts

The pinna functions to localize sound and augment delivery of sound to the ear canal and tympanic membrane. Unfortunately, injury is common because of its protuberant position. Perhaps more important than its function is its appearance. The configuration of a normal ear is unique in nature, and it may draw little attention to itself; the same may not be said of an auricle deformed by trauma or the complications thereof. Trauma to the pinna may be thermal or mechanical. The former includes frostbite and burns, whereas the latter group of injuries may be subdivided into those related to birth, pierced ears, blunt trauma, sharp trauma, and avulsions. Chondritis is a very serious complication of several of these conditions, and I include methods for its management

■ THERMAL INJURIES

Frostbite

The pinna may rapidly develop frostbite when exposed in severe winter weather. Initially, it may be very difficult to assess the true extent of injury. Typically, the ear exhibits pallor and numbness. Rapid rewarming should be immediately instituted using wet cotton balls that have been soaked in saline at 38° to 42° C. Because of the ice crystals initially present within the soft tissues, extreme care needs to be taken to avoid manipulation of the pinna during the rewarming process. Rewarming is continued until complete thawing has occurred. Sedatives and parenteral analgesics may be required. As the frostbitten area thaws, fluid extravasates from damaged vessels and may eventually lead to formation of bullae and vesicles. Somewhat later, one notes areas of hyperemia, demarcating healthy tissues from those exhibiting frostbite damage. Hemorrhage, edema, and necrosis may occur days later. Tissue is not debrided until it is known to be dead in order to minimize cosmetic deformity.

Burns

Burns of the auricle are classified in the same way as elsewhere on the body. They are nearly always associated with extensive burns in the head and neck area. Treatment again is directed at caring for the acute problem, but with an eye toward preventing complications and minimizing tissue loss. First-degree burns manifest erythema and mild to moderate discomfort and may be carefully observed. Second-degree burns exhibit formation of vesicles and bullae, which if possible should be left intact. The ear is gently cleansed daily. If areas of rupture are small, they may be treated on an outpatient basis with applications of silver sulfadiazine cream. If dressings must be applied, this is to be done with minimal pressure. The patient should use a headrest for sleep to prevent any pressure on the ears. With extensive vesicle disruption in second-degree burns, or in third-degree burns, prevention of infection becomes most important. In addition to these measures, the patient should be treated with both anti-pseudomonal drops in the ear canal and parenteral antibiotics that have good coverage of *P. aeruginosa* and *S. aureus.* This can usually be arranged to be done at home by a visiting nurse, who is also often very capable of performing the local ear care once or twice a day; the patient or family can perform the rest of the ear care. The patient should be seen by the treating physician very frequently. It has been found beneficial to inject a solution of gentamicin (40 mg per cubic centimeter) into several areas on the anterior and posterior surface of the ears when the opportunity presents itself, such as at the time of debridement. It is recommended that not more than 1 mg per kilogram of body weight of gentamicin be used for these injections. When minimal debridement is begun, it is most often done under local anesthesia (without epinephrine), and exposed cartilage is treated with cleansing, sulfadiazine, and protection from pressure. If the cartilage exposure is minimal, granulation tissue will form, and the area will epithelialize from the wound edges; or grafts can be applied when the wound bed is healthy. Meshed grafts are to be avoided because of the poor cosmetic results. Upper eyelid skin, if available, provides an excellent texture match. With more extensive cartilage exposure, it may be necessary to provide coverage by placing it in a postauricular pocket, or even at a distant site for later reconstructive efforts.

■ MECHANICAL INJURIES

Birth Injuries

When an infant is born with a deformed but complete pinna, it may often be treated within the first week of life with very satisfactory results. The ear may have been in an abnormal position in utero, or it may have become deformed with the application of forceps during delivery, or it may have suffered some other birth trauma. Because of circulating maternal estrogens in the infant's bloodstream, the ear remains very pliable for a few days after birth. Moist cotton is placed in the areas of concern to mold the ear into a normal configuration, and the cotton is then secured with benzoin and tape and left for 10 days. Once maternal estrogen levels have decreased within a few days after birth, this process will be ineffective.

Blunt Trauma

When a hematoma or a seroma results from blunt trauma, treatment must be instituted. A hematoma is usually the result of shearing forces that separate the lateral perichondrium from the underlying cartilage, often seen in wrestlers, boxers, or those who have suffered unprotected seizures.

The presentation is of a mildly painful swelling of the lateral aspect of the pinna that obliterates some or all of the normal contours of the auricle. Even when these injuries are adequately evacuated with aspiration, they will most often recur when treated in this fashion. Therefore, all but the smallest, most discrete hematomas or seromas should be treated with incision and drainage under local anesthesia. This accomplishes two purposes: first, it eliminates the probability that the hematoma will become organized, and possibly replaced with dense fibrous tissue or neocartilage; second, it allows reapposition of the perichondrium and the cartilage to re-establish the nutritional source to the cartilage and also to prevent chondritis. Pressure must typically be applied for at least a week to prevent recurrence.

Treatment is easily accomplished in the outpatient clinic. After application of local anesthesia, drainage is effected under scrupulous sterile technique through an incision placed over the hematoma in such a fashion that it will not be very obvious after healing, such as parallel to a natural fold. Incision should be wide enough to ensure complete removal of the hematoma. An antibiotic ointment such as mupirocin is applied to the incision; then a 3–0 or 4–0 monofilament, nonabsorbable suture is used to secure dental rolls placed on both sides of the pinna as bolsters. Depending on the size of the hematoma, several pairs of dental rolls may need to be placed in order to assure that the elevated perichondrium is in secure, gentle contact with the underlying cartilage. An oral anti-staphylococcal antibiotic is prescribed for the duration of time that bolsters will be in place. The area should be kept clean, and some surgeons advocate that antibiotic ointment should be applied to the areas where the sutures enter the skin three times daily, or that anti-pseudomonal drops should be applied to these areas at a similar frequency.

The use of dental roll bolsters allows the patient to be active, and if a wrestler, he may return immediately to that activity with the use of protective head gear. The bolsters are removed after 7 days.

When the physician is dealing with a late, deforming, fibrotic, or neocartilaginous mass within an auricle, or if a hematoma has occurred in such an ear, the ear must usually be opened to remove the fibrotic tissue and/or neocartilage. This procedure is often best done under general anesthesia, because it is typically quite time-consuming. Treatment is then as described previously with dental rolls and so forth.

Split Lobule

The split lobule is usually a result of prolonged traction from wearing heavy earrings, but this condition may occur acutely when an earring is suddenly caught or pulled. In the acute situation, the skin edges may simply be reapproximated using 5–0 nylon after aseptic preparation of the area and administration of local anesthesia. When the split has existed chronically and has epithelialized, the skin on the opposing sides of the split must be removed, and the edges should then be accurately realigned. If the lobule tip is small and the surgeon is concerned about notching, a Z-plasty may be done on the most inferior aspect of the lobule. If the position is appropriate, and the patient wishes to continue to wear pierced earrings, a post may be left in place in the most superior aspect of the repair, or, alternatively, the ear can simply be pierced again at a later date.

Keloids

Keloids are a cosmetic and sometimes painful problem in susceptible individuals. After careful excision, injection of triamcinolone acetonide is carried out in the immediately surrounding tissues. Reinjection should occur every week or two for 2 to 3 months, and then again if recurrence is noted.

Lacerations

Lacerations span the spectrum from abrasions to amputation of the auricle. After creating a sterile field around the area and applying adequate local anesthesia, abrasions should be meticulously cleaned of all foreign material, which, if left in place, may lead to permanent tattooing of the skin. Gentle scrubbing may be adequate, or power irrigation may be required, in addition to using surgical instruments, loupes, or a microscope. A topical antibiotic is applied to prevent secondary infection. The patient should be instructed to cleanse the ear and reapply the antibiotic two to three times daily until the ear is healed, typically in 1 to 2 weeks. Alternatively, fine mesh gauze impregnated with antibiotic ointment can be placed on the cleansed ear, followed by a loose mastoid dressing that is left in place for 48 hours. At this point, the fine mesh gauze is dried, and it may be left in place until it separates on its own as re-epithelialization occurs. The patient should be informed to watch for symptoms and signs of perichondritis: pain, fever, swelling, or progressive erythema.

Lacerations, whether simple or complex, require meticulous realignment of wound edges in order to assure the most normal postinjury configuration or appearance of the auricle. After thorough cleaning, minimal debridement is carried out. The repair proceeds from known landmarks toward areas of more significant tissue disruption. When questions exist, it is often helpful to study the uninjured ear, in order to help the surgeon establish the appropriate alignment of tissue fragments. Atraumatic soft-tissue techniques are required in accurately bringing the tissues together in layers: cartilage, perichondrium, and skin. Minimal suturing of the cartilage should be done, because blood supply here is virtually nonexistent, and foreign material will predispose to infection. A very small amount of cartilage may need to be resected at the wound edges in order to allow approximation of the perichondrium. In many areas on the lateral surface of the pinna, the perichondrium and skin are firmly attached to each other and often are best closed together as one layer. Undyed, absorbable 6–0 sutures are usually an excellent choice for the cartilage and perichondrium. If permanent sutures are required, clear or white material should be used. Skin is reapproximated with 6–0 nylon. If through-and-through sutures are required for placement of a bolster to prevent formation of a hematoma, nonabsorbable, monofilament suture is chosen.

Near-total avulsions should be repaired immediately if there is any remaining pedicle at all. The pinna has an excellent blood supply, and it is sometimes surprising how little of a remaining pedicle is required to allow survival. Gentle manipulation is needed to protect the pedicle. Strict avoidance of vasoconstrictors is imperative. Landmarks are accurately approximated as noted previously. A nonocclusive dressing that applies no pressure to the pedicle or repair is applied to allow frequent observation for venous stasis. If venous congestion becomes a problem, limited areas may be treated by making multiple small skin incisions over the affected area; alternatively, a leech or two may be applied. The leeches draw off blood, but also, what is more important, they inject vasodilators and anticoagulants, which allow the site of the leeches' attachment to continue to ooze for many hours after their removal. Leeches are available through medicinal or biologic supply houses.

Successful reattachment of amputated auricles has been reported with interrupted sutures, but there are undoubtedly many failures of this technique that have gone unreported. If this technique is attempted, it probably should be reserved for those situations in which the detached ear is immediately cooled and then cleansed and reattached within 4 hours of injury. The skin edges of the avulsed segment and the avulsion site should be freshened by removing no more than 1 mm on each side. Reattachment failure is most likely due to venous congestion, hypoxia, and acidosis, so techniques noted previously will very likely be needed. The final result is at best hyperpigmented and mildly deformed, but this is usually superior to total auricular reconstruction. With partial amputation, fragments less than 2 cm in size that are repaired within 2 hours have a good chance of survival.

An additional technique that may be used in this circumstance is to de-epithelialize the medial surface of the fragment as well as the postauricular skin over the mastoid. In addition to then suturing the amputated segment into its place, it is secured to the de-epithelialized postauricular area with sutures tied over Xeroform bolsters. Approximately 6 weeks later, the auricle is elevated off of the mastoid, and a skin graft is placed. Alternatively, if the ear is mangled, or if other unfavorable factors exist, such as a several hour delay before presentation, extreme contamination, and so forth, the pinna is de-epithelialized both laterally and medially, and is placed in a pocket created through a postauricular incision. Two weeks later, the pinna is removed from the pocket and is allowed to re-epithelialize.

Microvascular reanastomosis may become the standard method for repair of auricular amputation; however, the vessels are very small and inconstant, and have often been badly damaged. Vein grafts may be required. This technique may, of course, be used in conjunction with some of the de-epithelialization techniques discussed previously, as well as those for control of venous congestion. Heparinization of the patient is initially accomplished with 10,000 units intravenously, and then a drip is continued to keep the partial thromboplastin time approximately two to two and one-half times normal until the avulsed segment appears viable and venous congestion decreases, usually approximately 7 to 10 days.

Dextran and vasodilators do not seem to be necessary. High-dose glucocorticoids have been shown to increase composite graft survival in the animal model, but this has not been demonstrated adequately in humans.

In situations in which reattachment is not possible under any of the aforementioned circumstances, cartilage is dissected from all of the overlying soft tissue, and it may be implanted subcutaneously for later reconstructive efforts. Placing this under postauricular skin would be the preferred option, but it may live in another location for later transplantation. Placing the cartilage under radial forearm skin to allow free flap transfer of the preserved auricular cartilage and the overlying radial forearm skin has led to somewhat disappointing results, because flap edema obscures the architecture of the cartilage.

■ CHONDRITIS

Chondritis is a serious complication of any auricular trauma, but it is most often seen in association with burns or after multiple aspirations of auricular hematoma or seroma. Symptoms and signs include relatively rapid development of pain, swelling, erythema, and tenderness. Before abscess formation, this condition is more appropriately referred to as perichondritis. It is an aggressive, inflammatory, and/or infectious process, with positive results from culture for *P. aeruginosa* in all but the tiny minority of cases. *S. aureus* is present in the majority of cases as well. If the process progresses to the development of fluctuance and abscess, it is most appropriately referred to as chondritis. Involvement of cartilage is now assured, and parenteral antibiotics alone will not be able to reverse the process. If not treated rapidly and aggressively, the entire auricular cartilage may be lost, leaving a very small, deformed pinna. Hospitalization is required for topical and parenteral antibiotic treatment as well as for parenteral pain medicines. After drainage of the abscess, multiply perforated catheters are placed between the cartilage and the perichondrium in the abscess cavities, and anti-pseudomonal antibiotics are used as irrigations through these catheters five times daily. It is suggested that the surgeon use 100 to 200 mg of gentamicin in 1 L of normal saline and irrigate with approximately 200 ml five times daily for a minimum of 5 days. Further drainage and/or debridement may be required if the infection does not subside. Although there is often some loss of cartilage, the result is usually satisfactory.

Iontophoresis is an alternative treatment with which some treatment centers are gaining experience. The area to be treated is submerged in a solution of the antibiotic to be applied. A direct current power source is required in order to drive positively charged gentamicin into the tissues by applying a positive electrode to the solution, and a negative electrode at a distant site (such as the chest). Typically, a current of 4 mA is applied for 15 minutes three times daily.

In summary, to prevent the dreaded complications of auricular trauma, the tissue must be treated promptly and atraumatically, with strict attention to asepsis and a vigilant eye to signs of inflammation.

Suggested Reading

deChalain T, Jones J. Replantation of the avulsed pinna. Plast Reconstr Surg 1995; 95:1275-1279

Henrich DE, Logan TC, Lewis RS, Shockley WW. Composite graft survival. Arch Otolaryngol Head Neck Surg 1995; 121:1137-1142.

Khalak R, Roberts IK. Cauliflower ear. N Engl J Med 1996; 335:399.

Templer J, Renner GJ. Injuries of the external ear. Otolaryngol Clin North Am 1990; 23:1003-1018.

Schiavon M, Cagnoni G. Salvage of an amputated ear temporarily lodged in a forearm. Plast Reconstr Surg 1995; 96:1698-1701.

NASAL FRACTURE

The method of
J. Gregory Staffel

Most patients who have a broken nose come to the emergency room with a significant amount of pain and swelling. Immediate management follows the ABC protocol for any trauma case as well as ruling out any significant neck trauma. Evaluation then proceeds for any associated facial bone fractures, and appropriate consultation (ophthalmology, neurosurgery) is obtained. I limit discussion in this chapter to my technique for managing the fractured nose.

Once the patient is stable, a photograph should be taken. Nasal radiographs do not change management and should therefore not be ordered. A photograph is quicker, less expensive, and provides better documentation. If the patient will be in any legal forays, the photograph is crucial to the repudiation or justification of any claims made.

The next step in the evaluation involves ruling out a septal hematoma, which appears as a submucosal swelling on one or both sides of the septum. The swollen area is usually pale, instead of dark or bluish as one might expect. The treatment is incision with light packing to prevent reaccumulation.

If no septal hematoma is present, the patient is treated with head elevation and ice to the nose. Oxymetazoline nasal spray prevents bleeding and shrinks the nasal mucosa, allowing the sinuses (which are often filled with blood) to drain. An antibiotic that covers *Staphylococcus aureus* is given because this is the most common organism to infect a septal hematoma, and also to prevent infection of any open skin wound. The patient is seen in the office 5 to 7 days after the fracture, when the swelling has subsided.

It should be noted here that some surgeons advocate immediate reduction in the emergency room. Although this undoubtedly can be done, patient comfort and physician capability are often compromised. rendering this (in the words of Tardy) a more traditional than useful procedure.

■ OFFICE EVALUATION

Once in the office, a complete set of photographs is taken. In my practice, the patient is then scheduled for an open reduction of a nasal and septal fracture.

Many surgeons have been trained to perform a closed reduction of any nasal fracture, with reservation of a future septorhinoplasty for those patients who fail closed reduction. As I have gained experience with closed reduction, I have learned several things. First, I have learned that closed reduction often fails to straighten a crooked nose. This lesson has come at various poignant moments, such as in the operating room when I turn around after retrieving the softening cast from the warm water to find the nose listing precariously toward its original deformity after being "reduced." Alternatively, the unveiling of the (still crooked) nose when the cast is removed brings new vistas of creativity to the use of the word *swelling*.

This is not to say that a closed reduction will never work; it is just to say that often a closed reduction alone is not enough. Happily, with a little experience one learns which patients undergoing a closed reduction will fail, and under the appropriate conditions further measures can be taken. The literature confirms that the more experienced and comfortable with nasal surgery a surgeon is, the more aggressively that surgeon will treat nasal fractures.

In my practice, therefore, all patients are taken to the operating room after they have signed permission for me to perform whatever procedures are necessary to straighten their noses. A prefracture photograph is obtained if possible.

■ OPERATING ROOM TREATMENT

After the patient is anesthetized (local or general), a closed reduction is performed. If the nose snaps back into place, and the patient has had no difficulty breathing since the fracture, a cast is applied, and the procedure is over. If, as is much more commonly the case, the nose is corrected somewhat, but still incompletely, or if it slowly drifts toward its previous deformity after closed reduction, closed reduction will not work! A cast placed at this point in hopes of straightening the nose is a triumph of hope over experience. If the nose does not sit perfectly straight, with no drift, tilt, list, or curve after the procedure but before the cast, it will not end up being straight.

Because of this, I follow a straightforward, graduated protocol to straighten the broken nose. If, after closed reduction, the nose is still not straight, a septoplasty is performed. It is very common that the septum is fractured as well as the external nasal skeleton, and a septoplasty may release the forces that are holding the nose in a crooked position, as well as help the airway.

If the nose is not straight after a closed reduction and septoplasty, medial and lateral osteotomies are performed. If the nose is fractured along an osteotomy line, the fracture is used as an osteotomy. If only one side of the nose is fractured, bilateral osteotomies are performed. Although this may seem counterintuitive, my empiric observation is that this helps create symmetry.

If the nose is still not straight after closed reduction, septoplasty, and osteotomies, the upper lateral cartilages are released from their attachment to the septum. This procedure is performed before osteotomies because these attachments, if straight, can help to splint a crooked nose into good position after osteotomies. Sometimes, however, these same attachments can serve to splint the nose in a crooked position, and therefore at this point they are severed.

The osteotomies and release of the upper lateral cartilages may be performed without elevating the skin off the dorsum of the nose. If the nose is still crooked after all these maneuvers, the central complex is fractured by applying adequate pressure with the thumb to cause the entire nose to overcorrect. Although this is a dramatic maneuver, it rarely causes any complications. If the nose is still crooked at this point, camouflaging bruised or crushed cartilage grafts are placed along the sidewalls in order to make the nose appear straight.

Thus, my protocol involves a stepwise graduated approach to straightening the broken nose. The broken nose has been equated thus far with the crooked nose because usually they are the same. Rarely, a broken nose is a crushed nose, with destruction of dorsal support. In this case, cartilage is harvested from the septum and used to augment the dorsum. I believe it is easier to operate on a crushed nose (with an accordioned septum) early rather than waiting for scarring to mature before later corrective rhinoplasty. Microplating or conchal cartilage may also be necessary to reconstruct the dorsum.

The subject often arises about taking down a hump during an open reduction. In general, a small hump may be removed before the osteotomies, unless one of the fracture lines is so close to the hump that removal is precarious. The danger is the avulsion of a larger amount of hump than was intended. Still, if the fracture lines are not too close, a small hump may be carefully removed.

Tip work is usually not performed in the setting of an acutely broken nose. Swelling is still present, and the patient usually has not thought about changing the tip before this nasal procedure. Some surgeons do perform tip work acutely, and in the hands of a good surgeon this is not unreasonable. Obviously, tip work is only very rarely related to the trauma itself, and thus it is not billed to a third party unless this is the case.

Pediatric nasal fractures elicit perhaps even more concern than do fractures in adults. This concern is on the part of both the parents and the surgeon. Many surgeons fear operating on a child thinking that removal of any septal cartilage and performing osteotomies may inhibit future growth of the nose. A thorough review of the literature, as well as my own experience and that of many more experienced surgeons, suggests that these fears are to a certain extent unfounded. If a child has a fractured septum, a septoplasty can be performed. The minimum amount of cartilage necessary to correct the deformity is removed, and the rest is preserved. Likewise, if straightening the nose requires osteotomies, they are performed. These procedures have not led to altered growth in my patients.

Patients and third parties are billed only for what is done. If the nose snaps back into place and no other procedure is performed, it is coded as a closed reduction nasal fracture. If osteotomies, release of the upper lateral cartilages, repair of the septum, central complex fracture, and a camouflaging graft have to be performed, the procedure is coded as an open repair of a nasal and septal fracture.

Performing all these procedures takes some training in nasal surgery, but usually it is not lack of knowledge about how to do a procedure in the nose as much as lack of knowledge about which procedure to do that leads to dissatisfied surgeons. (The patients are almost always satisfied.) I have had superb results with this protocol and offer it to you until your own experience either confirms it or grows beyond it.

Suggested Reading

Sheen JH, Sheen AP. Aesthetic rhinoplasty. 2nd ed. St. Louis: CV Mosby, 1987.

Staffel JG. Basic principles of rhinoplasty. Washington, DC: American Academy of Facial Plastic Reconstructive Surgery, 1996.

Tardy MR Jr. Rhinoplasty: The art and the science. Philadelphia: WB Saunders, 1997.

ZYGOMATIC FRACTURE

The method of
Michael G. Stewart
by
W. Douglas Appling
Michael G. Stewart

Zygomatic fractures are relatively common in patients who have midface trauma. Zygomatic fractures have been given many different names, including malar complex and tripod, trimalar, and tetrapod fractures. Typically, zygomatic fractures consist of four fracture components: the frontozygomatic (FZ) suture, the zygomatic arch, the zygomaticomaxillary (ZM) buttress, and the inferior orbital (IO) rim. In addition, most zygomatic fractures also cause an orbital floor fracture. The maxillary portion of the fracture typically includes the infraorbital foramen and extends inferolaterally along the anterior wall of the sinus toward the ZM buttress, which usually fractures inferiorly near the maxillary tooth roots. The action of the masseter muscle on the zygomatic arch tends to displace the fractured malar eminence inferomedially, and the zygomatic arch is usually depressed in its middle portion—which impinges on the temporalis muscle and causes pain with chewing. The cosmetic deformity caused by a zygomatic fracture may not be apparent until after the soft-tissue swelling has diminished, usually a few days following injury.

The management of zygomatic fractures has changed in recent years. Use of computed tomography (CT) scan has significantly improved the clinician's ability to assess the extent of zygomatic fractures preoperatively. In addition, microplates and miniplates have gained wide acceptance for open reduction and internal fixation of facial fractures. Further, the use of "hidden" incisions, such as sublabial, transconjunctival, and extended hemicoronal and bicoronal approaches, allows excellent visualization and mobilization of zygomatic fractures without the need for a visible skin incision.

■ EVALUATION

The clinical assessment of a patient who has a zygomatic fracture includes evaluation of facial symmetry, orbital function, and mouth opening and chewing. The characteristic cosmetic deformity is a "flattening" or depression of the malar eminence on the affected side, although this may be obscured initially by soft-tissue swelling. Step-off fractures may be palpable at the FZ suture and inferior orbital rim, although these may also be obscured by soft-tissue swelling and pain with palpation. If the orbital floor has been significantly fractured, the patient may have enophthalmos; entrapment of either the inferior rectus or inferior oblique muscles, or the fibrous septae that attach to these muscles; or diplopia. Even with a significant orbital floor fracture, however, these symptoms may not be present early in the postinjury course. In cases of suspected orbital fracture, an ophthalmologic consultation, including a dilated retinal examination, is probably indicated. Depressed fractures of the zygomatic arch may impinge on the temporalis muscle and cause pain on mouth opening and chewing; this should be assessed clinically.

A plain roentgenogram facial series, including a Caldwell view, a Waters view, and a submentovertex ("bucket handle") view will identify the presence of a zygomatic fracture, although plain films usually do not adequately assess the orbital floor or the degree of fracture dislocation. Although axial and coronal CT scans of the midface and orbits will give the otolaryngologist a more detailed view of the extent of fractures, CT scans may not always be necessary in patients with obvious cosmetic deformity who will undergo surgery anyway. In most cases, a CT scan with both axial and coronal views is needed to fully assess a zygomatic fracture. Axial views are best for assessing the zygomatic arch and IO rim, and coronal views are preferred for assessment of the FZ suture, the ZM buttress, and the orbital floor. As a general rule, fracture displacement of more than 2 mm will result in noticeable cosmetic deformity, and therefore fractures with at least 2 mm of displacement should be reduced.

■ MANAGEMENT

The indications for surgical reduction of zygomatic fractures are (1) cosmetic deformity; (2) orbital floor fracture causing enophthalmos, restriction of upgaze, or diplopia; and (3) trismus or pain with chewing.

Zygomatic Arch Fractures

Isolated fractures of the zygomatic arch that cause a cosmetic deformity or pain with chewing can usually be reduced using a closed technique. A Gilles approach, with a 2 cm incision just behind the hairline and dissection in a plane deep to the superficial temporalis fascia down to the level of the zygomatic arch, is typically used. This dissection deep to the temporalis fascia avoids injury to the frontal branch of the facial nerve. The depressed portion of the arch may then be elevated using any heavy, blunt instrument. We prefer to use a large urethral sound, although a heavy clamp works equally well. Typically, the arch "snaps" or "pops" back into position and remains in place after reduction; if not, an open reduction will be necessary, but this is unusual in our experience. The surgeon should be careful to palpate the skin overlying the zygomatic arch *during* reduction to avoid overcorrection. It is important for the surgeon to remember that the midportion of the zygomatic "arch" is actually fairly straight in most patients (review of axial CT scans will illustrate this point). A common mistake is to overcorrect the zygomatic arch until it actually assumes an archlike shape; this will usually result in asymmetry with the opposite side.

In patients for whom a Gilles incision is unacceptable (e.g., patients who are bald or prefer very short haircuts), an intraoral approach for closed reduction of the zygomatic arch is also possible. A 2 cm incision is made in the gingivobuccal sulcus approximately over the first molar, and blunt dissection is carried superiorly toward the arch in a submucosal plane. When the inferior surface of the arch is reached, the arch is elevated in a similar fashion, and the surgeon is careful not to overcorrect the depressed portion.

If adequate reduction is achieved and the patient still has significant pain on mouth opening or chewing, consider a missed fracture of the coronoid process of the mandible. If a symptomatic, isolated zygomatic arch fracture cannot be reduced using a closed technique, the arch may be exposed using an extended hemicoronal approach, and plates and screws can be used for open reduction and fixation. This approach is discussed in more detail next.

Nondisplaced and Minimally Displaced Fractures

Nondisplaced and minimally displaced zygomatic fractures without orbital findings may be safely observed for the development of delayed complications. If the patient remains asymptomatic for 7 to 10 days after injury (e.g., after the soft-tissue swelling has significantly decreased), reduction is not necessary. If, however, cosmetic deformity becomes apparent, or the patient has developed new symptoms, the bones should still be mobile enough to allow reduction and fixation. During the immediate postinjury period, the patient should be kept on a soft diet to minimize the pull of the masseter muscle on the zygoma.

Displaced Fractures

For displaced zygomatic fractures, we typically perform open reduction and internal fixation 3 to 7 days after the injury to allow soft-tissue swelling to decrease. This allows intraoperative comparison of the symmetry of the malar complexes to ensure appropriate reduction. We believe that mobile zygomatic complex fractures should be repaired with at least two points of fixation, and a plate at the FZ fracture should always be incorporated. Even if displaced, the zygomatic arch can usually be reduced using a closed technique such as a Gilles approach, a sublabial incision, or a transcutaneous hook placed through the cheek. Although fixation using wires at one or more fracture points is acceptable in many surgeons' experience, we typically use titanium microplates or miniplates with 1.0 to 1.5 mm screws for internal fixation. Although the management of patients should be individualized, in general the relative order of importance for internal fixation of fracture sites is, from most important to least important, (1) the FZ suture, (2) the ZM buttress, (3) the IO rim, and (4) the zygomatic arch. The decision on which fractures to plate is usually made based on the CT scan, although the surgeon should be flexible enough to add additional plates as needed based on intraoperative findings. For instance, if the zygoma is still mobile with movement at the IO rim after the FZ and ZM fractures have been plated, the rim should then be exposed and plated. We usually use plates with 1.0 mm screws at the IO rim, and 1.3 or 1.5 mm screws for FZ or ZM fractures and the zygomatic arch.

An important technical point is to expose and reduce all fracture sites that are displaced *before* any fracture site is plated. In very thin patients whose inferior orbital rim can be easily palpated, palpation through the skin alone may suffice to confirm reduction if the rim is minimally displaced (e.g., the rim does not require plating). To expose the fracture sites and apply plates, we typically use a lateral brow incision or the lateral portion of an upper lid blepharoplasty incision for the FZ fracture area; a sublabial incision for the ZM buttress, if necessary; and a transconjunctival approach to the IO rim (Figs. 1 and 2). The transconjunctival approach may be extended (using a lateral canthotomy for improved exposure) to perform an orbital floor exploration and repair, if necessary. The transcutaneous hook technique—using a stab wound through the cheek skin made with a No. 15 blade—is a safe and effective way to reduce the zygomatic complex before plating. Because the malar eminence is typically displaced inferomedially, the pull on the hook (and zygoma) should be superolateral to achieve reduction.

If there is a linear fracture along the orbital floor, usually rotation and reduction of the zygomatic complex is sufficient to reduce the orbital floor fracture. If there is missing or depressed bone that requires reduction, we typically use one of the following techniques for reconstruction. For defects with sufficient stable bone on either side and posteriorly, we use either thin Teflon or Medpor sheeting, custom-cut to a size slightly larger than the defect—typically about the size of a guitar pick. We routinely close the periosteum of the orbital rim to minimize mobility of the implant, and we have had very few problems with extrusion of alloplastic implants. For near-total floor defects or combined medial wall and floor defects, we use either manufactured titanium orbital floor plates or custom-cut titanium mesh, affixed to the orbital rim with screws.

Complicated or Comminuted Fractures

Patients who have multiple other facial fractures in addition to a zygomatic fracture can be treated using extended approaches to the facial skeleton. For instance, if a concomitant frontal sinus fracture is present, an extended bicoronal approach to the zygomatic arch may be used, or a midface degloving approach may be used if concomitant maxillary medial buttress fractures are present. Similar techniques can be used for exposure if the zygoma is comminuted and requires multiple plates—for instance along the lateral orbital rim—or if the zygomatic arch requires open reduction. Again it is important to close the periosteum over the plates.

In the extended bicoronal technique a subperiosteal plane is developed first along the superior orbital rim. Next, dissection is carried down to the periosteum of the zygomatic arch, in a plane just deep to the superficial layer of the deep temporal fascia (e.g., along the lateral surface of the temporal fat pad). Using this approach, the frontal branch of the facial nerve remains lateral to the temporal fascia, and therefore is preserved with the forehead flap. The periosteum of the zygoma is first exposed in its posterior portion, and then extended forward and connected with the superior orbital rim periosteum; the surgeon is careful to dissect along the superior edge of the arch. Once the periosteum of the zygoma is exposed, it can be elevated extensively for wide exposure and plating of all displaced fractures, including the zygomatic arch.

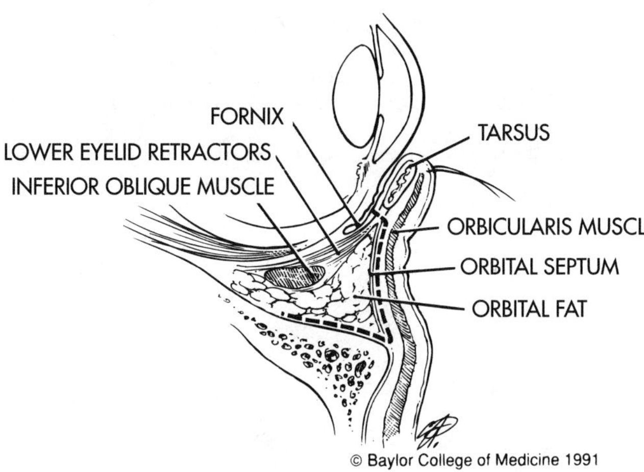

Figure 1.
Anatomy of the lower eyelid. The dotted line represents the direction of dissection to reach the orbital floor. *(From Appling WD, Patrinely JR, Salter TA. Transconjunctival approach versus subciliary skin-muscle flap approach for orbital fracture repair. Arch Otolaryngol Head Neck Surg 1993; 119: 1000–1007; with permission.)*

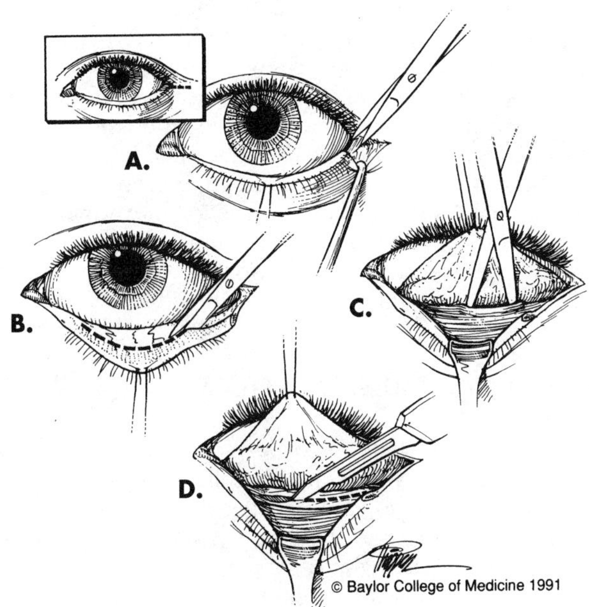

Figure 2.
Operative technique for transconjunctival approach to the orbital floor. The lateral commissure is incised (inset), and the inferior limb of the lateral canthal tendon is severed *(A)*. The conjunctiva is incised just beneath the tarsal plate *(B)*, and the dissection proceeds in a preseptal plane *(C)* to the level of the orbital rim, where the periosteum is incised *(D)*. *(From Appling WD, Patrinely JR, Salter TA. Transconjunctival approach versus subciliary skin-muscle flap approach for orbital fracture repair. Arch Otolaryngol Head Neck Surg 1993; 119:1000–1007; with permission.)*

■ POSTOPERATIVE COURSE

Patients are given ice packs to place on the cheek, and they are advised to keep their heads elevated in the immediate postoperative period to minimize soft-tissue edema. We typically do not use drains for lateral brow incisions, although a small suction drain is used in hemicoronal incisions. If a sublabial incision is used, patients are kept on liquid diet for the first 2 days, then advanced to a soft diet for the next week.

■ COMPLICATIONS

The most common complication after reduction of a zygomatic fracture is malar depression. This may result from inadequate fracture reduction, as well as bone loss from the injury itself. Inadequate fracture reduction is usually due to unrecognized rotation of the malar eminence around one of its axes. Remember that there are usually four components to a zygomatic fracture, and all of these fractures should be properly aligned before plates are applied. A common source of error is exposure and reduction of only the FZ and IO rim components of a zygomatic fracture; even when these fracture lines are in contact, the zygoma may still be malrotated and depressed because the zygomatic arch and ZM buttress fractures are not approximated. The key to avoiding this complication is adequate exposure and reduction of *all* displaced components of a zygomatic fracture. Stable reduction may be achieved with two-point fixation only as long as all components are reduced and the zygoma remains stable to direct pressure.

If postoperative malar depression is present despite adequate rotation and reduction, it is usually due to bone loss. This problem can be treated with malar augmentation using a bone graft or prosthetic implant; split calvarium is a good source of donor bone.

Other complications of zygomatic fractures include enophthalmos, diplopia, and orbital entrapment. A small amount of enophthalmos or diplopia with extreme upward or lateral gaze may occur despite adequate reduction, probably from tissue loss. However, these complications may be the result of an inadequately treated orbital floor fracture. These problems are invariably difficult to treat several weeks or months after the injury, and care should be taken to prevent these problems. Enophthalmos may be treated using bone grafts along the orbital floor; this technique has varying degrees of success. Entrapment and diplopia should be managed with re-establishment of the orbital floor using the same techniques as previously described.

Ectropion and permanent inferior scleral show are potential complications after exposure and reduction of IO rim fractures. In our experience, these complications are less common with a transconjunctival approach than with a subciliary incision. Oroantral fistula is possible after a sublabial incision is made if there was a significant fracture into the maxillary sinus. This complication can be avoided by using meticulous closure techniques for the sublabial incision. Infraorbital nerve anesthesia and dysesthesia are possible after a zygomatic fracture, but this is typically caused by the initial injury. Care should be taken, however, during reduction of

IO rim and ZM buttress fractures to avoid excessive traction or injury to the infraorbital nerve.

Suggested Reading

Appling WD, Patrinely JR, Salter TA. Transconjunctival approach versus subciliary skin-muscle flap approach for orbital fracture repair. Arch Otolaryngol Head Neck Surg 1993; 119:1000-1007.

Davidson J, Nickerson D, Nickerson B. Zygomatic fractures: Comparison of methods of internal fixation. Plast Reconstr Surg 1990; 86:25-32. Holmes KD, Matthews BL. Three-point alignment of zygoma fractures with miniplate fixation. Arch Otolaryngol Head Neck Surg 1989; 115:961-963.

Zingg M, Chowdhury K, Ladrach K. Treatment of 813 zygoma-lateral orbital complex fractures: New aspects. Arch Otolaryngol Head Neck Surg 1991; 117:611-620.

FRONTAL SINUS FRACTURE

The method of
Lanny Garth Close
by
Jose N. Fayad
Lanny Garth Close

Frontal sinus fractures are uncommon and are usually the result of severe trauma. Complete naso-fronto-orbital fractures comprise between 5 percent and 10 percent of all facial fractures. Motor vehicle accidents, criminal assault, industrial accidents, sports, and suicide attempts are the most common causes of frontal sinus fractures. Due to its proximity to the intracranial structures, inadequate treatment of a frontal sinus fracture can lead to significant early and late complications including meningitis, encephalitis, cerebral abscess, cerebrospinal fluid (CSF) leakage, mucopyoceles, osteomyelitis, meningoencephaloceles, and significant aesthetic deformities.

Management of these fractures is still controversial. The indication, timing, and mode of treatment remain debatable. Following the procedures outlined in this chapter, we have been able to minimize complications and obtain satisfactory anatomic and clinical results.

■ ANATOMY AND PHYSIOLOGY

The frontal sinus results from the pneumatization of the frontal bone and is not fully developed until age 20 years. Growth of the frontal sinus over a long period of time explains why the incidence of frontal sinus fractures in the adult group is twice the incidence in the pediatric group, as well as why the incidence of frontal sinus fractures increases with age. The frontal sinus configuration is roughly triangular in the sagittal plane, with the apex directed superiorly and the base inferiorly. The anterior wall of the sinus is by far the strongest. Most of the floor is made up by the orbital roof, which is thin bone, as is the posterior wall of the sinus. Riding in the midline of the posterior wall is a thickened triangular ridge into which inserts the superior sagittal sinus. The frontonasal duct or frontal sinus ostium is found in the anteromedial extent of the frontal sinus floor. This duct or ostium opens into the anterior ethmoid sinuses or into the infundibulum of the middle meatus. These openings are found on either side of the intersinus septum of the frontal sinus. When exposed to trauma, the mucosal lining of the frontal sinus tends to form cysts that secrete mucus into their lumen and cause the erosion of bone as a result of pressure on the sinus wall. They can become infected and form a mucopyocele that may result in an osteomyelitis of the frontal bone and, worse, an intracranial infection. The spread of the infection from the sinus into the subarachnoid space is facilitated by the presence of the foramina of Breschet, sites of imbrication of the sinus mucosa, and vascular pits for the passage of veins from the subepithelium of the sinus mucosa into the subarachnoid space.

■ CLINICAL PRESENTATION

Motor vehicle accidents are the leading cause of these fractures. In polytrauma patients, controlling the airway, stopping the hemorrhage, and assessing the neurologic status take priority. These patients usually are evaluated initially with a computed tomography (CT) scan of the head to rule out a central nervous system injury and a facial CT scan to delineate the extent and complexity of the fracture. Many patients remain unconscious after the accident and might experience amnesia for the period surrounding the accident.

The complaint of frontal headache and nosebleed is common. Forehead numbness may go unnoticed. Anosmia should raise the suspicion of a possible contiguous fracture of the frontal sinus and the anterior fossa floor. The presence of clear fluid drainage from the nose raises the suspicion of CSF rhinorrhea. A deformity created by a depressed anterior wall fracture may be hidden by hematoma formation. Lacerated forehead skin and protrusion of bony fragments and brain tissue is obvious in comminuted and severely displaced fractures. Frontal sinus tenderness is of no help in the comatose patient and is often missing in isolated frontonasal duct, floor, or posterior wall fractures.

The accurate diagnosis of frontal sinus fractures is more difficult in the pediatric population. Failure to identify physical findings suggestive of frontal sinus fracture is twice as common in the pediatric age group. Also, there is a major discrepancy between the CT findings and operative findings in 25 percent of pediatric frontal sinus fractures. The severity of injury and associated injuries are similar for the pediatric and adult populations. In this chapter, we classify frontal sinus fractures based on site and severity to explain the treatment modalities specific for each one of those sites. Fractures are classified as anterior wall, posterior wall, frontonasal duct, and through-and-through, although it is uncommon for fractures to be limited to one specific site.

■ THERAPY

Nearly all fractures of the frontal sinus need to be explored surgically. The goals of surgical treatment are to (1) isolate and protect the intracranial structures and stop any CSF leak, (2) prevent early and late complications, and (3) restore facial aesthetics. Surgical access should be wide. It is usually afforded by the bicoronal scalp incision unless direct exposure of the sinus can be obtained via skin and soft-tissue traumatic defects.

When the sinus is to be obliterated or cranialized, meticulous mucosal lining removal has to be achieved. We prefer the use of autologous materials to fill frontal sinus defects; the use of alloplastic materials should be avoided. The key to optimal management of frontal sinus fractures is the handling of the nasofrontal duct. In selected cases, the patency of the nasofrontal duct can be achieved using the endoscopic technique. Long-term follow-up of patients who have sustained fractures of the frontal sinus is mandatory due to late complications that can become clinically apparent many years after the initial injury.

Anterior Wall Fractures

The anterior wall of the frontal sinus is the most common site of fracture. These fractures may be undisplaced or displaced, simple or compound, and with or without missing bone. Patients who have undisplaced fractures complain of pain and have swelling over the forehead; they do not, however, have a palpable step-off of the bone of the anterior sinus wall. CT scan confirms the nondisplaced nature of the fracture.

No surgical intervention is needed for these "greenstick" fractures of the anterior wall in the absence of local soft-tissue injuries. The possibility of a complication from such an injury is very small.

Displaced fractures of the anterior wall show an obvious indentation in the forehead if the patient happens to be seen soon after the accident; otherwise the space will be occupied by a hematoma. Usually a step-off of the bone can be palpated and can be confirmed on CT scan. Displaced fractures should be operated on for two reasons: (1) to avoid an inevitable significant deformity once the swelling and hematoma disappear, and (2) to prevent mucocele formation due to entrapment of swelling and mucosa in the fractured segment. Surgical access to repair a displaced fracture can be obtained through a butterfly incision or through a bicoronal scalp incision. If the skin over the sinus is lacerated, the incision can be extended into a wrinkle of the forehead and used to expose and repair the fracture. The bony fragments are exposed and left attached to the periosteum. The mucosa is stripped away from the bone. A cutting bur can be used to thin the bone at the site of mucosal removal. Trauma to the area of the frontonasal duct should be avoided. No sinus packing is required. We try to avoid stenting of the nasofrontal duct. The fragments are approximated and fixed together using microplates. The wound is closed in layers, and the patient is told to avoid sleeping in the prone position and to avoid direct trauma to that area.

If there is significant missing bone, the sinus is approached through a bicoronal flap incision, and a split calvarial graft is harvested and used to bridge the defect. Other surgeons have used iliac crest bone.

Posterior Wall Fractures

The treatment of posterior wall fractures is somewhat controversial. These fractures are usually displaced and may have associated torn dura and CSF drainage. The majority of posterior wall fractures are explored because the morbidity associated with missing a displaced fracture of the posterior wall is significant (i.e., intracranial mucocele, mucopyocele, meningitis, and brain abscess). We prefer approaching these fractures with a wide exposure through a bicoronal flap. An osteoplastic flap of the anterior wall of the sinus is done in the usual fashion in order to access and evaluate the severity of the posterior wall fracture. Lacerated dura is repaired. Small lacerations are sutured. Larger dural defects are repaired using lyophilized dura, a graft of temporalis fascia, or fascia lata. A pericranial flap should be used as a second layer of closure if there is any concern regarding a watertight closure. In cases of severely comminuted posterior sinus wall fractures, the bony fragments are removed as well as the mucosal lining; the nasofrontal duct is obliterated using muscle or pericranium; and the sinus cavity is cranialized, which allows the intracranial contents to occupy it. In sinuses with minimal bone loss, fat obliteration is the treatment of choice. Fat obliteration of frontal sinuses with a significant amount of missing bony walls often results in reepithelialization, infection, and mucocele formation because of graft absorption. If we do choose to obliterate the sinus, we prefer to fill the sinus with cancellous bone harvested from the iliac crest. If the mucosa of the nasofrontal duct is intact and there is a small dural tear, the dura is sutured, and the sinus is neither cranialized nor obliterated. In cases of nondisplaced fractures and intact mucosa, the sinus is neither cranialized nor obliterated.

Frontonasal Duct Fractures

Frontonasal duct fractures are usually in continuity with a frontal sinus floor fracture. The floor may be displaced or nondisplaced into the sinus cavity, the ethmoid sinus, or the orbit. It is very difficult to diagnose an isolated fracture of the duct. An opacified sinus is often the only radiologic sign. Trephination of the sinus and injection of dye or contrast material makes it possible to check the patency of the duct.

Taking down the intersinus septum is one way of dealing with a unilateral blockage of the nasofrontal duct. This can be achieved through a wider trephination or using an osteoplastic flap. One common method of dealing with this problem is to obliterate the sinus. In selected cases, we prefer the endoscopic approach to re-establish the patency of the nasofrontal duct. The floor of the sinus can be drilled away through an endoscopic approach, thus obviating the need for an obliteration procedure and the long-term sequelae that follow.

Through-and-Through Fractures

Through-and-through fractures are the most devastating fractures. Both anterior and posterior walls are fractured. The skin is lacerated, as is the underlying dura, with exposure of the brain to the outside. Many of these patients die before they reach the hospital. Because of the intracranial injury, these patients should undergo a frontal craniotomy. The neurosurgical team debrides necrotic brain tissue, controls central bleeding, and repairs the frontal dura. The calvarial bone fragments recovered from the site of injury are cleaned. Mucosa is eliminated, and the anterior wall is burred down to remove every vestige of mucosa. The posterior wall of the sinus is completely eliminated, and the nasofrontal duct opening is abraded and obliterated with muscle, temporalis fascia, or bone. The anterior wall of the sinus is reconstructed using the recovered calvarial bone. In this way, the sinus is cranialized. In our hands, the cranialization technique has been found to be reliable, highly effective, and minimally morbid. Ablating the frontal sinus as described by Reidel for these severe injuries is not done anymore due to major aesthetic deformities.

Suggested Reading

Close LG, Lee NL, Leach JL, Manning SC. Endoscopic resection of the intranasal frontal sinus floor. Ann Otol Rhinol Laryngol 1994; 103: 952-958.

Donald PJ. Frontal sinus ablation by cranialization: A report of 32 cases. Arch Otolaryngol 1982; 108:142-146.

Donald PJ, Bernstein L. Compound frontal sinus injuries with intracranial penetration. Laryngoscope 1979; 88:225-232.

Donald PJ, Ettin M. The safety of frontal sinus fat obliteration when sinus walls are misssing. Laryngoscope 1986; 96:190-193.

Ioannides C, Freihofer HP, Friens J. Fractures of the frontal sinus: A rationale of treatment. Br J Plast Surg 1993; 46:208-214.

Wallis A, Donald PJ. Frontal sinus fractures: A review of 72 cases. Laryngoscope 1988; 98:593-598.

Wright D, Hoffman HT, Hoyt DB. Frontal sinus fractures in the pediatric population. Laryngoscope 1992; 102:1215-1219.

MIDFACE FRACTURE

The method of
John L. Frodel, Jr.
by
Allyson M. Ray
John L. Frodel, Jr.

Fractures of the midface may aptly be described as fractures involving the maxilla, a pyramid at the center of the face that provides support to all neighboring structures. It is the horizontal link between the zygomatico-orbital regions, comprising part of the orbit and supporting the globe, and is the vertical link between the cranium and the occlusal plane of the mandible. In an anterior-posterior direction, the maxilla also provides the necessary projection to give form and function to the middle third of the face. Consequently, injuries to the midface, as commonly seen in high-velocity motor vehicle accidents, may result in a variety of fracture patterns involving the orbit, nasoethmoid complex, zygoma, or alveolus; these injuries result in globe malposition or immobility, midfacial retrusion, or malocclusion. The primary goal in repairing these injuries is to re-establish the maxillary buttress system that, in turn, restores form and function to the midface and its neighboring structures. Included in this chapter is our approach to the evaluation and treatment of midfacial injuries according to the current principles of maxillofacial fracture management. Isolated fractures of the nose, zygomatic arch, and frontal sinus are discussed in other chapters.

■ PREOPERATIVE EVALUATION

The most important consideration in the evaluation of all traumatic injuries, but especially in severe facial trauma, is establishing a safe airway. Many of these patients will have additional injuries that may endanger their airway or decrease their respiratory drive, although this condition may not be immediately apparent. Intracranial injury, cervical spine injury, and associated mandibular fractures are not uncommon and should be suspected in all cases of severe facial trauma. If these injuries are not addressed immediately, the patient may experience sudden deterioration of mental status with obtundation due to intracranial hemorrhage or edema. Moreover, upper airway obstruction from a flail mandible or tooth fragments is a constant threat.

Emergency intubation may be made even more difficult if cervical spine stabilization is required. To prevent such a disastrous scenario, the patient should be immediately evaluated with these injuries in mind, and if any doubt exists as to the stability of the airway, oral endotracheal intubation or tracheotomy under local anesthesia can be performed in a controlled manner. Traditionally, nasotracheal intubation has been contraindicated in complex midface fractures because of concern for cribriform plate injuries and intracranial complications from a blindly passed endotracheal tube. In experienced hands, fiberoptic visualization techniques, however, allow safe passage of the tube, and it is an ideal method to use in the controlled setting of the operating room, such as when intermaxillary fixation is planned and a tracheotomy is otherwise unnecessary.

After the cervical spine has been stabilized and the airway assessed, the next concern is injury to the globe. Many studies have estimated that approximately 25 percent of all maxillofacial injuries include ocular injury as well. Visual acuity, pupillary function, and extraocular mobility can easily and immediately be tested. However, full ophthalmologic evaluation with anterior chamber and funduscopic examination is indicated if the fracture involves the orbit, or if associated eyelid injuries are present. Direct ocular trauma may occur that causes hyphema or a ruptured globe, and indirect injury to the orbital apex may result in optic nerve compression. Inspection for telecanthus should also be performed, and this condition is suspected when the intercanthal distance measures more than half the interpupillary distance. A diagnosis of naso-orbital-ethmoidal (NOE) fracture with medial canthal tendon displacement can be confirmed using bimanual palpation with a blunt instrument placed intranasally. A complete head and neck examination is essential, with attention to oral mucosal lacerations, open alveolar fractures, loose dentition, and occlusion. This also includes the testing and documentation of *all* cranial nerves, especially hypesthesia in the infraorbital nerve distribution, which is a common finding.

Midface mobility is assessed by grasping the anterior alveolus with thumb and forefinger of one hand and gently lifting while observing mobility of the midface. According to the classic Le Fort's patterns of fracture, if the palate is free floating, the alveolar process is completely separated from the body of the maxilla, and the fracture line extends through the piriform aperture, which indicates a Le Fort's fracture; if the maxilla is free floating, the nasal pyramid will move with the alveolus as the fracture line passes bilaterally across the nasal bone, the infraorbital rim, zygomaticomaxillary buttress, and lateral wall of the maxillary sinus, and then posteriorly to the pterygoid plates, completing a Le Fort's II fracture; if the entire midface is mobile, craniofacial disjunction or Le Fort's III fracture is present, and the fracture lines may be easily palpated at the zygomaticofrontal and zygomaticotemporal regions. Classically, a Le Fort's III fracture involves the nasofrontal suture and crosses the orbital floor bilaterally but does *not* disrupt the inferior orbital rim as it passes posteriorly to the inferior orbital fissure and extends laterally to the lateral orbital wall and posteriorly to the pterygoid plate.

Most fractures of the midface do not strictly adhere to one of these three classification schemes but may display incomplete features of some or all types, unilaterally or bilaterally, with variation from one side to the other. Also, zygomatic and NOE fractures commonly exist in combination with other midface fractures.

Imaging

Computed tomography (CT) is the imaging mode of choice, and should be obtained in 3 mm bone windows, axial and coronal views, if possible. This modality is an invaluable part of the preoperative evaluation, because it allows precise identification of all fractures and their degree of displacement, and thus aids the surgeon in the decision-making process. For instance, if a fracture is nondisplaced, direct reduction and fixation are often unnecessary; or if the orbital floor is intact, the surgeon can avoid intraoperative exploration. Patients should be shown their scans so that the extent of their injuries can be visualized and better appreciated. Also, intraoperatively the surgeon may refer to the scans for fracture localization or re-evaluation. Three-dimensional formatting of CT scans is now available in many medical centers; however, current opinion favors the use of this type of CT scan only in severely comminuted injuries with bony defects such as gunshot wounds. These scans are of limited benefit in most fractures of the face, which are derived from blunt trauma.

Treatment Planning

The timing of repair has often been a source of controversy, because many surgeons believe that facial edema should be resolved before any skeletal repair. This concept has been gradually discarded in favor of early repair, which may actually reduce the amount of edema that the patient experiences by restoring the natural contours of the face sooner. In general, open reduction with rigid internal fixation should be performed as soon as possible unless the patient's condition is so unstable as to preclude any elective surgery. This is often the case with concomitant closed head injury. A low Glasgow Coma Scale (GCS) score and intracranial hemorrhage with cerebral shifting is associated with poor prognosis, and these patients are at high risk of developing complications when undergoing general anesthesia. If the GCS score is relatively high and the intracranial pressure can be maintained at less than 25 mm Hg, acute repair of facial fractures can be performed without additional risk. Consultation with a neurologist or neurosurgeon is obviously warranted under these circumstances.

Additional considerations in the preoperative management of patients who have maxillofacial trauma include perioperative prophylactic antibiotic therapy that provides coverage for the most common oral and sinus pathogens. In addition to the proven benefit of prophylactic antibiotics in clean-contaminated surgery of the sinonasal and oral cavities, many patients who have maxillary and ethmoid fractures experience ostial occlusion, which, although temporary, theoretically predisposes to sinusitis. We recommend beginning treatment with oral antibiotics and nasal decongestant spray from the time of initial presentation until 24 to 48 hours postoperatively. If orbital injuries are present, the use of perioperative steroids is considered as well.

PRINCIPLES OF REPAIR

As with any skeletal fracture, the primary goal is to reduce or realign the fractured segments into normal anatomic position, and then to fixate or stabilize these segments to allow bone union to occur. The least invasive method of repair involves manual disimpaction with closed reduction and external fixation by means of intermaxillary fixation (IMF) and craniofacial suspension wires. Traditionally, suspension wires were used to prevent a common sequela of untreated maxillary fractures—the triad of midface retrusion, facial elongation, and anterior open bite deformity. Results of treatment with IMF and suspension wires were not uniformly successful, however, because overzealous tightening of the wires produced midface retrusion and facial *shortening*, a loss of projection, and vertical height. Facial plating techniques have now replaced these external techniques as the method of choice for complex maxillary repair, offering many advantages with proven lower morbidity, earlier rehabilitation, and faster healing. With a combination of three craniofacial incisions, the entire maxilla can be visualized, and all fractures can be exposed and reduced openly. After the occlusion is established with IMF, the fragments are plated in rigid fixation. The patient can then be released from IMF immediately and be maintained on a soft diet. Although more invasive and time-consuming, the combination of open reduction with internal rigid fixation allows optimal bone healing, with complication rates comparable to external methods.

Essential to the application of rigid internal fixation techniques to the midface is knowledge of the maxillary buttress system. Three well-defined, paired vertical buttresses—nasomaxillary (NM), zygomaticomaxillary (ZM), pterygomaxillary (PM)—bear the load of mastication, and are therefore key structures to reconstitute in any midface fracture. They are also reinforced by horizontal buttresses that resist any horizontal compressive forces. These buttresses include the frontal bar and cranial base, the zygomatic arch and temporal process of the zygoma, the maxillary palate and alveolus, and the greater wing and pterygoid plates of the sphenoid. Understanding the altered anatomy that is produced by traumatic forces will thus direct the vectors of disimpaction. In order to restore facial height, the vertical buttresses must be aligned, and in order to restore horizontal symmetry, the infraorbital rims and palate should align properly. The anteroposterior dimensions are primarily defined by the zygomatic arch, and any unrecognized fracture dislocation of the arch or its temporal root may prevent proper reduction. After all fragments are reduced and IMF is performed, plating should proceed from stable to unstable, meaning peripheral to central, or cephalic to caudal. By working from the stable cranium, Le Fort's III fractures are repaired first; then the order of repair is any Le Fort's II fractures, and finally Le Fort's I.

Currently, standard craniofacial plating systems for rigid internal fixation are comprised of titanium plates in a variety of shapes and admitting screws ranging in diameter from 2.0 mm to 1.0 mm. Unlike the mandible, the midface skeleton is not as significantly affected by forces of tension and compression, and biomechanical concerns are limited to proper fixation and stabilization. There is no need for dynamic compression plating, and therefore most midfacial plates are available only in noncompression, or neutral, mode. “Miniplates” refer to 2.0 mm, 1.5 mm, or 1.3 mm screw applications, whereas “microplates” use the smallest 1.0 mm screws and are ideal in providing a low profile for areas with thin soft-tissue coverage.

METHODS OF REPAIR

Le Fort's I Fractures

Traditionally, Le Fort's I fractures were managed with IMF alone if the fracture was stable, or IMF combined with circumzygomatic suspension wires if the fracture proved unstable after closed reduction. This method required the patient to remain in IMF with a liquid diet for 4 to 6 weeks. In contrast, open reduction with internal fixation allows direct visualization when reducing the fracture, temporary intraoperative placement in IMF, and then after rigid plating of the fracture immediate release from IMF. Postoperatively, the patient is allowed a soft diet for 6 weeks before returning to a full masticatory diet. We favor this latter technique for all displaced or unstable Le Fort's fractures due to its many advantages as previously mentioned, namely, lower morbidity, earlier rehabilitation, and faster healing. In Le Fort's I fractures, rigid internal fixation can be provided with a 1.5 mm or 2.0 mm diameter noncompression plating system via standard sublabial incision. It is best to place the mucosal incision approximately 1 cm from the gingivolabial sulcus on the labial side in order to provide an adequate wound edge for closure and to allow for scar contracture. The dissection is carried through muscle down to bone, and then continued in the subperiosteal plane superiorly. All fracture sites should be exposed and then reduced if necessary with disimpaction forceps. Arch bars are placed, and the occlusion is established with IMF before plating the fracture in rigid fixation. Care should be taken to avoid drilling through tooth roots, of which the canine is the longest. Proper plating techniques should be strictly followed, and the wound should be irrigated copiously with sterile saline before closing muscle and mucosal layers with a heavy absorbable suture. The patient can be released from IMF before extubation.

Le Fort's II Fractures

Classically, Le Fort's II fracture is the only Le Fort's fracture to extend across the infraorbital rim, and therefore requires a second incision, either transconjunctival or subciliary, in order to gain access to the rim. Both methods have proven reliability in infraorbital rim repair, as well as orbital floor exploration and repair, if required. The transconjunctival approach with dissection in the preseptal plane appears superior in limiting postoperative ectropion and scleral show. However, it usually requires a lateral canthotomy and inferior cantholysis to provide better orbital exposure and minimize retraction on the eyelid. The transconjunctival incision is limited medially by the inferior punctum, and if excessive traction is applied in this area, the inferior canaliculus may be inadvertently avulsed. If medial exposure is a concern, then the subciliary incision may be preferable.

The fracture line often passes through the infraorbital

foramen on its way across the zygomaticomaxillary buttress. The infraorbital nerve almost always remains intact, although contused, and should be identified and carefully preserved. The standard sublabial approach is extended subperiosteally to the orbital rim, where it meets the previous orbital rim incision, and thus exposes the full length of the fracture. After disimpaction and reduction, the maxillary fragment is placed in occlusion to the mandible, and IMF is applied. At this point, it is wise to apply closed reduction to the fractured nasal bones; if unstable, the fracture requires rigid fixation of the nasofrontal area, preferably via the coronal approach. It is important to determine whether the unstable segments actually represent an NOE complex with disruption of the medial canthal tendons, and to perform the repair at this time. If the nasal fracture is stable, further fixation is not required other than an external cast for stabilization. Plating can then proceed using the 1.0 mm system for the infraorbital rim and the 1.5 mm or 2.0 mm system for fixation of the zygomaticomaxillary buttress. Again, when positioning plates in the maxilla, avoid drilling into tooth roots and avoid compression of the infraorbital nerve.

Le Fort's III Fractures

Le Fort's III fractures, or craniofacial disjunction, represent the most serious and complex of the Le Fort's injuries. Some variation of intracranial injury is usually present, and these patients often require immediate airway protection. The basic tenet in repairing these fractures is to begin stabilization at the cranium, with the nasofrontal and frontozygomatic fractures, and work caudally from there. In reality, the isolated Le Fort's III fracture is rarely encountered, but it is associated with other Le Fort's and zygomatic fractures. Rarely, all fracture sites may be minimally displaced and necessitate IMF alone, but in most instances the fractures require disimpaction, placement in IMF, and reduction of all segments with rigid internal fixation.

The coronal incision is the ideal approach for Le Fort's III fractures because it provides adequate exposure for plating of the nasofrontal, zygomaticofrontal, and zygomatic arch areas and avoids direct facial incisions. The incision begins in the pretragal crease and extends across the scalp in the coronal plane to the opposite pretragal crease; dissection proceeds in a subgaleal fashion until periosteum is incised over the nasofrontal and frontozygomatic fractures. Access to the zygomatic arch requires careful avoidance of the frontal branch of the facial nerve by incising deep temporalis fascia 2 cm above the temporal root of the zygoma and dissecting subfascially until the zygomatic arch is encountered; the periosteum over the arch can then be incised, and the fracture segments can be exposed with the nerve branch safely reflected laterally. The low-profile 1.0 mm microplating system is preferred for fixation of these three areas and usually provides adequate stabilization.

If a concomitant NOE fracture is present, repair is performed at this time. This fracture pattern most commonly involves dislocation of the central fragment to which the medial canthal tendon is still attached. Additional exposure is gained through subciliary and sublabial incisions, and the fragment is stabilized to the nasomaxillary buttress and orbital rim, as well as nasofrontal region. If the medial canthal tendon is partially or totally avulsed from the central fragment, or if the central fragment is severely comminuted, repair requires transnasal wiring. If the injury involves severe nasal bone impaction with comminution and collapse of septal supporting structures, bone grafting of the nasal dorsum should be considered in order to prevent a saddle nose deformity. This deformity comprises a functional as well as cosmetic debilitation that is much more difficult to correct secondarily than primarily. Primary repair entails a split-calvarial bone graft that is cantilevered to the frontal bone with microplates.

Non–Le Fort's Fractures

As emphasized earlier, most fractures of the midface do not strictly adhere to the three patterns described by Le Fort, but may also incorporate other sites in the maxilla. *Alveolar* fractures may result in a displaced, unstable segment of the maxillary alveolus, and may be associated with dental injuries. Rigid internal fixation with a screw and plating system is often impractical, and even contraindicated in some situations because of the proximity of the fracture line to tooth roots. Reduction and stabilization with an arch bar may suffice, or further fixation via IMF or intraosseus wiring may be required. Any tooth that is injured and determined to be nonvital should be extracted, especially if located in the fracture line, where the risk of infection is greatest. If the tooth is fractured or avulsed but is in excellent condition without extensive caries or periodontal disease, it may be preserved during the initial fracture repair; however, this tooth requires subsequent evaluation and close follow-up by a dentist or endodontist to ensure its potential viability. *Medial* maxillary fractures involve the medial wall of the maxillary sinus and frontal process of the axilla and can occur as an isolated injury or in association with nasal or inferior orbital fractures. Nasal obstruction can result from displacement of the medial segment into the nasal cavity, and epiphora may occur from injury to the nasolacrimal duct. Closed reduction via the nasal cavity may be attempted, but this procedure usually requires stabilization with intranasal packing. Alternatively, fixation with miniplates via the sublabial degloving approach provides better success in unstable, complex fractures,

Sagittal Maxillary Fracture

One type of fracture that is generally associated with severe injuries of the face and mandible is the *sagittal* maxillary fracture, or *palatal split.* A high-velocity frontal impact force is required to produce this fracture, which is also likely to produce a symphyseal mandible fracture, Le Fort's, and NOE fractures. If the palatal mucosa remains intact, the fracture can easily be missed, and occlusal difficulties will arise when IMF and repair of associated injuries is attempted. In these situations, reconstituting prior occlusal relationships requires three-dimensional adjustments that IMF alone cannot accomplish. Stabilization should also be provided at the anterior alveolar arch and posterior palatal arch. Miniplates or intraosseous wire fixation can be used for the anterior arch, and a palatal splint can be used for stabilization of the posterior arch. In edentulous patients, the dental prosthesis can be fixed temporarily to the palate with screws to provide a similar function. Obviously, obtaining proper reduction with good bone-to-bone contact and maintaining optimal stabilization is a primary concern.

■ COMPLICATIONS

Malunion or Nonunion

Complications arising from the skeletal repair of maxillary fractures may involve aesthetic as well as functional deficits. It is well recognized that rigid fixation using plates and screws is an "unforgiving" technique, because it maintains the position of the bone and allows very little interfragmentary motion to occur. Precise realignment of all fractured segments should be achieved before plating, or the fracture will heal as a *malunion.* This may be evident postoperatively with malocclusion, such as a cross-bite or open bite deformity, and consequently may also result in midfacial retrusion or facial asymmetry. If a significant degree of malocclusion is noticed early in the postoperative period, the patient should probably undergo a revision procedure to realign the fragments, with attention to the proper occlusion for that individual. If only a mild degree of malocclusion is noticed, IMF or other orthodontic maneuvers may correct the problem. Otherwise, once a malunion has occurred, osteotomies and possibly bone grafts are required to correct these functional and aesthetic deformities.

Nonunion is a rare occurrence in the midface, but can occur in the presence of inadequate reduction with poor fixation, infection, or repeated trauma. In our experience, nonunion is more likely to occur from gunshot wounds to the face rather than from blunt trauma. Resorption of bone can occur that requires bone grafting. Extensive defects will require vascularized bone and soft-tissue replacement.

Dental Injury

Other complications involving rigid internal fixation techniques include injury to the tooth roots by a screw placed inappropriately close to the alveolar edge. In general, sufficient distance of at least two times the height of the crown will estimate the length of the root, and drilling should be avoided in this area. Also, the proper length of screws should be chosen to avoid penetration through sinus mucosa; any exposed screw or plate will predispose to infection, and only the minimum number of screws and plates needed for adequate fixation should be used.

Sinusitis

Sinusitis may occur as a sequela of treated, or untreated, maxillary fractures due to the inflammation, bleeding, and bony disruption caused by the injury or its repair. Traditionally, nasoantral windows were routinely performed at the conclusion of the surgical repair; however, we find this procedure unnecessary in most instances. In uncomplicated maxillary fractures, our preferred method of management is the prophylactic, perioperative use of both topical nasal decongestant and antibiotic coverage. If severe comminution of the medial wall of the maxillary sinus or ethmoid sinuses is present, ethmoidectomy and enlargement of the natural maxillary ostium may be necessary at the initial surgical repair, or may be performed as an elective endoscopy.

Nasolacrimal System Injury

Nasolacrimal system injury with subsequent obstruction and epiphora may occur in association with medial maxillary or NOE fractures, or it may occur as a complication of such fractures. It is a rather uncommon injury, and can usually be repaired more easily as a secondary procedure rather than an attempt at primary repair that may compromise reconstruction of the medial canthal tendon and NOE complex. A full understanding of the nasolacrimal system anatomy is essential before attempting repair of any injury involving the medial maxilla and naso-orbital area, and meticulous intraoperative attention is necessary to prevent inadvertent injury to the canaliculi, lacrimal sac, or nasolacrimal duct.

Orbital Injury

Fracture repair involving the orbital rim or orbital floor potentially includes a spectrum of complications concerning the globe and its surrounding structures. Often, techniques that gain exposure to the inferior orbital rim may result in postoperative scleral show or lower lid ectropion, especially if lid laxity existed preoperatively. Using a transconjunctival approach, or performing a concomitant lateral canthoplasty, will limit the development of this problem. Other problems include impairment of globe motility caused by muscle entrapment, or globe malposition (enophthalmos, hypoglobus) if an increased orbital volume has not been addressed. One clinical symptom of severe disruptions in motility or position is diplopia, although diplopia may also exist transiently secondary to postoperative edema. Any change in visual acuity should be immediately assessed, because it may indicate an intraocular disturbance. Although rare, the complication of blindness from retinal detachment, ruptured globe, or optic nerve injury has been reported in orbital fracture repair.

Neural Injury

Other cranial nerve injuries that may occur more commonly include those involving the infraorbital nerve and facial nerve. During sublabial degloving, the infraorbital nerve is exposed and can be severely contused or injured by traction. If inadvertently severed, the ends should be cleaned sharply and reapproximated with interrupted 8–0 nylon suture, because partial sensory function will return. The frontal branch of the facial nerve is also at risk during the coronal flap exposure for Le Fort's III fractures. It is often not visualized during exposure, and injury may not be apparent until a frontalis muscle paralysis is noted postoperatively. This may be temporary or permanent, either due to stretching or severing the nerve branch when raising the flap. Exploration and repair of this nerve branch is rather impractical, and therefore attention is focused on proper intraoperative techniques that avoid nerve injury.

Suggested Reading

Frodel JL. Primary and secondary nasal bone grafting after major facial trauma. Facial Plast Surg 1992; 8:194-208.

Kellman RM. Midfacial fractures. In: Gates GA, ed. Current therapy in otolaryngology—Head and neck surgery. 4th ed. St. Louis: Mosby–Year Book, 1990:114.

Kellman RM. Principles of facial plating techniques. In: Papel ID, Nachlas NE, eds. Facial plastic and reconstructive surgery. St. Louis: Mosby–Year Book, 1992:460.

Markowitz BL, Manson PN, Sargent L, et al. Management of the medial canthal tendon in nasoethmoid orbital fractures: The importance of the central fragment in classification and treatment. Plast Reconstr Surg 1991; 87:843-853.

Mathog RH, ed. Atlas of craniofacial trauma. Philadelphia: WB Saunders, 1992.

Mathog RH, Schmidt RN, Scapini DA. Le Fort fractures. In: Papel ID, Nachlas NE, eds. Facial plastic and reconstructive surgery. St. Louis: Mosby–Year Book, 1992:496.

Meleca RJ, Mathog RH. Diagnosis and treatment of naso-orbital fractures. In: Mathog RH, Arden RL, Marks SC, eds. Trauma of the nose and paranasal sinuses. New York: Thieme Medical Publishers, 1995:65.

Paskert JP, Manson PN. The bimanual examination for assessing instability in naso-orbitoethmoidal injuries. Plast Reconstr Surg 1989; 83:165-167.

Robinson KL, Marks SC. Maxillary trauma. In: Mathog RH, Arden RL, Marks SC, eds. Trauma of the nose and paranasal sinuses. New York: Thieme Medical Publishers, 1995:50.

Rohrich RJ, ed. Advances in craniomaxillofacial fracture management. Clin Plast Surg 1992; 19(1).

Shumrick KA, Kersten RC, Kulwin DR, et al. Extended access internal approaches for the management of facial trauma. Arch Otolaryngol Head Neck Surg 1992; 118:1105-1112.

Stanley RB. Maxillofacial trauma. In: Cummings CW, et al. Otolaryngology—Head and neck surgery. Vol. 1. St. Louis: Mosby–Year Book, 1993:374.

TRAUMATIC OPTIC NEUROPATHY

The method of
Robert A. Sofferman

The discovery of the ophthalmoscope and extension of its clinical use by Helmholtz in 1851 directed clinicians away from the eye itself in traumatic blindness. The normal appearance of the retina in the circumstance of traumatic visual loss and identification of optic atrophy several weeks later are characteristic funduscopic sequences in traumatic optic neuropathy. The patient who presents to the emergency room with substantial head trauma, loss of consciousness, and traumatic optic neuropathy is at risk of failed recognition of the condition. It is critical for emergency physicians, neurosurgeons, and maxillofacial surgeons to understand these issues and pay strict attention to pupillary responses. The swinging flashlight test for afferent pupil, or Gunn's pupillary sign, is an extremely important examination tool. In the simplest form of this test, the pupil of the injured eye does not respond to direct light stimulus, but does constrict with light stimulation of the contralateral retina. When the light stimulus is returned to the injured eye, the pupil dilates (the normal pupil would ordinarily constrict with this maneuver). This represents failure of light stimulus to induce an afferent signal for reflex bilateral pupillary constriction and thereby localizes injury to the optic nerve. This important sign is critical to early recognition and treatment of traumatic optic neuropathy. A lack of appreciation of the intensity for saturation of the color red is another important indication of optic nerve deficit. This sign is much more useful in circumstances in which some vision is preserved.

The optic nerve extends from the posterior pole of the globe through orbital fat to the orbital apex. It is surrounded by subarachnoid space contained by a dural sheath and is somewhat S-shaped and redundant in length. The nerve then enters the optic canal, a complete osseous channel within the lesser wing of the sphenoid. Here the sheath is adherent to bone, and the nerve itself is more vulnerable to injury. In injury to the frontal bone, concussive forces are transmitted to the orbital apex roof at the orbital end of the optic canal. Discrete maximum bone deformation of the orbital roof near the optic canal is confirmed experimentally by studying the surface of the orbital roof through holographic interferometry after application of frontal loading forces. When fractures of the canal are identified on computed tomography (CT) scan, compression of the nerve from depressed bone fragments or regional hematoma can be obvious explanations for the neuropathy. Usually there are no identifiable fractures and the nerve injury is probably due to either axonal stretch or shearing of the microvasculature. The latter is the most likely explanation, because the nerve sheath is most adherent superiorly where direct vessel penetration into the nerve occurs. Many patients who have partial traumatic visual loss demonstrate inferior altitudinal field defects, which reflects pathology of the upper half of the optic nerve.

Evaluation

It is apparent that physical examination is the most important element in arriving at a diagnosis of traumatic optic neuropathy. Visual evoked responses (VER) can confirm deficits in optic nerve transmission, but the test is no more reliable than a well-performed alternating flashlight test in pursuit of an afferent pupillary defect. The most important imaging study is a fine-cut axial CT scan on a plane coaxial with the optic canal. Bausberg and co-workers studied optic canal relationships to the sphenoethmoid sinuses in 48 patients using 1.5 mm CT sequences. In 48 percent of patients, the optic canals were in direct contact with the posterior ethmoid cells, and in 8 percent of patients, there was actual projection well into the posterior ethmoid labyrinth. In 25 cadaver sphenoid sinuses, Fuji and co-workers demonstrated that 8 percent of carotid arteries and 4 percent of optic nerves were completely dehiscent of bone. These issues have important implications in endoscopic sinus surgery, because the optic nerve is vulnerable to injury in overly aggressive or poorly conceived intervention.

■ SURGICAL THERAPY

The modern management of traumatic optic neuropathy has evolved over several decades of simple observation and poorly controlled studies. Hughes accrued experience of 90 patients over 22 years and reviewed many pertinent series from the time period spanning 1916 to the end of World War II. In these series, 72 percent of patients had traumatic optic neuropathy secondary to frontal trauma, and skull fractures were identified in 64 percent of patients. However, only 6 percent of patients with traumatic optic neuropathy had identifiable optic canal fracture. Most important, of the patients who had absent light perception, only 6 percent regained useful vision. The dismal spontaneous recovery of the eye without light perception after trauma was hardly improved by many earlier attempts at optic nerve decompression via transfrontal craniotomy. In 1969, Walsh and Hoy reviewed these experiences and expressed pessimism about the efficacy of surgical decompression. In retrospect, there were so many timing and technical variables in these studies that meaningful scientific conclusions could not be established. Even today, no single surgeon or center in Western medicine has accrued enough cases to allow meaningful comparative information.

The process of optic canal decompression achieved new interest in the mid 1960s and early 1970s through the independent works of Niho and Fukado in Japan. Both researchers reported successful improvement in vision after traumatic optic neuropathy and decompression via the external ethmoid approach. Niho described his experiences with 20 cases and reported a visual recovery rate of 85 percent. In 1972, Fukado published a series of 353 patients who had optic canal decompression after traumatic optic neuropathy; Fukado reported achieving a 55 percent recovery rate in patients who reached surgery by 1 week from the time of injury. It is interesting that in several cases there was visual return in patients whose surgery was delayed for 3 months. An interesting comparison of patients observed versus those committed to surgical decompression was reported in 1990 in two studies from the same institution. Joseph reported improvement in 11 of 14 patients who were managed with surgical decompression and concomitant steroids. Lessell reviewed a parallel series of 25 traumatic optic neuropathy patients who were treated conservatively, and only five of these patients experienced visual improvement.

■ SURGICAL APPROACHES

The most common recognized surgical techniques are as follows: (l) transfrontal craniotomy, (2) external ethmoidectomy, (3) sublabial septal translocation, and (4) endoscopic sphenoethmoid. The transfrontal approach is time-honored and may in some ways have been responsible for a declining interest in surgical management before the 1970s. Because this approach inserts a major neurosurgical procedure into the management pattern, delays in performing the procedure, or more likely reluctance of neurosurgeons to recommend the procedure based on dim historical success, may adversely affect the outcome. The extracranial procedures offer several advantages over the transfrontal craniotomy: (1) frontal lobe elevation is avoided; (2) anosmia, a common bilateral complication of frontal lobe elevation, is avoided;

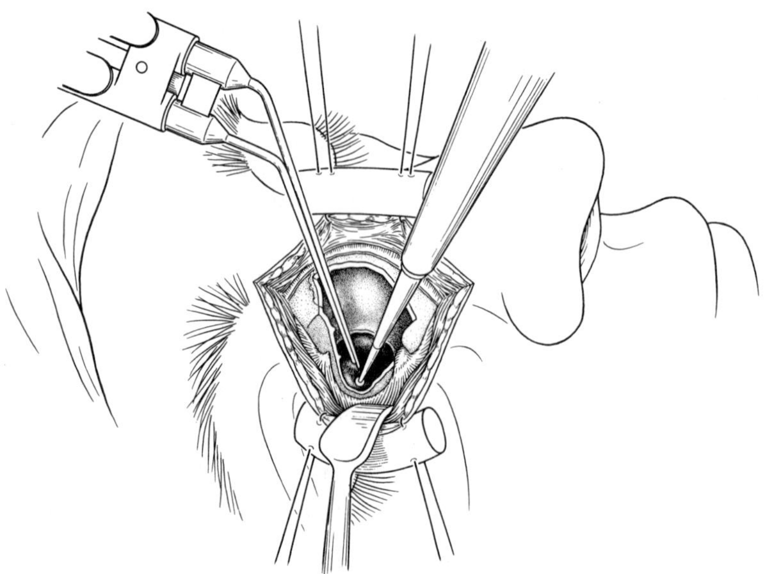

Figure 1.
External ethmoid approach to the optic canal.

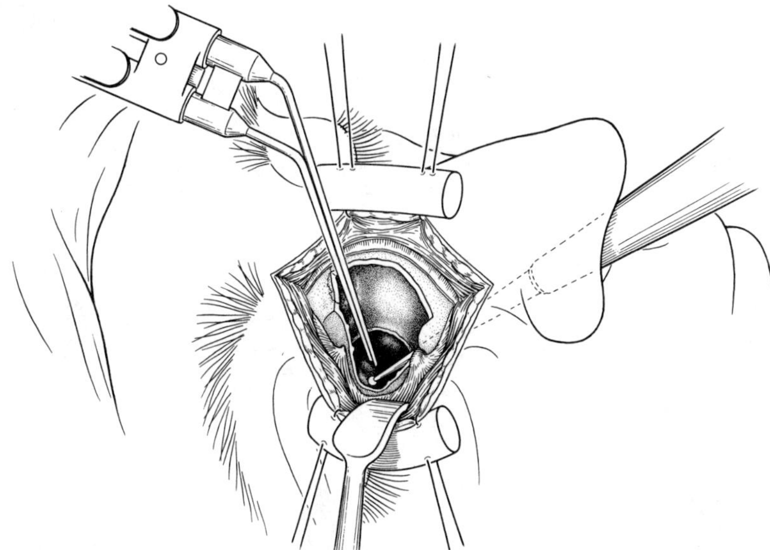

Figure 2.
Improved exposure with drill employed transnasally and suction irrigation through the medial canthal incision.

(3) it is a short, relatively simple procedure with limited blood loss; and (4) it involves no intracranial entry, thus reducing complications such as meningitis.

The external ethmoidectomy is performed through a medial canthal incision and allows the surgeon to follow two straightforward landmarks to find the orbital apex and optic canal (Fig. 1): the anterior ethmoid artery marking the position of the frontoethmoid suture and cribriform plate and a 14 to 16 mm measurement to the start of the optic canal and the medial periorbita. Once the orbital end of the optic canal is identified, suction irrigation and removal of the medial osseous canal with a diamond bur allow exposure of the annulus tendineus and optic nerve sheath (Fig. 2). The annulus and optic nerve sheath should be incised to expose the nerve itself. Uemura demonstrated the benefits of sheath incision in four patients. Walsh and Guy in separate publications discussed the presence of hemorrhage in the sheath subarachnoid space and the fact that visual improvement occurred after evacuation of the sheath hematoma or traumatic cyst.

The sublabial technique is a modification of the transseptal sphenoidectomy approach to the pituitary gland. It is technically very different from the pituitary approach in that the septum is mobilized from the maxillary crest, and the retractor blades are not placed into the septal pocket. Thus, the self-retaining retractor, placed sublabially, produces an ipsilateral wide nasal aperture for the use of suction, drill, and coaxial illumination. This is accomplished by the retractor actually pushing the septum into the opposite nasal passage (Fig. 3). This technique requires an extra-long drill and suction irrigation, but it delivers some important advantages. Whereas the external ethmoidectomy suffers from a narrow angle of approach to the canal (approximately 36 degrees), the sublabial method allows a wider, 72 degree angle with improved visualization of the entire canal length (Fig. 4). This method does require special practice and planning in advance of clinical application. Last, the endoscopic

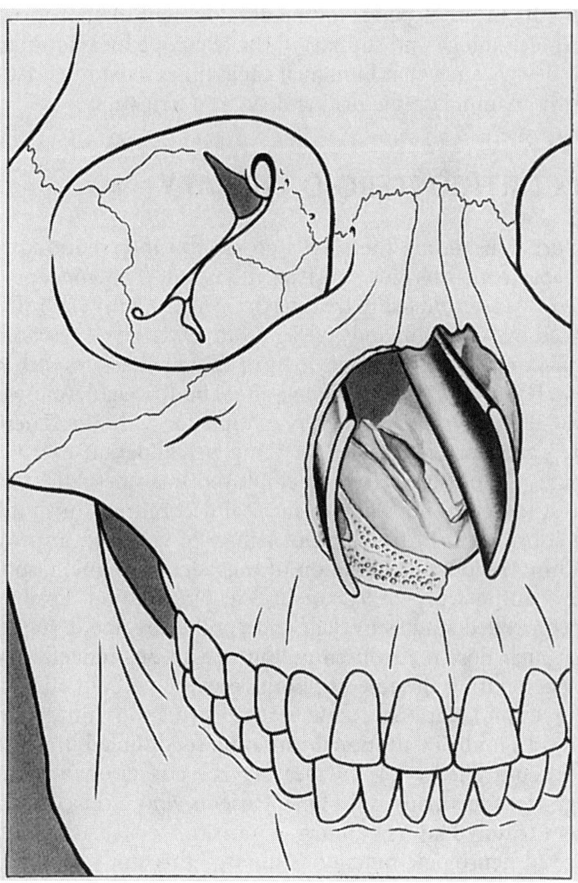

Figure 3.
Septal translocation in preparation for transnasal approach to the optic canal.

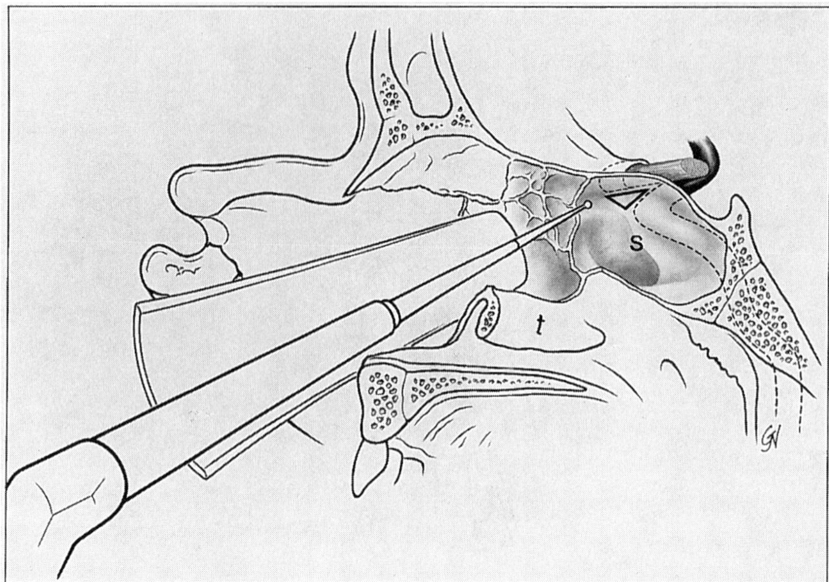

Figure 4.
Sublabial approach demonstrating important carotid artery–optic canal relationships.

approach is in its infancy, but conceptually it may become the optimum procedure for treating traumatic optic neuropathy. Its future depends on the development of appropriate drill technology and support of the telescope by a nonmanual device, such that bimanual capabilities exist to concurrently manipulate the drill and suction irrigation.

■ CORTICOSTEROID THERAPY

Before considering the results of surgical intervention, the use of corticosteroids must be discussed, The concept of high-dose steroid use in treating optic neuropathy was introduced by Anderson and colleagues in 1981. These researchers recommended massive doses of dexamethasone, with an initial dose of 0.75 mg per kilogram of body weight, followed by 0.33 mg per kilogram every 6 hours for 24 hours. Thereafter, the dose is reduced to 1 mg per kilogram every 24 hours. Steroid use has been employed in some patients as a test to determine whether surgical decompression should be considered. In the event of failure of vision to improve within 12 hours of initiation of megadose dexamethasone, these authors proceeded to surgical intervention. Limited, uncontrolled studies by Seiff and another by Spoor suggest that high-dose methylprednisolone might be quite effective in accelerating the rate of vision recovery without surgery. The Second National Acute Spinal Cord Injury Study employed a multi-institutional, randomized, double-blind, placebo-controlled study to measure the effects of the same high-dose methylprednisolone. Patients who received treatment within 8 hours of injury demonstrated statistically improved neurologic function. Although this study measured the therapeutic manipulation of spinal cord white matter, it probably suggests that treatment for traumatic optic neuropathy should optimally be administered early, preferably within 8 hours of the time of injury.

The results of optic nerve decompression with or without concurrent steroids are difficult to standardize. No single surgeon or even institution deals with significant numbers of cases to allow a meaningful comparative study. Thus, we are still left to review small series with basically anecdotal results. The larger studies of Niho and Fukado have been difficult to reproduce in this country. Joseph and associates have accrued substantial experience with the external ethmoid procedure and concomitant high-dose steroids. Najak and co-workers from India reported on 63 patients, with 30 percent demonstrating improvement in vision after extracranial decompression. Von Waltrand Winter and co-workers from Germany reported a 60 percent success rate with surgery in 50 patients compared with a 30 percent rate of spontaneous recovery. For 10 of my patients with traumatic optic neuropathy who underwent extracranial surgery (usually the sublabial technique), 70 percent demonstrated significant visual improvement. When visual fields were obtained preoperatively, 60 percent demonstrated significant expansion of the field. In this series, all four patients with desperate bilateral blindness experienced sufficient improvement with surgery to allow return to independent living and reasonable visual acuity.

■ INDICATIONS FOR SURGERY

The indications for surgery are not universally agreed upon. It is critical to determine whether the patient had any time of preserved acuity from the point of injury. The patient who has absent light perception from the time of injury has a desperate problem and will not be likely to achieve recovery by observation alone The patient who has some preserved vision after trauma can be managed expectantly with steroids; surgery remains in reserve for stable, marginal, or progressively deteriorating vision. Two patients who had light perception only and no improvement over 6 weeks were submitted to desperate surgical decompression. They both developed remarkable improvement in vision over the 2 to 4 week period after surgery, which suggests that restoration of axoplasmic flow and/or remyelination of the optic nerve were responsible for the visual recovery.

Within the sphenoid, the optic nerve maintains a close anatomic relationship to the cavernous carotid artery. The precise relative anatomic position of each structure must be understood, and if there is any anatomic confusion, an image intensifier can be used as an assistive aid. Postoperative development of cavernous carotid artery aneurysm has been described, which suggests that the artery and not the optic nerve might have been decompressed. The dura of the anterior fossa can be opened, which produces a cerebrospinal leak and the risk of meningitis. Last, the nerve can be injured through overzealous drilling and nerve manipulation, but this would go unrecognized in most cases requiring surgery with the poor preoperative acuity.

■ DISCUSSION

In summary, the management of traumatic optic neuropathy has received new surgical attention with the evolution of extracranial and endoscopic techniques. Although many relevant inquiries about this condition and management are unanswered and demand a well-crafted, prospective, multi-institutional, controlled study, the experiences of many clinicians justifies the use of steroids and extracranial decompression. One patient with a severe head injury and complete afferent pupillary defect underwent transfrontal craniotomy and concomitant optic canal decompression and removal of compressive bone fragments 4 hours after the time of injury. She recovered visual acuity to 20/25 with optic atrophy; her success was ascribed to early intervention. Until future assessment better clarifies the role of surgery in treating traumatic optic neuropathy, early and decisive intervention is the best opportunity for recovery. At the very least, early institution of megadose steroids should be fundamental to the management of all patients who have significant traumatic optic neuropathy. The patient with some preserved acuity has the best prognosis for recovery as temporary interruption of axoplasmic flow is reversed. An interval of preserved vision from the time of injury preceding complete monocular blindness offers some hope and demands aggressive medical and probably surgical management. The recovery of the eye with no light perception from the time of injury is less certain. The poor results with observation alone or steroid therapy suggest that a combination of optic nerve decompression and steroid use may be the proper early management option.

Suggested Reading

Anderson RL, Panje WR, Gross CE. Optic nerve blindness following blunt forehead trauma. Ophthalmology 1982; 89:445-455.

Bausberg SF, Harner SG, Forbes G. Relationship of the optic nerve to the paranasal sinuses as shown by computed tomography. Otolaryngol Head Neck Surg 1987; 96:331-335.

Bracken MB, Shepard MJ, Collins WF, et al. A randomized controlled trial of methylprednisolone or naxolone in the treatment of acute spinal-cord injury. N Engl J Med 1990; 322:1405-1411.

Fuji K, Chambers SM, Rhoton AC. Neurovascular relationships of the sphenoid sinus. J Neurosurg 1979; 50:31-39.

Fukado Y. Results in 350 cases of surgical decompression of the optic nerve. Trans Fourth Asia-Pac Cong Ophthalmol 1972; 4:96-99.

Gross CE, Dekock R Jr, Panje WR, et al. Evidence for orbital deformation that may contribute to monocular blindness following minor frontal head trauma. J Neurosurg 1981; 55:963-966.

Guy J, Sherwood M, Day AL. Surgical treatment of progressive visual loss in traumatic optic neuropathy. J Neurosurg 1989; 70:799-801.

Hughes B. Indirect injury of the optic nerves and chiasma. Bull Johns Hopkins Hosp 1962; 3:98-126.

Joseph MP, Messell S, Rizzo JR, et al. Extracranial optic nerve decompression for traumatic optic neuropathy. Arch Ophthalmol 1990; 108:1091-1093.

Lessell S. Indirect optic nerve trauma. Arch Ophthalmol 1989; 197:382-386.

Najak SR, Kirtane MV, Ingle MV. Transethmoid decompression of the optic nerve in head injuries: An update. J Laryngol Otol 1991; 105: 205-206.

Niho S, Murakami I, Sato T. Decompression of the fractured optic nerve by the transethmoid route. Pac Med Surg 1965; 73:237-240.

Osguthorpe JD, Sofferman RA. Optic nerve decompression. Otolaryngol Clin North Am 1988; 21:155-169.

Pringle JH. Atrophy of the optic nerve following diffused violence to the skull. Br Med J 1922; 2:1156.

Seiff SR. High dose corticosteroids for treatment of vision loss due to indirect injury to the optic nerve. Ophthalmic Surg 1990; 21:389-395.

Sofferman RA. The recovery potential of the optic nerve. Laryngoscope 1995; 105.

Sofferman RA. Transnasal approach to optic nerve decompression. Op Techniq Otolaryngol Head Neck Surg 1991; 2:150-156.

Spoor TC, Hartel WC, Lensink DB, et al. Treatment of traumatic optic neuropathy with corticosteroids. Am J Ophthalmol 1990; 110:665.

Stankiewicz JA. Blindness and intranasal endoscopic ethmoidoscopy: Prevention and management. Otolaryngol Head Neck Surg 1989; 101:320-329.

Uemura T, Iisaka Y, Kazuno T, et al. Optic canal decompression—The significance of simultaneous optic canal sheath incision. Neurol Med Chir (Tokyo) 1978; 18:151-157.

Von Waltrand Winter W, Ritter J, Gerhardt H, et al. Die mikrochirurgische transethmoidale optikusdekompressionaus ophthalmologischer sicht. Folia Ophthalmol 1988; 13:351-356.

Walsh FB. Pathological-clinical correlations: I, Indirect trauma to the optic nerves and chiasm. II, Certain cerebral involvements associated with defective blood supply. Invest Ophthalmol 1996; 5:433-449.

Walsh FB, Hoyt WF. Clinical neurophthalmology. 3rd ed. Baltimore: Williams & Wilkins, 1969.

MANDIBULAR FRACTURE

The method of
William D. Clark
Eric J. Simko

We assume that the reader is familiar with the anatomy of the teeth and facial skeleton, the pathology of maxillofacial trauma, and the genera] principles of its management. A detailed history and complete physical examination should be done for every patient who has a mandibular fracture. All possible associated injuries should be fully evaluated, and specialty consultations should be obtained when appropriate.

GENERAL TREATMENT CONSIDERATIONS

Bed rest, elevation of the head and neck, and cold packs will decrease the patient's discomfort and lessen swelling. We have not found Barton's bandages and similar devices to be particularly useful. Early immobilization of fractures will greatly reduce the patient's discomfort and the incidence of complications. It is usually desirable to accomplish these ends by application of maxillomandibular fixation (MMF) or definitive rigid internal fixation. In the occasional case for which this is not practical, Ivy loops, Kazajian buttons, or similar temporary wiring techniques may prove useful.

The patient's status regarding tetanus immunization should be explored and managed appropriately. This is especially important if the patient has recently emigrated from an area where routine immunization is not practiced.

Almost all mandibular fractures communicate with the oral cavity or skin and are therefore open fractures. Prophylactic antibiotics are indicated in all of these cases. We use an oral suspension of penicillin, cephalexin, or clindamycin in an age-appropriate dose.

Moderate-strength analgesics will be necessary for the first 5 to 7 days. Acetaminophen with codeine elixir is convenient for this purpose. Requests for stronger analgesics beyond the first 48 hours should alert one to the possibility of a pending complication or a drug abuse problem.

Nutrition is an important consideration for those treated with MMF. A blenderized, regular diet is prescribed with the realization that it will not be practical for all meals. Liquid diets of the type used for head and neck cancer patients are convenient sources of supplemental feedings and for meals taken away from home. Ideally, elderly and chronically ill patients are weighed at each postreduction examination. This patient group can often benefit from supplemental feeding with commercially available canned products.

We recommend half-strength hydrogen peroxide oral rinses, brushing with a soft toothbrush, and an oral irrigation device set at low pressures for maintenance of oral hygiene.

Weekly examinations are routine for the postreduction patient. Examinations should assess the following: (1) dental occlusion, (2) state of nutrition, and (3) condition of MMF or other hardware.

Patients who have mandibular fractures are a litigious group. Therefore, it is especially important to document informed consent, not only as it relates to the initial treatment, but also as it relates to the importance of follow-up care. If the patient refuses treatment, informed consent is also a major consideration. With increasing frequency, the courts are awarding damages to patients who claim that they were not adequately informed as to the consequences of refusing treatment.

TREATMENT OPTIONS

No Treatment

Isolated fractures of the coronoid process do not require specific treatment. Analgesics, reassurance, and follow-up are all that is needed. Antibiotics are not necessary.

Dietary Restrictions

A unilateral fracture of the subcondylar area of the mandible with minimal displacement and normal occlusion in a reliable patient may be treated with liquid-to-soft diets and weekly examinations. Patients who develop malocclusion and/or persistent pain at the fracture site should be managed with MMF.

Maxillomandibular Fixation

Simple MMF requires the presence of adequate dentition. Most stable fractures can be treated with MMF alone. Unilateral and bilateral subcondylar fractures can be so managed. Alveolar process and body-of-mandible fractures can also be managed by MMF.

Open Reduction and MMF Fixation

Most fractures that are not amenable to MMF alone may be managed by combining open reduction with internal fixation and MMF. Injuries that typically require this or another of the more aggressive approaches include (1) angle-of-mandible fractures, (2) symphyseal or parasymphyseal fractures, (3) multiple fractures, and (4) fractures associated with midface instability.

As with most problems in medicine and surgery, it is difficult to provide a complete cookbook approach to the decision-making process. Factors that weigh on the side of using open reduction include (1) poor dentition, (2) unstable fractures, (3) multiple fractures, (4) presence of Le Fort's fracture in the same patient, and (5) badly displaced fragments.

Factors to be weighed against open reduction include (1) young, healthy patient, (2) good dentition, (3) stable fracture sites, and (4) minimal fracture displacement.

In borderline situations, the physician may wish to pursue a staged approach. A closed reduction with MMF is performed, and the patient is closely observed. If good, stable occlusion and fracture reduction are not obtained over a 2 to 3 day observation period, the physician can proceed with open reduction.

External Pin Fixation

The major indications for use of external pin fixation are injuries involving significant tissue loss at the fracture site and injuries that require prolonged immobilization for the treatment of nonunion. This technique also has potential application in the following circumstances: (1) patient who has seizure disorder, (2) patient who cannot tolerate MMF, and (3) edentulous patient for whom splinting techniques are not practical. In each of these instances, dynamic compression plate (DCP) fixation is also a viable option.

Rigid Internal Fixation

The use of rigid internal fixation in the treatment of mandibular fractures has become increasingly popular in the United States over the past 15 years. The advantages are (1) improved patient comfort, (2) lack of airway concerns, (3) ease of oral hygiene, (4) ease of clearance of secretions and vomitus, (5) maintenance of temporomandibular joint (TMJ) mobility, and (6) reduced rates of delayed union and nonunion. The disadvantages are (1) implantation of a large amount of foreign material, (2) reduction of blood supply at the fracture site due to the extensive exposure required, (3) decreased periosteal coverage at the fracture site, and (4) greater probability of producing occlusal disharmonies than procedures with MMF alone. Although some proponents of rigid internal fixation claim a reduced incidence of infection as an advantage, our experience has not supported this claim.

Lag Screws

Lag screws are used by some physicians as the sole treatment of selected angle-of-mandible and symphyseal or parasymphyseal fractures. These are advanced techniques that should be undertaken with caution by those surgeons who lack extensive experience in mandibular fracture treatment.

Dynamic Compression Plates

A DCP can be used as the sole treatment of most body-of-mandible, angle-of-mandible, symphyseal or parasymphyseal, and ascending-ramus-of-mandible fractures. Limitations include traumatic bone loss, extensive comminution of fragments, and severe bony atrophy. Where they can be used, DCPs have become the treatment of choice for many physicians who treat mandibular fractures.

Reconstruction Plates

A reconstruction plate (RCP) is an excellent device to obtain rigid internal fixation when there is traumatic bone loss, extensive comminution, or a series of several mandibular fractures.

■ SPECIAL PROBLEMS

Pediatric Patients

Fortunately, facial fractures are not common in children. From age 3 to 5 or 6 years, a child normally has a full complement of deciduous teeth. Using careful techniques, stable MMF is possible by the application of arch bars. From ages 6 to 12 years, the dentition is fixed (some deciduous, some permanent teeth); these patients present difficulties in securing MMF. Routine arch bar application alone is rarely adequate for these patients, but combinations of the following adjunctive techniques are useful: (1) circum-mandibular wiring to stabilize arch bars and/or splints, (2) zygomatic arch suspension with or without piriform aperture suspension for stabilization of maxillary arch bars and/or splints, (3) custom-fabricated splints of acrylic or cast metal from a dental laboratory, and (4) open reduction with interosseous wiring.

The most common mandibular injuries that we have encountered in children have been body and condylar area fractures. Isolated body fractures are treated with acrylic splints attached to the mandible via three-point circum-mandibular wiring. These patients are allowed to take a liquid or soft diet. Displaced condylar area fractures in this population require MMF. Because children are more prone to problems with TMJ mobility, the duration of MMF is reduced to 2 to 3 weeks.

Edentulous Patients

The following techniques are useful for managing the edentulous patient who has a fractured mandible: (1) use of dentures as splints to achieve MMF, (2) open reduction with interosseous wiring, (3) open reduction with DCP fixation, and (4) use of Gunning's splints.

Removal of MMF in Adults

The recommended duration for maintenance MMF varies with the site of fracture(s), the patient's age, and the overall health of the patient. When fractures are limited to the subcondylar area(s) of healthy young patients, 3 to 4 weeks of immobilization is often sufficient. Six weeks is the usual period of immobilization for fractures at other sites in healthy patients. In the elderly and infirm, 6 to 8 weeks is the usual period of immobilization.

After the appropriate time interval, intermaxillary elastics or wires are removed, and Bernstein's tongue blade test is applied. The patient is asked to bite on a wooden tongue blade placed between the dental arches, in a place remote from any fracture site. Pain at a fracture site indicates the need for further immobilization. Elastics or wires are reapplied, and the test is repeated in 1 week.

If the tongue blade test is passed, the elastics or wires are left off, and the patient is instructed to eat a soft diet. If the patient has no problems when examined a week later, the arch bars may be removed.

Tooth in the Fracture Line

A tooth in a mandibular fracture line should be extracted if it is fractured into the pulp cavity, associated with periapical or periodontal pathology, loose in its socket, or interfering with fragment reduction. An exception is a fractured and impacted third molar. We believe that these teeth should be left in place until the fracture heals if there is reason to believe that removal will be the least bit difficult.

Open Reduction of Condylar Area Fractures

It is uncommon that condylar area fractures require an open reduction and internal fixation. Indications include displacement of the condylar head into the middle cranial fossa, embedded foreign body, lateral extracapsular displacement of the head of the condyle, and inability to reduce the fractures by other means.

■ COMPLICATIONS

Infection

Infection is a relatively common complication of mandibular fractures. The following factors have been identified as predisposing to infection: (1) delayed reduction, (2) fracture through tooth socket, (3) lack of prophylactic antibiotics use, (4) pre-existing dental disease, and (5) poor oral hygiene.

Infections that occur early after a fracture are usually managed by antibiotics, local wound care, and possible extraction of involved teeth. Late infections often require (in addition to the aforementioned) surgical debridement of the fracture site, including removal of any hardware.

Malocclusion and Malunion

Malocclusion is a reflection of malunion. Minor degrees of malocclusion may be managed by precise spot-grinding of the teeth. This should only be done by a dentist who has expertise in problems of occlusion.

Major degrees of malocclusion may require one or more of the following: (1) surgical repositioning of malunited fragments, (2) orthodontic treatment, (3) major rehabilitative dental treatment, and (4) orthognathic surgery.

Nonunion is usually associated with advanced age, atrophy of the mandible, major systemic illnesses, and/or loss of bone at the fracture site. The usual treatment is debridement of the fracture site, autogenous bone grafting, and prolonged immobilization.

■ TECHNICAL CONSIDERATIONS

Arch Bar Placement

Local anesthesia is sufficient for placement of arch bars in the cooperative adult. General anesthesia is preferred under the following circumstances: (1) extensive manipulation of fragments is required, (2) open reduction is anticipated, (3) the patient is a child or uncooperative adult, (4) use of circummandibular wiring is anticipated, (5) the surgeon is not experienced in arch bar placement, and (6) the patient requests it.

Erich arch bars are cut to length and contoured to the dental arch. Each arch bar is secured by dental wire ligatures of 26 gauge stainless steel and are applied to the canine, premolar, and molar teeth. When the arch bar crosses the fracture line, the fracture should be reduced before ligatures posterior to the fracture are secured. It is occasionally necessary to section an arch bar where it crosses the fracture line in order to avoid its interfering with fracture reduction. Once fracture reduction is accomplished, it is often possible to rejoin the cut arch bar segments with wire ligatures.

Accurately contoured, securely fixed arch bars are the cornerstones of MMF. Poor results in the treatment of mandibular fractures can often be traced to the lack of attention to details in the application of arch bars.

Open Reduction with Nonrigid Internal Fixation

External approaches are generally preferred over intraoral approaches, especially for the occasional operator. A transverse incision is placed in a relaxed skin tension line 2 to 3 cm inferior to the mandibular border. Care is taken to avoid injury to the mandibular branch of the facial nerve. The fracture site is cleaned of soft tissue, and the fragments are brought into anatomic reduction. One drill hole is made on each side of the fracture, approximately 7 to 10 mm above the inferior margin of the mandible (5 to 6 mm in the child), and approximately the same distance from the fracture line. A figure eight ligature of 22 to 24 gauge stainless steel wire is placed. Final tightening of this ligature is best delayed until MMF has been established. This avoids the problems of minor errors in fragment reduction interfering with obtaining ideal occlusal relationships; it also avoids breaking the figure eight wire by intraoral manipulations. The trade-off is difficulty in avoiding gross contamination of the external wound.

Fractures of the angle are usually oblique, and there is a tendency for the posterior fragment to be pulled superiorly and anteriorly by the pterygoid and masseter muscles. When a two-hole figure eight ligature does not hold the reduction, a four-hole figure eight often accomplishes this task. A useful alternative is simple wire ligature through two holes with the posterior drill hole being placed superiorly and as nearly vertical in relationship to the anterior as conditions will permit. This reduces the propensity of the posterior fragment to "slide up the incline."

Open Reduction with Rigid Internal Fixation

Drill holes for lag screws should be perpendicular to the plane of the fracture, not the external surface of the mandible. The outer hold is overdrilled and the inner hole is tapped to allow the fragments to be compressed.

DCPs should be overcontoured by 3 to 5 degrees to avoid producing distracting forces on the lingual surface of the mandible. It is also important to recognize that compression at the lower border of the mandible produces distracting forces at the superior border. This problem may be overcome by applying tension banding (e.g. arch bars) at the superior border of using eccentric dynamic plates (EDCP). EDCPs have an extra set of holes that direct forces in a superior direction, thereby compressing the superior border.

When compared to the traditional techniques of treating mandible fractures, rigid internal fixation requires a much more exacting technique and leaves less margin for error. There is merit to first mastering the traditional techniques before undertaking the more technically challenging approaches of rigit fixation.

Dentures as Splints

Intact dentures can be modified to serve as splints for MMF. The mandibular incisors are removed to allow space for postoperative feedings. A segment of arch bar is wired to each side of the denture, leaving the incisor areas uncovered. Each denture can then be wired to the patient. Circumandibular wires are used for the mandibular denture, and zygomatic arch wires with or without piriform aperture suspension wires fix the maxillary denture to the patient. Repair of fractured dentures can easily be performed by dental laboratories. Denture teeth removed to facilitate feeding should be saved, as a dental laboratory may be able to later repair dentures used as splints.

The edentulous patient who requries MMF, but who has no dentures, may be managed with Gunning splints. A dentist knowledgeable in prosthetic techniques and a dental laboratory are required to produce adequate splints.

Suggested Reading

Clark WD. Management of mandibular fractures. Am J Otolaryngol 1992; 13:125-132.

Clark WD, Bailey BJ. Management of fractures of the mandible. In: Mathog RH, ed. Maxillofacial trauma. Baltimore: Williams & Wilkins, 1984:162.

Clark WD, Morehead JM. Mandibular fractures—what to do when. In: Lucente FE, ed. Highlights of the instructional courses. St. Louis; Mosby-Year Book, 1995:3.

Farris PE, Dierks EJ. Single oblique lag screw fixation of mandibular angle fractures. Laryngoscope 1972; 102:1070-1072.

Niederdellman H, Shetty V. Solitary oblique lag screw osteosynthesis in the treatment of fractures of the angle of the mandible: a retrospective study. Plast Reconstr Surg 1987; 80:68-74.

Zide MF, Kent JN. Indications for open reduction of mandibular condyle fractures. J Oral Maxillofac Surg 1983; 41:89.

THE CROOKED NOSE

The method of
Fred J. Stucker
by
Fred J. Stucker
Paul C. Drago

The crooked or twisted nose represents a dilemma to the rhinoplasty surgeon because of its combination of functional and cosmetic problems. Its frequent recurrence following attempted corrections attests to this dilemma. By definition, the crooked nose shows an appreciable deviation from the normal, straight vertical orientation. The crooked nose has a lateral orientation that is a result to varying degrees of soft-tissue, scar-tissue, cartilage, and skeletal deformities and their attachments.

Correcting (straightening) the crooked nose remains a formidable challenge for the surgeon despite considerable advancements in nasal surgery. Both the functional and cosmetic aspects of correction must be dealt with as appropriate and simultaneous surgical corrections. Most crooked or twisted noses occur from trauma. To repair the nose correctly, in the face of previously uncontrollable fractures, requires expert planning and precise surgical execution.

As with all deformities, the proper management commences with an accurate assessment of the problem. The desired result is a straight nose, which depends not only on surgical expertise, but also on the knowledge of predictable aspects of soft tissue, cartilage, and wound healing. We believe that a consideration of all these aspects will produce an acceptable result in most circumstances. Unsatisfactory results are usually a result of failing to understand these principles, faulty execution, or an inexperienced surgeon. It is to be emphasized, however, that even the most accomplished surgeon is not immune to creating an undesirable result.

■ DEFINING THE ANATOMIC COMPONENT

External Nasal Findings

The position of the nasal bones and frontal process of the maxilla is of critical importance in determining if the nose is crooked. Because most trauma to the nose is delivered from one side or the other, there is usually a side that is deflected, and the opposite side is depressed. The C-shaped and scoliotic noses have the same fundamental bony deformity. Without understanding and appreciating the bony contribution to the pathology, any hope for correction is extremely difficult.

The cartilaginous vault (upper lateral cartilages) is intimately attached to the underside of the bony dorsum. The upper lateral cartilages and the septal cartilage are attached not only to the external nasal bones, but also to the endonasal skeleton. These are generally very firm attachments and must be corrected if malaligned. The lower lateral cartilages and the caudal septum are often twisted and result in the various C- and S-shaped deformities. This results from a hypertrophic skeletal frame fitted into a restrictive periosteal or perichondrial envelope.

Endonasal Findings

Endonasal deformities are next evaluated. In the past, it was very difficult to examine all but the most caudal deformities in cases where the septum was twisted, thickened, or gnarled. Nasal endoscopies have greatly improved the preoperative evaluation of posterior endonasal deformities. Good topical vasoconstriction and topical anesthesia are helpful and often essential for an adequate preoperative evaluation.

A dislocated quadrilateral cartilage is commonly associated with a spur. The cartilage is usually not slotted in its normal position in the maxillary or vomerine groove. Spurs do not necessarily adversely impact function or cosmesis, and unless the reconstructive surgery necessitates modification or removal, spurs can be ignored. The septal deformity in a crooked nose cannot be ignored and is best dealt with by employing removal of strips of cartilage or larger resections. Sufficient dorsal and caudal struts must be retained to maintain the necessary nasal support. If the septal deformity is ignored, it is very likely that a recurrence of the twisted nose will result.

The perpendicular plate of the ethmoid is usually malaligned. Because it is attached to the nasal bones and septal cartilage, any deformity of one is likely associated with a deformity of its attached member. This ethmoid plate is a thin piece of bone and is often fractured (and overlooked) when the nasal bones are fractured. The perpendicular plane may be telescoped and is universally dislocated laterally with most nasal fractures. Inadequate recognition of the injury and failure to refracture the perpendicular plate of the ethmoid can result in early postoperative spreading of the nasal bones. Refracturing the perpendicular plate of the ethmoid is a preliminary step in our recommended technique and mitigates against this type of recurrence. This is generally done with a Sayer elevator using a gentle rocking motion, superiorly to inferiorly on both sides. This tends to fracture the PPE in an eggshell fashion and has successfully been performed over 6,000 times by the senior author without one known incident of cerebrospinal fluid leak.

The vomer is the least critical component of the twisted nose. It is often midline in all but the most severely twisted noses. Posterior spurs are often not a significant cause of airway obstruction and can, in the absence of associated pathology, be ignored. Spurs in this region result from the bony and cartilaginous septum being dislocated from the vomerine groove.

The mucosa, with its perichondrial and fibrous attachments, can be unyielding to the midline repositioning of the septum. In these cases, it is necessary to incise the soft tissue to allow free positioning of the septum.

Surgical Technique

After the nose has been anesthetized, the initial maneuver is directed at completely mobilizing the bony septum. The Sayer elevator is our instrument of choice for this purpose. With the rocking motion from superior to inferior on both sides of the bony septum, eggshell fractures occur, and repositioning of the ethmoid is accomplished. If needed, the vomer is also repositioned. This action improves the septal cartilage position and sets the tone for a proper straightening. It must be remembered that bone binds cartilage to an abnormal position—not the other way around.

The three basic approaches to gain access to the structural components of the nose are inter- and intracartilaginous incisions and the open rhinoplasty, The open rhinoplasty is the appropriate method for managing the most difficult of twisted noses. A No. 15 scalpel blade is our preferred method of opening the nose and separating the skin and soft-tissue envelope from its underlying structures, which are often scarred in the crooked nose. Because there is often much scarring and normal planes may be lost, the scalpel is the most propitious instrument for dissecting the soft-tissue envelope from the skeletal structures.

Following elevation of the skin and soft-tissue envelope, the septoplasty is performed. Usually, a unilateral mucoperichondrial or periosteal flap is elevated. There is no anatomic plane that allows an easy elevation where the septum abuts the premaxillary crest. This area of fibrous decussation is often an area of inadvertent mucosal tears. Our technique carries the mucosal elevation inferiorly to where the plane ceases (where the fibers decussate to the other side) and incises the inferior mucoperichondrial or periosteal flap with a scalpel or scissors in a horizontal fashion. This provides an unparalleled vista of the septum, avoids the common mucosal tear, and affords a postoperative drainage site. The remainder of the septoplasty is carried out in the usual manner.

The upper lateral cartilages are separated from the septum, if required. If possible, it is prudent to leave the mucosa attached to the septum and underside of the upper lateral cartilage. This again illustrates an advantage with the open technique. If after both upper lateral cartilages are severed and a widening occurs, one can suture the cartilages back to the septum.

In cases in which the septum is markedly thickened or reduplicated, we employ a diamond bur to thin the septal cartilage. This is performed under direct visualization, which enables the septum to be literally shaped to a proper midline position.

After the septoplasty and before commencing the bony skeletal surgery, a whip stitch is employed to coapt the mucosal flaps (Fig. 1). This is done with a 4–0 chromic suture on a straight or straightened needle (P-3). Universally, this suture alleviates the need to pack the nose, but equally important, it provides architectural integrity to the septum. Routinely, we do not employ any type of nasal packing. This suture effectively eliminates the dead space and prevents hematoma formation. It is important to pull the needle through areas of dehiscent cartilage to prevent over-riding of the cartilage fragments.

The bony dorsum is addressed, and the hump, if present, is removed using the surgeon's instrument of preference. The medial osteotomy on the depressed side is carried out first by using a curved 4 mm osteotome. When the bony cut is complete, the depressed nasal bony wall is elevated. A medial osteotomy is done on the opposite side just to fracture and separate the apical portion of the PPE. If an intermediate osteotomy is required, it is done next. Last, the lateral osteotomy is performed on the deflected side using the 2 mm osteotome. The senior author has never found it necessary to do a lateral osteotomy on the depressed side of a crooked nose in order to elevate the bony plate.

The lateral osteotomy is begun immediately caudal to the inferior turbinate. The osteotome is advanced by using the mallet in a superolateral direction, aimed at the lateral canthus until it encounters the thicker bone of the nasomaxillary groove. The chisel is repositioned and advanced superomedially in the bony nasomaxillary groove, which completes the lateral osteotomy.

■ DISCUSSION

Careful analysis of both the internal and external components of the crooked nose ensures the accuracy of the diagnosis. As with all problems, the correct diagnosis is the critical first step in attempting appropriate treatment. The crooked nose is best managed, and many in the field think

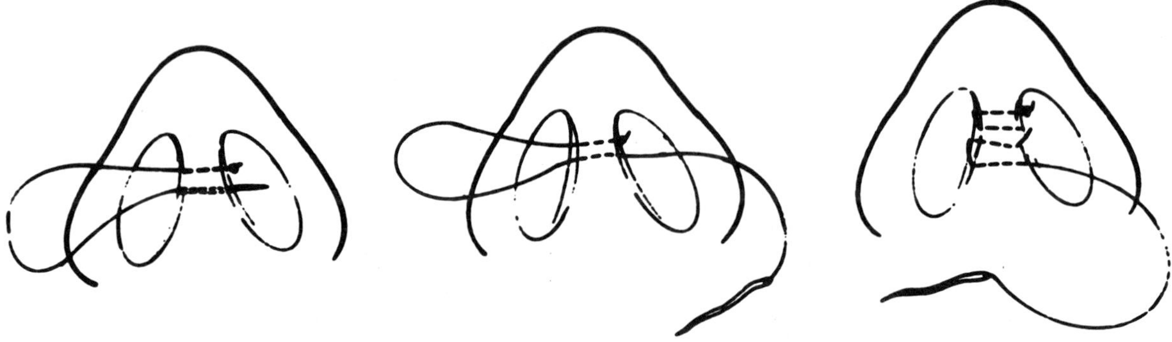

Figure 1.
Diagrammatic illustration of septal whip stitch.

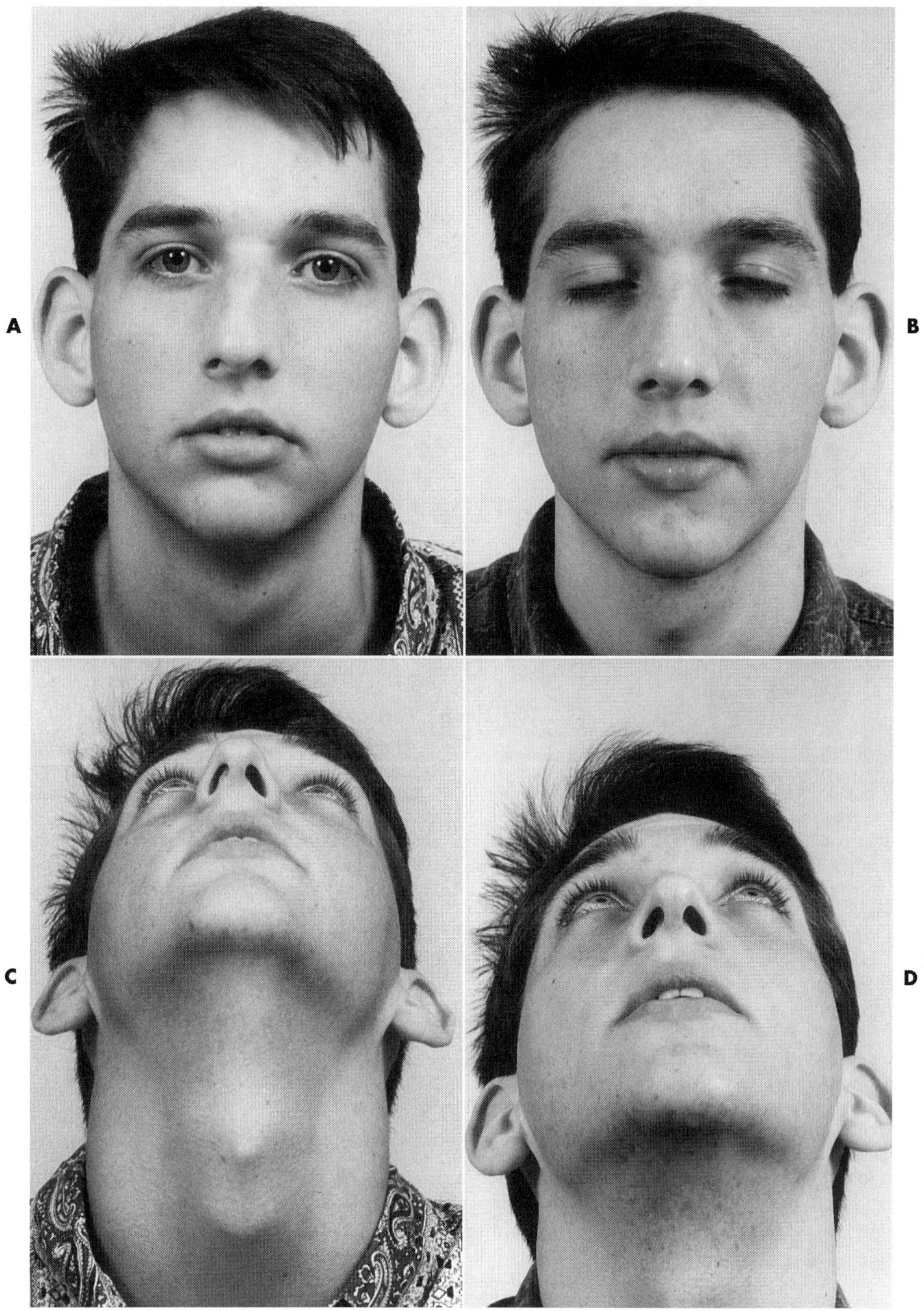

Figure 2.
A, Preoperative full-face view of crooked nose. *B,* Two years postoperative full-face view. *C,* Preoperative submental view. *D,* Two years postoperative submental view. *Continued*

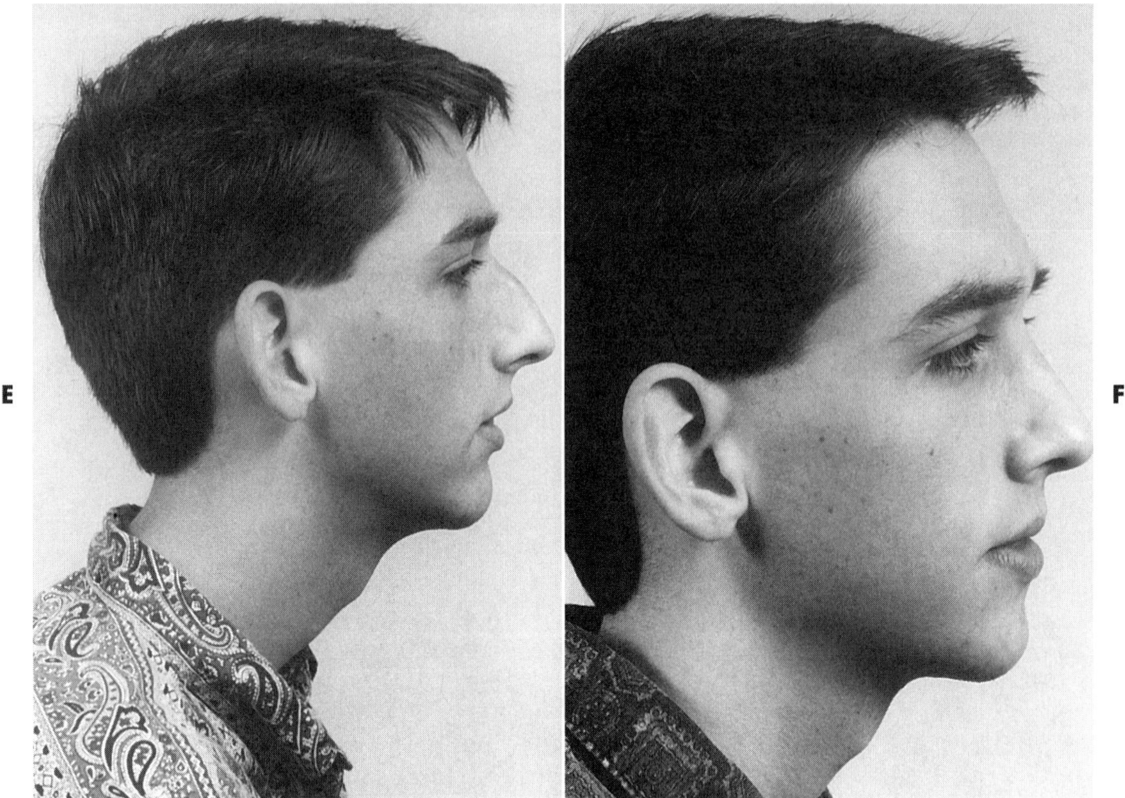

Figure 2, cont'd.
E, Preoperative right lateral view. *F,* Two years postoperative right lateral view.

can only be managed, in one operation because of the relationship of the septum and nasal bones.

Septal surgery can be achieved via a unilateral or bilateral mucoperichondrial flap; we prefer, when possible, the unilateral flap, which maintains the mucosal integrity. As mentioned previously, this is not always possible, especially with a redundant, gnarled septum. A running whip stitch is always employed to coapt the mucosal flaps, whether a unilateral or bilateral flap is developed. This suture increases the septal stability and has eliminated the need for nasal packing in a majority of cases. Nasal packing is not innocuous and can contribute to increased edema, swelling, and patient discomfort. Packing can also cause toxic shock and vasovagal reactions when it is removed. Packing can also tear the mucosa when removed and, when present, can potentially spread the nasal bones.

Attention to the depressed and deflected nasal bones is critically important. Outfracturing of a unilateral depressed nasal bone can be universally achieved after a medial osteotomy without the need for a lateral osteotomy. Recognition and repair via mobilization of the perpendicular plate of the ethmoid bone greatly increases the chance of success when the crooked nose is realigned (Fig. 2).

Our experience with more than 7,000 nasal repairs and corrections emphasizes the need for accurate diagnosis. A one-stage repair is successful in more than 85 percent of cases. Less than 15 percent of our patients require a secondary procedure.

Suggested Reading

Kian H. The twisted nose. In: Gates GA, ed. Current therapy in otolaryngology—Head and neck surgery. 5th ed. St. Louis: Mosby–Year Book, 1994:164.

Stucker Fred J. Management of the scoliotic nose. Laryngoscope 1982; 92:128-134.

Toriumi DM. Open rhinoplasty. In: Bailey BS, ed. Head and neck surgery—Otolaryngology. Philadelphia: JB Lippincott, 1993:2128.

THE LARGE NOSE

The method of Norman J. Pastorek

The most commonly requested facial plastic surgery procedure is reduction rhinoplasty. It is difficult to say how long in human history the large nose has been an aesthetic problem. Prior to the description of a controlled aesthetic procedure to change the size and shape of the large nose, the nasal appearance was assimilated into the physical and cultural heritage of the individual. The large nose was passed down to generations of sons and daughters as part of a familial or cultural heritage. The dorsal hump was a hallmark of nobility in certain European families. The ability to choose rhinoplasty seems commonplace today, but it represents a triumph of the individual to control his or her personal identity rather than "settle for the genetic cards they have been dealt." In a way, this option for changing nose size is a metaphor for the expression of the individual that has been evolving in Western civilization and culture for most of the twentieth century.

Much of facial plastic surgery, for example, facelift, blepharoplasty, forehead lift, chemical peels, laser abrasion, and brow lift, represents rejuvenation surgery. This surgery returns the face to a youthful but recognizable appearance. Rhinoplasty (and to a lesser degree, chin and malar augmentation) has the ability to change the facial image so that it is unrecognizable to the patient, his or her peers, relatives, or significant others. It is a powerful aesthetic and psychological tool. The facial plastic surgeon will find that motivational investigation is very important in the rhinoplasty patient.

The initial patient-physician encounter is very important. In most medical circumstances, the history, physical examination, and appropriate laboratory evaluations direct the physician to the diagnosis and course of treatment. The aesthetic surgery consultation attempts to integrate the psychosocial elements without which the diagnosis has no meaning. The patient expects the aesthetic surgeon to be as much a sensitive artist as a technical expert. The surgeon who demonstrates a sincere involved interest in the whole patient and a genuine enthusiasm for his or her craft will establish an enduring and trusting relationship. Although detection of the psychologically unsuitable patient is obligatory, the number of patients in this category is small. The vast majority of preoperative rhinoplasty patients are psychologically suited for surgery. The consultant should be aware that these normally motivated persons are watching, listening, and sensing to determine if he or she is a suitable surgeon.

■ PREOPERATIVE ASSESSMENT

Motivational and Psychological Evaluation

Simple observation of the patient's affect, appropriateness of dress, voice, hygiene, and general appearance can reveal important clues to the mental state. The surgeon silently asks himself or herself, "Can aesthetic surgery help this patient?"

Even though the surgeon may know that the patient has come for a rhinoplasty consultation, it is best to ask, "What can I do for you?" Patients can then express briefly what they would like corrected. The patient usually mentions what is most important first. A mirror should not be available at this point, or the discussion will quickly evolve into the details of the surgery. It is important that the motivational factors be evaluated first. Three groups of patients are characteristically good candidates for rhinoplasty (or any facial plastic surgery):

1. The patient who has considered aesthetic correction for some time, but because of social, cultural, or financial reasons, was unable to follow through.
2. The patient who is successful, whose livelihood involves public exposure with expected good appearance (as in theater, television, public relations, sales, courtrooms, or other activities), and who wants to maintain a good image.
3. The patient with an overwhelmingly obvious aesthetic problem that dominates the appearance, but who has not fixed upon the abnormality as the basis for his or her problems.

Patients in the following groups are considered questionable:

1. *Revision surgery.* This is an entirely separate subject technically, but the motivation of these patients is also quite a separate issue. A poor result by a surgeon with a poor reputation must by handled differently from a poor result at the hands of a skilled surgeon. The former may be the result of technical mistakes; the latter may be secondary to healing problems. The expectations are always high, whereas the possibilities are usually limited. Although not the subject of this chapter, revision cases require considerable surgical experience.
2. *Unusual motivation.* Patients who come for surgery because of pressures from family, peers, spouses, or significant others are not good candidates unless the surgeon can be certain that the patient independently desires surgery. A patient who feels that his or her life or something in the world will change in some way because of the surgery is not a good candidate.
3. *The sudden decision.* The patient who makes a sudden decision about surgery may not be a good candidate, even if the physical features could reasonably be helped by aesthetic surgery. In such cases, a second consultation at an appropriately later date will separate the good candidate from the whimsical one.
4. *Previous psychiatric illness.* The patient who has previous psychiatric illness must be carefully evaluated. Usually, a formal psychiatric consultation is needed. Patients who demonstrate manic affect; paranoid responses to questions; hysterical reaction to minimal, nongraphic surgical description; or hygiene and clothing standards that are mismatched to the requested surgery may be displaying signs of overt or impend-

ing psychiatric illness. Cosmetic surgery must always be considered a major stress. Major life stresses like the loss of a loved one, loss of employment, divorce, and moving a residence are usually tolerable when they occur singly. When these life stresses occur in multiples, they can be difficult for a well-balanced person to handle. For a person who is emotionally fragile, a major life stress combined with cosmetic surgery may be intolerable. It is always best to delay surgery until there is less outside stress to interfere with the postoperative course.

Physical Evaluation

The nose must be evaluated as an entity and also in its relationship to the entire face. I have found it advantageous to have the patient withhold discussing the aesthetic goals until the examiner has completely evaluated the internal and external nose and formulated a plan for surgery that should be ideal for that patient. An experienced surgeon should be able to tell the patient, "Let me show you what I think would be the ideal nose for your face." This is a very different approach from the more familiar, "Tell me what you would like me to do for you." Almost invariably the surgeon's plan for the rhinoplasty is the same as the patient's plan. The patient will feel comforted by the surgeon's intuitive understanding of the aesthetic problem.

Examination of the nose requires an evaluation of all of the anatomic elements: (1) the tip, (2) the columella and nasal base, (3) the bony-cartilaginous vault, (4) the nasal skin, and (5) the septum and turbinates.

The most critical part of the evaluation is examination of the nasal tip. The size, shape, position, and strength of the lower lateral cartilages and the relationship of lower lateral cartilage domes will dictate the proper approach to the rhinoplasty and determine the degree of refinement possible. The most advantageous configuration of the lower lateral cartilages are cartilages that are resilient to palpation, posterior pressure, and those that have domes in close apposition so that no space is palpable between the domes. These cartilages easily retain their strength and resist long-term displacement following cephalic margin excision. The most disadvantageous condition of the lower lateral cartilages exists when they are palpably soft and easily retrodisplaced, and when the domes are either visibly separated or separate upon gentle fingertip pressure. These weak lower lateral cartilages require suture binding of the domes and/or cartilaginous strutting of the columella to support the tip and preserve an aesthetic appearance. Viewing the tip laterally, the examiner can estimate the amount, if any, of necessary aesthetic tip elevation. Ideally, the angle between the columella and lip should be 90 to 100 degrees in men and 95 to 110 degrees in women.

The columella should be positioned approximately 2 to 4 mm below the alar rim when viewed laterally. The columella, ideally, should occupy two-thirds of the nasal base, and the lobule should occupy one-third when viewed from below. The nostril should be almond- or pear-shaped, with the anterior aspect inclined medially. The nasal base width should be equal to the intercanthal width. If the lateral alar margin extends beyond the medial canthus by more than 2 mm, it may require alar base reduction. The length of the columella should be approximately the length of the upper lip.

The osseocartilaginous vault is examined for the length and position of the nasal bones and their contribution to the overall width of the upper two-thirds of the nose. Both the nasal bones and the upper lateral cartilages contribute to the nasal hump. An assessment is made of how much hump is to be removed to give the nose a "normal" appearance. Short nasal bones and long upper lateral cartilages may lead to a collapse of the middle third of the nasal pyramid following rhinoplasty. If recognized preoperatively, this outcome can be prevented. The area between the top of the nasal bones and the glabella is evaluated for depth. A deep nasion may require grafting to make the nose appear longer, and a very shallow nasion may require bone removal to give the appearance of a shorter nose. The nasofacial angle determines the projection of the nose. Ideally, this angle is 36 to 40 degrees. Beyond this ideal, the appearance of the nose becomes severe and austere. The position of the chin and the glabella also contributes to the overall appearance of nasal projection.

The texture and thickness of the nasal skin will play a major role in the final outcome of the surgery: both very thick skin and very thin skin present problems. Normal thickness of skin allows the skin to drape predictably over the altered bony-cartilaginous network. Thick sebaceous skin is overwhelmingly more common than is thin skin. Thick skin will preclude a refined nasal appearance, especially on the tip. Removal of the subcutaneous tissue at the time of rhinoplasty, especially of the tip and supratip, allows more postoperative definition than would otherwise be possible in thick-skinned individuals. The patient who has thick skin must always be aware of the aesthetic limitations caused by this condition. The thick-skinned individual is at risk for showing nasal irregularity of any minute flaw in the bony-cartilaginous framework following rhinoplasty. Care must be taken to be certain that the bone is absolutely smooth and that no sharp edges are present to any altered cartilage.

The nose must be considered the central feature of the patient's general facial anatomy. The height and slope of the forehead must be considered. A sloping forehead will give the nose a projecting appearance. A small receding chin will also give the nose an apparent projection. Augmenting the chin may be as important as the reduction rhinoplasty. A very wide face may dictate leaving the nasal pyramid fairly wide. The surgeon should see the face vertically as equal thirds, with the eyes and forehead as the upper third, the nose as the middle third, and the mouth and chin as the lower third. Horizontally, the face is seen as equal fifths, with the nose as the central fifth, the eyes as equal fifths adjacent to the nose, and the distance from lateral canthus to the malar arches are the lateral fifths. Most patients who seek reduction rhinoplasty complain of one or more of the following features: (1) a large nasal hump, (2) a wide nasal upper two-thirds, and (3) a large nasal tip. The surgeon's task is to reduce these features so that they are in balance with one another and the other facial features, as well as to leave the nose with no stigmata of the aesthetic surgery. Invariably, the patient seeking rhinoplasty today wants a conservative reduction of the nasal size. He or she is most concerned about having the nose "look operated," having the nose "too turned up," and having a final result that "does not look like myself." It is important that the surgeon listen to the patient's desires.

Preoperative Preparation

All patients are advised to avoid aspirin, nonsteroidal anti-inflammatory drugs, and vitamin E for 14 days before surgery. These medications all act as anticoagulants. The patient is encouraged to take vitamin C 2,000 mg per day for 14 days preoperatively. If the patient is a smoker, the dose must be 4,000 mg per day, because nicotine directly affects vitamin C levels. The patient is also advised to stop smoking. The patient is cautioned to avoid alcohol for at least 4 days before surgery. A prescription for vitamin K is given with instructions to take one tablet each day beginning 3 days before surgery.

Anesthesia

I prefer to perform most rhinoplasties on an outpatient basis using local anesthesia. The patient is given sodium pentobarbital, 50 mg orally, 1 hour before surgery; meperidine hydrochloride, 100 mg; and promethazine hydrochloride, 50 mg intramuscularly, 30 minutes before surgery. The effect of this combination of medications is very predictable and has been used without incident in more than 4,400 nasal procedures. In most cases, no additional intravenous (IV) medication is needed. Additionally, 4 cc of 10 percent topical cocaine is used on six cotton pledgets to anesthetize the nasal mucosa. Approximately 6 to 7 cc of lidocaine 2 percent with 1:100,000 epinephrine is used to anesthetize the external nose. Additional IV medication may be required, depending on the particular temperament of the patient or the surgeon. Appropriate monitoring is used, as with any surgical procedure.

Operative Technique

Because tip positioning is so important in rhinoplasty, this area is approached first in almost all cases. Once the surgeon has established the potential projection for the tip, the amount of osseocartilaginous reduction becomes clear.

Rhinoplasty for the large nose is *most commonly* performed through an endonasal cartilage delivery approach. A decision to deliver the lower lateral cartilages is made when the following nasal tip types are found by observing and palpating the nasal tip: (1) the domes are widely separate, (2), the domes are very weak, (3) the lateral ala of the lower lateral cartilages (LLC) of the arch far laterally, (4) the high point of the nose in profile is at the septal angle, (5) the LLC are asymmetric, or (6) there is nasal tip ptosis. All of these nasal tip configurations indicate a general weakness or inadequacy in the factors that maintain good tip support. These factors include the fibrous union between the LLC domes, the attachment of the LLC feet to the septum, the basic integrity of the LLC, and fibrous union of the LLC to upper lateral cartilages.

The other *less common* endonasal approach to rhinoplasty in the large nose is the intracartilaginous or cartilage splitting incision. When the nose is very straight in the frontal view, strong LLC are in tight unison at the tip, and in the lateral view, there is a bony hump with a well-defined supratip break, the rhinoplasty may be performed through an endonasal cartilage splitting. This type of nasal anatomy is found in many patients of Northern European heritage. These nasal configurations are in minority in the New York metropolitan area and rather common in the American Midwest. In this type of nose, the LLC cartilages may be altered without fear that distortion will occur over the years following rhinoplasty.

The least common approach to reducing the primary large nose is the open or external rhinoplasty. A large nose combined with serious traumatic asymmetry or a nose that has been previously operated on may be an indication for open rhinoplasty. I do not discuss the open rhinoplasty in this chapter.

The Endonasal Cartilage Delivery Approach

In the cartilage delivery approach, the LCC are delivered by using two incisions. The first incision is made along the cephalic margin of the LLC beginning at the lateral intercartilaginous area, 2 mm below the free margin of the upper lateral cartilage. This incision continues medially over the septal angle onto the caudal margin of the septum.. The lower incision hugs the inferior margin of the LLC. This incision begins laterally 3 to 4 mm medial to the piriform aperture attachment of the LLC and extends to the area of the soft triangle, and then onto the columella. A curved tenotomy scissors is then used to separate the LLC from the nasal tip skin (Fig. 1). In turn each of the two lower lateral cartilages is drawn down into the nares, and a MacKenty elevator is placed beneath the area of the dome. The tip of the elevator passes over the nasal tip. The dome of the LLC is presented for inspection. Some cephalic margin is removed if the height of the dome and the lateral ala immediately lateral to the dome is more than 6 mm. The cephalic margin of the dome and lateral ala are removed as a complete rim strip so that 5 to 6 mm of cartilage remains. This amount of remaining LLC gives an attractive refinement to most nasal tips. The underlying mucosa is preserved. Because the cartilage delivery approach is used in all those cases in which a lack of support or poor tip support has been demonstrated, all of these cases will require an intradomal binding suture at the conclusion of the procedure. In those cases in which LLC weakness will not allow the tip to project slightly above the dorsal line in profile, a columellar strut will also be necessary at the conclusion of the procedure. The dome suture and columellar strut are not placed at this stage of the procedure. Manipulation of the area during surgery on the septum or dorsum may disturb the final delicate balance of the tip. Occasionally, major overprojection of the nasal tip must be overcome. In these cases, the LLC are dissected to their insertion near the piriform aperture. The posterior margin of the LLC is excised in the amount necessary to reduce the overprojection millimeter by millimeter (Fig. 2). A small bridge of mucosa must remain intact at the most posterior attachment of the LLC to facilitate closure of the mucosal incisions. If the nasal tip is very ptotic with a downward thrust of the LLC, something more than a cephalic margin excision must be done to elevate the tip. A V-shaped excision of cartilage at the midlateral LLC will allow the tip to rotate superiorly. As the tip elevates, the V-incision will close to a vertical incision, with cartilage edges apposing each other. Most of the time, this incision can be

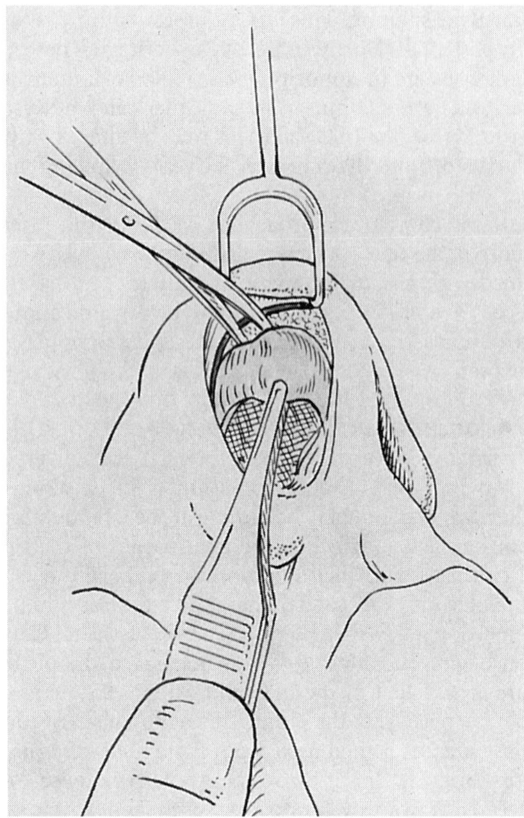

Figure 1.
Right lower lateral cartilage (LLC) shown being delivered into the nares. The cartilage is separated from the nasal tip skin as a bipedicle flap. It remains attached at the anterior columella and lateral ala. The mucoperichondrium remains attached to the posterior surface of the LLC.

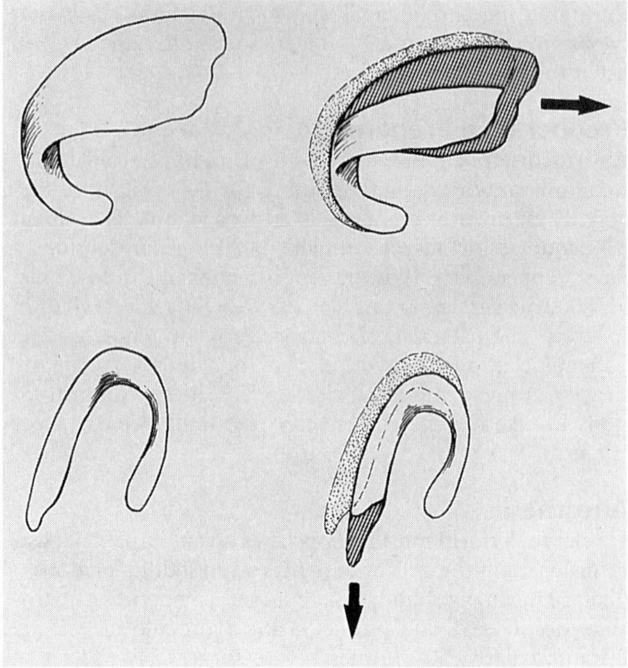

Figure 2.
In the nose with major tip overprojection, the lower lateral cartilage is separated entirely from its posterior attachment. A mucosal bridge remains intact at the posterior extent of the dissection for orientation. An amount of cartilage is removed from the posterior margin of the LLC equal to the amount of desired projection reduction. This allows for a reduced projection with minimal disturbance of the LLC.

stabilized by suturing the mucosal incisions that were made to deliver the LLC. If the vertical cartilage edges are not stable, a suture can be placed across the incision. The patient who has very thick tip skin will require a soft-tissue excision to give some refinement to the tip. A Brown-Adson forceps is used to avulse the soft tissue to the level of the dermis over the tip and down into the lateral ala if these are also thick.

Endonasal Intracartilaginous Incision Approach

This approach is limited to the nasal tip that demonstrates very strong LLC, little or no palpable separation of the domes, and a distinct supratip break. In these cases, the dome must be located precisely intranasally. The tip of a No. 15 blade is pressed gently into the apex of the mucosal surface of the dome, with just enough pressure to mark the mucosa. Cartilaginous excision takes place lateral to the mucosal mark on the internal surface of the dome. The LLC are inspected by pressing inward on the lateral ala. A mucosal incision is made from the dome mark extending laterally to approximately two-thirds the distance of the LLC. It is important that at least 5 to 6 mm of LLC remain intact following removal of the cephalic margin of the LLC. A lesser amount will not support the nasal tip and can lead to long-term postoperative deformity. It is also important that the mucosal lining of the excised LLC be preserved.

Bony-Cartilaginous Dorsum

The cartilaginous and bony dorsum are approached next. The middle third of the nose is exposed by elevating the nasal skin over the upper lateral cartilages (ULC). This is done simply with use of a No. 15 blade inserted into the incision at the intercartilaginous area and held parallel to the plane of the ULC. The loose areolar tissue separates easily with gentle pressure on the blade to the free margin of the nasal bones. The skin is elevated to the extent that it will allow the nasal bones to be viewed and to allow excision of an appropriate amount of dorsal septal cartilage. The periosteum is elevated from the nasal bones with a sharp MacKenty elevator just in the area of anticipated bony hump removal. If the periosteum is elevated lateral to the region of the lateral osteotomies, it will create a condition that allows the nasal bones to fall medially following the osteotomies because they have no lateral support.

The cartilaginous hump is removed first using an Aufricht elevator to observe the entire nasal dorsum. A long-handled No. 15 blade is placed at the bony-cartilaginous interface. With a single straight line pull, a portion of the cartilaginous hump is removed down to the septal angle. The section of cartilage should be in the shape of a tall thin isosceles triangle with its base at the septal angle. The area of the septal angle is then rounded to imitate the natural anatomy of this area. The nose is then inspected from the profile to determine if the tip is above the level of the septal angle. Additional increments of dorsal septal cartilage are removed to create an aesthetic supratip break.

In the nose with thick skin, the relationship between the position of the LLC domes and the height of the septal angle may be difficult to determine visually. Finger palpation of the supratip region will allow the surgeon to feel the level of the septal angle. Additional excision of the septal angle is counterproductive, because that action merely increases the dead space beneath the skin and encourages scar tissue formation.

Once the tip–supratip relationship is set, the bony hump is removed. A bony hump of 2 to 3 mm can easily be removed with a rasp. A No. 5 tungsten-carbide down rasp is used to remove most of the bony hump. The remaining 1 mm of bone is removed with the No. 3 tungsten-carbide down rasp to provide the smoothness necessary beneath the thin upper third dorsal nasal skin. Nasal bony humps larger than 3 mm are removed initially with the 16 mm fishtail osteotome. A few millimeters of the bony hump are left in place, which can be removed secondarily with the 3 mm rasp. In this way, the final level and smoothness of the bone can be determined precisely. Any resulting bone debris is removed with suction.

At this point, there is usually some residual elevation of the septal and upper lateral cartilages. This is determined by observation and palpation of the tip. Absolute smoothness is determined by wetting the gloved index finger and passing over the dorsum. The surgeon can be mislead by observing the dorsal septum and ULC directly, because the skin thickness varies from the tip to the nasion. Observing the nasal dorsum with the skin lying over the osseocartilaginous framework is a much more precise way to gauge the smoothness of the nasal dorsum. Small elevations of ULC are removed with the Joseph scissors. Care must be taken in the nose with short nasal bones. It is in these cases that removal of too much ULC can produce middle third collapse. For these situations, it is advisable to elevate the mucosa from beneath the junction of the nasal septum and the ULC. This will help prevent the ULC from falling medially,

If the nasion is not deep enough, the diamond carbide barrel rasp can be used to deepen it. If the nasion is very deep secondary to a frontal bossing, consideration should be given to placing a small cartilage graft beneath the periosteum of the nasion. By elevating the deep nasion, much less of the nasal hump will require removal. At this point, the dorsum should be lowered to a pleasing aesthetic level, and the tip should be at or just slightly above the dorsal line.

The Nasal Septum

At this point of the rhinoplasty, the dorsal septal excision is complete. Necessary septal and/or turbinate surgery is begun. Most septal resections, partial-thickness incisions, or manipulation, can be done by elevating the mucoperichondrium and mucoperiosteum on one side only. A columellar strut may be obtained at the time of septoplasty, or if there is no pathology the same approach can be used to obtain a portion of septum along the anterior vomer bone. This is the area of the septum where the cartilage is the thickest and strongest, even in those patients who have thin septums. If the lip-columella angle requires opening (because the tip needs elevating), a triangular base-anterior portion of the caudal septal border is resected. Any turbinate hypertrophy is handled with an elevation of the medial mucoperiosteal membrane through a small anterior incision in the inferior turbinate. Once the membrane is maximally elevated, the MacKenty elevator is used to finely comminute the turbinate bone. The turbinate is then widely lateralized. By maximally interrupting the bony scaffold, the turbinate cannot expand medially. Also, there is little bleeding caused by interrupting the mucosa at one small point anteriorly and eschewing removal of mucosa. At the conclusion of the procedure, the septum is closed with a single continuous mattress suture. The turbinate incision is not closed.

Osteotomies

A decision is made at this point concerning osteotomies. It is very rare that osteotomies are not done. Occasionally, a patient may have a large nasal tip and a very small nasal hump combined with a narrow nasal bony pyramid. In such a situation, reduction of the nasal hump with a few passes of the rasp and reduction of the tip may be all that is required. Usually, however, even modest lowering of the nasal dorsum gives the appearance of widening of the upper two-thirds of the nose. The cross-sectional anatomy is changed from a pyramid to a truncated pyramid. Osteotomies are required for this optical appearance of width. It is important that the periosteal elevation used to prepare the nasal dorsum for the hump removal not be carried down to the area of the lateral osteotomies, or the nasal bones can collapse medially. This very important caution was noted previously and is repeated here to reinforce the recommendation. Generally, osteotomies should be made as wide laterally as possible in the nasomaxillary junction. Occasionally, very wide outwardly arched nasal bones will require a double osteotomy. The most medial osteotomy of a double osteotomy is done first. The mucosa is incised at the piriform margin with inferior turbinate. This incision is not carried deeply to avoid interrupting the angular artery or vein. A MacKenty elevator is used to lift a single narrow submucosol tunnel from the area of mucosal incision to a point just medial to the lateral canthus. This serves as a pathway for the osteotome. It also lifts the vessels above the periosteum away from the osteotome. The osteotomy is generally done with a 6 mm osteotome. Much has been written about the advantages of small and guarded osteotomes to avoid bleeding and mucosal damage. The single most important feature of bloodless osteotomy is achieved in lifting the periosteum.

The osteotomy is begun just above the insertion of the inferior turbinate. It is curved at first laterosuperiorly, then superiorly, then more medially toward the medial canthus to an area just medial to the medial canthus. This preserves a triangle of bone at the nasal valve. Both lateral osteotomies are done before any attempt is made to infracture the bones. Medial osteotomies are also done in almost all cases to produce a true complete fracture. The osteotomy is directed from the free margin of the most medial aspect of the nasal bone as it joins the septum and then fades laterally to the level of the lateral osteotomy. A small bridge of intact bone between the distal ends of the medial and lateral osteotomies is easily fractured with an outward pressure of the osteotome beneath the nasal bone. Inward pressure with the surgeon's finger and thumb then moves the nasal bone medially to the desired position. It is important that the fracture be complete. A greenstick fracture from medial digital in-fracturing of the nasal bone is not enough. A consistent small percentage of greenstick fractures will lateralize, which causes unilateral or bilateral widening of the upper dorsum and necessitates secondary osteotomies. Any irregularities along the dorsum can be removed by gently dragging the No. 3 tungsten-carbide rasp downward over the nasal bones while stabilizing the bones laterally with the index finger and thumb. Any cartilaginous irregularity can be removed with the Joseph scissors.

Supporting the Underprojecting Nasal Tip

All underprojected nasal rips require suture binding of the LLC domes. The most underprojected and nonsupporting tips also require a cartilaginous strut. If dome binding alone brings the nasal tip above the dorsal profile in the lateral view, a strut is not necessary. If the tip is at the same level as the nasal dorsum, a strut will be necessary because all nasal tips fall by approximately 3 to 4 mm in the weeks following rhinoplasty. A strut of cartilage must be at least 2 cm in length to be effective. It is most easily placed by first delivering the right dome external to the nares. A pocket is then made with a blunt curbed tenotomy scissors along the medial surface of the medial crus down toward, but not to, the maxillary spine. The strut is then slid down into the pocket so that the anterior end is just below the domes. The tip of the nose is then pulled gently forward with a double-pronged hook. Several chromic sutures are placed individually through both medial crura, and a strut is sandwiched between them. The strut should not be placed directly against the maxillary spine. It will usually ride to one side, causing an irregularity at the columellar base. This maneuver will give great strength and some projection to the tip. It will prevent the tip from falling postoperatively.

The domes are brought into unison with a permanent suture (polypropylene) just between the medial curve of the domes, just at the lateral curve of the dome, or 1 to 2 mm posterior to the dome, depending on the particular nasal tip configuration. A suture is used between the medial surfaces of the domes when very little additional projection is needed, but the domes are slightly separated. The suture is placed just at the domes when the domes are widely separated; the domes arch is wide, and some additional projection is required. The most powerful suture results from the mattressing of the domes 2 to 3 mm posterior to the domes. This also gives maximum narrowing of the tip without the need to resect much of the lateral LLC (Figs. 3 and 4). The effect of the suture is to create a concave curve in the LLC to replace the convex shape that contributes to the bulbous appearance of the tip. The polypropylene suture is placed so that the knot always lies between the domes. An absorbable suture will not maintain the long-term tethering needed to maintain the tip shape. Absorbable sutures are much too reactive. Nylon sutures have an inherent reactivity that is not seen with polypropylene and are also not recommended. Additional chromic sutures are used between the columella and the caudal margin of the septum to further add to the projection of the nasal tip on the operating table. This additional projection is temporary, but may prevent losing some of the projection gained from the strut- and dome-binding sutures. As healing occurs, additional single chromic sutures are used to close the intercartilaginous incisions.

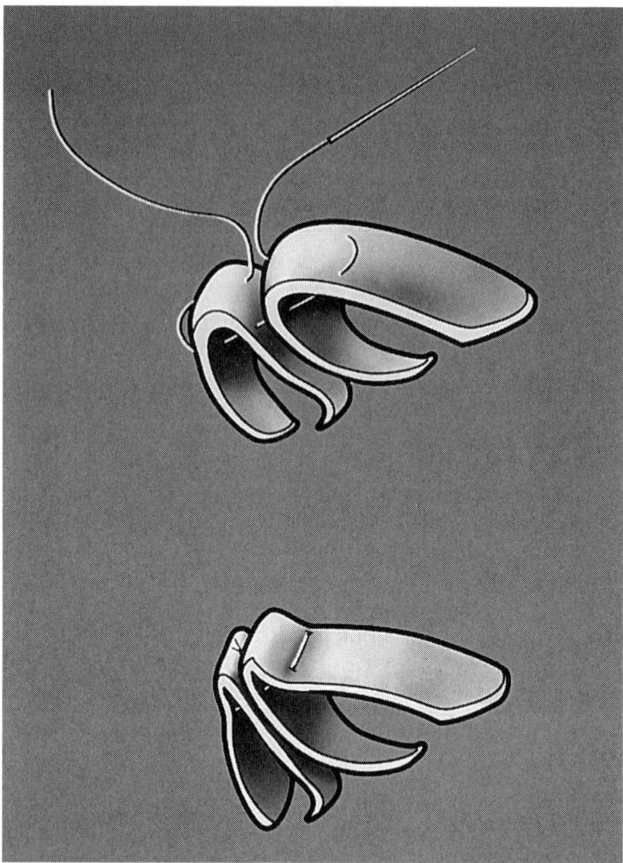

Figure 3.
The dome-binding suture gives improved strength and stability to the lower lateral cartilage in the many conditions that produce underprojection. The sutured domes resist posterior pressure, lateral flaring, and flattening.

The nasal tip judged to be adequately supported preoperatively will have been approached by the intracartilaginous incisions. No further work is necessary in the tip area. The transfixion incision in the anterior columella is closed with several sutures uniting the columella with the caudal margin on the septum. The intracartilaginous mucosal incisions are closed with multiple single sutures.

Alar Base Excision

The alar base is judged at the conclusion of the rhinoplasty. Alar base reduction should be considered if the ala have flared beyond a line dropped vertically from the medial canthus. Usually, an excision confined to the internal nares is sufficient to adequately move the ala to a more aesthetic position. Incisions that continue onto the external alar surface usually result in a scar that is difficult to improve and become a source of patient unhappiness despite an otherwise very good rhinoplasty result. This triangular or wedge-

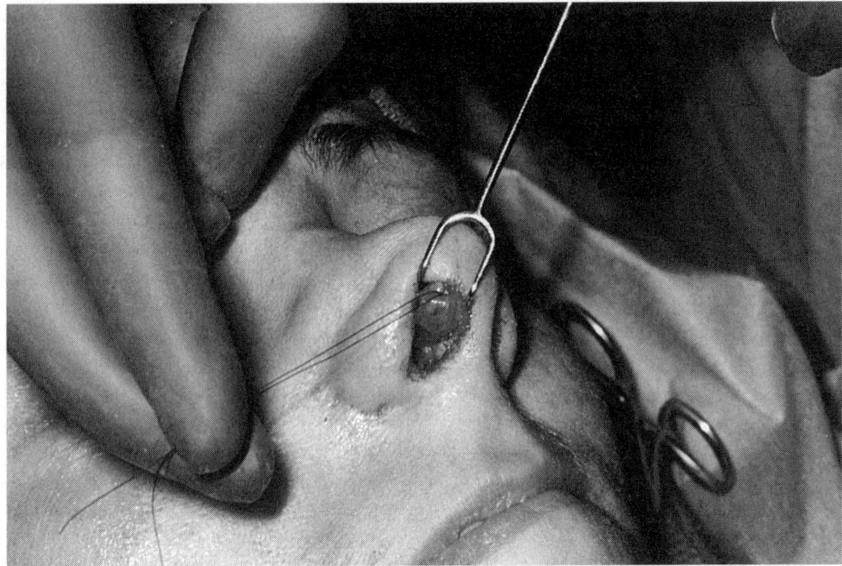

Figure 4.
A patient with an underprojecting tip. The domes are bound with a 4–0 polypropylene suture with the knot placed between the domes. The suture is cut at the knot so that no suture tail is present.

shaped skin excision at the nasal sill is closed with multiple 6-0 polypropylene sutures.

Splinting and Packing

At the conclusion of the procedure, the entire nose, but especially the tip, is compressed beneath a gauze sponge to squeeze out the edema. Then a small roll of Telfa (7 to 8 mm diameter × 2.5 cm) is placed just into and slightly internal to the nares. The purpose of this small wick is to prevent crusting at the confluence of incisions. Internal compression packing is not necessary. The continuous mattress suture of the septum precludes the need for posterior or heavy packing. The small Telfa wick is removed by the patient on the morning following the rhinoplasty. The Telfa is grasped with a tweezers and pulled downward. Ointment can find its way into the incisions and the subcutaneous space, so this is avoided with the small Telfa roll. Two layers of half inch surgical paper tape are applied to the external nasal skin and around the nasal lobule over an application of Mastisol. The taping begins at the supratip. This strip of tape defines the tip. The remaining strips are applied in shingle fashion, with the strips overlapping by 3 mm. This is continued to the nasion. The tape around the nasal lobule must be tight enough to compress the tip skin and hold it against the underlying LLC. It must not be so tight as to blanch the skin. An additional layer of Mastisol is applied over the paper tape. A thin Aquaplast trapezoid-shaped splint is heated in hot water until malleable, blotted, and applied over the paper tape. It is held firmly in place until it hardens. A mustache bandage is applied beneath the nares and changed as necessary.

The patient is instructed to remain essentially at rest until the morning following surgery, when the wick is removed. At that time, the nares are cleaned with a peroxide-soaked cotton-tipped applicator. Following the cleaning, a small amount of neomycin, polymyxin B sulfates, bacitracin (Cortisporin) ointment is used just inside the nares three times per day. Most patients use a methylprednisolone dose pack beginning on the first postoperative day. This appears to reduce the nasal edema quickly. The nasal splint remains in place for 6 to 7 days. It is removed by saturating the nasal splint with Detachol and carefully slipping a Freer elevator beneath the tape. The patient is told to anticipate edema and not the final result at the time of the splint removal. Patients who have thick or oily skin are treated immediately with an alpha-hydroxy acid solution 10 percent to 20 percent to reduce the oiliness. All patients who required soft-tissue excision at the nasal tip will require an injection of triamcinolone acetonide, 10 mg per 0.1 ml, into the supratip subcutaneous tissue with a 30 gauge needle to prevent accumulation of soft-tissue scar in the dead space. Any other patient with edema fullness of the supratip at the time of splint removal may also be a candidate for treatment with triamcinolone acetonide. Approximately half of the patients who require an initial triamcinolone acetonide injection will require a secondary treatment. Soft tissue of the supratip that is allowed to remain for a long time will eventually become mature scar tissue and will be unaffected by triamcinolone acetonide.

The patient can begin exertional activity 14 days following the procedure and progress to full activity at 30 days. During the first 7 days, exercise can induce bleeding; during the second week, exercise causes swelling.

Complications

The two functional surgical problems of infection and bleeding are very uncommon. Many surgeons who do not use antibiotics with routine primary rhinoplasty cases have an exceedingly low infection rate. Some bleeding occurs in all rhinoplasty cases. Significant bleeding requiring repacking of the nose usually occurs on the third or fourth postoperative day. It is usually associated with some inciting factor, that is, weight lifting, running, alcohol consumption, or bulimia. The bleeding usually occurs at the upper end of the lateral osteotomy site. I have encountered five significant bleeding problems in 4,400 patients during 26 years. Airway obstruction can occur from compromise of the nasal isthmus.

Aesthetic complications are far more familiar. These are the result of over-resection or under-resection of bone or cartilage, recurrent septal deviation, asymmetries secondary to scar retraction, or unequal matching anatomic landmarks, unequal osteotomies, or subcutaneous soft-tissue scar formation. The complication can also simply reflect differing aesthetic tastes between the patient and the surgeon. Consistency in rhinoplasty technique is only achieved after years of practice. Even the most accomplished surgeon knows better than to promise any patient—even one with an apparently easy case—that his or her result will certainly be good. An honest admission of the uncertainties of rhinoplasty surgery should always end each consultation.

Suggested Reading

Aarstad RF, Hoasjoe DK, Stucker FJ. Functional rhinoplasty. Facial Plast Surg 1994; 10:322-336.

Alkhairy F. Art and science in aesthetic rhinoplasty. Aesthet Plast Surg 1993; 17:37-41.

Berman WE. Reduction rhinoplasty. In: Krause, Mangat, Pastorek, eds. Aesthetic facial surgery. Philadelphia: JB Lippincott, 1991:74.

Daniel RK. The nasal tip: Anatomy and aesthetics. Plast Reconstr Surg 1992; 98:216-224.

Johnson CM Jr, Godin MS. The tension nose: Open structure rhinoplasty approach. Plast Reconstr Surg 1995; 95:43-51.

Tardy ME Jr. Rhinoplasty. In: Cummings C, ed. Otolaryngology—Head and neck surgery. St. Louis: Mosby–Year Book, 1993:807.

Toriumi DM, Johnson CM Jr. Open structure rhinoplasty. Facial Plast Surg Clin North Am 1993; 1:1-22.

THE DIFFICULT NASAL TIP

The method of
Ira D. Papel
by
Ira D. Papel
Theda C. Kontis

Surgery to refine the nasal tip is considered by many surgeons to be the most challenging aspect of rhinoplasty. Successful treatment of the nasal tip requires both knowledge of anatomy and experience with a variety of surgical techniques. Long-term follow-up is essential to understand the cosmetic and functional results of each technique. The ideal nasal tip should appear symmetric, producing a double light reflex when viewed frontally. The lateral view should present a tip with a double break, adequate projection, and proper rotation. Our preoperative analysis of the nasal tip involves critical review of tip projection, lobule definition, nasolabial angle, nostril shape and symmetry, columellar length, and the degree of columellar show. The functional patency of the internal and external nasal valves is also assessed. The nose is palpated to determine the strength of the lower lateral cartilages, the degree of tip support, and the presence of an elongated nasal spine. Preoperative analysis for nasal tip surgery requires the ability to "look through" the skin of the nose to determine the exact anatomy of the lower lateral cartilages (LLC). Deformed noses from trauma, congenital defects, or previous surgery may present unique anatomic challenges. Thin skin must be considered because minor irregularities will be obvious, whereas noses with thick skin require overcorrection to improve definition.

Historically, rhinoplastic surgeons aggressively resected both the upper and lower lateral cartilages in functional airway problems from collapse of the internal and external nasal valves, We urge conservativism in cartilage resection. The difficult nasal tip often requires augmentation of cartilage and tip support, especially in revision cases.

Preoperative counseling must include a discussion of the patient's cosmetic and functional goals and the surgeon's suggestions and expectations. The occasional need for minor revision surgery must be fully understood. If the external rhinoplasty approach is used, the columellar scar is described. The placement of internal and external nasal splints is explained; these splints are usually removed during the first postoperative week. Because edema of the nasal tip will resolve slowly, the patient must be aware that final results may not be apparent for several months to years.

Surgery is performed under either general or local anesthesia with intravenous sedation. We use prophylactic antibiotics (cefazolin intraoperatively, and cefadroxil postoperatively) on a routine basis. Dexamethsaone is empirically given intravenously at the start of the procedure.

■ SURGICAL EXPOSURE

The use of the external rhinoplasty approach in primary rhinoplasty is still a point of debate. Primary rhinoplasties in our practice are usually performed using the intranasal approach because it is unnecessary to produce an external scar with this technique. The delivery technique is ideal for patients who have wide nasal tips and thick skin, or those who have underprojected tips. The transcartilaginous incision with excision of cephalic lower lateral cartilage is also extremely useful.

The open approach is reserved for patients who have severe tip deformities, either congenital or acquired, who may require significant grafting. The open approach is also selected for patients who have had previous surgery with aggressive resection of the LLC. Such revision surgery often requires restoration of tip support, placement of multiple grafts, and correction of gross asymmetries. The columellar incision in the open approach is performed with an inverted "V" or a "stair-step" technique. Trauma to the columellar flap is avoided. Care in closure and minimal handling of the columellar skin will minimize postoperative scarring.

■ ASYMMETRIC TIP

In the aesthetic nose, the lower lateral cartilages are mirror reflections of one another, with domes juxtaposed to give a two point light reflex. Because of the central location of the nose on the face, and the eye's desire to view symmetry, nasal tip asymmetry is a glaring deformity. Nasal tip irregularities can arise spontaneously, be secondary to traumatic injury, or develop from iatrogenic causes.

Through the delivery approach, the lower lateral cartilages are analyzed and the irregularities in the cartilages are assessed. A cartilaginous strut sutured between the medial crurae of the LLC is used to both increase tip support and straighten the medial crurae, which may be buckled. The strut is placed in a pocket dissected between the medial crurae that lies above the nasal spine. The surgeon should avoid extending this pocket to the nasal spine itself, because the strut may sublux to one side of the spine, which results in asymmetry. The ideal placement of the strut should bring the domes into symmetric apposition. The domes should be separated by a distance of approximately 2 to 4 mm to preserve the double light reflex.

Tip symmetry can be restored with a variety of techniques. On occasion, portions of redundant LLC must be resected. Alar grafts may be necessary both to restore alar symmetry and to support the external nasal valve. These grafts may also function as onlay external nasal camouflage grafts, filling subtle depressions and giving the illusion of symmetry.

■ WIDE TIP

The wide or "boxy" tip results from domes that are far apart or LLCs that are flat and poorly projected. Tip definition is poor because the domes are widely separated by a soft-tissue bridge. A wide tip can occur naturally, or it may be a consequence of scar tissue forming either between the domes or subcutaneously after rhinoplasty.

The delivery approach is most often used in this scenario. The domes are delivered, and the interdomal area is defatted. When adequate tip projection is present, a double dome suture is placed. The domes are delivered through one nostril, and a through-and-through suture of 5–0 polydioxanone is placed. This serves to increase tip definition, but does not increase tip projection appreciably.

For some underprojected wide nasal tips, the modified Goldman tip technique as described by Simons is used. The LLC is divided vertically lateral to the dome, with preservation of vestibular skin. Each LLC is dissected medially, with lengthening of each medial crura. The two medial crurae are then approximated, with the cut ends of the LLC serving as the new domes, which provide increased tip definition and projection. Approximately 2 to 4 mm of separation between the new domes must be created to give the double dome appearance. This procedure should only be performed in patients who have adequate alar stiffness to tolerate a dome division. Lateral crural resection should be kept to a minimum.

In non-caucasian rhinoplasty, the LLCs are usually quite flat and weak. Division techniques are rarely useful in this situation. Increasing tip projection by cartilage grafts will also improve tip definition.

■ UNDERPROJECTED TIP

Analysis of nasal tip projection can be performed in a number of ways. Our routine tip projection analysis includes the Goode technique. This method formulates a ratio of the ala-tip distance to the nasion-tip distance. The ratio should ideally lie in the range of 0.54 to 0.59 (Table 1). Papel defined types I to IV of tip underprojection, ranging from mild tip underprojection (type II) to severe underprojection (type IV). Type I describes normal tip projection. We have developed a graduated method of tip graft fixation, depending on the degree of tip underprojection.

The delivery approach is selected, and often struts are used to increase tip support and projection. Type I (normal) projection may still require slight augmentation to create a double break, or minor asymmetries may be present that need camouflage grafting. Onlay grafts are used in such cases by placing a cartilage graft into a pocket dissected over the existing domes. Suture fixation is not used, because the pocket is designed to precisely secure the tip graft in appropriate position. Mild tip underprojection (type II) is also treated by tip onlay grafting. These grafts may be larger than those required for type I nasal tips, so graft placement may require wider undermining and percutaneous suture fixa-

Table 1. Good Classification of Nasal Tip Projection

TYPE	DESCRIPTION	PROJECTION RATIO*
I	Normal	0.54–0.59
II	Mild underprojection	0.51–0.53
III	Moderate underprojection	0.48–0.50
IV	Severe underprojection	<0.48

* Ratio of ala-tip distance to nasal-tip distance.

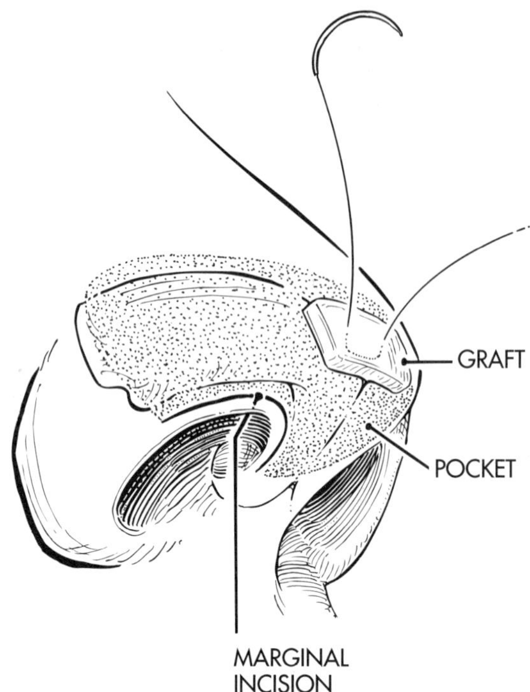

Figure 1.
Widely undermined tip with percutaneous suture fixation of tip onlay graft for type II underprojection. *(From Papel ID. A graduated method of tip graft fixation in rhinoplasty. Arch Otolaryngol Head Neck Surg 1995; 121:623–626; with permission.)*

tion (Fig. 1). The ideal position of the graft is determined, and a 6–0 polypropylene mattress suture fixes the position of the graft. The suture, placed with the knot externally, is removed 1 week postoperatively.

Moderate tip underprojection (type III) requires additional augmentation and more stable suture fixation. Wide tip undermining is required for this procedure, and both LLC are delivered (Fig. 2). A strut may be placed between the medial crurae, and a tip graft is sewn to the caudal margins of the LLCs using 5–0 polydiaxanone. If necessary, multiple grafts can be placed using this technique.

The severely underprojected nose (type IV) may occur after previous rhinoplasty and usually requires extensive augmentation. The external approach is selected to address such cases, which allows better display of the cartilaginous deformities. As described previously, a strut is often needed for increased tip support and tip graft(s) sutured directly to the LLC. When adequate septal cartilage is not present, auricular cartilage is harvested and used for grafting. These severely underprojected noses often have associated functional valve problems, alar collapse, over-resected dorsums, and so forth. Spreader grafts, alar batten grafts, and cartilaginous onlay grafts to the dorsum may be required for these difficult noses.

■ OVERPROJECTED TIP

Tip overprojection is usually caused by excessively long medial crurae or the presence of an extended intermediate crus (LLC cartilage present between the dome and medial crus). The delivery or open techniques may be used, depending on the severity of overprojection. When the delivery technique is chosen, the tip is widely undermined, and the domes are delivered. The intermediate crus is trimmed, if excessive. The LLC integrity is then restored by suturing the cut ends of the medial crurae together using 5–0 polydioxanone. If an intermediate crus is not present, excessive medial crurae are resected, and the cut ends are reapproximated. When dividing the LLC, the dome anatomy is preferably left undisturbed. The cut end of the medial crus can be tucked under the dome, and the cartilage is coapted with 5-0 polydioxanone, which preserves dome anatomy and decreases nasal projection.

A full transfixion incision diminishes tip support, and subsequent scar contracture can deproject the tip. When closing the transfixion incision, the surgeon can shift the alignment of the skin edges to further reduce tip projection. Alar wedge excisions may be necessary to prevent flaring when projection is decreased.

■ COLLAPSING ALAE AND/OR NASAL VALVES

The external nasal valve is supported by the lateral crurae of the LLC. The internal nasal valve is the angle formed by the junction of the septum and caudal margin of the upper lateral cartilage. These valves are key components of nasal airway patency.

Over-resection of the lateral crurae can result in collapse of the external nasal valve, especially when nasal skin is thin or the LLC is weak. We have seen patients who have undergone complete removal of the entire lateral crus of the LLC. This may result in a narrow, pinched tip, and severe nasal obstruction from external valve collapse.

The open approach is used in such patients. If complete transection of the LLC has been performed, and no lateral crus is present, a new lateral crus is created using conchal cartilage. Conchal cartilage has favorable shape and thickness, and septal cartilage is usually scant in these patients. If residual lateral crurae are identified, a cartilage graft is sutured to the caudal remnant as a batten to increase support of the ala and reduce valve collapse with inspiration.

When the internal nasal valve is narrowed and compromised, spreader and/or batten grafts are required. Spreader grafts are strips of cartilage positioned between the medial aspect of the upper lateral cartilage and septum. These grafts lateralize the upper lateral cartilages and widen the valve area. Although these grafts can be placed by an endonasal approach, we find that the open approach facilitates exact placement of these grafts. Septal cartilage is preferred for these grafts, and often enough cartilage can be harvested even from a previously dissected nose.

Tip and valve collapse often requires measures to increase tip projection and support, as previously described.

■ THICK SKIN OR PTOTIC TIP

Elderly patients often complain of diminished nasal airflow due to loss of tip support. These patients will characteristi-

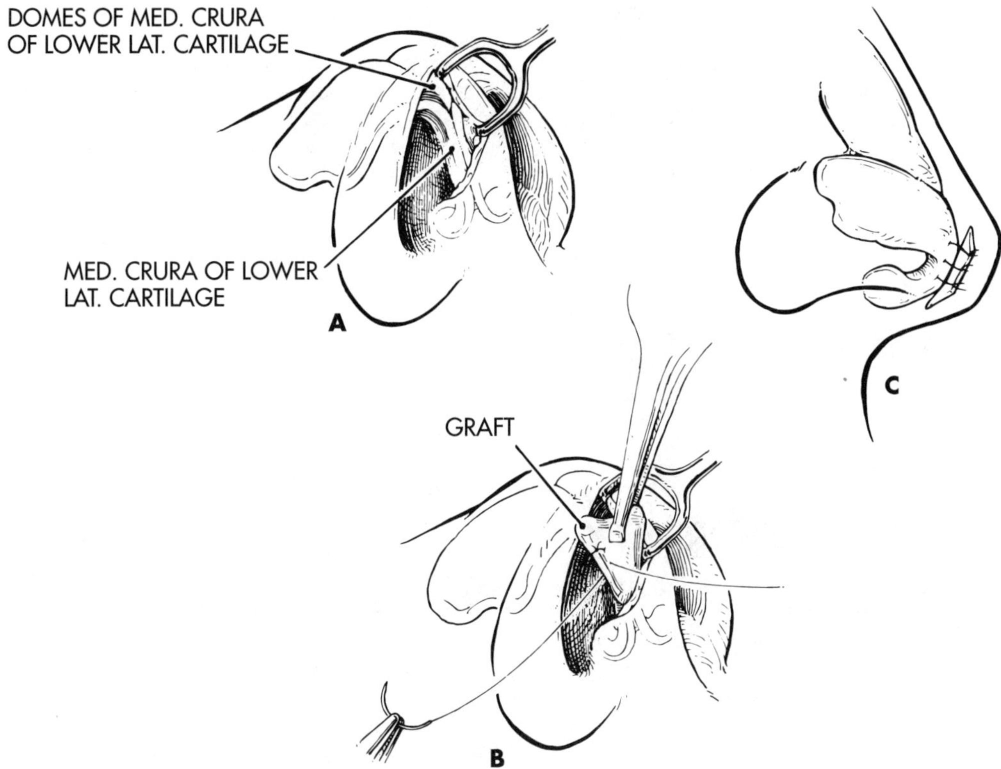

Figure 2.
Dome delivery technique with direct fixation of tip graft for type III underprojection. *A,* Exposure of LLC. *B,* Placement of tip graft. *C,* Position and fixation of tip graft. *(From Papel ID. A graduated method of tip graft fixation in rhinoplasty. Arch Otolaryngol Head Neck Surg 1995; 121:623–626; with permission.)*

cally lift up the tip of their noses to show the surgeon how they breathe better. Often, these patients are men who have thick, sebaceous skin.

A closed approach to these nasal tips is often selected, because we try to avoid external scars in these patients who have sebaceous skin, which is prone to scarring. The delivery technique is used, and the supratip area is defatted using an Brown-Adson forceps. Tip grafts and a strut are needed to augment tip support and projection. Tip grafts will increase projection and help stabilize the nasal valves. Large or multiple grafts may be required with such thick nasal skin. Alar battens may be necessary to support the alae and improve the airway. Overcorrection of these deformities is often required to maintain nasal patency. In severe cases, the lateral crural overlay technique may be necessary to help rotation.

During the postoperative period, these patients are monitored for the development of supratip fullness. If early supratip fullness is noted, injection of steroid (triamcinolone acetonide, 10 mg/mL) may be helpful. Edema may resolve slowly, and patients should be counseled appropriately.

■ DISCUSSION

In conclusion, an individualistic approach to the nasal tip is necessary for each patient. The anatomy and aesthetics of the LLC must be analyzed before and during surgery, and the appropriate technique should be selected to restore or improve form and function. Cartilage resection should be conservative. The surgeon must be facile with both closed and open approaches to rhinoplasty. In the most difficult tip cases, augmentation with cartilage grafts is necessary. We use autologous tissue at all times in the nasal tip. If septal cartilage is not available, auricular cartilage is used. Temporalis fascia may be used at times for nonstructural augmentation or camouflage of tip defects.

Suggested Reading

Adamson PA. Refinement of the nasal tip. Facial Plast Surg 1988; 5:115-134.

Constantin MB. The incompetent external nasal valve: Pathophysiology and treatment in primary and secondary rhinoplasty. Plast Reconstr Surg 1994; 93:919-931.

Constantin MB, Clardy RB. The relative importance of septal and nasal valvular surgery in correcting airway obstruction in primary and secondary rhinoplasty. Plast Reconstr Surg 1996; 98:38-54.

Goldman IB. The importance of the mesial crura in nasal tip reconstruction. Arch Otolaryngol 1957; 63:143-147.

Goode RL. Surgery of the incompetent nasal valve. Laryngoscope 1985; 95:546-555.

Johnson CM, Toriumi DM. Open structure rhinoplasty. Philadelphia: WB Saunders, 1990.

Kridel RWH, Konior RJ. Controlled nasal tip rotation via the lateral cru-

ral overlay technique. Arch Otolaryngol Head Neck Surg 1991; 117: 411-415.
Papel IP. A graduated method of tip graft fixation. Arch Otolaryngol Head Neck Surg 1996; 121:623-626.
Peck GC. The onlay graft for nasal tip projection. Plast Reconstr Surg 1983; 71:29-37.
Sheen JH. Spreader graft: A method of reconstructing the roof of the middle nasal vault following rhinoplasty. Plast Reconstr Surg 1984; 73: 230-237.
Sheen JH, Sheen AP. Aesthetic rhinoplasty. St. Louis: CV Mosby, 1987.
Simons RL. Vertical dome division techniques. Facial Plast Surg Clin North Am 1994; 2:435-458.
Toriumi DM. Management of the middle nasal vault in rhinoplasty. Op Tech Plast Reconstr Surg 1995; 2:16-30.

SADDLE NOSE DEFORMITY

The method of
Craig S. Murakami
Robert Guida

The term *saddle nose deformity* is a nonspecific description of a nose with a depression over its dorsal surface. The actual depth of depression, the degree of nasal obstruction, and the physical findings may vary considerably from patient to patient. The literature is filled with a wide range of treatment recommendations for the saddle deformity. This vast array of treatment options corresponds with the wide spectrum of deformities that fall under this title and the difficulty surgeons often encounter when treating severe saddle deformities. The spectrum of deformity ranges from a patient who has a mild supratip depression and a normal airway to a patient who has a massive depression of the entire bony-cartilaginous nasal complex associated with severe nasal obstruction. The treatment techniques for correcting saddle nose deformities obviously vary and range from simple onlay grafting to complex reconstruction that might require bone grafts with internal fixation, cartilage grafts, composite grafts, or soft-tissue flaps. In this chapter, we review the workup, analysis, classification, and the options available for treating the various types of saddle nose deformities.

■ HISTORY AND PHYSICAL EXAMINATION

A successful outcome in medicine and surgery always begins with a thorough history and physical examination. The surgeon must determine each patient's aesthetic concerns and also define the functional goals in terms of the nasal airway.

The etiology of the saddle nose deformity may be congenital, traumatic, iatrogenic, infectious, or pathologic. It is important to determine the etiology because the deformity may be one that progresses or fluctuates, and there may be an ongoing pathologic process that requires medical management. The most common cause of saddle deformity is trauma. Iatrogenic causes can be included within this group because the saddle is essentially the result of surgical trauma.

The patient's general health should be reviewed to rule out systemic causes of saddle nose deformity, such as relapsing perichondritis, Wegner's disease, syphilis, T-cell lymphoma (lethal midline granulomatous disease), or a paranasal sinus malignancy. These systemic diseases and malignancies are destructive processes that lead to perforation of the septum and loss of dorsal nasal support. Obviously, a diagnosis of this nature requires medical management before reconstructive surgery.

Reviewing the records of previous surgery(ies) may be helpful to determine the position of previous grafts and incisions. The surgeon should know the previous cartilage donor sites so that healthy cartilage can be obtained with minimal risk of septal perforation, ear deformity, or pneumothorax.

During the examination, the surgeon must determine the status of the bony pyramid, the septum, the upper lateral cartilages and nasal valve region, and the lower lateral cartilages and nasal tip. Intranasally, the surgeon must pay particular attention to the nasal valve and its effect on the nasal airway. The general health of the tissue in this region is also assessed to determine whether there is a great deal of scar contracture or tissue thickening. In general, patients who have small saddle depressions in the supratip region have normal airways. However, even patients who have small external deformities may have significant airway obstruction if nasal valve collapse is present. It is important to determine the status of the nasal valve, because placing a dorsal onlay graft to correct the supratip saddle may not adequately address the nasal valve collapse and may actually exacerbate and stabilize the nasal obstruction.

One must determine whether the nasal valve collapse is secondary to loss of cartilaginous support or secondary to nasal stenosis caused by scar contraction of the inner nasal lining. In cases of nasal stenosis, the collapsed valve is fixed in position, and during examination the nasal airway will not improve with lateral traction on the cheek or manual rotation of the nasal tip superiorly. Many patients who have nasal stenosis have had previous surgery. Often, they have undergone multiple attempts at reconstruction in which numerous incisions have been used with inadequate grafting techniques that fail to open the nasal valve.

The septum is examined, and if a septal perforation is present, the surgeon must carefully inspect the margins of the perforation to assess the general health of the remaining septal cartilage and mucosa. The margins of the perforation are gently palpated with a cotton-tipped applicator to determine the size and stability of the dorsal and caudal struts, because they are vital support structures. The condition of the remaining septum and the size of the perforation will determine whether the perforation is repairable.

■ CLASSIFICATION

Once the history and examination is completed, we find it helpful to classify the saddle deformity into one of five broad types.

Type 1

A type 1 deformity is a mild supratip saddle with a normal airway. Supratip depression of 1 to 2 mm from the tip defining point is generally acceptable, but depressions beyond that are considered to be a mild saddle deformity. For these patients, the deformity is usually secondary to trauma or previous surgery, but occasionally it is congenital.

Type 2

In a type 2 deformity, there is moderate depression of the dorsal septum and upper lateral cartilages, with mild collapse of the nasal valve. In these patients, the collapse of the nasal valve will cause nasal obstruction, and a simple onlay graft may not improve the nasal airway.

Type 3

Type 3 deformity consists of moderate depression of the dorsal septum and the upper lateral cartilages with nasal stenosis. In these patients, the inner lining of the nose is also contracted; additional lining may be required along with cartilage grafts.

Type 4

In a type 4 deformity, there is depression of the cartilaginous and bony nose, with an intact but deviated septum. These patients require large onlay grafts of bone and cartilage, or both. The status of the nasal valve must be addressed, as is the case for the other types. The deformity in these patients is usually secondary to severe nasoethmoid-complex trauma and may be associated with traumatic pseudotelecanthus.

Type 5

The most severe deformity is a massive depression of the cartilaginous and bony nose without a septum. These patients will require large bone grafts that may need to be cantilevered to provide dorsal support, because the graft cannot be placed in an onlay fashion. In some patients, the inner mucosa and the external skin of the nose is deficient or contracted, and in some of these patients, a forehead flap may be necessary to provide additional skin to correct the saddle deformity.

Although this classification scheme is broad, it helps to clarify the extent of the deformity and assists in surgical planning. Accurate evaluation and planning will lead to a satisfactory cosmetic and functional result.

■ THERAPY

Once the classification has been determined, the surgeon has roughly established the level of surgical complexity that is necessary to correct the deformity. This information is helpful to both the surgeon and the patient in terms of perioperative and operative planning.

Type 1

For mild supratip saddle deformities, a simple onlay graft of septal or conchal cartilage placed into a small pocket through an intercartilaginous incision is generally recommended. For larger depressions that do not affect the nasal valve, we still prefer using layered autologous cartilage, although some surgeons prefer synthetic implants such as solid silicone or Gore-Tex. Dorsal augmentation of Asian or African-American noses are examples where synthetic implants are commonly used.

Type 2

For moderate-sized depressions associated with nasal valve collapse, the nose is approached using an open technique and a transcolumellar incision. Others may prefer to use an endonasal approach. In type 2 cases, the upper laterals are separated from the dorsal septum, and the mucosa is elevated from the septum bilaterally. In our technique, a single onlay spreader graft is designed from conchal or septal cartilage. It is cut into a trapezoid shape approximately 3 to 4 mm along the superior margin, 5 to 8 mm along the inferior margin, and 15 mm in length (Fig. 1). The onlay spreader straddles the depressed dorsal septum and is sutured to the margins of the upper lateral cartilages. This single spreader onlay graft serves to open the nasal valve and simultaneously elevate the depressed saddle deformity. Occasionally, bilateral medial osteotomies are done before placement of the onlay spreader graft to outfracture the nasal walls and help open the nasal-septal angle. Multiple trans-septal sutures are then placed beneath the onlay graft to reapproximate the mucosa to the septum and support the graft. This also prevents webbing of the nasal valve mucosa at the nasal-septal angle. Intraoperative improvement of the nasal-septal angle should be observed. If the dorsal profile is still undercorrected, a simple dorsal onlay graft can be placed over the onlay spreader graft. The single onlay spreader graft in the type 2 deformity is preferred over two separate Sheen-type spreader grafts, because the dorsal septum is depressed in the saddle nose deformity, and placing separate spreader grafts on either side of the depressed septum will not increase dorsal projection. The single onlay spreader graft not only increases the dorsal projection, but also lateralizes and dorsally elevates the medial margin of the upper lateral cartilages.

Type 3

For cases of moderate depression with nasal stenosis, we use the same external approach and separate the upper lateral

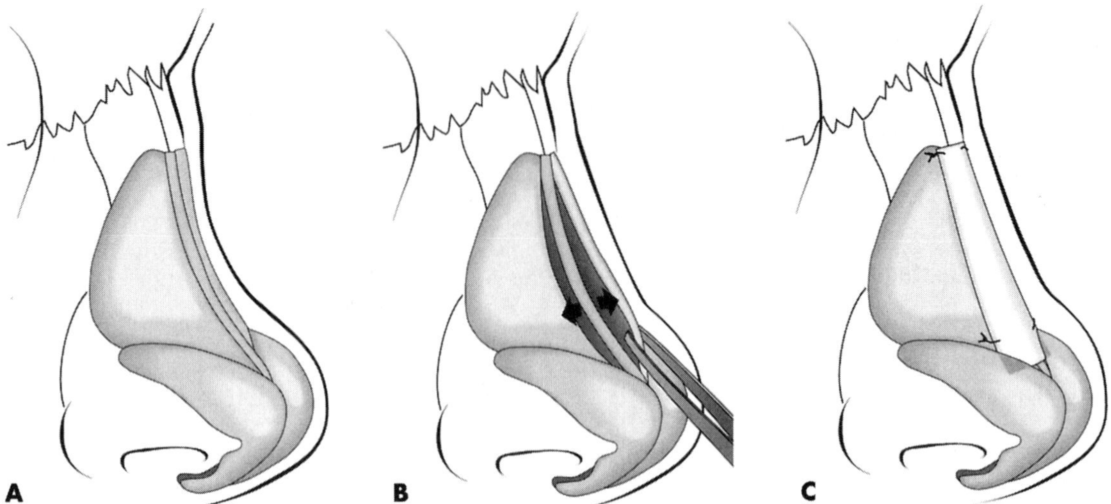

Figure 1.
Type 2 saddle nose deformity. *A*, Collapse of the nasal dorsum and narrowing of the upper lateral cartilages and nasal valve. *B*, The upper lateral cartilages are separated from the dorsal septum to open the nasal-septal angle and expand the nasal valve. *C*, Placement of the onlay spreader graft stabilizes the nasal valve and projects the dorsal profile.

cartilages from the septum. The mucosa is mobilized, and if the stenosis improves or resolves, the reconstruction is done using the onlay spreader technique as described in type 2. However, if the stenosis remains, the nasal valve stenosis is opened by making an incision through the mucosa on either side of the septum. An elliptical composite graft of skin and cartilage is harvested from the posterior conchal bowl. The skin on the graft is vertically transected across the short axis, creating two islands of skin fixed to the cartilage. The composite graft is then straddled over the dorsal septum and sutured into position. The nose is packed with a soft sponge dressing for 3 to 5 days. In many of these patients, the nasal tip has also lost projection due to collapse of the septum and the septal angle. This problem is addressed in the standard manner using columellar struts and tip grafts.

In cases in which there is massive loss of the dorsal cartilaginous and bony support, a graft of sizable dimensions is required. Our first choice is autologous septum and conchal cartilage (sometimes bilaterally) and pieces of the vomer or perpendicular plate. However, these defects often require larger grafts, and we generally prefer using split calvarial bone or rib. If rib is selected, the graft is harvested at the bony-cartilaginous junction so that the graft is part cartilage and part bone. The cartilaginous portion is placed distally over the cartilaginous septum, which gives the nose a more natural texture on palpation. The bony portion is placed under a subperiosteal pocket to enhance fixation and prevent displacement of the graft. The bone grafts may be layered to provide additional volume, and occasionally the grafts are secured with a single lag screw placed through a percutaneous incision. The nasal valve may have to be addressed, as is the case for Types 2 and 3.

Some surgeons may prefer using implants in type 4 cases. Acceptable implants include Gore-Tex (expanded polytetrafluoroethylene), or Medpor (high density polyethylene polymer), and Mersilene mesh (polyethylene mesh). These grafts have pores that allow fibrous ingrowth and stabilization of the grafts, which reduces the incidence of infection and extrusion compared with solid silicone implants.

Type 5

This category is reserved for massive saddle nose deformities where there is complete loss of bony-cartilaginous support, and the dorsum of the nose is essentially parallel or flush with the plane of the anterior maxilla. The soft-tissue envelope of the nose is often contracted and atrophic, which makes using this tissue for reconstruction difficult. Many of the patients in this category are cancer patients who have undergone extirpation of large intranasal or paranasal sinus carcinomas. Postoperative radiotherapy is often part of their treatment protocols, which makes overlying tissues exceptionally fragile.

It is essential that structural support of the nose is recreated using bone grafts. Unfortunately, it is often impossible to place cantilevered bone grafts between the fragile skin and the atrophic inner lining of the nose without risking eventual graft exposure and extrusion. In these cases, the surgeon may be forced to transfer healthy soft tissue from distant sites such as the forehead to protect the grafts. The skin overlying the dorsum and nasal tip of the saddle deformity is de-epithelialized, and cantilevered bone grafts are placed over this surface and secured to the frontal bone using a microplating system. A full-thickness (including galea) forehead flap is transferred to cover the reconstructed framework of bone grafts. The galea is partially separated from the skin flap and wrapped around the undersurface of the bone grafts to fill in dead space and protect the grafts.

Occasionally, the surgeon may need to replace the inner lining of the nose with healthy tissue in addition to the overlying skin. In these cases, we have been using a number of techniques with variable success. If large amounts of tissue are necessary, a staged radial forearm flap is used with a skin graft, followed by de-epithelialization of the skin graft, bone grafting, and forehead flap reconstruction. If smaller amounts of inner lining are needed, a turbinate mucosal flap or staged melolabial flap is used.

REVISION RHINOPLASTY

The method of
M. Eugene Tardy, Jr.
by
M. Eugene Tardy, Jr.
Steven H. Dayan

The patient requesting secondary rhinoplasty presents both complex psychological and anatomic problems to the nasal surgeon. Having experienced one or more failed procedures, disenchantment with the surgical process (and even the surgeon) represents a common preoperative psychological condition. Permanent alteration of the nasal tissues (scar formation, obliteration of surgical tissue planes, alteration of skin thickness and elasticity) dictate significant limitations in the process of reconstruction. It is essential, therefore, that patients understand and accept the potential limitations inherent in revision surgery.

■ GENERAL PRINCIPLES

Secondary rhinoplasty embodies different, as well as many of the same, surgical principles involved in primary rhinoplasty. Because the nasal soft tissues and skeletal support foundations have been disturbed, removed, or reoriented, new approaches and procedures must be invoked after a thorough palpation and inspection of the anatomic conditions encountered. The presence and magnitude of inevitable scar tissue influences planning for the type and extent of surgical intervention, and may limit possible improvement. In particular, any damage to or thinning of the investing skin–subcutaneous tissue complex plays a vital role in what can and cannot be accomplished. Decisions must be made about whether it may be more appropriate and safe to engage in a major dissection and exploration of the nasal anatomy via the external approach, or whether more limited incisions and dissection created through endonasal approaches place the damaged tissues, and therefore the patient, at less risk by improved control of healing. It is axiomatic that each successive revision rhinoplasty procedure may render the anticipated outcome less predictable, due to the vagaries of scar tissue healing and diminished blood supply. Thus, accurate preoperative diagnosis is vital to correction of the problem in a final restorative procedure.

The vast majority of revision rhinoplasties can be categorized as operations in which less was accomplished (underoperation) than was required, more was carried out (overoperation) than necessary, or a combination of these two scenarios. Common among secondary cases are those noses in which an incomplete primary operation has occurred (Fig. 1). The surgeon must accurately diagnose the deficiencies and create a plan to complete the procedure in order to produce a more finished project. Equally common are those noses in which overaggressive surgery has produced deformities, requiring at the very least restoration of supportive structure by grafting and augmenting with appropriate materials to restore balance, function, and harmony (Fig. 2). In addition, asymmetric noses often displease patients and require reoperation. Rhinoplasty is, after all, the consequence of two operations carried out on opposing sides of the nose in an attempt to produce a single symmetric midline organ of refinement and elegance. Finally, copious combinations of the previously described surgical shortcomings are encountered, in which attention must be devoted to adding to, subtracting from, and regularizing the previously operated nose to achieve an acceptable outcome.

■ GUIDELINES IN SECONDARY RHINOPLASTY

Three decades of experience in rhinoplasty have illuminated significant principles and guidelines that are deemed useful in secondary rhinoplasty. This arduous learning curve may be significantly shortened by religiously studying the evolving dynamics of the nasal healing process through graphic records coupled with longitudinal standard and uniform photographs (Fig. 3). The "Ten Commandments in Secondary Rhinoplasty" are offered as a helpful guide to surgeons involved and interested in the nuances of revision rhino-

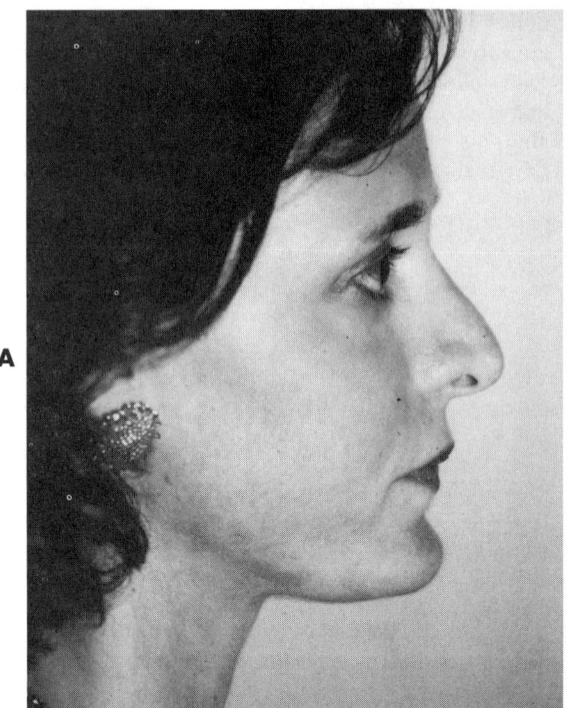

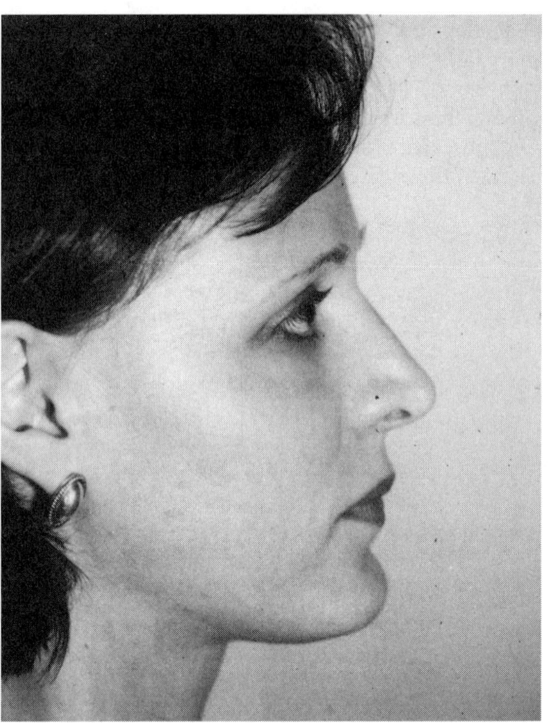

Figure 1.
A, Classic example of rhinoplasty complication in which an incomplete and unfinished operation has occurred, requiring further reduction rhinoplasty to effect improvement. *B,* Following revision correction.

plasty (Table 1). Clearly, additional principles will occur for treating individual and unique noses.

Ensure That Improvement Is Possible

It is always tempting to attempt to revise every nasal deformity, no matter how difficult or problematic. Not all rhinoplasty deformities can be satisfactorily corrected, and in fact some may be made worse by surgical intervention. The wise surgeon distinguishes, by psychological evaluation and painstakingly precise diagnosis, between those problems that can be reasonably helped and those that clearly cannot ("in the first place do no harm"). Noses that are still twisted after multiple operations represent very difficult challenges to straightening, which may only be realized by cartilage grafting to provide the "illusion" of straightening.

Make an Accurate Diagnosis

This principle is essential for assuring the first principle. Palpation of the suppleness, mobility, and scarring of the skin–subcutaneous tissue complex is equally important to visual inspection of the topography and internal airway of the nose. Determining which anatomic components of the nose require repair (reduction, augmentation, or reorientation) and, just as important, which do not, is vital. Determinations must be made about which regions of the nose require additional reduction, and which require supplemental augmentation. In deviated noses, the elements creating the deviation must be clearly identified before effective repair is possible. The presence or absence of residual septal cartilage, confirmed by palpation and/or transillumination, provides information about the need for cartilage grafts from the auricle or rib if septal cartilage is absent.

Of even greater importance in the diagnostic process is the psychological determination of whether the patient's expectations can be realized, which is a task often more difficult than that of physical diagnosis.

Instill Realistic Patient Expectations

The over-riding goal of every rhinoplasty, primary or secondary, is to make the patient happy. Unless a clear comprehension of the patient's concerns and expectations is understood, it is unlikely that any outcome, no matter how well achieved in the surgeon's mind, will be successful. Because of differences in experience as well as aesthetic preferences, the surgeon and patient may harbor entirely different expectations about revision surgery. It is mandatory to place the patient in front of a three-way mirror and require a detailed description of what is disliked and what is expected. Because it is not always possible to correct every complication of rhinoplasty, it is useful to gently demand of the patient, in order of preference, a ranking of what problems are most disturbing. Nowhere in aesthetic facial surgery is true informed consent more important. Limitations of reparative surgery must be stressed, with realistic acceptance by the

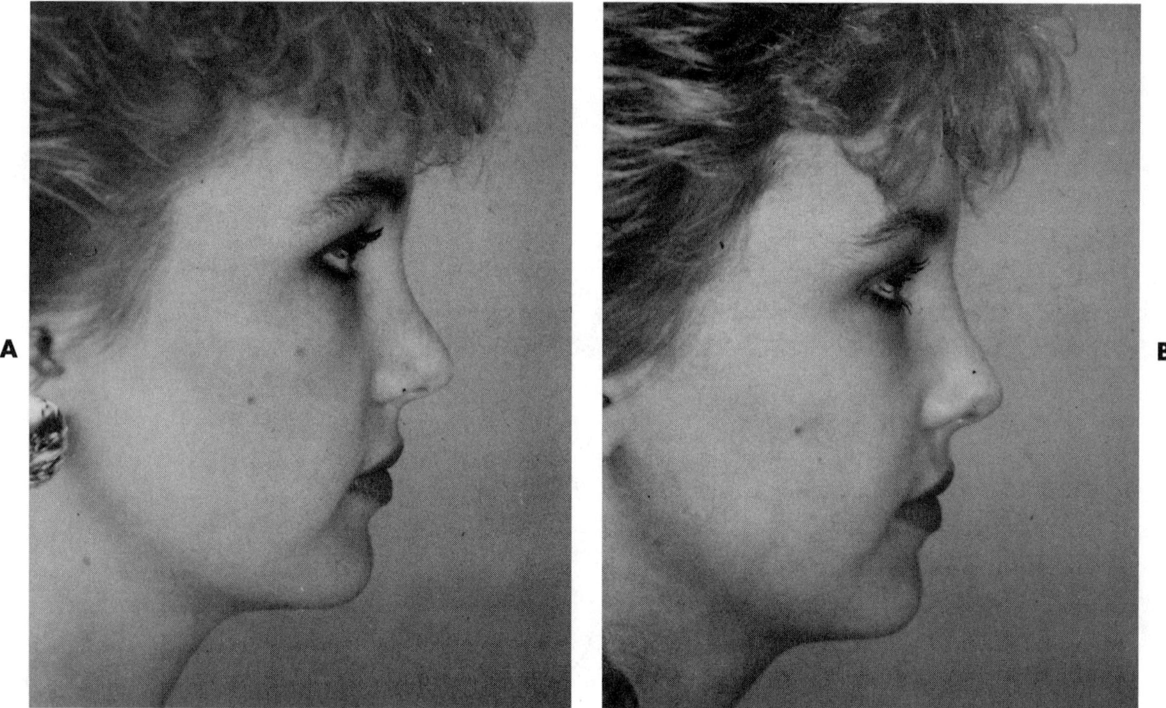

Figure 2.
A, In this patient, an overaggressive reduction of the dorsum has led to serious visible disharmony of proportion; *B,* Correction of over-reduced profile with cartilage onlay grafts.

patient being the passport to undertaking surgical attempts at revision.

Consider Surgical Timing Carefully

Surgical textbooks commonly recommend a delay of at least 1 year before undertaking revision rhinoplasty. Certainly, it is true that at least this period must elapse before scar tissue is sufficiently mature to withstand additional repair without worsening the complication. Depending on the amount and degree of trauma created by the first operation, a delay of more than 1 year may be necessary to ensure safety and predictable healing. Exceptions to this temporal principle exist and, properly diagnosed and understood, they will allow revision much sooner than 1 year and promote earlier patient satisfaction without undue risk. An incomplete, inadequate, or lateralized greenstick osteotomy may be safely and effectively infractured early after detection. Alar base reduction, deferred at the primary operation, does not require months of healing to carry out for ultimate improved refinement of nasal proportion. Likewise, alar retraction in the early postoperative period may be safely corrected with internal alar composite grafts. Rasping of an asymmetry or minimal elevation of the nasal bony profile is generally safe and effective within several months after primary rhinoplasty. Other modest corrective procedures, if they involve minimal and limited tissue dissection, may be safely performed. All major surgical revisions, particularly those requiring structural grafting, should always be delayed until the tissues are pliable, scar tissue is supple and mature, and few further healing changes are anticipated. In general, patients who have thin skin may be safely reoperated earlier than those patients who have thick, sebaceous skin quality.

Table 1. Ten Commandments in Secondary Rhinoplasty

1. Ensure that improvement is possible
2. Make an accurate diagnosis
3. Instill realistic patient expectations
4. Consider surgical timing carefully
5. Diagnose and correct functional problems
6. Plan reconstruction options and alternatives
7. Limit surgical dissection
8. Implant autogenous tissue only
9. Maximize concepts of "illusion" in revisions
10. Avoid irreparable deformities

Diagnose and Correct Functional Problems

A common indication for revision surgery is failure to correct nasal obstruction from septal deviation or deformity. Thorough rhinoscopy following shrinkage of the nasal mucosa should reveal the majority of obstructive problems. Also necessary may be correction of nasal valve collapse, turbinate hypertrophy, alar collapse after over-reduction of alar cartilages (Fig. 4), and overnarrowing of the nasal bony pyramid.

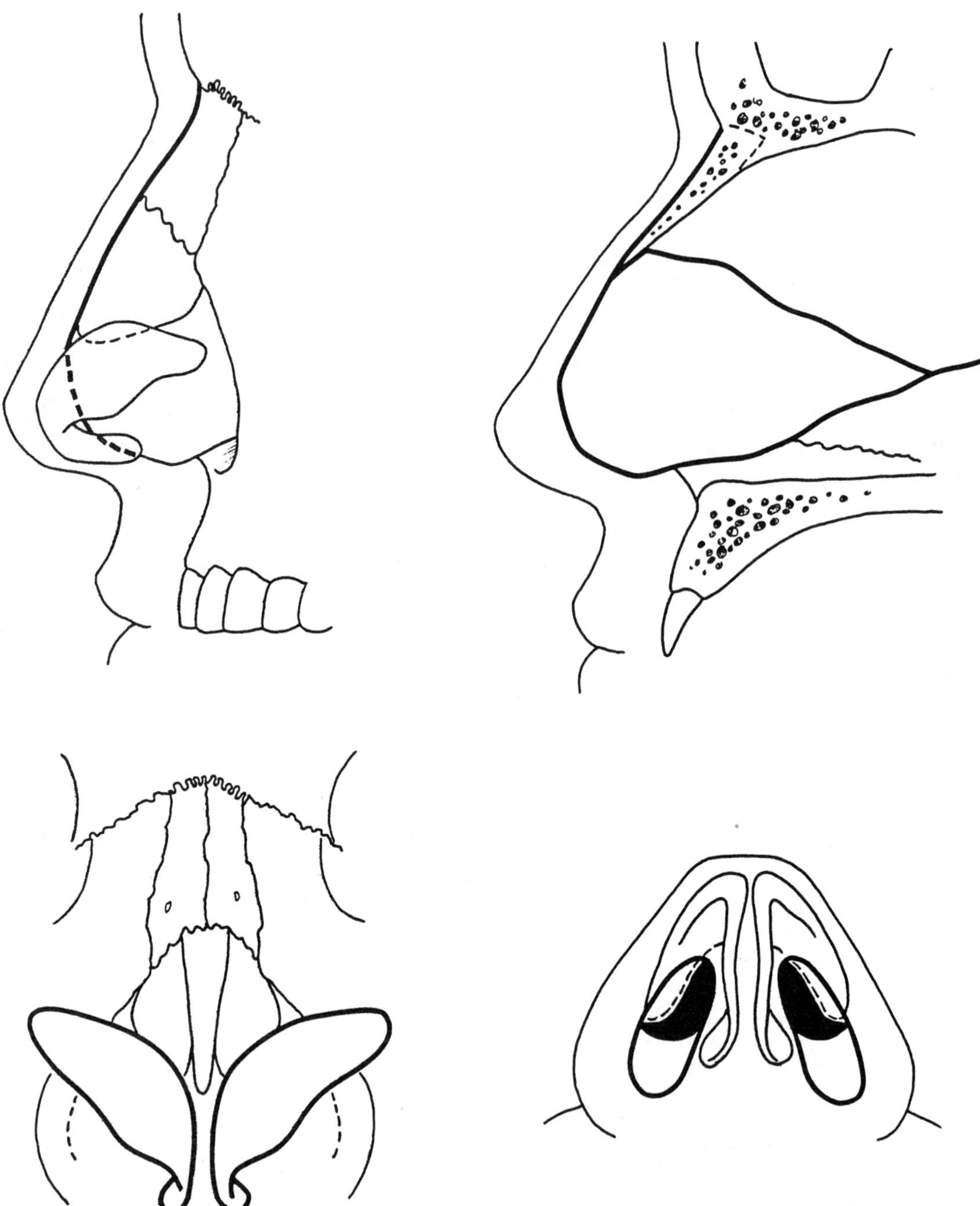

Figure 3.
Graphic record of rhinoplasty procedure completed immediately after surgery and used as an important adjunct to standardized photographs to analyze long-term postoperative outcomes.

A 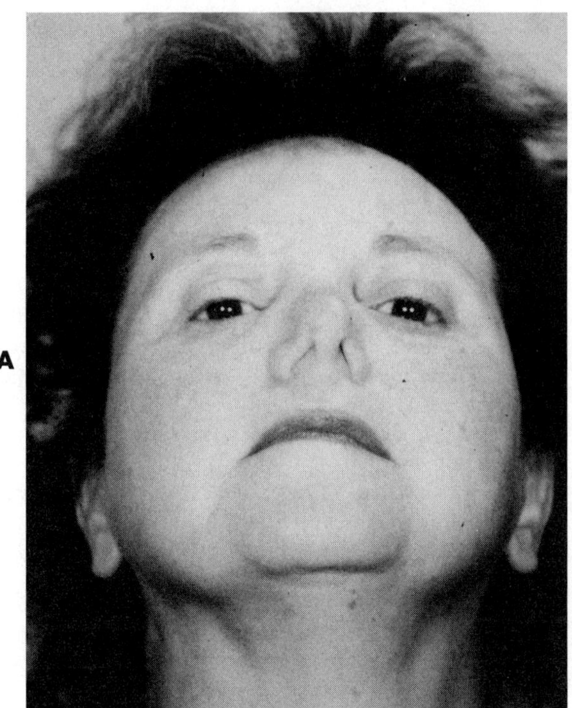

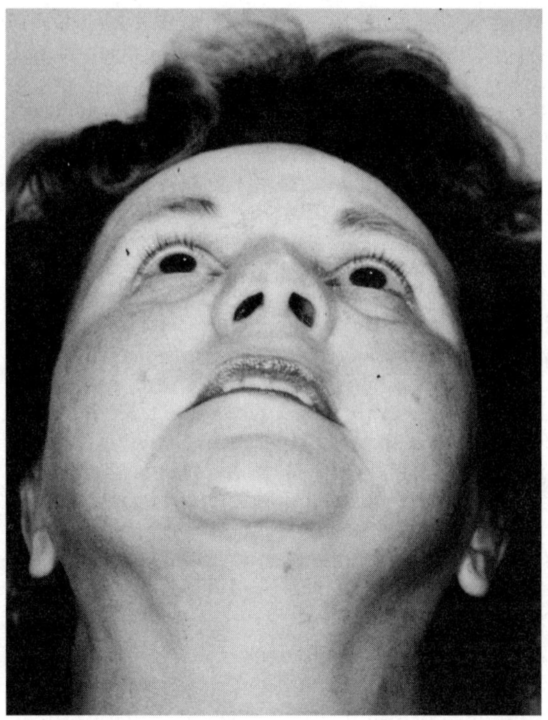 B

Figure 4.
A, Inspiratory alar collapse after over-reduction of supportive lower lateral cartilages, which is a commonly encountered postoperative complication; *B*, After insertion of convex alar batten graft from auricle.

Plan Reconstruction Options and Alternatives

Unlike primary rhinoplasty, where studious inspection and palpation reveals for the experienced surgeon a clear understanding of the surgical needs to be employed, revision rhinoplasty not uncommonly leads to surprises upon entering the nose. Subcutaneous scar tissue often imparts unpredictable contours to the external cutaneous topography, which may change significantly when undermining of the soft-tissue sleeve is undertaken. Dense scar likewise hinders accurate palpation of the skeletal support of the nasal tip. During revision rhinoplasty, the surgeon must remain flexible as the dynamics of the operation unfold differently than might be expected. In particular, plans for grafting with cartilaginous or soft-tissue autografts are essential in the majority of secondary procedures. Surgical improvisation, based on experience and good surgical judgment, requires that the successful revision rhinoplasty surgeon possess mastery of a wide variety of reconstruction techniques to manage the myriad number of complications possible after rhinoplasty.

Limit Surgical Dissection

The blood supply of the scarred nose is tenuous and unpredictable; extensive dissection and undermining involve increasing risk of poor healing. In the majority of reconstructive revision rhinoplasties, it is judicious to limit dissection of nasal tissues to the minimum possible to gain exposure. Less additional scar is produced, unpredictable healing is minimized, and the visual results of tissue grafting are readily and more quickly apparent. If dissection in several regions of the nose is required, we prefer to create several different precise tissue pockets, through limited incisions, to gain access to the nose for either reduction or augmentation surgery.

The exposure provided by the external rhinoplasty approach is unparalleled and provides the surgeon with the twin benefits of binocular vision and bimanual surgery. We reserve this approach, which requires extensive tissue dissection, for those revision patients who require exploration for unexplained deformities and severe distortion of the nasal tip, and when large grafts require suture-fixation for long-term stabilization.

Implant Autogenous Tissue Only

The previously operated nose, especially if blood supply is compromised and the skin–subcutaneous tissue complex is damaged, scarred, or attenuated, supports all forms of alloplastic implants poorly. Respected surgeons worldwide are near unanimous in their preference for autogenous tissue implant reconstruction in secondary rhinoplasty. We prefer autogenous cartilage (septal, auricular, rib); bone; fascia (temporalis or facial superficial musculoaponeurotic system); dermis; and occasionally mature scar tissue (if available) for nasal reconstruction. Particularly in the young patient undergoing revision rhinoplasty who has a life expectancy of 60 to 70 years, the demonstrated long-term safety of autogenous materials is deserved. In the near future, biogenetic engineering will undoubtedly be able to provide unlimited quantities of cloned nonimmunogenic cartilage for effective and safe reconstruction of damaged noses.

Maximize Concepts of "Illusion" in Revisions

In many secondary rhinoplasties that are chosen with care, elegant refinement can be achieved by creating visual illusions from changing nasal proportions or by grafting. Difficult deviated noses may be "straightened" by carefully designed cartilage grafts on or along the nasal dorsum. The over-rotated nose may be visually "lengthened" by dorsal onlay grafting combined with cartilage grafts to the infratip lobule (Fig. 5). Recessing the dependent "hanging" columella may render an apparently overlong nose proportionate. Wise surgeons recognize that not every revision patient requires a complete secondary rhinoplasty; improvement is often best achieved with more conservative but equally effective surgery.

Avoid Irreparable Deformities

Every rhinoplasty surgeon will encounter from time to time patients who have deformities of such serious nature that no amount of surgical skill or ingenuity can hope to provide satisfactory correction. Although often difficult, it is always judicious to gently refuse operation to such patients, because the outcome will undoubtedly be unsatisfactory to both patient and surgeon alike.

■ ILLUSTRATIVE CLINICAL EXAMPLES

To demonstrate the usefulness of many of the aforementioned principles and guidelines, four clinical examples are examined that incorporate the thought processes and techniques previously expressed.

Case 1

A 25-year-old schoolteacher underwent primary rhinoplasty 11 years previously elsewhere (Fig. 6). The immediate and long-term outcome has led to increasing dissatisfaction and negative comments by friends and colleagues. Immediately after the initial surgery, she voiced concerns to her surgeon about over-reduction of the nasal dorsum and low nasal bridge. As healing progressed over the years, tip asymmetry and bossae became more evident. Nasal breathing was difficult due to a significantly deviated septum to the right.

Analysis

A marked disproportion between the upper nose and the tip is immediately apparent. The dorsum appears wide and "washed out." Prominent asymmetric bossae exist, with tip bifidity apparent as a consequence of diverging intermediate crura. Exquisitely thin skin accentuates the tip abnormality. Clefting exists between the crura. A significant alar-columellar disproportion exposes an excess of vestibular skin and membranous columella, with the appearance of a "hanging" columella.

A 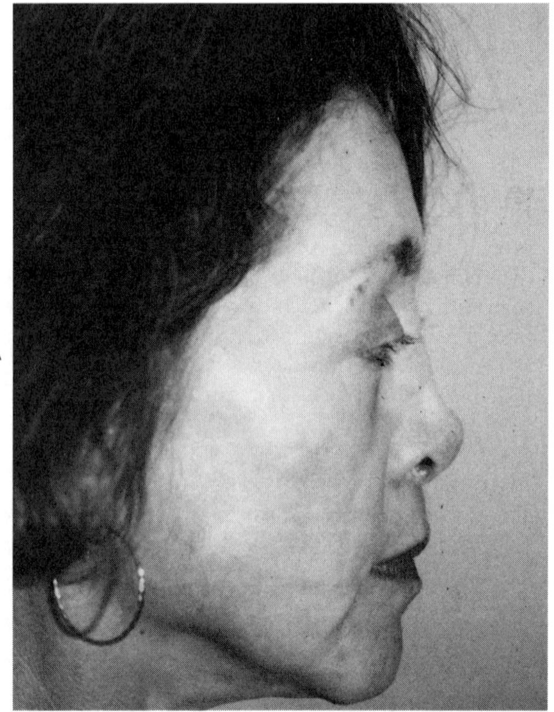

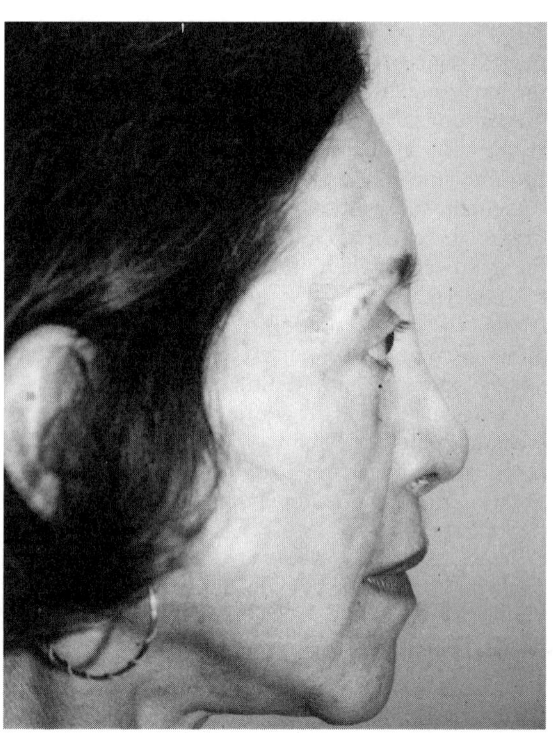 B

Figure 5.
A and *B*, Pre- and postoperative view of favorable lengthening of nose with cartilage grafts placed in infratip lobule.

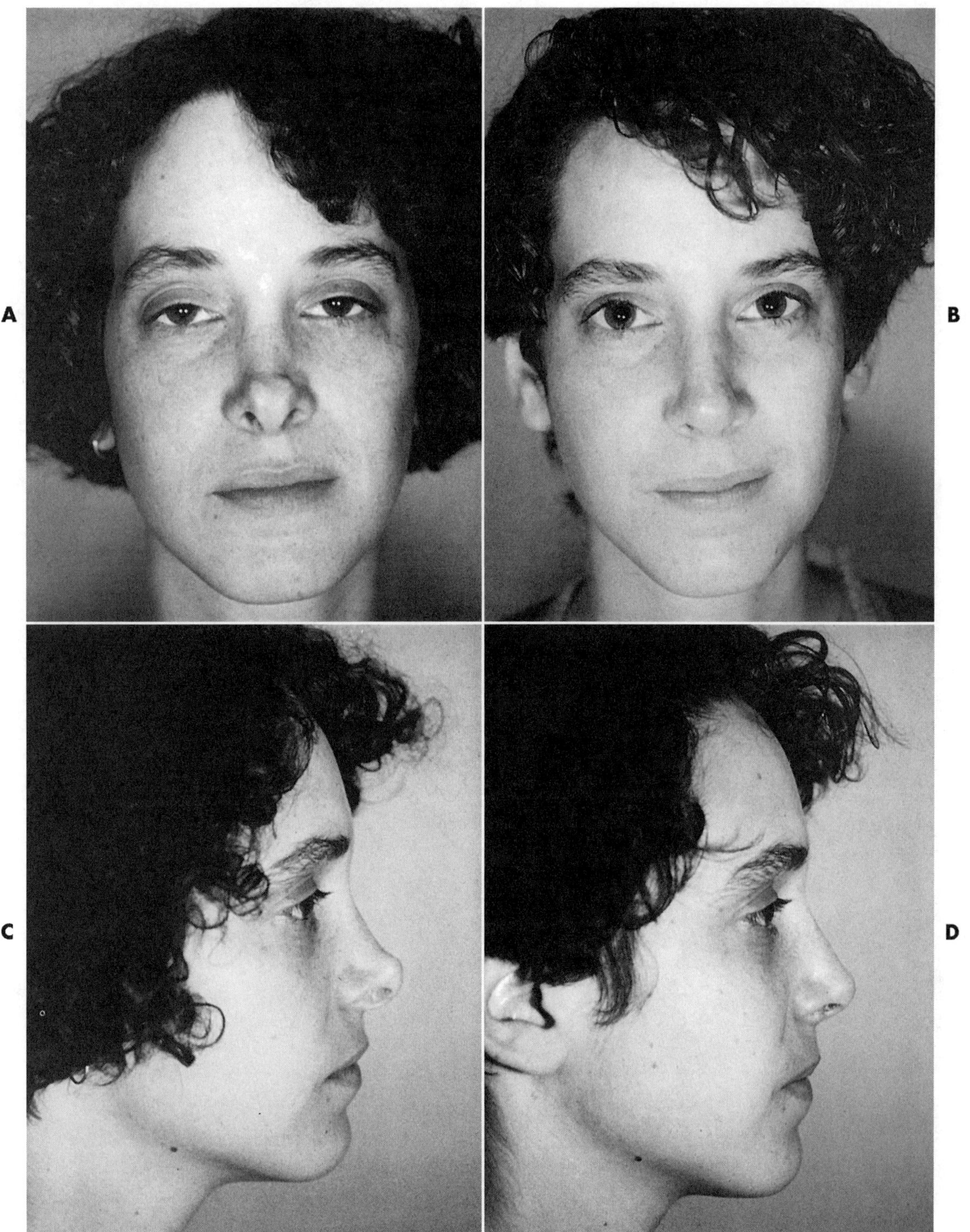

Figure 6.
Two year outcome of secondary rhinoplasty by technique described in text. *A*, Frontal view preoperative: Thin skin–subcutaneous tissue complex; wide, flat dorsum; hanging infratip lobule; asymmetric tip; prominent bossae; tip bifidity; *B*, Frontal view postoperative; *C*, Lateral view preoperative: Shallow, over-reduced dorsum and radix; indistinct profile "starting point"; slightly overprojected tip; overly convex columella; alar-columella disproportion; excess membranous columellar exposure; *D*, Lateral view postoperative.

Continued

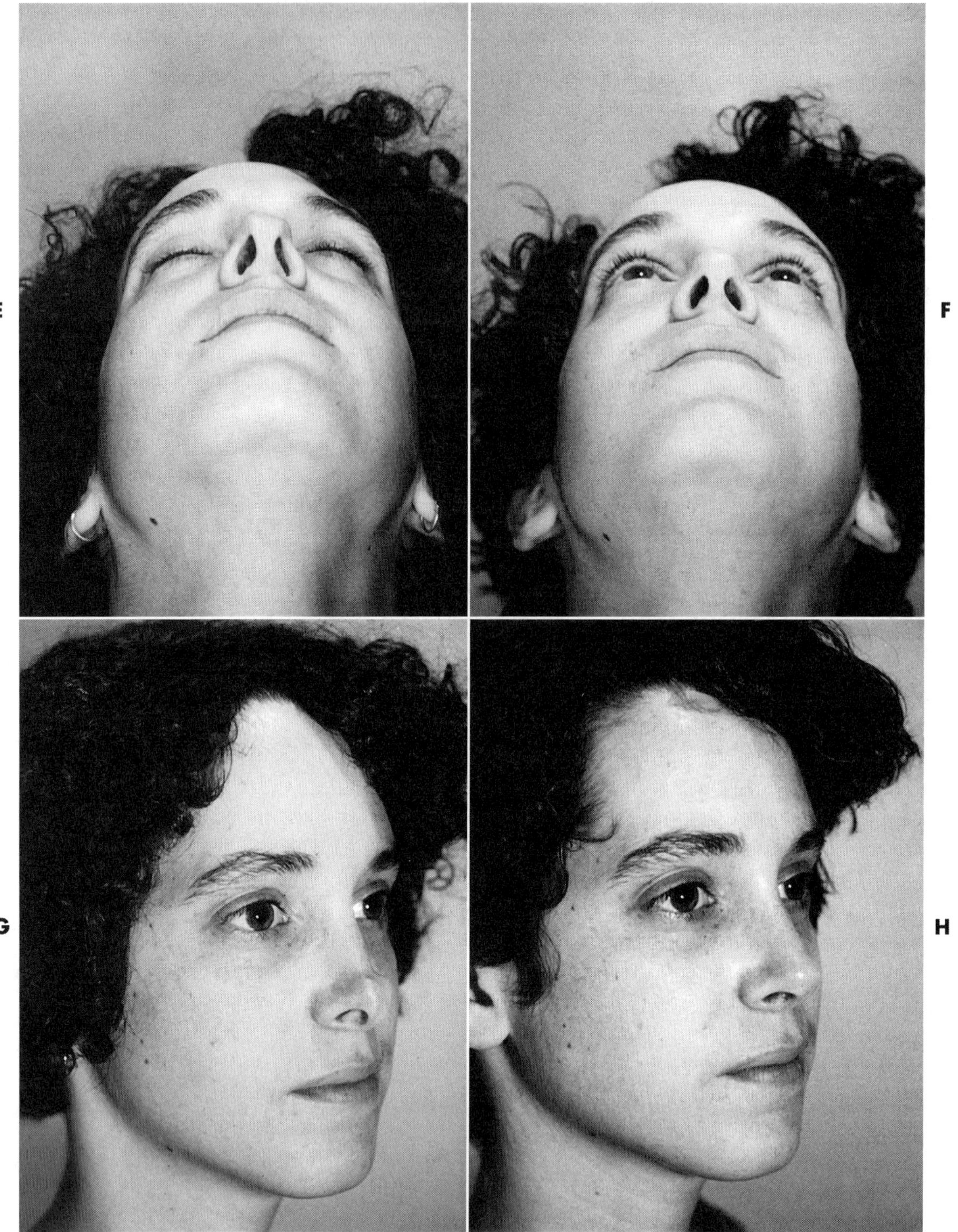

Figure 6, cont'd.
E, Base view preoperative: Prominent bossae; wide, bifid tip; intercrural clefting; prominent medial crural footplate; elongated medial crura; asymmetric tip defining point; *F*, Base view postoperative; *G*, Oblique view preoperative: Confirms other views; *H*, Oblique view postoperative.

Overall, the nose is significantly unbalanced and reveals the classic stigmata of an operated appearance.

Rhinoscopy reveals an intact deviated septum to the right, obstructing 80 percent of the nasal airway. The nasal mucosa and turbinates are normal.

The exquisitely thin skin with sparse underlying subcutaneous tissue makes coverage of cartilage grafts, which is essential for reconstruction, difficult.

Psychosocial Evaluation

This pleasant young woman is acutely aware that her nasal appearance is abnormal and invites negative comments from her pupils and associates. Confidence in her original surgeon was lost early on; she had requested revision surgery shortly after becoming aware of the surgical appearance shortfalls. Inadequate finances had prevented her from seeking corrective surgery heretofore.

Her psychological evaluation revealed a stable, pleasant, realistic young woman who easily understood the risks inherent in secondary surgery and was eager to breathe better as well as to improve her appearance.

Surgical Technique and Strategy

The principles involved in the reconstruction of this problem primarily involve an augmentation of the shallow dorsum, reduction-refinement of the nasal tip bossae, and repair of the deviated septum. Augmentation of the dorsum will help restore proportion to the upper and lower nasal structures as well as to provide the illusion of narrowing. The scarred contracted bossae must be reduced by removal and reconstitution, thus creating the indicated retroprojection. Tip narrowing by transdomal suturing is mandatory. Finally, the alar-columellar disproportion must be regularized. Crushed cartilage autografts of septal cartilage provide a softening buffer between the scarred strong alar cartilages and the thin tip skin.

Operative Technique and Sequence

The following text outlines the operative technique and sequence (Fig. 7).

1. Harvest of right auricular cartilage grafts
2. Left Killian septal incision
3. Elevation of light septal mucoperichondrial–periosteal flaps; septal reconstruction by:
   a. Disarticulation of ethmoid from quadrangular cartilage (followed by trans-septal quilting mattress suturing of septal flaps)
   b. Excision obstructing ethmoid plate and tail of septal cartilage
   c. Excision 3 mm strip of cartilage along floor of nose
   d. Harvest septal cartilage grafts
   e. Suture caudal septum to periosteum of spine
4. Delivery of alar cartilage through intercartilaginous and marginal incisions; complete transfixion incision to retroproject tip
5. Amputation of scarred domes (bossae) and suture-repair of cut cartilage margins to reconstitute complete strip
6. Narrowing of bifid tip with transdomal sutures
7. Resection of portion of flared medial crural footplates
8. Resection of crescent of excess membranous columella and caudal septum
9. Elevation of narrow pocket over dorsum for graft insertion
10. Onlay grafting of shallow dorsum with dual-layer cartilage grafts
11. Insertion of multiple crushed cartilage; septal cartilage grafts to tip and infratip lobule
12. Bilateral curved low lateral osteotomies for bony pyramid narrowing with 3 mm micro-osteotome
13. Suture-repair all incisions with 5–0 chromic catgut suture
14. Application of Denver splint

Retrospective Analysis and Critique

At 1 year, balance and proportion has been restored to the nose and face, which provides an improved relationship between the nasal dorsum and tip by profile augmentation and tip retroprojection. The bifidity, apparently unappreciated at the patient's initial surgery, is now corrected, with improved triangularity and symmetry on base view (the diagnostic triad of thin skin, strong cartilages, and tip bifidity or divergence of the domes must always be recognized in primary rhinoplasty, and the domes should be brought closer together). The bossae have been excised, and the alar cartilage dome integrity has been restored with fine suture-repair. The nose, which appeared overshort and excessively rotated, now demonstrates proper length. The visually distracting alar-columellar disproportion is corrected.

The most important long-term consideration is whether the thin skin–subcutaneous tissue layer will allow the onlay grafts to become visible with continued epithelial thinning. Margin shave-excision and edge beveling of grafts aids in preventing visible graft edges

Case 2

This 37-year-old housewife underwent rhinoplasty on two occasions in the past by two different surgeons. The normal appearance has worsened progressively over the intervening years, with increasing bilateral airway obstruction. She requests repair of her external deformities (primarily the profile and tip abnormalities), and wishes to breathe more comfortably.

Analysis

The surgical outcome of two procedures in this patient represents multiple problems of over-reduction of the bony dorsum; undercorrection of the cartilaginous dorsum; loss of tip support with bilateral alar collapse; and bilateral bossae formation, with tip bifidity clearly apparent. The bony dorsum is low and discontinuous from the cartilaginous dorsum, which demonstrates both a cartilaginous and soft-tissue pollybeak. Internally and externally, the alar sidewalls are flail and collapsed inward, which contributes to the nasal obstruction. The asymmetric tip bossae have developed as a consequence of failure to initially diagnose and subsequently properly treat the triad of thin skin, strong cartilages, and crural bifidity. The overall nose is unbalanced, disproportionate, and appears distinctly surgical.

Psychosocial Evaluation

This attractive mother of two children suffers from loss of self-esteem as a consequence of the surgical-appearing nose, examination of which reveals several complications. She confides that she has felt "stared at" in public, and that her children have commented negatively about her nose. As the alar collapse has progressively worsened, breathing through the nose has worsened, leading to constant mouth breathing.

She realistically accepted the limitations and risks inherent in an additional procedure and was eager for airway and appearance improvement.

Operative Technique and Strategy

This patient's nose represents overaggressive surgical reduction in some areas of the nose, with undercorrection in other regions. Balance of the upper and lower nose must be restored by onlay grafting of the upper nose combined with reduction of the cartilaginous–soft-tissue pollybeak deformity (Fig. 8). The bifid nasal tip requires refinement and narrowing by shave-excision of the scarred bossae as well as suturing the divergent crura and domes closer together. Bilateral curved cartilage battens from the auricle are necessary to resupport the alar sidewalls and prevent inspiratory collapse, thus favorably improving the nasal airway.

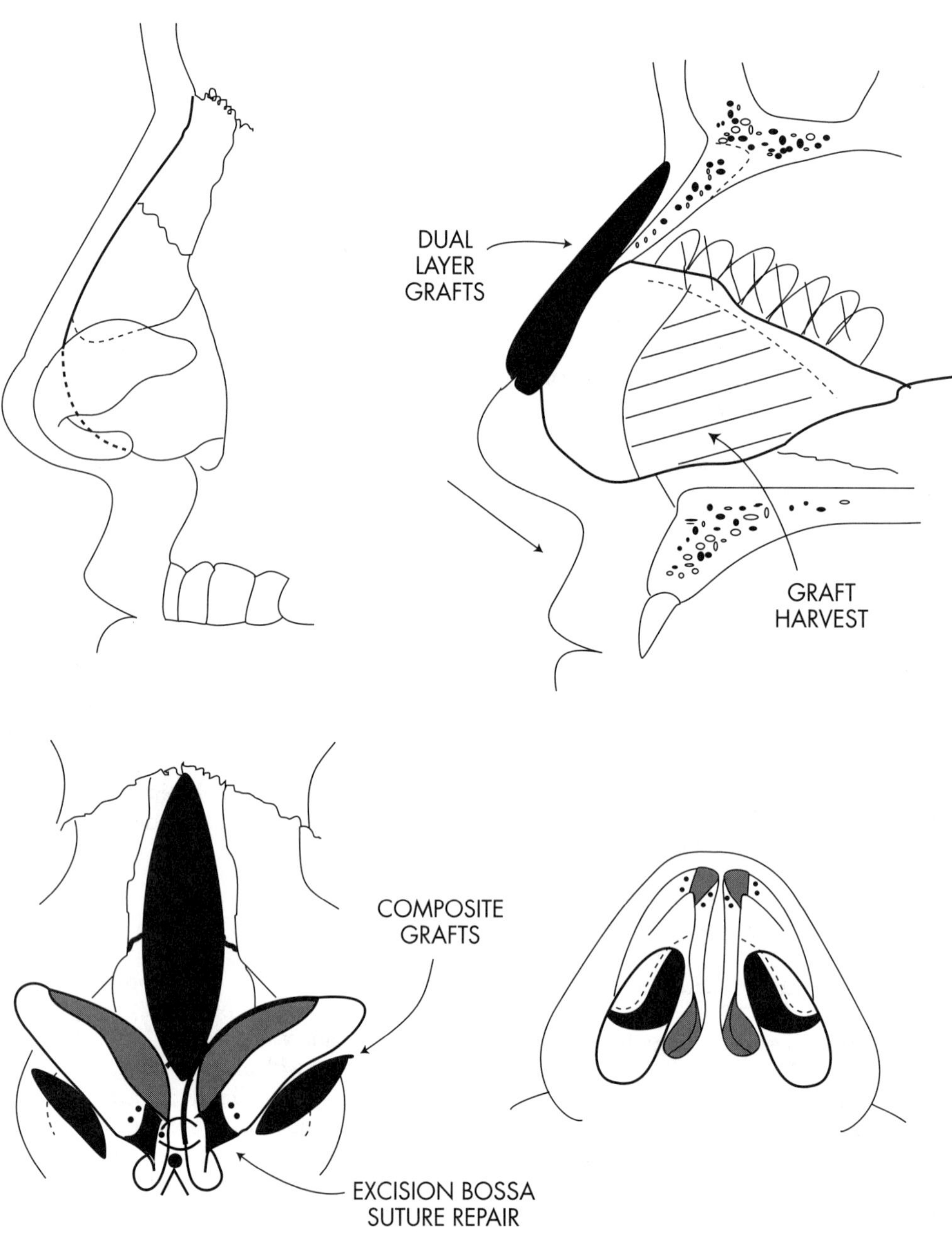

Figure 7.
Graphic representation of surgical techniques employed in Case 1.

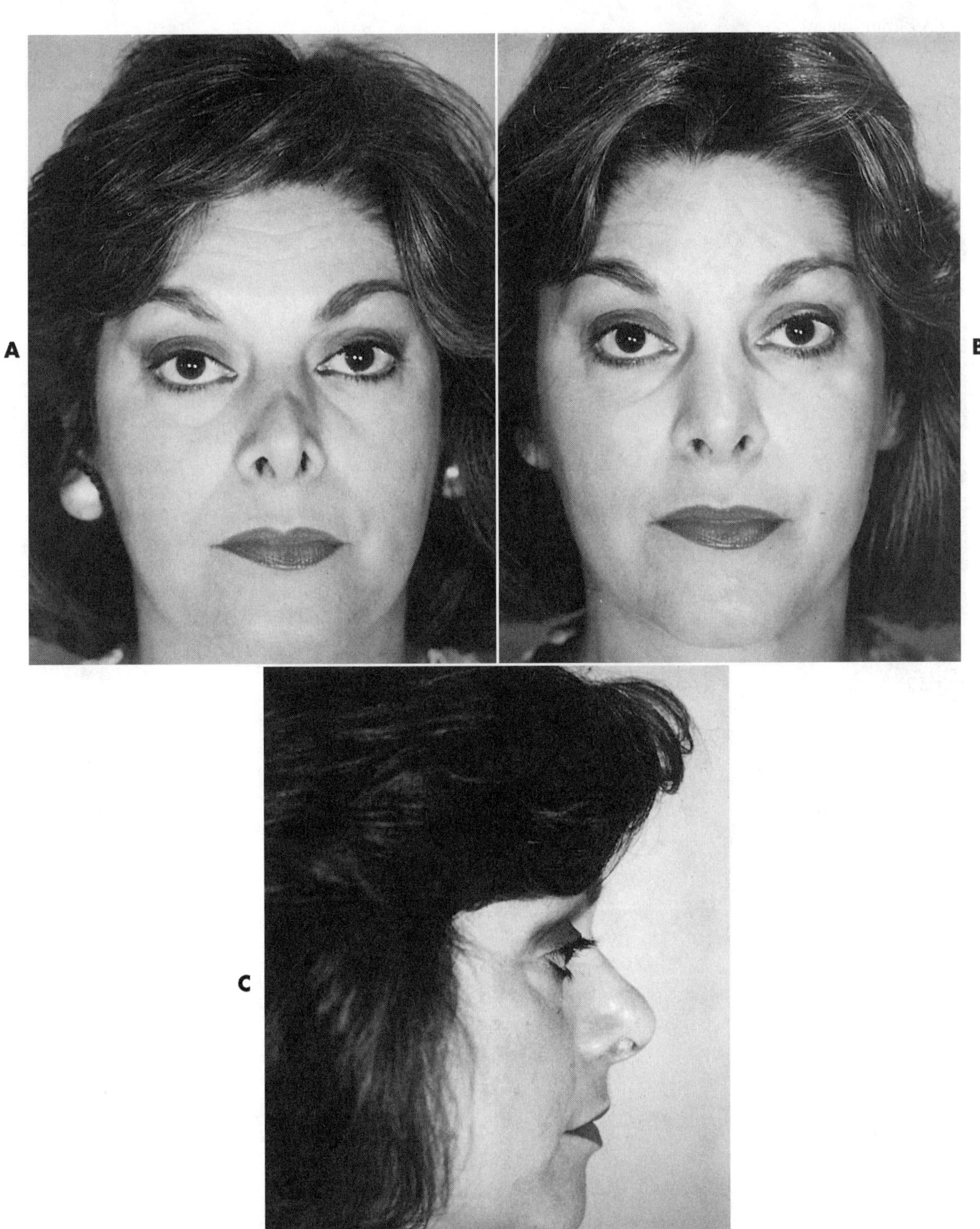

Figure 8.
Two year representation of secondary rhinoplasty by techniques described in text. *A*, Frontal view preoperative: Indistinct, washed-out bony dorsum; inverted "V" deformity; upper lateral cartilage collapse; discontinuous aesthetic lines from brow to tip; collapsed supratip regions bilaterally; prominent tip bossae; intermediate crural bifidity and divergence; thin skin; *B*, Frontal view postoperative; *C*, Lateral view preoperative: Over-reduced bony dorsum—nose appears short; under-reduced cartilaginous dorsum, with tip–supratip disproportion; tip ptosis with loss of support; supra-alar depression; bossae evident; unbalanced, disproportionate nose.

Continued

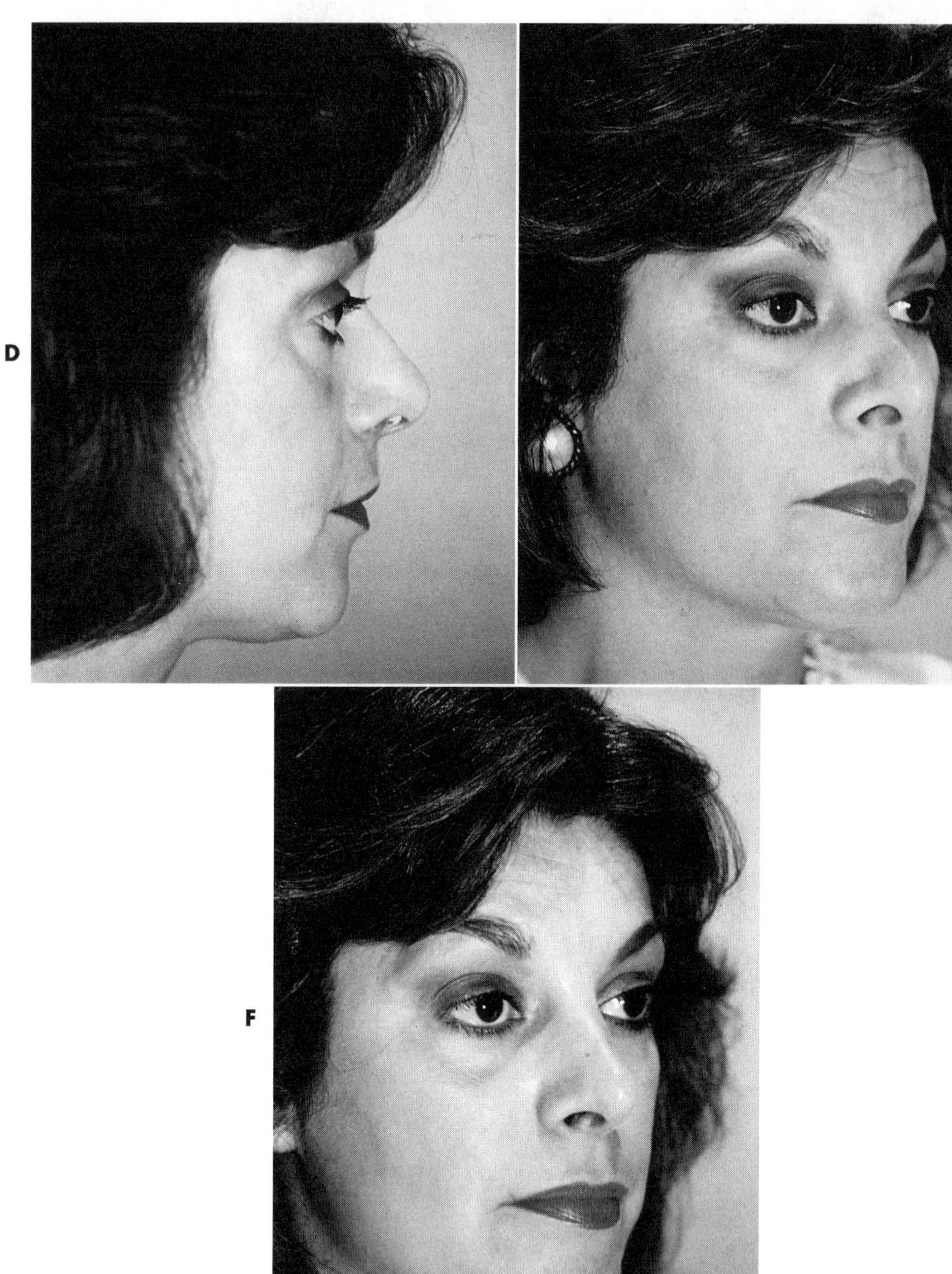

Figure 8, cont'd.
D, Lateral view postoperative; *E*, Oblique view preoperative: Confirms other views; *F*, Oblique view postoperative.

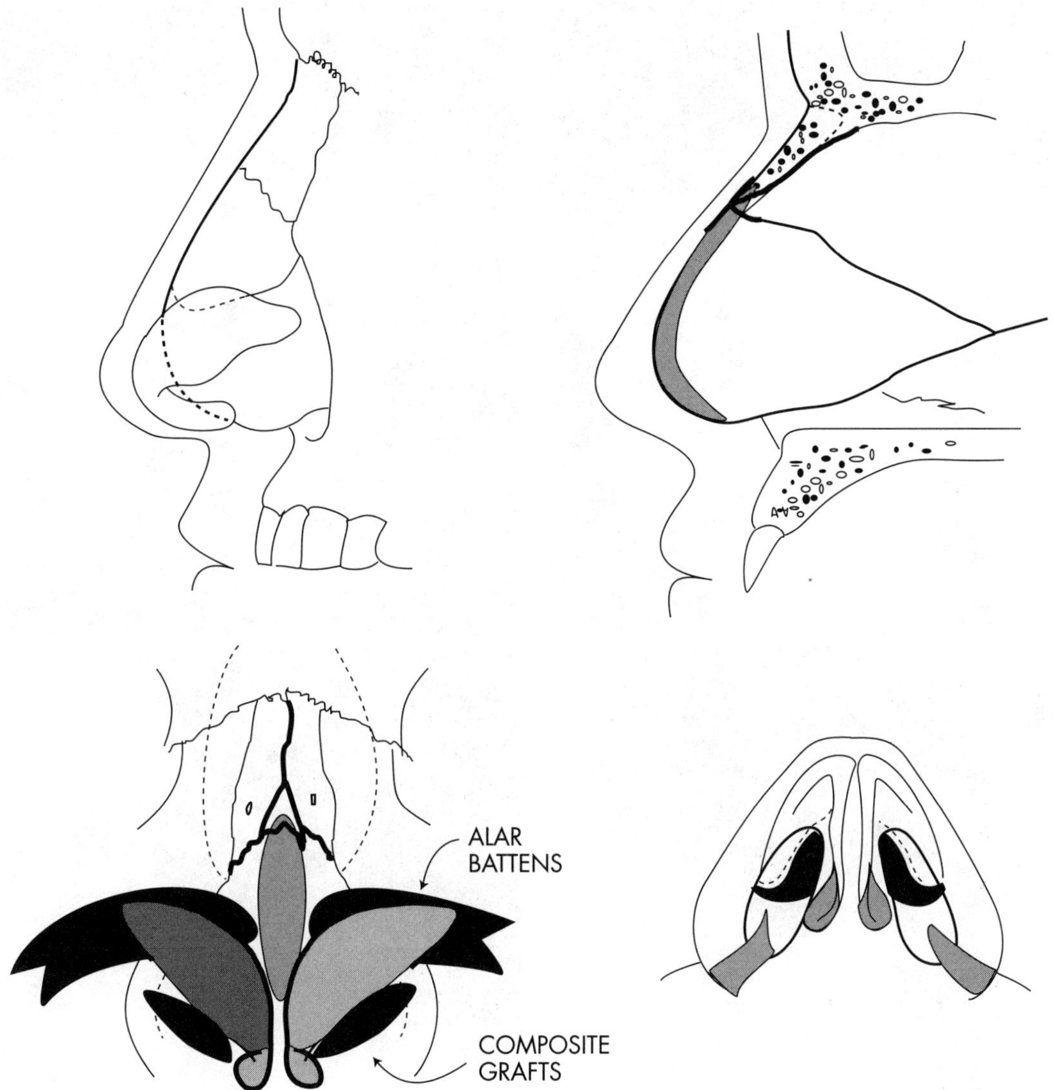

Figure 9.
Graphic representation of surgical techniques employed in Case 2.

Operative Technique and Sequence

The following text indicates the operative technique and sequence (Fig. 9).

1. Harvest of auricular cartilage from cavum and cymba conchae
2. Delivery of alar cartilage remnants through intercartilaginous and marginal incisions
3. Removal of soft-tissue interdomal area
4. Shave-excision of sharp edges of bossae
5. Transdomal suture narrowing of bifid domes with 4–0 PDS suture
6. Elevation (wide) of skin–subcutaneous tissue complex of cartilaginous dorsum
7. Knife excision of cartilaginous–soft tissue pollybeak with excision of excess supratip scar
8. Creation of limited (narrow) pocket in midline over bony dorsum
9. Onlay grafting of bony dorsum with two-layer sandwich graft of auricular cartilage
10. Creation of precise subcutaneous pockets in supra-alar regions bilaterally in exact areas of alar collapse
11. Insertion of bilateral convex auricular cartilage battens into supra-alar pockets
12. Suture-repair all incisions with 5–0 chromic catgut suture
13. Insertion of layer of crushed cartilage into tip lobule subcutaneously
14. Bilateral curved low lateral osteotomies with 3 mm micro-osteotome

Retrospective Analysis and Critique

A combination of augmentation and reduction revision surgery characterizes this procedure, which has produced a more balanced, proportionate, and natural nose. Attention is thus drawn to attractive eyes and away from the nose. Aesthetic lines are improved on all views, and the alar collapse is corrected with airway improvement. Reorienting and grafting the scarred tip structures has restored appropri-

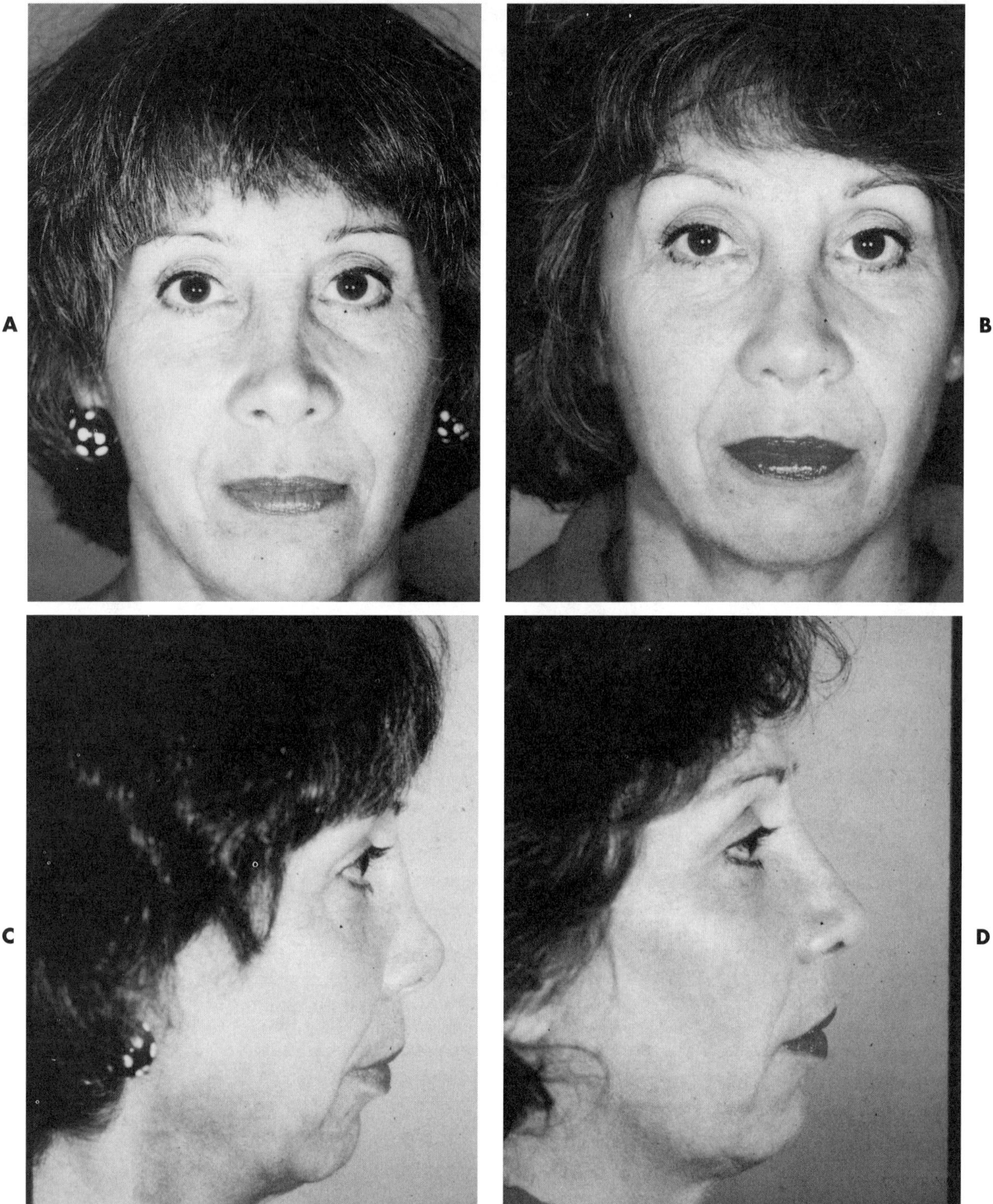

Figure 10.
Three year outcome of secondary augmentation rhinoplasty carried out employing techniques described in the text. *A,* Frontal view preoperative: Thick, sebaceous skin with rhytidosis; asymmetric lateral sidewall lines; supratip depression; overshort nose; excessive nostril exposure; wide alar base; *B,* Frontal view postoperative; *C,* Lateral view preoperative: Significant supratip saddling; bony pyramid profile irregularity; severe nasal over-rotation; abnormal columellar "double-break"; obtuse columellar-labial angle; *D,* Lateral view postoperative.

ate triangularity to the tip. The nose now appears longer and balanced to the face.

Case 3

Now in midlife, this patient underwent primary rhinoplasty many years ago. She immediately noted over-rotation of the nose, with slow but progressive collapse of the supratip region resulting in a saddle nose. Recent comments by family and acquaintances about the nose being too short and excessive nostril show have prompted her to seek secondary surgery.

Analysis

The overdeep dorsum is apparent on frontal view, with asymmetry of the opposing lateral sidewalls. It is apparent that the nose is clearly over-rotated, which allows the observer to look directly into the exposed nostrils. The alar base is overwide, making the nose "bottom-heavy." Laterally, a distinct supratip saddling exists. Combined with over-rotation of the tip, with an excessively extreme columellar "double-break," the nose appears snubbed and too short. The skin is thick, demonstrates high sebaceous gland activity, and reveals rhytidosis near the nasal root.

Palpation and transillumination of the nasal septum reveals almost totally absent cartilage.

Psychosocial Evaluation

The patient demonstrates excellent motivation for secondary rhinoplasty. Her life is stable, fulfilled, and happy except for the increasing concern about the "snubbed" appearance to the nose, which is worsened by the progressive saddling. Comments from friends and family have prompted her to seek reconstruction. She particularly dislikes the extent of visible nostril from frontal and oblique views. Her understanding of the limitations and risks associated with augmenting and lengthening the nose is realistic and appropriate.

Operative Technique and Strategy

The surgical goal in this attractive middle-aged woman is to augment the nose to restore a strong, elegant dorsum while lengthening the overshort nose (Fig. 10). Ear cartilage grafts will be necessary if insufficient septal cartilage remains for harvest. The central segment nasal length will require true elongation by adding cartilage grafts to the infratip lobule, which will produce the added benefit of restoring a normal columellar inclination. The lateral sidewalls, because of heavy alar lobules, are of adequate length. Finally, the bottom-heavy alar base will benefit by bilateral alar base reduction procedures, which will narrow the excessive horizontal width of the nasal base.

Operative Technique and Sequence

The following text indicates the operative technique and sequence (Fig. 11).

1. Harvest of auricular cartilage from cavum and cymba conchae
2. Exploration of nasal septum through left Killian incision—thick cartilage harvested from junction at maxillary crest (majority of septal cartilage absent)
3. Elevation of limited midline skin–subcutaneous pocket over entire nasal dorsum
4. Rasp of bony dorsum prominence

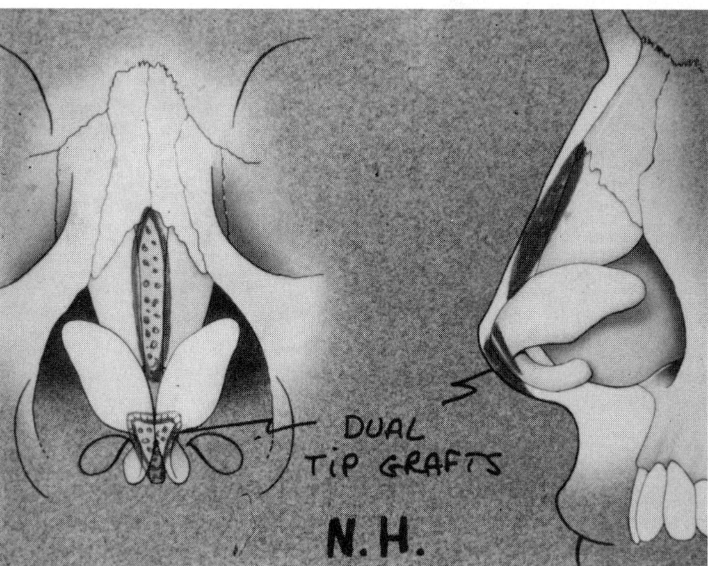

Figure 11.
Graphic representation of techniques utilized in Case 3. Tip grafts are used here to lengthen nose and not to increase tip projection.

5. Insertion of double-layer auricular cartilage grafts, stabilized in place by cephalic and caudal transcutaneous pullout sutures of 5–0 mild chromic catgut
6. Creation of precise pocket below infratip lobule with small bilateral infradomal marginal incisions
7. Insertion of two-layer triangular-shaped auricular cartilage grafts to lengthen central segment of nose
8. Bilateral alar base reduction with wedge excisions
9. Suture-repair of all incisions with 5–0 chromic catgut
10. Application of Denver splint for 5 days

Retrospective Analysis and Critique

Balance and proportion has been restored to the nose of this patient by making the nose larger and longer (well-proportioned large noses are infinitely more attractive than malpositioned small noses). Both actual length and the illusion of lengthening have been achieved. No longer can the observer gaze directly into the nostril. Alar base reduction aids in balancing the upper two-thirds and lower third of the nose. The frontal aesthetic lines are improved and more symmetric, although not perfect. In retrospect, a longer dorsal graft might have provided improved frontal lines. In addition, modest chin augmentation would have provided improved facial balance, but this was not desired by the patient.

Suggested Reading

Goin JM, Goin MK. Changing the body: Psychological effects of plastic surgery. Baltimore: Williams & Wilkins, 1981.

McKinney P, Cunningham BL. Rhinoplasty. New York: Churchill Livingstone, 1989.

Meyer R. Secondary and functional rhinoplasty. New York: Grune & Stratton, 1988.

Tardy ME. Rhinoplasty: The art and the science. Vols. I and II. Philadelphia: WB Saunders, 1996.

Tardy ME. Surgical anatomy of the nose. New York: Raven Press, 1992.

Tardy ME, Cheng EY, Jernstrom V. Misadventures in nasal tip surgery. Otol Clin North Am 1987; 20:4.

Tardy ME, Thomas JR, Brown RJ. Facial aesthetic surgery. St. Louis: Mosby–Year Book, 1994.

Tardy ME, Toriumi D. Alar retraction: Composite graft correction. Vol. 6. Facial Plastic Surgery Monographs. New York: Thieme-Stratton, 1989.

Thomas JR, Tardy ME. Complications of rhinoplasty. In: Complications in otolaryngology—Head and neck surgery. Vol. 2 (Head & neck). New York: BC Decker, 1986.

CHIN DISPROPORTION

The method of
Gary J. Nishioka
by
Gary J. Nishioka
Wayne F. Larrabee, Jr.

The facial profile is principally defined by the forehead, nose, chin, and to some extent the lips. Improvement in profile disharmony can be achieved by making changes in the nose and/or chin. Chin disproportion can be categorized as anteroposterior (AP) deficiency or excess, vertical deficiency or excess, asymmetry, or a combination of these. By far, the most commonly encountered situation clinically is AP deficiency, with or without vertical deficiency of the lower third of the face (see Fig. 1). We discuss in this chapter the evaluation and management of deficiency of the chin, also known as microgenia. The reader is directed to the literature on variations of the genioplasty procedure for management of the other types of chin disproportion.

■ PREOPERATIVE EVALUATION

The first step in evaluating a patient with microgenia is to determine if he or she has an AP deficiency of the mandible. A patient who has a class II malocclusion associated with a retrusive-appearing chin should be informed that optimal correction of this dentofacial deformity may require orthodontics and orthognathic surgery. A consultation with an orthodontist or an oral and maxillofacial surgeon should be offered. If this consultation is declined, the preoperative evaluation can continue, but careful documentation is recommended.

In patients who have no AP deficiency of the mandible, that is, the problem is an isolated microgenia, an evaluation of chin projection is then performed. One method that is simple and can be adapted to computer imaging is the zero meridian of Gonzales-Ulloa.

With the dentition in occlusion and lips at rest, have the patient look directly at his or her own eyes in a mirror placed 2 or more feet away. This places the patient's head into the "natural head position" and assures that the Frankfort horizontal line parallels the floor. Using the morphing feature of the computer imager, advance the chin to the desired position. Ideally, this should be at or just behind a vertical line dropped from the nasion (Fig. 1). The desired distance of soft-tissue advancement can then be measured using the computer imager.

If a computer imager is not available, a photograph taken of the patient in natural head position with a ruler taped to

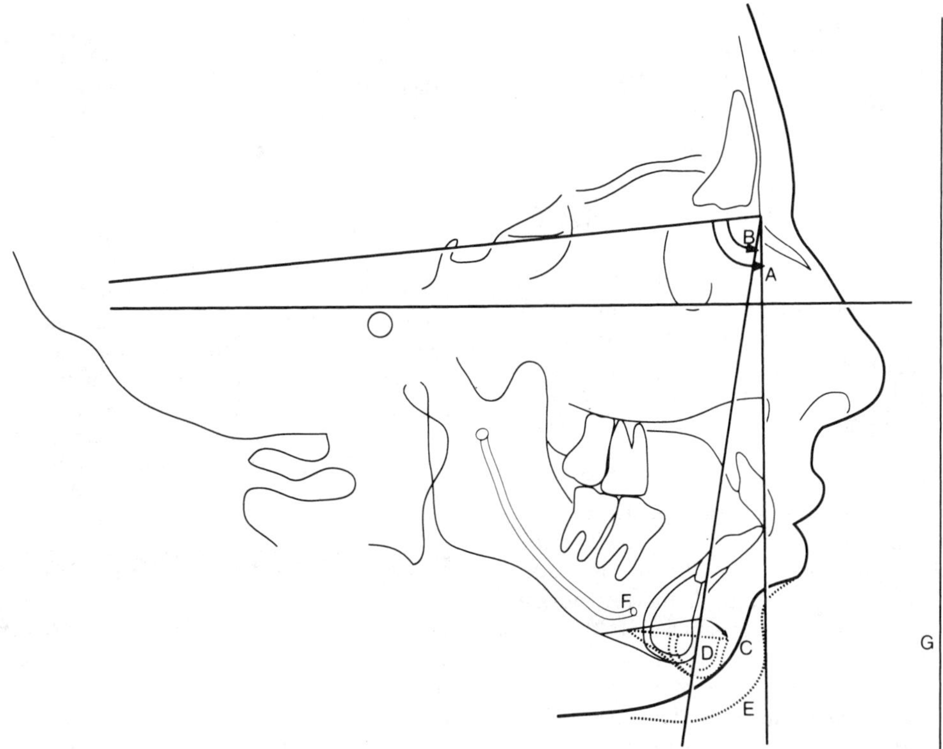

Figure 1.
Eighteen-year-old female who has both anteroposterior and vertical deficiency of the mandible. *A,* SNA; in this case, the NA line coincides with a vertical line drawn from the nasion; *B,* SNB; *C,* Preoperative soft-tissue chin profile demonstrating microgenia with an associated vertical height deficiency of the lower third of the face; *D,* Chin segment advanced 9 mm and rotated 4 mm; *E,* Prediction of postsurgery soft-tissue chin profile; *F,* Inferior alveolar nerve canal and mental foramen; *G,* Hanging chain for vertical reference.

the face can also be used. In this situation, the surgeon can estimate the desired soft-tissue advancement by measuring from the chin just to or slightly behind a vertical line drawn from the nasion. The photographed ruler serves as the means of measurement. It is important to understand that all methods of evaluating the chin aesthetically are only guides. The surgeon's aesthetic sense must be the final judge.

■ SELECTION OF SURGICAL TECHNIQUE

In general, we use alloplastic implants for advancements of 7 mm or less (mentoplasty), and the horizontal mandibular sliding osteotomy (genioplasty) for larger advancements, or if an increase in vertical height of the lower third of the face is desired, or correction of an asymmetry is needed.

In order to properly select the appropriate implant size, one needs to know the ratio of soft-tissue advancement as a function of the anterior-posterior thickness of the implant. For most implants this ratio is 0.7:1.0. Thus, a 10 mm implant will provide a 7 mm soft-tissue advancement. For the advancement genioplasty, most studies show the ratio between soft-tissue advancement and bone movement is 0.9 to 1.0:1.0.

If a genioplasty procedure is selected, a panorex lateral cephalogram and mandibular incisor periapical radiographs are obtained. For asymmetry cases, an anteroposterior cephalogram is also obtained. The panorex provides a survey of the mandible that excludes dental or bone pathology. The periapical radiograph of the mandibular incisors allows the surgeon to measure the length of these teeth such that the osteotomy cut can be made at least 5 mm below the root apices. This will prevent inadvertent tooth root injury and maintain an adequate blood supply to the teeth.

The lateral cephalogram is used to develop the treatment plan. After the cephalometric tracing is completed, a prediction tracing is made by drawing a template along the planned osteotomy site. The osteotomy is dictated principally by the position of the mental foramen. The chin segment is advanced and rotated inferiorly if an increase in vertical height is needed. The magnitude of bony movement is limited by the need for central overlap of the proximal and distal segments. The lingual cortex of the distal segment (bony chin segment to be moved) cannot be advanced beyond the anterior cortex of the proximal segment (remaining bony portion of the mandible) Bone contact in the central portion is not necessary as long as there is contact of the bone flanges laterally, but these segments must overlap centrally to ensure bone fill-in (see Fig. 1). A prediction tracing is drawn.

If greater advancement is needed than this prediction will

permit using a single piece genioplasty, a multiple piece or "stair-stepped" genioplasty, or placement of an alloplastic implant in addition to the single piece genioplasty, is considered. It is beyond our scope in this chapter to discuss these options.

■ GENIOPLASTY OPERATIVE TECHNIQUE

This procedure can be performed using intravenous (IV) sedation; however, general anesthesia is recommended. When the genioplasty is combined with other procedures, it is performed first. The principal drawback when combined with a rhinoplasty is that a nasal endotracheal tube is required, which must be switched to an endotracheal tube for the rhinoplasty.

As soon as the IV line is placed, 10 mg of dexamethasone and a first-generation cephalosporin are administered. Local anesthesia using 1 percent lidocaine with 1:100,000 epinephrine is generously infiltrated transorally over the anterior chin and its lingual surface. Using a diathermy cautery, an incision is made approximately 1 cm anterior to the buccal vestibule from canine tooth to canine tooth. Care is taken to look for branches of the mental nerve as they begin to pass just under the mucosa lateral to this point. The dissection is continued at a 45 degree angle toward the mandible through the mentalis muscle; the surgeon leaves a cuff of muscle superiorly to assist in closure.

A subperiosteal dissection is carried inferior to the planned osteotomy, with the surgeon maintaining as much soft-tissue attachment as possible. The osteotomy cut is generally made 5 mm or more below root apices of the teeth, as determined by the periapical radiograph. Posteriorly, the mental nerves are exposed and identified. Using a small fissure bur, a midline mark bisected by a mark at the planned level of the osteotomy is made. Using a thin long V-shaped sagittal saw, the planned osteotomy is scored on the bone. It is important that the planned osteotomy is 5 mm below the mental foramen to prevent injury to the nerve, which often dips in this area. It is also important that the planned osteotomy is symmetric on both sides, because any asymmetry will be magnified following advancement and will undoubtedly require further correction. Under irrigation the osteotomy is made. One can judge the depth of the saw blade tip by tactile sense. The tip should be just through the lingual cortex to prevent laceration of the deeper soft tissues.

Once the osteotomy is completed, the chin segment is mobilized. Careful release of soft-tissue tethering is done until the segment can be positioned with minor tension. Rigid internal fixation using preformed chin bone plates is performed. A custom-bent 2.0 mm bone plate system or lag screws can also be used. Increase in vertical height is achieved by bending the plate appropriately to rotate the distal chin segment. A small bony gap centrally will fill in with bone as long as there is overlap of the segments. However, if a large gap is present, placement of demineralized bone should be considered. The wound is closed in layers using 3-0 polyglactin 910 for deep tissue, and 4-0 chromic gut for the mucosa.

A chin dressing to support the lip is placed and maintained for 5 days. The chin dressing consists of a 2 inch Elastoplast cut to 5 or 6 inches in length and split at each end for 2 inches. Mastisol is applied to the skin. The dressing is applied with the upper portion placed at the level of the mental sulcus, with the lower cut limbs sweeping up over the inferior border of the mandible. This dressing is designed to prevent inferior retraction of the lip. Oral antibiotics are prescribed for 5 days. A lateral cephalogram is obtained the following day, and at 6 months and a year.

Possible complications of genioplasty are listed in Table 1.

Table 1. Genioplasty Complications

Malposition	Bone plate/screw exposure
Mental nerve injury	Inferior contraction of the lip
Injury to teeth	Bone healing problems

■ MENTOPLASTY OPERATIVE TECHNIQUE

One of three types of implants is selected: a preformed Gore-Tex or Silastic implant, or a custom-trimmed implant made from a block of Gore-Tex. If desired, sizers are available for these preformed implants. A custom Gore-Tex implant is fabricated if a suitable preformed implant is not found for the patient's needs. At this time, we prefer preformed Gore-Tex implants to Silastic. This technique discusses placement of preformed implants, and is applicable for Gore-Tex or Silastic.

This procedure is easily performed under intravenous sedation. When combined with a rhinoplasty or facelift, the implant procedure is performed first. Placement of a long-acting local anesthetic such as bupivacaine is recommended, with intravenous sedation for pain control. General anesthesia obviates this need, but can still be of value in the early postoperative period.

Once an IV line is established, 10 mg of dexamethasone and a first-generation cephalosporin are given. Local anesthesia is infiltrated in the mental nerve region, submental incision site, and over the anterior soft tissue of the chin. A skin incision 10 to 15 mm long is made, with dissection carried to the level of the periosteum. The periosteum is then incised using a No. 15 scalpel blade for 2.5 to 3.0 cm and elevated using a small periosteal elevator such as a Joseph or St. Louis 7 elevator. Superior midline elevation is carried to the midportion of the mandible, but care is taken to stop short of entering the buccal vestibule. If the vestibule is disrupted, the implant can migrate superiorly, which effaces the vestibule. As an added safeguard against migration, a suture can be placed from periosteum to the inferior border of the implant.

The subperiosteal elevation is continued laterally under direct vision to prevent injury to the mental nerve. An Aufrich or Senn retractor works well. Efforts are made to create a precise pocket. The implant is inserted subperiosteally by placing one end in first with lateral retraction of the periosteum. It is inserted more than halfway past the midline to facilitate insertion of the other end. The implant is then centered. When using a Silastic implant, a groove placed in the center of the implant helps to verify its midline position.

Preformed Gore-Tex implants already have midline perforations for suture placement and readily serve as a midline reference. A 4–0 polyglactin 910 suture is placed from the periosteum to the inferior border of the implant to add further stability if the surgeon believes that this is necessary. It should be noted that glove talc should be removed before handling the implant to help reduce the risk of chronic inflammation.

The closure is performed in two layers. The periosteum is closed with 4–0 polyglactin 910 suture. The skin is closed with 5–0 or 6–0 nylon. A two-layer dressing is applied. The first layer is $\frac{1}{2}$ inch paper tape, alternating from superior to inferior, and conforming the soft tissue around the implant in a gentle compressive fashion. A strip of 2 inch Elastoplast, with a horizontal slit through which the implant protrudes, is placed. The dressing and sutures are removed in 5 days. Oral antibiotics are prescribed for a week.

Possible complications of implants are listed in Table 2.

Table 2. Implant Complications

Implant displacement	Mental nerve injury
Infection/chronic inflammation	Poor scarring
Bone resorption	Improper size selection

Suggested Reading

Bell WH, Gallagher DM. The versatility of genioplasty using a broad pedicle. J Oral Maxillofac Surg 1983; 41:763-769.

Calhoun KH, Gibson FB. Chin position in profile analysis: Comparison of techniques and introduction of the lower facial triangle. Arch Otolaryngol Head Neck Surg 1992; 118:273-276.

Glasgold AI, Glasgold MJ. Mentoplasty. Facial Plast Surg Clin North Am 1994; 2:285-300.

Krekmanov L, Kahnberg KE. Soft-tissue response to genioplasty procedures. Brit J Oral Maxillofac Surg 1996; 30:87-91.

Ritter EF, Moelleken BRW, Mathes SJ, Ousterhout DK. The course of the inferior alveolar neurovascular canal in relation to sliding genioplasty. J Craniofac Surg 1992; 3:20-24,

BAGGY EYELIDS

The method of
Frank M. Kamer

The eyelid, globe, and orbit contribute much to the overall expression and individual characteristics of the human face. It is essential that inappropriate surgical changes not result in an unnatural or abnormal appearance in this central area of facial expression. The achievement of optimal aesthetic and functional results in blepharoplastic surgery requires that the surgeon develop a clear understanding of the functional and anatomic characteristics of the presenting problem.

■ UPPER BLEPHAROPLASTY

Preoperative Evaluation

The position of the upper tarsal crease is a very important consideration in the aesthetics and surgical management of the upper eyelid. The lid crease is created by the fusion point of the levator aponeurosis and the orbital septum. The position of this fold greatly influences the individual expression and ethnic characteristics of the face. Genetic, environmental, and age-related changes in the skin, fat, muscle, and tarsus are determined during the initial consultation. The position of the eyelids and any asymmetries of the eyelid, globe, or orbit are pointed out to the patient preoperatively in front of a well-lit mirror. It is wise to have any suggestion of lid ptosis or visual field defects evaluated and documented. The extent of skin, muscle, and fat to be excised is dictated by the anatomy of the individual eyelid and orbital complex. Perfect symmetry is rare, but conservative upper lid surgery can improve both the function and the cosmesis of heavy or baggy eyelids, with or without brow or tarsal repositioning.

Surgical Technique

After prepping the face, I have the patient sit on the operating table so the position of his or her eyes is approximately level with mine. I elevate the brow with one hand and have the patient open and close his or her eyes so I can clearly define the position of lid crease devoid of redundant skin. A surgical marker outlines the fold from the medial canthal region to an appropriate crow's foot laterally. The amount of skin to be excised is conservatively determined by depressing the brow and having the patient look down. The upper limb of the incision is outlined to include the redundant eyelid skin and a few lateral crow's feet. The incision tapers laterally, often extending lateral to the orbital rim, especially in those patients who have low brows and well-formed crow's feet to hide the incision. This presentation is often seen in the aging male population. Perinasal or infrabrow skin is not included in the incision, because healing can be less predictable in these areas of thicker dermis.

The patient lies down and is sedated. Although light intravenous sedation can be used, I prefer a controlled intravenous infusion of propofol administered by an anesthesiologist. Local anesthesia consisting of 1 percent lidocaine with 1:100,000 epinephrine is infiltrated subcutaneously with a No. 30 gauge needle. Care is taken not to stick any small vessels that tend to bleed, which would obscure the surgical field and create ecchymosis. I begin my incision in the middle of the lower surgical marking and by two-point traction extend it laterally to meet the upper incision at an acute angle. The incision is completed from medial to lateral before raising the skin. Four-point traction and good local anesthetic hydrodissection facilitate lifting the skin by scalpel dissection without injuring the underlying orbicularis muscle (Fig. 1).

I rarely change the position of the upper lid crease, except to "westernize" an Asian eye. Tarsal fixation can deepen the fold, but it can drastically alter the expression of the upper lid. I often use muscle and fat resection to subtly deepen and contour the upper lid crease and fold without changing their position. I estimate the amount of redundant muscle by pinching a few millimeters of orbicularis muscle with a forceps where it is obviously redundant. An elongated muscle ridge is raised and pinched with a fine curved hemostat. The muscle strip is then excised with a fine straight scissors, beginning laterally and extending to the medial extent of the wound. Bleeding is controlled by bipolar cautery of the small submuscular vessels. Most of the smaller bleeders will coagulate without the need for cauterization.

Fat removal also changes the depth but not the position of the upper lid crease. The amount of fat to be excised is determined by the preoperative condition of the lids in relationship to the globe and orbital rim. A deeply set eye with a prominent globe can look even deeper if only a little fat or muscle is removed. There is a very fine line between leaving some unwanted fat behind and hollowing the eyes by too much fat removal.

To expose the fat, I apply gentle pressure on the upper lid and underlying globe while spreading the orbicularis fibers between my fingers. I use a No. 15 scalpel, cutting in the direction of the muscle fibers while applying light counterpressure against the globe. The herniated fat slowly emerges with repeated deeper passes of the knife blade through the orbital septum. Usually, individual incisions are made to expose the central and medial fat compartments. Fine iris scissors can facilitate separating the fat from the surrounding orbital septum. In some cases, especially older patients with considerable muscle resection, the entire fat compartment is opened. Redundant fat is determined by applying gentle pressure on the globe while teasing the fat out of the wound. The base of the fat is clamped with a hemostat, the excess is removed, and the stump is cauterized before removing the clamp. Subcutaneous as well as suborbicularis fat can contribute to lateral hooding. I remove the subcutaneous fat by elevating the eyebrow in order to expose the redundant fat, which is excised with a straight scissors. In some patients, a subluxated lacrimal gland can also contribute to lateral hooding. In those cases, I anchor the lacrimal gland to the periosteum on the inferior surface of the supraorbital rim with a 5–0 polydioxanone (PDS) suture.

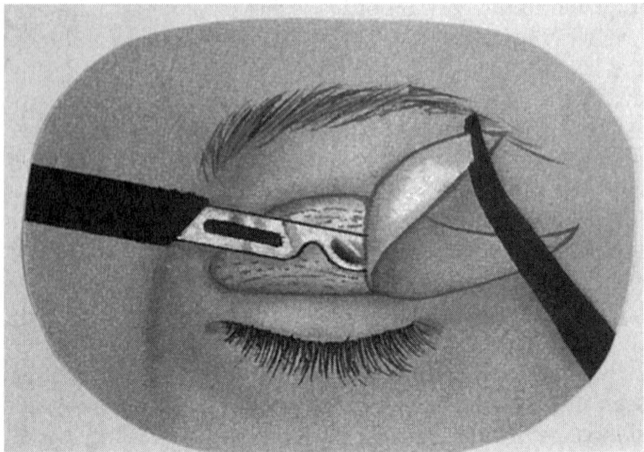

Figure 1.
Upper blepharoplasty.

After ensuring adequate hemostasis by pinpoint bipolar electocautery, I irrigate the open wound with sterile saline solution and begin skin closure at the lateral extent of the incision. To facilitate closure, a fine hook is placed in the skin a few millimeters lateral to the incision and left in place to retract the apex of the wound laterally. The skin between the apex and the lateral canthal region is closed with interrupted 6–0 fast-dissolving catgut sutures, augmented by butyl-2-cyanoacrylate (Histacryl). I place a similar single interrupted suture at the apex of the medial wound near the nose and tag it with a hemostat, which I use to retract the wound medially. Another clamp is set on the most medial of the lateral canthal sutures and likewise used to retract the wound laterally. This maneuver facilitates a straight line closure with a continuous "baseball" stitch of the same suture material. Knots are tied loosely so as not to strangulate any tissue, and bacitracin ointment is applied to the suture line.

Patients are instructed to apply iced compresses to their eyelids for 2 days, and to use petroleum jelly on the incisions until the crusts of adhesive and dissolving suture material come off, which is usually approximately 1 week.

■ LOWER BLEPHAROPLASTY

The choice of the best surgical technique is subjective; it is influenced by the surgeon's skill, training, knowledge, and overall aesthetic judgment. As a rule, it is best to obtain the optimum result with a minimum of surgery, because complications often rise with an increase in surgical intervention. A conservative approach aids in preventing radical alterations in the normal aging eyelid. Compromises must frequently be made between the "ideal" eyelid and a more individualized surgical result. Certain conditions cannot be significantly improved or changed by lower blepharoplasty. For example, rhytidosis of the lower lid skin can rarely be improved by blepharoplasty alone. Attempting to eliminate these wrinkles and fine lines by removal of excess skin often results in pulling of the lower lid margin downward, causing unacceptable scleral show, if not frank ectropion. An ounce of prevention is worth a pound of cure, especially as it relates to the aesthetic unit of the eyelid, globe, and orbit.

Preoperative Evaluation

Preoperative assessment of the problem is essential. The patient is made aware during the initial consultation of those conditions that can be helped by surgery and those that require other modalities of treatment. Asymmetry, fine lines, malar edema, and dark discolorations present limitations to the surgical result. I show these conditions clearly to the patient in front of a mirror.

Both trancutaneous and transconjunctival approaches are used to remove fat, but the transcutaneous route affects the muscle and skin of the anterior eyelid. Although I sometimes use a chemical peel or laser resurfacing for the skin with a transconjunctival approach, I never do it at the same time if the anterior lamella is violated, because this can cause further contraction of the skin and lead to scleral show, or even frank ectropion. I advise such patients to return in a few months to have the aforementioned skin treatments if they so desire.

Pinch Technique

The pinch technique has been my workhorse transcutaneous method for many years. Fat is removed by making stab wounds through the preseptal orbicularis, while maintaining the integrity of the pretarsal orbicularis. By splitting the orbicularis oculi muscle in this fashion, maximum support of the lower eyelid is preserved by keeping the tarsoligamentous complex intact. This tarsoligamentous complex is of particular surgical importance. It is composed of the pretarsal orbicularis oculi muscle, the medial and lateral canthal tendons, and the fibrous tarsal plate (tarsus). Lower eyelid position and tone are related in great part to the integrity of this anatomic unit. The increase in lower lid laxity with age has been attributed to stretching of the lateral canthal tendon. Preservation of the tarsoligamentous complex as a single unit aids in resisting contractile forces placed on the lower lid.

The amount of lower lid skin to be excised is estimated by pinching prior to the skin incision. Hyaluronidase (3 U per milliliter) must be added to the local anesthetic solution in order to enable the skin to adhere as a ridge after being pinched. The patient is asked to look superiorly and open the mouth if he or she is under light sedation; otherwise a conservative estimate of the amount of redundant skin to be excised is made. The skin just inferior to the lower lashes is pinched with a small Brown-Adson forceps, followed by a curved hemostat, which forms a ridge extending from the lateral canthus to the medial limbus (Fig. 2). If the shape of the lower eyelid is altered by pinching, the ridge of skin formed can easily be flattened by gentle traction, and pinching can be repeated until no change in lower lid shape results. I frequently extend the ridge laterally into an appropriate crow's foot line if some lateral skin redundancy is present. However, any significant lateral skin redundancy as well as crow's feet and laugh lines will not be changed by the pre-excision blepharoplasty. These are best handled by a skin flap or skin-muscle flap with lateral extensions.

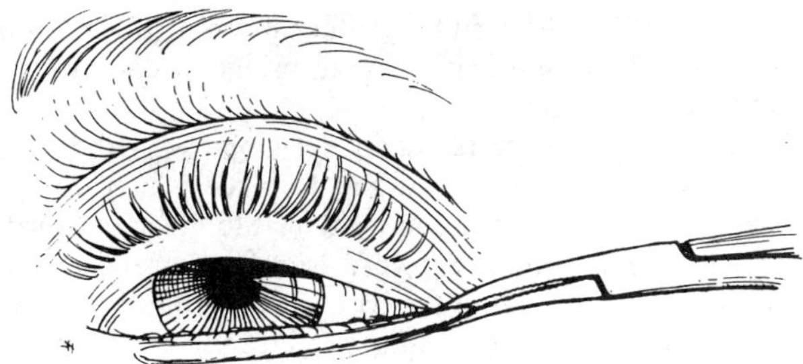

Figure 2.
Lower blepharoplasty: pinch technique. *(From Kamer FM, Milaelian AJ. Pre-excision blepharoplasty. Arch Otolaryngol Head Neck Surg 1991;117:996.)*

I make the incision just inferior to the ciliary line. Placing the incision lower and preserving the pretarsal skin as advocated by some surgeons adds little if any support to the lower lid and makes for a more visible scar that can be difficult to camouflage, even with cosmetics. The ridge of skin formed by pinching is easily excised using fine straight scissors. I place a 5–0 nylon suture in the pretarsal tissue and apply traction in a superior direction. Inferior countertraction is applied with a finger on the cheek below the orbital rim. Using a No. 15 blade, I dissect the pretarsal skin from the pretarsal orbicularis muscle. Although a small amount of hypertrophic orbicularis oculi muscle can be judiciously reduced, it is best to preserve the bulk of pretarsal orbicularis oculi muscle because it maintains the integrity and support of the tarsoligamentous complex, thus helping in prevention of ectropion and rounding of the lower lid. Individual incisions are made through the preseptal orbicularis and orbital septum, which exposes the three lower fat compartments. The fat is identified and dissected free of the septal fibers. I clamp the bases, excise the excess fat, and cauterize the stumps. Hemostasis is obtained by judicious cautery, trying not to disturb the orbital septum, which can contract if exposed to excessive surgical or electrocautery trauma. The skin is redraped over the surgical site and carefully approximated with Histacryl. Iced gauze compresses are applied for 48 hours, and the patient is encouraged to institute eye closure exercises within 72 hours. Petroleum jelly is lightly rubbed on the incision twice a day until the adhesive comes off, usually in approximately 1 week.

Skin Flap

Although the pre-excision (pinch) technique is quite useful in removing pseudoherniated fat, hypertrophic orbicularis muscle, and some redundant skin, a medially based skin rotation flap is employed for more severe dermatochalasis with deep furrowing, especially if there is redundant skin laterally upon animation. A skin flap can contract approximately 10 percent to 15 percent, so much care and judgment must be exercised to assure conservative excision. The incision is made with a No. 15 blade in a laterally based crow's foot or laugh line. It is continued medially just inferior to the lashes in a subciliary line. I place a 5–0 nylon suture in the pretarsal subcutaneous tissue and retract the lid superiorly in order to apply countertraction on the skin flap, which I raise by sharp dissection inferiorly to about the level of the orbital rim. Care is taken to leave the underlying muscle intact. After adequate hemostasis by bipolar cautery, three separate incisions are made through the preseptal orbicularis oculi muscle. The pseudoherniated fat is then isolated, clamped, excised, and cauterized (Fig. 3). Some hypertrophic muscle can be conservatively removed, but it is best to leave the tarsoligamentous complex intact to aid in lid support. A sharp hook is placed in the lateral extent of the wound to aid in lateral retraction. The skin flap is rotated

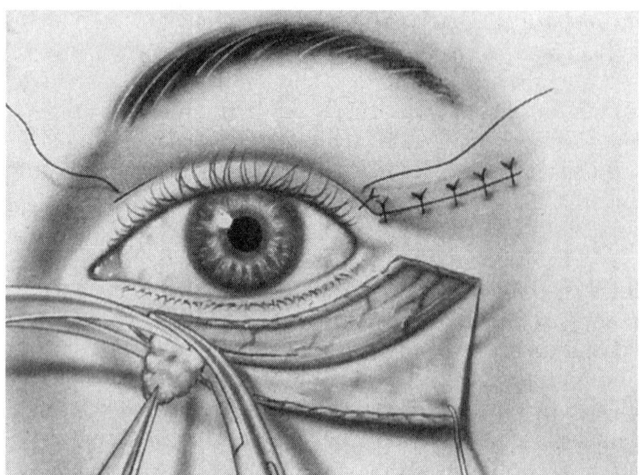

Figure 3.
Lower blepharoplasty: skin flap.

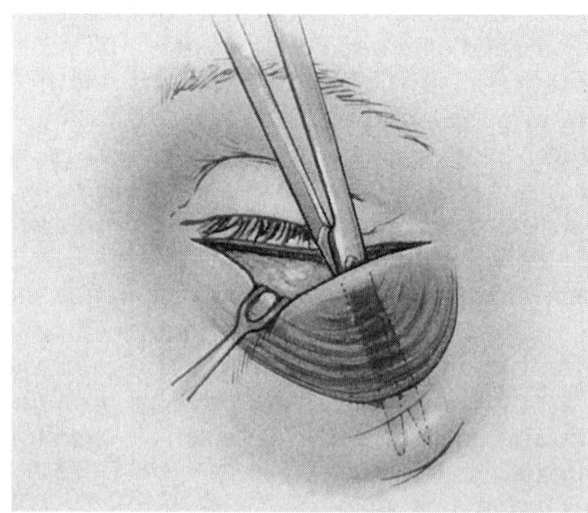

Figure 4.
Lower blepharoplasty: skin-muscle flap.

superiorly; the hook creates the point of rotation. I estimate the amount of redundant skin by conservatively scribing with my eye, and with a scalpel begin the excision laterally at the hook. Fine 6–0 fast-dissolving sutures are placed lateral to the canthus, and after conservatively removing skin from the eyelid, the wound is carefully closed with Histacryl. Care after surgery is as described previously. These patients tend to have more ecchymoses in the postoperative period.

Skin-Muscle Flap

Although many surgeons prefer this technique for their standard approach to blepharoplasty, I reserve it for more advanced presentations. Severe attenuation and stretching of all the elements of the lower lid can create festoons that hang over the infraorbital rim. To adequately improve these advanced conditions, a submuscular dissection is necessary. This technique seriously compromises the integrity and support of the lower lid by severing the pretarsal orbicularis oculi muscle and interrupting the continuity of the tarsoligamentous complex. It can drastically alter the shape, contour, and aesthetics of the eyelid. Although the flap will not contract as much as a skin flap, much care is taken to reapproximate the tissues and reconstitute the support with a lateral suspension suture.

The incision is outlined laterally as in the skin flap, but in a deeper plane, down to the periosteum of the lateral orbit. By placing fine curved scissors in the wound, undermining proceeds medially deep to the orbicularis oculi muscle until the entire area is free. The subciliary incision is then made with the scissors, just inferior to the lashes. As this is a sub–superficial musculoaponeurotic system dissection, there is little bleeding. I use scissors dissection to carefully undermine over the infraorbital rim, freeing the thick flap of skin and muscle medially and laterally (Fig. 4). The pseudoherniated orbital fat is completely exposed and adequately excised and cauterized. In order to strengthen support, I place a 5–0 PDS suture through the orbicularis muscle and anchor it firmly to the periosteum of the orbital rim. This sometimes creates a dimple, but it subsides with time. The flap is trimmed and sutured carefully as described previously.

Transconjunctival Technique

The transconjunctival approach to inferior orbital fat was described by Bourget in 1928. However, it has only gained popularity over the past 10 to 15 years. Because the anterior lamella is not violated, the tarsoligamentous complex remains intact and lid support, position, and contour are unchanged. Only the fat is removed. The skin and overlying tissues conform to the new outline without any chance of ectropion or scleral show unless excessive fat is resected. It is a quick and safe technique, with no skin incision or visible scar. For these reasons, it has become my most frequently performed lower lid procedure for baggy eyelids over the past few years.

The fat compartments are marked with a surgical marker as the patient sits upright and gazes superiorly. After adequate sedation, a couple of drops of tetracaine are placed in the cul-de-sac. An assistant pulls the lid down to expose the cul-de-sac, and a few milliliters of 1 percent lidocaine with 1 :100,000 epinephrine are injected transconjunctivally with a No. 30 gauge needle into the three fat compartments. The surgeon places a small vein retractor in the lid, making sure it remains anterior to the inferior orbital rim. Gentle pressure is applied to the upper lid and globe to expose the redundant fat, which presents as a bulge deep to the conjunctiva. I do not use eye shields, because the upper lid can protect the globe. I make two small incisions, one overlying the lateral fat and the other more medially. I do not connect them, but leave a small bridge of conjunctiva intact between them.

As I apply gentle pressure on the globe with the vein retractor in proper position, a No. 15 blade is used to cut through the conjunctiva and allow the fat to bulge outward. The fat is grasped with a Brown-Adson forceps and teased out of its position. I clamp the base with a hemostat, excise the excess, and cauterize the stump. All three compartments are exposed and treated. The central compartment lies more anteriorly at the infraorbital rim, and it can be frustrating to expose. It is essential to be conservative in the fat removal, because overzealous excision can leave the eye with a hollow appearance and, in extreme cases, some degree of scleral show, or even entropion. I do not suture the incisions, which allows for natural drainage and closure. Iced compresses are placed for 24 to 48 hours, and the patient can then resume relatively normal activities.

Although this technique is safe and quick, it has some distinct limitations. Because the skin and muscle of the anterior lid are not altered, the final result depends on skin draping. Fine lines can be treated simultaneously with peeling or laser resurfacing, but deeper lines with redundant skin or muscle will require reconstruction with an external skin incision as previously described. I am very cautious with patients who present with hypertrophic orbicularis oculi muscle, especially seen on such animation movement as smiling. Transconjunctival fat removal in these cases can exacerbate the problem and lead to the necessity of secondary surgery on the skin and muscle by an external approach. Thus, it is important to correctly analyze the problem preoperatively.

Vertical wedge resections, lateral canthotomies, and similar reconstructive procedures are often performed in attempting to correct all the anatomic variations and perceived deformities of the aging lower eyelid. These techniques, however, radically alter the support and integrity of the eyelid, changing not only the anatomy but also often the individual expression and characteristics of the eye. These complications can be prevented by a more conservative surgical approach. In developing our surgical philosophy and technique, each of us must decide how radically to alter a normal but aging eyelid in pursuit of an aesthetic ideal. Because patients have such a wide variety of individual eyelid characteristics, well-performed blepharoplastic surgery requires that routine not become one's master in the pursuit of improved functional and aesthetic results.

Acknowledgment
I would like to thank Patrick G. Pieper, M.D., for his editorial assistance with this chapter.

Suggested Reading

Bourget J. Notre traitement chirurgical de 'poches' sous les yeux sans cicatrice. Arch Gr Belg Chir 1928; 31:133.

Kamer FM, Joseph JH. Histacryl: Its use in aesthetic facial plastic surgery. Arch Otolaryngol Head Neck Surg 1989; 115:193-197.

Kamer FM, Mikaelian A. Pre-excision blepharoplasty. Arch Otolaryngol Head Neck Surg 1991; 117:995-999

Ousterhout DK, Weil RB. The role of the lateral canthal tendon in lower eyelid laxity. Plast Reconstr Surg 1982; 69:620-622.

THE AGING FACE

The method of
Calvin M. Johnson, Jr.
by
Calvin M. Johnson, Jr.
Mark J. Yanta

A facelift, when properly performed, can be an incredibly satisfying procedure for both surgeon and patient. Few procedures restore a patient's sense of youth and beauty as much as a facelift. Recent advances in deeper place facelifting techniques have enabled surgeons to reposition more of the elements of the aging face and obtain better flap vascularity. By carefully selecting the patient and paying meticulous attention to detail, it is possible to perform a procedure that will have a profound effect on the patient for years to come.

■ INITIAL EVALUATION

The initial consultation period is essential for developing a rapport with the patient and evaluating whether he or she would be a good facelift candidate. The patient must be allowed to communicate his or her expectations and desires to the surgeon, and the surgeon must decide whether these expectations can be met. During this visit, one must determine whether the patient is self-motivated and psychologically prepared for a facelift. Many patients are not aware of and are not prepared for the investment in time and effort that a facelift demands of them. Only with open and honest communication are we able to decide whether the patient is appropriate for the procedure.

In our office, the initial consultation begins with a written patient questionnaire. After the patient has taken a tour of the facilities, both slide film and Polaroid photographs are taken in the standard planes. During this time, the questionnaire is reviewed, and a brief medical history is taken. It is extremely important to know what procedures the patient has already undergone. We also carefully review any medical conditions that may make the patient a poor surgical candidate. In the examination room, the patient discusses areas for improvement. The patient is examined in front of a mirror, with the physician standing behind with fingers placed where the incision lines would be; a lifting motion will demonstrate the effect of a facelift. The Polaroid pictures can also be used to demonstrate areas that can be improved with the facelift procedure. We must not allow our enthusiasm for the procedure to raise the level of patient expectations. The amount of change demonstrated is only that which can be reasonably delivered. It is most common that all elements of the face age simultaneously. Thus, operating on only one aspect of the face tends to leave the patient with an "operated" look. At our center, this is explained to the patient as engaging in the New Orleans custom of painting the front of the house while leaving the back and side untouched. For the purpose of this chapter, however, only the facelift procedure is discussed.

■ PREOPERATIVE INSTRUCTIONS

After the patient has decided to have a facelift, our office nurse gives written and oral preoperative instructions. We ask that the patients refrain completely from using cigarettes and alcohol for a minimum of 2 weeks before and after the procedure. The patients are also instructed to avoid any product containing aspirin or nonsteroidal anti-inflammatory agents during this period. We encourage patients to take a multivitamin before surgery, and also urge them to take a high dose of vitamin C supplement (2,000 mg per day) to aid in the postoperative healing phase. Prescriptions for postoperative medications are also given at the preoperative visit.

■ PROCEDURE

Performing a good facelift is a lengthy and difficult task. We believe that patient movement and varying levels of sedation only complicate the process. Thus, at our center, we perform facelifts under general anesthesia unless a patient's medical evaluation prohibits this. As soon as an intravenous (IV) line has been started, dexamethasone, 6 mg, is given. We also administer cefazolin, 1 g IV, before the procedure begins. In patients who are allergic to penicillin, clindamycin, 600 mg, and gentamicin, 80 mg, are given. Upon the induction of a sufficient level of anesthesia, the entire surgical field is prepped and draped in a sterile fashion. The anesthesia tubing is also draped in a sterile fashion with a stocking.

The facelift portion of aging face surgery is done after the other areas (forehead and eyes) have been addressed. In this way, we are able to place a hemostatic dressing immediately at the conclusion of the facelift procedure. The incisions are marked with a sterile surgical marker. We use a 1:1 mixture of 0.5 percent bupivacaine with 1:200,000 epinephrine and 2 percent lidocaine with 1:100,000 epinephrine to infiltrate the incision lines and the areas of surgical dissection.

Figure 1 demonstrates our incision placement. The temporal incision runs in a curvilinear manner just superior to the ear. This avoids the loss of the temporal hairline that the classic vertical incision creates. The preauricular incision is at the exact junction of the auricle and face. It is important to make a curve in this incision to avoid scar contracture along a straight line. We prefer to make a pretragal incision, unless a previous scar dictates otherwise. A pretragal incision avoids bringing heavy facial skin onto the relatively thin skin of the auricle. Placing the incision behind the tragus can also distort the appearance of the tragus and produce an "operated" look. The incision follows the attachment of the lobule to the facial skin inferiorly. Posteriorly, the incision follows the postauricular crease before gently curving posteriorly into the occipital hairline. This curve starts at the level of the inferior crus of the auricle. The orientation of this incision roughly bisects the angle formed by lines drawn along the hairline and a posterior extension of Frankfort's plane. This placement allows reconstitution of a normal hairline and avoids a step-off deformity in the postauricular area (Fig. 1).

After the facial incisions are made, Stille Original Supercut scissors are used to dissect the preauricular flap in the subcutaneous place. Medial skin traction by the surgical assistant as well as "backlighting" of the flap help maintain the proper dissection plane during this portion of the procedure, In the temporal region, it is important to stay just deep to the hair follicles to avoid any hair loss. Too deep a plane endangers the frontal branch of the facial nerve, which courses superficially in the temporal region before entering the posterior aspect of the frontalis muscle. This dissection proceeds anteriorly until the lateral aspect of the orbicularis oculi muscle is reached. This same plane is lifted inferiorly down past the inferior border of the mandible and into the cervical area. Again, in the occipital area, care must be taken to remain deep to the hair follicles to avoid hair loss.

Next, we elevate the cervical flap. The level of dissection over the sternocleidomastoid muscle must avoid injuring the greater auricular nerve. This cutaneous sensory nerve originates posterior to the sternocleidomastoid muscle and

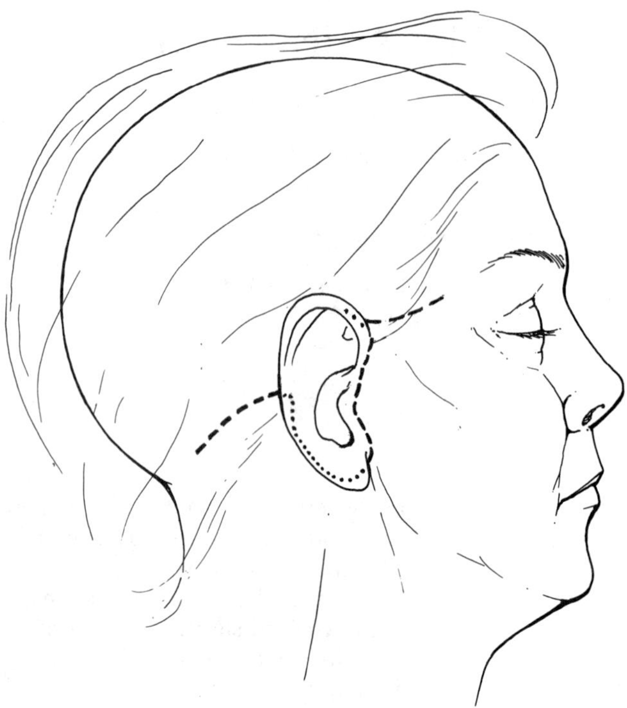

Figure 1.
Placement of incision lines.

runs anteriorly toward the angle of the mandible. Anteriorly, we identify the posterior border of the platysma muscle. Dissection then continues in a preplatysmal plane as far anteriorly as the exposure allows. Metzenbaum Supercut face-lift scissors are used for this portion of the procedure, and the motion is a vertical spreading action (Fig. 2). The superior margin of this dissection is the inferior border of the mandible, and the inferior limit is below the level of the hyoid bone. Staying in a preplatysmal plane protects the marginal mandibular nerve as it courses below the mandible near the notch of the facial artery. Excessive traction or direct damage to the lateral platysma muscle can also cause a pseudoparalysis of the marginal branch, as described by Ellenbogen. If needed, we perform liposuction of the underside of the cervical flap under direct visualization at this time. We do not extend our level of liposuction superior to the inferior border of the mandible, because marked asymmetries of facial contour and skin dimpling are too often the result here.

When the cervical dissection is complete, we return to the facial dissection. An incision is made in the superficial musculoaponeurotic system (SMAS) and parotid fascia extending from just anterior to the angle of the mandible to the junction of the body and arch of the zygoma. The consistency of this layer varies from patient to patient and can range from a fairly defined muscular layer to a thin fascial sheet. We prefer to use a No. 10 blade to dissect underneath this fascial plane. The motion involves a scraping of the underside of the fascial layer with the knife blade. Essential to this portion of the dissection are the use of a lighted, serrated breast retractor and medial countertraction by the assistant.

Superiorly, we have already identified the lateral and inferior portion of the orbicularis oculi muscle. This marks the superolateral border of the deep dissection. We do not perform extensive dissection or resuspension of the orbicularis in order to avoid postoperative ectropion or other changes in eyelid position. At a slightly deeper level and somewhat more inferiorly, we identify the origins of the zygomaticus major and minor muscles. Scissor dissection through the zygomatico-cutaneous ligaments in this area allows skin and soft tissue to redrape over the body of the zygoma and restores the youthful appearance of the cheeks. We continue our medial facial dissection by pushing down on these muscles and lifting the skin and soft tissue off of them. As dissection continues anterior to the parotid gland, facial nerve fibers are often seen coursing just over the masseter muscle. These fibers course superficially to the buccal fat pad and innervate the intrinsic muscles of the mouth and midface (Fig. 3). This dissection continues anteriorly to just lateral to the nasolabial fold.

In patients in whom there is excessive jowling, the buccal fat pad is addressed. We make a small buttonhole incision just superior to the inferior border of the mandible in the area of the jowl fat. The incision parallels the orientation of the facial nerve fibers, and care is taken that they are not injured. Buccal fat is then "teased out" through this incision. A bipolar cautery is used to trim excessive buccal fat and ensure hemostasis. It is important to avoid cauterizing the fascial layer, because the facial nerve fibers may be injured in this manner. Once dissection has been completed, we irrigate the cavity with a lincomycin solution. After carefully attaining hemostasis with bipolar cauterization, we place

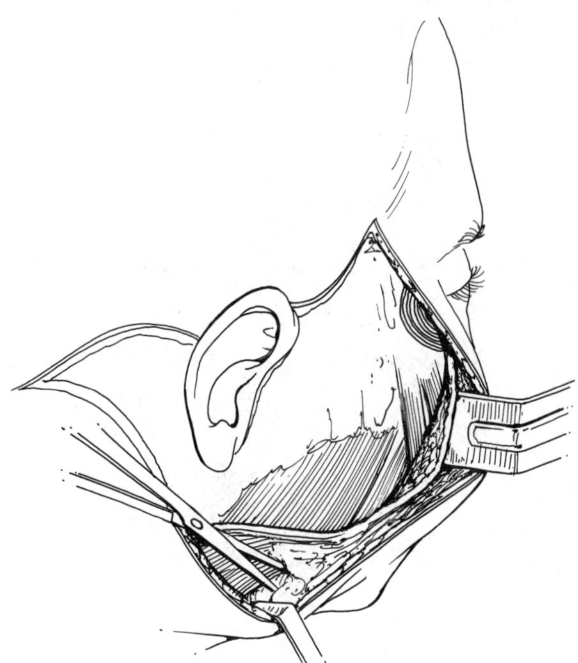

Figure 2.
Lateral aspect of orbicularis oculi muscle and origin of zygomaticus muscles. Preplatysmal dissection with vertical spreading in the neck.

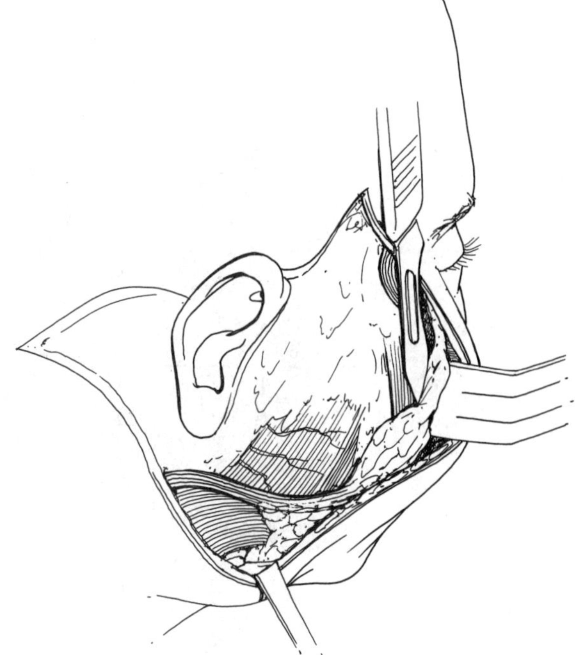

Figure 3.
Deep-plane dissection over zygomaticus muscles. Facial nerve fibers are seen coursing over masseter muscle.

gauze packs lightly into the cavity and turn our attention to the opposite side.

When both sides of the face have been dissected, the submental portion of the dissection is performed. We make a separate 2 to 3 cm incision in the submental area. This incision is placed parallel to the submental crease unless a previous surgical or traumatic scar dictates its position elsewhere. If indicated, a chin augmentation or ptotic chin repair procedure can be performed at this point. These procedures are not discussed in this chapter. For an excellent review of the ptotic chin repair, please refer to Hamra's textbook (see Suggested Reading). Using a retractor for exposure, we perform sharp scissor dissection in a preplatysmal plane. This extends inferiorly below the hyoid bone and over the thyroid cartilage, if possible. The two side of the dissection are thus connected across the midline in this plane. The medial edges of the platysma are then grasped with an Allis clamp. Excessive platysma muscle is trimmed, as well as any excess submental fat. It is important to be conservative in this fat and muscle removal in order to avoid adhesions between the platysma muscle and the skin edges. After obtaining hemostasis with a bipolar cautery, we suture the medial edges of the platysma muscles to each other using interrupted buried 3–0 Prolene sutures (Fig. 4). At the conclusion of the entire procedure, we close the incision with interrupted 5–0 Prolene sutures placed in a vertical mattress fashion. Care is taken to ensure that the wound edges are sufficiently everted.

We then return our attention to the preauricular area. A shelf of tissue has been created by dissecting in two separate planes anteriorly (see Fig. 3). The SMAS edges are then resutured to the preauricular tissues using buried, interrupted 3–0 Prolene sutures. A total of five or six sutures is needed to complete this closure. Figure 5 demonstrates the approximate direction and location of these SMAS–suspension sutures. As can be seen, the manner of redraping is in a superior and posterior direction. Excessive posterior redraping will give a "wind tunnel" appearance. If necessary, the edges of the fascia can be trimmed to avoid making a bulge in the skin. Before skin closure, we insert a 10 Fr round drain in the dependent portion of the cervical dissection field. This drain is brought out through a separate stab incision in the occipital region.

We then redrape the facial skin flap in a superior and posterior direction. We make an incision with a knife in the area that will drape over the ear. A tacking suture is placed in the posterior corner of this incision, using 5–0 Prolene.

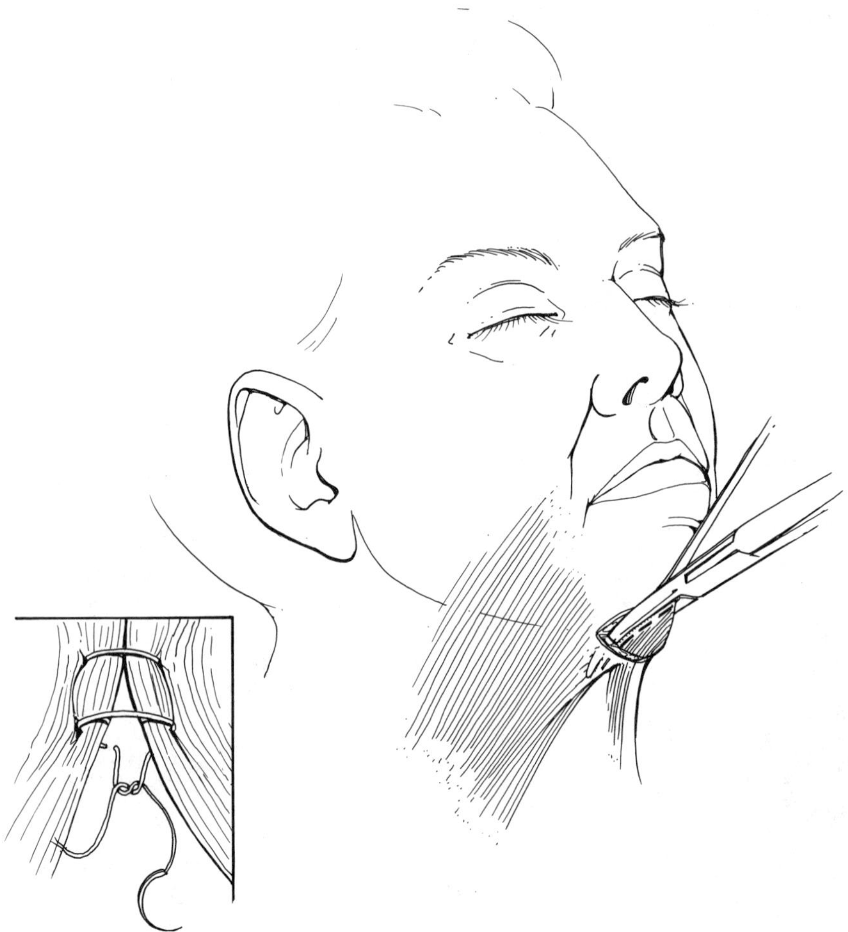

Figure 4.
Removal of medial platysma and submental fat. Inset shows suture reapproximation of platysma in midline.

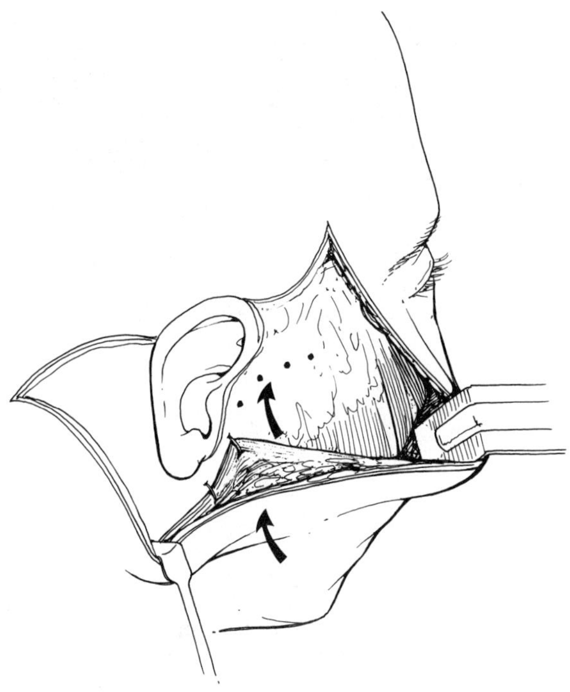

Figure 5.
Resuspension of superficial musculoaponeurotic system and deep tissues in a superior and posterior direction.

Excess temporal skin is removed to match the incision lines. We then trim excess preauricular skin to match the natural curvature of the pinna. Because we have already suspended the SMAS, these closures will be tension-free. In the postauricular area, the redraping is mainly done in a superior direction. Before trimming postauricular skin, we tack the superior and anterior corner of this incision using a Prolene suture. Scissors or a knife blade are then used to remove excess occipital skin. We approximate areas of hair-bearing skin in the temporal and mastoid areas with staples, and close the remaining areas with 5–0 Prolene sutures in an interrupted or running fashion. Care is taken to resuspend the lobule in a natural position to avoid an "operated" look.

At the conclusion of the procedure, we place antibiotic ointment over the suture lines, and nonadherent Telfa gauze over the submental and periauricular incisions. We place a bulky pressure dressing over the face, and place the drains to bulb suction. In order to minimize postoperative bleeding, the patient is extubated at a deep level of anesthesia and carefully observed in the operating room before being transferred to the recovery room.

■ POSTOPERATIVE CARE

Patients are admitted to the facility overnight, and are closely supervised by a nurse. Careful attention is paid to the level of patient anxiety, blood pressure, and activity level. The drains are stripped and emptied as needed. All of these measures are aimed at preventing postoperative hematoma formation. The patient is seen by the surgeon on the first postoperative morning. We take down the bulky dressing and remove the drains. Any cleaning of the incision lines is performed before a light dressing is replaced. We advise the patient to engage in very minimal activities, and we provide them with adequate sedative and analgesic medications.

We next see the patient on postoperative Day 3 or 4. At this visit, we remove the preauricular and submental sutures. We place Collodion and flesh-colored Micropore tape on the skin surface after removing the sutures. We remove staples and postauricular sutures on the seventh postoperative day, and these incisions are similarly taped. The tape is left on for approximately 7 to 10 days, after which time it is removed with the aid of an acetone solution. Prolonged taping is done to prevent wide or pigmented scars. Occasionally, the postauricular incision will require one or two injections of a steroid solution if a hypertrophic scar develops. We use approximately 0.1 ml amounts of triamcinolone acetonide, 10 mg per milliliter, to manage this.

■ THE MALE PATIENT

In many ways, the male patient is not as good a candidate for the facelift procedure as is the female patient. The typically heavier skin does not drape as well, and the extra vascular supply to the bearded skin leads to a higher incidence of postoperative hematoma formation. Men who are unable to limit their level of activity postoperatively are also at risk for this complication. The skin may also have a more sebaceous quality to it that does not tend to heal scars as well. The male facelift patient must also understand that he may need to shave behind the ear postoperatively. The procedure, however, differs little from the operation in the female. The preauricular portion of the incision is moved slightly more anteriorly in order to prevent bringing hair-bearing skin onto the auricle. Similarly, the postauricular incision is placed away from the crease if hair-bearing skin would otherwise be transferred onto the posterior portion of the auricle.

■ REVISION PROCEDURES

The majority of patients who are followed up long-term do not request a revision facelift at a later date. Of those who had surgery elsewhere or had surgery many years ago, the sub–SMAS planes have often not been dissected. Thus, there is little or no scar tissue in these areas, and the procedure differs little from the primary procedure. Where possible, old scars are used for the revision procedure. In a subset of patients requesting revision procedures, the facial tissues have continued to age out of proportion to the cervical portion of the facelift. In these patients, an anterior facelift can be performed. This is performed in a manner similar to the standard facelift procedure, with the incision ending just inferior and posterior to the inferior attachment of the lobule. This procedure can also be used in a very young patient who has aging of the cheek and jowl area with preservation of a youthful-appearing neck.

RESULTS

The senior author's experience with more than 300 deep-plane rhytidectomies has been reviewed by Dr. Neil Gordon. In this review, overall patient satisfaction was 97 percent. Temporary facial nerve paralysis occurred in 0.7 percent, with no permanent paresis or paralysis. The overall hematoma rate was 5 percent, and there was a 1 percent limited skin loss rate. Infection rate was similarly low at 0.3 percent.

Acknowledgment
The authors would like to give special credit to Dr. Sam T. Hamra for his description of deep-plane facelifting techniques.

Suggested Reading

Ellenbogen R. Pseudoparalysis of the mandibular branch of the facial nerve after platysmal face lift operation. Plast Reconstr Surg 1979; 63: 364.

Hamra S. Composite rhytidectomy. St. Louis: Quality Medical Publishing, 1993.

Owsley J. Aesthetic facial surgery. Philadelphia: WB Saunders, 1994.

PROTRUDING EARS

The method of
Thomas Romo III
by
Thomas Romo III
Sarah A. Stackpole

Excessively prominent auricles have inspired many surgeons to devise corrective techniques for these complex defects. The earliest noted method was that of Ely, who described anterior excision of a full-thickness crescent. Further modifications were described by Converse, who delineated a planned cartilage excision from a postauricular approach, and Mustardé, who described reshaping the cartilage with permanent sutures. Stenstrom popularized an anterior cartilage scoring method. Conchal setback has been advocated by Furnas, and Farrior has combined this technique with posterior cartilage scoring. Many techniques are thus available to reshape and reposition excessively prominent auricles. We delineate in this chapter a safe and reliable technique that has produced consistent results.

The goal in otoplastic surgery is the creation of an auricle that appears normal in its position and configuration. This may require creation of new folds in the cartilage, which should be soft and smooth in appearance like those of a normal auricle. Avoidance of sharp edges is very important in achieving a natural appearance.

Our priority in otoplastic surgery is to use a cartilage-sparing technique when possible, while achieving adequate medialization. Cartilage reshaping may be accomplished by cartilage scoring or cartilage excision. Techniques that excise cartilage achieve reduction of protrusion by direct removal, but the sharp edges produced often show through the delicate overlying skin. These sharp angles result in an unnatural appearance. Cartilage scoring softens the spring of the existing cartilage, which is then reshaped by multiple sutures (conchal setback and Mustardé) to achieve a new position. This technique avoids the sharp edges of direct excision.

The repositioning of the auricle as well as the creation of a natural antehelical fold requires an accurate analysis of the defects present in the existing cartilage framework. Inspection will reveal the absence or inadequate angulation of the antehelical fold. Manual folding of the ear posteriorly against the mastoid process will disclose conchal excess and will also define the area for creation of an absent antehelical fold. This soft transition area will be sculpted into a defined antehelical curve by the placement of Mustardé sutures. These permanent mattress sutures cause the cartilage to fold or buckle, without creating unnatural sharp edges.

Many types of postauricular incisions have been described, and these incisions are usually located at or near the sulcus. Violation of the postauricular sulcus can result in webbing, hypertrophic scar, or keloid formation. The design of a posterior skin flap that avoids distortion of the sulcus, as well as eliminates any wound closure tension, has been previously described by the senior author. The following is a description of our technique, which uses a postauricular skin flap approach for a cartilage-sparing, but cartilage-scoring, otoplasty. The unique aspect of this technique is the use of the posterior skin flap, which is described in detail.

PREOPERATIVE EVALUATION

The ears are inspected for symmetry as well as for specific individual defects. Particular attention is paid to the extent of conchal excess and the presence or lack of antehelical fold development. The lobule is also evaluated for its extent of protrusion. It should be kept in mind that the ears may not protrude to the same extent, and therefore each side must be individually tailored to produce a symmetric result.

The timing of surgery is generally planned for when the child is 5 to 6 years old. This timing is important for three reasons. First, the visible deformity is corrected before the child starts grammar school, where peer ridicule may adversely affect him or her. Second, the child is old enough to participate in the postoperative surgical care without disturbing the wound or injuring the reshaped auricle. Third, by age 6 the auricle has achieved 90 percent of average adult size, which allows the surgeon to judge the anticipated result in a nearly adult-sized auricle. Therefore, the reconstruction is highly accurate for long-term stability. Surgery is routinely performed under general endotracheal anesthesia due to the child's age. Procedures on older adolescents and adults may be performed using local anesthesia and intravenous sedation techniques.

Photographic analysis is an important aid in surgical planning. Preoperative photographs are obtained that illustrate the deformity from the anterior, lateral, and posterior directions. The hair should be drawn away from the ears using headbands or clips. Preoperative photos also allow comparisons of postoperative results.

Measurements are performed at four points along the helix, which are repeated on the day of surgery, and compared for adequacy of correction on both sides (Fig. 1). Four marks are made. The primary point is the first marked, and it serves as the reference for the additional markings. The first point (point 1) is marked at the edge of the helix on a level at the top of the external canal meatus (i.e., along a continuation of the Frankfort horizontal). The second point is marked 2 cm below the primary point, along the helix, and the third point is marked 2 cm above the primary point.

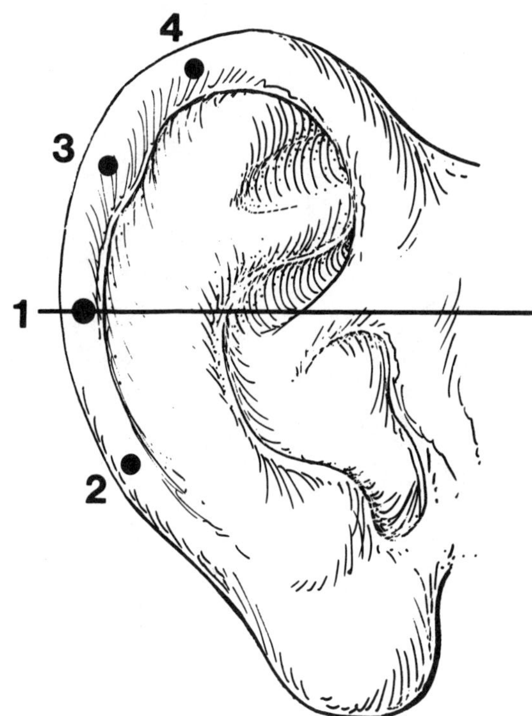

Figure 1.
Marking of the measurement points.

Finally, a fourth point is marked at the site of the greatest helical height, usually 1.5 to 2 cm above point 3. Measurements are made from the lateral skull to each point and recorded. The goal is to produce a final measurement of 15 to 18 mm of helical protrusion for points 1 and 2, and 18 to 20 mm for points 3 and 4. The concha must be set back adequately to produce a pleasing alignment, generally at least 3 to 4 mm less (i.e., more medial) than the primary point along the helix. The conchal protrusion thus is usually 12 to 15 mm after adequate repositioning.

■ OPERATIVE TECHNIQUE

This technique uses a unique approach to the posterior auricular skin incision. A skin flap is designed to expose all areas of suture placement and cartilage scoring. The design thus prevents complications of scar placement in the postauricular sulcus. The posteriorly based skin flap allows excellent exposure, yet remains cosmetically pleasing due to its location behind the helical rim.

Most procedures are performed under general anesthesia. The ears are prepped with Techni-Care surgical prep solution. Both ears are draped into the field so as to allow head rotation. The face may be covered with a transparent drape or fully included in the surgical field.

The procedure begins with marking of the primary point along the helical rim, which serves as a reference for additional markings. As in Figure 1, point 1 (primary point) is marked on the helix at the level of the top of the external canal (i.e., on a continuation of the Frankfort horizontal). Point 2 is marked on the helical rim 2 cm below the primary point, and point 3 is marked 2 cm above the primary point. Point 4 is the final point marked, at the site of greatest helical height, usually 1.5 to 2 cm above point 3. For each ear, measurements of the amount of protrusion are made for each point. These measurements are recorded for further comparison so that the surgeon can easily see them, either on a marking board or on the drapes.

The superior helix is manually medialized, which indicates the naturally occurring crease that will become the newly created antehelical fold. The desired amounts of conchal and helical medialization are determined by manual positioning. Once the desired position is stabilized, the new distances to points 1, 2, 3, and 4 are measured, and the planned protrusion measurements are recorded. The sites of the Mustardé sutures are also noted while the medialized position is maintained. These sites are marked anteriorly and posteriorly using marking pens; the final position will be slightly adjusted with the placement of each individual suture.

The ear is then folded anteriorly to mark the posterior skin flap (Fig. 2). The skin flap is based on the mastoid skin and has no disruption at the posterior sulcus. The marking is begun superiorly, beginning 1 cm above the edge of the superior sulcus. The marking is then carried onto the posterior ear skin close to the edge of the helix. The marking must include the areas of all planned Mustardé sutures, including the most superior and most inferior sites. The planned flap may be marked to continue onto the lobule if lobule medialization is planned. The marking is then carried posteriorly onto the mastoid skin, crossing over the posterior sulcus, but not lying within it.

Local anesthetic is injected along the planned incision line, as well as infiltrated under the marked flap and adjacent mastoid and temporal skin. A dilute solution of 0.5 percent lidocaine with 1:200,000 epinephrine is routinely used, which creates adequate vasoconstriction and hydrodissection. The routine 1 percent lidocaine solution (with 1:100,000 epinephrine) is diluted with an equal volume of sterile water. This allows a larger volume to be injected, which may be especially beneficial in small children.

The skin incision is made with a No. 15 blade, and then fine curved Stevens scissors are used to dissect the posterior skin off the perichondrium. Double-pronged skin hooks are used to gently retract the ear as well as to hold the skin flap. The skin flap is retracted by the surgeon onto the ball of his supporting finger so as not to puncture the delicate flap. The perichondrium is preserved in this dissection, because the plane is developed just superficial to the perichondrium. The skin is elevated off the entire posterior aspect of the ear all the way across the posterior sulcus. This allows easy redraping of the skin at the conclusion of the medialization. A 5 to 6 mm skin margin is preserved intact at the helical rim. The excess soft tissues are carefully trimmed from the skin flap to prevent bunching and step-off deformities with the skin closure (Fig. 3).

After adequate exposure has been achieved, hemostasis is achieved with electrocautery. Fine-tipped jeweler's forceps are used to grasp the bleeding vessels, and then a limited current is applied to the forceps to minimalize thermal dam-

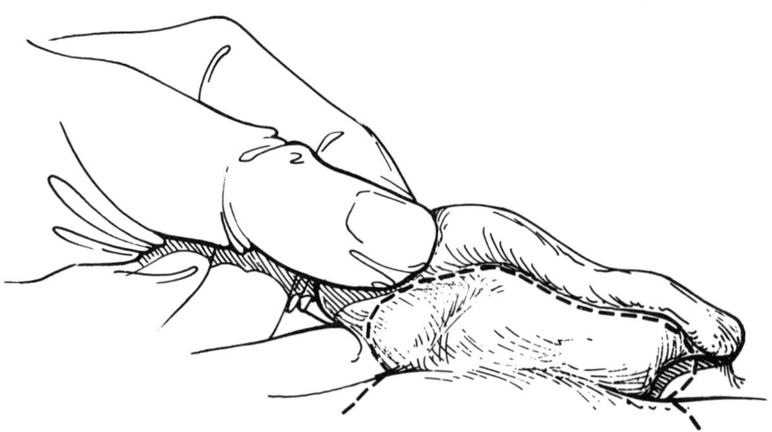

Figure 2.
Marking of the skin flap.

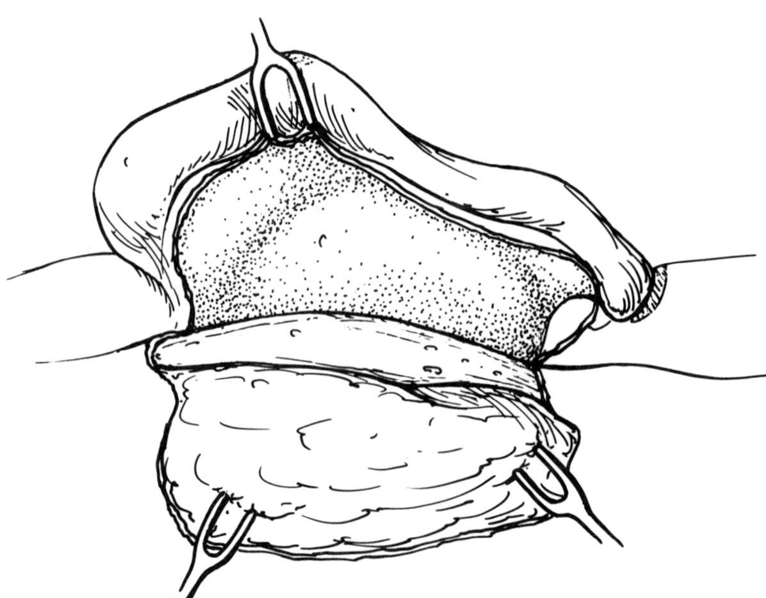

Figure 3.
Elevated postauricular flap.

age to the delicate flap and perichondrium. Then, the medialization is begun. To weaken the spring of the conchal cartilage, a No. 15 blade is used to score the cartilage in parallel strokes along its posterior surface. Several parallel cuts are made from superior to inferior in a gently curving pattern. The first cut is made near the external auditory meatus, and further incisions are made fanning outward parallel to it (Fig. 4). The anterior perichondrium should not be violated with these scoring incisions. Additional scoring is performed on the posterior surface of the scaphoid cartilage. These incisions are directed parallel to the planned curve of the antehelical fold.

Further medialization of the concha may be performed by relaxing incisions, if necessary. These incisions are made extending the conchal scoring inferiorly and superiorly, very close to the attachment of the cartilaginous canal. Relaxation of this tightly tethered area will allow the whole cartilage to settle into a more gentle medial curve.

After adequate scoring is completed, conchal setback sutures are placed (Fig. 5). Three sutures are placed from the

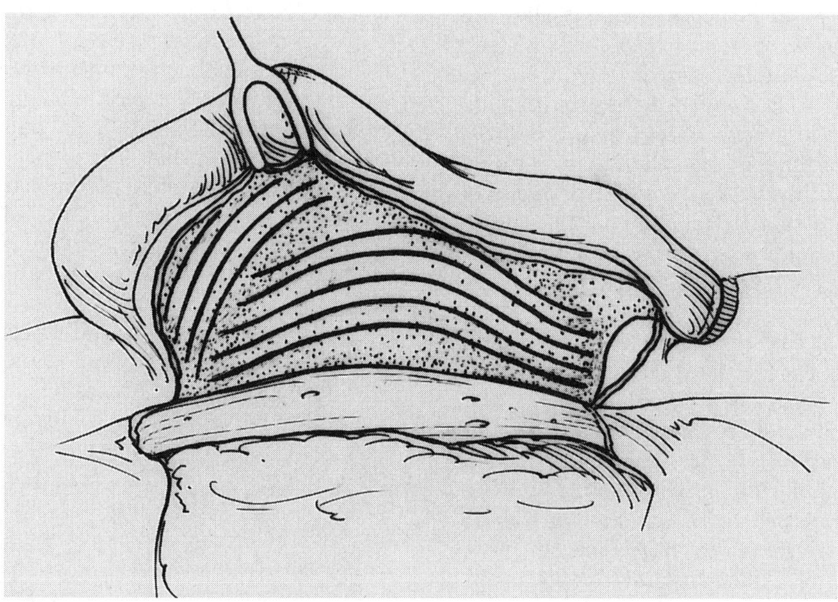

Figure 4.
Scoring pattern.

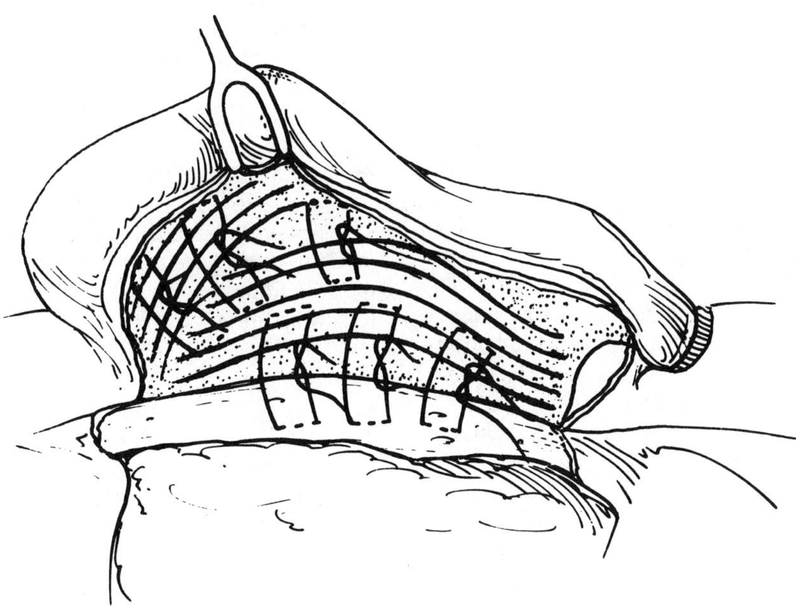

Figure 5.
Conchal setback and placement of Mustardé sutures.

most posterior edge of the conchal cartilage to the mastoid periosteum, which is accessible due to the prior posterior flap dissection. Mersilene 3–0 sutures are used to draw the concha down to the mastoid, reducing the protrusion of the entire pinna from the side of the skull. The sutures are placed from the edge of the conchal cartilage to the deep mastoid periosteum. A central suture is placed primarily, and then an inferior and a superior suture are added. A single long suture is used for each setback stitch. Each suture is secured with multiple primary throws of an extended surgeon's knot, but not tied down. Each initial throw is tightened down to medialize the concha, but not knotted. The sutures are left long, and secured with a fine hemostat clamp, to allow for further adjustment. Once all sutures are tightened into their final position, the knots are fully secured.

After the conchal setback is completed, the external auditory meatus should be inspected. Excessive suturing may cause rotation of the cartilage at the meatus, which results in a stenotic opening. If this is noted, the sutures should be released and placed so as to maintain an adequate meatal opening. The concha should be set back at least 3 to 4 mm more medially than the helical rim, as measured at the new antehelical fold.

After adequate scoring has been completed, the Mustardé sutures are placed (Fig. 5). Usually three sutures are used in a mattress pattern to form a new curved antehelical fold, but sometimes four or five may be necessary to achieve good definition. White or undyed 4–0 Mersilene is used because it does not show through the thin auricular skin. All sutures are placed before they are tied down, and then each is adjusted to the appropriate tightness to create a smooth curvature to the antehelical fold. The Mustardé sutures are intended to create a new antehelical fold, and are thus concentrated in the upper half of the auricle, at the level of the marked primary point and above this area. Generally, no Mustardé sutures are necessary below this point.

The first Mustardé suture is placed on the posterior surface of the cartilage, medial to point 3 on the helical rim. The lateral bite is performed first, and the suture edges are grasped with a Brown-Adson forceps and drawn medially to test the ideal placement of the medial site. After the optimal position has been ascertained, and the front of the auricle has been inspected for the adequacy of the antehelical folding, the second bite of the mattress suture is placed. Again, a multiple-throw surgeon's knot is made, and the ends are clamped. Additional Mustardé sutures are placed to form a new antehelical fold, and they are similarly cinched down. The second and third Mustardé sutures are placed above and below the first suture in a fan-shaped pattern radiating outward from the upper half of the conchal bowl. The tightening of these sutures will buckle the cartilage to create a gently curved antehelical fold. After all final adjustments have been made, each suture is fully tied down.

If excessive lateralization of the lobule is still noted after the cartilage is adequately addressed, medialization of the lobule may be performed. Usually, an elliptical excision of skin from the posterior lobule will provide sufficient posterior positioning of the lobule. However, if this is insufficient, the soft tissue of the lobule may be sutured to the mastoid periosteum or overlying muscular fascia. A 4–0 Mersilene suture is used. If a protruding lobule is not addressed, the postoperative result will be marred by its abnormal orientation to the rest of the repositioned pinna. If the position of the lobule is not improved by elliptical excision of posterior skin, the protrusion may be due to the persistent force of the cauda helicis. This inferior extension of the helical cartilage toward the lobule may need direct trimming. This area of cartilage is accessible due to the wide exposure of the posterior skin flap. The excess knuckle of cartilage is gently exposed and carved smoothly on its inferior surface using the No. 15 blade.

After adequate medialization of the cartilage framework and soft tissue has been achieved, the posterior skin flap is draped over the sulcus and the posterior surface of the ear. The skin is carefully positioned without tension, and excess skin is marked and excised. The emphasis in this step is avoidance of tension, just as in the redraping of skin in a lower lid blepharoplasty. The management of this skin flap is very important to avoid postoperative complications such as webbing or keloid formation.

The skin is then closed in two layers over a drain. The subcutaneous layer is closed using 5–0 undyed polyglactin 910, and the skin edges are closed using interrupted 5–0 Poligiecaprone 25. A small rubber band drain is positioned at the inferior edge of the closure, and this is removed when the dressing is changed on postoperative Day 5. The suture line is covered with topical bacitracin ointment.

A conforming dressing is placed to support the ear in its new configuration. Cotton strips impregnated with mineral oil are carefully tucked into the creases along the antehelical fold and into the concha, as well as behind the ear to support the postauricular skin flap. A bilateral mastoid dressing is applied, using fluffs and a wrapped ear dressing (2 inch Kling). Both ears are wrapped while the head is supported by an assistant. Care is taken to keep the dressing high on the forehead, and this area is secured with adhesive tape to prevent the dressing from slipping down over the eyes.

All patients receive preoperative intravenous antibiotics and postoperative oral antibiotics for adequate gram-positive coverage. Minimal oral analgesics (usually acetaminophen) are used. If the patient develops excessive pain, this may herald a hematoma or skin necrosis. All patients who experience new or excessive pain should have the dressing removed and the ears inspected.

The mastoid dressing is removed on postoperative Day 5. A wide headband is used to maintain the ears in a medial position during the early weeks of healing. The headband is used 24 hours per day for 2 weeks, and then only at night for an additional 6 weeks.

■ COMPLICATIONS

Complications of otoplasty may be grouped into early and late occurrences. Early complications include hematoma, skin necrosis, cellulitis, and perichondritis. Prophylactic preoperative and postoperative antibiotics are routinely used to minimize the chance of infectious complications. The use of a drain as well as a gentle compressive dressing similarly minimizes the likelihood of hematoma formation. Skin necrosis may occur at points of excessive pressure, but wound inspection in any patient who complains of excessive pain should catch this uncommon problem early on. The gentle redraping of the postauricular skin also avoids excessive tension.

Late complications include keloid formation, posterior sulcus webbing, suture protrusion, and hypesthesia as well as inadequate correction or other poor cosmetic results. This postauricular skin flap technique is designed to eliminate tension on the postauricular closure. Thus far, no instances of webbing or keloid formation have been seen in patients treated with this approach. Any extruded sutures should be removed as atraumatically as possible. Once adequate healing and fibrosis has occurred, the extrusion of a Mustardé or conchal setback suture should not significantly affect the final result. Inadequate correction or poor cosmetic results must be analyzed individually to determine the cause, and revision surgery will probably be required to achieve the desired result.

Suggested Reading

Farrior RT. A method of otoplasty. Arch Otolaryngol 1959; 69:400-408.

Furnas DW. Correction of prominent ears by concha-mastoid sutures. Plast Reconstr Surg 1968; 42:189-193.

Mustardé JC. The correction of prominent ears using simple mattress sutures. Br J Plast Surg 1963; 16:170.

Romo T III, Sclafani AP, Shapiro AL. Otoplasty using the postauricular skin flap technique. Arch Otolaryngol Head Neck Surg 1994; 120: 1146-1150.

MICROTIA: RECONSTRUCTIVE METHODS

The method of
John K. Niparko
John L. Frodel, Jr.
by
Allyson M. Ray
John K. Niparko
John L. Frodel, Jr.

The term *microtia* refers to complete hypoplasia of the pinna, the most common type of congenital auricular deformity. Classically, the defect is unilateral and comprises a longitudinal peanut-shaped vestige of skin and deformed cartilage that occupies the position of the external meatus. The external auditory canal may be partially or completely atretic. Because this deformity represents abnormal development of the first and second branchial arches, one should be aware of other anatomic anomalies that may be manifest, such as those of the middle ear, facial nerve, or temporomandibular joint, and syndromes with hemifacial microsomia, mandibulofacial dysostoses, or cleft palate. Hereditary factors and intrauterine assault from drugs or infections have been linked to microtia, although these etiologies are not well defined. There does appear to be a preponderance of unilateral cases; the right ear is affected more frequently than the left, and males have this condition more than females.

Microtia is a deformity readily apparent at birth that can be very distressing to families. A great deal of counseling and support should be provided at this time, as well as involving a team of specialists. Emphasis must always be placed on audiologic rehabilitation as the first priority in the management of the child who has microtia, and audiometric evaluation should be obtained as early as possible. If surgical repair of the aural atresia is to be performed, close collaboration with the otologic surgeon is essential, because timing with the microtia repair should be coordinated. In rare instances, some families may choose *not* to have their child undergo microtia repair, either by surgical reconstruction or prosthetic rehabilitation. However, the psychological impact of this deformity is often readily apparent as the child becomes socially interactive, as when he starts school. For this reason, most surgeons agree that repair of microtia can start as early as age 6 years. At this age the normal ear has reached nearly 85 percent of its adult size, and rib size is sufficient for graft purposes if surgical reconstruction is proposed.

■ GOALS OF REPAIR

After the decision has been made to repair the defect, the surgeon should spend a significant amount of time discussing each of the two options, surgical reconstruction versus prosthetic rehabilitation, and the goals of repair for each. If the patient is a child, both child and parents must understand that each of the methods has advantages and disadvantages, each entails multiple stages, and neither one will create a "perfect match" to the normal ear. The aim of both options is to restore facial symmetry and to provide a structure that closely approximates the size, position, and projection of a normal ear. If surgical reconstruction with a costal cartilage graft is being considered, the patient and family should have realistic expectations and acknowledge that surgically re-creating the intricate folds of the helices is a complex process that does not solely reside in the technical—or artistic—abilities of the surgeon, but also on the properties of skin thickness and its healing capabilities. Precise, natural-looking contours are rarely achieved, and scar tissue is always present to some degree. On the other hand, an auricular prosthesis with fine, elegant folds can easily be fashioned, but it is synthetic, and can easily be distinguished as such upon close inspection. Psychologically, some patients also may be reluctant to rely on a prosthesis rather than their own tissue.

SURGICAL RECONSTRUCTION

The greatest success in surgical repair of microtia has been seen when using sculpted costal cartilage graft in a multistaged procedure. A summary of this method is included here, but for a detailed description, one can refer to the published works of Brent, who has mastered and refined this technique. Again, the ideal age to begin this process is age 6 to 7 years, and in most cases microtia repair should precede aural atresia repair. The best results are obtained when the cartilage framework is inserted under virgin skin, and not under scarred tissue that has previously been violated by surgical repair of the atresia. Only in cases of bilateral microtia with atresia where audiologic rehabilitation is inadequate should one ear be explored first in order to correct the hearing loss.

Stage I: Creation and Insertion of Cartilaginous Framework

Preoperatively, the size and shape of the proposed auricle is measured by outlining the opposite, normal pinna using transparent radiographic film. The inverted image then is used to design the rib graft and its placement at the defective site. In patients who have bilateral microtia, the ear must be created according to standard anatomic measurements and landmarks. The position of the ear is most easily determined by the distance to the lateral canthus of the eye and the corner of the mouth, whereas the longitudinal axis of the ear should align with the nasal dorsal profile. When harvesting costal cartilage, one should take advantage of the rib configuration inherent on the side *contralateral* to the microtia defect that is being repaired. The first free-floating rib can be used to form the helix, and the synchondrosis of the above two ribs is ideal for the body of the framework (Fig. 1). The helix and body are sculpted according to template dimensions and then secured together with nonabsorbable sutures. A carving curet can be used to excavate the scaphoid and triangular fossae (Fig. 2, *A*). Finally, a three-tiered structure is constructed by the addition of an extra block of cartilage sutured to the medial aspect of the body (Fig. 2, *B*).

Fabrication of the framework requires an understanding of the healing properties of skin, because skin thickness and tension will alter the ultimate appearance of the cartilaginous framework. The details of this crucial portion of the procedure are well described in the literature; however, the

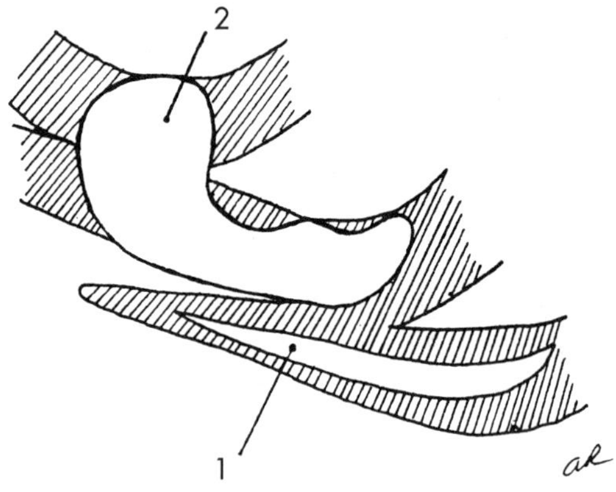

Figure 1.
Method of surgical reconstruction: harvesting costal cartilage using synchondrosis of lower ribs to create the body (2) of the framework, and the first free-floating rib as the helix (1).

surgeon should possess technical expertise in sculpting these complex frameworks before use of these techniques in the operating room. A preauricular incision and subcutaneous pocket is created, and any vestigial cartilage is removed before inserting the framework. Vestigial skin and soft tissue, including the misplaced lobule, is left in place at this time. If the hairline extends low over the helix and scapha, the problem can be dealt with at a later date, either when a skin graft is applied in stage III or with electrolysis. Continuous suction drains are applied, and a protective head dressing is placed.

Stage II: Lobule Transposition

Two months after healing is complete, the lobule can be rotated and spliced onto the cauda helicis, with lifting of the tip of the framework away from the skull at the same time. The lobule defect can usually be closed primarily, but if this is not feasible, a skin graft can be placed. A full-thickness skin graft can be placed after further soft tissue is removed, and after conchal excavation is performed. If no earlobe exists, it should be incorporated in the cartilaginous framework and lifted later when the entire postauricular sulcus is created.

Stage III: Detachment of the Auricle

A posterosuperior sulcus is formed by incising just below the hairline along the helix and detaching the upper margin of the auricle from the temporal bone. The hair-bearing scalp is thus reflected behind the ear, and a split-thickness skin graft is applied to the newly created sulcus and superior helical margin. This procedure simply detaches the auricular framework from the skull and does not compensate for a lack of projection caused by insufficient depth of the framework.

Stage IV: Tragus Construction

After several months, the final stage includes construction of a tragus using a composite conchal graft from the normal ear when available. If there is inadequate projection of the

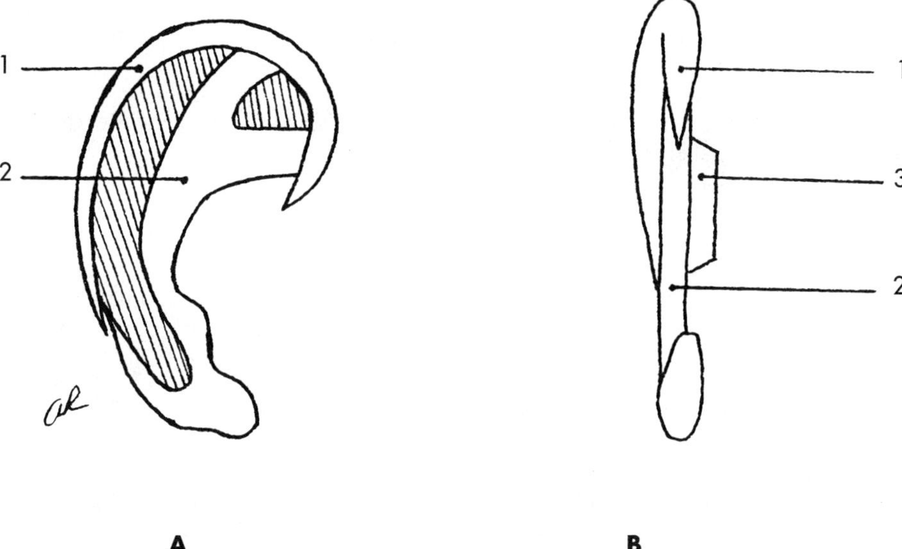

Figure 2.
Method of surgical reconstruction: creating a three-tiered, cartilaginous framework. *A*, Lateral view: helix (1) is secured to the body (2), and the scaphoid and triangular fossae have been shallowed with a curet. *B*, Frontal view: additional block of cartilage (3) is sutured to the medial aspect of the framework to provide projection from the skull.

reconstructed auricle, one can set back the normal auricle at this time while harvesting the conchal graft, in order to achieve frontal symmetry. The illusion of a meatus is created by excavating the conchal site of soft tissue, if this has not been performed previously. The shadow cast by the newly formed tragus and the deepened conchal bowl will mimic the external ear canal.

Clinical Results

Complications of surgical repair with costal cartilage may involve either the graft site or the insertion site, but these are rare occurrences if the surgeon adheres to proper techniques. Pneumothorax is a potential complication that should be recognized intraoperatively and easily dealt with before closing the chest wound. Atelectasis is the most common postoperative problem, which can be prevented with perioperative instruction and respiratory therapy. Infection, hematoma, and skin necrosis with cartilage exposure may cause devastating wound care dilemmas that threaten graft survival and result in severe scar formation. These problems are best addressed by preventing their occurrence. Experience has shown that strict attention to sterile technique and hemostasis and the use of suction drains rather than bolster sutures appears to decrease the incidence of skin slough. During the first 2 weeks postoperatively, one should also carefully monitor the wound and all head dressings for early signs of these problems.

After healing is complete, perhaps the most common problem is a less than satisfactory result. Because of the inherent limitations in cartilage graft survival as related to skin thickness and vascularity, wound healing is unpredictable. Even in experienced hands, scar formation and contracture are present to some degree in all reconstructions, and an inexperienced surgeon may actually create a structure more devastating than the unrepaired defect. To limit untoward results, one must adhere to known principles of auricular reconstruction and meticulously attend to these details intraoperatively. Again, preoperative counseling is essential in preparing a patient and the family for realistic expectations and the possibility of unsatisfactory results. It is not uncommon for patients to require multiple revision procedures.

On long-term follow-up, the durability of auricular reconstruction with sculpted costal cartilage has been effectively demonstrated by Brent in an extensive series of patients. There appears to be little or no resorption, with most reconstructed ears growing to keep pace with the normal ear, and these ears retain their detail without blunting or softening. Even when subjected to trauma from sports injuries and insect bites, the reconstructed ears have healed without incident. The psychological and emotional benefits that accompany this procedure have also been observed with long-term follow-up. With satisfactory results, parents and patients indicate a greater level of extroversion, with increased participation in social, athletic, and academic activities.

■ PROSTHETIC REHABILITATION

An alternative to surgical reconstruction of the auricle with autogenous tissue, prosthetic rehabilitation methods use alloplastic polymers to create an aesthetically acceptable auricle that can be fixed to the mastoid bone. In the past, prosthetic rehabilitation was limited by problems with fixation; however, current use of osseointegrated tissue techniques has proved very successful. The concept of osseointegration is based on the ability of bone to grow directly into the oxide surface of titanium. When the implants are surgically placed in atraumatic fashion, there is absence of fibrous tissue ingrowth, and true osseointegration is feasible. Experience in fixating auricular prostheses percutaneously has shown this method to be a reliable option for patients. In particular, patients who are either predisposed to hypertrophic scar formation or have previously undergone unsuccessful reconstructive procedures with resultant scarring and disfigurement may benefit from tissue-integrated prosthetic rehabilitation.

Methods

Surgical methods have been described in detail previously; however, a summary of each stage is presented here. Two surgical stages are involved, each performed easily under local anesthesia in an outpatient setting unless they are planned in conjunction with external ear canal reconstruction. First, the implant fixture is anchored to the mastoid cortex and covered with soft tissue. Three months later, the second procedure involves fitting with percutaneous abutments. After 2 weeks of healing, the external retention unit and prosthesis are applied at the third stage.

Stage I: Placement of Intraosseous Implants

Preoperative consultation with the prosthetic sculptor is obtained before planning the location of the implants, because these sites determine the eventual location of the retentive unit. During the initial surgical stage, atraumatic and precise preparation of the implant sites is observed in accordance with principles that preserve bone viability. Pilot holes are drilled 10 to 20 mm from the external meatal center to correspond to the projected antihelix. For the left mastoid, these positions correspond to 1 and 4 o'clock, and for the right mastoid, 11 and 8 o'clock (Fig. 3, *A* and *B*). Depth-limiting burs are used to assess cortical thickness and detect underlying dura or sigmoid sinus (Fig. 3, *C*). When the pilot holes demonstrate at least 3 mm of cortical bone thickness, the hole is enlarged and countersunk in order to increase the surface area contact with the implant flange (Fig. 3, *D*).

Preparation of the implant site now involves low-revolution rotary drilling and liberal amounts of irrigation. The wall of each drill hole is threaded with the titanium tap at speeds of 8 to 15 rpm (Fig.3, *E*). At this point, the tap surface and titanium fixture must be kept free from any non-titanium contaminants. The fixture is then driven into the tapped hole, again at low revolutions and with copious irrigation (Fig. 3, *F*). The implanted fixture is capped and covered with soft tissue as the incision is closed (Fig. 3, *G*).

Stage II: Seating of Percutaneous Abutments

Three months later, the implants are exposed through the same incision and fitted with 3.0 to 5.5 mm abutments that perforate the overlying skin and soft tissue. Subcutaneous fat is excised from the flap in order to facilitate direct seating of the dermis onto the mastoid periosteum. This allows for reduced soft-tissue mobility (Fig. 3, *H–J*). At this stage, cartilaginous remnants should be removed or, in the absence of a tragus, these remnants can be used for reconstructing the tragus. The presence of a native or reconstructed tragus is helpful in camouflaging the anterior margin of the prosthesis. A gauze dressing is wrapped around the abutments to compress the skin against the mastoid during the 2 week healing phase.

Stage III: Assembly of Retention Unit and Prosthesis

The external retention unit and prosthesis are assembled and anchored using a bar-clip system (Fig. 3, *K–M*). Because chemical adhesives are unnecessary, skin reaction to the prosthesis is uncommon, and the prosthesis may be designed with thin, translucent margins. This produces a more natural skin-to-prosthesis transition and understandably a superior aesthetic result.

Clinical Results

Presently, many authors worldwide have documented their experience with osseointegrated prostheses in auricular rehabilitation, and their overall success rate is encouraging. Several criteria are available for assessing the success of these implants, including implant longevity, patient morbidity, and cosmesis. The technique of osseointegration in the mastoid cortex is easily performed in two surgical stages, with success rates exceeding 95 percent and reliably maintained long term. Morbidity, which occurs in less than 10 percent of patients, appears limited to adverse skin reactions at the percutaneous abutment sites. The incidence of these skin reactions can be lowered by thinning the soft tissue surrounding the abutments, avoiding hair-bearing areas, and maintaining good hygiene at the wound site. Because the prosthesis is securely fixed without the need for skin adhesives, this method provides far better function and cosmesis when compared to traditional prosthetic fixation techniques.

■ DISCUSSION

Microtia is a congenital auricular deformity that results in psychological and emotional distress to patients and their families. In most instances, aural atresia is an associated deformity and requires early audiologic evaluation, parental counseling, and collaboration with an otologist. Hearing rehabilitation is always the primary concern, and after that has been achieved, attention can be turned to elective repair of the microtia defect. Current options include either surgical reconstruction with costal cartilage or prosthetic rehabilitation using osseointegrated implants. Both options will restore facial symmetry and provide a three-dimensional structure that closely resembles an external ear, and have demonstrated low morbidity and long-term durability. Each has advantages and disadvantages, however, and are perceived quite differently by each individual.

In experienced hands, reconstruction with sculpted costal cartilage has been considered the traditional standard since it has the advantages of creating an auricle using autogenous tissue, thus providing significant psychological benefits. The procedure has the disadvantage of entailing at least four surgical procedures and a donor morbidity site. The final result will always have a less refined appearance than a normal ear. The physiologic properties of wound healing and the expertise of the surgeon are factors that directly influence

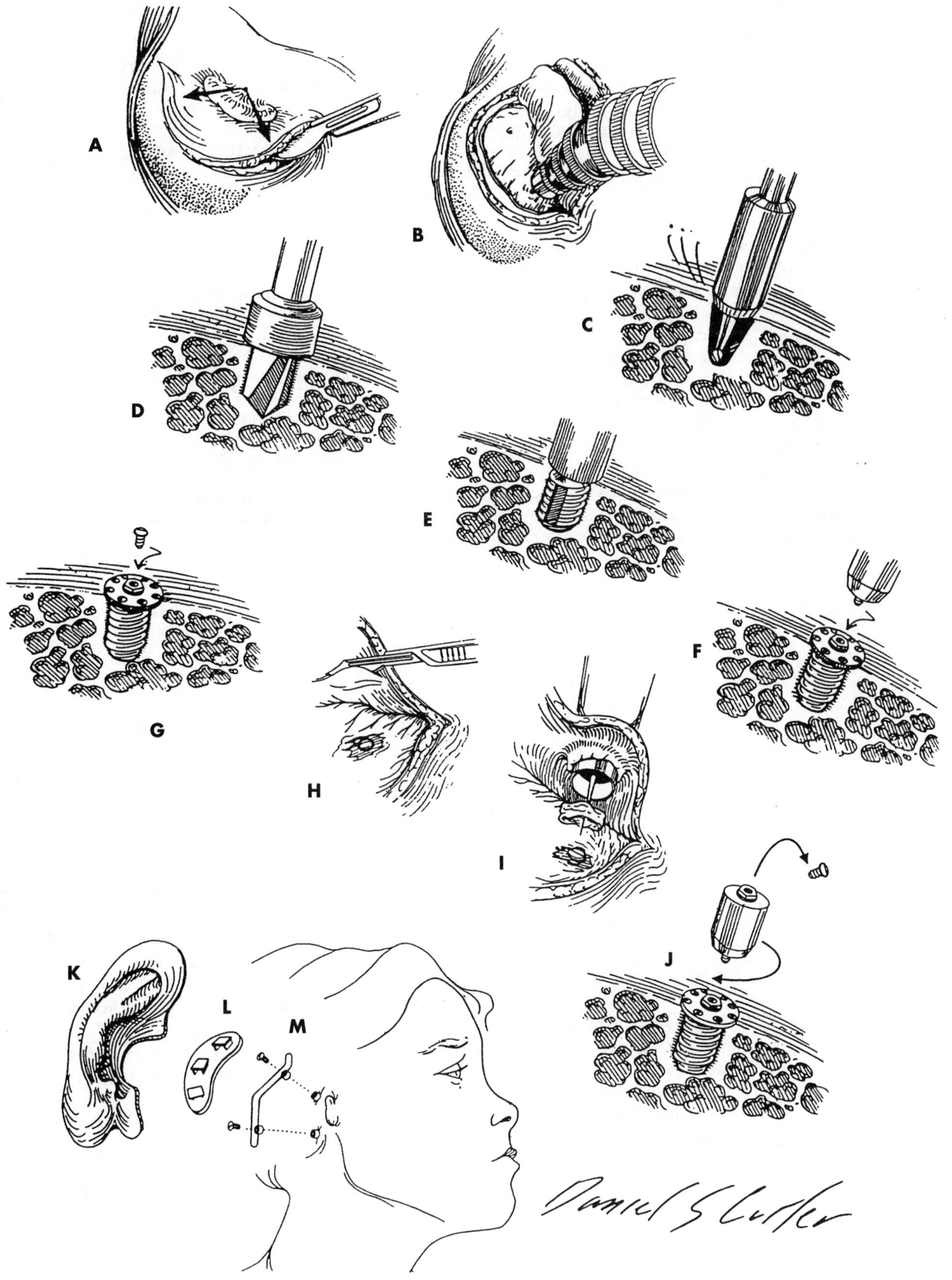

Figure 3.
Method of prosthetic rehabilitation: *A–G,* Placement of osseointegrating fixture. *H–J,* Seating of percutaneous abutments. *K–M,* Assembly of retention unit and prosthesis. *(From Niparko JL, et al. Tissue-integrated prostheses in the rehabilitation of auricular defects: Results with percutaneous mastoid implants. Am J Otol 1993; 14:343–348; with permission.)*

this result, and should be carefully considered when recommending this procedure. Perhaps the ideal situation would be a 6-year-old child without prior surgical violation, parents with realistic expectations, and a surgeon with requisite knowledge and experience.

On the other hand, prosthetic rehabilitation with osseointegrated implants has the advantage of entailing only two surgical procedures and producing a structure with a greater level of artistic refinement than what cartilage grafts could ever achieve. Also, it has the added advantage of being used as a salvage option when autogenous surgical reconstruction has failed. The major disadvantage is the technique's inherent prosthetic nature; patients perceive a synthetic structure and not their own flesh. Prosthetic rehabilitation is indicated in adults who are predisposed to hypertrophic scar formation, have extensive scarring and disfigurement from prior surgeries, or simply elect to undergo this option. It is also a viable option for children in similar situations; however, once performed, the prosthesis violates the bed of skin and soft tissue that is essential in auricular reconstruction with costal cartilage insertion.

Understandably, there is much contoversy to microtia repair with regards to the treatment options, timing and coordination with aural atresia repair, and variations in technique.

Suggested Reading

Brent B. Auricular repair with autogenous rib cartilage grafts: Two decades of experience with 600 cases. Plast Reconstr Surg 1992; 90:355-374.

Brent B, Total auricular construction with sculpted costal cartilage. In Brent B, ed. The artistry of reconstructive surgery. Vol. 1. St. Louis: CV Mosby, 1987:113.

Burton MJ, Niparko JK, Johansson CB, Tjellstrom A. Titanium-anchored prostheses in otology. Otolaryngol Clin North Am 1996; 29: 301-310.

Niparko JK, Langman AW, Cutler MS, Carroll WR. Tissue-integrated prostheses in the rehabilitation of auricular defects: Results with percutaneous mastoid implants. Am J Otol 1993; 14:1-6.

Niparko JK, Schuller DE. Reconstructive surgery for congenital and acquired malformations of the auricle. In: Cummings C, et al., eds. Otolaryngology—Head and neck surgery. Vol. 4. St. Louis: Mosby–Year Book, 1993:2772.

Tanzer RC. Bellucci RJ, Converse JM, Brent B. Deformities of the auricle. In: Converse JM, ed. Reconstructive plastic surgery. Vol. 3. Philadelphia: WB Saunders, 1977:671.

THE WRINKLED FACE

The method of
W. Gregory Chernoff

Current demographic studies suggest that by the year 2000 more than half of our population will be aged 45 years or older. With improved health care, patients are living longer lives, and in doing so they realize that they do not feel their chronologic ages, nor do they accept their chronologic looks. As patients strive to look as good as they feel, they also seek minimally invasive cosmetic surgery with low risk, little pain, short healing time, and maximal benefit. The development of such procedures continues to be at the forefront of facial plastic surgery and in high demand by our patient population.

■ PATIENT EVALUATION

The initial workup of a patient who has a wrinkled face involves delineating the pathophysiology involved. It is prudent to evaluate the face in thirds: upper, middle, and lower. Within each third of the face, the physician should decide whether gravitational forces, dynamic folds, or static rhytids are the source of the problem. This information gives a concise treatment plan that can then be adhered to, with specific modifications proportional to each patient's needs.

As we age, quantitative as well as qualitative changes occur in the skin. Gravitational forces act on the upper third of the face. As the brows fall, blepharochalasis and dermatochalasis appear, and the midface then falls, yielding deep nasolabial and melolabial folds. Patients also exhibit loss of bulk to the upper and lower lip, as well as loss of definition to the Cupid's bow region of the upper lip. The nasal tip then reveals excess ptosis. Jowling becomes evident along the mandibular border, with submental fullness and platysmal banding evidenced in the neck.

Patients with excessive dynamic folds who have been treated with therapies more appropriate for static rhytids are dissatisfied with the results. Dynamic folds such as the region of the glabella, crow's feet, and nasolabial and melolabial folds are regions in which the dermis has connection to the underlying facial musculature. These regions can be softened through various techniques that shall be mentioned; however, resolution of dynamic folds will not be achieved with the same success rate as that for static rhytids. Static rhytids, such as the fine lines around the mouth or eye visible when there is no expression on the face, can be very meticulously softened or removed in some patients.

Table 1 summarizes contemporary techniques used in

the treatment of the aforementioned problems affecting patients in each third of the face.

The procedure to be used will be revealed in the preoperative consultation. Computer imaging has gained widespread acceptance among contemporary facial plastic surgeons and is used as an honest tool to allow a patient to decide which procedures would be of benefit. Current philosophy favors performing complete facial rejuvenation of the upper middle and lower third of the face at the same operative setting so that the patient can heal once and avoid having to undergo repeat procedures. This also saves costs for the patient. It makes little sense to rejuvenate the upper third of the face and leave the lower third of the face looking its chronologic age, or vice versa.

It behooves the treating physician to delineate the patient's expectations of aesthetic surgery. The best surgical candidate is the patient who has no pre-existing expectations and who wishes to look better, not different. A general psychological profile should also be obtained by the treating physician, because some patients seek aesthetic surgical improvement to correct psychological problems. If such problems are not discovered preoperatively, a stressful physician-patient relationship can result.

Table 1. Treatment of the Wrinkled Face

PREVENTION AND MAINTENANCE	
Diet: Multivitamins, vitamin C, vitamin E, antioxidants	
Sun block	
Smoking cessation	
Stress coping	
Skin care	
Facial wash (hydroxy acid)	
Toner	
Moisturizer	
Sunblock	
GRAVITATIONAL FORCES	
Brow fall	Endoscopic brow lift
Blepharochalasis	Blepharoplasty
Dermatochalasis	Blepharoplasty
Midface falls	
Nasolabial folds	
Melolabial folds	Endoscopic midface lift
Nasal tip ptosis	Rhinoplasty
Jowling	
Submental fullness/platysmal folds	Rhytidectomy
Loss of lip bulk/definition	Gore-Tex
DYNAMIC FOLDS	
Glabellar	Gore-Tex, Softform
Crow's feet	Isolagen
Nasolabial/Melolabial	
STATIC RHYTIDS	
Alpha-hydroxy acid, tretinoin, wash/toner/moisturizer/serum	
TCA peel/phenol	
Laser exfoliation, YAG, holmium, CO_2	
Isolagen	
PIGMENTED NEVI	
4–8% HQ/Alpha-hydroxy acid/Retin-A	
Q-switch ruby laser	
Alexandrite laser	
TELANGIECTASIA	
Vitamin K cream	
Pulsed dye laser	
Long pulsed green laser	

TCA, trichloroacetic acid; HQ, hydroquinone.

■ THERAPY

Skin Care

The treatment of the wrinkled face begins with preventive maintenance. Most contemporary aesthetic surgeons view their practices as wellness centers aimed at counseling patients on everything including diet therapy, exercise therapy, stress management, and building positive self-esteem.

Table 2 lists the common histologic changes associated with aging skin. The physician should have a good working knowledge of the pathophysiology of aging, because this will help correlate recommendations made to the patient regarding preventive maintenance. Preventive recommendations begin with proper diet and multivitamin therapy to keep collagen and elastin tissue healthy. Counseling to avoid sun exposure and other deleterious factors leading to cutaneous cancers such as melanoma should be enforced. Patients should be instructed to wear sunblock with a minimum of a 15 to 30 sun protection factor on their faces. It has been scientifically shown that smoking and the associated oxygen free radicals act directly to prematurely age skin. Avoiding smoking is stressed to the patient seeking aesthetic improvement. New therapies are emerging subsequent to scientific studies showing that antioxidant medications have a positive effect on collagen regeneration and collagen maintenance. These products are also offered to the patient as part of the complete maintenance package. A patient's ability or inability to cope with stress is also reflected in the skin. The treating physician should have a working relationship with a psychologist to provide this form of therapy, if needed.

Using some form of skin care product is better than not in maintaining a youthful-appearing skin. The facial regimen should be kept simple, usually consisting of a facial wash

Table 2. Histologic Correlates of Aging Skin

Epidermis↓
Dermis↓
Elastin↓
Collagen↑
Ground substance↓
Dermal cells↓
Microcirculation↓
Cutaneous nerves↓
Appendages
Eccrine glands↓
Apocrine glands↓
Sebaceous glands↓
Hair↓
Nails↓
Subcutaneous tissue↓

with alpha-hydroxy acid or glycolic acid bases, a facial toner, a moisturizer, and a sunblock.

Selection of Procedures

It is the physician's responsibility to delineate those ancillary procedures for which the patient would benefit when undergoing facial rejuvenation surgery. The most common combination of facial rejuvenation procedures includes an endoscopic brow lift, upper lid laser-assisted incisional blepharoplasty, lower lid laser-assisted transconjunctival blepharoplasty, endoscopic mid- or lower face lifting, rhytidectomy with extended neck, a filling substance to the nasolabial and melolabial folds such as Gore-Tex or Softform, and a rhinoplasty. Six weeks later, the patient is offered therapy for the qualitative changes to the skin, most commonly by cutaneous laser exfoliation. Six weeks after healing of the laser exfoliated skin, the patient is offered therapy for any residual benign pigmented nevi or telangiectatic regions of the face. This encompasses for pigmented lesions topical applications, such as 4 percent to 8 percent hydroquinone, 10 percent alpha-hydroxy acid, and 0.1 percent tretinoin. Pigmented geared lasers such as the Q-switched ruby laser or the Alexandrite laser can also be used. Telangiectatic lesions are approached by using topical vitamin K preparations or vascular laser such as pulsed dye lasers or long pulsed green lasers.

■ CUTANEOUS LASER EXFOLIATION

The use of aesthetic lasers to exfoliate skin has arisen from improved delivery systems and has been largely consumer led. With improvement in laser technology, the concept of selective photothermolysis is now a reality. The introduction of lasers that respect the thermal relaxation time of skin, allowing tissue exfoliation while leaving residual adnexal structures healthy to heal, has made this possible.

Resurfacing skin is not a new concept. Dermabrasion and chemical peeling have been used for centuries. It is now generally accepted that the new-generation lasers allow greater depth and linear control in exfoliation than do chemical peeling and dermabrasion. The thermal effect of the carbon dioxide (CO_2) laser in particular has a specific effect on collagen fibers. Type one collagen is exquisitely sensitive to temperatures as low as 50 to 60° C, which results in contraction and rearrangement of collagen fibers parallel to the surface of the skin. Beyond 60° C, irreversible destruction of collagen occurs, which leads to new collagen production.

The ultimate success of cutaneous laser exfoliation is proportional to the depth of injury. It is clear that sufficient depth of epidermal or dermal injury is necessary to remove pathologic changes such as rhytids; however, excessive depth is undesirable because the surgeon does not want to inflict coagulative necrosis to the deep adnexal structures, which can lead to scarring. With any of the laser systems on the market, a treatment protocol exists that can enable a physician to exfoliate to the epidermal basal layer to effect a superficial exfoliation or to the superficial reticular dermis, thereby effecting a deeper exfoliation. Patients who have superficial actinic changes will benefit from a more superficial exfoliation, whereas those who have deeper rhytids will require a deeper level of exfoliation to achieve a satisfactory clinical result. Current laser studies are examining other wavelengths such as that of the erbium Yag laser as well as the holmium laser in an effort to effect more dermal changes with fewer epidermal changes. I have completed work on an instrument that automatically measures epidermal and dermal thickness, computer-integrates this measurement into any available laser on the market, and automatically sets the treatment parameters from forehead to chin on the patient. This instrument should be commercially available within the next 5 years.

Indications

Patients of all skin types can undergo CO_2 laser resurfacing. Those individuals of Fitzpatrick skin types 4 to 6 will experience postinflammatory hyperpigmentation and should be pretreated and postoperatively treated accordingly to downregulate the tyrosinase pathway.

Static rhytids due to actinic damage respond best to the CO_2 laser, whereas deeper furrows respond only temporarily because of postoperative inflammation. Those rhytids ideal for laser resurfacing include periorbital rhytids, static crow's feet, perioral rhytids, static forehead lines, and midcheek wrinkles. False promises of tremendous resolution of dynamic crow's feet, nasolabial folds, or marionette lines should not be made.

Acne scars are also amenable to laser exfoliation. Mild and moderate scars show softening with exfoliation alone. Scars that are deeper have yielded best results with excision and subsequent closure or excision with postauricular punch grafting. I have used a new form of therapy called Isolagen for acne scars and rhytids, which uses the patient's own cultured fibroblast for reinjection. Injecting viable fibroblasts that begin to produce collagen while stimulating collagen with the thermal effect of the laser has had a synergistic effect on softening acne scars. This treatment modality is also gaining widespread acceptance.

Exophytic skin lesions, including benign epidermal nevi, seborrheic keratoses, dermatoses, papulosa nigra, syringomas, xanthelasmas, solar keratoses, trichoepitheliomas, and sebaceous hyperplasia, are amenable to this new therapy. If there is any concern as to the malignancy of a nevus, the lesion should be excised and sent for pathologic evaluation.

Postsurgical and post-traumatic scars are blended if a laser resurfacing is performed 6 to 8 weeks after initial injury. This is the most important time for collagen remodeling. Older scars will show some response, but the response is less dramatic than that for younger scars. Other lesions such as rhinophyma and actinic cheilitis are also amenable to this therapy

Contraindications to CO_2 Laser Exfoliation

Patients who have recently taken oral isotretinoin for the treatment of acne are not suitable candidates for laser exfoliation. Isotretinoin alters appendage structure and function; hence, the normal mechanism for re-epithelialization is temporarily impaired. This can persist for at least 2 years after drug use has ceased. The physician should determine whether normal skin moisture and oiliness has returned subsequent to isotretinoin use.

Another contraindication is loss of the appendages due

to scarring such as burns, chemical peeling, and scleroderma. This can also apply to patients who have had excessive electrolysis in specific regions. A lack of dermal appendages is another contraindication. In areas where appendages are scarce, such as the neck and hands, excess scarring can result. Finally, patients who have unrealistic expectations are also a cause for concern. Patients must realize that re-epithelialization will take 7 to 10 days, with residual erythema lasting 8 to 12 weeks. During this time, careful sun avoidance and the use of ultraviolet sunscreens containing titanium dioxide are essential to minimize postoperative hyperpigmentation.

Patients undergoing rhytidectomy procedure should not be resurfaced simultaneously on the skin flap because impaired blood supply can cause abnormal healing. Resurfacing can be performed in regions where skin is not undermined. Typically, the surgeon should wait 6 weeks after undermining of a skin flap before performing resurfacing.

Patients who have red lip liner tattoos with high iron contents should not undergo CO_2 laser exfoliation because the tattoo can be oxidized to a permanent purple color.

Patients who have a history of shingles or herpes zoster can be a problem if they have experienced significant neuralgia with the shingles. These patients may experience severe prolonged pain and swelling.

Preoperative Preparation

The concept of pretreating patients before laser exfoliation has been controversial. Pretreating patients who are prone to increased postinflammatory hyperpigmentation allows the melanin-producing pathways to be downregulated. The pretreatment includes placing the patient on 4 percent hydroquinone, 0.1 percent tretinoin, and kojic acid. Alphahydroxy acid facial washes are also used. This pretreatment continues for 6 weeks preoperatively. Some authors believe that this pretreatment stimulates more rapid healing and decreases postoperative milia. I have not found this to be the case. I find that emphasizing the importance of pretreatment is a method of training the patients for their postoperative maintenance program, which can prolong the results. Patients should be given a loading pretreatment dose of an antiviral drug, and they should also be kept on this for 10 days postoperatively.

Technique of CO_2 Cutaneous Exfoliation

The level of anesthesia should be left to the patient to decide. The procedure can be performed under anything from regional blocks with subcutaneous infiltration to intravenous sedation to general anesthesia. All appropriate laser safety protocols should be followed, and proper eye protection for the patient and ancillary staff should be rigidly enforced.

Table 3 delineates the common accepted safe treatment parameters for the various laser systems available. The success of cutaneous laser exfoliation is technique dependent. Far too much emphasis has been placed on how many passes are required to achieve what depth of exfoliation. With differing epidermal and dermal thicknesses, and differing laser parameters, it is more important that the physician understand where he or she is with each pass of the laser. A biopsy-proven study has revealed a chamois yellow color to indicate a lower dermal position with the laser, and this marker should be utilized as an end point. An exception is the patient who has a large amount of solar keratosis; in this case, a chamois yellow color will be evident after the initial pass. If in doubt, treat less.

The technique can be summarized as follows:

1. Exfoliating a full face is preferred. Otherwise adhere to a cosmetic unit. Avoid exfoliating single rhytids only.
2. Feather the wound appropriately with appropriate settings.
3. Remove exfoliated or coagulated tissue after each pass.

Table 3. Laser Exfoliation Treatment Parameters

	LASER TYPES				
FACIAL REGION	COHERENT ULTRAPULSE COMPUTERIZED PATTERN GENERATOR	SURGILASE XJ DUAL MODE SCANNER	SHARPLAN SILKTOUCH 220 MM HANDPIECE	LUXOR NOVAPULSE	PALOMAR TISSUE TECHNOLOGY
Eyelid (intraorbital) Vermilion lip	150 mj/100 W Density 3%, Size 5 1 pass	200 mj Density 30%, Size 0.5 1 pass	6.0 mm Spot 16 watts 1 pass	1 cm^2 6 W D = 0.0 1 pass	300 mj 1 pass
Cheeks, forehead Perioribital White lip	150–250 mj/100 W Density 5%, Size 9 1–3 passes	400 mj Density 40%, Size 2 cm^2 1–3 passes	6.0–9.0 Spot 18–20 W 1–3 passes	15 W D = −0.3 1–3 passes	400 mj 2–4 passes
Feathering	150 mj/100 W Density 3%, Size 7 1 pass	150 mj Density 20%	Feathertouch Mode 6.0–9.0 Spot 28 W 1 pass	6 W D = −0.3 1 pass	300 mj 1 pass

D, density; mj, millijoules.

4. Rehydrate remaining tissue after each pass.
5. Remember that exfoliation depth is proportional to laser energy, power, and the number of passes.
6. Leave dermal adnexal structures intact.
7. Visualize an end point.
8. Occlude the wound.

The most time-efficient method of exfoliating a full face is to feather the entire area to be treated first. Typically, I commence at the earlobe, continue around the turning edge of the mandible, and extend to the opposing earlobe. The hair is then moistened with saline and feathering continues in the preauricular region up through the temple over the forehead and to the opposing earlobe.

The laser is then again set for an exfoliation depth, and beginning on one side of the face at the oral commissure the exfoliation on one-half of the face is completed. The periorbital region and perioral regions are left to be treated last. The alternate side of the face is then exfoliated to the appropriate exfoliation depth. Caution is always taken to wipe previously exfoliated tissue away before delivering another pass. This avoids tissue debris acting as a thermal conductor yeilding dermal coagulative necrosis. The forehead is then exfoliated around the previously feathered region. The laser spot size is then reduced for greater control around the perioral and periorbital regions. The eyelids can be resurfaced to the eyelashes, although it is rare to find significant rhytids in the pretarsal region.

The five most common regions yielding scarring during treatment for which fluence levels should be decreased are:

1. The lateral temporal region lateral to the crow's feet.
2. The junction between the nasal complex and the malar complex.
3. The lower eyelid.
4. The vermilion border.
5. The turning edge of the mandible.

Before the periorbital region is exfoliated, testing should be performed to identify any potential lid laxity. If there is any question as to preoperative lid lag, a lid-shortening procedure should be performed before exfoliation.

Common adjuncts to laser exfoliation include simultaneous placement of perioral Gore-Tex, particularly in the upper lip wetline, the lower lip vermilion, the nasolabial folds, and the melolabial folds, Clinical studies have revealed a synergistic approach to improved profilometric results. Simultaneous injection of Isolagen has also yielded a superior result, particularly with resurfacing profilometric rhytids greater than 0.5 mm or acne scars measuring greater than 0.5 mm. It is common to perform laser exfoliation of the perioral region and periorbital region simultaneously with transconjunctival blepharoplasty and rhytidectomy. If the subperiosteal plane is used in an endoscopic brow lift, the skin can also be exfoliated.

Postoperative Care

The use of specific semiocclusive dressings has revolutionized postoperative wound care following exfoliation procedures. A moist environment allows rapid re-epithelialization to occur, and this reduces the risk of scarring and infection. Another advantage is minimal postoperative pain experienced by patients when these semiocclusive dressings are used compared with open air treatment of the treated skin.

A variety of dressings are available, including Vigilon, Biobrane, and Sialon. Some authors also prefer the use of semiocclusive ointments such as Vaseline or Aquaphor. I currently use Vaseline in patients who I believe will not cope well with wearing an occlusive dressing. For patients I believe will have a problem with pain, I use the Sialon dressing. If a semiocclusive dressing is used, it is imperative that it be removed and the wound cleansed within 24 hours. This avoids staphylococcal, pseudomonal, and candidal infections within the occlusion period.

The occlusive dressing can then be reapplied for 2 to 3 days, or the patient can be switched to a semiocclusive ointment. Antibiotic ointments should be cautioned against because contact dermatitis is a common sequela to use of these preparations.

All patients receive oral antiviral medications for 10 days postoperatively. If the patient develops active herpetic outbreaks, the maximal allotted dosage is recommended. Most patients are also placed on an oral antibiotic for 10 days.

Postoperative edema can occur with extensive exfoliation. This can be minimized with the use of 0.5 mg per kilogram of dexamethasone, up to a maximum oral dosage of 8 mg twice daily for 5 days.

Postoperative analgesia is patient specific. The physician should ensure that the patient remains comfortable.

After-Care

Once epithelialization has occurred, several measures are recommended. These include sun protection for a minimum of 3 months postoperatively. The patient should also be advised to use a nonperfumed, nonocclusive cleanser. This acts to remove heavy cosmetics that the patient may have worn in the past. Patients should be introduced to hypoallergenic water-soluble cosmetics that can also provide excellent sunscreen protection ranging from the ultraviolet B through the ultraviolet A and visible light ranges. Traditionally, patients are instructed to apply a green foundation under their makeup to neutralize the erythema. A yellow foundation can also yield a natural look.

The most important element for the patient in the postoperative phase is the use of a moisturizer. Moisturizers that contain fragrances or preservatives should be discouraged; a nonperfumed moisturizer is recommended.

The intensity and duration of erythema is proportional to the depth of exfoliation, degree of thermal injury, and degree of inflammation. Erythema can last anywhere from 1 to 6 months, so patients must be educated on this condition before treatment. Topical 1 percent hydrocortisone cream can reduce erythema and can be continued for 10 days.

Postinflammatory hyperpigmentation is common following exfoliation; combinations of 4 percent hydroquinone, 0.1 percent tretinoin, and kojic acid can be used to remedy this problem. To date, there have been no incidents of permanent hyperpigmentation, although if it occurs, this condition can last anywhere from months to 1 year.

The physician's greatest ally in the postoperative period is a makeup artist. All resurfacing patients should be provided with a makeover at the physician's expense to help the patient cope in the postoperative phase.

Complications

An increasing number of hypertrophic scars have occurred because of overaggressive therapy. This can be minimized by always taking an overly conservative approach. Patients are more accepting if the physician has to re-treat in 6 months rather than initially cause an area of unnecessary scarring.

If an area remains erythematous while the surrounding area has resolved, the physician should consider this area to be a hypertrophic scar until proved otherwise. A topical silicone gel called Kelocote has proved tremendously beneficial in reversing potential hypertrophic scars at this stage. This silicone polymer is placed daily for 1 month to help reverse potential hypertrophic scars. Other topical treatments such as intralesional triamcinolone acetonide or topical silicone sheeting can be applied. The use of the pulsed dye laser for early hypertrophic scars has been tremendously efficacious for reversing these troublesome problems.

The most common causes of hypertrophic scars have been the use of low-energy density, overlapping laser pulses, lasing too deeply, infection, wound crusting, isotretinoin therapy, or previous electrolysis.

Patients should be warned that not all the wrinkles will disappear and that this treatment is meant to soften their appearance overall.

SKIN CANCER

The method of
Karen H. Calhoun
by
Karen H. Calhoun
Luke K.S. Tan

Basal and squamous skin cancers, referred to as nonmelanotic skin cancer (NMSC), are increasingly common. The approximately 600,000 new cases diagnosed each year include a yearly 4 percent to 8 percent increase over the preceding year. Conservative estimates are that the risk of having a recurrent NMSC is one in six for whites. Other studies have placed this figure as high as one in two.

Although deaths from NMSC are uncommon, the morbidity of these tumors can be significant. The mainstay of treatment is complete surgical excision. Because NMSCs occur mainly in the head and neck region, the resulting defects can cause profound functional and aesthetic problems. Successful treatment includes functional and cosmetic reconstruction. Less commonly, radiotherapy is employed. Chemotherapy is not useful at present in the initial treatment of NMSC.

In the future, increasing awareness of NMSC by clinicians and the general public should result in better prevention and early detection, which will lead to uniform cures, with excellent functional and cosmetic outcomes.

RISK FACTORS

The primary risk factor for developing NMSC is damage to the skin from sun exposure. The degree of sun reactivity in each person's skin is inversely related to the degree of pigmentation. Fitzpatrick's classification of skin type (Table 1) is useful in estimating risk. The blonde or red-headed person with fair skin who burns easily (types I or II) is at greatest risk for developing NMSC. Freckling, male gender, older age, and having one or more previous NMSCs are also associated with greater risk. Women who had six or more severe sunburns during childhood are at greater risk of developing squamous cell skin cancer.

The cumulative daily sun exposure is greater as one nears the equator. In the white population, the incidence of NMSC in the Northern Hemisphere increases the further south one lives. No similar increase is found in persons who have darker pigmentation, including persons of African and Indian descent. Previous medical irradiation is another risk factor for developing NMSC, and smoking may also contribute to the risk of cutaneous malignancy.

Cutaneous exposure to actinic damage is ameliorated by the ozone layer. As this ozone layer has been reduced, the risk of skin cancer has risen. There may be as much as a 2 percent to 4 percent increase in risk with each 1 percent reduction in the ozone layer.

Table 1. Fitzpatrick's Sun-Reactive Skin Types

SKIN TYPE	SKIN COLOR	TANNING RESPONSE
I	White	Always burn, never tan
II	White	Usually burn, tan with difficulty
III	White	Sometimes mild burn, tan average
IV	Brown	Rarely burn, tan with ease
V	Dark brown	Very rarely burn, tan very easily
VI	Black	No burn, tan very easily

MECHANISM OF PHOTOCARCINOGENESIS

Exposure of the skin to the sun results in photodamage to the proliferative cells of the skin. The molecular mechanisms involved in the process of carcinogenesis are presently being elucidated. Ultraviolet rays can cause alterations to DNA sequences by cross-linking of the adjacent pyrimidine bases, for example, thymine dimers. These genetic alterations, described as "UV signatures," can result in the inactivation of tumor suppressor genes or activation of oncogenes. For example, the activity of tumor suppressor gene p53 increases in response to UV exposure. The p53 gene normally allows for repair of the damaged DNA or destruction of the damaged cell (apoptosis), thus preventing proliferation of altered DNA that could ultimately lead to carcinogenesis. Inactivation of this gene, by as of yet some unknown mechanism, increases the possibility that damaged DNA will be replicated, eventually resulting in NMSC. The precise mechanism of actinic carcinogenesis remains to be completely unraveled.

PREVENTION

Ultraviolet rays reaching the earth are divided into UVA and UVB, the latter being the shorter wavelength generally responsible for the carcinogenic effects. Sunscreens are substances that are placed on the skin to partially block the transmission of these damaging rays to the skin. Sun protection factor (SPF) is a measure of the effectiveness of sunscreen against UVB. A product with an SPF of 15, for example, theoretically permits the user to spend 15 hours in the sun while sustaining only the sun damage that would usually be expected from 1 unprotected hour in the sun. A dry white T-shirt provides an SPF of between 5 and 9.

Sunscreen products are clearly marked with their SPF, usually between 15 and 30. Use of higher SPF is recommended for those who have fairer skins and those with a history of premalignant photodamage or previous skin cancers. The use of these products should follow the manufacturer's suggestions, especially with respect to reapplication intervals and reapplication after swimming.

DIAGNOSIS

Skin cancer is diagnosed by histopathologic patterns. Assessment of each patient begins with history, including the rate of growth of the lesion, other lesions on that patient, family history of skin cancers, and sun exposure or tanning history. Although this chapter focuses on the head and neck skin cancers, the trunk and limbs are other common sites for NMSC, and these areas should be thoroughly inspected in each patient who is seen with skin cancer.

Clinical presentation often allows establishing the diagnosis of basal or squamous cell carcinoma with fair certainty, but the final diagnosis is histologic. Clinically, squamous cell carcinomas are usually irregular in shape with raised edges and significant central ulceration that may bleed. Depending on their size and site, they may invade surrounding and underlying muscle, cartilage, and bone. Although less common, poorly differentiated squamous cell carcinomas of the skin can be biologically aggressive, with a short tumor doubling time and a propensity to metastasize. Actinic keratosis presenting as red scaly patches over sun-exposed areas is estimated to have up to a one in five chance of becoming malignant.

Basal cell carcinomas, on the other hand, are usually nodular in appearance, with rolled-over regular edges, a pearly sheen, and often surrounded by telangiectasias. A benign tumor, keratoacanthoma, has a similar appearance, and it can be difficult to distinguish the two clinically. Basal cell carcinomas usually have a well-defined margin and are non-pigmented in whites, but are pigmented in the majority of cases in patients of Hispanic or Asian descent. Basal cell carcinomas rarely metastasize. Although the majority of basal cell carcinomas are nodular, a diffuse form of the tumor exists that should be recognized because it has a high rate of recurrence. This is due to the involvement of the dermis with islands of tumors. When encased in dense fibrosis, these tumor islands are labeled as sclerosing or morpheic.

The "H" zone of the face is the skin around the eyes, nose, upper lip, ears, and a strip of preauricular skin between the angle of the mandible and the temple. Basal cell carcinomas occurring in the "H" zone often exhibit a more aggressive behavior. In the neck, the commonest site of basal cell lesions is at the superior aspect of the sternocleidomastoid muscle.

THERAPY

Surgical Excision

Surgical excision of NMSC is removal of a three-dimensional fusiform tumor with surrounding, apparently normal tissue. In treating basal cell carcinomas, a margin of between 3 to 5 mm is recommended for lesions less than 2 cm wide; up to 15 mm margins may be required for larger lesions. For squamous cell carcinomas of less than 1 cm, a 5 mm margin is sufficient, and larger lesions require up to 20 mm margins, because the incidence of local infiltration can be significant with these lesions. After removal of the lesion, the surgeon generally takes frozen section margins from the skin edges and deeper tissues. These are examined by the pathologist, and additional margins are taken if necessary.

A small and favorable wound can heal by second intent, or it can be closed primarily. Larger and more complex wounds require surgical reconstruction.

The 5 year cure rate for standard surgical excision of basal cell carcinomas is 90 percent to 93 percent. For previously treated basal cell carcinoma, the 5 year recurrence rate can be as high as 20 percent. The risk factors associated with a higher recurrence rate include sclerosing and morpheaform histologic variants; tumor size of greater than 3 cm; and high-risk locations, including the nose and the auricular and preauricular regions of the "H" zone.

Recurrence of squamous cell carcinomas is a reflection of tumor size. After standard surgical excision, smaller lesions have 5 year control rates of approximately 87 percent, whereas lesions larger than 3 cm have recurrence rates of greater than 40 percent. Histologic evidence of perineural invasion is associated with higher risk of recurrence and mortality. Neck dissection is recommended for advanced lesions with aggressive histologic features such as perineural invasion. In the presence of clinically positive nodes or extracapsular spread, adjunctive postoperative radiotherapy is also advised.

Mohs' Micrographic Surgery

Mohs' micrographic surgery (MMS) is a method often used for removal of NMSC. It differs from conventional surgery (with frozen section sampling of the margins) in that the entire interface between the tumor and underlying normal tissue is mapped and examined histologically, which allows immediate re-excision of areas showing residual tumor. The technique was developed by Dr. F.E. Mohs, a general surgeon from the University of Wisconsin, in 1930, when he was a medical student.

The technique was originally known as chemosurgery, because zinc chloride paste was applied directly to the wound after tumor excision. The Mohs' defect is usually saucer-shaped. After the zinc chloride paste causes tissue fixation, a complete "saucer" 2 to 3 mm thick, including skin margins, is excised. The tissue sample is shaped something like the intact peel of half an orange. This specimen is inverted, and divided into precisely marked quadrants, which correspond to exact marks left on the patient. Each quadrant of the specimen is then sectioned in a horizontal fashion, so that the whole undersurface of the original saucer can be microscopically examined by the pathologist.

If residual tumor is noted in this saucer, the pathologist can tell from the tissue markings in exactly which quadrant the section with positive findings originated. This is followed by application of additional zinc chloride paste, and excision of additional tissue from the positive quadrants only. Again, the 2 to 3 mm thick partial saucer interface between the tumor and normal tissue is excised, oriented, marked, horizontally sectioned, and examined. If necessary, additional excisions are carried out, each one involving only re-excision of the area shown to have positive findings (Fig. 1).

A very similar process is used today, with the zinc chloride chemosurgery replaced by frozen sectioning of the entire sample. The advantage of this technique is its ability to detect narrow fingers of tumor extending out from the margins that might be missed by the sampling technique usually used with frozen sections; this technique is achieved with maximum preservation of uninvolved tissue.

Mohs' micrographic techniques have lowered recurrence rates, with control rates for primary basal cell carcinomas now as high as 99 percent, and recurrence rates for basal cell carcinomas as low as 8 percent. The 5 year recurrence rate for primary squamous cell carcinoma is 3 percent using Mohs' technique compared with 13 percent using other techniques. Although the Mohs' technique is an effective method of ensuring clear margins and attaining high local cure rates, it does take significantly longer than do other techniques, with a 2 to 3 hour lag between stages of the procedure. The procedure is performed under local anesthesia, which some patients find unpleasant. The time-consuming, labor-intensive character of this approach has definite cost implications. Other potential risks of this technique are shared with any surgical approach, including the quality of frozen section specimens, interpretation of frozen specimens, tissue orientation difficulties, tumor transection with risk of tumor seeding, and inability to detect multifocal or skip lesions. As with any method of surgical removal, reconstruction of the resulting wound is often required.

Radiotherapy

Radiotherapy can be used as (1) primary treatment modality for NMSC, (2) postoperative adjunct, (3) treatment of regional nodal disease, or (4) reirradiation of recurrent skin cancer of the face. Irradiation for skin cancers has been delivered by both external beam and interstitial implants. The modality and dosage depends on the indications for irradiation and the nature of the lesion. Cumulative doses of up to 110 Gy have been used for reirradiation of patients who have recurrent skin cancers.

Radiotherapy for NMSC can be helpful in the head and neck areas, where results of reconstruction may be anticipated to be suboptimal, such as the pinna, nasal vestibule, and eyelid. Advantages of radiotherapy include avoidance of surgery, especially in very sick patients and those patients who have bleeding problems, such as the patient in whom anticoagulant therapy cannot be interrupted safely. In addition, for patients who have wound healing problems, such as heavy smokers, diabetics, and those who have severe vascular disease, radiotherapy may be a good choice. On the other hand, radiotherapy takes 4 to 6 weeks compared with the 2 to 4 days of surgical excision and reconstruction. Postirradiation skin necrosis, cartilage necrosis, and scarring may leave unsightly results with loss of function. Secondary reconstruction is difficult in these cases due to postirradiation scarring and compromised blood supply. The risk of carcinogenesis from the radiotherapy and the loss of a salvage modality must also be considered in young patients.

Photodynamic Therapy

Photodynamic therapy is the administration of a photosensitizing agent, followed by exposure of the tumor to a specific wavelength of light that renders the agent toxic to the cells. Some success has been reported in treatment of NMSC with photodynamic therapy. For example, hematoporphyrin derivatives have been used with light of 590 to 690 nm. The primary limitation of this therapy for NMSC is the prolonged systemic skin sensitivity, which means the patient cannot go out at all during daylight hours without the risk of sustaining a photosensitivity reaction, which usually lasts for 4 to 6 weeks and in some cases for months. This therapy is considered experimental at present.

■ DISCUSSION

For most basal or squamous cell carcinomas of the head and neck, either surgical excision or Mohs' micrographic surgery is the treatment of choice. Because the Mohs' technique has a slightly lower recurrence rate, we prefer the use of Mohs' surgery for treating recurrent cancers, morpheaform basal cell cancers, and many cancers occurring in the "H" zone of the face. Radiotherapy is usually reserved for unusual cases or use as an adjunctive treatment, if needed. Elective nodal dissections are almost never performed for basal cell

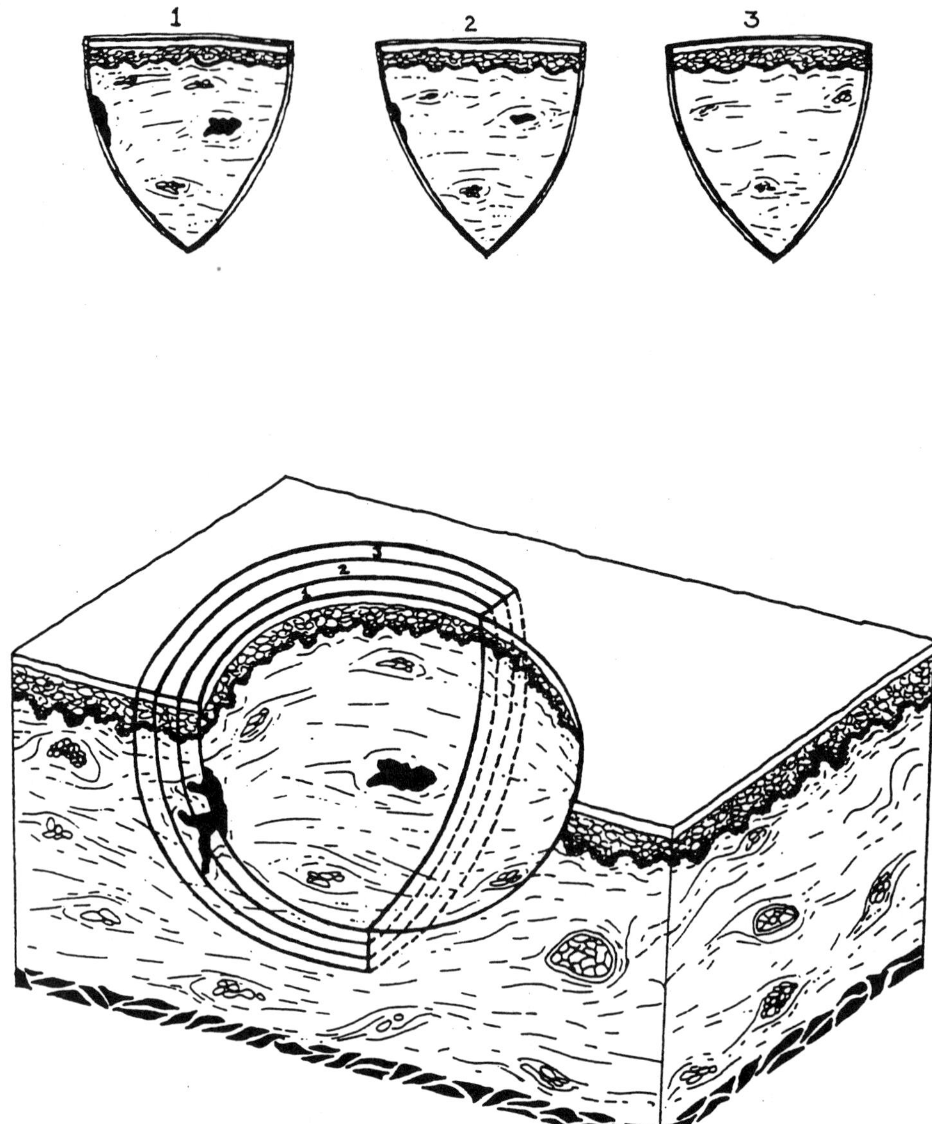

Figure 1.
Schematic diagram illustrating the principle of Mohs' micrographic surgery of serial section margins of the entire tumor bed, which allows for identification and removal of the relevant margins.

carcinoma. For large (> 3 cm) squamous cell carcinomas, consideration should be given to the staging and prognostic information gained by elective dissection of the primary draining nodes.

The most important part of treating NMSC is prevention. In our practice, sun exposure and sunscreen use is part of the initial history taking of every new patient, even one who has an earache or stuffy nose. These patients are counseled about the importance of minimizing sunlight exposure in the interest of preventing NMSC. We use more intensive counseling in patients who have NMSC, reminding them that their total sun exposure has already been enough to cause skin cancer.

Suggested Reading

Larrabee WF Jr, Sherris DA. Principles of facial reconstruction. Philadelphia: Lippincott-Raven, 1995.

Weber RS, Miller MJ, Geopfert H. Basal and squamous cell skin cancers of the head and neck. Baltimore: Williams & Wilkins, 1996.

MALIGNANT MELANOMA

The method of
Ronald C. Hamaker
by
Anna Maria Pou
Ronald C. Hamaker

The incidence of cutaneous melanoma is increasing throughout the world. In 1985, the risk of developing melanoma in white males in the United States was 1 in 150. Today, the risk has been estimated to be 1 in 87, and if this trend continues, the risk will be 1 in 75 in the year 2000. Despite the increase in incidence, the mortality rate has steadily decreased over the past 20 years. Early diagnosis and treatment of melanoma has probably had the most profound effect on cure rates, which is perhaps the result of increased awareness among the general population and primary care physicians regarding pigmented lesions.

Cancer statistics for 1988 to 1992 show that 82 percent of individuals with melanoma had localized disease at the time of diagnosis, 8 percent had regional metastases, and 46 percent had distal metastases. The overall 5 year survival rates for individuals with localized, regional, and distant disease were 95 percent, 61 percent, and 16 percent, respectively. Patients who have melanoma must be followed up indefinitely; it is not unusual for a patient with ocular melanoma to develop liver metastases 20 years later. This fact demonstrates the capricious nature of this disease as well as the probable effects of the immune system on manifestation of disease. We discuss in this chapter our philosophy of head and neck melanoma treatment.

■ PATIENT ASSESSMENT

Diagnosis

An excisional biopsy, which is defined as a biopsy that contains the original specimen free of tumor at all margins, remains the method of choice in diagnosing melanoma. However, excision of some lesions (lentigo maligna melanoma) may produce a deformity or loss of function due to their large size or location. In these situations, a punch biopsy of the most suspicious areas should be performed. Special stains, including S-100 protein and HMB (homotropine methobromide)-4, are helpful in determining the diagnosis of melanoma. Nevertheless, melanoma is occasionally misdiagnosed as undifferentiated carcinoma, reticular cell sarcoma, and malignant fibrous histiocytoma, because it is a great imitator. Once the diagnosis has been made, evaluation and definitive treatment should be rendered within 1 to 2 weeks. It should be noted that an excisional biopsy with negative margins is never considered to be definitive treatment for primary invasive melanoma.

Preoperative Evaluation

The preoperative workup for invasive melanoma includes a computed tomographic (CT) scan of the chest, liver function studies, and most important, a thorough physical examination of the entire body to look for subcutaneous nodules and palpable nodes in the neck. A CT scan of the neck should also be performed to identify nonpalpable cervical lymph nodes. If the patient has a specific complaint, a gastrointestinal (GI) series, magnetic resonance imaging (MRI), and/or bone scan should be obtained, depending on the complaint. In a review of 660 melanoma cases, it was extremely unusual to find an isolated metastasis to the brain, GI tract, bone, thyroid, kidney, or heart without involvement of the lungs, liver, subcutaneous tissues, or all three.

■ SURGICAL TREATMENT

The pathologist's interpretation regarding the depth of invasion in cutaneous melanoma is paramount to the appropriate treatment. Decisions regarding tumor margins and the need for nodal dissection are made according to the depth of invasion. We urge our pathologist to report both the Breslow and Clark levels of invasion. This is important because the same depth of invasion can demand a different treatment, depending on the location of the lesion. For example, a 1.5 mm lesion located on the skin of the eyelid can behave much differently than 1.5 mm lesion on the skin of the cheek; the eyelid lesion may extend to the level of the muscle, whereas the cheek lesion may extend only to the level of the papillary dermis.

Margins for Primary Excision

As a general rule, the deeper the lesion, the larger the margin (Table 1). The depth of dissection is to the underlying muscle (e.g., platysma, orbicularis oculi or oris, frontalis) or to the level of the superficial musculoaponeurotic system (SMAS) over the cheek and temporal areas. In the head and neck, cosmesis is considered in determining the margin of resection, but this consideration should not prevent the surgeon from performing the necessary oncologic procedure. Deformity is often caused by the need to excise branches of the facial nerve or hair-bearing skin. These cases must be individualized according to the biologic aggressiveness of the melanoma, which can be determined by the history, ulceration, or satellitosis of the lesion. In the neck, larger margins can be excised with primary closure, whereas in the region of the forehead, cheek, eyelid, or nose, flaps and grafts are frequently necessary to reconstruct the defect.

Melanomas of the scalp require larger margins (4 to 5

Table 1. Surgical Treatment: Margins for Primary Excision

THICKNESS (MM)	MARGIN (CM)
In situ	0.5
1.0	1.0
1.1–1.50	2.0
1.51–4.0	3.0
>4.0	4.0

cm) due to the extensive vascularity and lymphatics in this area, as well as the great potential for recurrent disease. The wound is typically closed using a skin graft that is placed on the periosteum. If periosteum is resected, the calvarial bone is drilled with a cutting bur, and the skin graft is then applied. Another choice of reconstruction involves using a scalp rotation flap, with a skin graft applied to the donor site.

Melanoma of the ear usually requires a resection of skin to or including the perichondrium. Many times a wedge resection is more cosmetically appealing. When there is deep invasion or involvement of cartilage, a 2 cm margin is required, and therefore subtotal auriculectomy may be necessary.

Recurrent local melanoma is treated as a Clark level V, or greater than 4 mm depth by the Breslow classification. Therefore, a 4 cm margin should be excised despite major cosmetic deformity. If a skin graft had been previously used to cover the defect, the entire graft should be removed at the time of resection, including the underlying tissue (i.e., periosteum, muscle). In treating recurrent melanoma of the ear, an auriculectomy is necessary.

Mucosal Melanoma

Mucosal melanoma of the head and neck constitutes 8 percent of all head and neck melanoma. The histologic staging systems of Breslow and Clark are of little use in assessing the extent of mucosal melanoma, mainly because of the lack of histologic landmarks analogous to the papillary and reticular dermis. Local control predicts better survival, and therefore aggressive resections should be performed when possible. A neck dissection is performed when nodes are either clinically palpable or are found to be positive by CT criteria (necrotic center, size greater than 1 cm). If nodal findings are histologically positive, postoperative radiotherapy is administered to the neck and retropharyngeal nodes. Adjuvant treatment with interferon alpha-2b is also recommended.

Intranasal melanoma involving the lateral nasal wall requires resection of the mucosa of the floor of the nose, unilateral septum, and medial maxillary wall. A septal melanoma requires a septectomy. Melanoma of the paranasal sinuses requires conventional resection for disease within that particular sinus. Laser treatment to the cribriform area has extended surgical margins in an occasional case. Melanoma of the palate, upper alveolus, and nasopharynx is treated by local resection. Melanoma of the lower alveolus is usually treated by marginal resection of the mandible and lateral neck dissection. Melanomas of the pharynx and glottis are managed by local resection and elective neck dissection.

Neck Dissection

Major controversy exists regarding treatment of the neck in melanoma, although the cervical lymph nodes are the most common and usually the initial site of metastases. Controversy surrounds indications for and the type of neck dissection to be performed. Melanomas 0.76 to 1.50 mm thick are associated with regional metastases in 25 percent of patients. A 60 percent incidence of regional metastases has been reported in melanomas 1.51 to 4.0 deep, and melanomas greater than 4 mm in depth.

A nodal dissection is performed on all patients who have clinically palpable neck disease but no distal disease. Having stated this, a dilemma exists in performing elective neck dissections in the group of patients who have melanoma greater than 4 mm in depth and a 72 percent incidence of distant metastases. This implies that the surgeon will be performing neck dissections on 75 percent of patients in this group without benefit. However, we believe that the dissection is useful as a staging procedure, because it identifies those patients with histologically negative nodes who have been found to have better survival rates compared with patients who have histologically positive nodes. Also, patients who have positive nodes may be eligible for treatment protocols and may also benefit by decreasing tumor burden and preventing unsightly tumor growth. On the other hand, we do not perform elective neck dissections on patients who have levels I and II (stage I) disease.

Computed tomography is invaluable in evaluating the neck for regional metastases. Ultrasound has also been found to be useful in detecting metastases in the parotid and cervical nodes. In patients with thin lesions (0.76 to 1.5 mm) who demonstrate no disease in the parotid or cervical nodes, the only primary lesion is resected. If the scan suggests nodal disease, that level of nodes in addition to the next echelon of nodes is resected with the primary lesion. If frozen section proves the node(s) to contain melanoma, then the next region of lymphatics is dissected and subjected to frozen section. Obviously, skip lesions can be missed, but this has been our treatment for lesions 0.76 to 1.5 mm deep that have positive CT scan findings.

In lesions measuring 1.51 to 4.0 mm without evidence of nodal metastases, the first and second echelon of nodes are resected (e.g., parotid and level II of the neck). Frozen section is performed on all suspicious nodes, and if disease is present, then levels III and IV, or III and V, are resected, depending on the location of the primary lesion and its presumed lymphatic drainage. This modified neck dissection is converted to a radical neck dissection when extensive metastases are present or more than two levels of nodes are involved with melanoma. It has been shown that the 5 year survival rate increases from 45 percent with excision alone to 72 percent if an elective neck dissection is performed in patients who have melanoma 1.51 to 4.0 mm in thickness.

Involvement of the parotid gland with regional melanoma always creates a dilemma for the surgeon; cosmesis, quality of life, and prognosis are all considered. For single metastases to the parotid, a parotidectomy with preservation of the facial nerve is performed. If a deep node is present, a total parotidectomy is performed, sparing the facial nerve. Intraoperative radiotherapy is then used in our practice. A dose of 15 to 20 Gy via a linear accelerator set at 5 MeV of energy is applied to the area of concern using a 10 cm port. We believe that this additional boost of irradiation to the parotid aids in preventing local recurrence. Time will prove this supposition to be correct or incorrect. Extensive disease in the parotid warrants a radical parotidectomy for clearance of disease.

Recurrent neck disease following a modified neck dissection carries a poor prognosis and should be treated aggressively. Recurrent disease is treated with a radical neck dissection, with resection of involved surrounding structures (i.e., marginal branch of cranial nerve VII, carotid). Following resection of recurrent neck disease, we again use intraoperative radiotherapy up to 20 Gy through a 10 cm port via a 5 MeV linear accelerator. Postoperative radiotherapy and/or interferon alpha-2b therapy is given for all recurrent cases.

Lymphoscintigraphy

Lymphoscintigraphy is being used by some clinicians for a more selective approach to the neck with clinically negative findings in patients who have cutaneous melanoma. This method has been developed to detect the sentinel node, which is defined as the first node in a particular nodal group to receive regional lymphatic flow from the tumor site. Alex and Krag introduced this technique, which uses a gamma-probe to localize a sentinel node labeled with technetium 99m sulfur colloid. Lymphoscintigrams are taken following injection of the primary lesion, and the skin is marked overlying the sentinel nodes. This method has been found to be as sensitive as the intradermal injection of blue dye in the intraoperative mapping of lymphatic drainage, and lymphoscintigraphy is easier to use.

It has been found that 21 percent to 84 percent of sentinel nodes are detected in areas that are outside the clinically predicted sites of drainage. When this occurs, the pattern of nodal dissection must be modified in order to remove these nodes that would have been missed following standard dissection. Therefore, the use of lymphoscintigraphy may forever change the way that we approach the treatment of cutaneous melanoma in the neck. At the present time, this method seems most applicable for midline or vertex lesions of the scalp. In these lesions, spread of disease can be bilateral, that is, to bilateral anterior and posterior triangles of the neck and parotid glands. Identifying sentinel nodes in this case may prevent a patient from undergoing bilateral neck dissections and parotidectomies, with their associated morbidity, when the biopsy results of these nodes may be histologically negative. On the other hand, the use of this method in the parotid remains an enigma, because removing a node from the parotid for frozen section without a formal parotidectomy places the facial nerve at risk of injury.

Multiple sentinel nodes can be identified in a single patient. It is time consuming to biopsy multiple sites, and there is an increase in morbidity and an increase in recurrent disease if more than one site is biopsied.

At present we believe that lymphoscintigraphy will ultimately prove to be beneficial in selecting the areas of nodal dissection in specific situations. Because of these reasons, we continue to treat the neck based on the most likely pattern of lymphatic drainage at the time of wide local excision.

Unknown Primary Lesion

Neck disease found with unknown primary lesions is resected in the conventional manner following complete evaluation. Spontaneous regression of primary lesions does occur, and good history taking may elicit a potential site. Resection of this site may be beneficial in isolating disease in the dermis or subcutaneous tissue, despite a normal-appearing surface. If the node has been removed for diagnosis (excisional biopsy) before consultation, a radical neck dissection, including platysma and the previous surgical incision, is performed. These patients then undergo intraoperative radiotherapy as well as postoperative radiotherapy.

Distal Disease

Distal disease is usually associated with a dismal prognosis. However, an isolated lesion to the cavernous sinus, lung, brain, GI tract, bone, or other site should be considered for resection, whether it is associated with an unknown primary or is a single distant metastasis of known disease. The extent of palliation or curability following resection of isolated distal metastasis is unpredictable, because treatment outcome in all aspects of regional and distal disease is unpredictable. However, a reduction in tumor volume is always desirable in treating melanoma.

■ NONSURGICAL THERAPY

Radiotherapy

Melanoma has the capacity to repair sublethal radiation damage, and therefore this condition was once thought to be radioresistant. However, it has been found that radiation given in high-dose fractions (400 to 500 cGy) is effective in treating patients who have bulky disease, residual or recurrent disease, unresectable lesions, or those who are too ill to undergo surgical resection. Because treatment of the primary lesion in widespread melanoma results in deformity or decrease in function, it is frequently best to treat locally with radiotherapy. Superficial lesions such as lentigo maligna melanoma may also be treated with radiotherapy in cases in which surgery would be disfiguring or debilitating. The 5 year cure rate for lentigo maligna melanoma using radiotherapy is approximately 80 percent. Radiotherapy is given adjunctively in situations in which the risk of recurrence is high, such as disease in the neck. To prevent recurrent disease, we use postoperative radiotherapy in addition to a single fraction of radiotherapy given intraoperatively to patients undergoing therapeutic neck dissection. Radiotherapy given in conventional doses, not hyperfractions, has been successful in treating microscopic disease in the neck, thereby preventing regional recurrence. Distal disease, particularly metastases to bone, can be palliated with radiotherapy.

Chemotherapy and Immunotherapy

Although different regimens of cytotoxic agents, biologic response modifiers, and melanoma vaccines have shown an improvement in disease-free interval and overall survival in limited groups of patients, the overall median survival of those who have advanced melanoma has not been significantly improved. We have enrolled a few of our patients in these protocols, but at present efficacy of treatment is unknown.

At this time, melanoma vaccines, combined with immunologic adjuncts such as bacille Calmette-Guerin, Detox, and Saponin fraction QS-21, which enhance the efficacy of the vaccine, are being used in patients who have metastatic disease. The use of vaccines was prompted by the clinical observations that the immune system plays an important role in melanoma. Although preliminary results are encouraging, these vaccines have not proved to be highly effective in protocols across the nation.

The biologic response modifier interferon alpha-2b has also been reported to increase the disease-free interval and overall survival in those patients who have high-risk primary melanomas and regional node metastases. The 5 year survival was increased by 20 percent in the Eastern Cooperative Oncology Group study. The dosage required is toxic, and treatment costs approximately $35,000. There is little doubt that the future treatment of melanoma will be immunologic, but at the present time melanoma is a surgical disease.

Suggested Reading

Alex JC, Krag DN. Gamma probe guided localization of lymph nodes. Surg Oncol 1993; 2:137-143.

Conley JJ. Melanomas of the mucous membrane of the head and neck. Laryngoscope 1989; 99:1248-1254.

Conley JJ, Hamaker RC. Melanoma of the head and neck. Laryngoscope 1977; 137:760-764.

Kirkwood JM, Strawderman, Ernstoll MS, et al. Interferon alpha-2b therapy of high-risk resected cutaneous melanoma: The Eastern Cooperative Oncology Group trial est 1684. J Clin Oncol 1996; 14:7-17.

Medina JE, Canfield V. Malignant melanoma of the head and neck. In: Myers EN, Suen JY, eds. Cancer of the head and neck. 3rd ed. Philadelphia: WB Saunders, 1997:160.

O'Brien CJ, Peterson-Schaefer K, Ruark D, et al. Radical, modified, and selective neck dissection for cutaneous malignant melanoma. Head Neck 1995; 17:232-241.

O'Brien CJ, Uren RF, Thompson JF, et al. Prediction of potential metastatic sites in cutaneous head and neck melanoma using lymphoscintigraphy. Am J Surg 1995; 170:461-466.

Storper IS, Lee SP, Abemayor E, Juillard G. The role of radiation therapy in the treatment of head and neck cutaneous melanoma. Am J Otolaryngol 1993; 14:426-431.

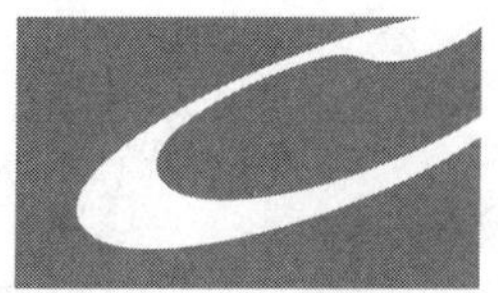

THE HEAD AND NECK

CANCER OF THE TEMPORAL BONE

The method of
Donald B. Kamerer
by
Donald B. Kamerer
Barry E. Hirsch

Malignancies of the external ear and temporal bone are relatively rare, and their true incidence is probably not known. Several factors are known to predispose this anatomic area to malignant transformation. The first of these is solar radiation, which causes squamous and basal cell carcinomas of the pinna and the external auditory meatus. Another common precursor of cancer in the temporal bone is long-standing otorrhea and inflammation secondary to chronic otitis media or chronic dermatitis. The chronicity of these conditions and their accompanying discharge of long duration often leads to a significant delay in the correct diagnosis of malignancy.

Most cancers arise from the pinna and cartilaginous portion of the external auditory canal. The bony portion of the external auditory canal is less frequently the site of origin, and primary malignancies of the middle ear and mastoid are rare. Basal cell carcinoma is the most common tumor of the pinna. Tumors of the external auditory meatus and canal are most frequently squamous cell carcinomas. Neoplasms may also arise from cerumen or sebaceous glands and develop into adenocarcinoma, acinic cell carcinoma, or rarely, adenoid cystic carcinoma. Melanoma is occasionally encountered originating from the skin of the external auditory canal. Primary sarcoma of the temporal bone is rare and occurs more frequently in the pediatric age group.

Symptoms of cancer of the ear are indistinguishable from those of chronic otitis media or chronic dermatitis until the development of pain, cranial nerve involvement, or regional adenopathy. For this reason, a high index of suspicion must be entertained when the physician is presented with any chronic, exophytic, draining, or bleeding lesion. Biopsies must be taken from multiple sites to avoid false-negative results. The bony external auditory canal is a relatively strong barrier against tumor invasion, but the skin and cartilage of the outer external canal provide little resistance to tumor spread. It is for this reason that parotid, conchal, and skin involvement are commonly seen when the diagnosis is made. Once tumor has invaded the middle ear, mucosal extension to the carotid artery, infratemporal area, and dura are seemingly met with little resistance. Lymphatic drainage from the external auditory canal extends inferiorly to the internal jugular chain, whereas anterior and posterior spread extend to the parotid and mastoid nodes, respectively.

■ EVALUATION

The principles of en bloc resection for cancer of the temporal bone have been applied for more than 40 years. Parsons and Lewis were pioneers in describing the principles and results of surgical management. Many subsequent authors have used improved technology and skills to extend the margins of dissection for primary treatment and to provide aggressive surgery and salvage from adjunctive therapy. Despite this, the overall survival rate for cancer of the temporal bone remains poor, except for the earliest of lesions. The chief deterrent to successful management until recently has been the failure to adequately determine the spread of disease medially and along the skull base. Since 1990, however, we have used the tumor, nodes, and metastases (TNM) system devised by Arriaga and co-workers to evaluate these lesions preoperatively in a similar fashion to other cancers of the head and neck. This system depends on high-resolution, thin-cut computed tomographic (CT) scanning in axial and coronal planes and examines 12 separate areas for evidence of tumor involvement or spread. It must be stressed that the strategy is no better than the radiologist who reads the films; experience is a necessity.

Based on this information, a T_1 lesion is limited to the external auditory canal without bony erosion or soft-tissue extension. A T_2 lesion is one with limited bony extension

Table 1. Carcinoma of the Temporal Bone Tumor Staging System

T_1	Tumor limited to the EAC; no bony erosion or soft-tissue extension
T_2	Tumor with limited bony erosion to EAC or <0.5 cm soft-tissue involvement
T_3	Tumor with full-thickness EAC bony erosion; <0.5 cm soft-tissue involvement; or tumor in middle ear, mastoid, or facial nerve
T_4	Tumor eroding the chochlea, petrous apex, medial wall of middle ear, carotid canal, jugular foramen, or dura; or >0.5 cm soft-tissue involvement

EAC, external auditory canal.
From Arriaga M, Cutin, Takahashi H, et al: Staging proposal for external auditory meatus carcinoma based on preoperative clinical examination and computed tomography findings. Ann Otol Rhinol Laryngol 1990; 99:714–721; with permission.

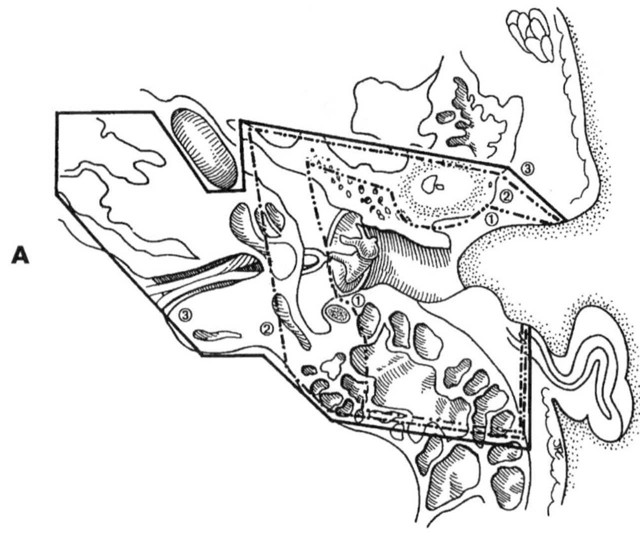

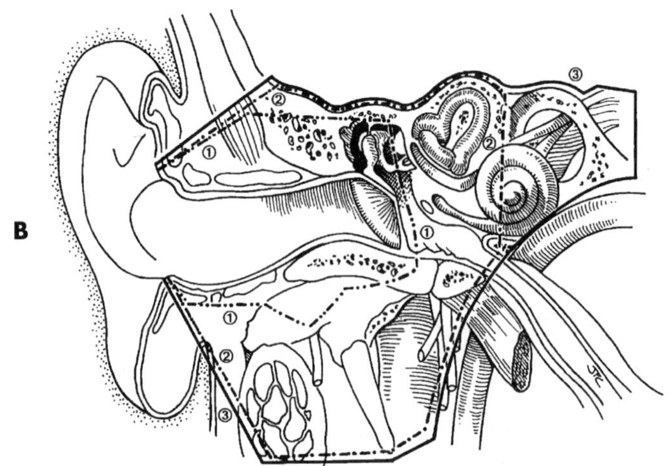

Figure 1.
A, Axial and *B*, Coronal illustrations demonstrating (1) Lateral resection of the temporal bone; (2) Subtotal resection of the temporal bone; and (3) Total resection of the temporal bone. The carotid artery is preserved in these illustrations. *(From Myers EN, et al. Operative otolaryngology—Head and neck surgery. Philadelphia: WB Saunders, 1997; with permission.)*

or soft-tissue involvement of less than 0.5 cm. Tumors with full-thickness osseous erosion in the external auditory canal or involving the middle ear and mastoid or with facial paralysis are considered to be T_3 lesions. Finally, those neoplasms that invade the otic capsule, petrous apex, carotid artery, jugular vein, or dura are considered to be T_4 lesions. Any lymph node involvement is associated with a poor prognosis, and for that reason, even an N_1 lesion is considered stage III. Distant metastases are rare; any evidence of such would be classified as stage IV disease.

Using this system (Table 1), we were able to show 2 year survivals with no evidence of disease in 100 percent of patients who had T_1 and T_2 lesions. Conversely, patients with T_3 lesions had a 56 percent survival rate, and those with T_4 lesions had only 17 percent survival. The utility of this staging system has proved itself, not only for determining prognosis, but also in planning the surgery that is appropriate in each case. In addition, a poor prognosis based on CT scanning has allowed for better preoperative counseling of patients and the avoidance of highly morbid surgical procedures when palliation would better serve these patients. Alternative treatment modalities such as radiotherapy, chemotherapy, or immunotherapy should be realistically considered when extensive disease is identified.

■ PREOPERATIVE PLANNING

Surgical planning depends on the results of careful analysis of CT scans plus physical examination. The en bloc resections that are recommended vary in their extent medially and along the skull base, depending on the results of tumor classification and staging. The extent of disease can then be defined, and a tumor "map" can be created. The en bloc procedures include lateral temporal bone resection, subtotal temporal bone resection, and total temporal bone resection. Figure 1 shows the general outline of these procedures.

Those individuals who have cancer limited to the pinna or external auditory canal (T_1, T_2) are candidates for lateral resection of the temporal bone along with superficial parotidectomy. The facial nerve is preserved in these cases. Malignancies that invade the middle ear or mastoid (T_3) are recommended for subtotal temporal bone resection. This also entails sacrifice of the facial nerve and inner ear and includes parotidectomy and superior neck dissection. Lesions extending to the dura, the carotid artery, or infratemporal fossa (T_4) require total temporal bone resection with anterior extension to the infratemporal fossa if surgery is deemed to be appropriate. Potential sacrifice or compromise of the internal carotid artery must be anticipated. In these cases, preoperative evaluation of contralateral arterial blood supply is mandatory and is accomplished by means of balloon occlusion testing combined with xenon flow studies. Following these tests, approximately 10 percent of patients fall into the "poor risk" category. For these individuals, primary carotid repair or bypass grafting to the middle cerebral artery must be an integral part of their surgical procedure.

The presence of lymph node involvement in the neck is unusual in cancer of the temporal bone, but parotid node involvement is more common. In a similar fashion, distant metastases are rare, and therefore chest and liver scans are not usually indicated, except for highly malignant tumors such as melanoma.

Extension of tumor to the dura or carotid artery signals the need for neurosurgical collaboration. When confronted with T_3 or T_4 lesions, or those with nodal involvement or distant metastases, the surgeon must assess other factors such as age, general health, and the patient's willingness to accept major cranial nerve deficits. A frank discussion of these matters is necessary for patients to arrive at an informed decision as to treatment and potential survival.

■ OPERATIVE TECHNIQUES

Lateral Resection of Temporal Bone

This procedure is advocated for T_1 and T_2 lesions without metastasis or nodal involvement. It begins with a long postauricular incision that allows forward retraction of the pinna and exposure of the parotid gland. A circumferential incision of the external auditory meatus and concha is made, depending on the size and location of the cancer. Frozen sections of the margins can be obtained if there is any question as to their adequacy. A complete mastoidectomy is next performed without undue thinning of the posterior canal wall. Extension of the mastoid dissection is carried anteriorly to the zygomatic root and inferiorly to expose the digastric ridge. An extended facial recess is next developed for visualization of the middle ear and separation of the incudostapedial joint. The facial recess is continued inferiorly, staying lateral to the vertical facial nerve and then continuing anteriorly. The inferior canal wall of the tympanic ring is dissected from the hypotympanum. Dissection through the root of the zygoma is continued with a small cutting bur to connect the anterior epitympanum with the temporomandibular joint capsule. A small curved osteotome is inserted through the facial recess and used to make the final cuts through the anterior canal wall. The entire external auditory canal, along with the tympanic membrane and malleus and conchal skin, are now mobilized. Superficial parotidectomy is then performed to complete the en bloc dissection. Split-thickness skin is placed over the bony defect and sutured to the remnant of the pinna. Bolster packing is placed over the skin graft and held in place with retention sutures. Finally, the postauricular incision is closed after suction drainage is placed.

Subtotal Resection of Temporal Bone

Tumors invading the middle ear, mastoid, hypotympanum, facial nerve, or otic capsule require the added dimensions provided by this technique. Once again, the success rate for these T_3 lesions is further compromised in the face of preoperatively known adenopathy or remote metastases. The intended margins in a subtotal temporal bone resection are the middle fossa dura superiorly, the sigmoid sinus and posterior fossa dura posteriorly, the carotid artery anteriorly, the jugular bulb inferiorly, and the petrous apex medially. The medial extent of dissection depends on the depth of otic capsule involved. Any extension of tumor discovered beyond these margins signals an extremely poor prognosis for the success of this surgical procedure.

A subtotal resection is begun in the same manner as a lateral resection. En bloc dissection is technically difficult to achieve in this situation, so some degree of piecemeal removal must be accepted. Removal of bone overlying dura is necessarily segmental, and this allows for frozen section examination of the soft tissues adjacent to the bone. In this manner, the dissection may be extended as necessary.

A decision must be made regarding facial nerve preservation in this procedure. Although the general margins of this resection would dictate sacrifice of the seventh nerve from its labyrinthine portion to the extratemporal nerve trunk, the surgeon may elect to preserve the nerve when preoperative function is normal and there is no visible sign of tumor involvement. Skeletonization of the nerve will permit its anterior or posterior mobilization in order to facilitate access to the otic capsule and retrofacial area. When facial function is compromised preoperatively or when tumor invasion is discovered, frozen sections of both proximal and distal ends of the nerve should be obtained to ensure clean margins.

Tumor involvement of the jugular bulb mandates ligation of the inferior jugular vein and proximal control of the sigmoid sinus. The superior sigmoid sinus may be packed or ligated. Extension of disease to the pars nervosa necessitates sacrifice of the lower cranial nerves, and therefore tracheostomy is indicated. Repair of the residual dural defect following removal of the sigmoid sinus and jugular bulb must be anticipated as well. This can be accomplished with fascia or homograft dura.

When tumor advances anteriorly into the protympanum or eustachian tube, the superior limb of the skin incision is extended anteriorly in order to expose the carotid artery and infratemporal fossa. The temporalis muscle is reflected anteroinferiorly, and the zygomatic arch is exposed and removed. After total parotidectomy, the mandibular condyle is also removed. If the intratemporal facial nerve has been preserved, the extratemporal nerve can be retracted inferiorly (except for the temporal branch). Dissection of the infratemporal fossa is begun posteriorly and extends anteriorly, with identification of the lateral pterygoid plate, the foramen ovale and V3, and the middle meningeal artery. The internal carotid artery, having previously been skeletonized, forms the posterior extent of the infratemporal fossa dissection. The carotid artery can be mobilized for removal of disease medial to it, and the cartilaginous eustachian tube can be sectioned and packed with muscle. Tumor exposing the dura renders a subtotal temporal bone resection inadequate.

Total Temporal Bone Resection

There is reason to question whether total temporal bone and carotid artery resection is ever justified, based on the poor survival rate of patients who have T_4 lesions. It has been the universal experience that cancers reaching the dura, dural sinuses, carotid artery, or nerve foramina have a poor cure rate despite seemingly adequate margins of resection and adjunctive therapy. Nevertheless, there are few alternative choices, especially for younger patients and those in good general health. Careful counseling is needed to assure that patients are realistically prepared for the significant morbidity of this operation. Vascular assessment, as previously described, must be done because of probable resection of the carotid artery, and tracheostomy is also planned to compensate for tenth and possibly twelfth nerve sacrifice.

An anteriorly based C-shaped flap is created to include the pinna. This exposes the parotid gland and also allows for extension of the lower incision into the neck. Control of the sigmoid sinus at its junction with the transverse sinus is accomplished, as well as ligation of the internal jugular vein. This allows for the posterior osteotomy to be made along the occipitomastoid suture line. Superiorly, after subtemporal craniotomy, the temporal lobe must be gently retracted in order to avoid injury to Labbe's vein. Dura of the floor of the middle fossa is preserved unless tumor invasion is seen. In that case, intradural dissection should proceed medially along the petrous apex; the dura should be kept attached to the specimen. The carotid artery is exposed posterior to V3, and clips are applied for distal control. Section of the greater superficial petrosal nerve is necessary, as well as division of the eustachian tube. Anterior dissection proceeds from the root of the zygoma toward the foramen ovale. V3 is preserved if possible, but the mandibular condyle is included in the specimen. Ligation of the middle meningeal artery permits completion of the anterior skull base dissection to the carotid canal. Parotidectomy and neck dissection are carried out in an attempt to keep the entire specimen intact. The medial osteotomy is performed via the subtemporal exposure and extends from the medial carotid canal to the jugular bulb. Lower cranial nerves are usually included in this portion of the specimen. The seventh and eighth cranial nerves are sacrificed, and bleeding from the inferior petrosal sinus is controlled with packing.

Dural defects are grafted with fascia and the facial nerve may be grafted with sural nerve. The use of vascularized tissue for obliteration of the bony defect is preferable because of the routine use of postoperative radiotherapy. Temporalis muscle may be used, as well as free musculocutaneous flaps from the abdomen. The cutaneous portion of these flaps is used to close the conchal defect, or split-thickness skin grafting can be used if temporalis muscle has been sufficient for bony obliteration. Layered closure to avoid cerebrospinal fluid leaks is performed and is supplemented by means of an indwelling lumbar subarachnoid catheter.

Postoperative head elevation and the use of spinal drainage continues for 3 to 5 days. Perioperative broad-spectrum antibiotic coverage is maintained for 7 to 10 days. Tracheostomy care and frequent suctioning are necessary to prevent aspiration, and routine eye care including implantation of a gold weight is done. Doppler monitoring of free flaps may be necessary in the immediate postoperative period, and careful attention is given to the pinna if surgery has compromised its blood supply. The use of medicinal leeches has proved helpful in salvaging this tissue when venous engorgement is observed.

■ COMPLICATIONS

Cerebrospinal fluid leakage is common when dura and dural sinuses are resected. Head elevation and spinal drainage are of great help in the resolution of this complication. The risk of stroke from internal carotid artery ischemia is minimal when preoperative balloon studies indicate a favorable prognosis. However, cerebral infarcts are occasionally noted secondary to temporal lobe or cerebellar retraction. Aspiration pneumonia is a potential danger following loss of lower cranial nerve function.

■ ADJUNCTIVE THERAPY

Radiotherapy is routinely recommended for every patient, with the exception of the smallest T_1 lesions. External beam, high dosage therapy is thought to increase survival in epithelial malignancies and is probably the most important modality in treating sarcomas. Chemotherapy is also used in these cases but has been questionably effective for cutaneous cancers. Palliative resections have also been followed by radiotherapy, but efficacy is difficult to judge.

■ DISCUSSION

Cancer of the temporal bone has traditionally been difficult to manage. Survival statistics continue to lag in comparison to soft tissue malignancies of the head and Neck. Failure is usually seen in the form of local recurrence. Certainly, this is due to the typical delay with which the diagnosis is made and the technical difficulty in extirpating bone involvement. The use of a TNM staging system has helped in the selection of the appropriate procedure, as well as confirming our knowledge of the prognosis with this difficult and unusual lesion.

Suggested Reading

Arriaga M, Curtin H, Takahashi H, et al. Staging proposal for external auditory meatus carcinoma based on preoperative clinical examination and computed tomography findings. Ann Otol Rhinol Laryngol 1990; 99:714-721.

Arriaga M, Hirsch B, Kamerer D, Myers EN. Squamous cell carcinoma of the external auditory canal. Otolaryngol Head Neck Surg 1989; 101: 330-337;

Parsons H, Lewis JS. Subtotal resection of the temporal bone for cancer of the ear. Cancer 1954; 7:995-1001.

Pensak ML, Gleich LL, Gluckman JL, Shumrick KA. Temporal bone carcinoma: Contemporary perspectives in the skull base surgical ear. Laryngoscope 1996; 106:1234-1237.

BENIGN PAROTID TUMORS

The method of
Michael J. Kaplan

The management of the clinically benign, small, apparently solid mass in the parotid gland is usually straightforward. Most would agree that if the surgeon thinks a benign tumor is the likely diagnosis in a patient who does not have significant operative risk factors, a superficial parotidectomy with dissection and preservation of the facial nerve is appropriate. Many clinicians would do no further evaluation of the mass. Why then read this chapter? Several issues warrant discussion.

Surgical Evaluation. What would make the surgeon suspicious that a "clinically benign tumor" might not be a tumor at all, or might be malignant? For whom should a nonoperative approach be considered? How long should a mass exist before a surgeon excludes reactive periparotid lymphadenopathy from the differential diagnosis? What is the role of fine needle aspiration (FNA)? What is the role of magnetic resonance imaging (MRI) or computed tomography (CT)? What about ultrasound or radionuclide scans? Does the size of the tumor affect any management decisions?

Operative Management. Is resection of the tumor with a cuff of normal parotid tissue adequate, or is removal of all parotid tissue lateral to the plane of the facial nerve (VII) branches necessary? What is the role of facial nerve monitoring? What is the role of intraoperative frozen sections? Would finding a low-grade malignancy alter the operative approach? If first-echelon nodes are found and demonstrate malignancy on frozen section, how comprehensive a neck dissection should be done? Are perioperative antibiotics indicated? How best can the more common complications (hematoma, infection, salivary leakage) be avoided? Why do some benign mixed tumors recur: is it the result of surgical technical error, or is it related to the genetics of the tumor?

Postoperative Management and Complications. Are active drains better than passive drains in preventing hematoma? Under what circumstances should the nerve be re-explored when postoperative facial paralysis is seen? What is the best way to treat recurrent pleomorphic adenoma? What are the indications for postoperative radiotherapy in low-grade malignancies?

■ PREOPERATIVE EVALUATION

Although 80 percent of parotid masses in adults are benign tumors, a complete history complemented by physical examination and radiologic and cytologic examinations may help select patients in whom a parotidectomy is not necessarily the next approach. If the mass is less than 2 cm and has been present for less than 3 to 6 weeks, especially if it is tender, it may be prudent to observe initially, possibly with a course of antibiotics. Although tenderness and a short history do not exclude a tumor etiology, such a history suggests a possible inflammatory origin such as reactive lymphadenopathy or an infected branchial cleft cyst.

A patient who has had a known recent malignancy that may have metastasized to the parotid gland warrants an FNA to exclude this possibility. A patient who is human immunodeficiency virus–positive has an increased risk of lymphoma as well as parotid cysts. If a FNA was insufficiently diagnostic, an MRI (or CT) scan may identify these cysts or identify an enlarged node. Such a node or cyst would be associated with fewer perioperative risks than would a parotidectomy. An FNA diagnosis may also prove useful in an older patient with increased surgical risks who might opt for clinical observation of a benign tumor rather than undergo a parotidectomy.

In addition to the already mentioned indications in deselecting patients for parotidectomy, are there other indications for FNA? Some surgeons believe that they would always like to know the diagnosis in advance. They would suggest that even in apparently straightforward cases the information obtained from FNA warrants the cost of the study, even if only to reassure an anxious patient that it is likely that the histology is benign. These surgeons would also correctly point out that a small low-grade malignancy is clinically indistinguishable from a benign tumor. In experienced centers, it is rare that an FNA is misleading (malignant tumor is read as benign or vice versa), although a descriptive diagnosis may be as much as the cytopathologist can make. Cystic or lymphoid lesions, rare histologies, mucoepidermoid carcinoma, and cellular mixed tumors without stroma or with nuclear atypia are the more common situations that may pose difficulty in allowing the cytopathologist to make a complete and accurate diagnosis. I believe that an FNA may be avoided in straightforward cases when an experienced surgeon, after discussion with an informed patient, would proceed to surgery as the next step in management; this situation is often true for either a benign tumor, a cyst, or a small parotid malignancy. In practice, many patients will have had an FNA done, and this too is highly reasonable.

For larger tumors (> 3 to 4 cm), where the suspicion of malignancy is higher or when there are clear indicators that malignancy is likely (such as skin involvement, facial nerve paralysis, or enlarged nodes), an FNA as well as an MRI may be helpful in planning surgical approaches and postoperative irradiation ports. Although benign and low-grade malignancies usually demonstrate low signal intensity on T1-weighted MRI images and high signal intensity on T2-weighted images (reflecting their higher seromucinous secretions), imaging for *small* parotid masses usually does not affect decision making and hence is unnecessary. Other imaging techniques similarly have little role in this setting. Because Warthin's tumors (and oncocytomas) are detected with technetium 99m radionuclide imaging, this technique had been advocated as a diagnostic tool; however, FNA is more specific. Plain radiographs may demonstrate a stone, and ultrasound may suggest an abscess, but clinically these situations are unlikely to be confused with a benign parotid tumor.

■ OPERATIVE MANAGEMENT

What is meant by a "superficial parotidectomy," and is that all that is involved in the surgical treatment of a small parotid mass? It is adequate and appropriate to remove a tumor with a cuff of normal parotid tissue around it. In practice, a tumor mass frequently is immediately adjacent to a branch of the facial nerve, which leads the pathologist to conclude that there is a close margin at that location. As we would all accept this close margin rather than sacrifice facial nerve VII, it follows that it is unnecessary to dissect at all branches of facial nerve VII distant from the tumor; in particular, a tail of parotid tumor often does not need much dissection of the superior branches distal to the pes.

Although recent literature on the genetics of pleomorphic adenoma suggests that there may be underlying reasons why some tumors may have a higher propensity to recur, surgical technical error has been suspected to be a contributing factor. Tumor spillage has been cited by some as correlating with a higher recurrence rate, as has the presence of positive margins. (Tumor spillage per se as a reason for recurrence sounds mechanistically simplistic given what we are learning today about what a tumor cell must successfully accomplish in order to implant and grow, but it is likely that tumor spillage correlates with larger tumors and positive margins.)

Adequate exposure, identification of anatomy, and meticulous hemostasis are key elements in a successful procedure. Usually, the facial nerve may be found directly in the small triangle bound by the tympanomastoid suture superiorly, digastric muscle posteriorly, and the styloid process anteriorly. The nerve usually lies 4 to 8 mm inferior to the bony suture, running an anterior-inferior course. Using a McCabe or similar dissector, adjacent tissue is dissected, tested with a portable facial nerve stimulator if there is any question in the surgeon's mind, and bleeding is completely controlled with a fine bipolar cautery forceps. This process is serially continued until the nerve is located. The nerve is then followed distally by lifting tissue just lateral to it, testing as previously described, and bipolar electrocautery is used for hemostasis and division. If the main branch cannot be dissected in this way because of an overlying large tumor, either a distal branch may be located and followed retrogradely, or in rare circumstances a mastoidectomy may be needed to locate the descending portion of facial nerve VII. Interfering as little as possible with the blood supply to the nerve branches may decrease the incidence of postoperative facial weakness. For instance, if the tumor is inferior, it may be possible to maintain some minimal surrounding tissue around the buccal branches and eye branches rather than dissecting directly lateral to them; certainly try not to lift branches unnecessarily.

Is facial nerve monitoring using a two-channel (or greater) device today the standard of care? No. In patients with a small parotid mass who have had no prior surgery of the parotid, the incidence of facial nerve paralysis is low; when paresis occurs, it is usually transient. Few would dispute an argument by an experienced surgeon that he or she finds that even the disposable facial nerve stimulator rarely adds anything to the case in this setting. In patients who have recurrent parotid masses where finding the nerve at all may be most challenging, I have found that external cranial nerve VII monitoring is extremely helpful; there have been times when that is the only indication of where the facial nerve VII branches lie.

It is prudent to look at and feel adjacent nodes in the parotid field, biopsying any that are enlarged (> 1.5 cm) or hard. It is more likely that larger tumors or those producing facial nerve paralysis will have involved nodes (and these are discussed in another chapter), but a low-grade malignancy may also spread to adjacent nodes. A modified radical neck dissection would be indicated if nodes are involved by mucoepidermoid carcinoma, squamous cell carcinoma (SCC), adenocarcinoma, melanoma, or undifferentiated tumor; there is no indication for elective neck dissection (except possibly in the case of SCC if one believes that SCC in the parotid is a metastasis from a possibly undetected skin site or unknown primary). In practice, however, this situation rarely arises in apparently straightforward small parotid tumors. It is a helpful practice to have previously discussed this unlikely event with the patient so as to avoid either having to discuss it de novo intraoperatively with a family member or recommending postoperatively a second surgical procedure.

Is there a role for frozen section diagnosis of the primary tumor? Usually not. Because FNA is at least equal to frozen section diagnosis and there is some advantage in knowing the diagnosis in advance, just to obtain an initial diagnosis intraoperatively is inadequate reason. If a decision to sacrifice a significant nerve branch or not would be influenced by confirmation that the tumor is malignant, then that is one indication for a frozen section.

Should perioperative antibiotics be used? There is no definitive answer. The incidence of infection is low without antibiotics. In breast surgery, a controlled study has shown a statistically significant decrease in wound infection rates from approximately 3 percent to approximately 1 percent, but is that *clinically* significant? Is it offset by the disadvantages of antibiotic-associated diarrhea and drug allergy, and the cost of administration of the antibiotics? If antibiotics are used, perioperative prophylaxis is begun within the hour before incision and continued for no more than 24 hours.

■ POSTOPERATIVE MANAGEMENT AND COMPLICATIONS

The complications of parotid surgery include facial nerve injury, hematoma, sialocele, gustatory sweating, and recurrence of tumor. Rare complications include skin flap necrosis, neuroma of the greater auricular nerve, and wound infection. Numbness of the earlobe resulting from sacrifice of the greater auricular nerve is a usual sequela of the procedure and should be included in the preoperative discussion.

Facial Weakness

Postoperative facial nerve paresis or paralysis may occur, even after surgery for a small tumor by a highly skilled surgeon, and even when there has been apparently minimal retraction or devascularization of nerve branches. If the surgeon knows that the nerve is intact, there is no indication to re-explore the operative field. Some clinicians would consider using steroids in this setting; others would not. Certainly the patient needs reassurance regarding estimates of recovery time, and the several approaches to appropriate management of the eye should be discussed and begun.

Hematoma

Are active drains better or worse than passive drains in reducing postoperative hematoma? Hematomas occur with either type of drain. An active drain appears to be more comfortable than the dressing associated with a Penrose drain, but I believe this matter should be left to the preferences of the individual surgeon. Patients used to stay in the hospital more than one postoperative night. As changes in medical care have led to reconsiderations of a number of prior assumptions, I do think it is acceptable for selected patients to go home with an active drainage system and return in 24 to 48 hours to have the drain removed. If a wound hematoma occurs, it will be noticed by abnormal swelling in the wound, and the patient will likely experience pain. If an expanding hematoma occurs, the wound should be re-explored, and any bleeders should be tied or otherwise controlled, and a new drain should be placed.

Sialocele

When a sialocele (or an actual salivary fistula leaking clear fluid) occurs postoperatively, it usually is noted at the first postoperative return visit a week or two after surgery. A pressure dressing (possibly with incision and drainage of the sialocele) is an option, but it is difficult to maintain pressure at this location. Aspiration for culture (delaying institution of antibiotics until cultural results are available) is another option that is often sufficient, although a number of weekly serial aspirations may be required.

Gustatory Sweating

Gustatory sweating (Frey's syndrome, auricular temporal syndrome) is common (35 percent to 60 percent) beginning several months after parotidectomy. Most patients are not bothered by these symptoms enough to seek medical therapy, and treatment is generally supportive. Glycopyrrolate is a possibly effective roll-on antiperspirant with few anticholinergic side effects; more readily available nonscented antiperspirants topically applied to the side of the face may also work. Among the numerous surgical treatments that have been proposed—including tympanic neurectomy, subdermal insertion of fascia lata grafts, and rotation of a sternocleidomastoid muscle flap into the parotid—none have convincingly been helpful and worthwhile.

Neuroma

Occasionally months or even years following surgery, a small (<1.5 cm) mass, often painful, may be palpated over the sternocleidomastoid muscle at the amputated end of the greater auricular nerve. The sole initial presentation of this neuroma may be radiating pain from a trigger point in the area. Excision of a symptomatic neuroma should relieve the pain. Because the differential diagnosis includes recurrent tumor, FNA may assist in making the diagnosis, particularly if a surgical procedure is not planned.

Recurrent Tumor

The management of recurrent pleomorphic adenoma requires judgment by and communication between doctor and patient. The patient's health, occupation, and desires are important considerations in choosing intervention. The incidence of recurrence is 2 percent to 30 percent. Time to recurrence is measured in years, with a significant percentage occurring more than 10 years after initial surgery. Once recurrent, more than 25 percent of excised pleomorphic adenomas will recur again, often in a shorter interval than after the first recurrence. The possibility of carcinoma ex pleomorphic adenoma should be considered in evaluating a patient with a possible recurrent benign mixed tumor. Hence, FNA is often indicated, especially if nonsurgical treatment is being considered. An MRI will help evaluate the extent of tumor, including possible multicentricity. Multicentricity is unusual initially, but it is increasingly common with recurrences.

Management options include re-resection with facial nerve monitoring, irradiation with or without repeat surgery, and careful clinical follow-up without intervention. If there is to be surgery, a total parotidectomy is likely to be needed. The facial nerve can usually still be dissected from the tumor, but the incidence of postoperative paresis is much greater than at the initial operation. For this reason, irradiation as an alternative should be discussed. Radiotherapy does appear effective in retarding subsequent growth of pleomorphic adenomas, but the side effects, including a low rate of radiation-induced malignancy, need to be considered. Hence, the third option of "watchful waiting" is often employed, especially when tumor appears adherent to a functioning facial nerve. A baseline MRI establishes the current extent of the tumor, and an FNA (to the extent possible) confirms benignity. Periodic clinical and radiologic examinations are needed. Intervention is postponed until either the rate of tumor growth suggests that intervention soon will be required or other events, such as facial nerve VII involvement, raise the suspicion of malignancy. Obviously, the decision for each particular patient must be clearly and thoroughly discussed. In subgroups of pleomorphic adenoma, if the correlation between identified cytogenetic differences and their clinical course strengthens, it may become appropriate to investigate whether a particular subgroup would achieve a disproportionate benefit from radiotherapy to treat recurrences.

■ DISCUSSION

The appropriate management of patients who have benign parotid tumors stems from a subset of management principles of salivary gland masses in general, both benign and malignant. Familiarity with the potential role and limitations of diagnostic and evaluation aids such as fine needle aspiration, magnetic resonance imaging, and electromyographic nerve monitoring is helpful in assessing the appropriate roles of additional evaluation, as well as effective counseling of patients. Understanding of the pathophysiology of inflammatory and infectious processes augments the evaluation and differential diagnosis. Prevention of complications begins with a thorough understanding of their etiology, as well as the various methods of identifying and preserving branches of the facial nerve. Complications that do occur are usually successfully managed conservatively. Corneal lubrication is key in transient facial nerve paresis. Permanent facial paralysis should be rare following surgery for benign tumors. Superficial parotidectomy, the usual procedure for benign tumors, should be associated with low morbidity and a short hospital stay of no more than 48 hours.

The surgeon experienced in the evaluation, surgery, and care of patients who have benign salivary gland tumors can effectively counsel and reassure patients without minimizing or exaggerating risks, choose additional diagnostic or intraoperative tests when needed, and achieve excellent results with few complications.

Suggested Reading

American Society for Head and Neck Surgery and Society of Head and Neck Surgeons. Tumors of major salivary glands: Parotid. In: Clinical practice guidelines for the diagnosis and management of cancer of the head and neck. American Society for Head and Neck Surgery and Society of Head and Neck Surgeons, 1996:65.

Eisele DW, Johns ME. Complications of surgery of the salivary glands. In: Eisele DW, ed. Complications in head and neck surgery. St. Louis: Mosby–Year Book, 1993:183.

Kaplan MJ. Complications of salivary gland surgery. In: Weissler MS, Pillsbury HC, eds. Complications of head and neck surgery. New York: Thieme Medical Publishers, 1995:172.

Kaplan MJ, Johns ME. Malignant neoplasms [of the major salivary glands]. In: Cummings CW, et al, ed. Otolaryngology—Head and neck surgery. St. Louis: Mosby–Year Book, 1992:1043.

MALIGNANT TUMORS OF THE PAROTID GLAND

The method of
George L. Adams

Malignant parotid tumors represent a heterogeneous group of malignancies that account for 1 percent to 3 percent of all head and neck cancer. Because their presentation, classification, and response to treatment is so determined by their specific histology, they have become a favorite area of discussion. In the adult, approximately 80 percent of parotid tumors are benign; pleomorphic adenoma represents almost 90 percent of these benign parotid tumors. The remaining 10 percent includes a variety of tumors, but papillary cystadenoma lymphomatosum (or Warthin's tumor) is by far the second most common benign tumor. Because of the high preponderance of benign disease to malignant disease, the surgeon must be careful in approaching and discussing the operative procedure with the patient. Remember there is a 20 percent chance of malignancy. Hemangiomas and lymphangiomas are the most common parotid tumors in children. However, in children, almost half of the solid tumors are malignant (40 percent to 50 percent). The most common is low-grade mucoepidermoid carcinoma, but adenocarcinoma represents the second most common type, and in children this tumor can behave even more aggressively than in the adult. Thus, preoperative assessment with needle biopsy in the child is even more important to assist in the planning for a potential extensive operative procedure.

CLINICAL EVALUATION

The most common presenting early symptom of both benign and malignant tumors is a slowly progressive, painless mass in the parotid region (Fig. 1). Cervical adenopathy is a rare initial presentation and is associated only with certain specific histologic types. Pain, firmness, tightness of the overlying skin or actual ulceration, and older age increase the likelihood of malignancy. Facial paralysis *represents* late stage of disease and is associated with those tumors that tend to involve the perineural area: squamous cell carcinoma, adenoid cystic carcinoma, and malignant melanoma. The nerve can be invaded by any malignant tumor and still have normal clinical function.

Metastatic disease to the parotid gland may have a presentation similar to that of a primary malignancy, often with rapid progression of the size of the mass and facial paralysis (Table 1). The most common sites of malignancies that metastasize to the parotid gland are skin cancers from the temporal and cheek areas, the eyelids, and the conjunctiva. In fact, approximately 80 percent of the metastatic disease to the parotid gland arises from malignant melanoma of the head and neck area. Direct extension by malignancies such as adenoid cystic carcinoma of the external ear canal can invade the parotid gland. Metastatic carcinomas from below the clavicle, such as that from lung, gastrointestinal, and

Table 1. Indicators of Malignancy
Age
Under 18 years
Over 65 years
Pain
Rapid growth
Facial paresis (especially only one division, e.g., marginal mandibular)
Involvement of overlying skin
Long history of mass, now sudden growth (carcinoma expleomorphic adenoma)
Transplantation patient who has a history of facial skin cancer

renal cell carcinoma, also have to be included in the differential diagnosis.

IMAGING

Because of all the aforementioned factors, a thorough preoperative assessment before embarking on surgical resection is essential. In addition to the customary head and neck history and physical examination, computed tomography (CT) or magnetic resonance imaging (MRI) should be performed whenever malignancy is suspected and, more recently in the literature, for almost all parotid masses. The MRI will provide more information than the CT scan, but if a patient comes to my office with a CT scan in hand, I seldom recommend doing the additional test if the CT study is adequate. The scan is of value in determining extension of the tumor into the parapharyngeal space and toward the skull base. It does not determine whether surgery should be performed, but is valuable in planning the extensiveness of the operative procedure, for example, determining whether a mandibular swing or a mastoidectomy is going to be required.

NEEDLE BIOPSY

Fine needle aspiration biopsy (FNAB) is advised for all parotid tumors. This technique is extremely sensitive in determining the presence of pleomorphic adenoma and has a greater than 90 percent accuracy. It also has an 80 percent accuracy in determining the presence of malignancy. Granted, these numbers are not sufficient to inform the patient that there is no likelihood of a suspected benign tumor actually being malignant, because many tumors, even pleomorphic adenoma, and particularly adenoid cystic carcinoma, may have heterogeneous cell populations. The presentation of mucoepidermoid carcinoma may have a cystic component, and whenever the FNAB reveals only fluid devoid of cells, the possibility of mucoepidermoid carcinoma must be considered. In particular, if the needle biopsy is repeated and again acellular fluid is obtained, surgical resection based on a consideration of mucoepidermoid carcinoma is advised.

Acinic cell carcinoma is the most common malignant parotid tumor that is bilateral. Large cystic lesions presenting in a patient who has HIV disease are generally lymphoepithelial cysts and require FNAB to rule out the possibility of infectious process, particularly tuberculosis or lymphoma. If lymphoma or sarcoma lesions are suspected, an open biopsy for a tissue sample is recommended.

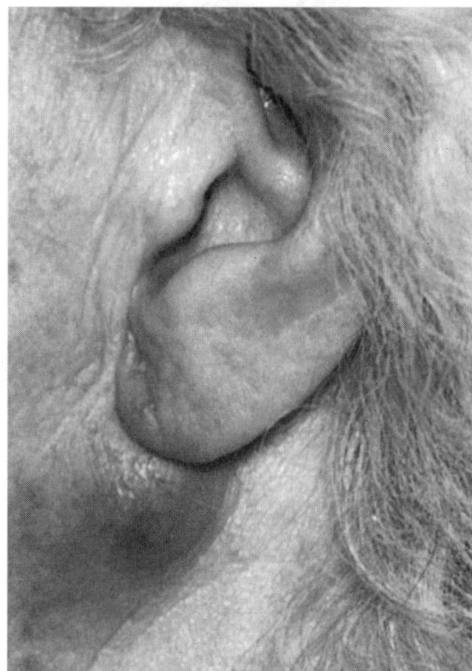

Figure 1.
Clinical appearance of parotid gland tumor.

CLINICAL PATHOLOGY

Parotid tumors have been divided into high and low grades (Tables 2 and 3). Biorklund and Enroth specifically list adenoid cystic carcinoma as a special intermediate group. That is because of the unique behavior of adenoid cystic carcinoma, and acinic cell carcinoma as well. Both tumors have initial excellent treatment results and are unlikely to metastasize to the neck. However, 15 and 20 year survival rates are poor, and distant metastases, particularly to bone and lung, may occur at that time even without local recurrence.

Table 2. Grading of Parotid Tumors*

T_x	Primary tumor cannot be assessed
T_0	No evidence of primary tumor
T_1	Tumor <2 cm in greatest dimension
T_2	Tumor 2–4 cm in greatest dimension
T_3	Tumor 4–6 cm in greatest dimension
T_4	Tumor >6 cm in greatest dimension
	All categories are subdivided: (a) no local extension (b) local extension

* Local extension is clinical and/or macroscopic invasion of skin, soft tissue, bone, or nerve. Microscopic evidence alone is not considered local extension for classification purposes.

Table 3. Parotid Malignancies

LOW-GRADE	HIGH-GRADE
Low-grade mucoepidermoid	High- and intermediate-grade mucoepidermoid
Acinic cell carcinoma	Adenoid cystic carcinoma
Low-grade adenocarcinoma	Adenocarcinoma
Terminal duct adenocarcinoma	Carcinoma ex pleomorphic adenoma
Basal cell adenocarcinoma	Salivary duct carcinoma
	Epithelial–myoepithelial carcinoma
	Undifferentiated carcinoma

Low-grade mucoepidermoid carcinoma is the most common malignant tumor in children, and acinic cell carcinoma is the second most common. Both of these low-grade tumors are treated by wide regional resection without facial nerve resection or postoperative radiotherapy. In adults, adenoid cystic carcinoma and low-grade mucoepidermoid carcinoma are the most common malignancies. The high-grade variant of mucoepidermoid carcinoma is one of the tumors most prone to metastatic disease in the neck. Thus, the high-grade carcinomas—squamous cell carcinoma; high-grade mucoepidermoid carcinoma; adenoid cystic carcinoma; high-grade adenocarcinoma, particularly ductal cell subtype; and carcinoma ex pleomorphic adenoma—are treated aggressively. They require both neck dissection and postoperative radiotherapy. Low-grade tumors are treated by complete or total parotidectomy, with preservation of the facial nerve when possible.

Metastatic malignancies to the parotid gland are treated by superficial parotidectomy, with preservation of the facial nerve. If the tumor is of the squamous cell type or melanoma and the nerve is involved, nerve preservation is not feasible. Often, in such cases, there is such extensive involvement of the area that the peripheral divisions are not available for cable grafting. Patients who have had solid organ transplantations may develop multiple squamous cell carcinomas of the skin. These patients have a particularly aggressive form of skin cancer secondary to immunosuppression. They may have a small squamous cell carcinoma of the skin (Fig. 2) and paralysis of one of the divisions of the facial nerve. Surgical resection includes not only the primary site on the cheek, but also total parotidectomy and, when possible, a facial nerve graft. Because of the poor prognosis, experience has demonstrated that postoperative radiotherapy is indicated in all such patients.

■ THERAPY

Before surgery, the patient and family should be aware of the possibility of malignant disease. Because even FNAB may give a false-negative result, the operative procedure begins with identification of the facial nerve at the stylomastoid foramen and performance of a complete lateral or superficial lobe parotidectomy. This is the biopsy. All divisions of the facial nerve are preserved unless it is apparent that the nerve and tumor are adherent. If the nerve disappears into a large tumor mass that is known to be malignant, that division of the nerve is sacrificed. When possible, the division to the lower eyelid is preserved. Because there is often considerable uncertainty as to the actual type of tumor or the grading of the malignancy, I describe the technique that I use.

A standard "lazy S" parotid incision is made (Figs. 3 and

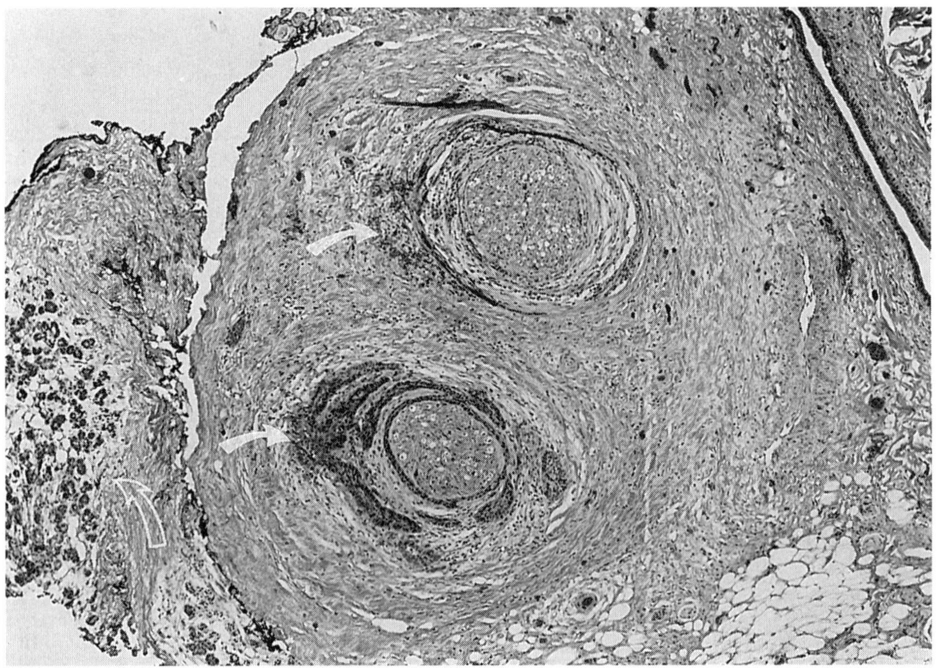

Figure 2.
Perineural invasion of the facial nerve in a patient who has metastatic squamous cell carcinoma to the parotid gland. Left-pointing arrow shows normal parotid, right-pointing arrows show perineural infiltration in two divisions of the facial nerve. Facial nerve function was absolutely normal preoperatively. At surgery, the nerve appeared mildly thickened and had no obvious tumor in it until a segment of the nerve was sectioned and examined. A negative margin was obtained in the vertical segment within the mastoid. Because of the possibility of skip lesions when perineural invasion is present, it is never certain that there is not more proximal involvement.

4). Parallel to this incision, a second incision is made, more anteriorly over the cheek, if the adherent skin is to be resected en bloc with the parotid mass. This includes excision of any previous incision in the area, because often the patient has had an open biopsy or a previous attempt at a superficial parotidectomy that was interrupted when it was determined that there was more extensive disease than had been initially anticipated. The superficial parotid fascia blends with the fascia overlying the sternocleidomastoid muscle. This fascia is divided, and the posterior belly of the digastric muscle is inspected. If the tumor is not adjacent to the main trunk of the nerve, the nerve is identified at this time, but no further dissection of the parotid is performed. The greater auricular nerve crosses the SCM muscle and approaches the parotid tail. Here, it often splits into two to three divisions. The direction and location of this nerve is noted, and it is incised at the parotid and laid back over the SCM muscle for possible future use as a nerve graft. The SCM muscle is retracted inferiorly, and the digastric muscle is retracted superiorly. This allows access to the jugulodigastric and subdigastric lymph nodes. The eleventh (accessory) cranial nerve lies deep, but in a path directly parallel to the more superficial greater auricular nerve as it approaches the jugular vein at the skull base. The jugular vein is identified as well as the carotid artery, and if the dissection is carried forward, the hypoglossal nerve is exposed.

Lymph nodes in this area are palpated and removed. Any suspicious lymph nodes are sent to the pathologist for frozen

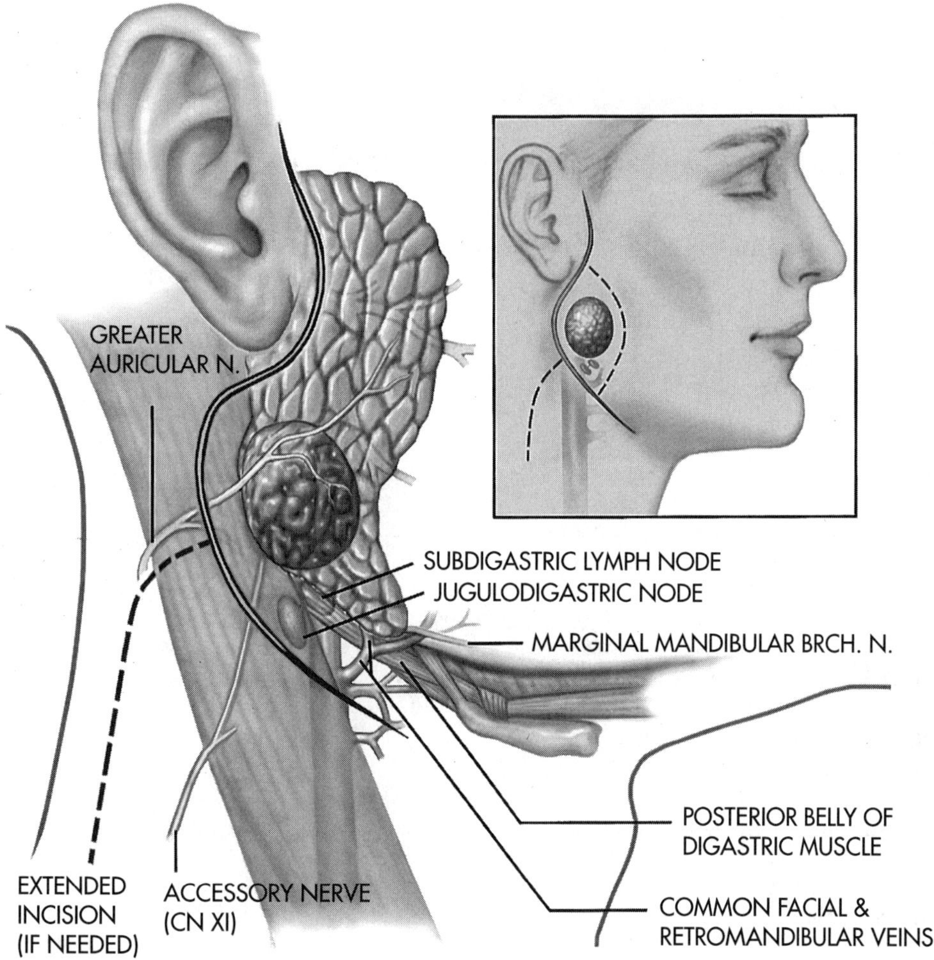

Figure 3.
A gentle S-curved incision is made. The skin is elevated in the preparotid fascial plane, exposing the parotid gland and the greater auricular nerve. This nerve is sectioned and preserved for possible grafting. Resection begins by identifying the posterior belly of the digastric muscle and examining the subdigastric and jugulodigastric lymph nodes. Metastatic involvement of these nodes affects the approach to the tumor and expedites its resection. Identification of positive nodes indicates a need for a modified neck dissection as well as total parotidectomy. If the facial nerve is definitely involved by tumor and it is known that this is a malignancy, no effort is made to save the involved nerve division, and preparation is made for a neural graft. If diagnosis is uncertain, the nerve is preserved until frozen section is complete.

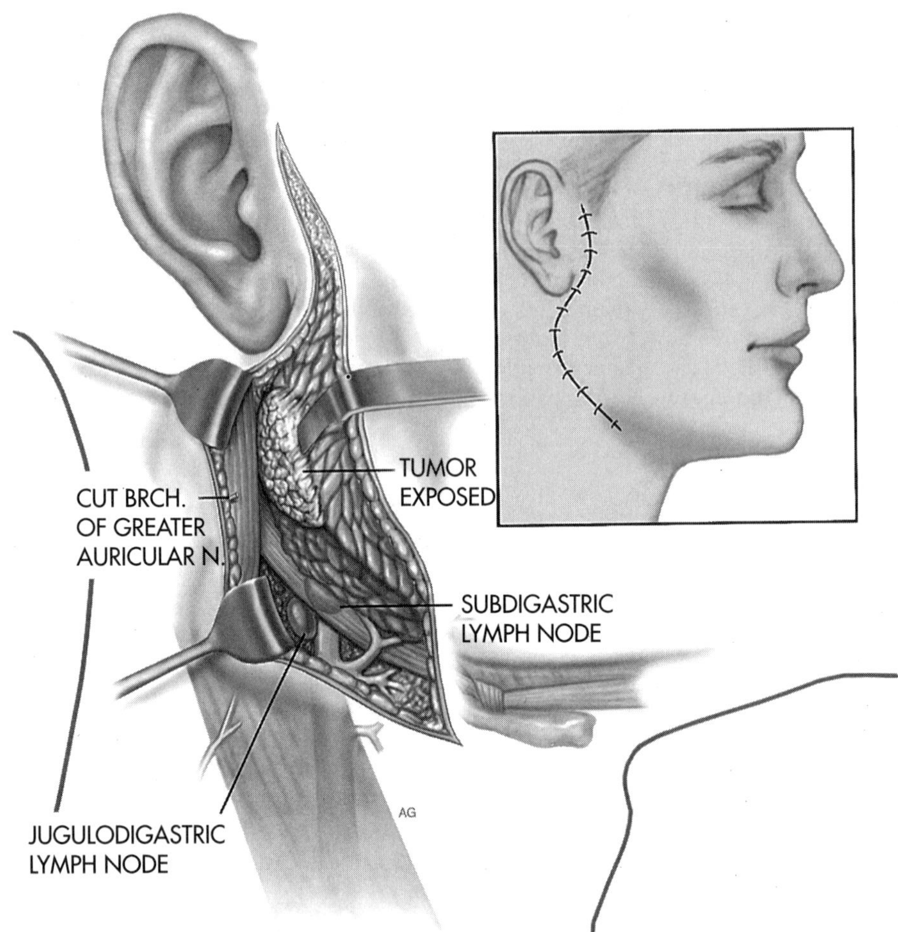

Figure 4.
Dissection begins posteriorly and inferiorly. The facial nerve is identified as it exits the stylomastoid foramen. In revision parotidectomies, it is perhaps easier to identify the marginal mandibular branch or the buccal branch and trace them proximally. If neck dissection is required, an extension of the initial incision is made. Even if skin is resected, it is often possible to perform a primary closure. Flap reconstruction may be required when more extensive overlying skin resection is necessary. Using this approach, there is rarely a need to return the patient to the operating room should there be a change in the pathologic diagnosis of the tumor.

section. At this time, a diagnosis of malignancy by metastases to the lymph node may be made. The histologic grade of the tumor is no longer relevant, because the determination is made that it is behaving clinically as an aggressive tumor. Thus, any tumor overlying or adjacent to the facial nerve that is not easily separable requires nerve resection and cable graft. Additionally, the need to perform a modified radical neck dissection is determined by the presence of a pathologically positive node. High-grade tumors may have positive nodes that are not clinically palpable and may not be apparent on either CT or MRI scan.

Now, facial nerve dissection is performed by first following the marginal mandibular division or the temporal and frontal divisions. Recall that this is not a facial nerve exploration, but a radical parotidectomy for malignancy. Thus, the nerve division farthest away from the tumor is identified first, and the actual tumor mass is approached by rolling the parotid gland forward toward the cheek. Eventually, the fascia overlying the masseter muscle is encountered. The entire superficial lobe is sent to the pathologist for frozen section evaluation. A small amount of deep lobe, usually only 20 percent of the gland, often lies deep to the first major division of the facial nerve. By using vessel loops for gentle retraction, the nerve is lifted, and tonotomy scissors are used to carefully dissect the deep lobe portion of the gland. Any divisions of the facial nerve that were intentionally sacrificed now undergo frozen section of the proximal and distal stumps. For adenoid cystic carcinoma, even this is not always adequate, because there may be skip areas extending along the nerve toward the brain stem. In such cases, one must be prepared to perform a mastoidectomy, identify the nerve, and remove it from the vertical portion of the facial canal. Again, frozen section, even this far from the tumor, is required to make certain the proximal stump is tumor free. It is technically easier to perform the cable graft from the midportion of the vertical portion of the mastoid, as only a single suture is required to stabilize the graft in the canal.

Malignant tumors tend to spread toward the skull base; they seldom spread peripherally. The previously dissected greater auricular nerve is useful as a cable graft for the buccal and lower lid divisions. The frontal and marginal divisions often are not reconstituted. My experience with nerve grafts in patients over 65 years of age has not provided satisfactory results. Therefore, at the same setting or at a second stage, under local anesthesia, these patients undergo a brow lift and gold weight implant in the upper eyelid. This can be performed before the initiation of radiotherapy. Fascial sling procedures for the lower face area can also be performed.

■ MANAGEMENT OF THE NECK

There has long been controversy over whether a neck dissection is indicated for parotid malignancies. In the past, all patients who had high-grade malignant tumors underwent radical neck dissection. Current practice is to administer postoperative radiotherapy to the primary tumor and neck of all patients who have high-grade tumors. This includes the clinically negative neck. If there are pathologically positive lymph nodes located as described earlier, the patient undergoes, as a minimum, a comprehensive neck dissection with preservation of the cranial nerves, SCM muscle, and jugular vein. Regardless, patients who have high-grade mucoepidermoid carcinoma, carcinoma ex pleomorphic adenoma, ductal carcinoma, and squamous cell carcinoma all undergo neck dissection. Patients who have acinic cell carcinoma or adenoid cystic carcinoma undergo neck dissection only when there is clinical or pathologic evidence of metastatic disease. As noted earlier, these tumors are capable of developing distant metastases.

■ ROLE OF RADIOTHERAPY

Radiotherapy is not used as a primary treatment unless the patient has recurrent disease, has disease that has been determined to be unresectable, or is of an age or general health status that prohibits surgical resection. As for other head and neck malignancies, radiotherapy is preferably started within 4 weeks to control microscopic disease. Indications for postoperative radiotherapy include (1) high-grade parotid malignancies; (2) close or microscopically positive margins; (3) preservation of the facial nerve when the tumor is close to, but not involving, that nerve; (4) recurrent disease; (5) invasion beyond the parotid capsule into the surrounding tissue; (6) deep lobe parotid malignancies; and (7) surgical "spill" of the tumor (cystic mucoepidermoid carcinoma).

■ SPECIAL SITUATIONS

The preceding discussion is the preferred management of malignant parotid tumors. Unfortunately, patients are often referred who have a more complex history and often have undergone previous surgery. Some patients have had a superficial parotidectomy and the initial diagnosis was believed to be pleomorphic adenoma, but the diagnosis was then changed on permanent section to adenoid cystic carcinoma, acinic cell carcinoma, or mucoepidermoid carcinoma. Should these patients undergo further surgery or postoperative radiotherapy? There is no question that the facial nerve is placed at greater risk with revision surgery, especially when there has been delay of 3 to 4 weeks. Additionally, these patients have some swelling and reaction in the parotid area, which makes surgery at that stage even more complex. I review the pathology slides, repeat the MRI scan, discuss the operative findings with the previous surgeon, and then discuss the risk with the patient. If it appears that there is extensive parotid tissue remaining, and a comparison can be made with the contralateral side or the preoperative MRI, and if the margins are grossly positive, then re-exploration is performed within 1 month after the initial surgery as soon as the postoperative wound inflammation is resolved. The facial nerve monitor is used to identify the facial nerve. Mastoidectomy is often required in order to identify the nerve and perform a nerve graft. In such cases, either the buccal division, which can be found 1 cm above and parallel to the parotid duct as it crosses the masseter muscle, or the marginal mandibular division as it passes lateral to the posterior facial vein, is identified, and the nerve is traced from distal to proximal. If nerve function remains intact, it is often possible to identify each of the peripheral divisions and gradually dissect the nerves toward the stylomastoid foramen. If a division of the facial nerve was removed earlier, it may be repaired at this time. However, it is difficult to count on being able to stimulate the peripheral divisions, and thus the patient should not be informed that repair is likely. On the other hand, if it is obvious what has happened and the divisions are apparent, immediate repair can be performed. As noted earlier, effective repair is more likely to occur in younger patients. As a minimum, a total parotidectomy is performed, including removal of sufficient surrounding tissue. The subdigastric lymph nodes are examined histologically, and neck dissection is determined on the basis of the findings of the preoperative MRI, clinical findings, and pathologic assessment of the adjacent lymph nodes. The previous scar is excised with 1 cm of margin on each side, and if there is any suggestion that the original tumor was close to the skin, that segment of skin is also resected. Postoperative radiotherapy is recommended to commence in 4 weeks.

■ TREATMENT RATIONALE

Surgery for parotid malignancy should be a single operative procedure. Few surgical procedures are more difficult than re-entering the parotid bed after a superficial parotidectomy and trying to resect residual tumor and preserve the facial nerve. The anatomy is distorted, the nerve is at risk, and there is substantial uncertainty on the part of the surgeon as to what tissues should be excised. By using the aforementioned approach of first performing an MRI, then an FNAB, as well as history and physical findings, there are strong suggestions as to whether the tumor is benign or malignant. However, none of the aforementioned are absolutely certain, and thus the additional time needed to identify and perform frozen section on the adjacent subdigastric lymph nodes, may, in the long run, be timesaving. The presence of a malignant node allows the surgeon to resect with confidence any division of the facial nerve that appears to be involved by tumor. This is preferable to trying to dissect the nerve division from the tumor, awaiting the frozen section, and then later, having to go back and re-resect that division. Most surgeons preserve all divisions that are not grossly involved with tumor. The fact that the nerve is still functioning does not mean it cannot be extensively involved with tumor. During dissection, the nerve may seem even easier to locate, and exposure may seem even easier, because the nerve will be very apparent due to its slightly enlarged diameter, but otherwise normal appearance. It is clinically very difficult to determine how far proximal the tumor has extended, and only frozen section will permit this. If the main trunk is involved close to the stylomastoid foramen, it is preferable to identify the nerve in the mastoid, because it is next to impossible to perform a satisfactory nerve graft adjacent to the stylomastoid foramen.

Too often, surgeons have experienced the telephone call from the pathologist a week later stating that the originally described benign tumor mass has been found to be malignant. Much discussion then evolves about whether the tumor bed should be reapproached surgically or radiotherapy alone should be administered. Further, many pathologists are tending to defer final diagnosis until special stains can be applied to the tissue. This further delays final pathologic diagnosis by several days. Although establishing the proper pathologic diagnosis is important and may determine whether postoperative radiotherapy is required, the frozen section is what is most useful to the surgeon, and although usually accurate, it too can be misleading. By using the aforementioned suggestions, the aggressive behavior of the particular tumor type is established early, and the appropriate surgery is then performed at a single stage. When the final pathology results are available, the need for postoperative radiotherapy can then be determined, but there is no need for additional surgery.

Suggested Reading

Atula T, Grenman R, Laippala P, et al. Fine-needle aspiration biopsy in the diagnosis of parotid gland lesions: Evaluation of 438 biopsies. Diagn Cytopathol 1996; 15(3):185.

Barnes L, Rao U, Krause J, et al. Salivary duct carcinoma: Part I–a clinicopathologic evaluation and DNA image analysis of 13 cases with review of the literature. Oral Surg Oral Med Oral Pathol Oral Radiol Endod 1994; 78(1):64.

Biorklund A, Eneroth CM. Management of parotid gland neoplasms. Am J Otolaryngol 1980; 1:155.

Byers RM, Piorkowski R, Luna MA. Malignant parotid tumors in patients under 20 years of age. Arch Otolaryngol 1984; 110:232.

Garden AS, El-Naggar AK, Morrison WH, et al. Postoperative radiotherapy for malignant tumors of the parotid gland. Int J Radiot Oncol Biol Phys 1997; 37(1):79.

Kelley DJ, Spiro RH. Management of the neck in parotid carcinoma. Am J Surg 1996; 172(6):695.

Shikhani AH, Johns ME. Tumors of the major salivary glands in children. Head Neck Surg 1988; Mar/Apr:257.

SUBMANDIBULAR GLAND TUMORS

The method of
Randal S. Weber

Tumors of the submandibular gland are rare and account for many fewer cases of primary salivary gland cancer than neoplasms arising in the parotid gland. Whereas most parotid neoplasms are benign (70 percent to 80 percent), 50 percent of neoplasms of submandibular gland origin are malignant.

When evaluating a patient who has a swelling in the submandibular triangle of the neck, the differential diagnosis should include inflammatory processes of the salivary gland, a salivary gland neoplasm, and inflammatory or neoplastic involvement of the facial lymph nodes. It is incumbent upon the physician to develop a differential diagnosis when evaluating patients who have masses in this area so that untimely incisional biopsy can be avoided. "Shelling out" the submandibular gland involved by tumor can result in tumor spillage, positive margins, a higher risk for recurrence, and in the case of malignancy the need for postoperative radiotherapy. To avoid an error in diagnosis, the physician must obtain a thorough history, physical examaination, and radiologic evaluation, and, at times, cytologic material on which to base appropriate intervention.

■ SURGICAL ANATOMY

The submandibular glands are paired salivary glands that are inferior to the horizontal ramus of the mandible and contain both serous and mucinous glandular elements. The gland is irregular and is composed of multiple globules. There is a superficial portion that lies lateral to the mylohyoid muscle and a deep portion that lies on the medial surface of this muscle and extends into the sublingual space. The superficial portion of the gland lies adjacent to the lingual plate of the mandible and abuts the medial pterygoid muscle. The superficial portion of the gland lies just deep to the superficial layer of the deep cervical fascia and is in close proximity to the marginal mandibular branch of the facial nerve. The anterior facial vein crosses the lateral surface of the gland, and the facial artery grooves the deep portion of the gland as it courses from inferior to superior. The deep portion of the gland lies between the mylohyoid muscle and the hyoglossus muscle. The nerve to the mylohyoid passes along the lingual plate of the mandible before entering the submandibular triangle. The nerve to the mylohyoid lies adjacent to the posterior border of the mylohyoid muscle and sends nerve branches to this muscle as well as to the anterior belly of the digastric muscle. Knowledge of the anatomic relationships between the seventh nerve and the fifth nerve is extremely important when managing tumors of the submandibular gland due to the propensity of some malignant salivary gland tumors to spread along peripheral nerves.

When the superficial portion of the gland is reflected inferiorly and the mylohyoid muscle is retracted anteriorly, the anatomic relationships between the deep lobe of the gland and the surrounding structures are visualized. The submandibular duct, which is 5 cm long, courses between the mylohyoid and the hyoglossus muscle anteriorly and passes into the genioglossus muscle, where it opens into the oral cavity at the lingual frenulum. The hypoglossal nerve lies deep to the duct, whereas the lingual nerve lies above the duct. The lingual nerve can be seen coursing from posterior to anterior and at its midportion gives off contributions to the submandibular ganglion.

The primary echelon of nodal drainage from the submandibular glands is to the preglandular, prevascular, and retrovascular facial lymph nodes. These nodes then drain to the upper jugular lymph nodes.

CLINICAL EVALUATION

As in the evaluation of any mass lesion in the head and neck, clinical signs and symptoms along with physical examination are extremely important for defining the most accurate differential diagnosis and ultimately arriving at the correct diagnosis. Important points from the history include the rapidity of onset, whether the symptoms are fluctuating or progressive, and antecedent exposure to infectious agents or trauma. Any history of cutaneous malignancy should be sought. Squamous cell carcinoma of the skin, melanoma, or adnexal tumors arising on the cheek, nose, or upper lip may metastasize to the facial lymph nodes within the submandibular triangle. At times, the patient may have forgotten that a skin lesion was previously present. Lymphoma is another consideration, but is usually associated with lymphadenopathy in other nodal basins. Metastatic squamous cell carcinoma from an intraoral primary carcinoma of the retromolar trigone, lower gum, or floor of the mouth is another potential source of lymphadenopathy in the submandibular triangle.

Inflammatory conditions such as cat scratch disease and atypical micobacterial infections may involve the facial lymph nodes and are associated with erythema of the overlying skin, constitutional symptoms, and at times fluctuance. Actinomycosis of dental origin may also result in suppuration of the facial lymph nodes, so any history of recent dental infection should be elicited.

Swelling of the submandibular gland is usually related to either inflammatory or neoplastic causes. A careful history can often differentiate between these two etiologies. Inflammatory swelling of the submandibular gland may be due to chronic sialadenitis with or without calculus formation. Patients who have chronic sialadenitis note intermittent swelling during salivary stimulation and often complain of a dull, aching pain. A salivary duct stone produces intermittent swelling that may occur with meals or result in complete obstruction, leading to acute sialadenitis. Symptoms may be abrupt, with fever, purulent drainage from the salivary duct, skin erythema, and marked tenderness. Patients may or may not relate a history of prior symptoms. Sjögren's syndrome, an autoimmune disorder, may produce symmetric swelling of the submandibular and parotid glands. Patients also complain of a dry mouth and dry eyes (sicca syndrome) as the disease progresses.

Neoplasms of the submandibular gland often appear as an asymptomatic progressive swelling that does not fluctuate over time and is not related to salivation. Pain and cranial nerve palsies have a strong correlation with the diagnosis of malignancy. Neurologic deficits may include weakness of the lower lip from marginal mandibular nerve involvement, numbness of the tongue in the distribution of the lingual nerve, or atrophy and fasciculations of the ipsilateral tongue due to invasion of the hypoglossal nerve. In previously untreated patients, invasion of the hypoglossal nerve is a rare finding. Table 1 provides the major differentiating features between inflammatory and neoplastic processes of the submandibular gland.

The physical examination is important for identifying the cause and site of submandibular triangle swelling. Palpation may reveal enlargement of the facial lymph nodes and define this as a separate pathologic process from the normal adjacent submandibular gland. Bimanual palpation of the submandibular triangle is valuable for localizing the mass to the submandibular gland. In inflammatory conditions, the entire gland will be firm and variably enlarged or atrophic. A calculus in the duct may also be palpated within the floor of the mouth. Bimanual or external palpation of the gland

Table 1. Submandibular Gland: Chronic Sialadenitis Versus Neoplasm

FEATURE	SIALADENITIS	NEOPLASM
Swelling	Intermittent	Progessive (slow/rapid)
Fever	Acute suppurative	—
Lymphadenopathy	Rare (reactive)	20–30% (malignant only)
Pain	With infection/during meals	Malignant tumors (20%)
Cranial nerve deficits	—	Marginal mandibular nerve, lingual/hypoglossal nerves
Plain radiographs	Sialoliths (90% radiopaque)	Intraglandular calcifications (pleomorphic adenoma)
CT/MRI	—	Mass/soft-tissue extension, bone/nerve involvement, poorly defined margins
Fine needle aspiration*	Negative for tumor	Positive or suspicious for tumor

CT, computed tomography; MRI, magnetic resonance imaging.
* False-positive findings for malignancy may occur in chronic sialadenitis.

should be performed to elicit the flow of saliva from Wharton's duct. The absence of saliva may suggest ductal obstruction and support the presence of a sialolith. A neurologic examination should include a sensory evaluation of the lateral tongue to light touch, the presence of tongue atrophy, or fasciculations and deviation on protrusion. The submandibular triangle and neck should be carefully palpated for the presence or absence of lymphadenopathy.

■ DIAGNOSTIC IMAGING

The principal modality for imaging in the submandibular triangle is computed tomography (CT) or magnetic resonance imaging (MRI). MRI has some advantages over CT by providing a multiplanar image and enhanced soft tissue detail. However, CT may be more beneficial for evaluating bone invasion and lymph node metastasis. The CT scan should be obtained in both the axial and the coronal planes with and without intravenous contrast. If fixation of the mass to the mandible is present, bone settings will be useful for evaluating cortical mandibular invasion. It is important to obtain the CT images before the administration of contrast in order to image calcifications within the gland or sialoliths within the duct. Regional lymph nodes involved by metastatic disease may demonstrate central hypodensity with peripheral ring enhancement. When perineural invasion is suspected, a gadolinium-enhanced MRI with fat suppression is more sensitive than CT for evaluating major nerve trunk invasion. A CT or MRI scan should be obtained for any patient who is suspected of having a submandibular gland neoplasm and will provide important information regarding extension into the floor of the mouth and muscles of mastication. Unfortunately, the radiographic appearance of the neoplasm is not often specific for differentiating benign from malignant tumors.

■ PATHOLOGY

Most benign neoplasms arising in the submandibular gland are pleomorphic adenomas. Other benign tumors may arise in the gland, but in general they are extremely rare. Examples include sebaceous adenoma, benign lymphoepithelial lesion, and oncocytoma. The most common malignant tumors are adenoid cystic and mucoepidermoid carcinomas. In decreasing frequency, adenocarcinoma, carcinoma ex pleomorphic adenoma, primary squamous cell carcinoma, undifferentiated carcinoma, acinic cell carcinoma, and malignant mixed tumors have all been reported to arise in the submandibular gland. It is important that the pathologist be well experienced with salivary gland tumors to avoid an error in diagnosis. For adenoid cystic carcinoma and mucoepidermoid carcinoma, the pathologist should attempt to assign a tumor grade. The low-grade mucoepidermoid carcinoma is predominately mucinous, whereas its high-grade counterpart is predominately epidermoid, with little mucinous component present. The adenoid cystic carcinoma has three grades: tubular, which is low grade; cribriform, which is intermediate grade; and solid, which is high grade. Recently, flow cytometry to determine DNA content of adenoid cystic carcinoma has been shown to correlate with tumor aggressiveness. Tumors with an aneuploid DNA content have a higher recurrence rate than their diploid counterparts. Salivary duct carcinoma has been recently described in the submandibular gland. This tumor resembles breast cancer, is highly malignant, and tends to metastasize early to regional lymph nodes and distant sites.

Malignant tumors of the submandibular gland may spread by direct extension from the capsule of the gland into the mandible or muscles of mastication. Direct extension into the medial pterygoid results in trismus. Extraglandular spread is one of the most important adverse histopathologic features predictive of recurrence and survival. Although tumor histology has not been shown to significantly predict overall outcome, patients with high-grade tumors have a worse overall prognosis. Other modes of spread include metastasis to regional lymph nodes. The sites of metastasis include lymph nodes in the submandibular triangle as well as the submental lymph nodes and jugular chain. Although adenoid cystic carcinoma of the parotid gland has a low incidence of metastasis, 25 percent of these tumors arising in the submandibular gland are associated with regional disease. Mucoepidermoid carcinoma, adenocarcinoma, and primary squamous cell carcinoma of the submandibular gland are also associated with a significant risk of Iymph node metastasis. Regional spread occurs with greater frequency in the presence of perineural invasion and extraglandular soft-tissue extension.

■ THERAPY

Prior to surgical resection, a fine needle aspiration (FNA) biopsy is obtained when a neoplasm is suspected or the diagnosis is unclear. FNA may indicate the presence of a neoplasm and allow the most appropriate surgical approach. An excisional biopsy of the submandibular gland (shell out) is inadequate surgical management for tumors. Although subcapsular gland excision for chronic sialadenitis is appropriate, neoplasms require an en bloc dissection of the submandibular gland and adjacent regional lymph nodes (submandibular and submental). This provides a histologic diagnosis and simultaneously removes the lymph nodes at greatest risk for metastasis. Regional nerves such as the marginal mandibular, lingual, and hypoglossal are not sacrificed unless they are directly involved by the cancer. Whenever a tumor is suspected, the patient is counseled preoperatively on the potential sequelae of cranial nerve palsies.

The patient is positioned on the operating table with a transverse shoulder roll to allow neck extension. With the patient under anesthesia, the submandibular triangle is carefully examined. This allows a better estimation of the tumor extent into the floor of the mouth, mandible, or pterygoid region.

Although a small incision can be used for inflammatory disease, when a neoplasm is suspected, a curvilinear incision extending from the sternocleidomastoid to the lateral aspect of the submental area is preferred. The flap is elevated in the subplatysmal plane, which leaves the superficial layer of the deep cervical fascia intact. The marginal mandibular nerve that courses from posterior to anterior lies beneath this fascial envelope. Provided there is no tumor extension to the superficial layer of the deep cervical fascia, the marginal mandibular nerve is identified and elevated from the lateral surface of the gland. The facial artery and vein are identified as they cross the horizontal ramus of the mandible and are individually clamped and ligated. The pre- and postvascular facial lymph nodes are then reflected inferiorly, which exposes the inferior edge of the mandible. As the dissection is deepened, the nerve to the mylohyoid muscle is identified and examined by frozen section, if perineural extension to this nerve is suspected. The superficial portion of the gland is then reflected off the mylohyoid muscle from the area just inferior to the mandible down to the tendon of the digastric muscle. The submental lymph nodes are dissected by removing the submental fat pad between the digastric muscles. These nodes are reflected inferiorly from the submental region and then across the ipsilateral anterior belly of the digastric muscle to remain in continuity with the submandibular gland.

Once the inferior edge of the mylohyoid muscle is exposed, this muscle is retracted anteriorly, which exposes the deep surface of the gland. The lingual nerve is readily apparent; provided there is no invasion or encasement of this nerve, the specimen is dissected inferiorly to expose the submandibular ganglion. With the ganglion identified, it is clamped and cut, and a portion is sent for frozen section to exclude the presence of perineural invasion. If the tumor lies in close proximity to the lingual nerve, a portion of the nerve or the main trunk is sectioned as dictated by tumor extent. The portion of the submandibular gland that extends anteriorly toward the floor of the mouth as well as the duct is then identified and dissected inferiorly.

Deep to the medial portion of the gland the deep layer of the cervical fascia, which overlies the hyoglossus muscle and the hypoglossal nerve, is identified. This fascial layer and the nerve are seldom invaded by tumors of the submandibular gland, especially in patients who have not had prior treatment. The lymph node–bearing tissue and the gland are then reflected posteriorly across the posterior belly of the digastric muscle, which exposes the facial artery that is again clamped and suture-ligated. This completes the entire regional dissection of the submental and submandibular triangles. If lymph node metastasis is present in the level I dissection, a complete neck dissection should be performed that includes levels II, III, and IV, with preservation whenever feasible of the sternocleidomastoid muscle, internal jugular vein, and spinal accessory nerve. If clinically evident metastasis or bulky disease exists in the remainder of the neck, a modified or radical neck dissection will be necessary.

In some instances of neglected, recurrent, or highly aggressive tumors, fixation of the mandible may be present. In these instances, the marginal mandibular nerve is sacrificed, and the tumor is reflected in the subperiosteal plane from the lateral surface of the mandible. The periosteum should be examined by frozen section and if invaded, the buccal plate of the mandible should be resected. If gross mandibular invasion is present, either clinically or radiographically, a segmental mandibulectomy is indicated. Fortunately, this is infrequently necessary for most primary operations. Table 2 shows surgical management of the primary tumor and neck for patients who have submandibular gland tumors.

■ RADIOTHERAPY

Adjuvant therapy is recommended for high-grade tumors and advanced or recurrent cancers that extend beyond the gland. Positive surgical margins; perineural invasion, either micro- or macroscopic; and lymph node metastasis are indications for postoperative radiotherapy. The radiation portals should include not only the surgical bed but also the entire ipsilateral neck. Unilateral treatment is frequently possible. If the main lingual nerve trunk is invaded, the entire distribution of V3 is treated, including the skull base. Before radiotherapy, the patient must undergo a thorough dental examination; any nonrestorable teeth should be extracted before administration of external beam radiotherapy. Appropriate use of radiotherapy provides excellent disease control in the head and neck; however, patients may subsequently succumb to distant metastasis 5 or more years following initial treatment.

■ OUTCOME

In a series from the University of Texas M.D. Anderson Cancer Center, Houston, among the 86 patients with malignant tumors, 45 percent developed recurrences. Twenty-one patients failed above the clavicle and 18 patients failed at distant sites. Overall survival rate was slightly less than 60 percent at 5 years. Adverse outcome was experienced among patients with extraglandular spread, lymph node metastasis, and invasion of a major nerve trunk. Although patients with adenoid cystic carcinoma had excellent control of their disease in the head and neck, many patients developed distant metastases 5 and 10 years after initial treatment.

Table 2. Surgical Management of Submandibular Gland Tumors

HISTOLOGY/GRADE	SURGERY FOR PRIMARY	CRANIAL NERVES	LYMPH NODES
Benign and low-grade*	Level I	Preserve	Level I only
Low-grade (N^+)	Level I	Preserve	Levels I–IV
High-grade (N_0)$^+$	Level I	Resect if involved	Levels I–IV
High-grade (N^+)$^+$	Level I	Resect if involved	Levels I–V (Functional RND, modified RND)

RND, radical neck dissection.
* Low-grade without lymph node metastasis.
$^+$ May require en bloc mandibulectomy, glossectomy, floor of mouth resection.

Suggested Reading

Andersen LJ, Therkildsen TM, Ockelmann HH. Malignant epithelial tumors in the minor salivary glands, the submandibular gland, and the sublingual gland: Prognostic factors and treatment results. Cancer 1991; 68:2431-2437.

Lucarini JW, Sciubba JJ, Khettry U, Nasser I. Terminal duct carcinoma: Recognition of a low-grade salivary gland. Arch Otolaryngol Head Neck Surg 1994; 120:1010-1015.

Luna MA, el-Naggar A, Batsakis JA. Flow cytometric DNA content of adenoid cystic carcinoma of submandibular gland. Arch Otolaryngol Head Neck Surg 1990; 116:1291-1296.

Seifert G, Sobin LH. The World Health Organization's histological classification of salivary gland tumors: A commentary on the second edition. Cancer 1992; 70:379-385.

Weber RS, Byers RM, Petit B. Submandibular gland tumors: Adverse histologic factors and therapeutic implications. Arch Otolaryngol Head Neck Surg 1990; 116:1055-1060.

NON-NEOPLASTIC DISEASE OF THE SALIVARY GLANDS

The method of
Richard D. Nichols

Treatment of tumors is usually considered the most interesting aspect of salivary gland disease. In fact, diagnosis and treatment of non-neoplastic conditions of these glands demands greater diagnostic acumen and a broader range of surgical techniques than are required in tumor management. I have designed this chapter to assist in diagnosis and successful treatment of selected salivary gland diseases.

■ FIRST BRANCHIAL CLEFT ANOMALIES

First branchial cleft anomalies are the most clinically significant congenital lesions of the parotid area. They should be considered in the differential diagnosis of any mass in the parotid, but particularly in the event of the occurrence of a cutaneous fistula or recurrent abscess in the region of the pinna, the parotid, or the immediately adjacent upper aspect of the neck. These lesions have an infrequent presentation as a chronically draining ear, and it is significant that they occur more commonly in females than in males.

First branchial cleft lesions are duplication anomalies of the external auditory canal. The presenting sign represents the visible or palpable aspect of the lesion that continues deeply as a tract lined with squamous epithelium. The tract has a characteristic relationship to the external auditory canal, parotid, and facial nerve.

There are two types of lesions. In type I, the mass or fistula is in the immediate area of the pinna. The deep aspect runs parallel and inferior to the external auditory canal, lateral to the facial nerve, terminating at the bony external auditory canal in the region of the tympanic membrane or middle ear. In type II, the visible or palpable aspect is generally lower in the neck, near the angle of the mandible or just below it, anterior to the sternomastoid, and above the posterior belly of the digastric muscle. The tract proceeds superiorly, intimately associated with the parotid or passing through it, with an inconstant relationship to the facial nerve, and terminating at the osteocartilaginous junction of the external auditory canal or continuing as a fistula into the canal. The latter fact explains the occasional presentation as a chronically draining ear. The epithelial tract passes superficially to the facial nerve in approximately 75 percent of cases, deep to the nerve in approximately 20 percent, and between the major branches in approximately 5 percent. This relationship was determined during embryogenesis when the mesoderm of the second arch, which forms the muscles of facial expression, migrates from caudal to the tract to points cephalad to it, accompanied by the seventh nerve filaments that serve them. Because this migration occurs after the tract has formed embryologically, the path of migration determines the relationship of the tract to the nerve.

Treatment is complete surgical excision. As with any surgical operation in this anatomic area, the ability to identify and protect the facial nerve and perform parotidectomy are requisite.

■ HUMAN IMMUNODEFICIENCY VIRUS (HIV)–ASSOCIATED SALIVARY GLAND DISEASE

HIV-positive persons often experience swelling of the salivary glands. This swelling is usually bilateral and almost exclusively involves the parotid. This swelling, which is sometimes accompanied by a complaint of dry mouth, has been termed *HIV-associated salivary gland disease* (HIV-SGD). The designation is, however, nonspecific. Although HIV-SGD includes a number of conditions seen more commonly or exclusively in HIV-positive individuals, the differential diagnosis includes all conditions that cause swelling of the parotid glands in the uninfected population. There are three HIV-related conditions of major interest.

The first condition is the occurrence of multiple intraparotid lymphoepithelial cysts that may be unilateral clinically but are usually bilateral pathologically. The finding is so characteristic as to be considered pathognomonic of HIV infection. It is nearly always associated with bilateral cervical lymphadenopathy. The pathogenesis of lymphoepithelial cysts, which may occur as single lesions in uninfected persons, is unknown. The precise reason for the proliferation of such cysts, which occur at any stage of the disease in HIV-positive persons, is unknown as well. These cysts are demonstrated best by computed tomographic (CT) scanning of the glands. CT may demonstrate bilateral lesions in patients who are thought, clinically, to have unilateral disease. Other diagnostic studies relative to the parotid pathology seem superfluous if typical CT findings are present. The cysts may decrease in size with zidovudine treatment. They can be removed surgically, but such treatment rarely seems indicated, except in very extreme cases where it may be justified on a cosmetic basis alone. Excision is not justified for diagnosis. Consideration for surgical removal must include all ramifications of the disease.

The second condition is the occurrence of a syndrome that is very much like Sjögren's, including bilateral parotid swelling, xerostomia, arthralgia, and dry eyes. Histopathology of tissue taken for biopsy from salivary glands is also characteristic of Sjögren's syndrome. This condition differs in that SSA, SSB, and rheumatoid factor serology results are generally negative. The designation HIV-SGD seems most appropriate for this entity.

The third condition relates to the fact that HIV-positive persons who have salivary swelling must be evaluated in the same manner as uninfected persons, except that the index of suspicion regarding the presence of certain intraglandular diseases must be higher in the former group. The diseases that occur at a higher incidence in HIV-positive persons are generalized lymphadenopathy, lymphoma, and Kaposi's sarcoma in intraparotid nodes. The B cell lymphoma seen more commonly in acquired immunodeficiency syndrome, however, is generally not within the salivary glands. Fine needle aspiration or open biopsy should be considered if the clinical picture suggests a malignant intraglandular process.

■ TRAUMATIC DIVISION OF THE PAROTID DUCT AND SIALOCELE

Division of the parotid duct should be suspected and excluded by careful examination of any facial laceration that crosses the course of the duct. The distal portion of the duct can be located by passing a lacrimal probe through the punctum into the wound. The proximal portion should be immediately posterior to that point. Repair is done with fine absorbable suture over a small polyethylene catheter (No. 90) passed from the oral cavity and secured intraorally with a silk stitch and left in place for 1 week.

Sialoceles can be managed by elimination of parotid function or re-establishment of flow to the oral cavity. Interruption of the parasympathetic supply to the gland by tympanic neurectomy does not completely and permanently eliminate salivation. This indirect approach is not recommended. Parotid function can be eliminated reliably with parotidectomy or radiotherapy. Re-establishment of flow to the oral cavity may be possible by intraoral incision of a sialocele and placement of a long-term drain, with the anticipation of epithelialization of the tract.

■ SALIVARY CALCULI

Stones are usually single and unilateral, but submandibular stones are sometimes multiple and of surprising size. Stones occur much more commonly in the submandibular than in the parotid duct and are more difficult to identify in the parotid because they are smaller, usually radiolucent (80 percent), and the duct is less accessible for examination. The majority of submandibular stones are radiopaque (80 percent) and can be palpated bimanually. Submandibular duct stones that are not fixed at the hilum of the gland can essentially always be expressed manually if the duct is opened adequately intraorally. The major vessels in the floor of the mouth are deep to the mylohyoid muscle, and the lingual nerve is 3 to 4 cm proximal to the punctum, passing underneath the duct. These structures are at little risk. For sialodochotomy, the duct is first cannulated with a lacrimal probe and opened over the probe; the stone is then manipulated and removed. Approximation of the mucosa of the floor of the mouth to the mucosa of the duct (sialodochoplasty) is not necessary. Removal of the caruncle should be avoided because it interrupts all continuity of the mucosa of the duct with the floor of the mouth, which risks stenosis. If caruncolectomy is believed to be necessary, sialodochoplasty should probably be done.

Symptomatic hilar stones require transcervical excision of the gland. It is important to identify the stone in the surgical specimen, because stones may erode the duct. If stones are undetected in the extraglandular soft tissue of the submandibular triangle, they may be left in the wound.

The parotid duct does not lend itself to extensive exploration so that stones, even if identified at the time of transoral sialodochotomy may be impossible to remove. Urology stone forceps may be helpful. Transcutaneous removal is possible because the duct proximal to the buccinator is a subcutaneous structure. It is paralleled by and in intimate association with the buccal branch of the facial nerve, which must be identified and preserved.

Extracorporeal shock wave lithotripsy has been applied to the treatment of salivary stones. Early instruments of the electrohydraulic and electromagnetic types had a shock wave focus too large to be considered for salivary stones because of the possibility of injury to intracranial and other structures in the head and neck. Piezoelectric and later models of electromagnetic and electrogalvanic instruments have been modified to produce a small focal zone that can be directed precisely at salivary stones using three-dimensional ultrasonography. Review of all English language reports of this technique indicate that the procedure is more successful in the parotid than in the submandibular ducts and is not associated with significant side effects. Successful treatment has sometimes been prolonged. Sialodochotomy to remove stone fragments has often been necessary.

Shock wave treatment of sialoliths is a natural extension of the interest and experience gained with that method of treatment for renal and gallstones, so this technique may prove to have a place in the treatment of *very* selected cases of salivary gland stones. The routine use of a treatment program that is sometimes protracted and requires the use of expensive equipment for this common clinical problem, which can nearly always be managed quickly and with minor surgical techniques in a standard examination room, seems to represent a poor use of medical resources.

■ SALIVARY DUCT STRICTURE

Narrowing of the submandibular duct occurs most commonly at the punctum. If there is still an opening present, dilation with progressively enlarging lacrimal probes should eliminate the problem. Generous sialodochotomy is an option. If the stenosis is complete or if the opening is so small as to prevent entry of the smallest dilator, a surgical procedure is necessary. The most direct approach is to excise the caruncle, but we prefer to, under anesthesia, locate the duct submucosally in the floor of the mouth and open it from that point to the normal location of the punctum. Sialodochoplasty is then done, extending proximal and distal to the extent necessary to relieve the stricture.

Because the parotid duct is smaller and less accessible than the submandibular, sialodochoplasty is more difficult and less likely to be successful. In general, stricture distal to the anterior border of the masseter can be managed with sialodochoplasty. Infiltration of lidocaine with epinephrine improves exposure. The duct is cannulated with a No. 90 polyethylene tube to facilitate location and dissection. The tube is sutured to the buccal mucosa anterior to the punctum. A horizontal mucosal incision is made beginning 1 to 2 mm posterior to the duct punctum, and that mucosal attachment is kept in place until suturing is begun, extending posteriorly to the area of the anterior aspect of the ascending ramus of the mandible. Soft tissue of the buccal area is then dissected, sharply and bluntly as necessary, to isolate the duct and identify the anterior border of the masseter. All soft tissue is cleared from the duct, leaving only its posterior attachment. This allows the duct to be "stretched" toward the oral cavity. An area of stricture may be associated with periductal scarring or granulation tissue. If such tissue is present, some should be removed for biopsy, because neoplastic stricture is possible. The duct is then incised on its medial aspect from distal to proximal. The buccal mucosa is approximated to the cut edges of the duct, using 6–0 absorbable suture; magnification is necessary. The polyethylene tube is left in place for 7 days.

If the duct stricture is inaccessible, excision of the gland may be indicated. The judgment is made on the basis of the patient's subjective and objective reaction to the pathologic condition.

■ SIALOGRAPHY

Sialography is an important diagnostic procedure that is often indicated in evaluation of obscure cases of what is clinically considered to be obstructive disease and in confirming a diagnosis of sialectasis. I use it essentially exclusively in parotid disease, because the submandibular area can be examined effectively with more direct methods.

■ SUPPURATIVE PAROTITIS

Suppurative parotitis occurs either as an isolated, acute event or is recurrent. Acute suppurative parotitis is related to acutely or chronically diminished salivary flow, dehydration, greater than normal susceptibility to infection, and poor oral hygiene. It is classically seen in elderly, hospitalized patients. However, a significant number of patients are those taking drugs that decrease salivation, particularly psychotropic drugs. The clinical presentation includes fever; painful parotid swelling; and creamy, purulent sialorrhea. Essentially all infections are staphylococcal, except in patients who have immunocompromise, where any organism may be responsible. Treatment includes anti-staphylococcal drugs and reversal of predisposing factors. Incision and drainage of acute suppurative parotitis, which is reserved for failure of medical therapy, is rarely indicated.

In our experience, recurrent, *nonobstructive,* suppurative parotitis occurs exclusively in patients who have sialectasis, although it has been reported by others in the field in the absence of that finding. Clinically, the patients experience recurrent, low-grade infection in one or both glands characterized by minimal swelling, minor discomfort, and sialorrhea that has a normal appearance except for tiny flecks of purulence. *Streptococcus viridans* is the usual infecting organism, and penicillin is the antibiotic treatment of choice. Adjunctive measures that will decrease the incidence of infections include sialogogues, more than adequate hydration, and mechanical emptying of the gland by masticatory exercise and massage of the gland toward the mouth. Benign lymphoepithelial disease (BLD) is the defining histopathologic lesion in this condition as well as in Sjögren's syndrome.

Recurrent parotitis may be a different disease in the pediatric age group, because it may remit over time. The episodes begin, characteristically, in the middle of the first decade, but sometimes in the first months of life. They tend to become less frequent over time, sometimes with spontaneous remission during or after adolescence. Some individuals continue to have recurrent infections into adulthood. There is one report of complete reversal of sialoectatic changes by adulthood.

Primary Sjögren's syndrome includes xerostomia, caused by the decreased salivary function of characteristic BLD, and xerophthalmia. Connective tissue disease is the third element of *secondary* Sjögren's syndrome, which is immunologically distinct from the primary form. The presenting symptoms with which such patients generally first see the otolaryngologist are recurrent infection, which is managed as noted previously; dry mouth; and salivary gland (usually parotid) swelling. In general, we concentrate on the management of these local complaints and request consultation with rheumatologists or general internists for treatment of systemic manifestations of the disease.

Dry mouth is managed most effectively with increased intake of water. Artificial salivas are expensive and do not seem to offer lasting benefit. Oral pilocarpine became available commercially after a study indicated subjective relief from dry mouth in a group of postirradiation patients. My experience with the effectiveness of this medication has been mixed. The suggested dosage is 5 mg three times per day, titrating to 10 mg, if necessary.

The parotid swelling is evaluated with regard to rate of growth, symmetry, homogeneity, and magnitude, Symmetric, homogeneous, mild or moderate swelling that is historically chronic generates little concern about a histopathologic diagnosis other than BLD. However, BLD can coexist with or precede the occurrence of other parotid pathology, a fact that should encourage careful physician follow-up and patient education about the normal and possible altered course of the disease. For example, Sjögren's syndrome is part of a spectrum of lymphoproliferative diseases, the malignant extremity of which is lymphoma, and lymphoma is more than 40 times more likely to occur in persons who have Sjögren's syndrome than in the normal population. Although the lymphoma may affect the salivary glands, it is usually extraglandular.

From a clinical perspective, sialographic demonstration of sialectasis in persons who have both dry eyes and mouth confirms the diagnosis of Sjögren's syndrome. Histologic confirmation by removal of tissue for biopsy from the lip or major glands seems superfluous, except perhaps in a setting wherein objective histologic confirmation of BLD is important for investigational studies.

Complete parotidectomy can be done as a cosmetic procedure in patients who have massive parotid enlargement. Residual gland may act as a target organ for the autoimmune process and cause recurrence of the hypertrophy.

■ FACIAL PARALYSIS ASSOCIATED WITH PAROTITIS

Facial paralysis associated with parotid swelling is considered pathognomonic of a malignant process. However, I have seen facial paralysis or paresis caused by infection in five patients, and a literature search has revealed additional cases. The phenomenon is probably more common than reported. The majority of these patients had acute suppurative parotitis, sometimes with abscess. Some had previously existent intraparotid lesions that became infected, and some had necrotizing infections of the region. Return of facial function was usually seen, except in the patients with necrotizing infection, which resulted in permanent paralysis. Significant intercurrent systemic disease, such as diabetes or renal failure, and the age of patients who have parotitis may predispose to facial nerve dysfunction. There was a bimodal distribution, very young or old, in the group.

■ NECROTIZING SIALOMETAPLASIA

Necrotizing sialometaplasia is a disease that may simulate carcinoma clinically and is characterized by an ulcer (70 percent of patients) or a mass located on the hard palate or at the junction of the hard and soft portions of the palate. The lesion is painful (75 percent of patients) or painless and may follow palatal trauma, even very minor injury, such as an injection. Of most significance is that the squamous metaplasia seen in specimens taken for biopsy may be misinterpreted as either mucoepidermoid or squamous cell carcinoma. A clinical clue to the true nature of the lesion is that there are both destructive (ulcer) and reparative (granulation tissue) components. Consider the possibility of the existence of this lesion, and ask your pathologist to review the histopathology in any questionable cases.

■ GRANULOMATOUS PAROTITIS

Tuberculosis is the most common granulomatous inflammation of the parotid. It involves single or multiple nodes within the gland or the parenchyma itself and may simulate a neoplasm, as is the case with isolated intraparotid lymphadenopathy related to any pathology. Chest radiographic findings are characteristically normal. In my experience, the disease has been limited to the gland. Treatment is administration of systemic antituberculous drugs.

Sarcoidosis affects the parotid clinically in 6 percent of patients and in one-third if autopsy material is considered. It is a diagnosis of exclusion, because the noncaseating granulomas seen in histopathologic material are not pathognomonic of the disease. The diagnosis is supported by the presence of anemia, leukopenia, eosinophilia, thrombocytopenia, hypoalbuminemia, and hyperglobulinemia. Elevated erythrocyte sedimentation rate, serum angiotensin-converting enzyme (ACE), alkaline phosphatase, and calcium levels are also characteristic. Elevated ACE levels in the absence of elevated alkaline phosphatase levels are very suggestive of sarcoidosis.

The chest radiograph is normal in more than 90 percent of patients. Hilar adenopathy is seen more commonly than is parenchymal disease. The Kveim test is positive in 50 percent to 80 percent of patients. Nonreactive skin tests for tuberculosis and false-positive reactions for syphilis may be seen. Five percent of patients have neurologic manifestations. The most common, facial paralysis, occurs in 50 percent of those who have neurologic disease. The paralysis is bilateral in approximately one-third of patients and has a good prognosis for return of function, but it may recur. The cause of the facial paralysis is unknown. It is not caused by the parotitis because it may precede, follow, or occur otherwise independent of parotitis and may improve in the face of worsening parotid findings. The incidence of uveitis is four times greater in patients who have neurologic manifestations than in those without. Uveitis, parotitis, and cranial nerve palsies constitute classic Heerfordt's syndrome.

Most patients do not require treatment. Steroids are used for significant manifestations of the disease.

■ RANULAS

Ranulas (cystic lesions of the floor of the mouth) are either localized or extend along muscles and fascial planes of the floor of the mouth into the upper aspect of the neck. The former results from an obstructed minor salivary gland, and the latter results from an injury to a gland, usually the sublingual, with escape of saliva into interstitial spaces, forming a pseudocyst that may present in the upper aspect of the neck. Localized ranulas are managed most effectively by complete incision. There is little risk to the normal structures of the floor of the mouth. Marsupialization may result in recurrence.

Nonepithelially lined pseudocysts (plunging ranulas) may be extensive, involving both sides of the neck as well as both sides of the floor of the mouth. Attention is often directed primarily toward the cyst because it is the obvious part of the lesion. Complete excision of the thin lining cannot be successful and is unnecessary because it is not a secretory structure. The important part of the procedure is identification and removal of the abnormal gland feeding the mucous sac. Sublingual gland excision is begun by identifying the submandibular duct beneath the mucosa in the floor of the mouth. This can be done by cannulating the duct on the affected side with a flexible polyethylene cannula. This serves as an important anatomic marker to assist in locating the lingual nerve. The tube is held in place with a suture placed anteriorly to the punctum. An option is to locate the duct visually without the use of a catheter. The floor of the mouth is injected with lidocaine with epinephrine to reduce capillary bleeding. An incision is made just through the mucosa of the floor of the mouth, beginning 1 cm lateral to the submandibular punctum and proceeding posteriorly, roughly paralleling the body of the mandible for approximately 4 cm. This incision crosses the course of the submandibular duct. Medial and lateral mucosal flaps are developed, the submandibular duct and sublingual gland are identified, and the gland is removed. This is done with blunt and sharp dissection; the surgeon is careful to identify and preserve the lingual nerve as it "double crosses" the duct. The twelfth nerve, which is medial and inferior to the expected dissection, must be avoided as well. It should not be encountered if the dissection is confined to the area between the mylohyoid and hyoglossus muscles. A loose closure of the floor of the mouth with absorbable suture and without a drain is adequate.

Recurrence is still possible, even if these surgical principles are followed carefully. A more radical approach to consider is an en bloc combined intraoral-extraoral excision of the floor of the mouth, sublingual gland, and submandibular gland on the affected side. My patients have not experienced any recurrences when such an operation has been done as a primary procedure for plunging ranulas.

Suggested Reading

Abrams AM, Melrose RJ, Howell FV. Necrotizing sialometaplasia: a disease simulating malignancy. Cancer 1973; 32:130-135.

Belenky WM, Medina JE. First branchial cleft anomalies. Laryngoscope 1980; 90:28-39.

Brannon RB, Fowler CB, Hartman KS. Necrotizing sialometaplasia: a clinicopathologic study of sixty-nine cases and review of the literature. Oral Surg Oral Med Oral Pathol 1991; 72:317-325.

Daniels TE. Clinical assessment and diagnosis of immunologically mediated salivary gland disease in Sjögren's syndrome. In: Talal N, ed. Sjögren's syndrome. New York: Academic Press, 1989.

Iro H, et al. Shockwave lithotripsy of salivary duct stones. Lancet 1992; 339:1333-1336.

Johnson JT, et al. Oral pilocarpine for post-irradiation xerostomia in patients with head and neck cancer. N Engl J Med 1993; 329:390-395.

Schiodt M, et al. Natural history of HIV-associated salivary gland disease. Oral Surg Oral Med Oral Path 1992; 74:326-331.

Sulavik SB, et al. Specificity and sensitivity of distinctive chest radiograph and/or 67Ga images in the noninvasive diagnosis of sarcoidosis. Chest 1993; 103:403-409.

Talal N. Sjögren's syndrome. In: Talal N, ed. Sjögren's syndrome. New York: Academic Press, 1989.

TUMORS OF THE PARAPHARYNGEAL SPACE

The method of
William M. Keane

The parapharyngeal space space is an inverted cone or pyramidal-shaped space based at the skull base superiorly and reaching the hyoid bone inferiorly. Most of the volume of this potential space is taken up with loose connective and fatty tissue, but the internal carotid artery, jugular vein, cranial nerves IX to XII, and the cervical sympathetic chain pass through it. In addition, glomus tissue, lymph nodes, and ectopic salivary tissue may be found there (Fig. 1).

The contents and structures adjacent to the parapharyngeal space dictate the type of pathology contained within it. Tumors in this space are rare, representing less than 1 percent of all head and neck neoplasms. Eighty percent of lesions are benign, and 20 percent are malignant. Salivary gland tumors represent 50 percent of all parapharyngeal lesions and typically arise from the deep lobe of the parotid gland, and occasionally from ectopic salivary tissue. They are benign pleomorphic adenomas in most cases, but approximately 30 percent of such salivary tumors are malignant; mucoepidermoid tumors are the most common. Neurogenic tumors account for approximately 25 percent of tumors in the parapharyngeal space. They are typically benign schwannomas of the vagus nerve. Paragangliomas or

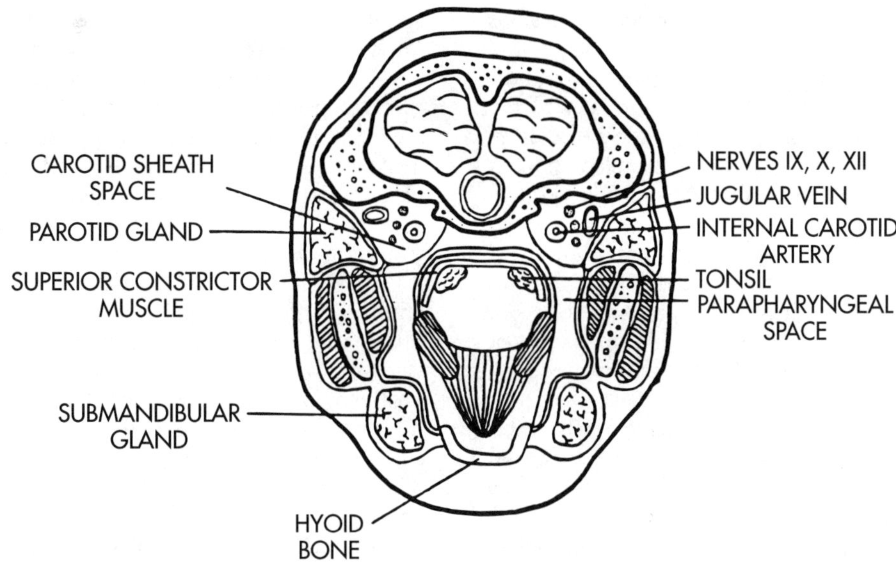

Figure 1.
Parapharyngeal space tumors.

chemodectomas often originate from the nodose ganglion of the vagus nerve near the skull base.

Carotid body paragangliomas arise at the carotid bifurcation inferior to the digastric muscle and do not normally extend superiorly into the parapharyngeal space. Malignant neurogenic tumors are rare and are most commonly malignant chemodectomas.

Malignancies involving the lymphoid tissue in the parapharyngeal space represent approximately 10 percent of lesions discovered here. Lymphoma is most common, but metastasis from nasopharyngeal, oropharyngeal, hypopharyngeal, or thyroid carcinomas are also found. The presence of cervical adenopathy associated with a lesion of the parapharyngeal space is highly suggestive of malignancy.

■ EVALUATION

Signs and Symptoms

The deep location of the parapharyngeal space and the rigidity of the mandible make early detection of lesions here unusual. They are typically greater than 3 cm in size when discovered. The most common presentation of parapharyngeal space tumors is as an asymptomatic mass near the angle of the mandible or as fullness at the soft palate or tonsillar area. Impingement on adjacent structures may produce vague symptoms of pain, fullness, or dysphagia. Clinical examination may reveal paresis of cranial nerves IX to XII or Horner's syndrome. Superior extension of lesions in this space may produce obstruction of the eustachian tube, with subsequent serous otitis media and symptoms mimicking temporomandibular joint dysfunction. It is not uncommon that lesions in this space are discovered on computed tomographic (CT) or magnetic resonance imaging (MRI) scans as incidental findings.

Given the slow growth pattern exhibited by these lesions, resultant vagal or hypoglossal nerve paralysis may produce minimal symptoms. Bimanual palpation of a parotid tumor may reveal the deeper portion of a dumbbell-shaped mass. Palpation of the tongue base may demonstrate induration consistent with a primary neoplasm, and nasopharyngoscopy may demonstrate a nasopharyngeal carcinoma. A complete head and neck examination is therefore critical.

Imaging

Radiographic imaging is central to the evaluation of parapharyngeal space lesions, and magnetic resonance imaging with gadolinium has become the cornerstone of these studies. MRI provides a multiplanar imaging technique with excellent resolution. The nature of the lesion may be defined by signal characteristics with T1 and T2 imaging, and the highly vascular nature of a chemodectoma may be well demonstrated. The differential diagnosis is best narrowed by demonstrating the effect of the tumor mass on adjacent structures. Salivary tumors represent the majority of lesions in the parapharyngeal space and may arise from parotid tissue or extraparotid ectopic salivary rests. Posterior displacement of the carotid artery with anteromedial displacement of the parapharyngeal space fat suggest a deep lobe parotid tumor. The preservation of the fat plane between the mass and the parotid gland suggests a lesion originating in the parapharyngeal space. Schwannomas demonstrate inhomogeneous signal intensity and typically develop in the poststyloid compartment. As a result, they typically displace the internal carotid artery anteriorly. Paragangliomas may develop within the parapharyngeal space from the nodose ganglion of the vagus nerve or reflect the superior extension of carotid body tumors. Magnetic resonance angiography (MRA) demonstrates the increased vascularity of these lesions. Anteromedial displacement of the internal carotid artery suggests vagal paragangliomas, whereas splaying of the internal and external carotid arteries is typical of a carotid body tumor.

Differentiating between benign and malignant lesions with MRI may be difficult. Obliteration of tissue planes and loss of distinct margins is suggestive of malignancy, but these observations may be seen in large benign lesions as well. CT scanning may be complementary to MRI, and better defines bone erosion of the pterygoid plates, vertebral bodies, or skull base. MRI best delineates dural involvement and intracranial spread.

MRI studies of a parapharyngeal space mass should extend from skull base to clavicle. This should allow for assessment of the cervical region for multiple paragangliomas or adenopathy suggestive of malignancy. In addition, the upper aerodigestive tract may be visualized. MRA has replaced routine angiography in most cases. When malignancy is suspected or when the tumor mass extends intracranially, arteriography better defines involvement of the internal carotid artery. In addition, carotid occlusion studies to determine the ability of the patient to tolerate carotid artery sacrifice may be accomplished. Arteriography also allows for a selective embolization of paragangliomas. We routinely embolize nearly all paragangliomas 1 day before surgery and have found that decreased blood loss is a reasonable trade-off for tissue reaction to the embolization.

Although most paragangliomas are nonfunctioning, patients may complain of a hypermetabolic state, with symptoms of tremulousness, headache, and labile hypertension. All patients should be tested for serum catecholamine levels, and a 24 hour urine collection should be obtained for measurement of vanillylmandelic acid. Those patients who have a secreting tumor are treated preoperatively and intraoperatively with adrenergic blocking agents such as propranolol and phenoxybenzamine and catecholamine-depleting agents such as alpha-methyl-P-tyrosine.

Needle aspiration is done when the lesion is not highly vascular, using a transcervical or transoral approach if the lesion is palpable. Ultrasound or CT-guided needle aspiration may be used in other cases. Incisional biopsy is to be condemned given the risk of tumor spillage with the increased incidence of recurrence. Incisional biopsy also creates an inflammatory reaction, which makes subsequent surgery more difficult.

■ THERAPY

Complete surgical excision remains the mainstay of treatment for tumors of the parapharyngeal space. A variety of techniques have been described, including internal and external approaches. Successful management requires adequate exposure of the tumor mass, as well as the neurovascular structures contained within the parapharyngeal space and their contiguous structures. For this reason, a transoral approach is rarely applicable.

Standard Approach

The external approach employs a horizontal incision placed at the level of the hyoid bone, with variable posterosuperior and anterosuperior extensions with or without mandibulotomy. A posterior limb is extended in the fashion of a standard parotidectomy incision. Subplatysmal flaps are elevated within the cervical region, and a subcutaneous skin flap is elevated over the parotid gland. The sternocleidomastoid muscle is reflected posteriorly away from the inferior portion of the parotid gland. Cranial nerves X through XII, as well as the internal and external carotid arteries and jugular vein, are identified inferior to the digastric muscle. The posterior belly of the digastric muscle is dissected posteriorly, and the parotid gland is bluntly dissected from the pretragal area. The styloid process is identified, and the tympanomastoid suture line is followed to the facial nerve.

The pes is identified, and the superficial portion of the parotid gland is reflected superiorly as the inferior division of the facial nerve is followed anteriorly. The facial artery and vein are divided and retracted superiorly with the posterior portion of the submandibular gland. The posterior belly of the digastric muscle is then divided, and the stylohyoid muscle is retracted anteriorly or divided. Cranial nerves IX to XII and the internal carotid artery are then followed superiorly to the apex of the parapharyngeal space. The stylomandibular ligament is divided, which allows for the anterior displacement of the mandible. The external carotid artery is ligated, and the neurovascular structures within the parapharyngeal space are followed further superiorly toward the skull base. Vessel loops around the proximal and distal limits of the internal carotid artery may be applied.

This approach allows for adequate exposure of most tumors involving the parapharyngeal space. Salivary gland tumors are typically well encapsulated and surrounded by a loose fibrofatty tissue plane. Removal is typically accomplished using blunt dissection, and finger manipulation is most useful. Excess pressure against adjacent bony structures is to be avoided, because rupture of the tumor capsule may take place. The styloid process may be removed to provide greater exposure, and care must be taken to reflect the internal carotid artery away from the tumor mass under direct visualization.

The preoperative embolization of paragangliomas and the use of an irrigating bipolar cautery allows for a relatively dry surgical field. Proximal and distal control of the internal carotid artery is accomplished, and the external carotid artery is typically ligated. Most carotid body chemodectomas do not reach into the parapharyngeal space and are resected with less extensive exposure.

Extended Approaches

Malignant lesions or large tumors with superior extension toward the skull base require greater exposure. In these cases, mandibulotomy is appropriate and is best accomplished in the midline between the central incisors. If an inadequate cleft is present between the dentition, extraction of an incisor is appropriate. We typically employ a stair-step mandibulotomy that will be reapproximated with a mandibular plate that has been prefitted and predrilled. A tracheotomy is accomplished at the beginning of the procedure. The horizontally placed midcervical incision is carried to the midline of the mandible, where the lip is divided centrally. A Z-plasty is placed in the submental portion of the incision to avoid bowstringing. Should the surgeon wish to avoid a lip split, the incision can be extended at the level of the hyoid to the contralateral cervical region and the mandible is then degloved.

Following the completion of the mandibulotomy, an incision is made intraorally between the opening of the submandibular ducts, and the ipsilateral submandibular duct is included in the lateral aspect of the incision. The incision is carried posteriorly along the gutter of the floor of the mouth toward the anterior tonsillar pillar. The tongue musculature is divided to the level of the hypoglossal nerve, which is preserved. The lingual nerve is identified and preserved as well. The mandible is then reflected laterally. Blunt dissection opens the plane between the pharyngeal constrictor muscles and the parapharyngeal space. The external carotid artery is divided, and the internal carotid artery and cranial nerves IX to XII are followed superiorly into the parapharyngeal space. This technique allows for excellent exposure of the upper limits of the parapharyngeal space, and with further superior extension, the skull base is readily exposed. The retropharyngeal space may also be dissected.

Tumors with intracranial extension or those reaching the temporal bone may require even greater posterosuperior exposure. These are typically paragangliomas of the vagus nerve or glomus jugulare tumors. In these cases, the superior limb of the incision is carried across the mastoid tip into the postauricular region. The external auditory meatus is divided at the bony-cartilaginous junction as the pinna is reflected anteriorly. A complete mastoidectomy is accomplished, and the facial nerve is identified. The bone over the jugular bulb is removed as the jugular vein and carotid artery are followed into the temporal bone. Cranial nerves X, XI, and XII are identified, and the bone overlying the facial nerve is skeletonized. Larger tumors require the transposition of the facial nerve, but smaller lesions may be approached using a facial recess approach. Tumors eroding the skull base may be approached through this incision in concert with a neurosurgical team. In those cases in which dural closure is suspect, a spinal drain is helpful. The mandibulotomy is reapproximated using premeasured miniplates, and suction drains are placed. The lip incision is closed with fast-absorbing 6–0 chromic sutures.

Complications

The location of the parapharyngeal space along with its contents makes surgery in this region potentially hazardous. The most common complications of surgery relate to the nerve structures contained within the space or contiguous to it. The majority of cranial nerve deficits are temporary in nature and typically occur from the dissection of tumor away from the nerves or while the nerves are retracted to provide greater exposure. A temporary paresis of the lower division of the facial nerve is the most common complication reported; this may be avoided by careful dissection and the maintenance of a soft-tissue buttress between the retractor and the nerve.

Resection of the vagus nerve within the parapharyngeal space typically takes place proximal to the nodose ganglion and is associated with significant morbidity. Loss of hypopharyngeal sensation and the absence of motor function of the superior and recurrent laryngeal nerves produce significant difficulties with voice and swallowing. The associated sacrifice of the hypoglossal nerve is particularly debilitating. These patients are best treated with a percutaneous gastrostomy and tracheotomy at the time of surgery. I do not routinely perform a cricopharyngeal myotomy. Temporary medialization of the affected hemilarynx is best achieved with fat injection, and more permanent medialization is best accomplished with a laryngoplasty. Postoperative swallowing rehabilitation is critical and is best achieved under the guidance of a skilled speech therapist. Depending on age and associated medical problems, rehabilitation may take months, but compensation is achieved in most patients.

The tracheotomy tube is maintained in position for pulmonary toilet until aspiration is no longer a problem. The tube is downsized so that it may be capped when the patient eats. We have not used cable grafts when cranial nerves are resected. In those rare cases in which the proximal and distal portions of the nerve are in close proximity, primary reanastomosis is appropriate. The use of monitors for cranial nerves VII and X are important adjuncts in decreasing the morbidity associated with surgery in this area. Most parapharyngeal space tumors are benign salivary gland lesions. These should be removed with minimal morbidity. Tumor recurrence is often related to rupture of the tumor capsule, which occurs when inadequate exposure is achieved or when overly aggressive blunt dissection is attempted.

The carotid artery may be inadvertently injured during the blunt dissection of a benign mixed tumor within the parapharyngeal space. This vessel is quite small and tortuous at the superior portion of the parapharyngeal space, so care must be taken not to injure it. The presence of carotid invasion by a malignant lesion may require carotid sacrifice. Such a resection should be a planned event, and its success should be predicted by the results of preoperative arteriography with balloon occlusion, technetium flow studies, and the concomitant monitoring of the electroencephalogram. In some cases, the carotid artery may be bypassed. Autogenous material such as saphenous vein should be used if there is contamination within the oral cavity. Care should be taken to avoid a hypoperfusion state in the early postoperative time frame.

A midline stair-stepped mandibulotomy is associated with few complications. Occasionally, a lower tooth may be devitalized or a malunion develops. Placing the osteotomy in the midline prevents injury to the inferior alveolar nerve. Overly aggressive retraction of the mandible laterally can result in temporary or permanent injury to the lingual or hypoglossal nerve. In those unusual cases in which a partial temporal bone or skull base resection is needed, a cerebrospinal fluid leak may develop, and watertight closure of the dural defect is critical. When closure is suspect; a spinal drain is necessary.

Infection is an unusual occurrence in those cases in which the oral cavity is not entered. We routinely use cefazolin parenterally in the perioperative time frame and add metronidazole when oral cavity contamination takes place.

Controversies

There is some controversy regarding the indications for surgical resection of tumors in the parapharyngeal space in elderly patients. Neurogenic tumors are typically slow growing and may be present for years with few or no symptoms. These lesions are nearly always benign, so following up a patient over the age of 70 with sequential MRI scans is appropriate. Intracranial schwannomas appear to be more radiosensitive than those tumors involving the cervical region.

For this reason, radiotherapy is not typically recommended in patients who have peripheral nerve sheath tumors. Paragangliomas, however, do respond to radiotherapy with cessation of growth and in some cases with return of cranial nerve function.

The high incidence of multiple paragangliomas presents a therapeutic dilemma. Those patients who have bilateral vagal paragangliomas are typically treated with surgical resection of the larger lesion and radiotherapy to the smaller one. The presence of a vagal nerve paralysis would also indicate the need for conservative treatment of a contralateral vagal paraganglioma and the use of radiotherapy. Some authors have argued that benign tumors of nerve sheath origin, such as schwannomas and neurofibromas, can be resected with preservation of the nerve of origin. These authors typically deal with peripheral nerve tumors and not those involving the cranial nerves. In my experience, neurogenic tumors of the parapharyngeal space cannot be completely removed with preservation of function of the nerve of origin. In some cases, I have performed a subtotal resection of schwannomas with preservation of the nerve of origin. These patients are subsequently followed up with sequential MRI studies, and should significant regrowth occur, then a complete resection with sacrifice of the nerve will be accomplished.

Salivary gland tumors are typically resected with minimal morbidity, and the potential for malignant transformation and persistent growth would support the argument for surgical resection in many patients over the age of 70. The violation of the capsule of benign mixed tumors is more common in the parapharyngeal space than in the parotid gland. Subsequent seeding of the surgical field leads to multifocal deposits within scar tissue. The combination of tumor and scar tissue adhering to important neurovascular structures within a confining space makes repeat surgical resection particularly difficult. Limited local recurrence is approached surgically. I have used radiotherapy in those cases in which complete resection would require sacrifice of cranial nerve X, when multiple sites of recurrence are present, and when disease recurs despite multiple surgical procedures. The incidence of malignant transformation in pleomorphic adenoma increases with recurrent disease, so histologic monitoring is critical. Long-term follow-up with MRI is important because recurrence or malignant transformation may not be apparent for more than 10 years.

Suggested Reading

Garrett CR, Pillsbury HC. Parapharyngeal space masses. In: Shockley WW, Pillsbury HC, eds. The neck: Diagnosis and surgery. St. Louis: Mosby–Year Book, 1996:313.

Olsen KD. Tumors and surgery of the parapharyngeal space. Laryngoscope 1994; 104:1-27.

ESTHESIONEUROBLASTOMA

The method of
Paul A. Levine

Although this tumor was originally reported in 1924 by Berger and co-workers, recognition of esthesioneuroblastoma has been more frequent over the past 25 years, probably because of an increased awareness rather than an acute increase in incidence. What has improved over the past 20 years has been patient survival, new approaches to treating more extensive disease, and the ability to differentiate this unique neoplasm from other small cell malignancies of the superior nasal vault.

■ HISTOPATHOLOGY

Although the presence of the Homer-Wright rosette is pathognomonic of esthesioneuroblastoma under light microscopy, the other light microscopic findings include (1) plexiform intracellular neurofibrils, (2) poorly defined to nonexistent cytoplasm, (3) round to oval nuclei, and (4) palisading sheets of neoplastic cells, separated by slender vascular septae, which creates a lobular pattern. Despite these findings, electron microscopy and immunohistochemical staining may be needed to make the definitive diagnosis. The typical staining profile for esthesioneuroblastoma is a positive finding for neuron-specific enolase and S-100 protein. Electron microscopy reveals dense neurosecretory granules in neuronal processes, with microtubules and neural filaments. The differential diagnosis for this neoplasm includes lymphoma, malignant melanoma, plasmacytoma, rhabdomyosarcoma, sinonasal undifferentiated carcinoma (SNUC), and neuroendocrine carcinoma. Of these, the one most difficult condition to differentiate that has the most impact clinically is SNUC. Although our original report (University of Virginia Medical Center) of 11 cases showed an aggressive behavior pattern and a very poor prognosis, a follow-up report by our institution has revealed that, if there was no distant metastatic disease or intracranial disease, aggressive combination therapy can provide a cure.

Despite alternative staging systems suggested by Biller and the modification proposed by Calcaterra, we still employ the Kadish system for the categorization of all superior nasal vault neoplasms (Table 1).

Table 1. Staging of Superior Vault Nasal Neoplasms

Stage A	Limited to nasal cavity
Stage B	Extension to one or more paranasal sinuses
Stage C	Extension beyond the sinuses to include the orbit, base of skull (cribriform plate) or intracranial cavity, cervical nodes, or distant metastatic sites

■ EVALUATION

Clinical Presentation

It should be remembered that a unilateral nasal mass is a neoplasm until proved otherwise. Although skull base defects with brain or intracranial components are more common in the younger population, it should be remembered that a unilateral mass can represent a neoplasm in this age group, because our youngest esthesioneuroblastoma patient was 9 years old. A functional endoscopic surgical procedure should not be done as the first diagnostic approach when evaluating these patients.

Although the tumor originates from the olfactory epithelium, patients rarely complain of anosmia. The usual tumor location, high in the superior nasal vault, as well as its vascularity, account for the two most common patient complaints, that is, nasal obstruction and epistaxis. Additional symptoms are based on the size of the lesion and the involvement of surrounding structures, which can lead to headache, proptosis, epiphora, cheek or tooth pain, diplopia, blurred vision, and cheek fullness. In differentiating esthesioneuroblastoma from SNUC, one of the most striking findings is the paucity of symptoms in those patients who have SNUC even in the face of very extensive disease.

Although an intranasal examination reveals a neoplasm in the superior nasal vault that is often friable, a biopsy should not be performed until the appropriate radiologic studies have been performed.

Imaging

The mainstay of diagnosis that usually shows the full extent of disease is the high-resolution computed tomographic (CT) scan. If the tumor margins are indistinct in the orbit or if there is cribriform plate erosion, a magnetic resonance imaging (MRI) scan with gadolinium enhancement is appropriate. Although the incidence of cervical metastases is only 10 percent to 15 percent, a complete head and neck examination that includes palpation of both sides of the neck is imperative. Additionally, a neuro-ophthalmologic examination in conjunction with radiation oncology, hematology-oncology, and neurosurgical evaluations is warranted to complete the full patient evaluation.

■ THERAPY

The addition of the craniofacial resection, first performed at our institution (University of Virginia Medical Center) in 1976, has made a great impact on the ultimate treatment outcome for patients who have this neoplasm. For both stage A and stage B disease, we employ preoperative radiotherapy (50 Gy), followed by a 4 to 6 week rest period, and then a craniofacial resection. The reason for preoperative versus postoperative radiotherapy is based on the better tumoricidal effects of radiotherapy when the blood supply has not been interrupted by surgery, the difficulty in obtaining significant clear surgical margins as in other head and neck regions due to the proximity of the brain and orbit, and, last, our approach to the orbit when the lamina papyracea has been eroded by tumor. For stage C disease, the patient is first treated with cyclophosphamide (650 mg per square meter) and vincristine (1.5 mg per square meter; maximal dose, 2 mg) given intravenously on Days 1 and 8 each month for 2 months. After 2 months, repeat CT scan is performed, and if the tumor has not responded, the chemotherapy is discontinued, and the 50 Gy of radiotherapy is begun for a 5 week period. If the tumor then responds, an additional month of chemotherapy is given.

The surgical management is a craniofacial resection, using a frontal sinus approach to the floor of the anterior cranial fossa and a transfacial approach either via a lateral rhinotomy or a midfacial degloving. Even with erosion of the medial orbital wall and possible periorbital involvement by tumor, it is our experience that an orbital exenteration almost never has to be performed. Using preoperative radiotherapy, frozen section analysis, and control of the periorbita, small and large sections of the periorbita can be resected with or without replacement, which provides good oncologic control of the tumor in the orbit and also gives the patient good functional results for the eye. Although others in the field have recommended bony reconstruction of the floor of the anterior cranial fossa following resection, we use a standard pericranial flap that is fashioned early on in the procedure, either based laterally on one side or both, in conjunction with an abdominal fat and Scarpa's fascia free graft to reduce the dead space between the anterior cranial vault and the sinonasal cavlty. This is then followed by a split-thickness skin graft, which is applied on the nasal side to reline the cavity. Tissue fibrin glue has provided a significant addition to sealing the dural openings, either from the reflection of the dural appendages into the cribriform plate or from resection of the involved dura and replacement with an autogenous fascial lata graft.

Positive cervical metastatic disease is now diagnosed by fine needle aspiration, and the neck disease is treated by radiotherapy without surgical resection (modified neck dissection), unless the tumor remains at the completion of the preoperative radiotherapy.

Results

Our 5 year disease-free survival rate for 23 esthesioneuroblastoma patients treated with the procedures just described from June 1976 to December 1992 was 90 percent. In this group, the vast majority of patients had stage C disease, and this 90 percent survival rate is in contrast with the poor prognosis espoused by Kadish. Although one-third of the patients treated developed recurrent disease, with those having stage C disease showing a higher rate of treatment failure, one-half of these patients were salvaged and exhibited no evidence of disease 5 years following completion of therapy.

■ DISCUSSION

The diagnosis of esthesioneuroblastoma is a favorable one in a group of patients with malignancies of the superior sinonasal vault that previously had a poor outcome. Our 5 year survival rate for esthesioneuroblastoma patients treated with combination therapy, including craniofacial resection, was 90 percent as compared with a 59 percent survival rate for the non-esthesioneuroblastoma patients. Our mortality rate has been 3 percent, with a 40 percent rate of minor and significant complications, which appears to be standard in the literature. The progress made in the treatment of esthesioneuroblastomas and most tumors of the superior nasal vault now makes this entity a curable malignancy.

Suggested Reading

Deutsch BD, Levine PA, Stewart FM, et al. Sinonasal undifferentiated carcinoma: A ray of hope. Otolaryngol Head Neck Surg 1993; 108:697-700.

Levine PA, Debo RF, Meredith SD, et al. Craniofacial resection at the University of Virginia (1976-1992): Survival analysis. Head Neck 1994; 16:574-577.

Levine PA, Scher RL, Jane JA, et al. The craniofacial resection—Eleven-year experience at the University of Virginia: Problems and solutions. Otolaryngol Head Neck Surg 1989; 101:665-669.

McCary WS, Levine PA, Cantrell RW. Preservation of the eye in the treatment of sinonasal malignant neoplasms with orbital involvement. A confirmation of the original treatise. Arch Otolaryngol Head Neck Surg 1996; 122:657-659.

Schuster JJ, Philips CD, Levine PA. MR of esthesioneuroblastoma (olfactory neuroblastoma) and appearance after craniofacial resection. Am J Neuroradiol 1994; 15:1129-1177.

ANGIOFIBROMA

The method of
Dale H. Rice

Juvenile nasopharyngeal angiofibroma is a benign but locally invasive vasoformative neoplasm occurring virtually exclusively in adolescent males. The classic presentation of this tumor in this age group is that of nasal obstruction, first unilateral, and then as the tumor enlarges, bilateral. It is frequently associated with epistaxis, which is episodic and generally does not involve trauma. It tends to occur into the nasopharynx and then into the pterygomaxillary fossa, which are the pathways of least resistance.

As the tumor enlarges, additional symptoms occur. These may include snoring, sleep apnea, facial asymmetry, and eye displacement, in particular proptosis and visual loss. Intracranial extension may also occur through the superior orbital fissure or through the roof of the infratemporal fossa. Rarely does the patient have intracranial symptoms, however.

■ THERAPEUTIC ALTERNATIVES

Treatment options may be single or in combination and include resection, radiotherapy, and chemotherapy. In the vast majority of patients, particularly for those who have no intracranial extension, resection is the procedure of choice. Radiotherapy is a viable alternative that is generally reserved for extensive tumors with intracranial extension or for tumors in such a location that complete resection seems unlikely (Figs. 1 to 3). The exact dose of radiation to administer is somewhat controversial, but it is generally believed to be between 3,000 cGy and 4,500 cGy. For very aggressive, recurrent angiofibromas, chemotherapy may be effective. Different treatment protocols have been used that typically involve multiple chemotherapeutic agents. In general, these techniques are expected to produce tumor regression and cessation of growth, but not total tumor eradication. Often, however, these patients remain asymptomatic indefinitely.

■ PREFERRED APPROACH

The preferred approach for management of angiofibroma is resection when that can be safely done. The approach chosen depends in large measure on the location and size of the tumor. For small tumors confined to the nasopharynx with no lateral extension, the commonly used transpalatal approach is quite satisfactory. If the tumor is in the nasopharynx with lateral extension into the pterygomaxillary space, then the transpalatal approach is not satisfactory. For this, the approach I prefer is through a facial degloving incision with osteotomies to remove the entire anterior face of the maxillary sinus with the piriform aperture in a single piece of bone. This bone is later plated back into position (Fig. 4). After removal of this bone, the surgeon has wide access to the nasopharynx as well as the pterygomaxillary fossa by removing the posterior wall of the maxillary sinus. In tumors with minimal intracranial extension, this latter approach is also satisfactory. Others prefer a Le Fort's approach. In tumors with extensive intracranial extension, particularly with tumor involvement around the cavernous sinus or the optic nerve, a combined facial degloving–transmaxillary approach with anterior craniotomy yields the best results.

■ PREOPERATIVE PREPARATION

All patients with this disease who are considered for resection should undergo preoperative angiography to first deter-

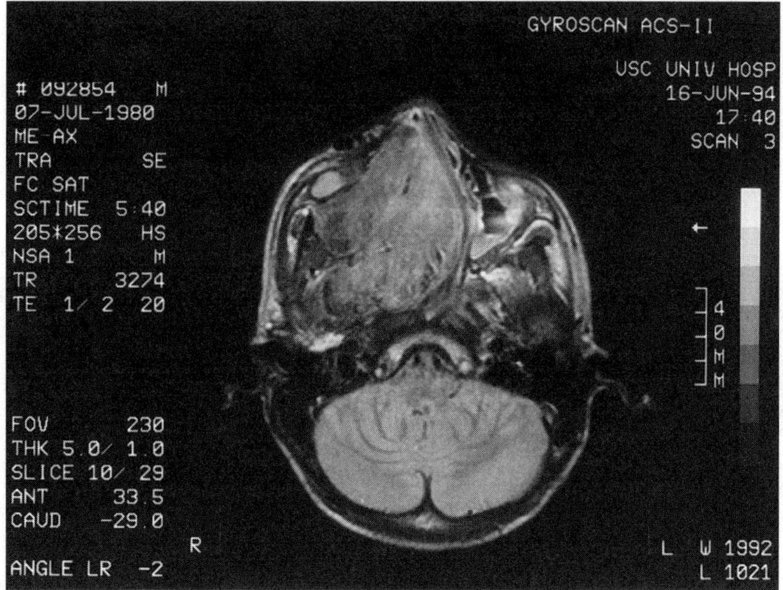

Figure 1.
Magnetic resonance imaging of patient who has large angiofibroma showing invasion into ipsilateral pterygomaxillary fossa.

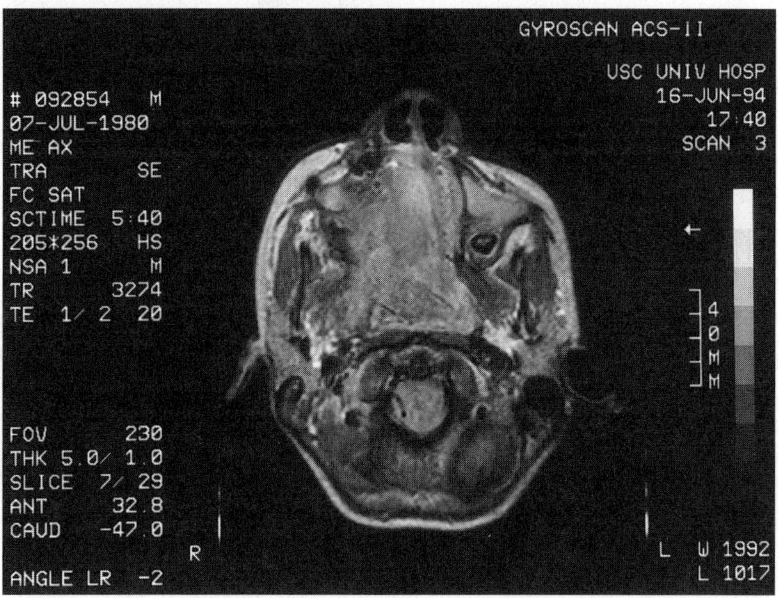

Figure 2.
Magnetic resonance imaging of patient from Figure 1 showing invasion into contralateral pterygomaxillary fossa.

mine the vascularity of the tumor—which is generally considerable—and at the same time to embolize all feeding branches of the external carotid system. This is best done the day before resection. Angiographic findings for large tumors will show feeding vessels from the internal carotid system, often branches of the ophthalmic artery, and occasionally unnamed vessels. Because these vessels are not part of the internal carotid system, embolization of these vessels cannot be done. Typically, the main feeding vessels are the internal maxillary and ascending pharyngeal on the ipsilateral side.

In addition, these patients should be typed and crossed for 4 U of blood, although rarely is transfusion necessary if embolization is thoroughly performed. I have on two occa-

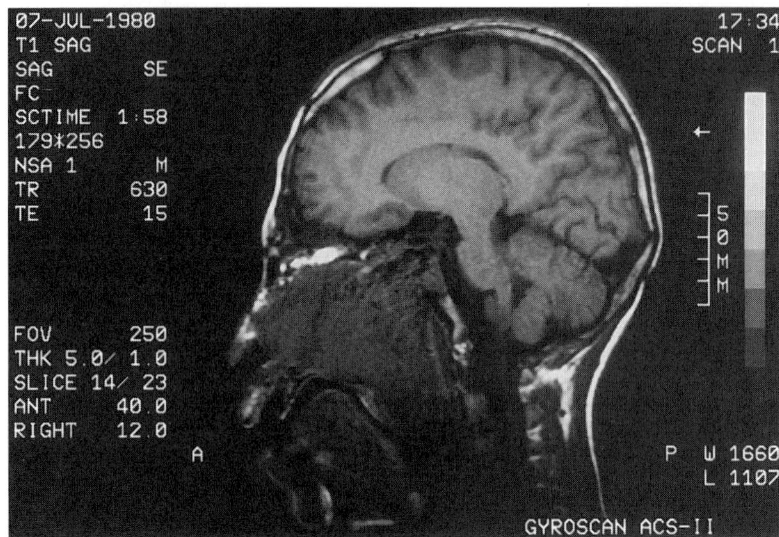

Figure 3.
Magnetic resonance imaging of patient from Figures 1 and 2 showing intracranial extension.

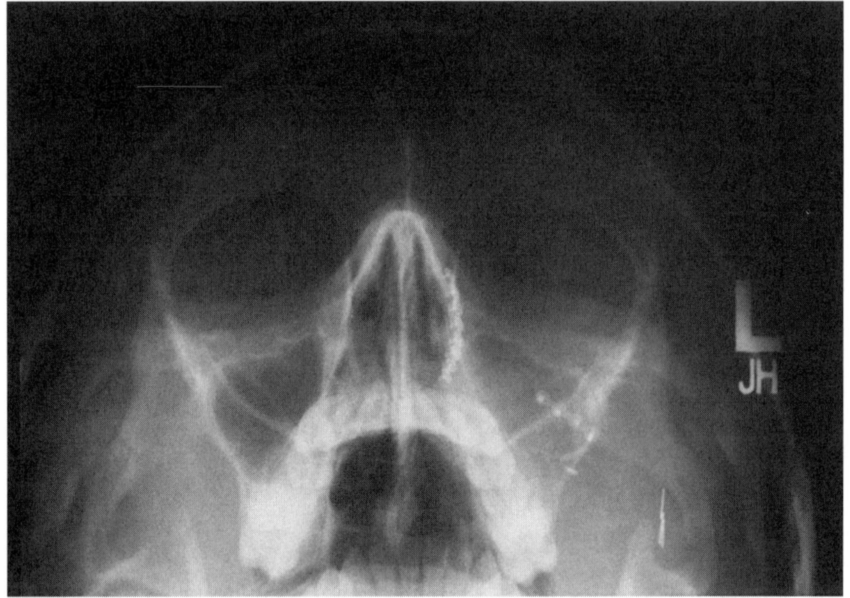

Figure 4.
Water views of patient after transmaxillary approach showing anterior one (anterior maxilla plus piriform aperture) plated back into place.

sions attended to a young patient with a massive tumor who was a Jehovah's Witness, and in that setting I used the cell saver as used in cardiac surgery to some advantage.

■ POSTOPERATIVE COURSE

At the termination of the resection, I prefer to pack the operative site with Gelfoam, coated with povidone-iodine ointment. I use no other packing. If the transmaxillary approach has been used, the anterior face of the maxillary sinus is plated back into position with microplates, and the facial degloving incision is closed. The patient is placed on antibiotics for approximately 3 days and then generally discharged on postoperative Day 3. The patient is generally seen 1 week later, at which time the remaining Gelfoam is easily suctioned out through the nasal cavity.

In the vast majority of patients, this procedure will be all that is necessary other than routine follow-up for possible recurrence. Recurrences are uncommon. An occasional patient will have a very aggressive angiofibroma, and these patients often require radiotherapy or chemotherapy to obtain satisfactory control.

■ COMPLICATIONS

In the past, the most important and worrisome complication from this procedure was excessive bleeding. With modern angiography and embolization in the hands of a good interventional radiologist, bleeding should be minimal, and in fact, rarely is transfusion required. It is important to have excellent hemostasis at the end of the procedure.

Postoperative wound infections are quite rare. In larger tumors, there is potential for injuring the optic nerve or the extrinsic muscles of the eye and their nerve supply. With careful technique, these injuries should be extremely rare; I have not seen one. In tumors with intracranial extension, whether they are done solely from a skull base approach or through a combined intracranial–facial degloving approach, there is risk of cerebrospinal fluid leak. Again, with careful attention to detail and repair of the dura as needed, this problem should be unusual; I have not seen it.

■ PROS AND CONS OF TREATMENT

For most patients with most types of this tumor, resection is the treatment of choice. This approach is generally definitive and can be done in a single stage with little or no morbidity. Although there is a risk of the complications cited previously, they are all extremely rare.

There is considerable controversy over the proper use of radiotherapy for this disease. Many in the field believe that all large tumors with intracranial extension should be treated with radiotherapy. Others think that radiotherapy should be reserved for recurrent tumors or tumors that have anatomically reached an area where total resection is unlikely to be accomplished. There is, of course, the possibility that radiotherapy may fail, but this seems to be unusual. There is a least a theoretic risk of the development of a malignant neoplasm in the field of radiation, but this too seems to be rare. If the eye is in the radiation ports, there will be damage to the eye.

Occasionally, very aggressive angiofibromas will require chemotherapy. Depending on the agents used, the short-term risks are quite variable, but they are generally manageable.

Suggested Reading

Gill G, Rice DH, Ritter FN, et al. Intracranial and extracranial nasopharyngeal angiofibroma: A surgical approach. Arch Otolaryngol 1976; 102:371-373.

Iannetti G, Belli E, De Ponte F, et al. The surgical approaches to nasopharyngeal angiofibroma. J Cranio-Maxillo-Facial Surg 1994; 22:311-316.

Moulin G, Chagnaud C, Gras R, et al. Juvenile nasopharyngeal angiofibroma: Comparison of blood loss during removal in embolized group vs. non embolized group. Cardiovasc Intervent Radiol 1995; 18:158-161.

Radkowski D, McGill T, Healy GB, et al. Angiofibroma: Changes in staging and treatment. Arch Otolaryngol Head Neck Surg 1996; 122:122-129.

Ungkanont K, Byers RM, Webber RS, et al. Juvenile nasopharyngeal angiofibroma: An update of therapeutic management. Head Neck 1996; 18:60-66.

Wiatrak BJ, Koopmann CF, Turrisi AT. Radiation therapy as an alternative to surgery in the management of intracranial juvenile nasopharyngeal angiofibroma. Int J Pediatr Otorhinolaryngol 1993; 28:51-61.

CARCINOMA OF THE NASOPHARYNX

The method of
William Ignace Wei

Carcinoma of the nasopharynx is common in Southeast Asia. Because the tumor is radiosensitive, the primary treatment modality is radiotherapy. The therapeutic external radiation fields usually cover not only the nasopharynx but also both sides of the neck, because the tumor has a high propensity for metastasis to the cervical lymph nodes. The probability of eradicating the tumor by radiotherapy depends on the stage of disease at the time of treatment. The overall success rate when all stages are considered ranges from 50 percent to 60 percent in most centers.

The pattern of treatment failure usually takes the form of persistent or recurrent tumor after initial external radiotherapy. When the disease is present in both the nasopharynx and the neck, curative therapy is unlikely to succeed. However, when carcinoma is present either at the primary site or in the neck, salvage treatment is still possible. All patients are initially managed with radiation, so a second course of external radiotherapy may lead to significant sequelae because the re-treatment dosage has to exceed that of the initial treatment regimen. The complications include neuroendocrinologic disturbance, otologic problems, and excessive fibrosis of surrounding soft tissues. Thus, surgical treatment, with or without the application of brachytherapy, is the usual recommended salvage procedure.

■ DIAGNOSIS

Disease in the Neck

Confirming the diagnosis of metastatic cervical lymph nodes is notoriously difficult. Palpation of the neck to detect pathologic lymphadenopathy after radiotherapy is not easy, because the induration and associated fibrosis make clinical examination difficult. Imaging studies such as computed tomography (CT) or magnetic resonance imaging (MRI) can identify only enlarged lymph nodes in the neck that are more than 1 cm in diameter. Even when a lymph node is identified, it is difficult with these imaging studies to confirm the exact nature of the enlargement.

Fine needle aspiration of the suspicious lymph node under ultrasound guidance also has limitations, such as sampling error and the accuracy of the cytologist on whom the interpretation of results depends. The success rate of ascertaining the presence of malignant cells in these suspicious lymph nodes is at most 50 percent. Preoperative radiotherapy also contributes to the low diagnostic rate. Serologic measurement of antibody titer against the Epstein-Barr virus is not useful in the diagnosis of cervical lymph node metastases.

Surgical salvage is carried out only when either a positive finding from cytologic or histologic sample is obtained from the lymph node, or the size of the suspicious lymph node has increased within a period of observation.

Carcinoma in the Nasopharynx

Imaging studies such as CT or MRI of the nasopharynx often detect abnormal signals that may suggest persistent or recurrent tumor, which can usually be confirmed by biopsy of the nasopharynx.

The examination of the nasopharynx can be satisfactorily carried out either with rigid or flexible endoscopy, and biopsies of any suspicious area can then be done under direct vision. When there is no obvious macroscopic abnormality, multiple blind biopsies should be taken; otherwise submucosal tumor cells, which are not uncommon in nasopharyngeal carcinoma, will be missed. Serologic measurement of antibody titer of Epstein-Barr virus is also not useful in the detection of persistent or recurrent tumor.

It will take 8 to 10 weeks after completion of radiotherapy for all the nasopharyngeal carcinoma cells to die. Thus, positive biopsy findings obtained before 8 weeks should be followed by sequential biopsies to determine the progression of the tumor. The diagnosis of persistent carcinoma is made only when positive biopsy findings are obtained more than 10 weeks after radiotherapy.

■ SURGICAL THERAPY

Cervical Lymph Node Metastasis

Before operation, patients undergo endoscopic examination of the nasopharynx to confirm the absence of tumor. Investigations such as liver and bone scans and chest radiographs are carried out to rule out distant metastasis. The patient should be medically fit to undergo surgery under general anesthesia.

The salvage surgical treatment for persistent or recurrent cervical lymph node metastasis is radical neck dissection. This operation is mandatory for curative eradication of neck disease even if there is only one palpable cervical lymph node.

Rationale

To study the extent of cervical lymph node metastasis in these patients, a "whole organ sectioning" study was carried out. After radical neck dissection, the specimen was streched and pinned onto a foam board. The whole specimen was immersed in 10 percent formaldehyde solution for fixation. After fixation, step serial sectioning was carried out for the whole specimen at 3 mm intervals.

Step serial sectioning of 43 radical neck dissection specimens showed no tumor-containing nodes on pathologic study of three specimens, although clinically the lymph nodes were 3 cm in diameter. In the remaining 40 specimens, more than 70 percent were found on pathologic study to contain more tumor-bearing lymph nodes in the neck than could be detected by clinical examination. Extracapsular tumor invasion was present in 73 percent of the tumor-bearing lymph nodes, and in another 25 percent of the specimens, tumor could be seen lying close to the spinal accessory nerve. In more than 35 percent of the specimens, tumor clusters could be identified among the muscle and soft tissue (Fig. 1). In view of the extensive pathologic behavior of the cervical metastasis, radical neck dissection is recommended as the salvage operation, with the acceptance of the chance that there may not be any tumor in 7 percent of the operations.

Technique

The radical neck dissection is carried out using a MacFee incision with the patient in the supine position. The sternomastoid muscle, internal jugular vein, spinal accessory nerve, and lymph nodes in all levels of the neck are removed. It is not necessary to dissect the retropharyngeal lymph nodes, because this region is included in the primary radiation field and falls within the high-dose zone. Ordinarily, unilateral neck dissection is carried out for lymph nodes localized on one side of the neck. If lymph nodes are detected subsequently in the contralateral neck, radical neck dissection can then be performed on the other side. When lymph nodes are present in both sides of the neck, bilateral radical neck dissection is carried out at the same time while preserving one internal jugular vein. Because the pharynx is not opened during the radical neck dissection, it is not necessary to mobilize the levator scapulae muscle for covering the carotid arteries to prevent contamination by saliva and subsequent rupture. The morbidity associated with radical neck dissection is usually limited, and this operation should be carried out as a salvage procedure whenever indicated.

Prognosis

Radical neck dissection carried out for persistent or recurrent tumor in the neck lymph nodes may achieve a local

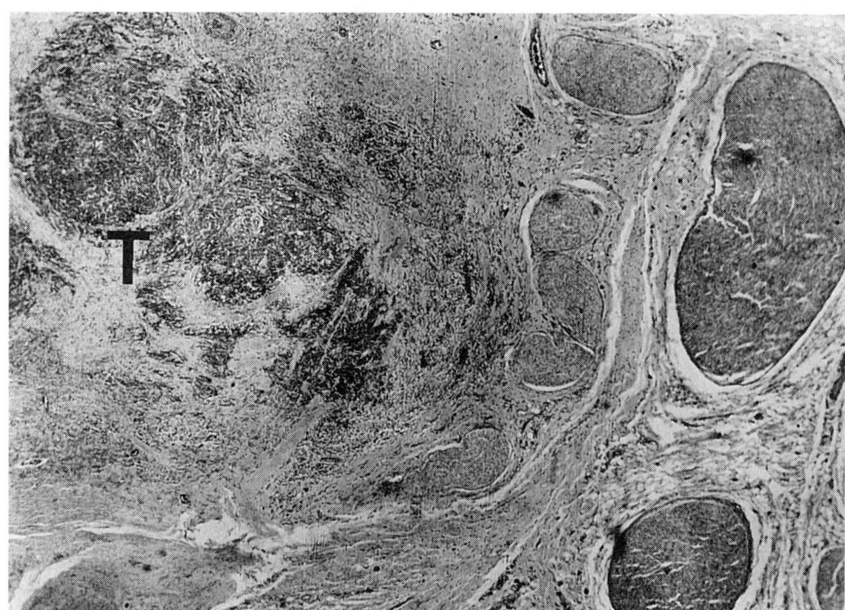

Figure 1.
Clusters of tumor (T) are present among soft tissue (hematoxylin and eosin × 100).

control rate of 66 percent at 5 years, although the 5 year actuarial survival for this group of patients is 38 percent.

Carcinoma in the Nasopharynx

When a persistent or recurrent tumor is detected in the nasopharynx after radiotherapy, the appropriate management depends on the size, location, and extension of the tumor into the paranasopharyngeal space. These factors are determined and assessed with endoscopic examination in combination with imaging studies such as CT or MRI.

Brachytherapy is one of the salvage options for tumors localized in the posterior wall of the nasopharynx without involvement of the fossa of Rosenmüller and less than 1.5 cm in diameter. However, the tumor should not affect the bone in the skull base and should not have extended to the paranasopharyngeal space. When the recurrent tumor is larger and/or has extended to the paranasopharyngeal space, nasopharyngectomy should be the salvage treatment.

Brachytherapy

In view of the location of the nasopharynx, the external beam radiation used for the treatment of the primary carcinoma has to traverse adjacent structures, including the temporal lobe, pituitary gland, brain stem, eye, and inner ear. A second dose of fractionated external radiation would cause additional insult to these important organs and lead to functional disturbances. Brachytherapy has the advantage of providing a high radiation dose to the tumor with a much lower dose delivered to the surrounding normal tissue. It also gives continuous slow, dose-rate irradiation that confers additional radiobiologic advantage over conventional radiotherapy.

Successful application of brachytherapy requires that the radiation source be implanted or placed directly into the carcinoma to effect a high tumoricidal dose; this can be achieved inferiorly with the split palate approach.

Technique

When a patient has trismus as a result of the radiotherapy, the interalveolar distance can be increased by passive stretching under general anesthesia. Successful operation can only be carried out when the interalveolar distance is greater than 3 cm. With the patient in the supine position, a mouth gag is inserted to displace the endotracheal tube inferiorly. The incision starts on one side of the uvula, and then goes over the soft palate in the midline. The incision continues onto the hard palate and stops approximately 1 cm from the central incisor. The soft plate and the mucoperiosteum of the hard palate are then retracted laterally with stay sutures to expose tumor in the posterior wall of the nasopharynx. Part of the posterior portion of the hard palate can be removed to gain additional exposure. While the tumor is under direct vision, radioactive gold grains (gold 198) are inserted with an applicator into the appropriate position. The palatal wound is then closed in layers. After insertion of the radioactive source, the surgeons and assistants should work behind a specially designed lead shield to minimize radiation dosage to the medical staff.

The patient ordinarily resumes oral feeding on the second postoperative day. Some patients experience some headache in the postoperative period, but this usually resolves a few weeks later. Palatal fistula occurs in approximately 10 percent of patients and, if present, is usually at the junction of the soft and hard palates. Palatal fistulas are managed conservatively with a dental plate, and the fistulas are closed surgically when indicated.

Prognosis

For this selected group of patients who have localized tumor in the nasopharynx, implantation of radioactive gold grains achieves an overall local tumor control of 75 percent at 5 years. The 5 year actuarial survival rate of this group of patients is in the region of 60 percent.

Nasopharyngectomy

After radiotherapy, when the persistent or recurrent tumor in the nasopharynx is larger than could be handled with brachytherapy, or if it has extended to the paranasopharyngeal space, nasopharyngectomy should be performed when there is no evidence of disease elsewhere.

Rationale

Because the nasopharynx is strategically situated in the center of the head, it is difficult to expose the region adequately for an oncologic procedure. Tumors situated in the posterior wall can be removed from the inferior aspect through the transpalatal, transcervical approach. Because most nasopharyngeal carcinomas originate from the pharyngeal recess, the recurrent tumor is usually in close approximation to the eustachian tube crural cartilage (Fig. 2). This cartilage should be included when an oncologic resection is performed. Furthermore, because some of the recurrent tumor also extends to the paranasopharyngeal space, wide exposure of the nasopharynx and its vicinity is mandatory to achieve adequate resection. Adequate exposure of the region for an oncologic resection can be obtained by the anterolateral approach, with the maxilla attached to the anterior cheek flap being swung laterally as one osteocutaneous complex.

Technique

The operation is performed with the patient in the supine position, under general anesthesia. Before the operation, a dental plate conforming to the patient's hard palate is made. Endotracheal intubation is performed through the nostril opposite to the side of the operation, or alternatively a tracheostomy can be carried out before incision.

An extended Weber-Fergusson-Longmire incision over the face is made, as for a maxillectomy. The incision over the lip is continued between the central incisors in the midline onto the hard palate. On reaching the junction between the hard and soft palates, the incision is turned laterally behind the maxillary tuberosity on the side of the swing. The facial incision goes through the soft tissues to reach the anterior wall of the maxilla, and only a strip of bone for osteotomy is exposed. Miniplates are placed at the zygomatic-malar bone region and in the midline, across the proposed line of osteotomy. Holes for the screws for these plates are drilled before the osteotomy, because this facilitates the accurate positioning of the maxilla bone on its return. An oscillating saw is then employed to divide the anterior wall of the maxilla just below the floor of the orbit. The osteotomy is continued onto the zygomatic arch and the medial wall of the nose. An additional osteotomy is also made over the midline of the hard palate. The pterygoid plates are separated from the maxillary tuberosity by a curved osteotome inserted transorally. After severing the bony connections, the whole osteocutaneous complex can be swung laterally to expose the nasopharynx and the paranasopharyngeal region (Fig. 3).

The posterior part of the nasal septum can be removed to enhance exposure. Tumor in the nasopharynx and/or the paranasopharyngeal region can be removed en bloc. The anterior wall of the sphenoid can be removed to give an additional margin of tumor clearance. In view of the wide exposure, the internal carotid artery pulsation can be felt, and soft tissues around the region can be cleared. With this approach, direct repair is possible should the artery be inadvertently injured (Fig. 4). After removal of the tumor, the

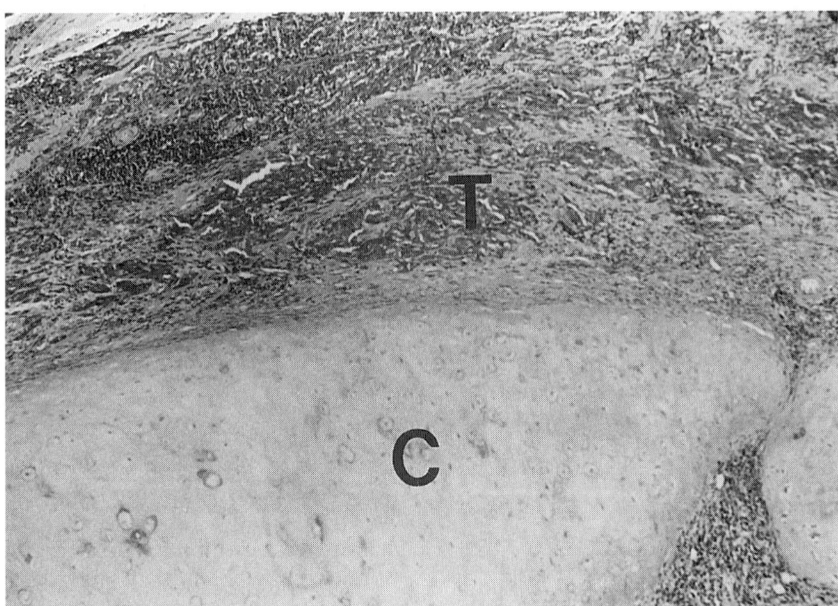

Figure 2.
Tumor (T) lying close to eustachian tube crura (C) (hematoxylin and eosin × 100).

raw area is covered by the free mucosal graft obtained following the inferior turbinectomy on the side of the swing. The maxilla is then returned to its original position and fixed to the rest of the facial skeleton with screws and miniplates. To provide additional stability, the prefabricated dental plate is then fixed onto the teeth on both sides (this is removed 6 weeks later). The nasal cavity is packed, and the facial wound is closed in layers.

Complications

Using the anterolateral approach to the nasopharynx, no necrosis of the maxilla bone was detected, and all patients survived the operation. The associated morbidity is limited and acceptable.

All 18 patients experienced a certain degree of trismus as the pterygoid region was disturbed by both radiotherapy and surgery. This could be prevented by early mobilization

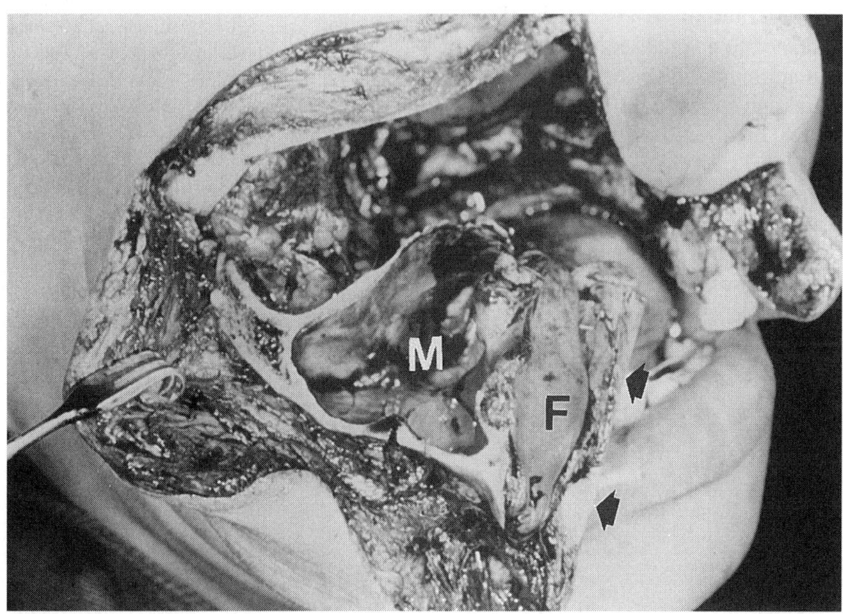

Figure 3.
The maxilla attached to the anterior cheek flap is swung laterally. Maxillary antrum viewed from above (M). Inferior turbinate (F), hard palate (arrowheads).

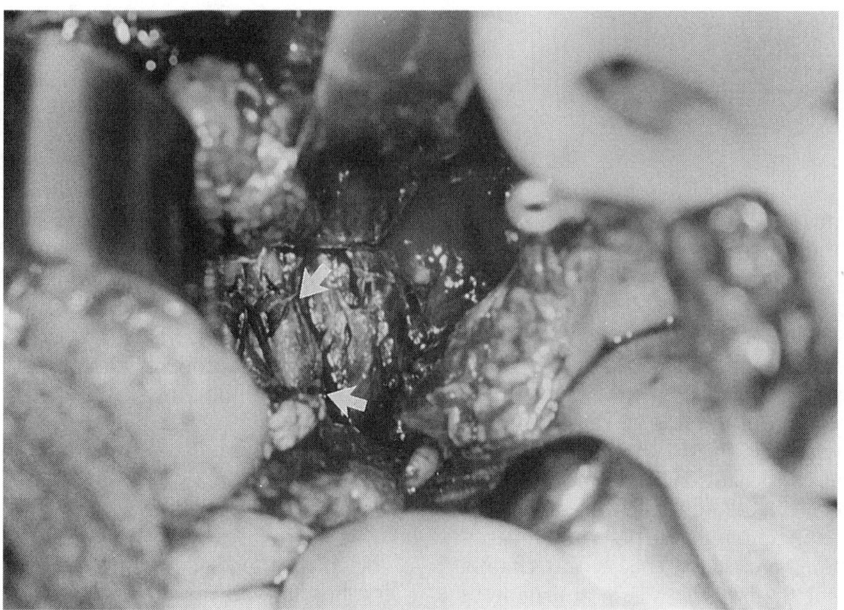

Figure 4.
Operative photo showing the internal carotid artery (arrowheads).

of the muscles of mastication in the postoperative period. If trismus becomes troublesome, active conservative management with stretching is usually effective to achieve an interalveolar distance that is functionally adequate.

Palatal fistulas were occasionally present, causing much inconvenience. Some patients developed fistulas at the junction of the hard and soft palate region in the midline, whereas in others the fistulas were behind the maxillary tuberosity and could be closed with palatal flap or managed conservatively with dental plates.

One patient developed a granuloma over the lateral aspect of the facial wound related to a small sequestrum lying close to the upper lateral miniplate. The sequestrum and these plates were removed under local anesthesia, and the wound healed subsequently. In the 17 other patients, the facial wounds healed primarily.

In the majority of patients, the facial wounds healed well. Occasionally, the contraction of the wound under the eyelid may result in ectropion, which can be corrected with another surgical procedure. A full-thickness skin graft taken from behind the pinna can be employed. Granulomas over facial wounds are uncommon and may be related to an underlying sequestrum. The treatment involves the removal of the bone and the associated miniplate.

Prognosis

The outcome of nasopharyngectomy depends on the size of the tumor and the extent of its infiltration. Overall, surgical salvage may provide an actuarial local tumor control rate of 45 percent at 5 years.

Suggested Reading

Choy D, Sham JST, Wei WI, Ho CM. Transpalatal insertion of radioactive gold grain for the treatment of persistent and recurrent nasopharyngeal carcinoma. Int J Radiat Oncol Biol Phys 1993; 25:505-512.

Sham JST, Wei WI, Zong YS, et al. Detection of subclinical nasopharyngeal carcinoma by fibreoptic endoscopy and multiple biopsy. Lancet 1990; 335:371-374.

Wei WI, Ho CM, Wong MP, et al. Pathological basis of surgery in the management of postradiotherapy cervical metastasis in nasopharyngeal carcinoma. Arch Otolaryngol Head Neck Surg 1992; 118:923-929.

Wei WI, Ho CM, Yuen PW, et al. Maxillary swing approach for resection of tumors in and around the nasopharynx. Arch Otolaryngol Head Neck Surg 1995; 121:638-642.

Wei WI, Lam KH, Sham JST. New approach to the nasopharynx, the maxillary swing approach. Head Neck 1991; 13:200-207.

CANCER OF THE LIP

The method of
Shan R. Baker

The incidence of carcinoma of the lip in the United States is 1.8 per 100,000 population. The male-female ratio is approximately 80:1 for the lower lip and 5:1 for the upper lip.

The vast majority of neoplasms of the lip are squamous cell carcinoma. Occasionally, a basal cell carcinoma will extend from the skin of the lip onto the labial surface. When basal cell carcinoma involves the lip, it is twice as common on the upper lip as the lower lip, and it is the most common form of cancer to arise in the skin of the upper lip. The remainder of malignant epithelial neoplasms of the lip are of minor salivary gland origin, predominately adenoid cystic carcinoma, adenocarcinoma, or mucoepidermoid carcinoma. Unless noted otherwise, statements in this chapter concerning carcinoma of the lip refer solely to squamous cell carcinoma.

Carcinoma of the lip is most commonly observed in the white male smoker who has a fair or ruddy complexion, light hair, and blue or gray eyes. The disease occurs primarily in men who are in the sixth decade of life; the average age of onset is approximately 60 years.

On the lower lip, cancer is most frequently found to originate on the exposed vermilion border. The tumor most often arises at a point approximately halfway between the midline and the commissure. Tumors arising from the commissure represent less than 1 percent of reported cases. When tumors occur on the upper lip, they frequently arise near the midline.

More than one-third of the patients who have carcinoma of the lip have outdoor occupations. Prolonged exposure to sunlight has been implicated as a major etiologic factor. Damaging effects of solar exposure are found in most patients who have lip carcinoma regardless of their ages. The lower lip receives considerable solar radiation under normal sunlight conditions, whereas the upper lip is by comparison shaded. This is probably the reason for infrequent occurrences of carcinoma involving the upper lip.

STAGING

The lip is defined as beginning at the junction of the vermilion border with the skin and includes only that portion of the lip that comes in contact with the opposing lip. It is classified as part of the oral cavity and is thus staged accordingly (Table 1).

Table 1. Staging of Cancer of the Lip	
T_{IS}	**CARCINOMA IN SITU**
T_1	Tumor 2 cm or less in greatest diameter
T_2	Tumor >2 cm but <4 cm in greatest diameter
T_3	Tumor >4 cm in greatest diameter
T_4	Tumor invades adjacent structure (e.g., through cortical bone, tongue, skin of neck)

■ TREATMENT OF PRIMARY TUMOR

Radiotherapy

Radiotherapy for carcinoma of the lip may consist of interstitial, contact, or external radiotherapy. Interstitial and contact applications of radium were once the standard technique of radiologic treatment. Surface or contact applications of radiation may be effective for early lip carcinoma that does not demonstrate deep invasion of more than 3 mm; however, deeply infiltrating tumors are more effectively treated by external therapy or a combination of surface and interstitial needle application.

Electron beam irradiation in the order of 7 to 18 MeV is frequently used for treating carcinoma of the lip. The advantage of 7, 9, or 11 MeV electron beams over conventional voltage radiotherapy is the additional depth of penetration. The electron beam results in 80 percent to 100 percent of delivered energy at a depth of 2 cm with 7 MeV and with 3 cm with 11 MeV. An added advantage of this form of irradiation is the rapid falloff in dose beyond those depths. Thus, the mandible receives very little irradiation in treating most lip carcinomas. Very small lip cancers subjected to electron beam irradiation may be treated with 2,000 rads delivered in 2 weeks or less. Large, deeply infiltrating tumors are treated with 7,000 to 8,000 rads in fractions over 6 to 7 weeks.

Surgery

The algorithm in Figure 1 displays my approach to the diagnosis and management of patients who have lesions of the lip. A history of prolonged sun exposure or smoking in combination with a typical appearing squamous cell carcinoma warrants incisional biopsy. Subsequent treatment would depend on the results of the histologic examination. Patients who have no predisposing factors for lip cancer and small lesions that do not have a typical appearance of malignancy should be managed by excisional biopsy of the area in question.

Small, less advanced carcinomas of the lip may be treated equally successfully by surgery or irradiation, and the results are cosmetically acceptable by both methods. In advanced tumors, surgery or a combination of surgery and postoperative radiotherapy is preferred (Fig. 1). Primary surgery offers eradication of disease, pathologic survey of margins, and reconstruction of the defect in a single procedure. Tumors that are 4 cm or less in greatest dimension and without evidence of cervical metastases should be treated by surgical resection. At least 0.5 cm of normal tissue margin should be obtained around the entire perimeter of the tumor. Tumors larger than 4 cm in size and without cervical metastases are best treated with surgical resection and flap reconstruction.

■ TREATMENT OF NECK METASTASES

Neck dissection is recommended for the treatment of neck metastases. Surgical treatment of cervical metastases offers a 5 year control rate of 50 percent. In patients who have nodes that develop after initial therapy, treatment by operation is approximately as successful as for patients operated on for nodes found on admission. Information is not available concerning the efficacy of combined radiotherapy and surgery for the treatment of cervical metastases from lip carcinoma. Presumably, combined therapy might allow greater control of neck metastases in cases in which metastatic nodes are large, multiple, bilateral, or have extranodal spread. I use radiotherapy after neck dissection to treat histologically positive lymph nodes.

Although metastases are usually confined to the submandibular and submental triangle areas for extended periods before extension to deep cervical lymph nodes occurs, supraomohyoid dissection is not recommended. Such an operation offers a higher recurrence rate than does a complete neck dissection. When lip cancer invades or approaches the midline, however, the therapeutic neck dissection on the affected side should include a prophylactic contralateral suprahyoid dissection. The presence of bilateral metastases calls for bilateral neck dissections.

Prophylactic neck dissection for occult metastatic disease is not indicated for two reasons. First, the percentage of patients who subsequently develop cervical metastases after treatment of their primary lesions is less than 10 percent. Second, the cure rate for therapeutic neck dissection compares favorably with the cure rate in patients undergoing a prophylactic neck dissection for confirmed occult metastases. The small group that eventually develop metastases thus have a fair chance of survival with adequate surgical treatment. Prophylactic neck dissection may be advised, however, for large undifferentiated tumors that involve the oral commissure and upper lip.

■ LIP RECONSTRUCTION

The lip plays a key role in deglutition, formation of speech, and facial expressions. Lip reconstruction offers a unique challenge to the surgeon. Few other sites require attention to such precise details of form and function. Over the last several years, emphasis has been placed on reconstructing lip defects with flaps contained within the aesthetic units of the lip or even aesthetic subunits, which for the upper lip are the philtrum and the two segments of the lip lateral to the philtrum. This principle can be applied in repairing smaller-sized defects of the lip and obviates the need to borrow tissue from the cheek and thus distort the melolabial sulcus.

Surgical procedures used to reconstruct the lip following tumor ablation may be classified as follows: (1) those that use remaining lip tissue, (2) those that borrow tissue from the opposite lip, (3) those that use adjacent cheek tissue, and (4) those that use distant flaps. The first two categories enable the reconstruction to remain within the aesthetic units of the lips and, when possible, are the preferred methods of surgical management. The algorithms in Figures 2 and 3 provide a helpful approach to reconstruction of the

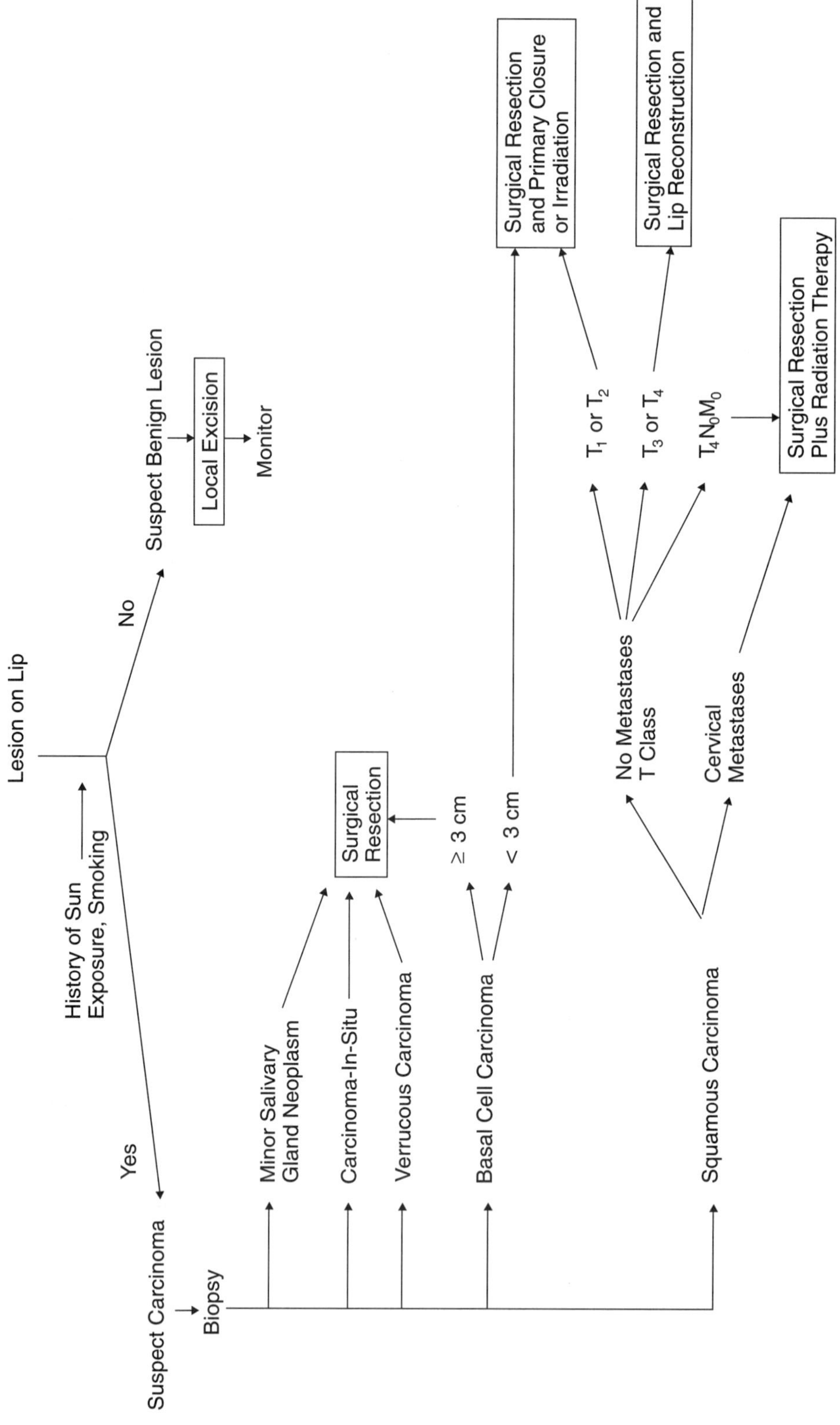

Figure 1.
Algorithm for management of lip tumors.

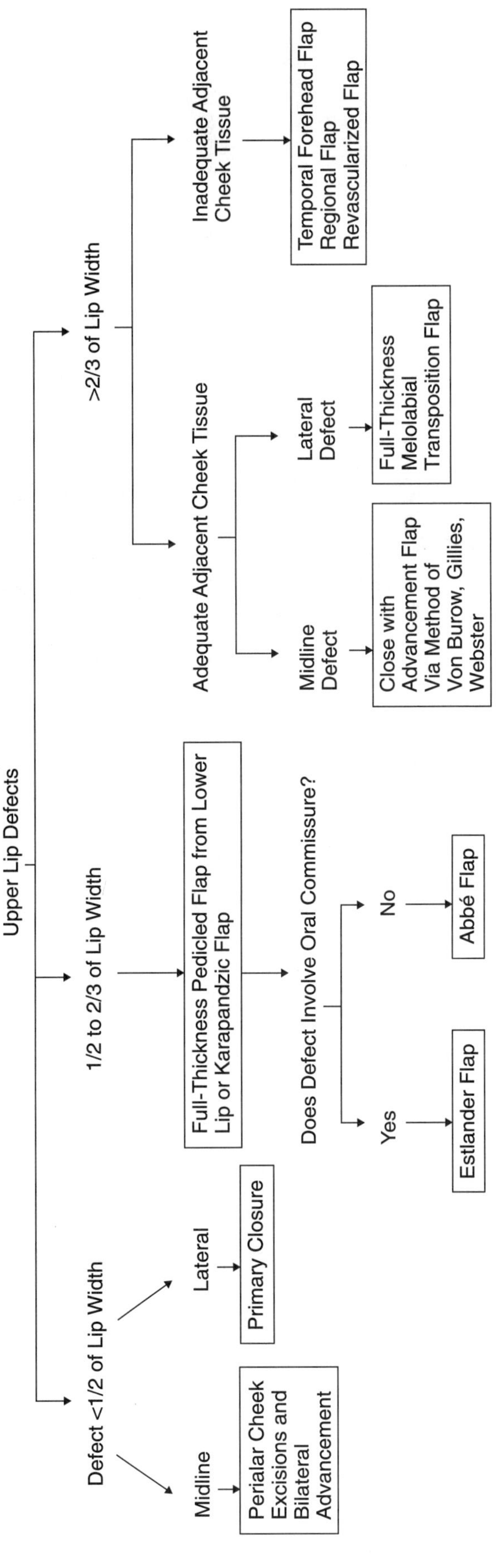

Figure 2.
Algorithm for reconstruction of upper lip defect.

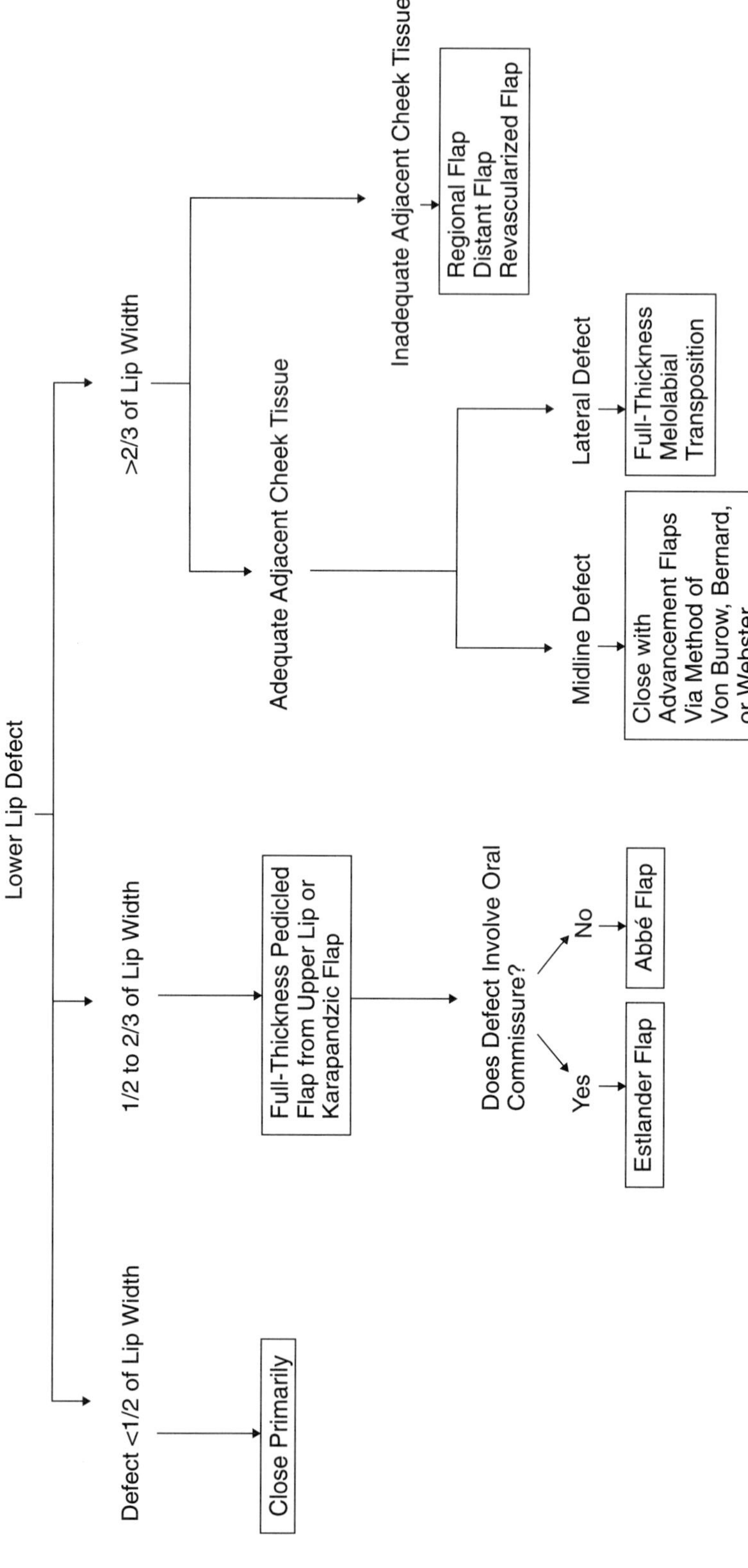

Figure 3.
Algorithm for reconstruction of lower lip defects.

lip for defects that are full thickness or represent loss of skin and muscle. This approach categorizes the size of lip defects into those less than one-half the width of the lip, those between one-half and two-thirds, and defects greater than two-thirds of the entire lip width. Defects of less than one-half of the lip width can usually be managed by primary wound closure or smaller local flaps confined to an aesthetic subunit of the lip. In the lower lip, conversion of the defect into a W-shaped configuration may be preferred, and in its simplest form this technique is usually adequate for primary closure, although modification to include lateral advancement flaps may be required when the defect base is broad. The W-shaped configuration maximizes conservation of tissue and prevents an unsightly pointed chin when it is necessary to extend the incision beyond the mental crease. Primary closure should be in four layers: mucosa, muscle, deep dermis, and skin. Care is taken to perform a precise approximation of the "white line" at the vermilion border on either side of the defect.

Primary wound closure of defects in the midline of the upper lip can be facilitated by excising a crescent of cheek skin in the perialar region. This method is similar to that described by Webster. Perialar skin excision allows advancement of the remaining lip segments medially and lessens wound closure tension after primary wound repair.

Reconstruction of defects consisting of one-half to two-thirds of the lip usually requires lip augmentation procedures. Closure can be most readily achieved by a full-thickness pedicle flap from the opposite lip (lip switch flap) or from the adjacent cheek. The Karapandzic flap may also be effective in closing medium-sized defects of the lip, and in some instances this flap may provide better functional results than other uninnervated or denervated flaps would. This technique consists of circumoral incisions through the skin and subcutaneous tissue, encompassing the remaining portions of the upper and lower lips. The orbicularis oris is mobilized and remains pedicled bilaterally on the superior and inferior labial arteries. The muscle also remains attached to the underlying mucosa. Adequate mobilization enables primary closure of the defect by rotating the portions of the remaining lips into the defect. The advantage of the Karapandzic flap is that it restores a continuous circle of functioning orbicularis muscle, which maintains oral competence. However, because no new tissue is recruited to aid in the reconstruction of the lip, microstomia may be a problem. Patients in the sixth decade of life or older will often develop laxity of the oral stoma following a Karapandzic flap closure and as a consequence will not require commissuroplasties to correct the microstomia.

Local flaps are preferable to regional flaps for closing defects of less than two-thirds of the lip width because of their close skin color and texture match and the availability of mucous membrane for internal lining. Defects located away from the commissure are best closed with an Abbé flap consisting of a full-thickness flap from the opposite lip pedicled on the vermilion border and containing the labial artery. The flap may be based medially or laterally, because the labial artery anastomoses with its counterpart to form a continuous circle of arterial loop. Estlander's original operation was devised for closure of a lower lip defect near the commissure of the mouth. This flap is now used to repair full-thickness defects of the upper or lower lip that extend into the lateral commissure. Since the original description of the Abbé and Estlander flaps, the operations have been modified in many ways to accommodate surgical defects located anywhere in the upper or lower lip.

The Abbé and Estlander flaps should be constructed so that the height of the flap equals the height of the defect. The width of the flap should be approximately one-half that of the defect to be reconstructed; however, when the entire philtrum is missing, the width of this groove should be completely replaced with the Abbé flap. This process will restore the total aesthetic subunit, which is preferable from the standpoint of cosmesis as well as function. The pedicle should be made narrow to facilitate transposition, and it should be positioned near the center line of the recipient site. The secondary defect should be closed in four layers, with accurate approximation of the vermilion border.

The superiorly based Estlander flap may be modified from its original description by designing the flap so that it lies within the melolabial sulcus. This provides better scar camouflage of the donor site and at the same time allows easy rotation of the flap into the lower lip defect. Oral commissure distortion is caused by the Estlander flap. This distortion, or microstomia, may be corrected with a secondary commissuroplasty when desired, but this procedure should be delayed for 2 to 3 months following initial transposition of the flap.

The pedicle of the Abbé flap crosses the oral stoma and may be severed in 2 to 3 weeks. During the interval between transfer of the flap and division of the pedicle, the patient is maintained on a liquid or soft diet that does not require excessive chewing. It is essential that precise approximation of the vermilion border be ensured at the time of pedicle severance.

Defects greater than two-thirds of the width of the entire lip and some smaller lateral defects are best reconstructed by using adjacent cheek flaps in the form of advancement or transposition flaps. Massive or total lip defects are best reconstructed by using regional or distant flaps or vascularized microsurgical flaps. Large defects of the upper lip may be reconstructed by excising crescent-shaped perialar cheek tissue and advancing bilateral cheek flaps medially. If wound closure tension is excessive, an Abbé flap may be added in the midline.

Similarly, midline lower lip defects may be closed by full-thickness advancement flaps as described by Bernard, Webster, or Gillies. These techniques may require excision of triangular-shaped standing cutaneous deformities (dog ear) in the melolabial sulcus to allow advancement of the cheek flaps. These excisions should follow the lines of the sulcus and should include only skin and subcutaneous tissues. The underlying muscle is mobilized to form a new commissure. The mucous membrane is separated from the muscle and advanced outward to provide a vermilion border. Incisions are made in the gingival buccal sulcus as far posterior as the last molar tooth if necessary to allow proper approximation of the remaining lip segments without excessive wound closure tension.

Melolabial transposition flaps consisting of skin and subcutaneous tissue only or full thickness consisting of skin, subcutaneous tissue, muscle, and mucosa can be useful in reconstructing lip defects as large as three-quarters of the width of the lip. Large skin only defects of the lateral lip are repaired nicely with melolabial flaps; however, keeping with the principles of maintaining borders between aesthetic units, I prefer to repair defects that extend from the lip onto the cheek with two separate flaps. A large rotation flap from the remaining lip segment is useful for repairing skin only defects of the upper lip that extend into the cheek. The cheek component of the defect is then repaired by a separate transposition or advancement cheek flap. This places nearly all the scars in the melolabial sulcus while maintaining the integrity of the border between the lip and cheek aesthetic units.

Adjacent cheek tissue may not be applicable or sufficient for reconstruction of near-total defects of the lip. In such cases, regional flaps may be used for reconstruction. Excisions of the lower lip, chin, and anterior section of the mandible for carcinoma often require such flaps for reconstruction.

The temporal forehead flap designed as a bipedicle advancement or unipedicle interpolation flap may be used for total upper lip reconstruction, but the unsightly secondary deformity precludes its common use. The flap may be lined with a split-thickness skin or mucosal graft. In males, hair-bearing scalp may be incorporated to provide hair growth for scar camouflage.

A number of regional flaps are used for repair of large defects of the upper and lower lip. The pectoralis major musculocutaneous flap has been used for lip reconstruction following extensive ablative surgery for malignancy of the anterior floor of the mouth involving large portions of the lip or skin of the chin. The pectoralis major musculocutaneous flap has the advantage of being an axial flap that may be elevated as a strip of muscle and an attached segment of overlying skin for a one-stage reconstruction of the lip. A portion of the flap may be turned on itself to provide tissue for the inner aspect of the lips and/or the anterior floor of the mouth. The flap has sufficient bulk to provide some structural support when a mandibulectomy is necessary for tumor exenteration.

The development of microvascular surgical techniques has allowed one-stage reconstruction of the lip, chin, and anterior mandibular arch by transferring free composite osteomusculocutaneous and osteocutaneous flaps that provide vascularized bone grafts for mandibular reconstruction and soft tissue for restoration of the lip and chin. Revascularized bone is advantageous because it heals more readily and has an overall better success rate than do conventional nonvascularized bone grafts. In addition, the simultaneous reconstruction of soft-tissue defects provides a superior rehabilitation technique for patients who have massive defects of the lip and jaw.

Suggested Reading

Baker SR. Malignancy of the lip. In: Paparella MM, ed. Otolaryngolgy—Head and Neck. Vol 3. Philadelphia: WB Saunders, 1991.

Karapandzic M. Reconstruction of lip defects by local arterial flaps. Br J Plast Surg 1974; 27:93.

Renner G. Reconstruction of the lip. In Baker SR, Swanson NA, eds. Local flaps in facial reconstruction. Philadelphia: Mosby–Year Book, 1991.

Webster RE, Coffey RJ, Kellcher RE. Total and partial reconstruction of the lower lip with innervated muscle-bearing flaps. Plast Reconstr Surg 1960; 25:360.

CANCER OF THE ANTERIOR TONGUE

The method of
Eugene N. Myers
by
Jeffrey N. Meyers
Eugene N. Meyers

Cancer of the oral tongue is one of the most common cancers of the head and neck. Approximately 3,500 new cases are diagnosed each year in the United States. This disease represents a major health care problem in some Eastern countries such as India, where cancer of the oral cavity makes up 30 percent of all newly diagnosed cancers. The vast majority of cancers arising in the oral tongue are squamous cell carcinomas. However, cancers of minor salivary gland origin or sarcomas may also occur.

Most patients (>95 percent) are over 40 years of age, with an average age at diagnosis of 60 years. There is an increasing incidence in patients under age 40. The etiology and clinical behavior of cancer of the tongue differ significantly between patients in the elderly and younger age categories. Squamous cell carcinomas in the older age group are positively associated with tobacco and alcohol use. Most patients under age 40 have no clearly identifiable risk factors, and a higher percentage of these patients are female. Poor dental hygiene has also been associated with the development and late diagnosis of cancer of the oral cavity. Some dietary factors are thought to protect against the development of these cancers.

These observations support the now well-accepted theory of multistep carcinogenesis in the development of squamous cell carcinoma, that is, that tumors arise as a result of multiple accumulated genetic alterations. Some of these genetic defects are inherited through the germline; the remainder are the result of repeated exposure to DNA–damaging molecules in tobacco and alcohol.

Cancer in younger patients without a history of exposure to tobacco and alcohol supports the concept that inherited germline defects play a role in the pathogenesis of squamous cell carcinoma of the oral cavity, although the specific molecular alterations in these cases have not been clearly defined. The detection of human papillomavirus DNA in cancer of the tongue suggests that viral proteins known to interact with molecules that are important for the regulation of cell proliferation may also contribute to the development of cancer.

■ EVALUATION

The presentation and clinical outcome varies with clinical stage and comorbidities. Localized pain and/or the presence of an ulcerated lesion on the tongue are the most common presenting complaints. Otalgia (referred pain), which generally indicates perineural invasion, weight loss, dysphagia, and/or a palpable mass in the neck are harbingers of more aggressive disease.

A thorough history should include how the lesion was first noted, previous biopsy and/or treatment, other medical illnesses, tobacco and alcohol use, and a family history of cancer. Assessment of the patient's nutritional status is also important. Patients who have lost greater than 10 percent of their body weight should be nutritionally replenished before treatment in order to optimize immune function and wound healing.

The candidacy of patients with more advanced cancer of the oral tongue who will require total glossectomy and laryngeal preservation can be assessed in part by their exercise tolerance. This can often be a more reliable test of pulmonary function than formal spirometry.

Physical examination of the tongue should include assessment of tongue mobility, general characteristics of the lesion, tumor thickness, and determination of extension of the lesion to surrounding structures, including floor of the mouth, base of the tongue, gingiva, tonsillar pillar, and mandible. Mobility of the tongue is best assessed by asking the patient to protrude and move the tongue from side to side. Deviation of the tongue to one side on protrusion and restricted mobility are signs of deep muscle or hypoglossal nerve invasion. Note whether the cancer is exophytic or ulcerative: ulcerative lesions are more infiltrative and have a greater tendency for cervical metastasis. Tumor thickness or depth of ulceration are correlated with lower rates of locoregional control and survivorship. The dimensions of the surface of the cancer are also important in order to properly stage the cancer by the tumor, nodes, and metastases system.

It is important to thoroughly examine the remainder of the oral cavity in order to rule out other areas of dysplasia or second primary cancers. In addition, the adequacy of the dentition must be established, and the need for dental extractions or restorations should be assessed, because timely dental management will aid in the prevention of osteoradionecrosis, in the event that the patient needs radiotherapy during the course of treatment. Removal of carious or fractured teeth and excision of areas of severe periodontal disease promote better healing of the operative site. In patients requiring total glossectomy, we recommend an evaluation by the maxillofacial prosthodontist to make impressions that will help in producing a tongue prosthesis that will assist in the rehabilitation of speech and swallowing. Speech therapists may also consult with the patient, because they will play a pivotal role in rehabilitation.

Careful palpation of the neck is essential to evaluate the presence of cervical lymph node metastases. Palpable cervical lymph nodes must be measured in order to assign a proper N stage to the patient. Examination of the remainder of the mucosa of the upper aerodigestive tract is essential to rule out second primary cancers. A chest radiograph and barium swallow esophagram are important for assessing the presence of second primary cancers.

Imaging studies of the head and neck with computed tomography (CT) or magnetic resonance imaging (MRI) help determine the full extent of the primary tumor and the stage of regional metastasis. Patients whose cancers are poorly demarcated on contrast-enhanced CT scans have a higher rate of local failure. Further, CT is very helpful in assessing whether there is involvement of the mandible before surgery. The Dentascan, a recent software modification of the CT scan, is very accurate in demonstrating invasion of bone. MRI has been useful in determining the extent of primary cancer of the tongue, particularly in delineating the relationship of the cancer to the midline or floor of the mouth. However, this modality is limited to identifying small superficial cancers and cortical invasion of the mandible. An unenhanced T1-weighted image is recommended for basic imaging of oral cavity lesions, and T2-weighted imaging or gadopentetate dimeglumine enhancement are suggested for use when tumor margins are not well delineated. MRI is useful for following up on a patient's response to radiotherapy.

A preoperative assessment by colleagues in internal medicine or cardiology is essential for patients who have significant cardiopulmonary or other comorbidities. All efforts to optimize the patient's general condition should be made in a timely way.

■ THERAPY

Treatment Options

Single-modality treatment with either surgery or radiotherapy has been the traditional mainstay of therapy for limited cancers of the tongue, whereas combined modality treatment is often required in the treatment of more advanced cancers. The use of brachytherapy and/or external beam radiotherapy in the treatment of early cancer of the tongue has been advocated in Europe and Asia. However, the high rate of complications has led to the use of surgery as the major modality for treating cancer of the oral tongue, followed by radiotherapy in patients who have specific indications.

The choice of the surgical approach in treating cancer of the oral tongue depends on the extent of the cancer as well as the patient's state of dentition and his or her general body habitus. Although transoral partial glossectomy is the optimal approach for treating most patients, patients who have a very large tumor, full dentition, or a thick, muscular neck may require a mandibulotomy approach.

Neck Dissection

Transoral excision of small cancers of the anterior tongue (T_1/T_2) yields very high control at the primary site. However, the limiting factor in improving the cure rate is the management of the N_0 neck, because most patients with T_1/T_2 cancers do not have clinically positive lymph nodes.

The high rate of metastases of cancer of the oral tongue to cervical lymph nodes as well as skip metastases indicates the need to address the neck in all patients undergoing treatment for cancer arising in this location. All patients who have early cancer of the tongue and an N_0 neck should undergo an ipsilateral level I to IV selective neck dissection for staging and treatment. Similarly, patients who have T_1/T_0 or T_2/T_0 lesions near or involving the midline should undergo bilateral neck dissections. For patients who have palpable or radiographically demonstrable neck metastasis, we recommend a modified radical neck dissection.

■ SURGICAL TECHNIQUE

These treatment techniques have evolved over the years in the Department of Otolaryngology at the University of Pittsburgh School of Medicine and reflect the methods developed by the senior author. The excision of T_1/T_2 lesions is usually done in discontinuity from the neck dissection. This method has withstood the test of time and has shown no disadvantages. The excision of the primary tumor is carried out first, and the neck dissection follows.

Partial and Hemiglossectomy

General anesthetia is preferred for most patients, although local anesthesia is used for high-risk patients. Nasotracheal intubation is used in those patients who do not undergo tracheotomy. Intravenous antibiotics are given before the start of surgery to decrease the incidence of wound infection.

Direct laryngoscopy and esophagoscopy are then performed to rule out synchronous primary cancers of the upper aerodigestive tract. If no additional primary cancers are identified, excision of the primary lesion and reconstruction are carried out before neck dissection. For most T_1 and T_2 lesions, transoral excision and primary closure are used, precluding the need for tracheotomy. For more extensive lesions or if a split-thickness skin graft is used for reconstruction, tracheotomy is performed after completion of endoscopy.

The patient is then positioned to fully extend the neck. After prepping and draping, a Jennings mouth gag and right-angled retractors are used to provide adequate exposure of the tongue. A 2–0 silk suture is placed 1 cm posterior to the tip of the tongue in the midline for retraction. The cancer is inspected and palpated to fully assess its size in three dimensions. The tongue is dried, and an elliptical incision is marked with at least 1 cm margins. A second 2–0 silk suture is placed at the anterior margin before resection, because proper orientation may be lost once the resection has begun, and the position of this marker is noted on the pathology form.

An electrocautery knife is used to make the mucosal incision. The best oncologic results are obtained when adequate margins are obtained initially, because muscle fibers of the tongue retract after transection, which makes complete re-excision of residual tumor difficult.

While hemostasis is obtained and before closure, the circumferential and deep margins of the specimen are analyzed by the pathologist using frozen sections. In our institution, the pathologist comes into the operating room to view the operative site and discusses the orientation of the specimen and what information the surgeons require, and then he or she returns to discuss the results of the frozen sections.

Once the adequacy of the resection has been verified, the dead space is obliterated with interrupted 3–0 chromic catgut, and the edges of the wound are approximated with vertical mattress sutures of 3–0 silk, which further close the dead space and evert the wound edges. Tracheotomy is performed in patients in whom extensive postoperative edema is anticipated or in patients who will have a skin graft requiring a large tie-on gauze bolster.

Hemiglossectomy is used for larger tumors that do not encroach upon the midline. A similar approach is used, except that the incision is begun at the tip of the tongue at the midline and carried through the median raphe in order to minimize blood loss. The specimen is delivered after posterior and lateral incisions are completed and is then sent for frozen section analysis of the margins.

Split-thickness skin grafting of the hemiglossectomy defect prevents debilitating restriction of tongue mobility that may result from primary closure of the defect. The individual taking the skin graft must regown and reglove before harvesting a graft 0.015 to 0.016 inch thick from the anterior thigh. The graft is sutured in place using a "pie-crusting" technique. In this method, interrupted 3–0 silk sutures are placed through the edge of the graft, then through the edge of the defect, and finally brought out again through the graft. Alternate sutures are left long in order to tie over a bolster dressing of impregnated gauze that will secure the skin graft in place, thus preventing shearing away from the underlying muscle. "Quilting" sutures of chromic catgut are also placed at several sites to fix the skin graft to the underlying bed before bolster placement in order to prevent hematoma formation or fluid collection under the graft that will ultimately lead to graft failure. This is of particular importance in healing because the tongue is in constant motion.

Neck Dissection

Following partial or hemiglossectomy and reconstruction, the surgical team regowns and regloves. The towel that had been stapled to the skin overlying the mandible is draped over the face. The neck dissection is then done without having to reprep and redrape. We perform the glossectomy first because the floor of the mouth will also be resected in some patients, and the neck may be entered. If this happens after neck dissection, it is difficult or impossible to close the defect without reopening the neck. If the neck is dissected after tumor resection, any dehiscence in the oral cavity can be repaired from below.

We use a selective neck dissection of zones I to IV for squamous cell carcinoma of the tongue with an N_0 neck. We carry out this procedure through what we refer to as a hockey stick incision, the vertical limb of which begins at the mastoid tip, extends almost to the clavicle, and then goes transversely to the midline. This flap provides excellent exposure, dependable circulation, and if the vertical limb is carried somewhat posteriorly, provides excellent cosmesis, because most of the incision is covered by either the patient's hair or clothing. Special attention must be paid to preservation of the ramus mandibularis in order to avoid weakness of the lower lip. The nerve must be identified and reflected superiorly. Oncologically, it is of utmost importance to excise the pre- and postvascular lymph node, which is in juxtaposition to the ramus mandibularis, because there is a high degree of positivity in this location. Zones I to IV are dissected because, as mentioned previously, there can be skip metastases (fast track) down to level IV, with nodes negative in zones I to IV that are not addressed by supraomohyoid dissection. At the completion of the surgery, the packet of lymph node–bearing tissue should be marked so that the pathologist can properly identify the levels of lymph node involvement. The wound is then closed over hemovac drains.

Total Glossectomy

Larger lesions of the oral tongue may require subtotal or total glossectomy for local tumor control, or alleviation of severe pain. Because total glossectomy will have a significant negative impact on deglutition, many patients will require total laryngectomy as well. However, in our experience, selected patients tolerate total glossectomy without laryngectomy and retain speech and swallowing function. Selecting well-motivated individuals without significant cardiopulmonary comorbidity is the key to success for this procedure. The criteria are similar to the selection of patients for supraglottic laryngectomy. These patients will always aspirate to some degree; therefore, they need adequate pulmonary reserve and an effective cough. Additional factors that contribute to success include good motivation and personal support systems, as well as a cognitive capacity adequate to learn and employ complex swallowing tasks. Ideally, the patient should also be ambulatory; wheelchair or bedridden patients generally do not tolerate aspiration well. In addition, a well-coordinated team consisting of a speech pathologist, maxillofacial prosthodontist, nutritionist, and social worker are essential in helping to maximize the patient's quality of life.

Additional considerations in treating patients who have advanced cancer originating in the oral tongue include management of the neck (both sides may be involved) and evaluation for possible mandibular involvement.

Even for those patients who are assessed to be suitable for laryngeal preservation, appropriate preoperative counseling about the possible need for total laryngectomy is required in the event that intraoperative findings demonstrate that resection of the larynx is required for oncologic control. Reconstruction of soft tissue using a skin graft, regional pedicled flap, or free tissue transfer is usually required, and on occasion, a defect in the mandible may need to be reconstructed.

There are several possible approaches to the resection of advanced cancer of the oral tongue that requires total glossectomy, including transoral, transhyoid pharyngotomy; midline mandibulotomy with mandibular swing; and lateral pharyngotomy. Unless midline mandibulotomy is selected, a large apron flap from mastoid tip to mastoid tip is preferred because it facilitates performance of bilateral neck dissections.

The surgical approach depends on the extent of the lesion and its proximity to other important structures. If the cancer has invaded the periosteum of the anterior mandible, a marginal mandibulectomy is recommended. In the case of direct involvement by the cancer of the cortical bone of the anterior mandible, anterior segmental mandibulectomy is performed. Proceeding posteriorly along the floor of the mouth, the muscles are detached from the hyoid bone, and the soft tissues of the base of the tongue and oral cavity are transected at the valleculae, thereby preserving the larynx. When laryngectomy is required in order to obtain an adequate margin, transhyoid pharyngotomy should be avoided in order to prevent entering the pharynx through the posterior aspect of the tumor. For lesions involving the tongue base, midline mandibulotomy or lateral pharyngotomy provide the best exposure of the posterior margin of resection and facilitate laryngectomy, if necessary.

While frozen section analysis of the margins is being carried out, a cricopharyngeal myotomy is performed. The larynx can be suspended anteriorly and superiorly with interrupted nonabsorbable sutures to the mandible in order to decrease aspiration. Reconstruction of the glossectomy defect is best accomplished with a pectoralis major myocutaneous flap or free tissue transfer using a rectus abdominis myocutaneous flap. Both of these methods provide for a bulky reconstruction that enhances swallowing. To avoid dehiscence related to gravitational pull on the myocutaneous flap, the flap should be suspended using circumdental sutures or sutures placed through holes drilled in the inferior aspect of the mandible.

Postoperative care requires careful attention to detail regarding the patient's wound, tracheostomy tube, and swallowing function. Suction drainage catheters must be observed for proper function, and the appropriate interventions should be made if evidence of a hematoma, seroma, chylous, or salivary fistula is noted.

Oral cavity care includes frequent suctioning of secretions, rinses of the oral cavity with half-strength peroxide three to four times per day, and cleaning the suture lines with peroxide. Early ambulation and frequent, vigorous suctioning of the tracheostomy tube are helpful in preventing pulmonary complications. Stepwise decannulation is achieved when patients are able to handle their oral secretions and tolerate occlusion of the tracheostomy tube.

If a portion of the flap is lost or if there is separation of the intraoral wound, efforts must be made to separate the flow of saliva from the neck to prevent deep neck infection and rupture of the carotid artery.

■ REHABILITATION

Once the patient has been successfully decannulated and the tracheostoma has healed adequately, swallowing rehabilitation can begin, which follows a course similar to that used for the patient who has undergone supraglottic laryngectomy. Swallowing function is severely impaired by total glossectomy, because this procedure combines the first two phases of swallowing into a single phase that cannot be controlled by the patient. Furthermore, current reconstructive options place an adynamic conduit between the lips and pharynx through which the bolus spills directly into the pharynx. Protective elevation of the larynx is also impaired due to excision of the suprahyoid musculature. In those patients in whom a portion of the supraglottic larynx has been resected as well, another tier of glottic protection is also lost, which further increases the amount of aspiration. Cricopharyngeal myotomy helps to decrease pooling of secretions in the hypopharynx, and thus may be helpful in preventing spillover into the glottis.

Patients must learn a new technique of swallowing in order to further minimize the degree of aspiration. When food is first taken into the mouth, the patient must initiate a form of Valsalva's maneuver in order to close the glottis. As the involuntary phase of swallowing begins, the glottis is cleared with a cough, and then the patient completes the swallow and exhales. The choice of foods of the proper texture helps the patient to achieve success in preventing aspiration. Thicker liquids and nonpourable pureed foods and carbonated beverages are better tolerated initially than are thin liquids, which often can be introduced later into the diet when swallowing function has improved. Another maneuver that is helpful to the total glossectomy patient is swallowing the bolus with the neck extended. Gavage feedings with a syringe and short rubber feeding tube or introduction of the meal directly into the pharynx with a spoon are other useful swallowing strategies.

Speech rehabilitation is achieved with the assistance of the maxillofacial prosthodontist and speech pathologist. A tongue replacement prosthesis fashioned by the prosthodontist facilitates speech and swallowing by decreasing the distance between the reconstructed floor of the mouth and the palate. Once the prosthesis has been properly fitted, the patient is observed to see what types of sounds he or she is able to make. Most often, labial sounds such as P, B, and M are preserved, but other consonants and vowels may be distorted or omitted, making intelligibility difficult. The speech pathologist can help the patient to improve upon this speech difficulty by introducing compensatory strategies such as bilablial closure to enhance the T and D sounds or partial pharyngeal constriction for clarifying the K and G sounds. With appropriate coaching and great motivation, the total glossectomee can achieve speech that is intelligible to most listeners.

■ COMPLICATIONS

A number of potential complications can occur when performing partial or total glossectomy. As discussed previously, wound complications can occur as a result of lapses in the planning or technical performance of the procedure. Examination of the wound for bleeding, chylous and salivary drainage, and proper suction drainage catheter placement before closure are invaluable for the prevention and management of wound complications.

Frequent pulmonary infections can be avoided by proper patient selection. Highly motivated patients who have a cognitive capacity adequate to handle complex swallowing tasks fare better with this procedure, and thus patients who have poor motivation, poor social support, organic brain syndrome, or certain types of mental illness are not good candidates for this procedure. Similarly, patients who have severe cardiopulmonary disease, neurologic disorders, or the inability to ambulate are also not appropriate candidates. Even under the best of circumstances, patients who are predicted to achieve a good performance status may have a difficult time dealing with the resultant chronic aspiration and may not be successfully decannulated. A feeding gastrostomy may be a useful method for maintaining adequate nutrition in some patients. Laryngotracheal separation or completion laryngectomy are more definitive methods of managing this problem and may need to be resorted to in severely debilitated patients.

Other complications can arise as a result of improper reconstructive flap selection, design, or placement. Selection of the wrong flap, a skin paddle that is the wrong size or malpositioned with respect to the underlying muscle and vascular pedicle, and failure to adequately close and reinforce the wound or failure to suspend the muscle from the mandible all can contribute to the development of wound dehiscence and orocutaneous fistula, with the potential for deep neck infection and/or vascular catastrophe to occur.

In light of the abundant and often conflicting data regarding prognostic indicators for cancers of the oral tongue, we find tumor size, margin status, and nodal status (including the presence of extranodal extension) to be the most reliable indicators, and therefore we recommend a form of glossectomy appropriate for the stage of the primary cancer combined with ipsilateral or bilateral neck dissection as the minimal treatment for squamous cell carcinoma of the oral tongue. Adjuvant treatment in the form of external beam radiotherapy with or without chemotherapy is reserved for patients who have advanced disease (stages III and IV), extranodal extension, perineural involvement, and close margins.

Suggested Reading

Boring CC, Squires TS, Tong T. Cancer statistics. CA 1993; 43:7-26.

Day GL, Blot WJ. Second primary tumors in patients with oral cancer. Cancer 1992; 70:14-19.

Myers EN, Cunningham MJ. Treatments of choice for early carcinoma of the oral cavity. Oncology 1988; 2:18-36.

Rubright WC, Hoffman HT, Lynch CF. Risk factors for advanced-stage oral cavity cancer. Arch Otolaryngol Head Neck Surg 1996; 122:621-626.

Sarkaria JN, Harari PM. Oral tongue cancer in young adults less than 40 years of age: Rationale for aggressive therapy. Head Neck 1994; 16: 107-111.

Shindoh MY, Sawada Y, Kohgo T, et al. Detection of human papilloma virus DNA sequences in tongue squamous-cell carcinoma utilizing the polymerase chain reaction method. Int J Cancer 1992; 50:167-171.

Spiro RH, Huvos AG, Wong GY. Predictive value of tumor thickness in squamous carcinoma confined to the tongue and floor of the mouth. Am J Surg 1986; 152:345-350.

FLOOR OF THE MOUTH CANCER

The method of
Jesus E. Medina
John R. Houck, Jr.

Despite the advances in surgical techniques, radiotherapy, and chemotherapy over the past 20 years, overall survival of patients who have squamous cell carcinoma (SqCC) of the floor of the mouth (FOM) remains approximately 55 percent. Survival is clearly related to stage at presentation. When the tumor is localized to the oral cavity, overall survival is approximately 80 percent; when regional or distant spread has occurred, survival is approximately 43 percent and 20 percent, respectively. Thus, early diagnosis and treatment are essential for optimum survival.

Likewise, prevention efforts are important. Tobacco use is the single most important risk factor for the development of SCC of the FOM. The risk in smokers is approximately six times that of nonsmokers. A growing concern today is the increasing use of smokeless tobacco, particularly among teenagers. Although attempts at eliminating tobacco use are often frustrating, physicians should not be dismayed in their efforts to educate patients about the association between tobacco and cancer of the oral cavity.

Alcohol has also been implicated as a risk factor, although its role has been difficult to study because most heavy drinkers also smoke. Approximately 75 percent to 80 percent of patients who develop oral cancer consume alcohol regularly. Poor oral hygiene, papillomaviruses, oral lichen planus, and syphilis may also be associated with FOM cancer.

ANATOMIC CONSIDERATIONS

The anatomic relationship of the FOM to the mandible and the neurovascular structures of the tongue and neck is important in planning and executing ablative surgery and reconstruction, as well as in planning radiotherapy for tumor in this region.

To avoid jeopardizing the blood supply to the tongue when resecting tumors of the FOM, it is crucial for the surgeon to have a working knowledge of the vasculature of the region. The principal blood supply of the floor of the mouth derives from the lingual artery. It arises from the external carotid artery and courses lateral to the middle constrictor muscle, and then medial to the hyoglossus. After entering the oral cavity, the lingual artery branches into the dorsal lingual branches, which supply the base of the tongue and tonsil, and the deep lingual branch, which supplies the anterior two-thirds of the tongue. Care must be taken not to injure the lingual arteries during surgery for anterior FOM tumors when the resection has to extend into the musculature of the ventral aspect of the tongue due to the risk of tongue necrosis. Of course, the artery has to be taken if necessary for adequate margins; however, careful identification and sparing of the artery can be done if margins permit. Similarly, during this kind of surgery, the lingual and hypoglossal nerves, which are located quite anteriorly near the ventral surface of the tongue, can be identified and spared if they are not needed for adequate margins.

The anatomic relationship of the FOM to the muscles of the ventral aspect of the tongue, that is, the genioglossus and hyoglossus, is such that a portion of these muscles must often be included in the resection to adequately encompass tumors of the anterior floor of the mouth. This can result in significant impairment in the ability to swallow, particularly in the elderly.

Thus, the surgeon must be aware of the anatomic relationships of the FOM, and the patient must be apprised of the possible functional consequences of inadvertent injury or resection of the various anatomic structures related to the FOM.

The anatomy of the lymphatics of the floor of the mouth is important in treatment planning. The lymphatic drainage of this region is continuous with the opposite side through vessels that cross the midline. The first echelon of lymphatic drainage for the FOM are the nodes of the submental, submandibular groups (particularly the preglandular nodes), and upper jugular groups (lymph node groups I and II). However, lymphatic drainage from the anterior FOM can occur directly to the jugulo-omohyoid lymph nodes (group III).

DIAGNOSTIC EVALUATION

When evaluating a patient who has FOM cancer, we perform a thorough head and neck examination using instruments and lighting that are adequate to visualize the mucosa of the entire oral cavity, pharynx, and larynx. If indirect laryngoscopy is inadequate, fiberoptic nasopharyngoscopy is used. Asking the patient to touch the roof of the mouth with the tongue aids in visualization of the floor of the mouth.

Careful palpation of FOM tumors helps determine thickness of the tumor and fixation to or invasion of the mandible. Examination under anesthesia may be necessary if the lesion is too painful for adequate assessment in the office.

Examination of the submental, submandibular, and jugular chain of lymph nodes is essential for accurate staging and treatment planning. However, in our hands, the false-negative rate for clinical evaluation of adenopathy in FOM cancers is 25 percent and the false-positive rate is 40 percent. The location, size, mobility, and relationship of enlarged nodes to adjacent structures is recorded.

A biopsy of the tumor is usually performed in the office with local anesthesia or may be performed during an examination under general anesthesia. Fine needle aspiration of suspected metastatic disease is performed in selected patients. Open biopsy of suspected metastatic disease is not indicated.

IMAGING STUDIES

The use of imaging studies such as computed tomography (CT) and magnetic resonance imaging (MRI) in the evaluation of FOM tumors is limited in our practice to those patients for whom the physical examination does not allow us to adequately answer specific questions about the extent of the primary tumor: depth of invasion and extension into the substance of the tongue. We also find these imaging studies helpful in determining whether enlarged neck lymph nodes are present in some patients who are obese, have thick necks, or have been previously irradiated.

MANDIBULAR INVASION

Physical examination continues to be the best method for assessing the relationship of an FOM tumor to the mandible, and thus in determining whether adequate surgical treatment will require a coronal mandibulectomy, that is, resection of the inner table of the mandible, or a segmental mandibulectomy. However, plain radiographs such as dental films and a submental vertex view may be helpful in this evaluation. They are inexpensive and can show erosion of the inner table of the mandible. The orthopantomogram (Panorex) is used for dental evaluation and to assess the inferior alveolar canal. Although radionuclide bone scans are used by some surgeons for evaluation of possible mandibular invasion, we do not use them routinely because of their high false-positive rate. In this regard, CT scanning is also limited by significant false-positive and false-negative rates. Only 75 percent of the patients in whom CT shows evidence of mandibular involvement actually have it histologically; and of those patients without CT evidence of bone invasion, 21 percent actually have it.

CONSULTATIONS

Patients who have FOM cancer are evaluated by a radiation oncologist in anticipation of the possible need for postoperative radiotherapy or for primary treatment of selected small lesions.

Consultation with a dentist who is familiar with the management of head and neck cancer patients is obtained in anticipation of the need for radiotherapy or dental rehabilitation. Speech therapy evaluation may be helpful for preoperative counseling in anticipation of the need for speech and swallowing rehabilitation.

STAGING

Tumor staging is outlined in Table 1.

Table 1. Tumor Staging in Floor of Mouth Cancer

T_x	Primary tumor cannot be assessed
T_0	No evidence of primary tumor
T_{is}	Carcinoma in situ
T_1	Tumor 2 cm or less in greatest dimension
T_2	Tumor more than 2 cm but not more than 4 cm in greatest dimension
T_3	Tumor more than 4 cm in greatest dimension
T_4 (lip)	Tumor invades adjacent structures (e.g., through cortical bone, tongue, skin of neck)
T_4 (oral cavity)	Tumor invades adjacent structures (e.g., through cortical bone, into deep [extrinsic] muscle of tongue, maxillary sinus, skin)

TREATMENT PLANNING

A number of factors are taken into consideration when planning therapy for a patient who has FOM cancer. Regarding the *primary tumor,* the following factors are considered:

1. Tumor size: In general, small tumors (stage T_1 or T_2) can be treated with a single treatment modality, either radiotherapy or surgery, thus minimizing morbidity and cost. Larger tumors (T_3 or T_4) may require combined therapy.
2. The relationship of the tumor to the mandible and the presence or absence of bone erosion: Tumors adherent to or invading the mandible are best treated with surgery. The same is true for patients who have prominent mandibular tori.
3. The condition of the patient's dentition.
4. Other factors include the patient's general condition, age, and to a lesser extent, the likelihood that the patient will stop excessive use of tobacco and alcohol.

Regarding the *cervical lymph nodes,* treatment decisions are based on the following factors:

1. The presence or absence of palpable adenopathy.
2. The likelihood of occult nodal metastases.
3. The need to enter the neck for surgical access to the primary tumor.
4. The reliability of the patient for follow-up clinic visits.
5. The therapeutic modality selected for the treatment of the primary tumor.

THERAPY

Primary Tumor

Early (T_1 to T_2) tumors of the FOM can be successfully treated with surgery or radiotherapy. We believe that surgery is the preferred modality because adequate treatment with radiotherapy often requires a combination of external beam and interstitial irradiation. This requires special expertise, which most radiation oncologists presently do not have. More important, such therapy is associated with osteoradionecrosis of the mandible in as many as 25 percent of patients.

In the surgical treatment of these tumors, the surgeon's judgment is called on to decide (1) whether adequate exposure, and thus the excision can be accomplished through the open mouth or will require a combined transoral-transcervical pull-through approach, and (2) whether a marginal or a coronal mandibulectomy is necessary to adequately resect the tumor.

Small lesions are approachable through the open mouth. Excision of very small tumors can be performed in the office or outpatient setting with local anesthesia and use of a CO_2 laser or electrocautery. Reconstruction of the resulting defect is often possible by primary closure. It can also be left to heal secondarily, with excellent results. However, if doing this will restrict tongue movement and potentially hinder speech and swallowing, then a split-thickness skin graft is preferable. Generally, a thicker graft (approximately 0.15 inch) gives an adequate base for prosthetic dentition. Local and regional soft-tissue flaps can also be used for mucosal reconstruction. The most popular is the nasolabial flap, which can reach the midline easily. The cosmetic result is excellent, especially in older patients. A second procedure is necessary 2 weeks later to transect the pedicle. If the excision involves the papilla and duct of the submandibular gland, the duct should be identified, mobilized, and stitched to a mucosal edge to improve function postoperatively.

For larger T_2 and some T_3 lesions, particularly those that invade deeply into the musculature of the root of the tongue, a combined transoral-transcervical (pull-through) approach may be necessary. This approach may also be necessary in patients who have a narrow anterior arch of the mandible and patients who have trismus due to previous treatment of other tumors or other conditions. Adequate resection of T_2 and T_3 tumors that abut the mandible or involve the periosteum—but without actual gross invasion of the mandible—requires a coronal, marginal, or combined coronal-marginal resection of the mandible for adequate margins. A coronal mandibulectomy consists of the removal of the inner or lingual table of the mandible (Fig. 1); this type of resection is used for the resection of tumors that involve only the floor of the mouth without extending to the alveolar ridge. A marginal mandibulectomy consists of the removal of the alveolar ridge and varying portions of the upper "edge" of the mandible (Fig. 2); this type of resection is commonly used in the resection of tumors of the lower gum. A combined coronal-marginal mandibulectomy (Fig. 3) is used to adequately resect tumors of the FOM that extend onto the alveolar ridge.

These mandibular resections deserve special technical consideration. They can be performed through the mouth, particularly the marginal type alone, or through the neck. To perform a coronal resection in the edentulous patient, a mucosal cut is made along the edge of the alveolar ridge, down to the periosteum; then a side-cutting bur, such as the MicroAire K-72, 1.2 mm, and the K-73, 1.6 mm, made by MicroAire Surgical Instruments (Charlottesville, VA), is used to perform the osteotomy by carefully drilling through the mandibular inner-table cancellous bone. In the patient who has partial or full dentition, we either remove all the teeth in the area of the osteotomy and carry out the drilling through the dental sockets, or we remove only the teeth at both ends of the anticipated osteotomy, and make a mucosal incision on the labial side of the gum, immediately below the level of the dental roots. Drilling of the mandible is then done first in a "horizontal" fashion, to outline the osteotomy and carry it through the outer table, then in a "vertical" fashion, angling the drill to perform the osteotomy through the inner-table cancellous bone. In our hands, both types of osteotomy can be accurately done through the mouth, care being taken to maintain the drill at a proper angle so as not to reduce the height of the outer table too much so that it would fracture and, more importantly, not to thin the inner table too much or actually enter the adjacent tumor with the drill. If the tumor is small and the exposure is adequate, the resection of the tumor can be completed through the mouth. Otherwise a combined peroral-transcervical approach is used. In such cases, we perform the neck dissection(s) first, then the appropriate mucosal incisions,

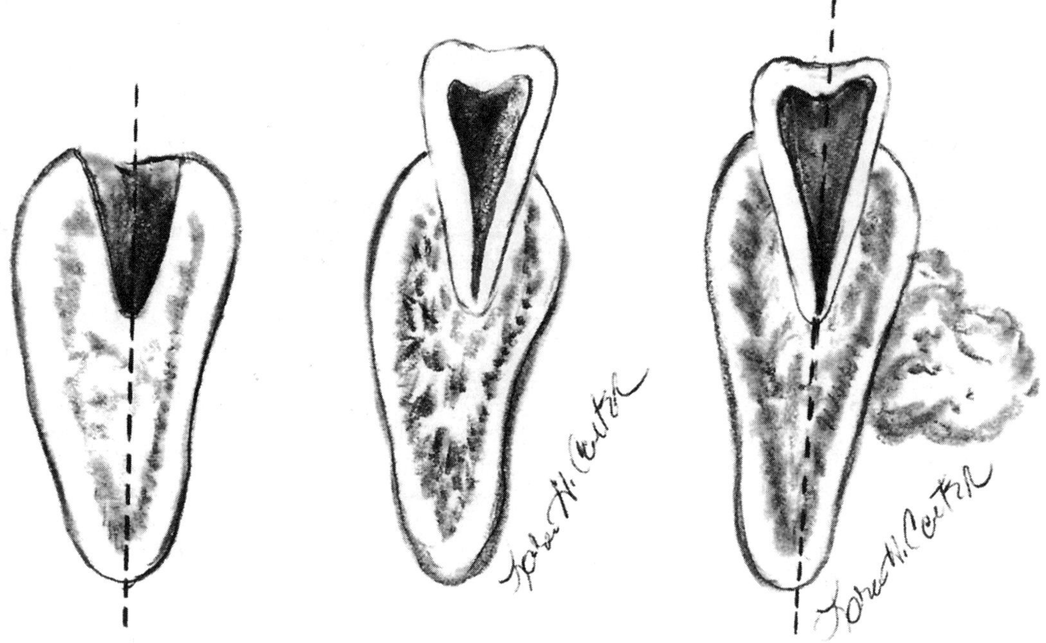

Figure 1.
Diagrammatic representation of a coronal resection of the mandible in edentulous and in the dentate mandible.

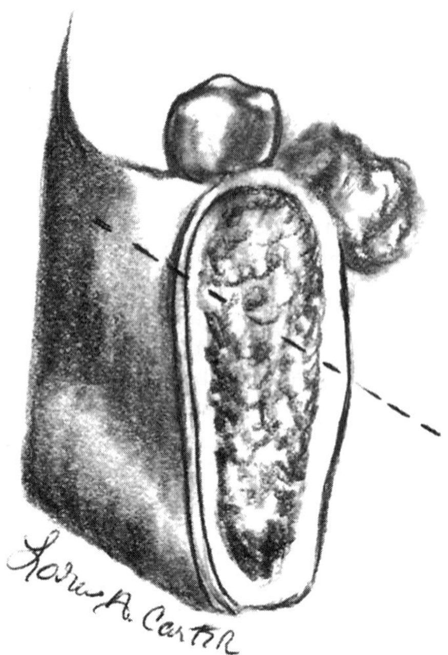

Figure 2.
Diagrammatic representation of a marginal resection of the mandible.

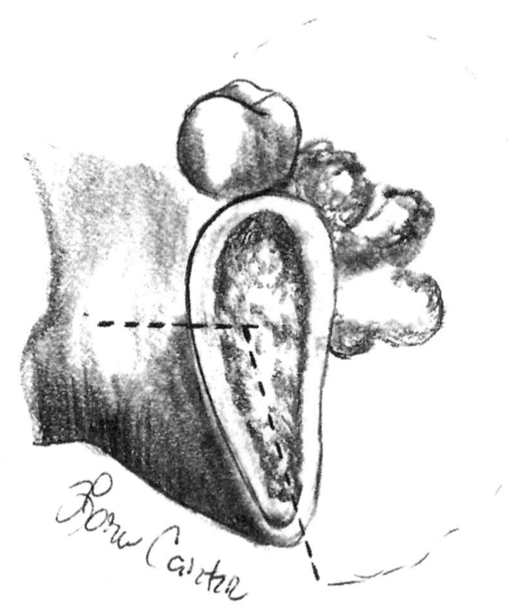

Figure 3.
Diagrammatic representation of a combined marginal-coronal resection of the mandible.

and, if necessary, bony cuts are made in the mouth. It is necessary to section the mylohyoid laterally and posteriorly without disturbing the tumor. The specimen with the attached bone is pushed backward and downward and delivered into the neck. This affords adequate visual and palpatory assessment of the "third" dimension of the tumor, which facilitates its resection.

Adequate resection of more advanced tumors requires a segmental mandibulectomy. The amount of mandible to be removed is still unsettled. Generally, the extent of the bone margins is based on clinical signs and radiographic findings. Three centimeters beyond macroscopic invasion is a reasonable guideline. The incidence of positive bone margins is quite low. However, if uncertain, bone marrow can be scooped from the mandible distal to the resection margin. This can be examined by frozen section by the pathologist. Alternatively, the pathologist can transect the mandible vertically using a band saw. Visual assessment of the gross extent of the tumor by the pathologist and surgeon is used to determine adequacy of the resection. Additional bone can be taken if the margins appear to be too close.

Reconstruction

The goals of reconstruction of FOM defects are (1) reliable primary healing of bone and soft tissue, (2) minimal contraction deformity, (3) minimal impairment of speech and swallowing, and (4) possible dental restoration.

Reconstruction of the resulting defect can often be easily accomplished by suturing the edge of the tongue to the alveolar mucosa. However, this type of primary closure usually causes anterior fixation of the tongue, which is aggravated by scarring and pronounced "dimpling" of the thinned anterior tongue. The result is a significant impairment of speech, cumbersome accumulation of saliva in the anterior oral cavity, and varying degrees of swallowing impairment. For these reasons, we prefer to use a skin graft or, if there is extensive exposure of bone or radiotherapy is anticipated, full-thickness flaps, such as unilateral or bilateral nasolabial flaps, provide excellent tissue coverage and better functional results. We do not favor using tongue flaps; they often result in tethering of the anterior tongue, with resultant difficulties in eating and speech. Tongue release and skin grafting may be required later. In a thin patient who has a large defect, a small radial forearm flap affords excellent reconstruction.

Vascularized bone free flaps may be harvested from the fibula, scapula, and radius. Success rates vary from 80 percent to 100 percent. Cosmetic appearance and functional outcome are better in primary reconstructions. Advantages of free flaps include a high success rate with experienced teams, good early function and cosmetic appearance, and the possibility of dental restoration. Disadvantages include the prolonged operative time involved and usually the need for two surgical teams. The procedures are technically difficult and are available only in medical centers that have experienced microvascular surgeons. In addition, free flaps may produce a significant donor defect and increase the blood loss.

Since the introduction of free bone flaps, vascularized bone pedicled flaps are used less often. The trapezius osteomyocutaneous flap has the advantage of a large piece of bone harvested from the crest of the shoulder blade; however, the venous return in the pedicle is variable and the arc of rotation of the flap is limited, often by the venous drainage. The pectoralis major muscle and attached rib suffers from a high failure rate because the blood supply to the rib from the muscle is minimal.

Mandibular Reconstruction Plates

In an effort to avoid donor site morbidity and reduce operative time, metal mandibular reconstruction plates can be covered by free or pedicled soft-tissue flaps. Titanium plates are better than stainless steel due to better biocompatibility and a hollow screw design that permits osseointegration, which lessens chances of bone atrophy and screw loosening.

Metal plates have problems with exposure during postoperative radiotherapy, including failure rates up to 40 percent. Increased scatter of radiation with plates of a high molecular weight metal increase the risk of osteoradionecrosis of the remaining mandible. Due to the pull of the soft tissue anteriorly, anterior plates have a higher failure rate and may fail even up to 6 years later. Lateral plates are more reliable, although the need for reconstruction of lateral defects, especially lateral to the mental foramen, is questionable.

■ TREATMENT OF THE NECK

Management of the N_0 Neck

Surgical treatment of the N_0 neck is preferred when surgery is selected for the treatment of the primary tumor, particularly when the expectations of controlling the primary tumor with surgery alone are reasonably good. In such cases (i.e., T_2 and selected T_3 tumors), appropriate dissection of the regional lymph nodes alone is, in most cases, sufficient to control the disease in the neck. However, postoperative radiotherapy may also be beneficial when the following features are found on histopathologic examination of the node dissection specimen(s):

- Presence of tumor in more than two or three lymph nodes
- Presence of tumor in multiple node groups.
- Presence of extracapsular spread (ECS) of tumor.

Surgical dissection of the cervical lymph nodes is also desirable when the neck must be entered, and certain structures, such as the hypoglossal nerve or the carotid artery, need to be exposed to facilitate adequate resection of the primary tumor.

In these cases we perform a *supraomohyoid neck dissection,* which consists of the en bloc removal of nodal regions I, II, and III. It is the preferred procedure for the surgical management of patients who have SCC of the oral cavity. The procedure is performed on both sides of the neck in patients who have cancers of the anterior tongue and floor of the mouth. A bilateral dissection is performed when the lesion is located at or near the midline.

Using the supraomohyoid dissection in this manner, the rate of recurrence in the neck ranges from zero when the nodes removed were histologically negative to 12.5 percent when there were multiple positive nodes or ECS.

Incorrect clinical staging of the N_0 neck occurs in approximately 20 percent of patients, even when imaging studies are used. Intraoperative palpation and inspection does not significantly improve the surgeon's ability to predict nodal stage. Thus, upstaging the neck without frozen section examination of suspected lymph nodes is not reliable. Although some authors recommend converting the selective dissection to a radical or modified radical neck dissection on the basis of the results of frozen sections, this is not necessary in our experience. Removal of the sternocleidomastoid muscle (SCM), the internal jugular vein (IJV), or the posterior triangle of the neck is not done unless these areas are obviously involved by tumor. The decision to extend a selective neck dissection to include the jugular vein, the spinal accessory nerve, or occasionally the hypoglossal or the vagus nerve is based on the findings at the time of surgery and on an objective assessment of the extent of nodal disease by the surgeon.

■ MANAGEMENT OF THE N^+ NECK

Surgery continues to be the mainstay in the treatment of patients who have palpable cervical lymph node metastases. The surgical treatment of the N^+ neck is, in our practice, a matter of surgical judgment, as we accept the premise that it is surgically feasible and oncologically sound to remove lymph nodes obviously involved by tumor, with the surrounding fibrofatty tissue of the neck, and without removing important uninvolved structures such as the spinal accessory nerve. In addition, with the judicious combination of surgery and radiotherapy, excellent tumor control in the neck can be obtained while preserving function and cosmesis. It cannot be overemphasized, however, that the main goal of the neck dissection is to *adequately* remove the tumor in the neck and that radiotherapy does not compensate for poor surgical judgment and technique. Preservation of adjacent structures should be pursued *only* when a clearly identifiable plane exists between the tumor and such a structure. Creation of a plane by cutting into the tumor and tumor spillage must be avoided.

Radiotherapy

Indications for radiotherapy of the primary tumor generally fall into four areas. First, T_1 or T_2 tumors can be safely treated for cure with radiotherapy. We tend to not recommend radiotherapy for smaller tumors because of the risk of osteoradionecrosis. Also, the high costs of the procedure and xerostomia are additional unfavorable features.

Second, T_3 or T_4 tumors usually require postoperative radiotherapy to improve the local control rate.

Third, surgical margins that are considered less than adequate require radiotherapy to improve the local control rate. However, we do not rely on radiotherapy to make up for poor surgical judgment. Every attempt should be made to ensure widely clear margins. The recurrence rate increases drastically when margins are microscopically positive.

Fourth, unfavorable pathologic findings, such as perineural or vascular (including lymphatic) invasion, also need radiotherapy to improve the local control rate.

Curative doses for the primary tumor are 65 to 70 Gy. They are usually delivered through opposing, bilateral cervicofacial fields that include the entire oral cavity and the upper echelon of regional lymphatics.

Brachytherapy, or interstitial irradiation, can be used after external beam therapy when indicated for unfavorable pathologic findings, such as close margins, but it increases the risk of osteoradionecrosis of the mandible.

Postoperative Radiotherapy of the Neck

Prophylactic irradiation of the N_0 neck can be accomplished with 50 Gy. Numerous studies have suggested that the rate of tumor recurrence in the N^+ neck is decreased by the addition of radiotherapy when multiple nodes are involved at multiple levels of the neck and when extra capsular spread

(ECS) of tumor is found. The timing and the dose of the radiotherapy is crucial if good regional control is to be achieved. Based on the results of a recent prospective clinical trial, it is recommended that patients who have advanced head and neck cancer be treated with daily fractions of 1.8 Gy, and receive a minimum postoperative dose of 57.6 Gy to the entire operative bed. Irradiation to sites of increased risk for recurrence, such as areas of the neck where ECS of the tumor was found, should be boosted to 63 Gy. Radiotherapy should be started as soon as possible after surgery. Some studies have suggested that a delay in the initiation of radiotherapy beyond 6 weeks may compromise tumor control.

Perioperative Care

Prophylactic antibiotics include, most often, an inexpensive second-generation cephalosporin such as cefoperazone. Coverage can be extended to anaerobes with clindamycin.

Generally, the patient is hospitalized for 3 to 10 days. Tube feedings are continued until the intraoral wounds have healed or the bolsters for skin grafts are removed. Low pressure is applied to the drains until the drainage is less than 30 cc per day for 2 days. Oral care with chlorhexidene gluconate rinses or toothettes should be done two to three times per day. Sutures are removed from the neck in 5 to 7 days; we remove them in about 10 days in previously irradiated patients.

Follow-Up

Follow-up visits are scheduled on an individual basis to observe for recurrence of the primary tumor; survey for development of second primary tumors; watch for morbidity from treatment (speech and swallowing problems, wound care); provide social and psychological support; and deal with comorbidity not directly related to the cancer itself. Regular visits should be scheduled during radiotherapy to help with pain control, nutritional support, and possible candidiasis.

Generally, visits should be every 1 to 3 months during the first year, 2 to 4 months in the second year, 3 to 6 months in the third year, 4 to 6 in the fourth and fifth years, and yearly thereafter. Yearly evaluations include chest radiographs (for detecting metastases, second primaries); liver enzymes; and thyroid function tests (for those who received radiotherapy).

Suggested Reading

Gulliamondegui O, Oliver B, Hayden R. Cancer of the anterior floor of the mouth—selective choice of treatment and analysis of failures. Am J Surg 1980; 140:560-562.

Medina J, Byers R. Supraomohyoid neck dissection: Rationale, indications, and surgical technique. Head Neck 1989; 11:111-122.

Mohit-Tabatabai M, Sobel H, Rush B, Mashberg A. Relation of thickness of floor of mouth: Stage I and II cancers to regional metastasis. Am J Surg 1986; 152:351-353.

Shaha A, Spiro R, Shah J. Strong E. Squamous carcinoma of the floor of the mouth. Am J Surg 1984; 148:455-459.

Spiro R, Huvos A, Wong G, Spiro J, Gnecco C, Strong E. Predictive value of tumor thickness in squamous carcinoma confined to the tongue and floor of the mouth. Am J Surg 1986; 152:345-350.

CANCER OF THE HARD PALATE

The method of
Edward C. Weisberger

Cancers of the hard palate are of two types—squamous cell carcinoma and minor salivary gland malignancies, the latter being slightly more common. A neoplasm of the minor salivary glands is more likely to be malignant than not, in contrast to neoplasms arising in the parotid gland. Seventy percent of salivary gland tumors of the hard palate are malignant, and most of these are adenoid cystic carcinoma. Mucoepidermoid carcinoma, the most common malignancy involving the parotid glands, is next in frequency for the hard palate. Malignant neoplasms seen far less frequently are lymphoma, extramedullary plasmacytoma, osteogenic sarcoma, melanoma, and Kaposi's sarcoma.

Adenoid cystic carcinoma involving the hard palate is usually seen as a nonulcerative submucosal swelling centered between the midline of the palate and the back of the maxillary alveolus and at the junction of the hard and soft palate. This corresponds to the area of greatest density of minor salivary glands on the palate.

There is no known cause or risk factor related to minor salivary gland malignancies of the palate. Their nonulcerative nature and frequent indolent growth pattern often give the clinician who first sees the patient a false sense of security, which can result in delayed biopsy and therefore delayed diagnosis.

In contrast, squamous cell carcinomas of the hard palate usually occur in cigarette smokers and may be preceded by leukoplakic or erythroleukoplakic changes of the mucosa. They can be located in the central portion of the hard palate or on the alveolus.

The hard palate is the bony roof of the oral cavity and consists of the premaxilla anteriorly, the palatine process of the maxilla behind the premaxilla, and the horizontal portion of the palatine bone. The bone is covered by mucosa that contains numerous minor salivary glands. The mucosa is tightly applied to the underlying periosteum with essentially no loose submucosal stroma. For this reason, any lesion originating in the minor salivary glands is, by definition, intimately related to the underlying bone.

It is worthwhile to briefly consider paths of egress from the hard palate. This aids in understanding the extension of tumor beyond this region. The greater palatine foramen is located between the midline and the second maxillary molar tooth and transmits the descending palatine artery and greater palatine nerve. The latter is a branch of the second division of the fifth cranial nerve. Neurotropic tumors, such as adenoid cystic carcinoma, can invade this nerve and extend to the skull base near the foramen rotundum and, through the latter, can be transmitted to the intracranial cavity in the region of the gasserian ganglion (Fig. 1). Malignancies arising near the alveolus can extend into the maxillary sinus superiorly, and from there they can extend to the inferior portion of the orbit. More posteriorly located neoplasms can gain access to the orbit through the inferior orbital fissure. Extension of tumor to the pterygomaxillary fissure provides access to the infratemporal fossa and therefore to the skull base.

■ EVALUATION

Evaluation of the patient who has a malignancy of the hard palate begins with the history and physical examination. Numbness of the palate or cheek may indicate involvement of V_2. If diplopia is reported, orbital involvement or even extension to the cavernous sinus may have occurred. The examiner should look for evidence of decreased sensation on the palate or cheek. The status of cervical nodes should, of course, be assessed, but metastatic nodes in the upper neck are quite unusual. Endoscopic evaluation of the nasal cavity and nasopharynx is performed. Tumor can be appreciated extending into the floor of the nose, indicating invasion through the bony palate. A computed tomographic (CT) scan of the head and neck is useful in evaluating for bony destruction extension to the maxillary, ethmoid or sphenoid sinuses; fovea ethmoidalis; cribriform plate; or orbit. Scrutiny of the skull base on CT scan can detect widening of the pterygopalatine canal or foramen rotundum. Magnetic resonance imaging (MRI) is more sensitive for detecting soft-tissue extension above the cribriform plate or fovea ethmoidalis to the dura and brain. MRI is also useful in assessing invasion of the second division of the fifth nerve, and extension into the orbit via the infraorbital fissure. Cavernous sinus involvement by more extensive tumors can often be best appreciated on MRI.

Diagnosis depends on adequate biopsy and histologic interpretation. Utilization of a disposable dermatologic punch (as made by Miltex Instrument Company, Lake Success, New York) provides a nontraumatized specimen that facilitates correct interpretation by the pathologist.

A standard chest radiograph should be obtained. Patients with squamous cell carcinoma usually have a history of smoking and may have coexisting bronchogenic carcinoma. Patients who have adenoid cystic carcinoma frequently exhibit pulmonary metastasis.

Pretreatment dental evaluation is an important adjunct. Inflammatory dental disease requiring immediate therapy, such as a periradicular abscess, is sometimes identified. If a through-and-through resection of the bony palate is contemplated, a dental impression is made, and a temporary prosthesis, usually of clear acrylic, is fashioned, to be placed in the operating room for immediate obturation of the defect, and to secure packing placed in the defect for hemostasis. Construction of a permanent prosthesis is delayed until contraction and final healing of the defect have occurred. Preoperative dental evaluation also initiates the patient into a vigorous program of dental hygiene that is especially important if radiotherapy is part of the treatment plan.

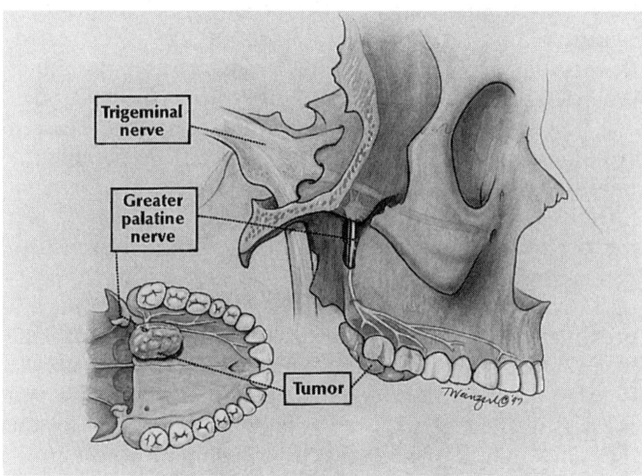

Figure 1.
Adenoid cystic carcinomas can involve the greater palatine nerve and therefore extend to the skull base at the foramen rotundum.

■ SURGICAL THERAPY

Transoral Local Resection

The treatment of cancer of the hard palate is primarily surgical. Superficial carcinomas of the hard palate that are minimally invasive carcinoma in situ or severe dysplasia on histologic evaluation often require resection of mucosa only, with an adequate soft-tissue margin, and preservation of underlying bone. This avoids a through-and-through defect and therefore the necessity for an obturating prosthesis. Squamous cell carcinomas of the hard palate usually occur in cigarette smokers and therefore may be part of a field cancerization phenomenon. Careful inspection of the entire mucosa of the oral cavity and aerodigestive tract is critical. This inspection can be augmented with magnification using loupes and/or the operating microscope to allow detection of mucosal abnormalities not appreciated with the naked eye. In a similar manner, toluidine blue staining can be used to detect subtle mucosal abnormalities that require biopsy or resection.

Salivary gland tumors originating in the hard palate almost always mandate resection of underlying bone. These neoplasms originate in submucosal minor salivary glands. The mucosa and submucosa of the hard palate are tightly connected to the underlying periosteum, forming a mucoperiosteum, and therefore any neoplasm arising in submucosal structures immediately abuts or invades the bony palatal plate. As previously mentioned, the most common site of origin for salivary gland tumors is the junction of the hard and soft palate just lateral to the midline. This places the neoplasm in close proximity to the greater palatine foramen, which transmits the greater palatine nerve. The histologic type is usually adenoid cystic carcinoma, which has a propensity for nerve invasion. For these reasons, the greater palatine nerve should usually be monitored by frozen section. If nerve invasion is identified, the greater palatine nerve is traced proximally to the foramen rotundum. If the second division of the fifth cranial nerve has positive findings at this point, or if preoperative enlargement of the foramen rotundum has been appreciated radiographically, resection of the distal portion of the gasserian ganglion may be required via a lateral frontotemporal craniotomy. When a nerve is invaded by adenoid cystic carcinoma, it is well documented that skip areas can occur. Therefore, invasion of any portion of the greater palatine nerve requires postoperative treatment with radiotherapy that includes the skull base.

Lesions that involve the palate more superficially or that invade only the inferior portion of the maxillary sinus can be approached transorally without an external incision. Adenoid cystic carcinoma that invades the inferior portion of the maxillary sinus requires resection of the mucosa of that sinus in its entirety, because microscopic submucosal spread is not infrequent.

Partial Maxillectomy

Extension of neoplasm to the roof of the maxillary sinus, ethmoid labyrinth, or pterygoid region requires a more formal partial maxillectomy performed through a Weber-Ferguson incision that follows the alar facial groove and splits the upper lip. The fundamental principles of this technique are well described elsewhere. It is necessary to transect the nasal lacrimal system to allow lateral retraction of the orbit. This should be done at the widest portion of the lacrimal sac to minimize postoperative stenosis. Another useful maneuver to prevent stenosis is the creation of a small incision in the anterior wall of the sac that parallels the long axis of the sac. This incision creates two anterior leaves of mucosa that can be tacked back to adjacent periorbita with a 4–0 resorbable suture. This technique, combined with the usually necessary resection of the bone of the medial maxilla and lamina papyracea, simply and effectively creates a dacryocystorhinostomy. A 4–0 polydiaxinone (PDS) suture is placed through the periorbita in the approximate location of the trochlea and then to soft tissues in the deeper portion of the opposite side of the alar facial incision. In a similar manner, the medial canthal tendon is sutured to deeper soft tissues on the apposing aspect of the incision. These maneuvers help avoid postoperative diplopia due to malposition of the trochlea and also postoperative rounding and deformity of the medial canthal region.

Orbital Reconstruction

In some instances, neoplasm involves the bony floor of the orbit but does not invade the orbital soft tissues. Preservation of the orbital contents can be accomplished if the inferior periorbita readily elevates from the surface of the bony orbital floor. When this situation arises, reconstruction of the orbital floor is readily accomplished with .040 Silastic sheeting used to create a hammock for the orbital contents. This is anchored medially using a 2–0 Prolene suture passed through a drill hole in the glabellar region and laterally, by a similar suture, passed around the remaining zygomatic arch. The Silastic hammock effectively prevents inferior displacement of the orbital contents, but does not allow synechial attachments to occur that would prevent movement of the globe and extraocular muscles. The latter is more likely to occur if autogenous material is used to reconstruct the orbit. The Silastic sheeting can be covered by a skin graft. Laterally it usually becomes exposed at the upper portion of the maxillectomy defect, but does not cause granulation tissue or infection, and virtually never needs to be removed.

Craniofacial Resection

More extensive tumors extending to the skull base may require craniofacial resection. Resection of the cribriform plate or fovea ethmoidalis is most safely accomplished if concomitant exposure of the anterior fossae is achieved from above via frontal craniotomy. As mentioned, resection of the gasserian ganglion and exposure of Meckel's cave is usually accomplished using a lateral frontotemporal approach. Resection of a portion of the cavernous sinus in the intracranial portion of the carotid artery can be technically achieved, but it is questionable whether this has an impact on survival.

Palatal Reconstruction

Maxillofacial Obturator

The nasal maxillary defect is packed. In large defects, a 36 inch roll of Xeroform gauze is used. The temporary prosthesis is very valuable in supporting this packing and allowing for early postoperative oral nutrition. The prosthesis is anchored by metal clasps to the maxillary teeth if most of these have been retained. If the patient is edentulous or a significant portion of the dental apparatus has been resected, the prosthesis is anchored using a circumzygomatic suture of No. 24 stainless steel wire or 2–0 Prolene passed through drill holes in the lateral lip of the prosthesis. These are passed around the zygoma using a wire-passing awl. Sometimes the inferior portion of the nasal septum or the inferior nasal turbinates prevent correct seating of the prosthesis. When this occurs, these structures can be conservatively resected.

Because the defect in the palate contracts during the postoperative period, a final prosthesis is not fashioned for approximately 2 months. A new dental impression must be made at this time to allow fabrication of this final prosthesis. If a significant portion of the maxilla has been resected and the patient is edentulous or has few remaining teeth on the maxillary arch, it may be difficult to retain an acrylic prosthesis. Sometimes an osseointegrated device permanently placed in bone can facilitate retention of the prosthesis in these situations. This may require secondary bone grafting to provide adequate bone for anchoring the osseointegrated device. Bone grafting and placement of an osseointegrated device are difficult to achieve if the oral cavity has been heavily irradiated.

Permanent Prosthesis

The most common method of rehabilitating a through-and-through defect in the palate is, as mentioned, using an acrylic maxillofacial prosthesis. Other options exist and include reconstruction employing a regional flap or free tissue transfer from a distant site. The ideal situation for prosthetic rehabilitation is a small to moderate-sized defect, with preservation of at least one-half of the teeth on the dental arch (the teeth being in relatively good condition). This permits solid retention of the prosthesis. If any postoperative trismus exists from fibrosis, intermittent removal of the prosthesis for cleaning and oral hygiene will be inhibited. If the surgical defect includes a significant portion of the soft palate, prosthetic rehabilitation becomes more challenging. A maxillofacial prosthesis readily rehabilitates the adynamic hard palate but cannot easily provide the dynamic changes that are an integral part of soft palate function. If the prosthesis is of inadequate length, velopalatal insufficiency will occur, causing interference with speech and deglutition because air and liquids intermittently escape into the nasal space. However, when the prosthesis is long enough to more adequately cover the soft palate defect, stimulation of the posterior pharyngeal wall sometimes occurs, with gagging and nontolerance of the prosthesis.

Flap Reconstruction

Flap reconstruction is an alternative, but again, dynamic function that completely rehabilitates a soft palate defect is not possible to achieve. With small to moderate-sized defects, a temporalis flap can be employed. Transfer of distant tissue, such as a free flap, can be accomplished if the appropriate microvascular expertise is available. Indications for free tissue transfer for reconstruction are a near-total palate defect with absent dentition precluding adequate retention of a maxillofacial prosthesis, and orbital exenteration performed concomitantly with maxillectomy. When orbital exenteration is combined with extensive resection of the ethmoid labyrinth and a portion of the malar eminence, free flap reconstruction is preferred. This permits obliteration of an unsightly orbital sinus defect, restores facial contour, and obliterates the defect in the palate. It should be noted that obliteration of the defect with a free flap prevents inspection of the cavity and surveillance for recurrence by this method. On the other hand, after such an extensive resection of soft tissues, usually combined with postoperative radiotherapy, recurrence is usually at the skull base and is not often amenable to further treatment for cure.

Radiotherapy

Radiotherapy can be used as primary treatment for more limited lesions. Superficial but invasive squamous cell carcinomas that occupy a significant portion of the soft palate may be best treated with external beam radiotherapy to avoid the significant morbidity attendant with surgical resection of the dynamic palate. Also problematic are squamous cell carcinomas that involve the gingiva and extend into the interdental spaces. In such cases, it can be difficult to be confident of a total surgical resection of disease if the teeth are preserved. An alternative is external beam radiotherapy employing a spacer that pushes the tongue inferiorly while radiation is being delivered, thus avoiding the morbidity of irradiation of the lower portion of the oral cavity and submandibular salivary glands. Another alternative for a superficial lesion that extends between the teeth is the construction of a maxillofacial prosthesis from a dental impression that will carry a radiation source, such as that used for brachytherapy of neoplasms. Usually, hollow tubes are incorporated into the prosthesis that are later afterloaded with iridium. Such brachytherapy is accomplished in a period of 2 days, during which time the patient is hospitalized for purposes of radiation quarantine. A rather intense initial mucositis, often with fibrinous changes, occurs. This condition diminishes over the next 3 to 4 weeks. Most of the salivary glands of the lower oral cavity are spared, minimizing xerostomia. Preservation of a good portion of the salivary output also diminishes the likelihood of severe dental caries. A significant drawback is heavy irradiation to the bone around the teeth, which increases the likelihood of future dental problems.

Indications for combined surgery and external beam therapy, given pre- or postoperatively, are tumors with a high-grade histology, large lesions over 3 cm in diameter, bone destruction, large nerve invasion, cervical metastasis, and extension to adjacent anatomic areas such as the upper maxillary and ethmoid sinuses and the oropharynx. It is controversial whether small adenoid cystic carcinomas that exhibit none of the aforementioned adverse criteria require adjunctive radiotherapy. Favorable-prognosis adenoid cystic carcinomas of the hard palate seem to be more amenable to cure by surgical resection alone than when these tumors occur in other sites of the head and neck.

Complications of radiotherapy include xerostomia, trismus due to fibrosis of the muscles of mastication, osteoradionecrosis of the palate and maxilla, and dental caries. Complications of surgical therapy include the usual acute postoperative problems and velopalatal insufficiency (especially if a significant portion of the soft palate was concomitantly resected). Trismus from scarring and contracture in the area of the muscles of mastication can also be a postoperative problem. As was previously mentioned, resection of a major portion of the hard palate coupled with absence of teeth for anchorage can severely compromise attempts at rehabilitation of the defect with a maxillofacial prosthesis.

Suggested Reading

Beckhardt RN, Weber RS, Zane R, et al. Minor salivary gland tumors of the palate: Clinical and pathologic correlates of outcome. Laryngoscope 1955; 105:1155-1160.

Kraut RA, Kabzenell J, Silken D, Ruben JS. Endosteal implants following tumor surgery and avulsive trauma. Laryngoscope 1994; 104:504-512.

CARCINOMA OF THE TONGUE BASE

The method of
Charles W. Cummings

Carcinoma of the base of the tongue is at the very least an unpleasant disease usually characterized by a delay in diagnosis or a frustrating therapeutic course and agonizing demise of the patient. Tumors of the tongue base are almost invariably squamous cell carcinoma, and they may frequently spill into other areas of the oropharynx. Although malignant tumors of the base of the tongue occur classically in older persons, there is evidence of some changes in pattern of incidence, such as an increased incidence in women and younger people, and—when considering all lingual malignant tumors—an increased percentage arising in the base of the tongue.

As pointed out by Callery, the overall cure rates for carcinoma of the tongue have not risen significantly in the past 25 years despite improvements in diagnosis as well as major therapeutic advances.

■ DIAGNOSIS

Certainly one of the pernicious aspects of carcinoma of the base of the tongue is the relative paucity of symptoms while the tumor is in an early stage. The hypopharynx may harbor a neoplasm in a most clandestine fashion until its sheer bulk heralds its presence. To be sure, a persistent sore throat, referred otalgia, and actual dysphagia may announce the presence of a lesion early in its course; however, this is not the usual pattern. More frequently, a mass in the neck signifying either direct extension or cervical nodal metastasis directs the patient's, and subsequently the physician's, attention to the hypopharynx. Compromise of the supraglottic airway or a minor impairment in the ability to speak usually arise in the later stages of the disease. Frequently, the patient knows that something is amiss and attempts to find a solution to the symptoms; and yet, because an indirect examination of the hypopharynx is not a routine diagnostic measure, the tumor is missed until the patient is referred to a head and neck surgeon for evaluation. It is also true that not all base of the tongue tumors are exophytic. Some may be deeply infiltrative yet produce limited distortion of the overlying mucosa. It is these tumors that are missed most frequently.

With respect to diagnosis, the symptoms point to the oropharynx if they are heard by a well-tuned clinical ear. A competent head and neck examination, including indirect laryngogscopy, most frequently divulges the tumor. Direct palpation remains an indispensable part of the physical examination. Unless the base of the tongue is palpated, previously described infiltrative submucosal tumor can elude visual detection. If suspicion is aroused, panendoscopy must be considered to biopsy the suspicious area and to ascertain that there are no other areas in the upper aerodigestive tract that house a second primary tumor. Computed tomography and magnetic resonance imaging contribute substantially to the seminal information needed for precise staging. Once the diagnosis of carcinoma has been established, a search for distant metastases should be made; if they are found, a radical therapeutic procedure would obviously not be entertained.

Characteristically, base of tongue tumors are exophytic and are represented by poor differentiation, which may account for the predictable therapeutic response to chemotherapy-radiotherapy, but may also account for the high incidence of recurrence at the primary site and for the high level of distant metastases. Certainly one of the most ominous histologic signs is perineural invasion by tumor.

■ THERAPY

Deciding which modality to use as primary therapy for these tumors is a multifactorial process. What must be taken into consideration are not only the age, general health, and lifestyle of the patient, but also the realities of cure. At what point is the choice of a surgically aggressive mode of therapy with a higher incidence of cure (in addition to an acknowledged short-term, surgically induced disability) indicated? When considering modalities of treatment, let us consider that the foe (tumor), unlike the surgeon, does not take into account anatomic limitations. An undertreated tumor of the tongue continues to proliferate, to the increasing despair of the patient. There is no doubt that primary radiotherapy alone, even when delivered solely from an external source, results in a low percentage of 5 year cures. However, some patients treated by primary radiotherapy whose tumors fail to resolve at the primary site may be salvaged by an aggressive surgical procedure. The total number of cures may, in fact, approximate the number of patients who are treated by extensive surgical resection and postoperative radiotherapy. Riley and associates have shown that the local control of tongue base tumors may be achieved 47 percent of the time with radiotherapy, and in Riley and co-workers' study, if surgery is used in combination with radiotherapy, the 5 year local control rate is 78 percent. On the surface, this would appear to be a stroke very much in favor of combined therapy. The overall survival figures for both groups, however, were the same, primarily because of the presence of second or third malignant tumors or distant metastases. This pattern of additional primary tumors or distant metastases is now well established in the literature. What, then, are the advantages of each modality when treating tumors at the base of the tongue? And what is the role of organ-preservation protocols?

Radiotherapy administered at curative levels in the base of the tongue results in a painful sore throat because of the associated radiation-induced mucositis, a diminution in salivary flow, and hence impaired deglutition secondary to relative absence of saliva, and frequently chronic mucosal changes and edema of the supraglottic larynx, which thereby causes hoarseness, local pain, and aspiration. Adjunctive use of interstitial irradiation increases the potential for local induration and increases the difficulty of adequate post-therapeutic follow-up. The proponents of radiotherapy as the primary modality point out that the anatomic abnormalities caused by extensive surgery can be avoided, and the dreaded side effects of pronounced impairment of speech may be mitigated. Perhaps the most compelling argument in my mind for surgical intervention is the ability to increase control of direct extension and cervical nodal metastases. This can less readily be accomplished by radiotherapy alone. The image of the patient with a partial mandibulectomy, subtotal glossectomy , and a radical neck dissection does not adequately, I believe, reflect the status of surgical therapy today. Advances in surgical technique, as reflected by the development of free tissue transfer, which contributes both epithelium to cover large raw surfaces and muscle to fill the surgically created void, allow for greater ease in alimentation, and even articulation, despite very large alterations in anatomy.

Subtotal or total glossectomy obviously courts a much higher incidence of aspiration, and thus management of the larynx becomes an integral part of the surgical technique. Methods to suspend the larynx out of the main flow of foods, as well as diversionary procedures such as the epiglottic sew-down, allow preservation of this organ and its ability to function in the face of a markedly distorted oropharynx. Indeed, the total glossectomy formerly was a procedure to be considered only in concert with a total laryngectomy to prevent the dreaded problem of aspiration. Now, many in the field believe that the larynx may be spared because of ability to reconstruct with bulky myocutaneous flaps, such as that from the pectoralis muscle or rectus abdominis or latissimus free flap. The neural anastomosis has potential to enhance tone as well. The transferred bulk allows the patient to articulate to a level of intelligibility. Aspiration, although always present to some minor degree, is not severe enough in most cases to merit a conversion laryngectomy at a second setting.

A most significant surgical advance involves the method of exposure to a tumor at the base of the tongue. Unless the periosteum is involved by tumor extension, a composite resection need not be performed. Equal surgical access may be accomplished by performing a midline osteotomy and then swinging the mandible laterally as the dissection is carried posteriorly along the floor of the mouth. The use of this procedure or the alternative midline glossotomy has all but eliminated the need for a partial mandibulectomy for surgical exposure in the absence of periosteal involvement.

There is no quarrel with sacrifice of the spinal accessory nerve when it is ultimately associated with a nodal metastasis of the base of the skull. Preservation of the nerve, unless it is intimately involved with tumor, has, I believe, increased the postoperative functional status of the patient significantly, and as further results unfold, I predict a greater adoption of procedures that spare the spinal accessory nerve. If one is to employ postoperative radiotherapy designed to enhance the control of histologic residual disease, the rationale for accessory nerve preservation becomes yet more reasonable. Thus, we have many documented improvements in the technique of surgical treatment that aid in the cosmetic and functional rehabilitation of the patient.

Total glossectomy must be considered the most drastic surgical maneuver in the armamentarium of head and neck surgeons, and obviously the question arises as to whether this surgery is justified, and to what end. Razack and colleague noted a 25 percent 2 year survival, certainly an admirable cure rate for advanced-stage disease. Sixty percent of these 45 patients had, in addition, laryngeal preservation, and six of those 27 patients subsequently had a conversion laryngectomy because of uncontrollable aspiration, leaving 21 of 45 patients with their larynges intact. The head and neck surgeon must be assured that preservation of the larynx results in adequate surgical resection and must avoid the potential for leaving residual microscopic disease. Harrison has found histologic extension of infiltrating base of the tongue tumors into the pre-epiglottic space. Extension of tumor into the supraglottic larynx mandates a total laryngectomy in concert with total glossectomy. The decision to embark on such an aggressive therapeutic course rests with the surgeon, the family, and, above all, the patient. As painful as it may be, full disclosure of the sequelae of this disease and of the therapeutic maneuvers remains central to good patient management. The concept of organ preservation as the treatment of oropharyngeal carcinoma has emerged on the heels of the successful laryngeal protocols. Evidence is mounting now that advanced-stage disease may well respond as favorably as when surgery and radiotherapy are used primarily. Surgical rescue may be associated with escalated perioperative morbidity; however, preservation of function seems worth the risk.

Suggested Reading

Callery CD, Spiro RH, Strong EW. Changing trends in the management of squamous carcinoma of the tongue. Am J Surg 1984;148:449-454.

Cumming C, Goepfert H, Myers E. Squamous cell carcinoma of the base of the tongue. Head Neck Surg 1986;9:56-59.

Razack MS, Sako K, Bakamjian VY, Shedd DP. Total glossectomy. Am J Surg 1983;146:509-511.

Riley RW, Fee WE, Jr, Goffinet D, et al. Squamous cell carcinoma of the base of the tongue. Otolaryngol Head Neck Surg 1983;91:143-150.

SUPRAGLOTTIC CARCINOMA

The method of
Ernest A. Weymuller, Jr.
by
Brendan Curran Stack, Jr.
Ernest A. Weymuller, Jr.

Management of laryngeal squamous cell carcinoma has become more diverse in the last decade with the development of organ-sparing approaches. However, not all lesions are best treated by a chemotherapy-radiotherapy approach, even though avoiding surgery is an attractive option for many patients. Skill and judgment are required to balance the objective of tumor eradication against the therapeutic morbidity for any given modality. Nowhere in the head and neck are the challenges of therapeutic decision making better demonstrated than in the treatment of malignant lesions of the supraglottic larynx.

Discussion in this chapter is confined to the diagnosis and treatment of squamous cell carcinoma of the supraglottic larynx based on the treatment preferences of the senior author (Fig. 1). Boundaries of the supraglottic larynx are considered to be the volume of the larynx superior to the horizontal plane at the level of the junction of the laryngeal ventricle and the most lateral dorsum of the true vocal cord. Staging terminology uses the tumor, nodes, and metastases (TNM) system of the American Joint Committee on Cancer (1992).

■ PATIENT EVALUATION

An accurate history and detailed physical examination with an emphasis on the head and neck is the first step in managing patients who have supraglottic carcinoma (SGC). Elements of the history that may later prove significant in therapeutic decision making include functional status, vocation, socioeconomic resources, chemical dependency, coexisting medical illness, and the likelihood of compliance with therapy. Given the many options that exist to treat various stages of SGC, a thorough knowledge of each patient's unique circumstances is crucial in order to provide the best counsel. In instances of advanced disease, these considerations may not impact significantly the choice of therapy but will assist in the logistics of treatment delivery so as to maximize compliance and decrease morbidity.

Physical examination should focus on the status of the patient's airway and extent of locoregional disease. Flexible fiberoptic laryngoscopy offers the best view of the upper aerodigestive tract in the clinic. Occasionally, patients with advanced SGC have obstructive symptoms that require urgent or emergent airway management. Care should be taken with these patients to place a surgical airway at a distance away from the primary tumor to avoid violation of the tumor.

Imaging studies are particularly important in the evaluation of both the primary lesion and regional metastasis. Information obtained from computed tomography (CT) allows for more accurate staging (presence or absence of preepiglottic space involvement), operative planning regarding therapy for the neck, and determination of carotid artery involvement with tumor. Axial CT scanning with intravenous iodinated contrast is the preferred modality. Magnetic resonance (MR) scanning is usually reserved for assessment of recurrent disease or as a means of surveillance when the physical examination is somehow compromised by anatomic deformity, flap reconstruction, or fibrosis.

All SGC patients need a traditional operative endoscopy with biopsy for further assessment of disease extent, the presence of multiple primary neoplasms, and/or airway management issues. All patients require a basic metastatic evaluation, including a chest radiograph and liver function tests; some patients may also require a thoracoabdominal CT scan in cases of advanced locoregional disease or equivocal or positive findings on screening examinations.

■ THERAPEUTIC OPTIONS: PRIMARY DISEASE

Endoscopic Resection

Endoscopic resection of SGC offers a quick, cost-effective means to treat T_1-N_0 lesions of the suprahyoid epiglottic fold. Resection can be combined with diagnostic endoscopy and biopsy, which results in one operative encounter.

With a CO_2 laser, endoscopic excision offers decreased operative complexity and diminished postoperative edema. Microscopic laryngoscopy offers improved operative visibility, control of bleeding, enhanced adequacy of excision, and the likelihood of local control. A brief, effective, and oncologically sound procedure can be performed with decreased cost and morbidity for the patient.

Infrahyoid T_1 as well as T_2 and larger lesions of the supraglottic larynx are less suited to the endoscopic approach. Adequacy of excision margins is of primary concern because these tumors can be bulky, involve more than one anatomic subsite, and extend beyond the confines of the larynx (preepiglottic space). Frequently, the proximal (caudal) and deep margins are inadequately excised due to limited visibility or access. Moreover, because all T_2 lesions have a substantial risk of cervical node involvement, the best surgical plan is to resect the primary tumor in conjunction with bilateral neck dissection. Other treatment modalities that offer simultaneous treatment of the primary as well as the neck may be considered in these cases.

Conservation Laryngeal Surgery

Although endoscopic resection is a conservation-based approach to tumor excision, the term classically refers to open laryngeal procedures resulting in the removal of part of the larynx while maintaining a remnant of the organ capable of phonation and airway protection. In the treatment of supraglottic primaries, this approach takes the form of the

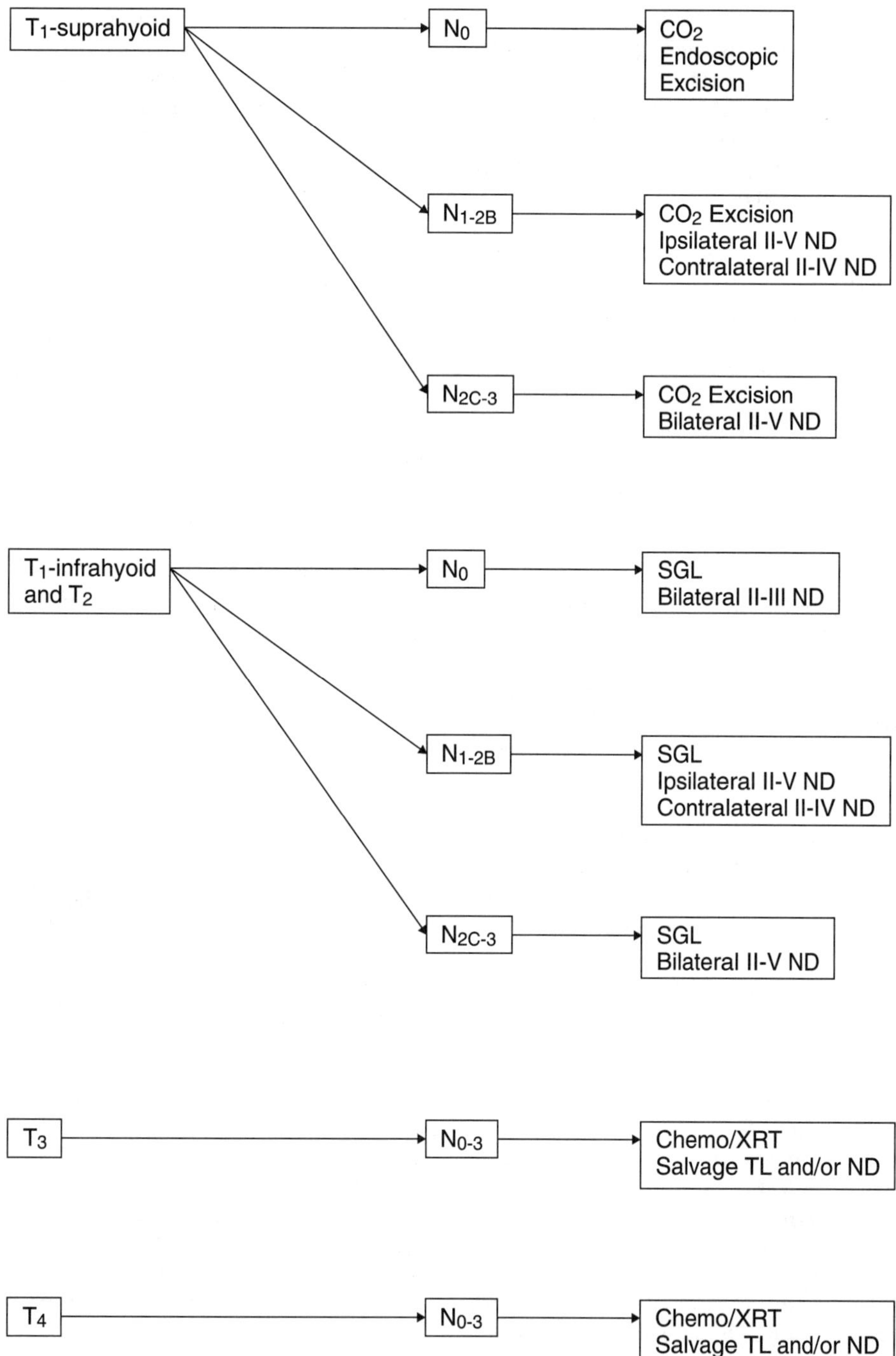

Figure 1.
Treatment preferences based on tumor (T) and node (N) status. SGL, supraglottic laryngectomy; ND, neck dissection; XRT, radiotherapy; TL, total laryngectomy.

supraglottic (horizontal hemi-) laryngectomy. Although this approach gives local control comparable to primary radiotherapy for T_1 disease and slightly superior control for T_2, its use has been limited in some centers by the superior swallowing results seen with primary radiotherapy. T_3 and greater disease as well as poor pulmonary function (forced expiratory volume < 1.0) are contraindications to supraglottic laryngectomy.

Recovery from this procedure is variable and can result in prolonged periods requiring tracheotomy or enteral nutrition. These considerations have been a disincentive for using this technique as a primary treatment for SGC. The morbidity from this procedure can be minimized by using a number of surgical maneuvers such as (1) preservation of at least one internal branch of the superior laryngeal nerve, (2) avoidance of arytenoid injury, (3) making laryngeal cartilage cuts under direct vision after the supraglottis is exposed, and (4) preserving and resuspending the larynx to the hyoid.

For N^+ and T_2 and higher disease, bilateral surgical treatment of the neck is recommended. Postoperative radiotherapy may be indicated in cases of angioinvasion, extracapsular spread, or involvement of resected margins with microscopic disease. If the primary margins are free of disease and the neck specimens are pathologically staged as N_{0-1}, radiotherapy may be held in reserve.

Conservation procedures may be used for early recurrences or small treatment failures following primary radiotherapy administered for T_{1-2} disease. Poor vocalization and aspiration are accentuated in the setting of irradiation failure, and permanent tracheostomy is often required. Occasionally, these patients will require a completion laryngectomy for intractable aspiration, chronic pain, or recurrent disease.

Primary Radiotherapy

Primary radiotherapy has been the principal nonsurgical treatment for SGC. When used for T_{1-2} N_{0-1} lesions, it offers the advantages of excellent control of locoregional disease (T_1 = 90 percent, T_2 = 76 percent), with minimal morbidity to voice and swallowing. The disadvantages of this therapy are its protracted length, single-use option, pharyngeal edema, mucositis, and the difficulties associated with postirradiation surgery.

Primary radiotherapy has been less effective for locoregional control of larger primary disease (T_3 = 61 percent, T_4 = 44 percent). It has generally been given with the understanding that total laryngectomy and neck dissection(s) are possible in the event of local or regional failure. Primary radiotherapy for treating these large lesions has largely been abandoned in favor of an organ-preservation approach modeled after the protocol for laryngeal SCC, VA-268.

Chemotherapy with Radiotherapy

The most recent development in the treatment of advanced SGC (T_{3-4}) has been the organ-sparing approach using concomitant chemotherapy with radiotherapy. The patient undergoes two to three cycles of cisplatin with 5-fluorouracil spaced at monthly intervals. Each cycle is 2 to 3 days in duration and is usually associated with moderate nausea and/or mucositis. Radiotherapy is delivered to the primary and bilateral neck sites. The patient is evaluated for locoregional response after 5,000 cGy of radiotherapy and two cycles of chemotherapy. If the patient has only a partial response, he or she is offered salvage surgery. If the patient has had a complete response at the primary site, radiotherapy is continued for an additional 2,000 cGy. Neck dissection is considered in these patients following radiotherapy if there is persistence of a neck mass on physical examination or CT scan.

By using primary response to chemo- and radiotherapy as the criterion for surgery, as many as 60 percent of patients retain their larynx as well as near-normal speaking and swallowing function. Some patients will, however, require tracheotomy either at the onset or during the course of therapy. Some patients retain their tracheotomies following successful treatment due to chronic edema or aspiration. Significant aspiration may require prolonged enteral nutrition as well. Long-term survival for patients treated with chemo- and radiotherapy appears comparable to that for total laryngectomy followed by radiotherapy.

Total Laryngectomy

Total laryngectomy has been the "gold standard" for the treatment of advanced SGC. Although native phonation is lost with this procedure, swallowing following this procedure is often excellent, and vocal rehabilitation with a Blom-Singer tracheoesophageal prosthesis offers an acceptable alternative. Total laryngectomy is accompanied by bilateral neck dissections due to the advanced disease stage and postoperative radiotherapy.

■ THERAPEUTIC OPTIONS: CERVICAL LYMPH NODES

N_{0-1} Neck Disease

Due to a high rate of occult and bilateral nodal metastases with early SGC, treatment of the cervical lymph nodes should be aggressive. In the case of the N_0 neck, suprahyoid T_1 disease does not warrant treatment. With infrahyoid T_1 or greater disease, both neck sites should be treated with either selective neck dissection or 5,000 cGy of radiation. N_1 nodal disease, regardless of the primary site, also requires definitive treatment.

N_{2-3} Neck Disease

Advanced neck disease requires aggressive therapy to maximize locoregional control. These patients will either undergo chemo- and radiotherapy or primary surgical therapy, including a neck dissection and followed by radiotherapy. Many organ-preservation–protocol patients have advanced neck disease that disappears during the course of therapy. We believe that these patients require close observation to monitor for residual disease. Neck dissection is reserved for patients who have residual mass, ambiguous physical or radiographic findings, or regional recurrence.

In SGC, local control is often more frequently achieved than is regional control. Many patients who are treated for SGC succumb to their disease through recurrence in the neck and distant metastases. For these reasons, cervical lymph nodes should be treated primarily, aggressively, and bilaterally.

■ POSTOPERATIVE REHABILITATION

The objective of organ-preservation therapy for SGC has been to minimize therapeutic morbidity and thus reduce the need for rehabilitation. Although many patients avoid total laryngectomy, organ-preservation therapies do affect vocal strength and quality. This has particular significance for patients who depend on their voice for their livelihood or the pursuit of a serious hobby.

The primary challenge encountered by many of these patients involves alteration of their swallowing. Progressive fibrosis following chemotherapy and/or radiotherapy results in restricted laryngeal elevation, which impairs the intricate involuntary events during the second phase of swallowing and increases the risk of aspiration. Many SGC patients deal with chronic low levels of aspiration following their therapy, and they are at risk for chronic bronchitis and pneumonia. Many of these patients have significant underlying chronic obstructive pulmonary disease, which further reduces their pulmonary reserve and places them at increased risk for aspiration-related complications.

Scarring after conservation treatment of SGC can also result in supraglottic or pharyngeal stenosis. This not only is a source of distress and potential malnutrition but also results in supraglottic pooling, which increases the probability of aspiration. Oropharyngeal secretions are often made tenacious as a result of radiotherapy, which further complicates the formation and transit of a food bolus.

For the same reasons as mentioned previously, patients may also experience airway obstruction during or following organ-sparing therapy, and chronic tracheotomy may be required. When supraglottic edema is a prominent and persistent feature, the possibility of residual or recurrent disease must also be considered.

PRACTICAL CONSIDERATIONS IN A MANAGED CARE ENVIRONMENT

Managed care and changes in reimbursement have brought increased scrutiny on treatment selection. Head and neck surgeons must provide leadership in the treatment of SGC by analyzing and reporting results of treatment in the context of cost, resource utilization, length and severity of disability, in addition to the traditional outcome measures of locoregional control and survival.

Decreasing expenditure of health care dollars while maximizing control of disease and minimizing side effects should guide our treatment of SGC. When using this framework for clinical decision making, some treatment alternatives may be eliminated to make this process less complex. For example, some in the field argue that given the cost and duration of radiotherapy, early SGC is better treated with endoscopic excision or glottic laryngectomy. This approach, however, may result in greater problems with dysphagia and voice quality, which must be considered as a cost of therapy and factored accordingly.

Another example of clinical decision making might be considering the uncertainty of long-term results for laryngeal salvage protocols. If many of these patients fail to demonstrate an adequate response to organ-preservation therapy, and others require salvage surgery for recurrence, when is it more expedient and cost-effective to proceed directly to surgery with postoperative radiotherapy? Not only would the expense and lost productivity resulting from the chemotherapy be saved, but also the risk of complications resulting from operating on an irradiation failure would be avoided. However, what is the value to patients and society for those who are spared laryngectomy as a result of the organ-preservation approach? Research for predictors of response to chemo- and radiotherapy is an obvious imperative in this setting.

Suggested Reading

American Society for Head and Neck Surgery. Clinical practice guidelines for the diagnosis and management of cancer of the head and neck. Pittsburgh: American Society for Head and Neck Surgery, 1996: 29.

Gregor RT, Oei SS, Hilgers FJM, et al. Management of cervical metastases in supraglottic cancer. Ann Otol Rhinol Laryngol 1996; 105:845-850.

Weber OC, Johnson JT, Meyers EN. Impact of bilateral neck dissection on recovery following supraglottic laryngectomy. Arch Otolaryngol Head Neck Surg 1993; 119:61-64.

GLOTTIC CARCINOMA

The method of

Byron J. Bailey

In most patients, carcinoma of the larynx originates on the true vocal cord; properly managed, this carcinoma is the most curable malignancy of the entire aerodigestive tract. The main issues in dealing with glottic carcinoma are local control, management of known or suspected cervical lymph node metastasis, and follow-up to detect residual carcinoma or second primary lesions. These are the points of reference to which I have oriented the following sections in this chapter; their importance derives from the fundamental issue of patient survival. Preservation of life takes precedence over the preservation of laryngeal function.

However, therapeutic morbidity, preservation of laryngeal function, and the quality of life after treatment are extremely important considerations. Unlike carcinoma of the lung, in which an all-out extirpative or radiotherapeutic attack may be routinely warranted, a more conservative approach can be successful for large numbers of selected patients who have glottic carcinoma. This is most fortunate in view of the vital role of communicative ability in our modern society.

The primary purpose of this chapter is to summarize my

current views regarding the management of glottic carcinoma, with an emphasis on surgical techniques. This is a rapidly changing area, and laser surgical management of early glottic cancer is an important recent advance.

■ PREOPERATIVE EVALUATION

On physical examination, most of these tumors arise on the membranous portion of the true vocal cord. Approximately 20 percent have some degree of supraglottic extension, approximately 20 percent to 25 percent extend to the anterior commissure, and approximately 20 percent have subglottic extension of 5 mm or more. I find that videostroboscopy is a valuable aid to precise diagnosis and staging of early glottic neoplasms.

Radiologic studies may be helpful in the preoperative evaluation, particularly computed tomographic scanning to demonstrate thyroid cartilage invasion or destruction. A number of clinical observations are helpful in preoperative planning. For example, when the primary lesion is confined to the true vocal cord, there is less than a 5 percent incidence of nodal metastases, but patients who have vocal cord fixation or extension of tumor outside the larynx are found to have a 30 percent to 40 percent incidence of positive cervical nodes and less than a 50 percent 5 year survival free of disease. A second primary will be present or develop in almost 20 percent of patients who have glottic carcinoma. In most cases, the second primary will be found in the head and neck region, lung, or gastrointestinal or genitourinary tract. A second primary will develop in the larynx or laryngopharynx in approximately 6 percent of patients. These second primary lesions are reported to occur twice as often following radiotherapy as in nonirradiated patients (8 percent to 14 percent) and are seen earlier after radiotherapy than after surgery (the range of detection of second primaries usually spans a period from 5 to 14 years following detection of the initial lesion).

■ THERAPY

Noninvasive Glottic Carcinoma (Carcinoma In Situ)

The diagnosis of noninvasive glottic carcinoma can be difficult to make with certainty. The spectrum of pathologic abnormalities may include keratosis, acanthosis, dysplasia, and atypia either singly or in various combinations. At some point, the orderly progression of cellular maturation becomes so disrupted, the cellular components become so atypical, and the presence of mitosis becomes so frequent, that a diagnosis of malignancy is made. This diagnostic point may vary with different pathologists, or with the same pathologist on different occasions. Confidence in making the diagnosis rests on a correlation of the gross appearance of the lesion with the microscope appearance and close communication between the surgeon and the pathologist.

When the diagnosis of carcinoma in situ is made, and when the lesion involves only the true vocal cord, microscopic suspension laryngoscopy with stripping of the epithelium and close observation of the patient is sufficient for initial treatment, provided that the patient discontinues smoking and ethanol intake and returns for indirect laryngoscopy every 3 to 6 months.

If the lesion recurs, the patient should undergo additional stripping procedures and must agree to cooperate fully with the follow-up program. The patient should also be informed that some practitioners would recommend radiotherapy after the first recurrence. I believe that radiotherapy is indicated when lesions extend to involve the supraglottic or subglottic area; those lesions confined to the membranous cord can be managed by repeat stripping or by endoscopic laser excision. I have begun to use laser excision in preference to repeat stripping because it allows more precise control of the depth of the excision.

Microinvasive Carcinoma

In recent years, considerable attention has been focused on that small number of patients who have superficially invasive glottic carcinoma where the cancer cells have extended through the basement membrane, but have not yet invaded the vocal muscle. This patient group ordinarily represents less than 5 percent of all patients who have glottic carcinoma.

At our institution, we use a structured protocol for the management of these patients that consists of microscopic suspension laryngoscopy and laser excision of the involved area down to a depth of the superficial portion of the vocal muscle and vocal ligament. The patients are then followed up with indirect laryngoscopy every 3 months. The appearance of any suspicious lesion triggers a repeat excision. This approach has been completely successful in 14 of 16 patients treated over the past 20 years in terms of eliminating all evidence of malignancy; one patient underwent a vertical partial laryngectomy, and another received radiotherapy. No patients have required total laryngectomy. None are alive with disease or dead from their disease.

In this patient group, great emphasis is placed on patient and family education with regard to smoking and alcohol ingestion and the early signs and symptoms of recurrent disease.

Invasive Epidermoid Carcinoma

Radiotherapy and Laser Excision

Although radiotherapy has historically been the treatment of choice for invasive epidermoid carcinoma of the membranous portion of the mobile true vocal cord, microscopic laser excision has now shown equivalent cure rates, with lower cost and less morbidity. Follow-up visits during the first year are at monthly intervals, bimonthly for the next 4 years, and quarterly for the subsequent 10 years. Late recurrence of carcinoma and the development of second primary tumors are issues of sufficient importance to cause me to adhere to this pattern of follow-up.

I also recommend postoperative adjunctive radiotherapy for any patient whose surgical management is associated with substantial doubt regarding complete excision. Postoperative radiotherapy should be instituted 4 to 6 weeks after the surgical procedure and should include a treatment field of sufficient size to deal with the region of known and suspected concern.

Radiotherapy reduces edema and fibrosis within the larynx that may result in post-treatment hoarseness, ranging in degree from mild and transient to marked and persistent. In most patients, the edema should diminish considerably within 3 months after the completion of radiotherapy, and the voice should improve. If hoarseness or edema is progressively worsening, or if edema persists 6 months after radiotherapy, a very high index of suspicion with regard to residual carcinoma should be present. Direct laryngoscopy with multiple deep biopsies in the area of the original tumor, including any other suspicious areas, is mandatory. On occasion, it has been necessary to repeat the diagnostic steps on as many as three occasions before biopsy proof of persistent carcinoma has been obtained. Only then, in my opinion, is further surgery warranted. However, some authorities maintain that persistent edema beyond 6 months, even in the absence of biopsy confirmation, is sufficient indication for total laryngectomy.

In the past, we viewed radiotherapy and partial laryngectomy procedures as the first line of treatment for early laryngeal cancer in patients at our medical center. We now believe that endoscopic treatment of early laryngeal cancer, including laser microscopic excision, is an acceptable alternative method for managing these patients. All three modalities are able to accomplish primary cure rates of 80 percent to 85 percent or more, and most reports indicate that the addition of secondary salvage efforts yield 90 percent and higher cure rates.

During the past 5 years, we have begun to use the advances and advantages associated with laser surgical techniques. Several specific operations have been described by Steiner, Thumfart, Ruder, and others for the resection of glottic carcinoma. These techniques are based on sound anatomic and embryologic concepts that were clarified during the middle of this century under the general heading of lymphatic compartments within the larynx. These compartments have been defined in terms of fibroelastic barriers and lymphatic drainage patterns that generally retard and channel the spread of glottic cancer to involve the cartilaginous skeleton of the larynx and the regional lymph nodes in predictable patterns.

Partial Laryngectomy

I prefer vertical partial laryngectomy procedures for treating patients who have glottic carcinoma that has extended to the vocal process of the arytenoid or to the anterior commissure and/or the contralateral true vocal cord.

I use vertical partial laryngectomy and its extended modifications in patients who have superficial (neither bulky nor deeply invasive) transglottic lesions, and even in patients who have extensive glottic carcinoma that involves the anterior commissure and both true vocal cords to such an extent that it is possible to preserve only the posterior commissure and one arytenoid cartilage. I have employed these techniques in patients who have N_1 regional metastases. My policy has been to perform the partial laryngectomy procedure in the usual manner, with a neck dissection that preserves the spinal accessory nerve. Postoperative radiotherapy is used routinely in this instance. It is uncommon to encounter the combination of a glottic carcinoma amenable to partial laryngectomy with a small palpable ipsilateral cervical lymph node. Others have had success with hemilaryngectomy for patients who have fixed cords, but I prefer total laryngectomy with neck dissection.

Vertical partial laryngectomy is contraindicated in the presence of bulky transglottic lesions, when the posterior commissure is involved, when there is evidence of invasion of the overlying thyroid cartilage, and when the tumor extends inferior to the superior margin of the cricoid cartilage or involves the cricothyroid membrane.

Postoperative function is enhanced by the use of a bipedicle sternohyoid muscle flap lined by perichondrium from the external surface of the thyroid cartilage to fill the surgical defect and line the laryngeal lumen. The central segment of the thyroid cartilage should be included with the surgical specimen when the tumor encroaches upon the anterior commissure in order to avoid persistent carcinoma at the anterior commissure that results from tumor growth into the point of attachment of the vocal tendons to the cartilage (Broyle's ligament region).

Frozen section analysis at the time of surgery of glottic carcinoma is mandatory. Because there are problems in interpreting frozen sections taken from the margin of the specimen, it is best to obtain for frozen section additional 3 to 4 mm specimens (margins) from the patient at each of the four quadrants and from the depth of the surgical bed. The original specimen should be oriented for the pathologist and should be pinned to cardboard to prevent shrinkage that might further confuse the histologic interpretation.

I have observed discrepancies between the frozen section report and the permanent section in 15 percent to 20 percent of cases. The scenario is almost always that a frozen section report indicates no tumor, whereas a permanent section report discloses the presence of tumor at the margins. When confronted with this dilemma, I recommend postoperative radiotherapy in the majority of instances. Although some surgeons embark on a program of careful observation rather than radiotherapy, the issue cannot be resolved without additional data.

Postoperative Care

When it has been necessary to employ bilateral laryngoplasty muscle flaps or to de-epithelialize the major remaining vocal cord, I employ a keel of Silastic, which is sutured into place with absorbable suture. The keel is removed endoscopically at approximately 3 weeks after surgery. An obstructive stent is unnecessarily dangerous with the described operative procedure. I rely on parenteral fluids until the patient has bowel sounds, at which time clear liquid feedings are begun, and the diet is slowly advanced until approximately the tenth postoperative day. In almost every instance, the patient can be discharged by approximately the twelfth postoperative day. When a keel has been placed, the patient is usually readmitted approximately 3 weeks after the surgical procedure, and with direct laryngoscopy the keel is removed, any granulation tissue present in the larynx is excised, and the patient is decannulated.

The appropriate utilization of conservative surgical techniques yields 5 year survival rates of 90 percent or higher. Our results are shown in Tables 1 to 3.

Total Laryngectomy

I select total laryngectomy less frequently than in the past, but it is still required for patients who have a bulky transglot-

Table 1. Site of Primary Lesion in Glottic Carcinoma, 1962 to 1983

SITE	NO. OF PATIENTS
Anterior commissure	84
Vocal process arytenoid	32
Mobile TVC (RT recurrence)	18
Transglottic	18
Total	152

TVC, true vocal cord; RT, radiotherapy.

Table 2. Mortality in Patients Treated for Glottic Carcinoma, 1962 to 1991

MORTALITY STATUS	NO.	PERCENT
Dead from cancer	9/152	5.9
Dead from other cause, 5 year follow-up	8/152	5.2
Laryngeal recurrence	15/152	9.9

Table 3. Results of Treatment of Glottic Carcinoma After Laryngeal Recurrence

PATIENT STATUS	NO. OF PATIENTS
Dead from cancer	5
Salvage by partial laryngectomy	3
Salvage by total laryngectomy	1
Total	15

tic carcinoma, a fixed cord associated with a large glottic lesion, extension of tumor to involve the posterior commissure or both arytenoids, thyroid cartilage invasion, and in most patients in whom there is subglottic extension of greater than 10 mm (especially when located anteriorly), or extension from the glottis to outside the larynx. In these circumstances, total laryngectomy is usually followed by radiotherapy.

Radical neck dissection is done along with total laryngectomy in any of the previously described circumstances in which there are palpable cervical lymph node metastases; or radiotherapy to the neck is given if there is no palpable cervical lymphadenopathy.

Patients whose glottic carcinoma is associated with airway obstruction obviously have an advanced malignancy; these larger tumors frequently have more infiltration and subglottic extension than usual. Some otolaryngologists perform total laryngectomy on an emergency basis within a few hours of the initial examination because many such patients have a high incidence of stomal recurrence. This high rate of residual disease has been attributed to the performance of a tracheotomy several days before the definitive surgery is accomplished, but may actually be related to occult cancer in paratracheal lymph nodes. There is no convincing proof on either side of this controversy at present. I believe that it is preferable to take 1 to 2 days to evaluate the patient, because it is almost always possible to control the obstructive problem by a combination of laser debulking, bed rest, and the administration of oxygen by mask during the workup. At the time of total laryngectomy, the tracheal stoma is created slightly lower than usual, and more attention is directed to dissection of the paratracheal nodes and inclusion of the ipsilateral thyroid lobe and isthmus with the tumor specimen. Postoperative radiotherapy includes a boost in the region of the stoma and inclusion of the mediastinum in the radiotherapy field.

RECURRENT CANCER

Managing Postradiotherapy Recurrence

Partial laryngectomy is a reasonable approach when the original lesion and the recurrence are both appropriate for partial laryngectomy surgery. I use the criteria outlined by Biller:

1. The contralateral cord must be free of tumor (anterior commissure may be involved).
2. The body of the arytenoid cartilage must be free of tumor.
3. There must be no more than 5 mm of subglottic extension.
4. Absence of cartilage invasion must be established.
5. Absence of cord fixation must be established.
6. Close correlation between the original primary lesion and the recurrence must exist.

However, the majority of patients who have recurrent carcinoma after radiotherapy require total laryngectomy for salvage. This is the strongest argument against using radiotherapy for all patients who have glottic carcinoma, observing them for evidence of recurrence, and then managing this situation surgically.

Managing Recurrence After Partial Laryngectomy

The incidence of residual and/or recurrent disease and second primaries is approximately 10 percent. About one-third of these patients have a superficial malignancy involving only the epithelial surface with minimal invasion. These patients can be managed with a second partial laryngectomy unless the recurrence involves an area such as the only remaining arytenoid cartilage or the posterior commissure, or unless adequate excision would result in an unacceptable compromise in terms of residual function. On rare occasions, radiotherapy can be used to salvage these patients.

Total laryngectomy is required for the salvage of most of these patients because of the depth of invasion at the time the recurrence is noted. The surgical specimen should be analyzed very carefully to avoid a resection that is less than adequate. Postoperative radiotherapy is used in almost every instance of this type.

Rehabilitation

Despite considerable effort expended in the rehabilitation of patients who have undergone total laryngectomy, complete return to preoperative levels of economic and social activity is exceedingly rare. Although the literature contains many optimistic references to the fact that the majority of patients undergoing laryngectomy can be adequately rehabilitated by means of esophageal speech or use of the external electrolarynx, in my experience only approximately one-third of patients are able to develop esophageal speech to the degree that they use it in social conversation. The percentage is slightly higher for individuals under age 60 and lower for those who are over age 60.

The electrolarynx is used by some of the remaining patients, but it produces speech that is disappointing to most patients, and the amount of their communication declines significantly after 1 to 2 years.

I rely on the Blom-Singer prosthesis for voice restoration after total laryngectomy. A tracheoesophageal puncture or fistula is performed at the time of the total laryngectomy. A red rubber catheter of the appropriate diameter is placed in the fistulous tract until it has healed sufficiently for the prosthesis to be inserted.

The role of speech pathology in the vocal rehabilitation of patients who undergo partial laryngectomy is also of considerable importance. Although the average patient will develop acceptable speech after these procedures, the quality and efficiency of vocalization after partial laryngectomy can be improved significantly by the therapeutic intervention of a skilled and dedicated speech pathologist.

Comprehensive rehabilitation of the patient who has undergone total laryngectomy is an area that must concern all laryngeal surgeons. This is a team effort involving the surgeon, nurse, speech pathologist, psychologist, nutritionist, social service worker, physical therapist, and occupational counselor. We have a responsibility to exert a maximum effort in those cases in which the tumor has been successfully managed so that our patients are able to return to an adequate functional level in relation to employment, home life, and social activities.

Suggested Reading

Biller HF, et al. Hemilaryngectomy following radiation failure for carcinoma of the vocal cords. Laryngoscope 1970; 80:249-253.

Johnson JT, et al. Outcome of open surgical therapy for glottic carcinoma. Ann Otol Rhinol Laryngol 1993; 102:752-755.

Olsen KD, et al. Indications and results of cordectomy for early glottic carcinoma. Otolaryngol Head Neck Surg 1993; 108:272-282.

Peretti G, et al. Endoscopic laser excisional biopsy for selected glottic carcinomas. Laryngoscope 1994; 104:1276-1279.

Mahieu HF, et al. Carbon dioxide laser vaporization in early glottic carcinoma. Arch Otolaryngol Head Neck Surg 1994; 120:383-387.

McGuirt WF, et al. Comparative voice results after laser resection or irradiation of T1 vocal cord carcinoma. Arch Otolaryngol Head Neck Surg 1994; 120:951-955.

Zeitels SM, et al. Premalignant epithelium and microinvasive cancer of the vocal fold: The evolution of phonomicrosurgical management. Laryngoscope 1995; 105:1-51.

PHARYNGOESOPHAGEAL RECONSTRUCTION

The method of
Bruce H. Haughey
by
Wayne B. Colin
Bruce H. Haughey

Reconstruction of the circumferential pharyngoesophageal (PE) defect has as its primary goal the reconnection of the pharynx to the esophagus with an epithelial-lined conduit. A fasciocutaneous microvascular free tissue transfer will satisfy this end, with little donor site morbidity and no mortality. With a healed, well-vascularized, and pliable tissue tube in place, patients will predictably swallow by mouth after a single reconstructive procedure. Both primary and secondary PE defect may be treated with equal confidence.

Construction of the neopharynx will improve a patient's quality of life. Immediate reconstruction of a circumferential PE defect facilitates early oral alimentation and allows oral speech after a tracheoesophageal puncture. Connection of the pharynx with the esophagus prevents soiling of the neck and chest with saliva and food and eliminates maceration of the skin. Aspiration of saliva into the tracheostoma with pneumonia is also avoided. Elimination of a pharyngostoma avoids the requisite packing and dressing, with their attendant costs and social stigmatism.

The various techniques of PE reconstruction have used a hierarchy of tissues from all levels of the "reconstructive ladder," with skin grafts and local, regional, and distant tissues employed to form a tubular connection between the pharynx and the esophagus. The method of random cervical skin "turn-in" flaps was popularized by Wookey. This technique proved unpredictable because of the need for multiple staged procedures, as well as fistula formation and stenosis and flap failure. Although an improvement, the axial pattern deltopectoral flap of Bakamjian met with similar problems. The myocutaneous pectoralis major flap of Ariyan has been used successfully, but it can be difficult to tube in women who have overlying thick breast tissue or men who have muscle bulk. Pedicled enteric flaps such as transposition of the colon or stomach require a laparotomy and blunt dissection through the thorax; these flaps can be associated with significant complications and mortality. Microvascular free tissue transfer of jejunum was described by Seidenberg in 1959. This technique has donor site problems related to the laparotomy and segmental jejunectomy, and still carries a 5 percent mortality.

More recently, the microvascular transfer of a tubed fasciocutaneous flap has been popular and is the focus of this chapter. With this approach, there are several appropriate superficial donor sites, none of which necessitate an abdominal or thoracic procedure. Therefore, the morbidity of the donor tissue harvest is site-specific, and the mortality related to the donor site is essentially nil.

PREOPERATIVE EVALUATION

Generally, patients who require a total or partial laryngopharyngectomy have one or more major systemic illnesses. Derangement of the pulmonary, cardiac, renal, airborne, vascular, hepatic, or hematopoietic systems carries inherent perioperative risk. Tobacco and ethanol abuse, the usual etiologic factors for head and neck cancer, are commonly coupled with long-standing malnutrition. Timely general medical clearance is mandatory before surgery for risk assessment, intervention, and anesthetic treatment planning. A percutaneous gastrostomy (PEG) tube may be placed several weeks ahead of the anticipated procedure in order to fortify a patient's nutritional status. Dental evaluation is also a requisite, especially if the dentate oral cavity is within the intended radiation portal. Social service input is helpful for postoperative home care.

Site-specific problems of the neck are usually related to prior surgery and/or radiotherapy, but these problems may have systemic implications. Fifteen percent of head and neck cancer patients have occult hypothyroidism, which if untreated could precipitate a perioperative cardiopulmonary event or result in delayed or failed wound healing. Radiation-induced atherosclerosis may cause subtotal occlusion of the carotid vasculature, with possible cerebral ischemia after manipulation. External carotid donor vessels may be similarly diseased and require an alternate donor vessel for flap viability. A neck previously dissected on both sides should be considered for a carotid and/or aortic angiogram to aid in the search for appropriate donor vessels.

A fasciocutaneous donor site is selected based on defect size, patient age, gender, body habitus, hair pattern, occupation, and preference of both patient and surgeon. My preferred donor site is the radial forearm, but reasonable alternatives include the lateral thigh, lateral arm, and scapula (Fig. 1). The radial forearm free flap (RFFF) allows a two-team approach, leaves few donor site problems, and imports new skin for the neopharynx and/or neck closure; but this flap requires a skin graft for donor site closure. Recent reports recommend harvest within the subcutaneous plane to maximize tendon and sensory nerve cancer. The lateral thigh free flap (LTFF) is usually closed primarily, even for a large skin donor paddle, and does not have the same concern with adequacy of vascular perfusion of the extremity as does the RFFF. The LTFF may be relatively contraindicated in an obese patient because this donor site is a usual location for the accumulation of fatty "saddle bags," especially in women. The lateral arm free flap (LAFF) is less convenient

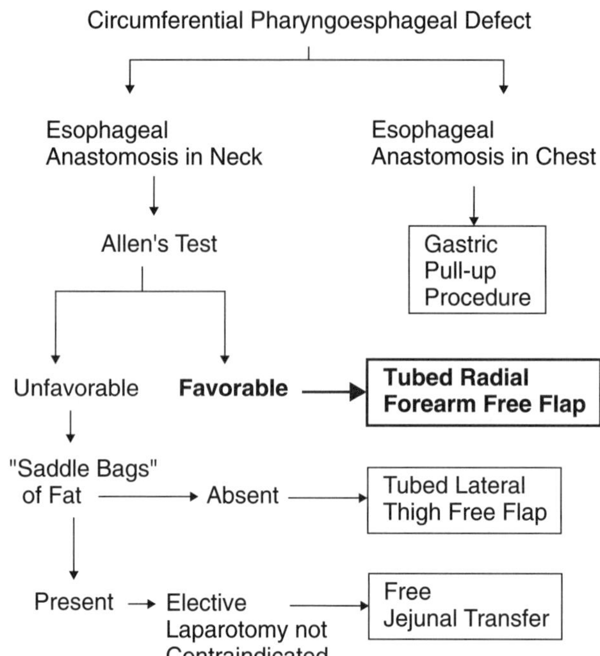

Figure 1.
Reconstructive options for the circumferential pharyngoesophageal defect are shown in the algorithm. The preferred reconstruction, shown in bold type, is the tubed radial forearm free flap.

to harvest simultaneously with the resection due to close proximity of the two operative fields, but it can generally be closed without a skin graft. The scapular and parascapular free flap donor sites pose the same problem as does the LAFF and require significant positioning maneuvers to obtain a workable surgical field. Vascular compromise of the extremity should be a minimal issue with the RFFF, provided that a favorable preoperative Allen's test is obtained, and intraoperative evaluation of vascular perfusion of the hand is performed after division of the radial artery. A compartment syndrome caused by an expanding hematoma, tight dressing, or splint is also possible. In contrast, without a laparotomy, there is no issue of a donor site–related ileus, abdominal abscess, enteric anastomotic leak, abdominal bleeding, or peritonitis.

Technique

The RFFF skin paddle typically measures 8 × 12 cm centered longitudinally over the radial artery. The distal edge stops 3 to 4 cm from the proximal wrist skin crease to allow for coverage with a shirt sleeve, and for a watch or jewelry to be worn over native wrist skin. Under tourniquet control for no more than 1.5 hours, the flap is elevated medially and laterally; the surgeon takes care to preserve the paratenon and epimysium for subsequent skin grafting. The superficial radial (sensory) nerve is preserved, and the cephalic vein is incorporated into the skin paddle. The radial artery is temporarily occluded on the distal end of the skin paddle with two microvascular clamps, and then the artery is divided. After release of the tourniquet, the hand and thumb are examined to confirm adequate vascular perfusion, and the distal radial artery backflow is assessed. Only then is the distal radial arterial stump suture ligated. If perfusion is inadequate, the radial artery can be reanastomosed, the hand is reperfused, and an alternate donor site is chosen. The pedicle is elevated from between the tendons and muscle bellies of the brachioradialis and flexor carpi radialis, with careful preservation of its attachment to the flap. The flap then remains attached only by the radial artery and veins, while the initial flap contouring is being done and perfusion continues in situ. The skin paddle is folded lengthwise upon itself, skin inside, thus forming an epithelial-lined tube on the forearm (Fig. 2); 3–0 polyglactin 910 interrupted vertical mattress sutures are used in this closure every half centimeter.

Recipient vessels are chosen and prepared in the neck in anticipation of the microvascular free tissue transfer. Branches of the external carotid artery are evaluated for diameter, length, patency, pulsatile flow, and lie of the vessel, including its relationship to any potential recipient vein. Typically, the linguofacial trunk or superior thyroid artery is chosen. The former vessel is turned beneath and then superficial to the hypoglossal nerve to help set up an unencumbered arterial anastomosis. A suitable recipient vein such as the external jugular or tributary into the internal jugular is selected and left in situ.

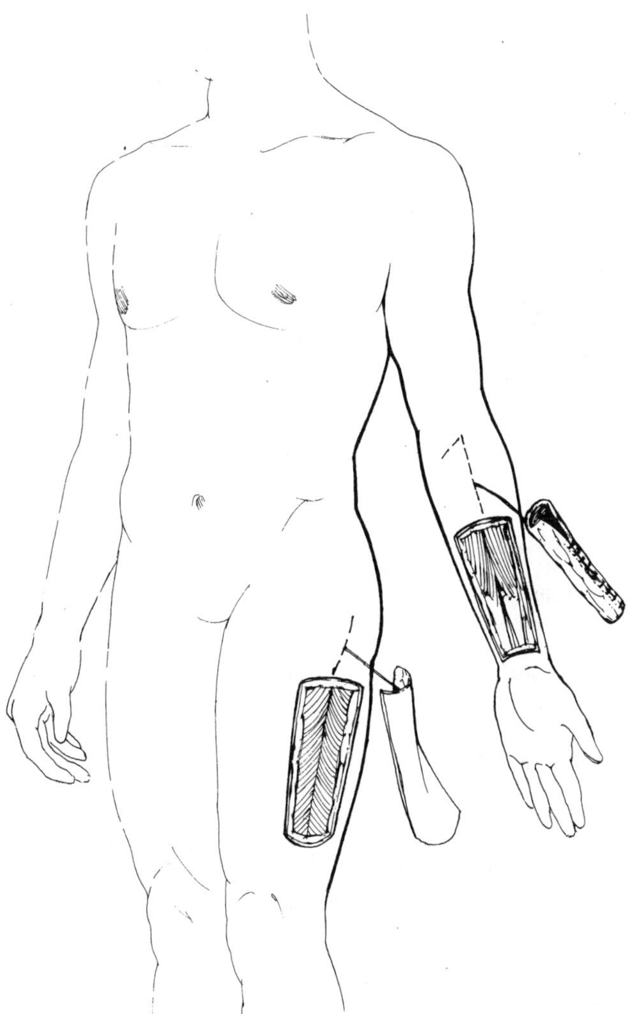

Figure 2.
The preferred donor sites for pharyngoesophageal reconstruction are depicted. The radial forearm free flap has been tubed while perfusion continues by the native radial vessels before transfer to the neck.

After flap harvest, the yet-to-be revascularized skin tube is oriented with the lengthwise suture line against the prevertebral fascia. Usually, the proximal part of the skin paddle can be made 2 to 3 cm wider than the distal paddle, which allows a wide open inlet to the prefabricated skin tube at the tongue base. The whole skin tube is then tacked to local tissue, and the vascular pedicle is properly draped. Attention is then directed to the microvascular anastomoses.

An interupted or running continuous 9–0 nylon suture is used to perform an end-to-end anastomosis of the artery, and a mechanical coupling device, such as the 3M Precise system, is used to perform the venous anastomoses. Ischemia time is routinely under 1.5 hours. The proximal and distal flap anastomoses to the pharynx and esophagus are performed usually over a nasogastric tube salivary stent. The longitudinal suture line uniting the sides of the flap into a tube is carefully positioned against the prevertebral fascia to ensure an immobile base (Fig. 3). The repair is then insufflated via the nostril with water or hydrogen peroxide, and the suture lines are assessed for leakage. Additional sutures are placed as necessary.

The neck flaps are reapposed over drains, and a marking suture is placed in the skin overlying a distal portion of the reconstruction where the Doppler signal is easily heard for postoperative monitoring.

Postoperative Care

Following the operation, the patient is sent to an intensive care unit for 1 to 2 days. Low doses of intravenous heparin (50 units per hour), aspirin per rectum (600 mg per day), hetastarch (500 milliliters per day), and dexamethasone (6 mg every 6 hours) are given for 3 days. The flap is checked hourly for clinical evidence of arteriovenous insufficiency by assessing the adequacy of the Doppler signal and by inspection, capillary refill, and needle prick testing of any visible paddle on the neck. The neopharyngeal reconstruction is also evaluated by daily inspection of the pharyngeal lumen using fiberoptic nasopharyngoscopy. The donor site is also evaluated to ensure adequacy of distal limb perfusion and to monitor for wound infection.

Patients are begun on oral feeding with clear liquids at 10 days after their reconstruction, or 14 days if there is a history of prior irradiation. If no fever or neck tenderness develops, then the diet is advanced daily as tolerated. A speech pathology consultation may be necessary for swallowing instructions.

Complications

The most common major complication of any type of PE reconstruction is the pharyngocutaneous fistula. A low cervical fistula carries risks of aspiration, mediastinitis, and erosion of the vessels of the neck and chest. Fistulas develop because of prior irradiation, residual tumor, nonhealing recipient tissue, flap tissue loss, or poor surgical technique.

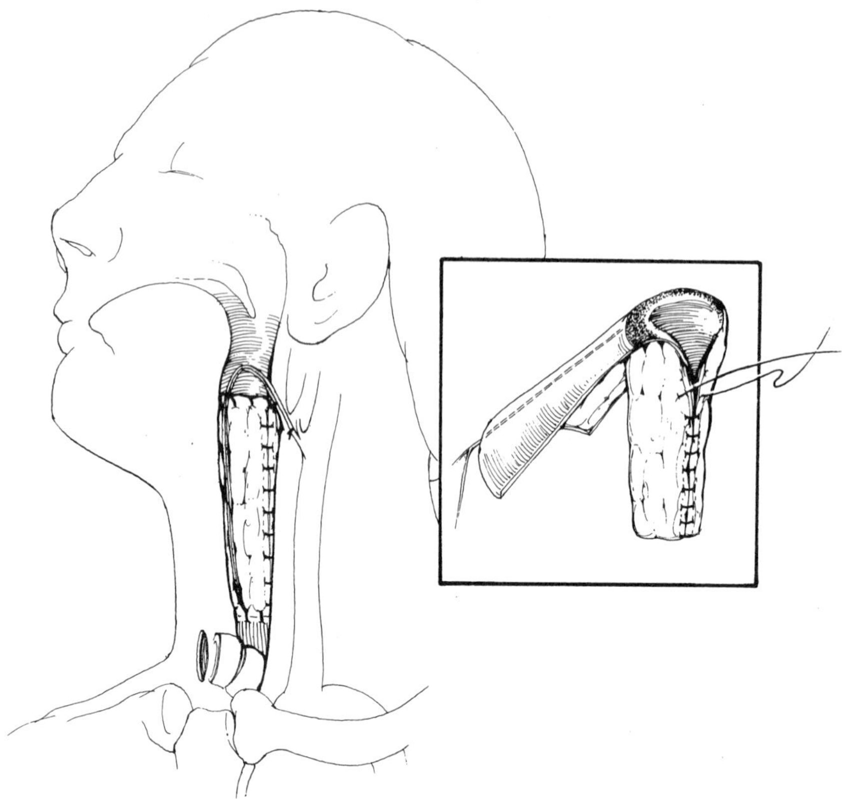

Figure 3.
The prefabricated fasciocutaneous tube has been inset to reconnect the pharynx and esophagus. Note that the vertical suture line is overlying the prevertebral fascia. The inset shows a tubed flap, a de-epithelialized skin segment, and an attached skin paddle. This technique allows pharyngoesophageal reconstruction along with resurfacing of deficient neck skin by a single free tissue transfer.

Tissue trauma, wound tension, mucosal inversion, hematoma formation, or infection contribute to development of a fistula. Once recognized, most fistulas will respond to conservative treatment. This requires protecting the airway with a cuffed tracheotomy tube, administration of culture-directed intravenous antibiotics, and possible biopsy to rule out recurrent disease. The fistula should be diverted away from the great vessels and tracheostomy by packing, wound revision, and pressure dressings. A suction drain, salivary bypass tube, or T tube may be helpful to reduce the amount of soilage of the neck tissues. If the fistula is persistent, relatively small, and not exposed to prior irradiation, local turn-in flaps may have value. For larger lesions, the time-honored technique is to create a controlled pharyngostomy or esophagostomy, which when matured can be closed with regional myofascial tissue such as the pectoralis major flap and covered with a skin graft.

Suggested Reading

Ariyan S. The pectoralis major myocutaneous flap. A versatile flap for reconstruction in the head and neck. Plast Reconstr Surg 1979; 63:73-81.

Bakamjian VY. A two stage method for pharyngoesophageal reconstruction with a primary pectoral skin flap. Plast Reconstr Surg 1965; 36: 173-184.

Brown MT, Cheney ML, Gliklich RL, et al. Assessment of functional morbidity in the radial forearm free flap donor site. Arch Otolaryngol Head Neck Surg 1996; 122:991-994.

Chang SC, Miller G, Halber CF, et al. Limiting donor site morbidity by suprafascial dissection of the radial forearm flap. Microsurgery 1996; 17:136-140.

Harii K, Ebihara S, Ono I, et al. Pharyngoesophageal reconstruction using a fabricated forearm free flap. Plast Reconstr Surg 1985; 75:463-476.

Haughey BH, et al. Vibratory segment function after free flap reconstruction of the pharyngoesophagus. Laryngoscope 1995; 105:487-490.

Hayden, R. Reconstruction of the hypopharynx. In: Cummings C, Fredrickson JM, Harker LA, et al., eds. Otolaryngology—Head and neck surgery. Vol. 3. 2nd ed. St. Louis: Mosby–Year Book, 1993:2178.

Seidenberg B, Hurwitt ES, Som ML. Immediate reconstruction of the cervical esophagus by a revascularized isolated jejunal segment. Ann Surg 1959; 149:162-171.

Wookey H. Surgical treatment of carcinoma of the pharynx and upper esophagus. Surg Gynecol Obstet 1942; 75:499-504.

TRACHEAL NEOPLASMS

The method of
Jack L. Gluckman
by
Jack L. Gluckman
Judith M. Czaja

Primary tracheal tumors are rare, with an overall incidence of 0.02 percent of all respiratory tract tumors. Although a wide variety of tumors may develop in the trachea (Table 1), the most common malignant tumors are adenoid cystic carcinoma and squamous cell carcinoma, and the most common benign tumor is squamous cell papilloma.

As a head and neck surgeon, one should always consider infiltration of the trachea by thyroid or cervical esophageal cancer because these lesions may mimic the findings of a primary tracheal tumor.

These tumors may manifest anywhere along the length of the tracheobronchial tree, but for the purposes of this chapter, we emphasize tumors of the cervical trachea.

PATIENT ASSESSMENT

Clinical Features

The clinical features are essentially dependent on the type, site, and behavior pattern of the tracheal tumor. Adenoid cystic carcinoma tends to grow slowly, whereas squamous cell carcinoma is more aggressive in growth. Thyroid cancer usually gradually infiltrates the tracheal wall (with the exception of anaplastic cancer); however, once it extends into the lumen, it progresses rapidly. Respiratory papilloma can be almost indolent, but occasionally it grows rapidly.

The earliest symptoms of a tracheal tumor are a persistent cough and occasionally mild dyspnea on effort, which may be quite insidious in onset. The patient is frequently misdiagnosed and treated for many months with a presumed diagnosis of asthma. Stridor at rest and hemoptysis develop late in the clinical course and usually signify extensive involvement or aggressive behavior. Hoarseness and aspiration indicate recurrent nerve involvement, and dysphagia is, of course, highly suggestive of involvement of the esophagus.

Physical examination is not particularly helpful in assessing these patients, particularly at an early stage. Remember that a patient may have over 60 percent of the lumen occluded with only minimal dyspnea, particularly if the patient leads a sedentary life-style. Palpation of the neck may reveal regional adenopathy or obvious thyroid cancer or features of superior mediastinal syndrome due to the primary tumor or nodal metastases. Fiberoptic endoscopy, including pharyngoscopy, laryngoscopy, and bronchoscopy using topical anesthesia, is tolerated by most patients. A true vocal cord paralysis or pooling of saliva in the piriform sinuses with aspiration may be apparent. It may occasionally be possible to visualize between the vocal cords and identify the tumor and degree of encroachment of the lumen by the tumor. This view is usually unsatisfactory, however, and further evaluation is now geared to determine the exact site, size (in terms of both encroachment on the airway and length of tracheal involvement), and histologic type without further compromising either the airway or any planned future therapy. Essentially this information can be obtained by imaging and direct visualization using fiberoptic or rigid bronchoscopy.

Table 1. Differential Diagnosis of Tracheal Tumors

PRIMARY
Benign
Squamous cell papilloma
Minor salivary gland adenoma
Granular cell tumor
Leiomyoma
Chondroma
Schwannoma
Vascular malformations
Paraganglioma
Malignant
Squamous cell carcinoma
Adenoid cystic carcinoma
Adenocarcinoma
Adenosquamous carcinoma
Small cell carcinoma
Melanoma
Chondrosarcoma
Spindle cell sarcoma
Rhabdomyosarcoma
EXTRATRACHEAL
Thyroid carcinoma
Esophageal carcinoma
Distant metastases

Imaging

Contemporary imaging is frequently able to supply much of the information necessary to make a rational decision regarding future therapy. Computed tomography (CT) using fine cuts is the most commonly used imaging technique for determining the site and extent of the tracheal involvement as well as identifying any extratracheal extension or regional superior mediastinal nodal metastases. Multiplanar magnetic resonance imaging is useful in determining subtle soft-tissue extension. Barium swallow may detect invasion of the esophagus.

Endoscopy

The best technique for assessing the extent of the tumor and obtaining a biopsy is bronchoscopy. If the lesion is not impinging on the airway to a great degree, this can be performed satisfactorily by means of a fiberoptic bronchoscope with sedation and topical anesthesia. If, on the other hand, the lesion is causing significant obstruction and any attempt at biopsy may further compromise the airway, in our opinion it is better to perform rigid bronchoscopy under general anesthesia in the operating room. In this situation, variously sized bronchoscopes should be available in order to assess the tumor as well as to insert beyond the tumor to permit ventilation, if necessary. In addition, the CO_2 laser bronchoscope should be available to permit debulking of the tumor. In cervical tracheal tumors, the neck should always be infiltrated with local anesthesia to permit an urgent tracheostomy if the airway should be compromised. Obviously, good communication with the anesthesia staff is essential to avoid disastrous complications. Deep inhalation anesthesia is used, and intravenous paralytics are avoided until a satisfactory airway has been secured.

After the tumor has been identified and the airway has been secured by any of the previously described techniques, the exact extent of the tumor needs to be assessed by measuring the distance from the carina below and the true cord above, as well as measuring the length of the tumor itself. In addition, particularly in dealing with high-grade malignancies, it is important to determine whether the tumor is circumferential or localized to the anterior aspect of the trachea. Posterior wall involvement should be noted, because if surgical treatment is contemplated, resection of the esophagus may be indicated. This can also be assessed by performing rigid esophagoscopy at the time of bronchoscopy. Biopsy is then performed.

■ THERAPY

As in dealing with all tumors, the ideal management of a particular tumor depends on tumor factors, patient factors, and physician factors. *Tumor factors* include type and extent of the tumor; for example, extensive high-grade malignancies may best be treated palliatively with radiotherapy after the airway has been secured. Smaller tumors, on the other hand, can be successfully resected, and, of course, benign tumors may be endoscopically ablated. *Patient factors* include general health, respiratory reserve, and so forth, which may affect any decision to perform radical resection. Finally, *physician experience* and *facilities available* may have a significant impact on the therapeutic options offered to the patient. In general, the cornerstone of treatment for tracheal tumors is surgery.

There are three possible surgical options: (1) endoscopic excision or ablation, (2) sleeve resection, or (3) wide radical resection.

Endoscopic Excision

Small benign and even low-grade malignant tumors that are very superficial may be treated by means of endoscopic excision. Although this can be done with sharp instrumentation, the instrument of choice is a CO_2 laser. This is best performed by using the CO_2 ventilating bronchoscope. Respiratory papillomatosis is the ideal tumor for this type of treatment, particularly if the trachea is involved at multiple sites. This procedure has the advantage of minimal trauma, good hemostasis, and can, of course, be repeated. It can also be used for palliative debulking of large obstructing tumors.

Sleeve Resection

The indications for this procedure are benign tumors, low-grade malignant tumors (e.g., chondrosarcoma), and high-grade malignant tumors, provided there has been no significant extension into the cervical esophagus or into surrounding soft tissues. In adults, 5 to 6 rings can be removed, and primary anastomosis can be performed if a suprahyoid release is done. The surgeon should not hesitate to perform a sternotomy and expose the whole length of the trachea if this will permit safe resection and reconstruction.

A collar incision and anastomosis is performed approximately two finger breadths above the clavicles in a natural skin crease. The strap muscles are retracted, and the trachea is identified. If one is fortunate, the superior and inferior extent of the tumor is clearly visualized. Frequently, however, particularly if there is no extraluminal spread, the extent of the tumor can be difficult to identify. To overcome this problem, needles are inserted through the anterior tracheal wall just distal and just proximal to the tumor under bronchoscopic control to ensure that excess trachea is not resected. The anterior and lateral aspects of the trachea are cleaned by a combination of sharp and blunt dissection. If the dissection plane hugs the tracheal wall, the recurrent laryngeal nerves are protected without identifying them.

Blunt and sharp dissection is then used to separate the esophagus from the posterior tracheal wall. The trachea is opened between the cartilaginous rings at the sites previously identified both proximally and distally. Careful intraluminal inspection through the tracheal incision is then performed to ensure adequate margins. The sleeve resection is performed after the previously placed endotracheal tube is withdrawn above the resection, and once resection is completed, the tube is reinserted into the distal tracheal segment. If a tracheostomy had previously been performed, this should be included in the resection. The previously placed nasal endotracheal tube, situated just above the tumor, is then advanced into the distal trachea following resection. Frozen sections are obtained to ensure adequate resection.

A suprahyoid release is performed, either through a separate skin incision or by extending the cervical incision. The lower trachea is mobilized by blunt dissection. Absorbable sutures (2–0) are used to perform the end-to-end anastomosis on the posterior wall, while on the anterior wall, 2–0 nylon is used, with the sutures being placed submucosally around the tracheal rings and the knots placed on the exterior of the trachea to decrease granulation formation.

After the wound has been closed in layers, a single 0 nylon suture is placed between the mentum and the sternum to prevent neck extension in the postoperative period. This remains in place for 5 days. A tracheostomy is not performed in combination with the sleeve resection. The patient may be extubated either immediately after surgery or remain intubated overnight, and extubation is then performed 12 to 24 hours postoperatively, with the surgeon in attendance. If there is any concern, the extubation should be performed over a flexible bronchoscope to permit inspection of the suture line and to allow for controlled reintubation, if necessary.

Extended Radical Resection

The indication for radical resection is a high-grade tumor that has extended beyond the confines of the trachea with or without nodal metastases. In this situation, tracheal resection is usually associated with cervical esophagectomy and total laryngectomy with or without superior mediastinal dissection and lateral cervical neck dissections as indicated. Division of the clavicular heads and manubrium sterni or a midline sternal split is frequently necessary to gain adequate lower clearance and facilitate reconstruction. Reconstruction is a significant challenge, which essentially necessitates suturing the distal tracheal remnant to the sternal skin and reconstructing the cervical esophagus with a free flap, usually a free jejunal graft. The great vessel needs to be protected by a muscle flap. It is very rare that this procedure can be performed without sacrificing the larynx.

Obviously, before embarking on such a radical procedure, very realistic expectations should exist for both the patient and the treating physician. Care should be taken to follow a regimented approach to ensure that the lesion is indeed operable before making the final irreversible cuts.

Suggested Reading

Gelder CM, Hetzel MR. Primary tracheal tumors: A national survey. Thorax 1993; 48:688-692.

Grillo HC, Mathisen DJ. Primary tracheal tumors. Ann Thorac Surg 1990; 49:69.

Regnard JF, Fourquier P, Levasseur P. Results and prognostic factors in resections of primary tracheal tumors. J Thorac Cardiovasc Surg 1996; 11:808-814.

CERVICAL METASTASIS

The method of
Bruce J. Davidson
Roy B. Sessions

The prognostic impact of metastatic squamous cell carcinoma to cervical lymph nodes is well known and is associated with a decrease in disease control and survival by approximately 50 percent as compared with similar primary lesions without regional metastases. Because of these associations, a major component in head and neck cancer treatment is the effort to determine whether metastases are present and what treatment is required. Treatment of metastases that are clinically obvious usually includes surgery in conjunction with radiotherapy. However, even in the clinically N_0 neck, surgery such as selected neck dissection may play a role in assessment of the neck for occult metastases. Thus, for necks with clinically negative findings, assessment may consist of neck dissection as a staging tool, whereas in the setting of clinically positive neck disease, neck dissection has a significant therapeutic role. The former should be minimally invasive and nondebilitating while obtaining accurate staging information. The latter must maximize treatment effectiveness without causing unnecessary morbidity. Many of the technical aspects of these neck dissections are the same, but their purposes are distinctly different.

■ OCCULT METASTASES

The likelihood of a neck having technically negative findings at the time of diagnosis varies relative to the primary site and stage, ranging from greater than 80 percent for T_1 oral cavity cancers to under 25 percent for T_3 and T_4 oropharyngeal or hypopharnygeal cancers. Several factors should be considered in these patients when deciding on the assessment and treatment of cervical lymphatics. Many historical data are available that help define the risk of metastases for tumors of various primary sites and stages. We have summarized selective data in Table 1.

Table 1. Relationship Between Primary Site and a Clinically Negative Neck at Presentation and the Incidence of Occult Metastases

PRIMARY SITE	% N_0*	% POSITIVE NODES IN ELECTIVE NECK DISSECTION†
Oral Cavity	50	23–34
Tongue	58	25
Floor of mouth	66	21
Gum		12
Retromolar	57	35
Oropharynx	34	31–35
Hypopharynx	29	17–55
Larynx		21–37
Glottic		16
Supraglottic	49	26

* Data derived from Lindberg R. Distribution of cervical lymph node metastases from squamous cell carcinoma of the upper respirratory and digestive tracts. Cancer 1972; 29:1446–1449.

† Data derived from Shah IP. Patterns of cervical node metastases from squamous carcinomas of the upper aerodigestive tract. Am J Surg 1990; 160:405–409; Byers RM, Wolf PF, Ballantyne AJ. Rationale for elective modified neck dissection. Head Neck Surg 1988; 10:160–167.

Clinical assessment of the neck can be supplemented by computed tomography (CT) or magnetic resonance imaging (MRI). Although clinical examination is approximately 70 percent accurate, CT and MRI show accuracy rates of approximately 90 percent for assessment of the neck for metastatic disease. The choice between CT and MRI is determined by the need for imaging of the primary lesion. CT is less expensive, and for cervical node imaging alone, this modality may be slightly superior to MRI. However, when primary lesions such as those in the nasopharynx or base of the tongue are present, MRI is preferred because enhanced imaging of the primary site is obtained. However, when primary lesions such as those in the nasopharynx or base of the tongue are present, MRI is preferred because enhanced imaging of the primary site is obtained.

After clinical examination and imaging studies, the decision regarding surgical assessment and treatment of the N_0 neck is made based on the treatment planned for the primary lesion. For early-stage pharynx and larynx carcinomas, the primary tumor usually is irradiated, and primary echelon nodal basins or any equivocal nodes that have been noted by CT or MRI are included in the treatment fields. For oral cavity lesions, however, surgical therapy is preferred, and pathologic findings are used to determine the need for adjunctive radiotherapy. In this circumstance, a staging procedure is performed incorporating selective neck dissection of levels I, II, and III. For midline or bulky lesions, bilateral neck dissection may be indicated. Postoperative radiotherapy is recommended for those patients whose pathology reveals more than one node with metastatic disease or evidence of extracapsular spread. For low-stage primary lesions, the use of selective neck dissection increases the staging accuracy and results in fewer patients receiving radiotherapy unnecessarily. Given an overall rate of microscopic cervical metastases in N_0 necks of approximately 30 percent, more than two-thirds of patients treated in this sequence may be spared unnecessary radiotherapy, provided, of course, that the primary lesion has been adequately treated by surgery alone.

For higher stage primary lesions, the use of surgical staging has not been validated by any prospective studies. Nevertheless, when access to the primary tumor requires a neck incision, a selective nodal dissection can be performed with little added morbidity. This will remove occult metastases and potentially direct the portals and dose requirement for postoperative radiotherapy.

■ CLINICALLY POSITIVE NECK DISEASE

When clinical disease is detected in the neck, intervention no longer requires an estimate of risk for nodal metastases These patients require surgery and radiotherapy, with chemotherapy used in selected cases.

Location of the nodal disease is an important feature. In the setting of an unknown primary tumor, location of the nodal disease may direct the surgeon toward the mucosal lesion. Low-level IV or V neck nodes imply an infraclavicular primary. Also, patients presenting with low neck nodes and an obvious head and neck primary have a poor prognosis and a higher likelihood of distant metastatic disease. The same is true of patients who have massive cervical metastases. Thus, in patients presenting with lower neck nodes or massive cervical metastases, we often obtain a chest CT either to rule out a lung primary or to evaluate for distant metastases, depending on the clinical situation.

Other nodal locations may require individualized approaches. These include retropharyngeal nodes, which are not addressed in classic radical neck dissections and require an extension of this procedure if surgical resection is carried out. High neck nodes may lie within the lower parotid gland and require parotidectomy in conjunction with treatment of the neck. Deeper nodes high in the neck may extend to the skull base along the jugular vein.

The N-staging system is based on the number and size of nodes. Moderate-sized metastases (3 to 6 cm), multiple nodes, or contralateral or bilateral nodes distinguish N_2 from N_1, whereas massive metastases (> 6 cm), regardless of number and location, are assigned an N_3 designation. The correlation between nodal size and prognosis led to the establishment of the N-stage definitions. A pathologic factor that likely explains this relationship is the finding of extracapsular spread in most large metastatic deposits. Extracapsular spread, metastatic disease that has grown beyond the capsule of the affected node, is present in one-quarter of small nodes and is found in more than 75 percent of nodes greater than 3 cm in diameter. Generally speaking, extracapsular spread is associated with a significant decrease in neck control and survival.

For resectable neck disease, a combination of neck dissection and radiotherapy is used. The order does not seem to matter from an oncologic standpoint. Nevertheless, we prefer surgery to precede radiotherapy, if possible. (As with selective neck dissection for occult disease, pathologic findings may direct adjunctive radiotherapy portals and dose to areas at greater risk of recurrence.) Practically speaking, treatment of the primary tumor often determines the timing of neck surgery. If surgical treatment of the primary is indicated (oral cavity, large oropharynx, and selected hypopharynx and larynx primaries), neck dissection will be performed at the same time. If radiotherapy is planned for the primary (nasopharynx, base of tongue, small tonsil primaries), however, neck dissection is performed after radiotherapy. For base of tongue primary tumors, neck dissection is performed at the same time as brachytherapy catheters are placed to boost the tongue base. When organ preservation using chemotherapy and radiotherapy is planned (larynx and hypopharynx primaries), the neck dissection will be carried out 3 to 6 weeks following completion of radiotherapy (Table 2).

Massive nodal disease may present significant therapeutic challenges due to the infiltration of surrounding structures. Growth may extend to skin and require modification of usual skin incisions and utilization of local or regional flaps for closure. Disease may be adherent to the carotid artery, deep muscles of the neck, or cranial nerves IX to XII. Surgical modifications that include any of these structures increase the risk of complications, ranging from increased shoulder morbidity from resection of the levator scapula muscle to cerebrovascular events after manipulation or resection of the carotid artery.

Preoperative imaging is particularly useful in massive adenopathy. Disease extending to the jugular foramen or occluding or significantly displacing the carotid artery may be identified before initiation of therapy. Attempting to down-

Table 2. Treatment Approach to Metastatic Squamous Cell Carcinoma to the Neck According to Primary Site and Neck Stage

SITE	T STAGE	N_0	N STAGE N_1 TO N_2	N_3	BORDERLINE/ UNRESECTABLE
Oral cavity	T_{1-4}	SND ± RT	MND + RT	RND + RT	Chemotherapy + RT ± RND
Nasopharynx	T_{1-4}	RT	RT	RT	RT
Base of tongue	T_{1-4}	RT/Brady	RT + MND/Brachy	RT + RND/Brachy	Chemo + RT ± RND/Brachy
Tonsil	T_{1-2}	RT	RT + MND	RT + RND	Chemo + RT ± RND
	T_3	RT alone vs SND + RT	MND + RT	RND + RT	Chemo + RT ± RND
	T_4	SND + RT	MND + RT	RND + RT	Chemo + RT ± RND
Hypopharynx	T_1–T_2	RT	RT + MND	RT + RND	Chemo + RT ± RND
	T_{2-4}	Chemo + RT	Chemo + RT + MND	Chemo + RT + RND	Chemo + RT ± RND
Larynx	T_{1-2}	RT	RT + MND	RT + RND	Chemo + RT ± RND
	T_{3-4}	Chemo + RT	Chemo + RT + MND	Chemo + RT + RND	Chemo + RT ± RND

SND, selective neck dissection; RT, radiotherapy; Chemo, chemotherapy; MND, modified neck dissection; Brachy, brachytherapy; RND, radical neck dissection.

stage such a tumor with chemotherapy or radiotherapy is often appealing, and we selectively use such an approach. It must be recognized, however, that a tumor that does not respond to such treatment is likely to be even more difficult to address surgically afterward.

Technical Details

Selective Neck Dissection

Supraomohyoid neck dissection is the most common selective neck dissection used. This operation selectively removes the submandibular gland and lymphatics of levels I, II, and III. The procedure is performed through a single transverse incision from the mastoid process to the submental triangle. Subplatysmal flaps are elevated superiorly to the body of the mandible and inferiorly to the omohyoid muscle. Care is taken to avoid injury to the marginal mandibular nerve when the superior flap is elevated. The posterior aspect of the inferior flap is raised over the sternocleidomastiod muscle to allow improved access deep to this muscle.

The investing fascia of the sternocleidomastiod muscle is used to begin the dissection posteriorly. The spinal accessory nerve is identified deep to the sternocleidomastoid muscle. The triangle posterosuperior to the spinal accessory nerve is included in the dissection to ensure that all level II nodes are removed. The value of this maneuver is questionable, however, because recent work has shown no evidence of isolated metastases to this area in clinically negative necks. As the dissection proceeds deep to the sternocleidomastoid muscle, the cervical nerve roots are noted and preserved. These mark the posterior border of the dissection.

As the specimen is mobilized anteriorly, a scalpel is used to expose the posterior aspect of the carotid artery and vagus nerve. Care must be exercised at the interior and superior aspects of the dissection, where the internal jugular vein can become compressed and twisted by traction on the specimen toward the midline. It is usually safer to identify the midportion of the internal jugular vein first, and then carefully approach the inferior and superior aspects of the dissection. Few veins are encountered along the posterior aspect of the internal jugular vein. A No. 15 blade can be used on the wall of the vein as the nodes of the dissection are mobilized medially. Two or three large tributaries will be noted entering the internal jugular vein anteriorly. These should be ligated far enough from the internal jugular vein to prevent compression of the jugular lumen. Once these branches are divided, the dissection can proceed deep to the jugular vein onto the anterior aspect of the carotid artery. The superior thyroid artery can be preserved in almost all cases. Dissection of the submandibular and submental triangles is carried out in the usual fashion either before or after dissection of the great vessels. Prior dissection allows identification of the posterior belly of the digastric and the hypoglossal nerve, and these steps may ease dissection of the anterior aspect of the carotid sheath structures.

After completion of the dissection, the specimen is marked with ties or tags at levels I, II, and III so that the pathologist has the proper orientation. The wound is irrigated, and hemostasis is obtained. Two closed suction drains are placed. The wound is closed with 3–0 polyglactin 910 and staples. No dressings are used on the neck wound. Staples are removed after 7 days in nonirradiated patients, 10 to 14 days in irradiated patients.

Comprehensive Neck Dissection

When a neck with clinically positive findings is treated, the dissection should include levels I to V. This may entail a classic radical neck dissection, but in many cases the spinal accessory nerve can be preserved. Other modifications, such as preservation of the internal jugular vein or sternocleidomastoid muscle, are used less often. Massive nodal disease may require extension of the radical neck dissection. This may involve resection of the posterior belly of the digastric, deep muscles of the neck, the hypoglossal or vagus nerves, or the external and/or internal carotid artery.

The incision for a comprehensive neck dissection is usually a bifurcating design, with the transverse component from the mastoid tip to the submental area, and an S-shaped vertical limb beginning where the external jugular vein reaches the transverse incision and extending to the midclavicle. It should be kept in mind when designing the neck incision that each of the flaps survives by random blood supply. The most vulnerable flap is usually the anteroinferiorly based flap. The blood supply to this flap can be jeopardized by a large S-curve in the vertical limb narrowing the blood supply to the trifurcation, a large tracheostomy incision, or excessively tight tracheostomy ties. Locating the trifurcation over the carotid artery can result in major and life-threatening complications from a minor wound breakdown.

We prefer to begin our dissection with the posterior triangle. The flap here is raised in the plane of the superficial fascia. The platysma is usually not present in the upper lateral neck, and care must be taken in raising this flap to remain at the proper depth; too superficial and the dermis will be encountered, too deep and the spinal accessory nerve can be inadvertently transected. Once the anterior border of the trapezius muscle is identified, dissection on the superficial aspect of the anterior border allows completion of the flap elevation without jeopardizing the spinal accessory nerve. At the superior aspect of the dissection, the posterior border is carried forward to the mastoid tip along the splenius capitis muscle.

The spinal accessory nerve can be preserved in most neck dissections for N_1 disease and many of those for N_2 disease. Its identification is often quite simple following elevation of the posterior flap. Often, the use of electrocautery during flap elevation will give an indication as to the location of the nerve. If not, careful inspection (before further dissection) of the posterior triangle may allow visual identification of the nerve below the fascia of the posterior triangle. In obese patients, location of the nerve can be more difficult, but careful dissection between Erb's point and the junction of the middle and inferior thirds of the trapezius muscle will usually lead to identification. Once located, dissection along the length of spinal accessory nerve is carried out from the trapezius to the posterior belly of the digastric. Depending on the course of the nerve and the neck disease at hand, the sternocleidomastoid muscle will either be divided from the mastoid tip and reflected interiorly to expose the digastric, or the muscle will be divided from Erb's point to the digastric directly over the spinal accessory nerve.

With the spinal accessory nerve freed throughout its course, the contents of the posterior triangle can be reflected anteriorly by raising these tissues from the deep layer of the deep cervical fascia, with care taken to preserve the neurovascular supply to the levator scapulae and other deep neck musculature. Posterior triangle tissues are elevated to the point of the cervical nerve roots and phrenic nerve.

At this point, the inferior neck is dissected with preservation or sacrifice of the internal jugular vein as dictated by neck disease and/or the need for venous anastomosis for microvascular reconstruction. The sternocleidomastoid is sacrificed in almost all cases of comprehensive neck dissection. The upper part of the neck dissection is carried out in a manner similar to the supraomohyoid dissection. Gross disease is usually dissected last, after exposure from above, below, and posteriorly. Following completion of the dissection, the wound is irrigated, and hemostasis is obtained. A sustained Valsalva's maneuver by anesthesia can assist in identifying small venous bleeders or open thoracic duct tributaries. Two closed suction drains are placed through stab incisions in the posterior skin flap. Closure is performed with 3–0 polyglactin 910 sutures and staples. To avoid masking a postoperative hematoma or seroma, a neck dressing is not used.

When extended neck dissection is performed in which skin is taken, closure by advancement of local flaps can usually be performed. Extensive disease along the jugular vein in the upper neck is often made more accessible by sacrifice of the posterior belly of the digastric. If the external carotid artery requires sacrifice, vascular clamps should be used, and the end of the artery oversewn with 6–0 Prolene. This is best done beyond the takeoff of the first branch of the external carotid in order to reduce the likelihood of thrombus formation and potential cerebral embolism. The sacrifice of both the hypoglossal and vagus during neck dissection can lead to significant morbidity in speech and swallowing. We usually do not intervene with immediate thyroplasty in these cases due in part to concerns about airway edema during ensuing radiotherapy. Also, we prefer to wait until there is a documented need for thyroplasty after a trial of adduction exercises. We then perform thyroplasty under local anesthesia during a separate procedure.

Complications

The most common complications after neck dissection alone are skin flap necrosis, hematomas, and seromas. Superficial skin necrosis is most commonly seen at the bifurcation along the posteroinferior or anteroinferior flap. Previous radiotherapy and elevation of these flaps in a subcutaneous rather than a subplatysmal plane may compromise the vascularity to this area. Other factors that may increase the risk of breakdown of the anteroinferior flap include a large incision for tracheostomy or excessively tight tracheostomy ties. Likewise, a sharp S-turn in the vertical limb of the skin incision may narrow the blood supply to the bifurcation. Once superficial necrosis is noted, little is done except periodic debridement and topical wound care. Topical collagenase can be used safely in this area, even if the carotid artery is exposed. Eschar can be debrided and scored with a scalpel, and then collagenase is applied once a day and covered with a dry dressing, which assists in debridement and appears to stimulate granulation tissue. When the carotid is exposed, keeping the wound moist and preventing desiccation of the carotid adventitia are of paramount importance.

Hematomas and seromas most commonly appear in the supraclavicular fossa and, when small, may be allowed to resolve spontaneously. When large, however, they should be drained because they can compromise the overlying skin flap and result in secondary wound breakdown at the trifurcation. Needle aspiration or incision and drainage are recommended in this situation. Increased wound drainage or collections that develop after initiation of enteral or oral feeding may indicate a chyle collection in the neck. Usually, these can be managed with a low-fat diet or one limited to medium-chain triglycerides and compression dressings to the supraclavicular fossa. When drainage fails to respond to these measures or when the volume exceeds 600 cc per day, neck exploration is indicated. Direct ligation of the thoracic duct is usually difficult due to extensive fibrinous exudate. Oversewing the duct with figure eight silk suture and coverage by local rotation of vascularized tissue (such as strap muscle) may be required.

Major vascular injury associated with neck dissection is usually recognized intraoperatively. If a branch of the internal jugular vein is avulsed with no residual stump, then simple ligation will not be effective. A 6–0 Prolene can be used to oversew the fenestration in the vein wall. Injury to the carotid artery is rarely seen during neck dissection. Occasionally, the external carotid artery must be oversewn to enable resection of a neck mass.

Neural injury may result from intentional sacrifice due to tumor proximity. Traction injury may occur when dissecting the vagus, spinal accessory, or hypoglossal nerves, and deficits are easily recognized postoperatively. Our approach to rehabilitation after vagus sacrifice has been described previously in this chapter.

Marginal mandibular nerve paresis is often missed by the casual examiner, but this condition is the most common nerve injury from neck dissection. Prevention of this injury depends on careful dissection of the superior neck flap. We recommend visual identification of the nerve and dissection and elevation of it up to the body of the mandible. If the nerve is identified and protected during surgery, then the only deficit should be related to sacrifice of the cervical branch of the facial nerve, with decreased motion of the platysma. If the nerve is known to be intact and not injured by inadvertent use of electrocautery, a postoperative marginal mandibular weakness can be expected to improve over 2 to 3 months follow-up.

■ RESULTS

The results of treatment for cervical metastatic squamous cell carcinoma are highly correlated with the stage of disease at presentation. N_0 neck disease addressed by staging neck dissection allows dichotomization into pathologically positive and negative subgroups. Those subgroups documented as pathologically negative have a risk of recurrence in the operated neck of approximately 5 percent after surgery alone. Contralateral metastases may rarely occur in these cases. Those subgroups who have pathologically proven subclinical metastatic disease will show excellent neck control after radiotherapy, with control of the treated neck in excess of 90 percent. Control of clinically obvious metastatic disease is greater than 80 percent for N_1 and approximately 70 percent for N_2 and N_3 neck disease after surgery and radiotherapy.

Suggested Reading

Byers RM, Modified neck dissection—A study of 967 cases from 1970 to 1980. Am J Surg 1985; 150:414-421.

Byers RM, Wolf PF, Ballantyne AJ. Rationale for elective-modified neck dissection. Head Neck Surg 1988; 10:160-167.

Kraus DH, Rosenberg DB, Davidson BJ, et al. Supraspinal accessory lymph node metastases in supraomohyoid neck dissection. Am J Surg 1996; 172:646-649.

Robbins KT. Neck dissection classification and TNM staging of head and neck cancer. Alexandria, VA: American Academy of Otolaryngology Head and Neck Surgery Foundation, Inc., 1991.

Shah JP. Patterns of cervical node metastases from squamous carcinomas of the upper aerodigestive tract. Am J Surg 1990; 160:405-409.

Spiro RH, Morgan GJ, Strong EW, Shah JP. Supraomohyoid neck dissection. Am J Surg 1996; 172:650-653.

DEEP NECK INFECTION

The method of
James N. Endicott

Infections of the head and neck may result in serious consequences despite antibiotic therapy. The modern head and neck surgeon may be challenged to make the diagnosis and properly manage the patient with this life-threatening infection when medical treatment has been inadequate. Successful management is based on a thorough understanding of the fascial planes and potential spaces of the neck, the etiology, bacteriology, diagnostic techniques, and possible complications of the deep neck infection. The deep neck spaces have a variety of names and descriptions that are relatively consistent throughout the literature (Table 1). The primary sources of space infections of the head and neck are isolated nodal abscess formation and dental, tonsillar, or pharyngeal infection sites. Pathologic organisms most commonly are streptococcus; staphylococcus in approximately 25 percent of cases; and anaerobic bacteria, the most common organism of dental origin.

Initially, the presentation of a deep neck infection may be local or systemic signs and symptoms of infection, usually swelling, with tenderness and pain in the involved area. There may be erythema of the skin over the infection and a pitting edema. Fluctuance is the exception rather than the rule. There may be an elevated temperature, leukocytosis, and general malaise. Trismus may be secondary to an abscess in several potential spaces: lateral pharyngeal, masticator, peritonsillar, submaxillary, temporal, and with Ludwig's angina. Torticollis, dyspnea, stridor, dysphagia, odynophagia, hoarseness, and aphonia may also occur, depending on the site of infection.

Systemic diseases such as diabetes, nephritis, tuberculosis, or acquired immunodeficiency syndrome (AIDS) may be associated with deep neck infections, and unless these conditions are diagnosed and, where possible, properly managed, they may result in a disaster.

Medical management includes hospitalization, high-dose

Table 1. Neck Spaces That Have Clinical Potential for Deep Neck Infections

I. Spaces involving the entire length of the neck
   A. Retropharyngeal space (posterior visceral space, retrovisceral space, retroesophageal space)
   B. Prevertebral ("danger" space)
   C. Visceral vascular space (within the carotid sheath)
II. Spaces above the hyoid bone
   A. Submandibular space
      1. Sublingual (medial)
      2. Submaxillary (lateral)
   B. Lateral pharyngeal (pharyngomaxillary, parapharyngeal space)
   C. Masticator space
   D. Parotid space
   E. Peritonsillar space
III. Spaces below the hyoid bone (anterior only)
   A. Anterior visceral (pretracheal) space

antibiotic therapy, and hydration, with observation of the airway and close monitoring of the infection response. The source of space infection may not be apparent. Cultures should be taken from the infected site or the abscess itself. Needle aspiration by computed tomographic (CT) scan technique may be necessary to obtain aerobic and anaerobic culture and Gram's stain. Blood cultures should be taken as well. Frequently, the patient has been receiving antibiotics before he or she has seen the specialist, thus preventing identification by culture techniques. Aqueous penicillin G, 20 million units intravenously (IV) daily, plus a β-lactamase–resistant drug such as clindamycin, chloramphenicol, or gentamicin are recommended.

The urgency of treatment is dictated by the severity and rate of progression of the signs and symptoms. No drainage attempts are necessary during the stage of phlegmon formation (cellulitis); however, an abscess should be surgically drained because it rarely will rupture spontaneously and drain externally. More than one space may be involved when the abscess breaks through a fascial barrier or follows an anatomic structure into an adjacent space. The patient who requires emergency treatment may have airway compromise, sepsis, or hemorrhage from the ear or pharynx.

The patient's airway may be at risk, and the surgeon must be prepared to establish a proper airway. The mucosa of the hypopharynx may be markedly edematous, and trismus may be present, making intubation extremely difficult or even hazardous. The intraoral examination may be troublesome or impossible because of trismus; however, a CT scan is very useful in monitoring the stage of infection.

We use a CT scan with 4 mm axial cuts to demonstrate, in most cases, whether the patient has only cellulitis of the soft tissues or whether the patient's space in question has an abscess that is displacing structures, thus requiring surgical drainage. The CT contributes to the indirect assessment of the site and extent of infection when one or more spaces are involved and may identify complications such as venous thrombosis. CT may be used for follow-up to determine the course of the infection when symptoms worsen or when there is progression of disease in the neck or chest. CT requires minimal positioning of the patient and allows examination of the critically ill patient. Although less expensive and less invasive than CT, ultrasound provides poor imaging beneath the clavicle and under the mandible and cannot detect a recent thrombus with low echogenicity. Magnetic resonance imaging (MRI), although avoiding IV contrast and radiation, is high in cost, and its limited availability makes it less attractive than CT for monitoring the patient.

Soft-tissue cellulitis may progress rapidly to a potential space abscess, in some cases in less than 24 hours, while the patient is receiving high-dose antibiotic therapy. In only 10 percent to 15 percent of adult patients will deep neck infections resolve with medical management. Establishment of a safe airway, vascular control, and adequate visualization are basic rules for surgery. The method of drainage varies according to the location of the deep space infection. If the source of the infection is a tooth, it should be removed at the time of the abscess drainage. Abscesses are drained by standard approaches described in the literature and based on anatomic relationships; however, drainage is not a cosmetic procedure. Enlarged incisions with well-loosened and retracted neck flaps are necessary, with the surgeon taking care to avoid cranial nerve injury. Airway management should be performed under local anesthesia by tracheostomy without relaxants or drying agents while the patient receives rapid intravenous hydration and antibiotics. Although marked swelling in the neck can distort landmarks during the operative procedure, elective tracheostomy under local anesthesia will avoid the emergency tracheostomy when ill-advised intubation attempts occur either by nasotracheal or orotracheal techniques. However, nasotracheal anesthesia in a patient who has trismus and a masseteric space abscess should be safe.

■ SPECIFIC SPACE INFECTIONS

Lateral Pharyngeal Space

The lateral pharyngeal space abscess characteristically has trismus with swelling at the angle of the mandible and parotid area. A plum-colored mucosa within the oral cavity may suggest that there is hemorrhage into the parapharyngeal space from either the carotid artery or one of its branches, and the surgeon should be prepared to deal with this complication during the drainage procedure. Intraoperatively, the posterior belly of the digastric muscle may be followed to its origin, where the styloid process can be palpated. The surgeon should slide the finger past the styloid into the pharyngeal space, which will then allow drainage out of the wound. The great vessels can be controlled through this incision, and vascular complications can then be managed. The transoral approach is contraindicated because of poor visibility and access.

Masticator Space

A masticator space infection is a subperiosteal abscess with cellulitis involving the mandible and surrounding soft tissue; this infection frequently involves the fascial sling containing the muscles of mastication (masseter, pterygoid, and temporal). The lateral facial swelling may resemble the lateral pharyngeal space abscess, and trismus is rather marked. CT scans may differentiate the site and whether both spaces may be involved. Drainage may be performed through a buccal sulcus incision after nasotracheal intubation. If the infratemporal space is involved, this site is drained above the zygoma, carrying the incision through the temporalis fascia, and taking care to avoid the frontal branches of the facial nerve.

A sublingual space abscess will respond to intraoral drainage, but when it progresses to bilateral submandibular space involvement, Ludwig's angina has developed. This infection is not a true abscess but a cellulitis that is very virulent and can cause rapid death from upper airway obstruction or mediastinitis when it descends past the level of the hyoid. A CT scan for this abscess has not been found to be helpful in management decisions. Trismus and hypopharyngeal mucosal edema contraindicate preliminary intubation, and a tracheostomy under local anesthesia is indicated through the edematous anterior neck tissue. During drainage of this abscess, frank pus is rarely encountered.

Parotid Space

The parotid space has many fascial septae running vertically throughout the gland that can result in multiple loculated abscesses within the gland when infection results in abscess. Massage of Stensen's duct may reveal a purulent flow, and adjacent neck spaces may be involved with spread of infection. Surgical drainage is through a preauricular Furstenberg incision, with skin elevation exposing the parotid capsule. Vertical incisions are made through the capsule into the gland with a blunt hemostat in a direction paralleling the branches of the facial nerve, breaking up the scattered foci of abscesses in the area of localized infection. This technique allows for drainage, yet protects the facial nerve. The most common pathologic organism is staphylococcus.

Retropharyngeal Space

The retropharyngeal abscess may also threaten the airway. In children under age 4 years, the abscess may be localized to a plane above the hyoid. This abscess in a child is usually secondary to suppurative retropharyngeal nodes draining the posterior two-thirds of the nose, paranasal sinuses, pharynx, and eustachian tube; the abscess usually is unilateral because of the midline raphe dividing the space, thus giving the appearance of a unilateral swelling of the posterior pharyngeal wall, which may push the palate forward. Signs include pain, drooling, dysphagia, and refusal to eat. Torticollis with the neck tilted toward the uninvolved side is a late sign. The voice may have a muffled sound, but no trismus is present. Palpation of the mass and aspiration with an 18 gauge spinal needle may be useful in examination and diagnosis of the causative organism. Classically, the lateral neck radiograph in a cooperative patient helps make the diagnosis. Measurements of the retropharyngeal space at the C-2 level greater than 7 mm in a child or adult are abnormal. Interpretation of this area in infants may be unreliable.

Management for the child is by transoral drainage under general or local anesthesia. The patient's head should be in Rose's position, with suction immediately available to prevent aspiration of purulent material. When the abscess is below the plane of the hyoid, as is commonly seen in adults and is usually secondary to ingested foreign bodies, gunshot wounds, or endoscopic trauma, an external drainage approach is indicated. The Dean approach, a lateral oblique incision anterior to the sternocleidomastoid muscle, is commonly used for the retropharyngeal abscess, as well as for abscesses of the prevertebral (danger) space, paravertebral space, pretracheal space, and visceral vascular space. CT scan of the neck that is correlated with physical diagnosis will help to localize the site of the abscess. Bilateral drainage may be required. The sternocleidomastoid and the great vessels are retracted laterally, whereas the larynx, trachea, and thyroid gland are retracted medially. The middle thyroid vein, the superior thyroid artery, and the omohyoid muscle may be sectioned for better exposure. Characteristically, the abscess may resemble a distended bag and lies between the carotid sheath and the paravertebral muscles behind the inferior constrictor muscles. The abscess then may be opened with a hemostat. If the abscess extends more inferiorly into the neck and upper mediastinum, the dissection is carried along the carotid sheath to the sternum, exposing the trachea and the esophagus, with care to avoid injury to the recurrent laryngeal nerve. A finger is inserted into the mediastinum beneath the esophagus to drain the space abscess. If the abscess has spread past the level of T-4 posteriorly or the tracheal bifurcation anteriorly, as determined by CT scan, drainage by external thoracotomy will also be necessary.

■ TECHNICAL CONSIDERATIONS

All abscess cavities should be irrigated vigorously and drained with Penrose drains sutured to the skin to avoid loss of drain on the first dressing change. Drains may be slowly advanced and then removed during the next several days as the patient's antibiotic coverage is continued. In the case of an esophageal perforation, the perforation site should be covered, if possible, with soft tissue, and a feeding jejunostomy or gastrostomy tube should be placed to allow the perforation to heal, which may take 6 months or more, depending on the size of the perforation and condition of the patient. After the patient has stopped drainage and the drains have been removed, IV antibiotics must be switched to the oral route for a 3 week period as the patient is followed up as an outpatient.

■ COMPLICATIONS

Complications of deep space abscesses vary with the site of abscess. The paravertebral space extends from the skull base to the coccyx. Trauma is a common cause of this space abscess and could result in a psoas muscle sheath abscess. A visceral space abscess (carotid sheath space) is the most common infection seen in patients with IV drug addiction who use the internal jugular vein as an access site. Jugular vein thrombosis with a spiking febrile course and secondary septicemia may occur, which would require either drainage or resection of the internal jugular vein. Heparinization has been suggested for the controversial role of anticoagulation therapy in internal jugular vein sepsis (Lemierre's syndrome). Most patients improve with antibiotics. Anticoagulants may be reserved for patients who have clinical evidence of propagating thrombus retrograde to the cavernous site. The anticoagulant regimen consists of 1 week of intravenous heparin, followed by 3 months of oral warfarin sodium. Thromboembolic metastasis is common, usually to the lungs, but may involve the joints, bones, meninges, and liver. The gram-negative anaerobic bacillus, *F. necrophorum*, is the common anaerobe. It is traditionally susceptible to clindamycin, benzathine penicillin G, and metronidazole. Mediastinitis may occur as a result of abscesses in the spaces running the length of the neck; this complication has a mortality rate of 35 percent to 50 percent.

Lateral pharyngeal space abscess may cause Horner's syndrome, hoarseness, unilateral tongue paralysis, dysphagia, thrombophlebitis of the internal jugular vein, and erosion of the carotid artery. A prevertebral space abscess may cause diaphragmatic and abdominal abscess. Ludwig's angina may result in loss of airway or mediastinitis when the abscess breaks past the hyoid barrier.

A paravertebral space abscess may result in osteomyelitis of the cervical spine, with secondary quadriplegia or subluxation of vertebrae. Instrumentation of pharyngeal abscesses without airway control may result in aspiration, lung abscess, pneumonia, empyema, and acute respiratory distress syndrome.

Carotid artery erosion may require ligation of the common carotid artery, with the potential consequences of stroke. Preliminary intraoperative arteriogram may localize the site of erosion to a branch of the external carotid in 20 percent to 35 percent of patients. The patient must be stabilized and hypovolemia and hypotension must be controlled if arteriogram is to be attempted.

■ DISCUSSION

Deep space neck infections often result in diagnostic or treatment dilemmas. There is a tendency for physicians to underestimate the potential severity of the infection. Unless the diagnosis is made early, abscess may result, and death may rapidly ensue as a result of asphyxia, hemorrhage, or septicemia. Antibiotics have greatly reduced the incidence of these infections; however, surgical drainage of a neck abscess is still mandatory to avoid complications. The CT scan and knowledge of cervical fascia help to guide the surgeon in evaluating an edematous, inflamed, and abnormally enlarged neck. Hospitalization, workup with imaging studies, and aggressive medical and surgical therapy will continue to be the standard of care in the modern health care environment.

Suggested Reading

Beck AL. The influence of the chemotherapeutic and antibiotic drugs on the incidence and course of deep neck infections. Ann Otol Rhinol Laryngol 1952; 61:515-532.

Brook I. Microbiology of abscesses of the head and neck in children. Ann Otol Rhinol Laryngol 1987; 96:429-433.

Dean LW. The proper procedure for external drainage of retropharyngeal abscess secondary to caries of the vertebrae. Ann Otol Rhinol Laryngol 1919; 28:566-572.

Endicott JN. Deep neck infections. In Gates GA, ed. Current therapy in otolaryngology—Head and neck surgery, 1982-1983. Trenton NJ: BC Decker, 1982:253.

Endicott JN. Infection of deep fascial spaces of the head and neck: Update of diagnosis and management. Vol. 3. (Instructional Courses). St. Louis: AAO-HNS Foundation, 1990.

Endicott JN, Molony TB, Campbell G, et al. Esophageal perforations: The role of computerized tomography in diagnosis and management of decisions. Laryngoscope 1986; 96:751-757.

Endicott JN, Nelson RJ, Saraceno CA. Diagnosis and management decisions in infections of the deep fascial spaces of the head and neck utilizing computerized tomography. Laryngoscope 1982; 92:630-633.

Holiger PH. Complications of esophageal perforations. Ann Otol Rhinol Laryngol 1941; 50:681-705.

Lewitt GW. The surgical treatment of deep neck infections. Laryngoscope 1971; 81:403-411.

Mosher HP. The submaxillary fossa approach to deep pus in the neck. Trans Am Acad Ophthalmol Otolaryngol 1929; 34:19-36.

Myers EM, Kirkland LS Jr, Mickey R. The head and neck sequelae of cervical intravenous drug abuse. Laryngoscope 1988; 98:213-286.

Rabuzzi DD, Johnson JT, Weissman JL. Diagnosis and management of deep neck infections. SIPAC, AAO-HNS Foundation, 1993.

CONGENITAL NECK MASSES

The method of
Charles F. Koopmann, Jr.

Congenital lesions must be considered in the differential diagnosis of neck masses in infants and children. A congenital etiology is suspected on the basis of the history and physical examination. These lesions are interesting not only because of their clinical manifestations but also because a knowledge of the embryology and anatomy is essential in the institution of appropriate initial therapy. Often, although these lesions are asymptomatic when first noticed, concerned parents or grandparents request immediate correction. In general, it is advisable to postpone surgery until the child is at least 2 years of age unless there are functional reasons to intervene, such as recurrent infections, feeding problems, or airway compromise. Surgical removal should be ideally done through an uninfected area, so any infection should be treated medically, if possible. If an abscess does form, aspiration and antibiotics or incision, drainage, and antibiotics are necessary. Any incision and drainage procedure should be planned so that the incision for definitive removal is not compromised.

I discuss in this chapter the following congenital lesions that present as neck masses: fibromatosis colli, cervical dermoids and teratomas, lymphangiomas and/or cystic hygromas, hemangiomas, thyroglossal duct remnants, and branchial cleft anomalies.

FIBROMATOSIS COLLI (CONGENITAL MUSCULAR TORTICOLLIS)

Fibromatosis colli is the unilateral involvement of the sternocleidomastoid (SCM) muscle in the newborn, which causes the head to be tilted toward the affected muscle, with a rotation of the head to the contralateral side. It is caused by fibrosis within the involved SCM muscle, with a resultant shortening to the muscle. This condition most likely occurs in the third trimester of pregnancy or in the immediate postpartum period and is usually noticed at birth or immediately thereafter. The etiology is believed to be secondary to venous occlusion. The presentation is usually within the first 10 to 14 days of life when a nontender mass is palpable in the lower third of the SCM muscle. The mass most commonly increases in size over the following 2 to 4 weeks, which causes the parents and referring provider to fear the presence of a malignant neoplasm. If left untreated, fibromatosis colli will usually regress and leave a contracted muscle, with the head tilted to the ipsilateral side and the chin tilted to the contralateral side.

For the patient who has a classic presentation, ultrasonography usually is sufficient to make the diagnosis. If doubt remains after the ultrasound, a computed tomographic (CT) scan, magnetic resonance imaging (MRI), or fine needle aspiration biopsy may be obtained, although these modalities are rarely needed now that sufficient experience exists in the ultrasound diagnosis of these lesions.

Once the diagnosis is made, the initial treatment consists of passive stretching exercises of the SCM after cervical spine radiographs have been obtained to rule out any concomitant anomalies. If conservative stretching fails to resolve the problem, surgery, consisting of division or partial excision of the sternal and clavicular heads of the muscle, followed by splinting of the neck, should be performed to prevent permanent contracture deformities. such as developmental asymmetry of the face.

CERVICAL DERMOIDS AND TERATOMAS

Cervical dermoids and teratomas come from pluripotential embryonal cells located in the neck that arise from germ layers buried in deep tissues formed from either failed fusion lines or buried pluripotential cells isolated in utero.

Dermoid cysts are most common and come from mesoderm and ectoderm covered with skin. They contain epidermal appendages such as sebaceous glands, hair follicles, or sweat glands. They occur along embryonic fusion lines; may be semisolid, cystic, or loculated; and often have an adipose matrix. They are painless masses that occur most commonly in either the submental area or the midline of the neck and may be confused with thyroglossal duct cysts or enlarged lymph nodes. Occasionally, these masses may become painful, especially when infected. Although submental dermoids are usually found inferior to the mylohyoid muscle, those arising superior to the mylohyoid may encroach upon the floor of the mouth and be mistaken for a ranula. The treatment for dermoid cysts consists of complete surgical excision of the well-encapsulated mass through a carefully planned incision placed in favorable skin creases. Incomplete excision will result in recurrence.

Teratomas are composed of poorly differentiated cells arising from all three germ layers. The lining of teratomas may be stratified squamous epithelium or ciliated respiratory epithelium and may contain calcified areas or tooth buds. Teratomas of the neck are usually present at birth and may be extremely large and lead to respiratory distress and/or feeding problems. Maternal polyhydramnios should make the physician suspicious of the presence of neonatal teratomas, which may be life threatening due to airway compromise. Prenatal ultrasound is important in the diagnosis. At birth, the airway must be secured, and then the mass should be excised. The mass is usually loculated and well-encapsulated. Recurrence and malignancy are rare in the neonate. However, the prognosis in neonatal malignant teratomas is poor.

LYMPHANGIOMAS AND CYSTIC HYGROMAS

Lymphangiomas and cystic hygromas have been variously described as developmental, hamartomatous, or neoplastic. For the purpose of this discussion, I consider them to be developmental anomalies of the jugular lymphatic sac or system that should eventually form connections to the venous system via the right-sided lymphatic duct and the left-sided thoracic duct. When this lymphatic system fails to connect to the venous system, the lymphatic spaces progressively enlarge, forming a lymphangiomatous malformation, which may be classified as lymphangioma simplex (made up of predominantly capillary-sized, thin-walled lymphatics); cavernous lymphangioma (made up of dilated lymphatics); cystic hygroma (made up of lymphatic cysts from a few millimeters to many centimeters); or lymphangiohemangioma (made up of all three vascular spaces: lymphatic, venous, and arterial).

These lymphatic lesions may occur anywhere in the head and neck, and often involve the intrinsic tongue musculature as well as the planes of the neck. Fifty percent to 60 percent are noticeable at birth, and up to 90 percent are visible by the age of 24 months. They may be asymptomatic or may involve various symptoms, from dysphagia to life-threatening airway obstruction. If left alone, they usually progressively enlarge at varying speeds, often fluctuating in size when upper respiratory infections occur.

Diagnosis is made by contrast-enhanced radiographic studies, with MRI being preferred. Such studies should display any large cystic components as well as venous or arterial contributions and any involvement of areas inaccessible to complete surgical removal, such as involvement of the intrinsic muscles of the tongue. Pure cystic hygromas may transilluminate.

Treatment goals should be directed at relief of symptoms, good cosmetic results, and preservation of function. It is my policy to attempt complete surgical removal whenever extirpation is achievable with preservation of function. When the lesion involves the deep tongue structures, I have found that surgical removal is usually not achievable if tongue function is to be preserved (due to the risk of bilateral hypoglossal nerve injury). Also, other cranial nerves, such as VII, X, and XI may be in great jeopardy, depending on the location and extent of the lesion. Radiotherapy and injection of standard sclerosing agents have been tried, but I do not support their use. In cystic lesions, injection of attenuated bacteria, which stimulates an inflammatory response and subsequent fibrosis, has been successfully tried and offers some hope if these solutions become readily obtainable. In three (of three) patients whose cranial nerve VII could not have been preserved with standard resection, I have successfully alleviated the cosmetic and functional complaints with the use of liposuction. This is not a standard modality of treatment, but it may offer either temporary relief from severe symptoms or, as in my patients, complete relief in highly selected individuals. Tracheotomy and limited resection may also be appropriate in certain patients.

HEMANGIOMAS

Hemangiomas are developmental vascular lesions that are present at birth or become noticeable within the first few months of life. They may be classified as capillary, cavernous, mixed capillary-cavernous, proliferative, or infiltrative (although this may just be an aggressive variation of a capillary or cavernous type), and may involve the skin, airway, deep musculoskeletal structures, or intracranial structures. Hemangiomas are the most common benign tumors of the head and neck in children. The large cavernous lesions should be evaluated with the use of contrast-enhanced CT and/or MRI (MRI angiograms may be very useful in select cases to rule out concomitant arteriovenous malformations). These studies should include not only the regional area but also often the brain or other areas.

Hemangiomas may pose life-threatening as well as cosmetic problems for the child, especially if they compress the aerodigestive tract or if they threaten vision.

Treatment should be directed at alleviating any emergent problem while at the same time preserving function. If the lesion grows rapidly and threatens the airway or interferes with alimentation or vision, systemic steroids should be administered in consultation with your colleagues who specialize in pediatrics. Congestive heart failure, bleeding diathesis, and rarely hemorrhage can occur and may require embolization or emergent surgical intervention. Tracheostomy and/or feeding tubes may be necessary in rare cases.

Most hemangiomas eventually regress with time and do not demand aggressive intervention but instead require conservative observation and patience on the part of both the parents and the physician. I counsel parents to expect an increase (often sudden) in size of the lesion over the first 1 to 2 years of life, followed by slow regression up until the ages of 5 years (50 percent of children) to 7 years (70 percent of children). After regression, cosmetic surgery may be necessary to remove redundant or discolored skin. However, early surgery may be necessary for hemangiomas of the nasal lid or periorbital areas. Although I have not used alpha-2a interferon or dye-directed laser applications, these modalities have been reported to be useful in selected cases.

THYROGLOSSAL DUCT REMNANTS

Thyroglossal duct remnants may persist anywhere from the foramen caecum of the tongue base to the thyroid gland, although most commonly they are located superficial and inferior to the hyoid bone. They are usually midline and move up and down when the patient swallows, but may indeed be lateral or quite superior or inferior to the hyoid bone. The cysts may first become noticeable or may enlarge in size when an upper respiratory infection occurs, and they may even become infected and require incision and drainage.

Treatment is surgical removal of the remnant during a period of relative quiescence (i.e., no active infection). Preoperative evaluation should include a complete history and physical examination. The need for a preoperative thyroid scan is controversial. I personally obtain a scan for medicolegal reasons only, although I am not aware of any case in which the entire functioning thyroid tissue was located in a remnant anterior to the hyoid bone or thyroid cartilage. Any patient who has a mass thought to be a possible thyroid remnant deep to the hyoid should always undergo a thyroid scan before any surgical procedure to avoid removal of lingual thyroid tissue, which could indeed be the patient's only functioning thyroid gland tissue.

Surgical excision should include any fistulous cutaneous opening; an ellipse of any involved skin (i.e., adherent to subcutaneous tissue after previous incision and drainage procedures); the cyst with a cuff of tissue surrounding it; the midportion of the hyoid bone (the Sistrunk procedure); any tract going to the thyroid gland; and the tract (or a central core of tissue if no discernible tract is present) between the hyoid bone and the foramen caecum. The surgeon must be careful to avoid injury to the superior laryngeal nerves at the level of the thyrohyoid membrane. and also to the hypoglossal nerves near the superior lateral region of the lateral cornu of the hyoid bone. Closure of the tongue mucosa must be carefully performed. The strap muscles are approximated to attempt to obliterate the dead space, the wound is drained, and a pressure dressing is applied overnight.

■ BRANCHIAL CLEFT ANOMALIES

Branchial cleft anomalies may occur due to anomalies from any of the branchial grooves, arches, or pouches. My chapter deals mainly with first, second, and third cleft lesions. Although first branchial groove anomalies may include aplasia, atresia, stenosis, or duplications, I cover only periauricular pits or sinuses. Most children who have these lesions are initially seen because of parental concern about appearance, drainage, or infection. Removal of noninfected pits or sinuses is not necessary unless there is extreme parental or patient concern regarding cosmesis or drainage. In the asymptomatic patient, I advocate conservative observation until the child is at least 2 years of age. However, if infection has occurred, total tract excision is advised.

Type I first branchial cleft anomalies are of ectodermal origin and are duplications of the membranous external auditory canal. They are typically medial to the concha, may extend to the postauricular region, and usually pass superior to the facial nerve and parallel to the external auditory canal. Type II lesions are duplications of the membranous external auditory canal, are both ectodermal and mesodermal in origin, have a tract that is at the level of the mandible, and have a varying relationship with the facial nerve. Although some surgeons believe that cysts superior to the external canal will not involve the facial nerve, I have found this concept to be misleading; thus, I counsel parents about the risk of facial nerve injury and prepare them for the possibility of nerve dissection under general anesthesia, often with intraoperative nerve monitoring. I attempt to cannulate the tract with a Fogarty catheter to aid in dissection. If the tract involves the parotid gland, a superficial parotidectomy with facial nerve dissection is completed.

Second branchial anomalies are the most common and may initially appear as a cyst, sinus tract, or fistula. These lesions may occur any time from birth to adulthood, often arising concomitant with or after an upper respiratory infection. The second branchial cyst is usually high in the lateral neck deep to the anterior border of the SCM muscle. I have found ultrasonography and contrast-enhanced CT scans to be most helpful, although others in the field prefer MRI. Surgical resection of the uninfected cyst is my treatment of choice. Care must be taken to place the incision in a skin crease while preserving the greater auricular nerve. Although the cyst will lie lateral to the carotid bifurcation, there may be a tract extending cephalad between the internal and external carotid arteries and ending in the region of the tonsillar fossa. If this occurs, complete dissection must be carried out.

A second branchial groove sinus tract usually appears with an external opening along the anterior border of the SCM muscle, although the surgeon may also find only a dimple or discolored spot. Although some surgeons believe that these tracts should be studied with contrast radiography, I do not believe that such procedures are necessary because of the need for general anesthesia in the young patient. Instead, I inject the tract with a contrast material at the time of surgery and thread an angioplasty or Fogarty catheter to aid in the identification of the tract. Again, the tract will usually run cephalad and medial to the bifurcation of the common carotid artery.

A second branchial groove fistula has an opening into the oropharynx and runs lateral to the hypoglossal nerve. These lesions have an external opening along the anterior border of the SCM muscle in the lower third of the neck, with the internal upper opening somewhere in the ipsilateral tonsillar fossa. The tract extends from the lower neck cephalad and medially, running between the internal and external carotid arteries, lateral to the hypoglossal nerve, and into the tonsillar fossa. Again, I usually do not perform preoperative radiographs because of the need for general anesthesia. At surgery, I do cannulate my patients with an angioplasty or Fogarty catheter. For tracts extending from the lower neck to the tonsillar fossa, it is necessary to make two or three short horizontal incisions in a stepladder fashion to follow the tract into the oropharynx. Such an approach is cosmetically superior to a single apron incision. This anomaly is drained with a suction drain and a light pressure dressing, as are all other branchial tract lesions.

Third branchial pouch sacs or sinuses and thymic cysts are rare but can cause management dilemmas. A persistent third pouch usually appears as an inflammatory mass in the lower anterior neck, which will either require an incision and drainage or forms a spontaneous fistula, causing a communication between the skin of the lower neck and the ipsilateral piriform sinus. The persistent third branchial pouch must be considered in recurrent lower neck abscesses. I have found that these often require more than one surgical procedure to remove due to the difficulty in identification of the complete tract after recurrent infections.

Cervical thymic cysts may appear as midline anterior neck masses. They are best evaluated by contrast-enhanced CT or MRI scans and may either cause respiratory distress or be relatively asymptomatic. Occasionally, these lesions may be associated with hypertrophy of the adjacent parathyroid gland, so an endocrinology evaluation may be needed if a cervical thymic cyst is diagnosed. Surgical excision with examination of the superior mediastinum is my preferred method of treatment.

Suggested Reading

Donegan JO. Congenital neck masses. In: Cummings CW, Fredrickson JM, Harker LA, Krause CJ, Schuller DE, eds. Otolaryngology—head and neck surgery. St. Louis: Mosby–Year Book, 1993:1550.

Johnson JT. Congenital neck masses. In: Gates, ed. current therapy in otolaryngology–head and neck surgery, 1982-1983. Trenton, NJ: BC Decker, 1982:250.

Karmody CS. Developmental anomalies of the neck. In: Bluestone C, Stool S, Kenna M. Pediatric otolaryngology. Vol. 2. ed 3. Philadelphia: WB Saunders, 1996:1497.

THYROID NODULE

The method of
Helmuth Goepfert
by
Elizabeth Blair
Helmuth Goepfert

Palpable or dominant thyroid nodules occur in about 4 percent of the population, more commonly in women, with the frequency increasing with age. The prevalence of thyroid nodules varies with the sensitivity of the detection method used, increasing with the application of high-resolution ultrasound, and further increasing with histologic analysis. However, thyroid carcinoma is an uncommon malignancy. The estimated 8,000 to 10,000 new cases in the United States each year represent less than 1.5 percent of all cancer cases, and fewer than 1,100 patients die from this disease annually. Of the multitudes of patients who have palpable thyroid nodules, approximately 5 percent to 10 percent have overt thyroid cancer. Despite the small numbers of new cases and the low mortality rates, thyroid cancer is not a benign disease. It remains a significant clinical problem for several reasons. Microscopic carcinoma in the thyroid can be identified in a large proportion of specimens obtained at autopsy in up to 40 percent of the population, depending on the age of individuals and the geographic location from which these samples are taken. The clinical significance of these microscopic tumors in an otherwise healthy individual remains to be determined. The accurate preoperative diagnosis of clinically relevant thyroid cancer remains a challenge; diagnostic tests need to have specificity and sensitivity to differentiate this malignant condition from the very common benign thyroid nodules and goiter. The difficulty in differentiating between benign and malignant processes requires the clinician's keen assessment of each individual patient. An additional consideration is the sometimes unpredictable nature and aggressiveness of these tumors. In the majority of patients, this disease follows a predictable course, but in others it is aggressive and deadly. The rarity of death from thyroid carcinoma does not imply that thyroid carcinoma is innocuous. It is often impossible to assess those patients who are at risk for aggressive, recurrent, or fatal disease. Patients who have aggressive thyroid cancers are more difficult to manage and suffer greater morbidity and mortality. The effective management of thyroid nodules has to be tailored to the type of disease in the individual patient.

In the last 2 decades, concerted efforts have led to advances in understanding some of the causes of thyroid carcinoma and in improving approaches to diagnosis and management. The specific molecular cause of clinically significant papillary and follicular cancer is largely unknown. But research in identifying cancer-causing genes has led to suggestions of molecular events likely to effect benign or malignant transformation of follicular or parafollicular cells of the thyroid gland. The most notable advance has been the discovery of the role of the RET proto-oncogene in the genesis of malignant transformation in follicular cells (papillary thyroid carcinoma [PTC]) and parafollicular or C cells (medullary thyroid carcinoma [MTC]). In differentiated papillary and follicular carcinoma and their variations, the clinical relevance of the RET proto-oncogene mutations has yet to be determined. Conversely, the identification of germ cell line mutations of RET proto-oncogene are very useful in the study of medullary thyroid carcinoma, especially in the search for causes of the familial syndromes associated with this cancer.

In assessing the risk of malignancy in a patient who has a thyroid nodule, it is important to consider features of an individual that contribute to the composite risk for cancer. Exposure to ionizing radiation, especially in childhood, predisposes an individual to development of parathyroid hypertrophy and adenoma formation, salivary gland tumors, and thyroid adenomas or differentiated carcinomas. Many studies have documented the increased risk of thyroid carcinoma with low-level radiation. Also, patients who have been exposed to atomic weapons and nuclear fallout accidents are at greater risk of developing thyroid cancer. The latent period from radiation exposure to the development of thyroid abnormalities is generally between 10 and 20 years. The unfortunate accident at Chernobyl in 1986 exposed a significant number of children to ionizing radiation. More than 100 cases of pediatric thyroid cancer were diagnosed in parts of Belorussia; the characteristics of these cases were as follows: a relatively rapid onset after exposure from up to 3 years and on; a much more aggressive behavior, with lymph node metastases in more than 75 percent of cases; and a poorly differentiated histology in more than 50 percent of the patients. It is suspected that the true radiation exposure in these patients may have been initially underestimated. Other factors implicated, but not well understood in PTC, are the roles of iodine, diet, and autoimmune thyroid disease.

Epidemiologic studies of the relationship of iodine consumption, diet, and iodine deficiency to thyroid cancer have been inconclusive. The evidence of genetic factors is increased in a small percentage of differentiated thyroid cancers, such as Gardner's syndrome (familial colonic polyposis) and Cowden's syndrome (familial goiter and hamartomas). PTC also seems to occur with greater frequency in some families with breast, renal, and central nervous syndrome malignancies.

■ REQUIREMENTS FOR ADEQUATE EVALUATION

Clinical Evaluation

The patient with thyroid carcinoma may have a thyroid mass or nodule or a mass in the lateral neck due to lymph node metastases. At the time of the patient's initial presentation, a thorough history is important in determining specific risk factors or features. A history of exposure to radiotherapy is important. Usually, this pertains to moderate to low doses, as were given in the past for treatment of tonsillar and adenoid hypotrophy or acne. Treatment for lymphoma, especially with the "Mantel" technique and accidental radiation exposure, such as from atomic plant disasters, need to be noted in the history. A family history of cancer is more likely to be present for a patient who has MTC. True familial PTC is rare, but 5 percent to 8 percent of patients describe another affected family member. Nevertheless, the reality is that most patients who have thyroid nodules and cancer do not have any known risk factors. In children, the most common presentation is a lateral neck mass, representing a regional lymph node metastasis. Other clinical features of concern are new-onset hoarseness and vocal cord paralysis, hemoptysis, and extensive lymph node enlargement. Children and adolescents rarely have solitary thyroid nodules, and if present these lesions should be thoroughly investigated for the possibility of cancer. People in their third to fourth decades of life, especially women, have a high incidence of thyroid nodules. But the majority of these are of a benign histology. In patients over 50 and 60 years of age, the incidence of carcinoma in isolated thyroid nodules increases progressively.

The initial examination usually reveals a solitary nodule in the thyroid gland. In a smaller percentage of patients, two or more nodules are palpated. A thorough evaluation also includes the larynx, tongue, and mobility of the cervical spine. The consistency of the mass and its relationship to surrounding structures affects treatment planning and prognosis. The lymph nodes of primary drainage for the thyroid, which lie in the central compartment of the neck (level VI), may be difficult to assess on physical examination. In the majority of patients who have lymph node metastases, the palpable metastatic adenopathy is most commonly found along the middle and lower portions of the jugular chain (levels II, III, and IV). Nodal disease may also be found lateral to the sternocleidomastoid muscle in the lower portion of the posterior triangle that overlies the scalenes (level V). Other physical findings that might point to a particular type of thyroid cancer include clinical feature of pheochromocytoma or hyperparathyroidism (multiple endocrine neoplasia, type 2A [MEN 2A] and MTC), mucosal neuromas and marfanoid features (MEN 2B and MTC), and colonic polyposis and PTC. Most patients have no physical indications specific to the diagnosis of thyroid cancer.

Functional Evaluation

The principal objectives are to (1) identify patients who need to be operated on for thyroid disease, (2) identify those who will benefit from medical management of the thyroid abnormality, and (3) correct any medical or metabolic abnormalities a patient may have before surgery.

The typical signs of thyrotoxicosis should be sought, but they may be absent in elderly patients. Similarly, clinical signs of hypothyroidism, usually secondary to autoimmune thyroiditis, may be subtle or absent in the elderly.

Biochemical assessment should include a determination of thyroid-stimulating hormone (TSH), with an assay sensitive enough to distinguish both a suppressed TSH level typical of hyperthyroidism and an elevated TSH typical of hypothyroidism. When hyperthyroidism is suspected or likely, serum for free thyroxine (T_4) index or radioimmunoassay and triiodothyronine (T_3) measurements should be added to confirm the diagnosis, stratify the operative risk, and monitor the patient's response to antithyroid drug therapy. Patients who have a diagnosis or suspicion of MTC must be evaluated for MEN 2A and 2B, which occurs 25 percent of the time. Determination of urinary catecholamine, vanillylmandelic acid (VMA), and metanephrine levels is necessary before surgery in all patients who have MTC. The presence of a functioning pheochromocytoma dictates initial therapeutic attention to the adrenal lesion. Hypercalcemia due to hyperparathyroidism is readily detected by measuring the serum calcium level, and the treatment of this condition would be coordinated with thyroid surgery.

■ FINE NEEDLE ASPIRATION

In the setting of unsuppressed serum TSH concentration, cytologic examination following a fine needle aspiration (FNA) is the most appropriate next diagnostic procedure. FNA is a relatively inexpensive procedure that provides an accurate diagnosis rapidly. It assists the physician in determining whether a patient should be observed, receive suppressive therapy, receive a repeat FNA, or proceed to surgery. In addition, it reduces the number of other diagnostic procedures.

Technical Details

It is safe to assume that in most settings the fine needle aspiration is performed by a clinician and then sent for interpretation to a clinical pathologist who has special expertise in cytology. In some instances, especially in a major cancer center, fine needle aspiration is performed by the pathologist who processes the specimen immediately and can render a rapid preliminary report.

The FNA technique is readily acquired, but both the processing of sample and accurate cytopathologic interpretation of its findings require practice and experience. Success of FNA requires a good sample. After sterile preparation of the neck, subcutaneous anesthesia with lidocaine may help the patient tolerate multiple aspirations. Aspiration is performed with a 22 to 25 gauge needle attached to a 10 to 20 mL syringe, which may be fitted to a syringe holder for easier use. For aspirations guided by palpation of the nodule, one hand operates the syringe and the other locates and "fixes" the target lesion. After the needle is inserted into the lesion, it should be passed back and forth through the lesion without applying any suction. If bright red blood is seen immediately in the needle hub, the procedure should be stopped, and the needle should be withdrawn. If nothing appears in the hub, then gentle suction should be gradually applied. The plunger is released prior to withdrawing the needle. Ideally, sufficient material is aspirated to yield one to two drops of fluid that are promptly smeared onto slides, which are then fixed or air-dried and stained.

For nonpalpable lesions and those that have yielded inadequate material on previous attempts, ultrasound-guided aspiration is appropriate. This is performed using an ultrasound probe to identify the nodule and to confirm the needle position in the nodule during aspiration. Ultrasound, the most sensitive procedure for identifying thyroid lesions, is capable of documenting solitary nodules in approximately 25 percent of symptomatic persons, and most of these nodules are benign.

■ ROLE OF IMAGING STUDIES

Before widespread application of FNA, routine evaluation of the thyroid nodule was commonly done by isotope scintigraphy. Radionuclide scanning, either iodine or pertechnetate, shows malignant lesions as hypofunctioning or "cold." Yet 90 percent to 95 percent of thyroid nodules are hypofunctioning, and therefore this finding is nonspecific and nondiagnostic. On the other hand, a "hot" nodule, defined as a hyperfunctioning lesion with suppression of the surrounding tissue, is rarely malignant.

Ultrasound, the most sensitive procedure for identifying lesions, is capable of finding lesion in approximately 25 percent of asymptomatic persons. Nodules as small as 2 to 3 mm can be demonstrated; however, the significance of most of these nodules is unclear, and most eventually prove benign. The advantage of ultrasound is its ability to measure nodule dimensions accurately and provide longitudinal follow-up. Many glands with apparent solitary nodules by clinical examination may accurately demonstrate multiple nodules consistent with multiple nodular goiter by ultrasound. Ultrasound may also help to localize a lesion and specifically direct a needle biopsy. Unfortunately, there are few sonographic findings pathognomonic of malignancy. Similarly, other imaging procedures, like computed tomography (CT) and magnetic resonance imaging (MRI), have no role in the routine diagnosis of thyroid nodules.

■ REPORTING OF CYTOLOGY AND DECISION MAKING IN THE MANAGEMENT OF THYROID NODULES

Because the major role of any diagnostic procedure is to identify benign nodules that do not require surgical excision, the following stringent criteria have been established for adequacy of the aspirated material to allow accurate cytologic exclusion of malignancy: six clusters of benign cells appearing on at least two slides that are made from two aspirations of different parts of the nodule. The presence of any number of malignant cells establishes the diagnosis of cancer. To minimize the number of false-negative results due to inadequate specimens, at least six separate cell clusters are usually necessary. The presence of a pathologist for simultaneous on-site cytologic review of adequacy of the diagnostic material can reduce the number of aspirates needed and improve diagnostic yield. Even in experienced hands, approximately 15 percent of all aspirations are inadequate or nondiagnostic, largely because of the aspiration of cystic, hemorrhagic, hypervascular, or hypocellular colloid nodules. Subsequent reaspiration may reduce this frequency by half. In one recent study of surgical diagnoses following repeated nondiagnostic aspirations, 4 percent of women and 29 percent of men proved to have malignant nodules. When fine needle aspiration is performed and evaluated by experienced practitioners, the sensitivity, specificity, and diagnostic accuracy are 83 percent, 92 percent, and 95 percent, respectively.

Clinicopathologic Correlations

The nomenclature used for the reporting of cytology varies among different centers. A straightforward diagnosis of cancer may be reported as papillary carcinoma, medullary carcinoma, anaplastic carcinoma, or large cell lymphoma. In other instances, just the term *malignant cells* may be used. When the report states "follicular cells," this in most cases represents a benign lesion, either goiter or adenoma. In certain instances, the report will read "benign" without any further specification.

Cytologic diagnoses following adequate aspiration fall into several categories. Benign or "negative" diagnoses, which occur in 60 percent to 90 percent of cases of adequate FNA, include hypocellular adenomatoid nodules (colloid nodule), hyperplastic nodules, thyroiditis, and cysts. The likelihood of malignancy (false-negative rate) in these cases is lower than 5 percent when surgical findings become available. Diagnoses of malignancy, including papillary (also follicular variant), medullary, and anaplastic carcinomas, as well as lymphoma, are made in about 5 percent of nodules. The false-positive rate is less than 5 percent. Occasionally, lesions are suspected to be malignant despite not meeting full diagnostic criteria, and most of these prove to be malignant. If MTC is suspected, a serum calcitonin is appropriate.

Other cases are cellular lesions that yield abnormal follicular epithelium of varying degrees of atypia and suspicion of malignancy. Diagnostic labels used to describe these lesions differ among cytologists, which makes comparison of results difficult. Follicular neoplasms are characterized by groups of crowded follicular epithelial cells with irregular nuclei, with the cells organized in microfollicles or rosettes rather than sheets. Follicular adenomas and carcinomas cannot be adequately separated without histologic demonstration of invasion. A similar diagnostic dilemma exists for oxyphilic or Hurthle cell neoplasms. Carcinomas can be found in approximately 15 percent of cytopathologically diagnosed follicular and oxyphilic neoplasms. One group examined patients for potential clinical features that might identify nodules at greater risk for malignancy, such as age, nodule size, and radiation exposure history. Only age greater than 50 years proved to be a significant predictor of malignancy among patients with follicular neoplasms; age increased this risk to 45 percent. It is interesting that the age factor did not contribute significantly to prediction of malignancy in nondiagnostic aspirates.

■ TREATMENT

Thyroid Suppression for Nodules with Benign Histology

The evaluation of the thyroid nodule is suitable for application of a diagnostic algorithm (Fig. 1). If the patient is hyperthyroid as defined by a suppressed TSH level, the workup should evaluate for thyrotoxicosis, and a radionuclide scan would be a suitable diagnostic test to look for a toxic nodule versus Graves' disease with a coexistent nodule. In most patients, the TSH level will be normal, and an FNA should

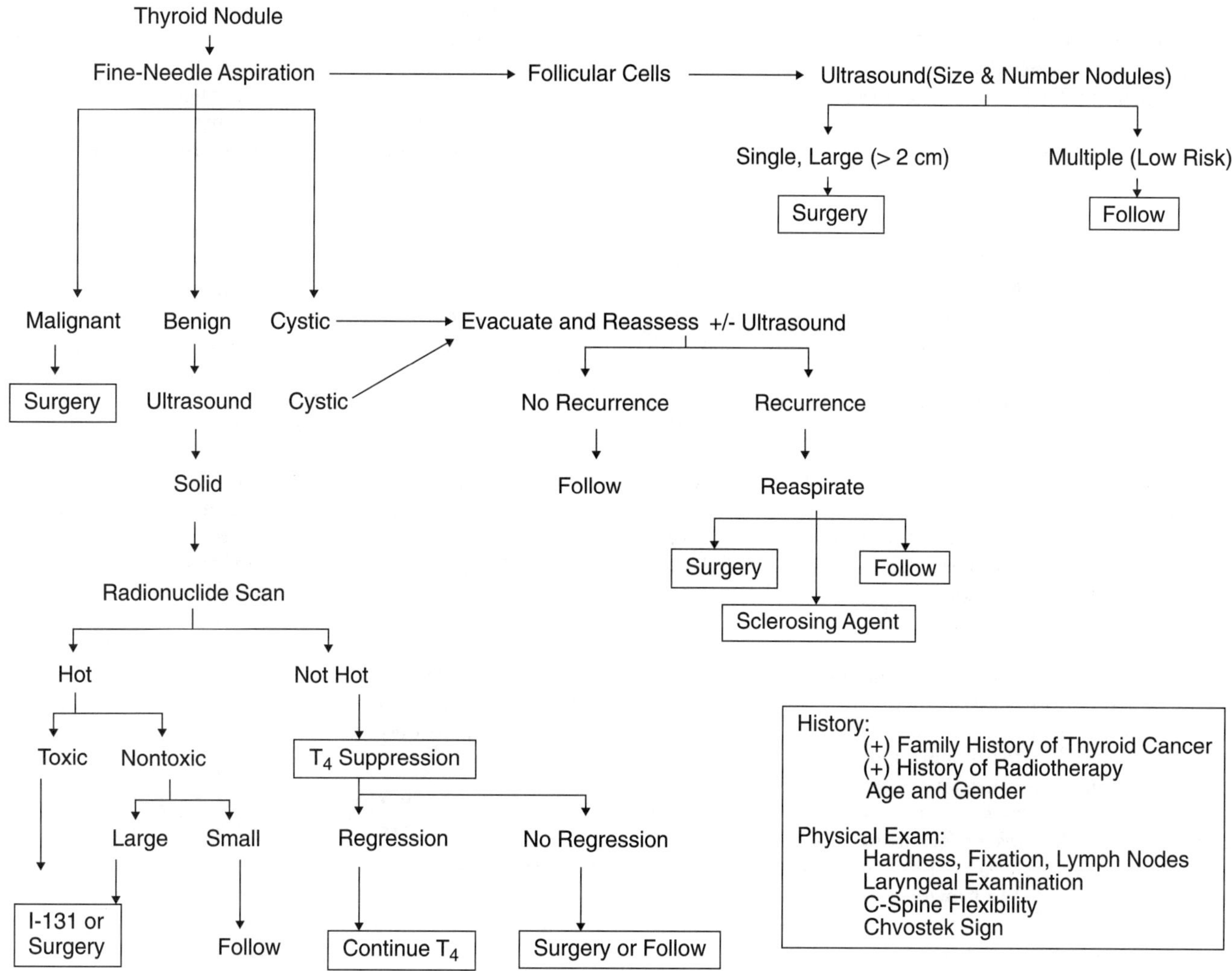

Figure 1.
Algorithm for the diagnosis and treatment of thyroid nodules.

be performed. Surgery should follow when the cytologic findings are either diagnostic or strongly suggestive of malignancy. When a nonoxyphilic follicular neoplasm is found, a radionuclide scan should be obtained to rule out a hot nodule; a thyroid hormone suppression scan may be necessary to demonstrate autonomous, nonsuppressible function. If the follicular lesion is hypofunctioning or oxyphilic, a decision must be made whether to operate. For patients over 50 years old, given their higher risk of cancer, surgery is definitely recommended. Similar recommendations may be given for men who have had multiple aspirations and whose cumulative yields remain nondiagnostic. In younger patients or those in whom a hyperplastic nodule cannot be distinguished from a follicular neoplasm, treatment with T_4 to suppress serum TSH levels to less than 0.1 mIU/L for 6 to 12 months may be recommended. A nodule that does not shrink significantly in this interval should be excised. Patients should be counseled about the relative risks and benefits of suppression therapy and surgery, so that they may participate in the therapeutic decision.

Patients who have solitary benign nodules, particularly men and premenopausal women, may also be treated with thyroid suppression therapy, as may women who have repeated nondiagnostic aspirations. The TSH level should be maintained at less than 0.1 mIU/L. A patient with a benign nodule that decreased in size during suppression may then be followed up without therapy, with adjustment of hormone dose to keep the TSH concentration near the lower limit of normal. Conversely, a nodule that grows during suppression therapy should be reaspirated or excised. The recommendations regarding the management of benign nodules continue to change as new data emerge about the efficacy of suppression therapy. Older studies suggested no benefit from suppression therapy, but recent placebo controlled trials have demonstrated levothyroxine suppression therapy as significantly more effective than placebo in shrinking colloid nodules, with nodule volume decreasing by at least 50 percent in up to 40 percent of patients. It is often argued that incidence of false-negative FNA diagnoses is too great to risk a trial of suppression therapy. Regardless, most large series that report the long-term outcome of patients following FNA suggest that malignancies not initially diagnosed by FNA but discovered during careful follow-up remain highly treatable, with a low risk of mortality.

■ THYROID LOBECTOMY

Before thyroid surgery for benign or malignant neoplasms, patients require both a general medical and thyroid-specific assessment to identify and minimize their perioperative risks. These assessments should include the patient's cardiovascular and pulmonary systems, medical history, and current medications.

Most patients undergoing thyroidectomy are euthyroid. The exceptions are patients who have coexisting Graves' disease or toxic nodular goiter, as well as the rare patient who has thyrotoxicosis caused by widespread metastatic follicular carcinoma.

Thyroid lobectomy is usually performed under general anesthesia, although local anesthesia may be used on selected occasions. The skin incision is usually placed two finger breadths above the medial epiphysis of the clavicles, and it is centered in the midline and placed in a natural skin crease. The skin, subcutaneous fat, and platysma muscle are elevated as a superiorly based flap to just above the thyroid cartilage or the hyoid bone. The inferior flap is elevated in a subplatysmal plane to the suprasternal notch and clavicles. The prethyroid strap muscles are then separated from the sternocleidomastoid muscle to expose the lateral portion of the gland and allow inspection of the lower jugular lymph nodes. The strap muscles are separated in the midline and rarely may be divided to provide better exposure. The thyroid compartment may then be approached laterally along the anterior border of the sternocleidomastoid muscle, or medially through the midline raphe. Dissection is carried between the posterior sheaths of the strap muscles and the thyroid capsule. Both the sternohyoid and sternothyroid muscles are separated from the underlying capsule. Any portions of muscle adherent to the gland are included with the resection of the gland.

The middle thyroid vein is ligated after dissection of the carotid sheath structures. Dissection then proceeds medially, with identification and dissection of the recurrent laryngeal nerve. Care is taken to identify a possible nonrecurrent vagal nerve on the right (or on the left in a patient who has transposition of the great vessels).

The superior thyroid vessels are isolated and individually ligated close to the thyroid capsule. The superior laryngeal nerve is identified as it crosses the constrictor muscle and enters the cricothyroid muscle. Great variability may be seen in the relationship between the superior laryngeal nerve and the superior thyroid artery. Meticulous dissection is necessary to avoid injury to the nerve when ligating the artery and branches. Downward traction on the thyroid lobe and dissection with a small right-angled hemostat can facilitate ligation.

Dissection of the thyroid gland is continued along the posterior aspect with incision of the visceral fascia that suspends the gland. The recurrent laryngeal nerve, if not previously located, is then identified in the tracheoesophageal groove inferior to the gland and dissected superiorly. The inferior thyroid artery is identified, and the vascular pedicle to the parathyroid glands is preserved. The branches of the inferior thyroid artery are individually ligated as they enter the gland, with avoidance of injury to branches of the recurrent nerve. All branches of the nerve are preserved as the dissection proceeds superiorly. Extreme variability may be encountered in the anatomic relationship between the recurrent nerve and the inferior thyroid artery. The lobe is completely mobilized, with division of the posterior suspensory (Berry's) ligament following dissection and preservation of the recurrent nerve to its entrance into the larynx. After the lobe is completely mobilized, the isthmus of the gland is divided, and the lobe is removed. In most patients who have a diagnosis of cancer or a history of irradiation to the thyroid gland, a similar lobectomy is performed on the contralateral side for a total thyroidectomy.

The technical details of total thyroidectomy as well as the prevention and treatments of complications are beyond the scope of this chapter. Meticulous dissection under optimum light and the optional use of magnifying loupes will allow for identification and preservation of laryngeal nerves and their branches as well as the parathyroids. Frankly invaded nerves should be removed, and parathyroid tissue that has impaired vascular supply should be reimplanted in the sternocleidomastoid muscle. The surgical report should be explicit as to gross findings and pertinent technical details.

■ WHAT TO EXPECT FROM SURGEON-PATHOLOGIST INTERACTION AT THE TIME OF SURGERY

Good surgeon-pathologist communication and interaction is vital to optimize the interpretation of a technically well done frozen section examination. In most cases, the distinction between thyroid carcinoma and benign nodules can be made with certainty. Papillary lesions of the thyroid gland present little difficulty in histopathologic diagnosis on frozen section. Papillary hyperplasia in adenomatous goiter and diffuse toxic goiter are easy to distinguish from papillary carcinoma. Papillary carcinoma shows infiltrative growth into the capsule, surrounding thyroid tissue, or lymphatics, and frequently contains psammoma bodies; most important, the nuclei have a characteristic ground-glass appearance. The distinction between follicular adenoma and well-differentiated follicular carcinoma may present greater difficulty for the surgical pathologist. This distinction is based on findings of capsular or vascular invasion. When the pathologist is faced with this dilemma at the time of surgery, at least four blocks from the capsule-thyroid interface should be examined. If this is inadequate, the diagnosis is deferred. If the pathologic evaluation is diagnostic or strongly suspicious of malignancy, then completion of the total thyroidectomy and appropriate neck dissection are done at the same time. If the pathologic examination is benign or equivocal, the wound is irrigated and closed. It may not need a closed suction drain. Frozen evaluation of thyroid neoplasms is subject to a final evaluation of the permanent specimen. The problem of accurately distinguishing between well-differentiated follicular carcinoma and a follicular neoplasm produces the most inaccurate results in the area of thyroid pathology; there are reports of only 61 percent of frozen section diagnoses being correct in these settings. The diagnosis of Hurthle cell carcinoma by frozen section examination involves the same type of dilemma. Only when a lesion is composed of large, granular oxyphilic cells with malignant characteristics such as anaplasia, high mitotic activity, and capsular or vascular invasion, should it be called a Hurthle cell cancer. A false-positive diagnosis will result in a patient's having total thyroidectomy for benign disease, and a false-negative diagnosis will require those patients to submit to additional surgery.

Suggested Reading

Blum M, Seltzer TF, Campbell CC, et al. Evaluation of euthyroid solitary autonomous nodule of the thyroid gland. Importance of scintillation scanning and thyrotropin-releasing hormone testing. JAMA 1982; 247:191.

Busseniers AE, Oertel YC. Cellular adenomatoid nodules of the thyroid: Review of 219 fine-needle aspirates. Diagn Cytopathol 1993; 9:581.

Cooper DS. Thyroxine suppression therapy for benign nodular disease. J Clin Endocrinol Metab 1995; 80:331.

Gershengorn MC, McClung MR, Chu EW, et al. Fine-needle aspiration cytology in the preoperative diagnosis of thyroid nodules. Ann Intern Med 1977; 87:265.

Gharib H. Fine-needle aspiration biopsy of thyroid nodules: Advantages, limitations, and effect. Mayo Clin Proc 1994; 69:44.

Hamburger JI. Diagnosis of thyroid nodules by fine needle biopsy: Use and abuse. J Clin Endocrinol Metab 1994; 79:335.

Hamburger JI. Solitary autonomously functioning thyroid lesions: Diagnosis, clinical features, and pathogenetic considerations. Am J Med 1975; 58:740.

Kini SR, Miller JM, Hamburger JI, et al. Cytopathology of follicular lesions of the thyroid gland. Diagn Cytopathol 1985; 1:123.

Mazzaferri EL. Management of a solitary thyroid nodule [see comments]. New Engl J Med 1993; 328:553.

McHenry CR, Walfish PG, Rosen IB. Non-diagnostic fine needle aspiration biopsy: A dilemma in management of nodular thyroid disease. Am J Surg 1993; 59:415.

Miller JM, Hamburger JI, Kini S. Diagnosis of thyroid nodules: Use of fine-needle aspiration and needle biopsy. JAMA 1979; 241:481.

Miller JM, Kini SR, Hamburger JI. Needle biopsy of the thyroid. New York: Praeger, 1983.

Papini E, Bacci V, Panunzi C, et al. A prospective randomized trial of levothyroxine suppressive therapy for solitary thyroid nodules. Clin Endocrinol (Oxford) 1993; 38:507.

Tyler DS, Winchester DJ, Caraway NP, et al. Indeterminate fine-needle aspiration biopsy of the thyroid: Identification of subgroups at high risk for invasive carcinoma. Surgery 1994; 116:1054.

Van Herle AJ, Rich P, Ljung B-ME, et al. The thyroid nodule. Ann Intern Med 1982; 96:221.

Vander JB, Gaston EA, Dawber TR. The significance of nontoxic thyroid nodules: Final report of a 15 year study of the incidence of thyroid malignancy. Ann Intern Med 1968; 69:537.

Walfish PG, Hazani E, Strawbridge HT, et al. Combined ultrasound and needle aspiration cytology in the assessment and management of hypofunctioning thyroid nodule. Ann Intern Med 1977; 87:270.

Wang C, Vickery AL Jr, Maloof F. Needle biopsy of the thyroid. Surg Gynecol Obstet 1976; 143:365.

HYPERPARATHYROIDISM

The method of
Larry A. Hoover
by
Larry A. Hoover
Daniel E. Bruegger

The diagnosis of hyperparathyroidism has become more common over the last decade. A significant amount of this increased prevalence is due to the routine use of serum calcium screening, which has greatly enhanced our ability to recognize the presence of hyperparathyroidism. A successful surgical strategy for the treatment of hyperparathyroidism requires a knowledge of parathyroid gland embryology and anatomy, as well as an understanding of parathyroid pathophysiology.

Enlargement of a single parathyroid gland, or benign adenoma, is sufficient to cause excessive hormone secretion. Eighty percent to 90 percent of primary hyperparathyroidism is due to a single adenoma and can be effectively cured by surgical removal. Multiple gland disease, or hyperplasia, is more likely if there is a family history of hyperparathyroidism or multiple endocrine neoplasia (MEN 1 or MEN 2A). Hyperplasia is believed to represent only 15 percent of patients who have primary hyperparathyroidism. Some studies, however, have shown a much greater prevalence of hyperplasia, and this generally is the case at institutions where all glands are typically biopsied. As it is essentially impossible to distinguish between adenoma or hyperplasia by either gross or histologic examination, histologic studies are unlikely to resolve this controversy. The fact that recurrence of hyperparathyroidism is rare after removal of a solitary enlarged parathyroid gland is good evidence that hyperplasia is less frequent than some would suggest.

Hyperparathyroidism affects 30 to 40 persons in every 100,000. A small percentage of these patients (0.5 percent to 4 percent) have parathyroid carcinomas. These masses often have significant adherence to surrounding structures. The etiology of parathyroid tumors remains unknown; however, there is an association with a prior history of local ionizing radiation.

Clinical manifestations of primary hyperparathyroidism have classically been described as "painful bones, renal stones, abdominal groans, and psychic moans." Now with routine screening tests many asymptomatic patients are being diagnosed. Hyperparathyroidism rarely causes death directly, but may result in significant morbidity. It may contribute indirectly as a risk factor for early mortality.

In early studies, renal involvement, especially recurrent stones, was reported in as many as 60 percent to 70 percent of patients. With earlier detection the incidence has now dropped to 5 percent to 20 percent. Likewise, bone disease is much more often subtle osteoporosis instead of the older classic osteitis fibrosa cystica. Twelve percent of my patients had bone pain or radiologic evidence of severe demineralization. Hypertension was present in one-fifth of my patients, as was emotional distress (most commonly manifested as lethargy, fatigue, and depression). One-third of my patients had gastrointestinal complaints, including constipation, a history of peptic ulcer disease, or dysphagia. Nearly half have had signs or symptoms of renal disease, with nephrolithiasis being most common. In general, the severity of renal disease has varied with the duration and severity of hypercalcemia.

The diagnosis of primary hyperparathyroidism is made by an increased parathyroid hormone (PTH) level, or at least an inappropriately on the high side of normal level in the face of elevated serum calcium levels. In my patient group, the average preoperative serum calcium level was 11.4 mg/dL (normal range, 8 to 10 mg/dL). The PTH level was elevated in 76 percent and in the high-normal range in the other 24 percent. The degree of elevation of serum calcium was directly related to the weight of abnormal parathyroid tissue found at surgery. Serum phosphorus level was decreased in 77 percent of my patients with primary hyperparathyroidism. Symptomatic patients who have primary hyperparathyroidism are surgical candidates, as are asymptomatic patients who have significantly elevated serum calcium levels, or markedly reduced bone density. Surgical treatment of symptomatic patients who have minimal calcium elevations remains controversial, and long-term studies of these patients for development of significant morbidity will probably be necessary to resolve this controversy.

■ PREOPERATIVE EVALUATION

The history should assess the patient's intake of antacids, diuretics, and vitamins, and include a family history, because hypercalcemia has many possible causes. Table 1 lists the most common causes of hypercalcemia. Hyperparathyroidism and malignancy account for more than 90 percent of all cases of hypercalcemia. A chemistry profile (including calcium, phosphorus, protein, albumin, blood urea nitrogen, creatinine), parathyroid hormone level, and 24 hour urinary calcium level (to rule out hypocalciuric hypercalcemia) are obtained for all patients. A minimum of two serum calcium elevations in association with a high level of parathyroid hormone and a low phosphorus level indicates hyperparathyroidism. Immunoassays can now differentiate between malignant conditions producing parathyroid hormone–related protein (PTHrP) and increased PTH production.

Localization of abnormal glands can be facilitated by computed tomographic (CT) and magnetic resonance imaging (MRI) scans, angiography, thallium-technetium scans, as well as the newer technetium 99m sestamibi imaging. The sestamibi imaging technique takes advantage of the fact that this contrast is preferentially taken up by tissue with large numbers of mitochondria. Parathyroid adenomas have large complements of mitochondria, which results in higher image activity and delayed release of sestamibi. This uptake is much greater in parathyroid than thyroid tissue, and results in a meaningful differential image. Sensitivity of more than 90 percent has been reported in the identification and localization of parathyroid adenomas. The use of all of these preoperative imaging techniques remains controversial. I use high-resolution, real-time ultrasonography initially, and have a 70 percent success rate in localization. I am present and actively involved in these studies. Real-time ultrasonography is inexpensive and particularly helpful in localizing the most common pathologic entity, solitary adenomas. This knowledge aids in informed preoperative consent from the patient and speeds surgical dissection. It is particularly helpful when the patient has had prior surgery or trauma to the neck, which would make exploration more difficult. Other imaging techniques are reserved for patients who have an initial negative neck exploration, or develop recurrent hyperparathyroidism and their site of disease cannot be identified by ultrasonography. Thallium-technetium scans have in the past provided useful information, but may be supplanted by sestamibi imaging. I have also successfully used digital subtraction angiography before mediastinal exploration.

■ SURGICAL STRATEGY

Parathyroid neck exploration is often a prolonged procedure that requires meticulous dissection and hemostasis. The pa-

Table 1. Causes of Hypercalcemia

PRIMARY HYPERPARATHYROIDISM	MALIGNANCY	RENAL	OTHER ENDOCRINE DISORDERS	DIETARY/DRUGS	OTHER
Adenoma	PTHrP production	Secondary HPT	Hyperthyroidism	Milk-alkali syndrome	Sarcoidosis
Hyperplasia	Bone metastases	Aluminum intoxication	Addison's disease	Vitamin D intoxication	Tuberculosis
Multiple endocrine neoplasia	Hematologic		Tertiary HPT	Vitamin A intoxication	Immobilization
				Thiazides	FHH
				Lithium	Infantile hypercalcemia

HPT, hyperparathyroidism; PTHrP, parathyroid hormone–related protein; FHH, familial hypocalciuric hypercalcemia.

tient is placed on the operating table with the head extended, and in a 30 degree reverse Trendelenburg's position. Anesthesiologists maintain the systolic blood pressure between 90 and 100 mm Hg, unless contraindicated, to decrease bleeding. Surgical loops and a xenon headlight are used to aid in microscopic dissection. A transverse surgical incision is made approximately 2 cm above the sternal notch and extending to the mid-sternocleidomastoid (SCM) muscle on both sides. Monopolar cautery is used for the skin and subcutaneous dissection. Bipolar cautery is used for dissection deep to the strap muscles. Subplastysmal skin flaps are elevated superiorly to the thyroid notch and inferiorly to the sternal notch. The strap muscles are separated in the midline, and the sternothyroid muscle is retracted, which allows palpation of both thyroid lobes and surrounding structures. If preoperative localization studies have not revealed a likely location for pathology, initial inspection for enlarged blood vessels often assists in determining a site for more favorable initial dissection. Improved exposure can then be obtained by dividing the sternothyroid muscle in the middle to upper third to avoid injury to the nerve supply from the ansa hypoglossi. Dividing the middle thyroid vein at the thyroid capsule assists in the medial rotation of the thyroid gland and exposes the tracheoesophageal groove where the recurrent nerve must be identified.

At this point, dissection is guided by normal parathyroid anatomy. It is often necessary to ligate the vessels of the superior pole of the thyroid gland at the thyroid capsule to aid in exposure of the upper pole. It is desirable to preserve the inferior thyroid artery because this is almost always the blood supply to the parathyroids. The lower pole, however, often needs to be completely exposed to demonstrate the inferior parathyroid gland. If the artery needs to be divided, it should be done as close as possible to the thyroid gland to avoid ischemic damage to the parathyroids. As the thyroid gland is dissected medially, adipose tissue between the carotid artery and the trachea is carefully examined for the characteristic oval, tan parathyroid glands.

The upper parathyroid glands arise from the dorsal part of the fourth brachial pouch. During embryologic development they have only a short descent, and more than 90 percent are found just posterior to the middle or upper third of the thyroid gland. They are usually posterior and lateral to the recurrent laryngeal nerve. The upper parathyroid glands are usually the most constant in position and generally, therefore, more easily located. When enlarged, however, they may become inferiorly displaced as far as the posterior mediastinum.

The lower parathyroids arise from the dorsal part of the third brachial pouch and have a much longer descent with the thymus. In fact, 17 percent of inferior glands are found within or near the thymus. Over half of the time, however, the lower parathyroid is found adjacent to the posterior or lateral surface of the lower pole of the thyroid gland. If the inferior parathyroid is not found in this location, surgical dissection should continue inferiorly, where an additional 10 percent to 20 percent of parathyroid glands are found within 2 cm of the inferior pole. Two percent to 5 percent of inferior parathyroid glands are located within the thyroid lobe, and some of these may be detected by careful inspection of the posterior surface of the thyroid gland with surgical loops and good illumination.

Enlarged glands are more likely to be found in aberrant locations than are normal glands. When a search in the normal locations previously described is unsuccessful, the retrotracheal and retroesophageal areas should be examined. We have found an inferior parathyroid adenoma within the carotid sheath (the artery supplying the third brachial arch). This vessel should be examined up to the carotid bifurcation. Likewise, the posterior-superior mediastinum and the anterior-superior mediastinum may contain upper or lower parathyroid glands, respectively. Meticulous microscopic dissection in these aberrant areas not only preserves normal structures, but also preserves the characteristic tan appearance of parathyroid tissue, which quickly becomes very similar to thyroid coloration with manipulation and hemorrhage.

Adenomas

The unilateral identification of one definitely hypertrophic gland and one normal gland (generally tan, oval, 5 to 8 mm structures) probably indicates a single adenoma. Multiple adenomas are highly uncommon (2 percent to 3 percent, but higher in elderly patients). A frozen section biopsy is performed on the normal gland only to confirm that it is parathyroid tissue, as pathologists have significant difficulty discerning normal parathyroid tissue from hyperplasia or adenoma. In this situation, after removal of a suspected adenoma, and biopsy of a normal second gland (with frozen section confirmation of parathyroid tissue in both specimens), a significant minority of experienced parathyroid surgeons would consider the procedure complete, with the expectation of postoperative normocalcemia. The argument in favor of unilateral exploration is a reduced rate of postoperative complications, such as recurrent laryngeal injury or hypoparathyroidism. Certainly, if the opposite side has been previously explored, this approach should be seriously considered. This is especially the case if preoperative imaging techniques were used and indicated that the pathology was limited to the side already explored. If there is not a clear differentiation between gland size on the side first explored, bilateral exploration must be performed. In patients over 65 years old, exploration of the second side should also be strongly considered because double adenomas can approach a 10 percent incidence in this age group. Our own approach is in keeping with the majority of parathyroid surgeons who would explore the opposite side, unless previous surgery or trauma has greatly increased the risk of complications.

Hyperplasia

If bilateral neck exploration reveals four enlarged glands, the diagnosis is hyperplasia. I treat primary hyperparathyroidism caused by four-gland hyperplasia with three and one-half gland resection and cryopreservation of resected tissue. The fourth gland is marked carefully with a nonferrous hemoclip. If there is recurrent hyperparathyroidism, the remaining gland can be excised. A portion of this excised tissue can be autotransplanted into the SCM muscle, where its position is again marked with nonferrous hemoclips and a silk suture. If persistent hyperparathyroidism dictates further removal, this can be done with local anesthesia and a small neck incision. More than 75 percent of parathyroid autografts briefly stored on ice in the operating room are successful. The success of cryopreserved autografts drops to as low as 50 percent but provides some significant hope for normal parathyroid function in the 5 percent to 15 percent of patients who experience permanent hypoparathyroidism following three and one-half gland removal.

Cryopreservation is performed by placing 10 small slivers of chilled parathyroid tissue into each of several vials containing cryoprotective solution. These are then placed in a liquid nitrogen freezer and frozen at a controlled rate to 50° C and stored permanently at 100° C. I have used autotransplantation of parathyroid tissue in patients who have secondary hyperparathyroidism following total parathyroidectomy, to salvage parathyroid gland tissue when their blood supply has been interrupted during surgery, and also in patients whose previous thyroid surgery left a question as to whether there was any remaining parathyroid tissue after excision of an adenoma. Approximately 50 mg of tissue is placed in an iced saline bath and cut into 1 × 3 mm slivers. Approximately 20 of these pieces are placed in two to three pockets in the SCM muscle, each of which is marked by a small nonferrous hemoclip and a silk suture.

Secondary and Tertiary Hyperparathyroidism

Advanced renal disease and chronic dialysis often results in secondary hyperparathyroidism with elevated levels of PTH. Autonomous hyperplastic parathyroid glands (tertiary hyperparathyroidism) can also develop, and when medical measures to control this process are unsuccessful, surgical intervention may be required. In this situation, a total parathyroidectomy and immediate autotransplantation into the SCM muscle or three and one-half gland subtotal parathyroidectomy with cryopreservation of removed tissue are performed. Total parathyroidectomy with autotransplantation is preferred because autotransplants have a high success rate in preventing permanent hypoparathyroidism. Reoperation for hyperparathyroidism is much easier on autotransplanted tissue into the SCM muscle and can generally be accomplished under local anesthesia, as described previously. These patients do not tolerate well the lengthy general anesthesia generally necessary for reoperation and removal of a residual hyperfunctioning one-half gland.

Parathyroid Carcinoma

In a small percentage (0.5 percent to 4 percent) of patients who have hyperparathyroidism, a parathyroid carcinoma is found. Carcinoma is more common in patients who have familial hyperparathyroidism. These patients usually have striking hyperparathyroidism and hypercalcemia, with resultant symptoms generally being more severe than those associated with parathyroid adenomas. Because these lesions are generally larger than adenomas, nearly half are palpable as neck masses. At surgery they appear gray-white to gray-tan and are quite firm. Local invasion or adherence to surrounding structures is frequently seen. If these lesions are completely removed, there is a 50 percent to 70 percent chance of finding no evidence of disease at 5 years. Because neck metastases are rare, a modified or radical neck dissection should be reserved for those patients who have positive neck nodes. All efforts should be made not to violate the tumor capsule when a suspicious, firm, and locally adherent lesion is found. Postoperative radiotherapy should be considered, especially when final histology reveals that capsular and blood vessel invasion is present, neck metastases are present, microscopic residual disease is suspected, or there has been violation of the capsule with tumor spillage.

Unsuccessful Exploration

The most frustrating result in parathyroid exploration is the inability to locate all four glands or significant pathology after meticulous neck and superior mediastinal exploration. If the carotid sheaths and areas dorsal to the esophagus and pharynx are also negative, and if fewer than two glands are found on one side by these means, a thyroid lobectomy is carried out on that side to rule out an infrathyroidal parathyroid. If four glands are not found after all these strategies are exhausted, the procedure is terminated, and the patient is assessed for persistent hypercalcemia. If hypercalcemia persists, digital subtraction angiography will assist in further localization. Two percent of all patients require a thoracotomy and mediastinal exploration.

■ POSTOPERATIVE CARE

Half-inch Penrose drains placed in both surgical beds are removed when significant drainage resolves. Blood pressure is monitored closely on patient awakening and in the postoperative recovery room, because significant hypertension greatly increases the possibility of postoperative hematoma, which can threaten the airway in the immediate postoperative period. A snug, Queen Anne style pressure dressing is applied for the first 24 to 48 hours.

Removal of an adenoma, carcinoma, or hyperplastic parathyroid tissue generally results in significant drop in the serum calcium level over the first 24 to 48 hours. Checks for muscular irritability (Trousseau's or Chvostek's signs) are performed regularly, and the patient is questioned about paresthesias of the fingers, toes, or in the circumoral area. When these symptoms are present, more frequent measuring of serum calcium and phosphorus is indicated. Rapid fall in serum calcium levels is significant in patients who were noted preoperatively to have radiologic evidence of bone resorption and postoperatively develop the "hungry bone syndrome." If symptoms of hypocalcemia are severe, they can generally be corrected by the infusion of 2 mg per kilogram of elemental calcium over 15 minutes. A longer infusion of 15 mg per kilogram of elemental calcium, which is given over 24 hours, with half the total administered in the first 6 hours, generally prevents the return of symptoms. Only 10 percent to 15 percent of patients require calcium replacement. Patients who have higher preoperative levels of calcium, PTH, alkaline phosphatase, the elderly, and those patients who have large adenomas or a large amount of parathyroid tissue removed, are the most likely to require such intervention. When hypocalcemia persists, vitamin D may also be required. If hypercalcemia persists despite identification of all four parathyroid glands, the possibility of the existence of more than four glands must be considered.

I routinely check for recurrent laryngeal nerve function by mirror or flexible nasal endoscopic examination of the true vocal cords as soon as the patient is awake in recovery. A normal examination ensures an intact nerve and nearly always indicates ultimate normal function, even if the nerve becomes temporarily paralyzed due to operative stretch or trauma in the later postoperative period. If hypercalcemia persists despite identification of all four parathyroid glands, the possibility of the existence of more than four glands must be considered.

■ COMPLICATIONS

The immediate postoperative development of a hematoma with airway compromise must be watched for closely, as alluded to previously. Hypoparathyroidism is best avoided, because medical management can be difficult. Meticulous dissection and preservation of parathyroid blood supply is crucial. Biopsies are carried out with small surgical instruments under microscopic control on the side opposite the blood supply. I normally perform a biopsy at most on only one normal-appearing parathyroid gland. If parathyroid gland blood supply is inadvertently compromised, autotransplantation should be considered. If the recurrent laryngeal nerve has definitely been sacrificed, as in the case of malignancy, and there is poor compensation or significant aspiration, cord medialization procedures are very helpful. Superior laryngeal nerve injuries are more difficult to repair and generally do not require treatment.

Suggested Reading

Fyfe S, Hoover L, Zuckerbraun L, et al. Parathyroid carcinoma: Clinical presentation and treatment. Am J Otolaryngol 1990; 11:268-273.

Hoover L, Blacker J., Zuckerbraun L, et al. Surgical strategy in hyperparathyroidism. Otolaryngol Head Neck Surg 1987; 96:542-547.

Lando M, Hoover L, Zuckerbraun L, et al. Autotransplantation of parathyroid tissue into sternocleidomastoid muscle. Arch Otolaryngol Head Neck Surg 1988; 114:557-560.

Sofferman R, Nathan M, Fairbank J, et al. Preoperative technetium Tc99m sestamibi imaging. Arch Otolaryngol Head Neck Surg 1996; 122:369-374.

Summers G. Parathyroid exploration. Arch Otolaryngol Head Neck Surg 1991; 117:1237.

Wells S, Cooper J. Closed mediastinal exploration in patients with persistent hyperparathyroidism. Ann Surg 1991; 555-561.

CAROTID BODY TUMORS

The method of
Thomas V. McCaffrey
by
Thomas V. McCaffrey
Mark C. Witte

The head and neck paraganglia are neural crest cell derivatives that are anatomically closely related to the arterial vasculature and vagus nerve. This location is related to their role as modulators of cardiovascular excitation and respiration. The best studied of the paraganglia, the carotid body, is well established as a blood hypoxia sensor that stimulates increased ventilation when arterial blood oxygen saturation falls. This function explains the high degree of vascularity and close proximity to the carotid artery that characterizes the carotid body, and thus the challenging nature of carotid body tumor surgery.

Located in the crotch of the carotid bifurcation, the oxygen-sensing cells of the carotid body reside in a vascular meshwork of collagen strands that condense at the organ's periphery into an ill-defined capsule that fuses with the adventitia of the carotid artery itself. Multiple microscopic arteries and feeding arterioles sprout directly from the carotid bifurcation and penetrate the carotid body to supply blood to this organ, which, for its mass, receives the highest blood flow in the body. This characteristic of normal carotid body architecture has surgical implications in carotid body tumor removal; namely, that the plane of tumor resection must separate the carotid adventitia from the muscular tunica media. This dissection may cross small feeding vessels and disrupt the wall of the carotid artery, requiring the surgeon to be prepared to repair the carotid artery during surgery.

The carotid body tumor is the most common of the relatively rare paragangliomas, accounting for 60 percent of the tumors of the head and neck paraganglia. Ten percent of patients with carotid body tumors will have multiple tumors of the paraganglia.

A familial form of paraganglioma has been identified. Forty percent of affected individuals are initially seen with more than one tumor, and in 95 percent of these patients, at least one of the tumors is of the carotid body. Pedigree analysis of affected families suggests that the disease is inherited as an autosomal dominant trait modified by genomic imprinting. Genetic researchers have postulated that the defective allele that predisposes to tumor growth is inactivated during oogenesis but not during spermatogenesis. Therefore, a paraganglioma will develop only if the defective allele is inherited from the father, who himself may not be affected (if he inherited the allele from his mother). The overall incidence of bilateral carotid body tumors in sporadic cases is

3 percent, whereas in familial forms the incidence approaches 30 percent. Additionally, the familial form carries an 8 percent association with other malignancies, particularly those of neural crest origin.

■ EVALUATION

The typical patient is in the fifth decade of life and is found to have a painless, slowly enlarging midlateral neck mass. It is not uncommon that the patient has noticed a lump for several months or even years before seeking medical treatment. It is uncommon that the patient may note hoarseness or dysphagia, which, particularly with large or long-standing tumors, may signify invasion or entrapment of the vagus nerve. Occasionally, the patient will describe variation or a rapid increase in the size of the mass. The family history is worth reviewing to determine the risk to other family members and the potential for multiple paraganglia. If positive, queries about tinnitus, hearing loss, dysphagia, voice change, or aspiration may direct attention to the possibility of multiple tumors. Prior or concurrent history of malignancy, particularly of neural crest origin, may occasionally be helpful in narrowing the differential diagnosis of the neck mass.

Physical examination should devote particular attention to potential sites of other paragangliomas; the tympanic membranes (glomus tympanicum or jugulare); lateral pharyngeal walls (glomus vagale); and opposite neck (contralateral carotid body tumor), in addition to the mass itself. Vocal cord mobility should be assessed by indirect fiberoptic laryngoscopy. Neck palpation typically reveals a smooth, firm, subcutaneous, noncompressible mass that may be resistant to superoinferior but not anterolateral displacement. The examiner should note the patient's reaction to palpation of the mass; feelings of anxiety or lightheadedness, flushing, or palpitations should alert the clinician to the possible presence of a rare functional (catecholamine-secreting) tumor. If the mass is of sufficient size, auscultation may reveal a bruit. In a patient who has a low clinical likelihood of head and neck squamous cell carcinoma (i.e., long-standing mass, limited smoking and/or drinking history, and normal-appearing oral-pharyngeal-laryngeal mucosa), it is wise to defer fine needle aspiration until after imaging studies have been obtained.

Although carotid angiography must be considered the classic definitive imaging study, head and neck computed tomography (CT) with contrast and magnetic resonance imaging (MRI) add valuable diagnostic information that can help determine the need for more invasive studies. The classic presentation on neck CT with intravenous contrast is of a regularly shaped enhancing mass at the carotid bifurcation interposed between and splaying the internal and external carotid arteries. Normal anatomic relationships should be verified along both vagus nerves, jugular bulbs, and middle ear spaces as well as in the opposite carotid artery. An MRI will show a mass in the carotid bifurcation with a characteristic "salt and pepper" appearance of flow voids within the mass.

If noninvasive imaging supports the diagnosis of carotid body tumor, digital subtraction angiography (DSA) of both carotid arteries is indicated. First, DSA provides for detection of multiple tumors that may not have been noticed on CT or MRI imaging (Fig. 1). Second, DSA allows documentation of collateral cerebral blood flow in the event that the carotid artery must be sacrificed during tumor removal. Third, DSA identifies preoperatively the vessels feeding the tumor, including the occasional branch from the vertebral artery or thyrocervical trunk. Where tumor size or angioinvasiveness suggests possible internal carotid sacrifice, arterial occlusion studies with cerebral blood flow monitoring should be performed at the time of angiography.

After completion of imaging studies, preoperative 24 hour urine tests for metanephrines and vanillylmandelic acid are warranted to rule out the 1 percent risk of a functional tumor or a concurrent pheochromocytoma. Should these tests have suspicious or positive findings, serum testing of norepinephrine and dopamine levels allows rapid confirmation of abnormal catecholamine levels before obtaining chest and abdominal CT with contrast. Paraxial abdominal or mediastinal masses discovered on CT may require evaluation for catecholamine secretion using selective venous sampling, particularly if the carotid body tumor itself is nonsecreting. Clearly, considerations of patient safety dictate surgical removal of the secreting tumor before removal of a nonfunctioning carotid body tumor.

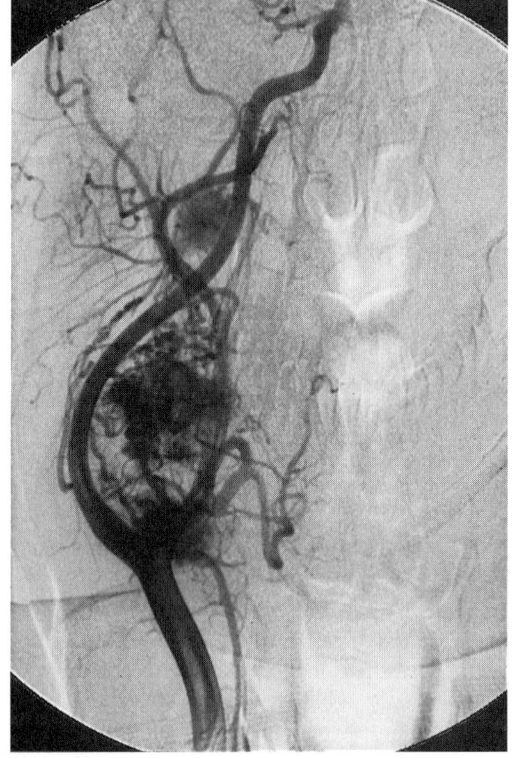

Figure 1.
Subtraction angiogram of the right carotid artery. This study demonstrates the typical appearance of a carotid body tumor splaying the internal and external carotid arteries at the bifurcation. In addition, a smaller glomus vagale tumor, that was initially unsuspected, can be seen.

THERAPY

The standard treatment of carotid body tumors in all but the elderly or debilitated patient is surgical excision. Despite reports of several small series to the contrary, external beam irradiation therapy does not always provide long-term tumor control. Indeed, several small surgical series have included up to 25 percent of patients who had failed radiotherapy; such cases entail significantly greater surgical difficulty and increased patient risk because of postirradiation fibrosis, with reduced carotid arterial wall blood supply and a higher risk of intraoperative or postoperative rupture. Nevertheless, the option of external beam irradiation or no intervention at all may be considered in elderly patients who are poor operative candidates or in patients with skull base invasion in whom achieving distal vascular control is likely impossible. Relative contraindications to surgery include poor cerebral collateral flow and significant carotid atherosclerosis, because arterial manipulation may result in showering of plaque fragments and cerebral infarction.

Preoperative Procedures

Preoperative embolization is usually only performed when the tumor shows indications of being difficult to resect, namely, very large or vascular tumors, or situations in which the tumor is likely to be quite fibrotic and adherent to surrounding structures, such as in revision or postradiotherapy cases. If selective arterial embolization is performed, it is essential to proceed to surgery within 24 to 48 hours before the tumor has had time to establish or augment collateral blood supply.

Two or three units of blood should be available for the operation; autologous donation can be used in most cases because the timing of the tumor removal is not critical. One unit of blood can be collected every 2 weeks before the surgery and stored in the blood bank until needed.

Surgical Technique

An oblique incision paralleling the anterior border of the sternocleidomastoid provides good exposure of the carotid proximal and distal to the tumor. Proximal and distal control of the common, internal, and external carotid arteries is ensured by prophylactic placement of vessel loops. The hypoglossal nerve is identified as it courses over the tumor mass; it is dissected from the tumor and retracted superiorly. The superior and inferior boundaries of the tumor are determined by blunt dissection. If the mass encases the external carotid artery, the artery may be ligated and mobilized to facilitate removal of the tumor from the internal carotid artery. As the dissection proceeds around the posterior aspect of the carotid sheath, special care is necessary to identify the vagus nerve and the sympathetic trunk in this region.

Using blunt dissection, a plane is developed between the internal carotid and its adventitia, which is adherent to the tumor. This is facilitated by gentle traction on the mass with a sponge under the surgeon's nondominant thumb. The tumor is usually supplied by several small vessels arising in the region of the carotid bifurcation. Evulsing these vessels may produce a rent in the carotid wall near the carotid bulb. The surgeon should be prepared to apply a patch graft if this should occur.

The internal jugular vein is ligated if it is encased or firmly adherent to the tumor mass; again, care must be taken at this vein's superior extent to avoid the trunks of cranial nerves IX to XII as they exit the skull base.

It is uncommon that transmural tumor invasion necessitates the resection of the internal carotid artery to ensure complete tumor removal. If preoperative occlusion studies suggest that cerebral ischemia is likely, a vascular shunt should be placed between the common and distal internal carotid arteries as the tumor mass is resected to permit uninterrupted cerebral perfusion. Once the tumor has been resected, reconstruction of the internal carotid should be undertaken. The saphenous vein is our choice for carotid reconstruction.

In the rare event of a functional carotid body tumor, exposure, manipulation, and removal of the mass must be carefully coordinated with the anesthesia team. In such a situation, multiple doses of intravenous nitroprusside or nicardipine, for example, may be necessary to control blood pressure and heart rate. Manipulation of the tumor mass should be minimized. Preoperative alpha blockade can be achieved over a period of several days and will mostly minimize these problems.

Postoperatively, the patient should be placed in the intensive care unit for 24 to 48 hours, and continuous blood pressure and hemodynamic monitoring should be instituted. In the event of ligation, grafting, or extensive intraoperative manipulation of the internal carotid, the surgeon should consider intravenous administration of heparin for 48 to 72 hours to inhibit thrombus formation. If the resected tumor is functional, maintaining the patient in the intensive care unit for 48 to 72 hours may be necessary to ensure hemodynamic stabilization; postoperative hypotension is possible following the removal of a catecholamine-secreting tumor.

As soon as practicable postoperatively, the patient's vocal cord function should be directly assessed. Initial oral intake postoperatively should include a trial of water sips in the presence of the otolaryngologist to ensure that no aspiration difficulties have arisen as a result of intraoperative vagus and/or glossopharyngeus nerve manipulation.

Alternative Treatments

Should radiotherapy be selected as the treatment modality, 4,500 to 5,000 cGy of external beam megavoltage photon or electron beam irradiation is considered standard treatment. Although multiple small series have reported 100 percent local tumor control, with arrest of progression and improvement of symptoms, there are numerous anecdotal reports of uncontrolled or recurrent carotid body tumor following radiotherapy. In elderly patients without evidence of rapid progression, no treatment is indicated. Patients should be observed at regular intervals to ensure stability.

PROGNOSIS

Overall, prognosis for carotid body tumors is excellent, particularly if the mass is resected while it is small. The realistic patient should not expect significant postoperative improvement of any cranial nerve palsies, and in cases of very large or very adherent tumors (e.g., previous biopsy or irradiation), the patient should be counseled that sacrifice of the involved nerves may be necessary to effect complete tumor removal. The surgical approach may be altered if other paragangliomas such as glomus vagale or jugulare are present concurrently.

Suggested Reading

Anand VK, Alemar GO, Sanders TS. Management of the internal carotid artery during carotid body tumor surgery. Laryngoscope 1995; 105: 231-235.

Balatsouras DG, Eliopoulos PN, Economou CN. Multiple glomus tumours. J Laryngol Otol 1992; 106:538-543.

McCaffrey TV, Meyer FB, Michels VV, et al. Familial paragangliomas of the head and neck. Arch Otolaryngol Head Neck Surg 1994; 120:1211-1216.

Mena J, Bowen JC, Hollier LH. Metachronous bilateral nonfunctional intercarotid paraganglioma (carotid body tumor) and functional retroperitoneal paraganglioma: Report of a case and review of the literature. Surgery 1993; 114:107-111.

Schild SE, Foote RL, Buskirk SJ, et al. Results of radiotherapy for chemodectomas. Mayo Clin Proc 1992; 67:537-540.

PHARYNGOCUTANEOUS FISTULA

The method of

Gerry F. Funk

by

Ross I.S. Zbar

Gerry F. Funk

An unplanned pharyngocutaneous fistula resulting from a communication between the upper aerodigestive tract and skin is a frustrating complication of head and neck surgery. All patients undergoing surgery of the upper aerodigestive tract are at risk for pharyngocutaneous fistulas; this complication may occur in patients who have obvious factors predisposing to compromised wound healing or in apparently healthy patients. As with any complication, the best management of pharyngocutaneous fistulas is prevention. However, if a fistula does occur, prompt treatment must be instituted to minimize the morbidity and potential mortality associated with this complication. In this chapter, we present our approach to the diagnosis, prevention, and management of pharyngocutaneous fistulas.

■ DIAGNOSIS

Pharyngocutaneous fistulas may be early or late complications of head and neck surgery. Fistulas that occur within 1 week of surgery frequently reflect problems related to the wound and its healing, including infection, poor surgical technique, inadequate perioperative antibiotic use, prior radiotherapy or prior surgery, distal pharyngeal stenosis, and poor nutritional status of the patient. Fistulas occurring 2 to 3 weeks after surgery may be due to these factors as well, but persistent cancer should be considered, particularly if a fistula persists despite appropriate management.

Early diagnosis of postoperative fistulas is beneficial before extensive spoilage of the neck wound and external skin breakdown occurs. The surgeon should carefully examine the neck skin flaps for erythema and induration, which may be apparent as early as postoperative Days 2 to 3. Erythema, tenderness, and palpable firmness of the skin flaps postoperatively may indicate early infection. The odor of anaerobic bacteria in drainage or on dressing material should be carefully sought, and this finding is very suggestive of impending fistulization. The intraoral and neck suture lines should be examined very carefully for evidence of nonhealing. If the suture lines are not healing together by postoperative Days 4 to 5, this is an indication of underlying infection, particularly if any of the previously mentioned findings are present. Palpation for fluctuance under the skin flaps is not adequate because inflammation and edema of the skin flaps will frequently obscure an underlying fluid collection. Leukocytosis is commonly found, and a white blood cell count that is trending upward in the presence of a poorly healing wound suggests infection and impending fistula.

The area of greatest erythema and swelling along the external suture line should be carefully opened under sterile conditions. Gentle digital exploration will usually be all that is needed to confirm the diagnosis of a localized infection or an infection with fistula. If a microvascular anastomosis is present, this suture line opening should be as far from the vascular pedicle as possible. Having the patient swallow dye is rarely needed to make the diagnosis of an early postoperative fistula, but this technique may be helpful to evaluate the healing of a fistula.

■ PREVENTION

Preventing a pharyngocutaneous fistula is much easier and less costly than treating one. This begins with a thorough preoperative history and physical examination to identify factors predisposing the patient to the development of a fistula. The preoperative and intraoperative management of the patient is then adjusted to maximize the chance of uncomplicated healing.

Systemic Considerations

Patients who have a history of heavy alcohol use may require aggressive, preoperative nutritional supplementation, including thiamine and vitamin B_{12} replacement. Preoperative admission for delirium tremens prophylaxis should be undertaken in the actively drinking patient, and aggressive management with chlordiazepoxide should be instituted. Postoperative delirium tremens may be life threatening and result in a prolonged stay in the intensive care unit. Poor healing during delirium tremens may result from severely compromised cardiopulmonary function or actual physical disruption of the wound by a thrashing, uncooperative patient.

Patients who continue to smoke up to the time of surgery are at increased risk for wound breakdown, and every effort should be made to prevent the patient from smoking in the preoperative and postoperative periods. Patients using long-term oral steroids may benefit from preoperative supplementation with vitamin A. Patients who have diabetes mellitus require tight perioperative control of blood sugar levels. There is some controversy surrounding the perioperative use of blood transfusions in head and neck cancer patients, and some evidence exists suggesting that perioperative blood transfusions increase the risk for cancer recurrence. However, these concerns must be balanced with the potential morbidity and poor healing associated with anemia. As a general guideline, we try to maintain a hematocrit in the 30 percent range for patients undergoing major clean-contaminated head and neck surgery.

When patients demonstrate evidence of malnutrition preoperatively (including hypoalbuminemia, hypoproteinemia, or greater than 10 percent unwanted weight loss), nutritional supplementation is indicated. Preoperative placement of a nasogastric tube or gastrostomy tube are the best methods to supplement poor oral intake. We do not perform percutaneous gastrostomy procedures on patients who have large, bulky hypopharyngeal or laryngeal cancers due to the reported risk of cancer seeding at the gastrostomy site.

Patients who have a history of radiotherapy to the head and neck should have thyroid function tests before surgery. Subclinical hypothyroidism (defined as a normal serum thyroxine level and an elevated serum thyroid-stimulating hormone level) may be associated with poor wound healing. Thyroid supplementation should be instituted in the hypothyroid patient before a major surgical procedure.

Local Considerations

Advanced cancer and use of a flap reconstruction are factors that have been associated with infection and fistula formation. Although stage is not within the surgeon's control, every effort should be made to select the most efficient reconstructive option that will meet realistic reconstructive goals. Longer surgery times are also associated with wound infection, and every effort should be made to minimize the operating time.

Most pharyngocutaneous fistulas are associated with a wound infection. With no antibiotic coverage, the wound infection rate in clean-contaminated head and neck surgery is between 30 percent and 80 percent. With appropriate antibiotic prophylaxis, the infection rate is reduced to between 5 percent and 30 percent. In order to be maximally beneficial, antibiotics must be in the circulation before the skin incision is made. The spectrum of coverage should include oral anaerobes, and the regimen we favor includes either cefazolin plus metronidazole or clindamycin alone. Ampicillin-sulbactam is also a reasonable perioperative antibiotic choice; however, we do not routinely use this drug combination. There is evidence that topical povidone-iodine, when rinsed in the mouth before incision, may reduce the incidence of postoperative wound infection following surgery of the oral cavity and oropharynx. For most routine cases, there is no additional benefit obtained by continuing antibiotic prophylaxis beyond the first postoperative day. In selected cases with anticipated healing problems, we may continue antibiotics beyond the first postoperative day; however, the benefit in doing this is unproved.

An increased incidence of wound infections and fistulization in head and neck cancer patients who have received preoperative radiotherapy has been reported in some studies and not demonstrated in others. In our experience, prior curative-dose radiotherapy clearly has a detrimental effect on wound healing and should be considered a risk factor for compromised healing. There is certainly evidence to suggest that wound breakdown or infection in the previously irradiated patient results in greater morbidity than in the nonirradiated patient.

In previously irradiated patients, the importation of vascularized tissue to protect vascular structures (great vessels and microvascular flap pedicles) and enhance wound healing should be considered. The pectoralis myofascial flap is rapidly harvested, and can easily be rotated into the head and neck defect to serve a variety of purposes. We do not hesitate to use this flap to replace compromised neck skin and separate the sutured pharynx from vascular structures in patients who have had prior radiotherapy. In all previously irradiated patients who have undergone pharyngectomy involving mediastinal dissection, the pectoralis myofascial flap should be used to obliterate dead space and separate the great vessels from the pharyngeal closure. Replacement of tenuous neck skin with healthy pectoralis muscle is particularly important near the trifurcation point of a Schobinger-type incision in a previously irradiated and previously operated patient. When used for external coverage, the exposed pectoralis muscle is skin grafted. The small additional time required to raise this flap is well worth the effort in the patient who is at high risk for the development of a fistula.

When closing the wound in an irradiated patient, meticulous care should be directed at obliterating dead space by closing the defect from the "bottom out." Internal raw surfaces should be opposed and sutured together wherever possible rather than simply closing the mucosa on the inside and the skin flaps on the outside. There must be no tension on the suture lines. One dose of preoperative steroid (8 to 10 mg dexamethasone) and a second postoperative dose appear to markedly decrease the swelling in previously irradiated patients. This may decrease the tension on suture lines, improve the microcirculation, and decrease the relative ischemia of mucosal and skin flaps.

In cases that require intraoral flap or mucosal closure adjacent to the dental arches, carious dentition with local gingivitis may predispose to wound infection. For patients with extremely poor dentition who will require dental extractions before radiotherapy, these teeth are best removed before or at the time of the primary surgery. Teeth abutting the tumor should not be removed before the definitive oncologic procedure. It is preferable to extract extremely carious teeth than to suture a flap adjacent to them.

A relatively rare but important local consideration predisposing to fistula formation, particularly in the partial laryngopharyngectomy patient, is pooling of saliva caused by resistance to flow through the pharynx. If the pharyngeal closure is tight enough that flow through the pharyngeal conduit is severely impaired, saliva will take the path of least resistance and may force through the suture line during swallowing. This problem should be dealt with by recruiting additional tissue for closure of the pharynx if the mucosa remaining after tumor removal does not easily close over a feeding tube. A pharyngocutaneous fistula in the presence of a distal tight structure will be very difficult to close until the stricture is corrected.

Careful planning of the neck incisions, and gentle handling of the neck flaps during the operation, may prevent wound breakdown and subsequent fistula formation. Skin flaps should be designed with trifurcation points (if needed) away from underlying mucosal suture lines and away from the carotid artery. Skin incisions in previously operated patients should use prior incisions when possible in order to prevent devascularization of skin islands. Neck flaps should be protected from pressure and kept moist during the procedure.

Meticulous care in drain placement, and ensuring continued function of the drains to prevent the collection of fluid or a hematoma, is crucial in the prevention of wound infection and subsequent fistula formation. A number of wound infections that occur following head and neck surgery are likely the result of localized fluid collections or hematomas becoming infected. Hematomas act as a tissue irritant, and the neck should be closely inspected for signs of this. A localized hematoma accumulation within the wound that does not continue to expand may not be obvious in the edematous patient. However, tissues overlying the hematoma will become erythematous, swollen, and somewhat firmer than normal. Without prompt drainage, the hematoma will prevent healing and likely become infected. Suction drains should be placed to maximally eliminate dead space in the wound. When possible, one drain should exit along what would be a safe course for a fistula to take, if one were to occur. It is best if drains exit the wound in a dependent position from a separate stab incision. Drains should remain in place until the output is less than 30 to 35 cc over a 24 hour period.

Waiting an appropriate amount of time before commencing oral feeding is important when a mucosal closure exists in the aerodigestive tract. Waiting 7 days before starting oral intake in a patient without prior radiotherapy is a proven technique. If the patient has received radiotherapy in the past, one additional day is added for each 1,000 cGy of radiation received. Obtaining a white blood cell count before feeding the patient who has had a complex closure that is not easily inspected is helpful as a baseline for comparison after the patient has begun an oral diet.

One way to prevent an unplanned fistula is to close the defect around a planned, controlled fistula. A controlled fistula is made by placing a large passive drain from the pharynx to the skin, with careful avoidance of the great vessels or any microvascular anastomoses. The channeled salivary flow will take the path of least resistance along the passive drain and be directed away from areas where healing is felt to be tenuous. The drain may be slowly removed, and the controlled fistula will significantly decrease in size with time. In most cases, a second surgical procedure will be required to close it.

■ MANAGEMENT

Pharyngocutaneous fistulas may occur despite the best preoperative planning and intraoperative technique. There are general principles to follow in the management of all pharyngocutaneous fistulas. However, pharyngocutaneous fistulas occur in a variety of clinical situations, each requiring a somewhat different approach to management. In this section, we discuss management of the more frequent clinical scenarios: (1) the patient with no prior radiotherapy in whom the carotid artery or a microvascular anastomosis is not threatened by the location of the fistula, (2) the patient who has had prior radiotherapy in which the carotid artery or a microvascular anastomosis is threatened by the location of the fistula, and (3) the massive pharyngocutaneous fistula.

The first step in management is to carefully open the wound and determine the extent of the infection or fistula. This gentle exploration of the breakdown site will allow a determination of whether vascular structures are at risk. When a fistula is diagnosed, the patient should receive nothing by mouth and be started on broad-spectrum antibiotics with anaerobic coverage. Aerobic and anaerobic cultures of fistulous drainage should be obtained, and the antibiotic therapy should be changed as needed when culture sensitivity results return. A method of nutritional support other than oral should be established, and it is useful to obtain a baseline white blood cell count.

No Prior Radiotherapy and Vascular Structures Not At Risk

In the patient with no prior radiotherapy in whom the carotid artery or a microvascular anastomosis is not at risk due to the fistula location, conservative treatment in general will be satisfactory. Meticulous wound care two or three times daily is required, with moist strip gauze packing of the fistula tract. The packing serves several purposes: it cleans necrotic debris from the tract, acts as a barrier to salivary contamination of the fistula, and provides a vehicle for the delivery of antibiotic solution to the wound. Packing the wound should be accompanied by daily, sharp debridement of all necrotic tissue from the wound. Removal of dead tissue from the wound will hasten healing more than any other local measure. Initially, the wound should be packed with saline-soaked iodoform gauze. Once granulation tissue has begun to line the wound, the packing material may be changed to strip gauze moistened with an extremely dilute povidone-iodine solution (1 cc povidone-iodine per liter of saline). After the fistula has closed, the packing is done with saline-soaked gauze. It is important that the healing wound be kept moist at all times. Healing will be retarded if purulence is allowed to build up under areas of crusting. In an otherwise healthy patient who has not received prior radiotherapy, the fistula should show significant healing within 7 to 10 days. If the fistula persists, biopsy of the fistula tract in the area closest to the prior tumor resection margin should be considered to rule out the possibility of persistent cancer.

Prior Radiotherapy with Vascular Structures At Risk

A pharyngocutaneous fistula in the patient who has received prior radiotherapy and has a carotid artery or microvascular anastomosis in the path of the fistula needs to be managed aggressively. Immediate plans should be made to return this patient to the operating room. Safe drainage and diversion of the salivary stream needs to be established, and in the majority of cases, the safest and most definitive management involves bringing healthy, vascularized tissue into the wound to protect the vascular structures and facilitate healing.

In the operating room, the neck is opened at the site of the fistula; the extent of infection and size of the fistula are determined. In general, vigorous probing and opening of healed tissue planes should be avoided. Most of the dissection can be done bluntly, and if the patient has a microvascular anastomosis, this should be manipulated as minimally as possible. Granulation tissue that has formed over a microvascular pedicle should not be disturbed. The wound should be copiously irrigated with half-strength povidone-iodine solution after removal of all nonviable tissues. When a microvascular pedicle is present, the irrigating solution should be warmed. In selected cases, the salivary stream can be safely directed away from the vascular structures and out through an unoperated side of the neck without the need to import vascularized tissue into the wound. A Penrose drain is placed along the safe course of the fistula, and the skin flaps are closed loosely over this drain. The Penrose drain is slowly backed out over 5 to 6 days, and the fistula is allowed to heal as the drain is withdrawn.

The sternocleidomastoid muscle should not be depended on for safe carotid coverage low in the neck. This is particularly true if the patient has had previous radiotherapy or a modified neck dissection in which the muscle was retained. Low in the neck the carotid may be exposed to salivary contamination, particularly in the laryngectomy patient who has a low fistula exiting adjacent to the tracheostome.

When the neck skin flaps are tenuous, the infection is relatively widespread, or a microvascular pedicle or the carotid artery are within the infection or fistula, vascularized tissue should be imported into the wound. This will allow definitive protection of the vascular structures, enhanced antibiotic delivery to the wound, replacement of tenuously viable neck skin, and faster healing of the underlying mucosal margins. In these types of cases, we prefer to use the pectoralis myofascial flap. The muscle can be rapidly harvested, and in females the cosmetic deformity is minimized with the use of an inframammary incision. In general, the pectoralis muscle on the side of the fistula is harvested and brought into the wound to cover the threatened vascular structure and separate it from the fistulous tract. In most pharyngocutaneous fistulas, the pectoralis muscle can be draped over the carotid artery or microvascular anastomosis and then sutured to the prevertebral fascia (Fig. 1). The drainage of the fistula is then directed along the course of a Penrose drain, with the muscle separating the fistulous tract from the carotid artery or microvascular pedicle.

When the margins of neck skin flaps are tenuous, the nonviable areas are excised, and the external surface is replaced with pectoralis muscle. In most fistulas, the mucosal opening will be surrounded with friable tissue, so suture closure of the mucosal defect is not possible. Attempting to close the friable edges of a mucosal defect may only make it larger. Pectoralis muscle that has been brought into the wound may be sutured to the tissue around the defect. In an infected neck with a large fistula, the goal is to bring healthy tissue into contact with the mucosal defect, not to create a watertight closure. The Penrose drain is slowly backed out over several days, and the fistula is allowed to heal as the drain is withdrawn. Bringing vascularized tissue into the wound offers a safe and definitive solution to this potentially severe problem, and it is usually the only procedure needed to facilitate complete healing. If any question exists regarding the safety of a microvascular pedicle or the carotid artery, these structures should be covered with nonirradiated vascularized tissue.

Massive Pharyngocutaneous Fistulas

Massive pharyngocutaneous fistulas most frequently occur in the severely compromised host and have been arbitrarily defined as fistulas that result in loss of greater than two-thirds of the pharyngeal wall circumference. In these cases, there is usually significant loss of overlying neck skin as well. Bringing vascularized muscle into the wound may be important for the protection of vascular structures, but may not be adequate for definitive closure of the fistula. When this type of fistula occurs, the first intervention should be to render the patient safe from vascular catastrophe by protecting the carotid artery through safe diversion of the salivary stream and coverage of the carotid artery, if required. Every effort should be made to address any correctable systemic conditions that may be contributing to the patient's poor healing. During this early period, the wound should be treated conservatively with iodoform strip gauze packing three times per day and daily debridement. In patients with massive defects who have previously received radiotherapy, hyperbaric oxygen appears to hasten the formation of healthy granulation tissue within the wound.

Treating the patient conservatively with packing for 2 to 3 weeks usually results in a considerable decrease in the size of the fistula. Once the patient has a safe wound, conservative management can be continued at home with the assistance of a visiting nurse. The goal of conservative treatment in these patients is a clean wound lined with healthy granulation tissue.

Definitive closure of the massive pharyngocutaneous defect requires replacement of both internal and external lining, and should not be undertaken until the wound is clean

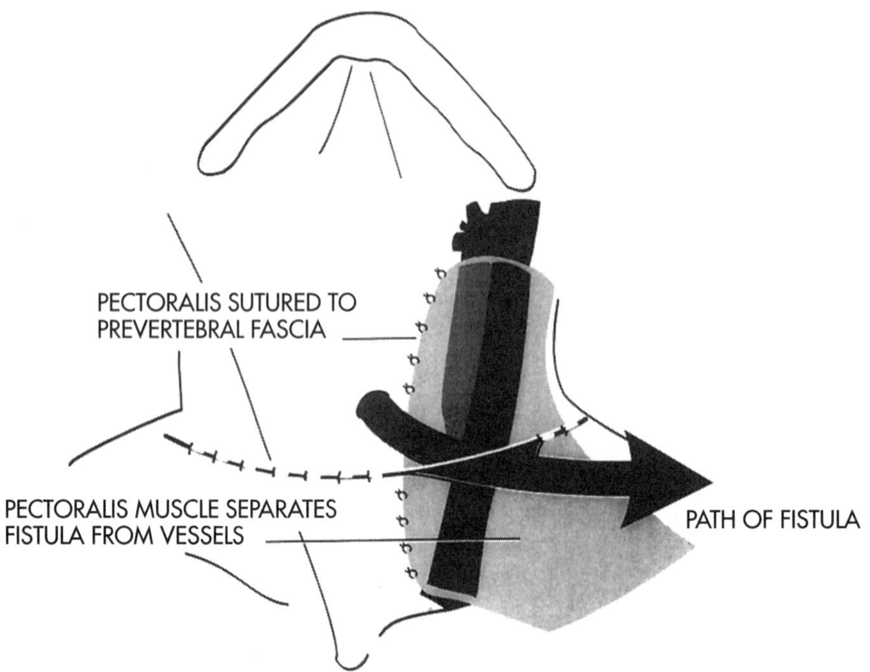

Figure 1.
Schematic representation of the position of the pectoralis myofascial flap when used to separate the carotid artery from the course of a pharyngocutaneous fistula. Suturing the pectoralis flap to the prevertebral fascia separates the vascular space from the pharyngeal space.

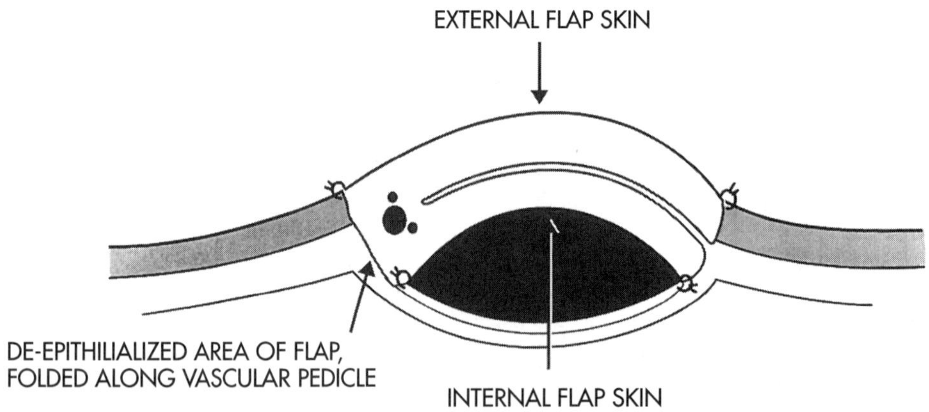

Figure 2.
Cross-sectional representation of the forearm free flap to replace both the pharyngeal mucosa and the external neck skin in the case of a massive pharyngocutaneous fistula. The fold in the forearm flap should be made lengthwise along the vascular pedicle.

and the patient's medical status is optimized. In these cases, the reconstruction must not only close the defect in the pharynx but also increase the circumference of the pharyngeal lumen. Several options are available, and the best choice depends on the anatomy of the defect, the medical condition and body habitus of the patient, and the availability of recipient vessels for microvascular anastomosis in the neck.

In the thin patient, a pectoralis myocutaneous flap is a good option, with the skin paddle used to resurface the pharynx and the pectoralis muscle covered with a skin graft externally. The deltopectoral flap is another locally available option best used in cases in which the external defect has decreased significantly in size. This flap may not be the most robust option when brought up into an irradiated bed and may require two or more procedures to achieve closure of the fistula.

In the patient who is able to tolerate a longer procedure and has a large defect involving a long segment of pharynx, the use of a forearm flap may be the best option for a single-stage closure. The forearm flap can be used in either of two ways for these reconstructions. With the first method, the forearm flap skin is used to replace only the internal lining of the pharynx, and the fascial surface of the forearm flap, which is then external, is covered with a pectoralis myofascial flap. This is the safest method to use when the neck skin flaps are not healthy and would offer questionable coverage for the underlying vascular pedicle. The second method uses forearm skin to replace both the internal pharyngeal and external surface by folding the flap 180 degrees and de-epithelializing a portion of it. This latter method must be done very carefully in order to prevent venous congestion distal to the fold. The fold in the forearm should be lengthwise along the vascular pedicle; the vessels should not be folded (Fig. 2). The latissimus dorsi as a free or pedicled flap is also useful in closing massive pharyngeal fistulas. When this flap is used, the skin paddle replaces the internal pharyngeal surface, and the external muscle is skin grafted. This flap allows a large amount of well-vascularized muscle to be brought into the wound. However, unless the patient is relatively thin, the skin paddle of the latissimus dorsi flap is fairly thick and may be difficult to work with.

Suggested Reading

Barra S, Barzan L, Maione A, et al. Blood transfusion and other prognostic variables in the survival of patients with cancer of the head and neck. Laryngoscope 1994; 104:95-98.

Becker GD. Identification and management of the patient at high risk for wound infection. Head Neck Surg 1986; 8:205-210.

Brook I, Hirokawa R. Microbiology of wound infection after head and neck cancer surgery. Ann Otol Rhinol Otolaryngol 1989; 98:323-325.

Celikkanat S, Koc C, Akyol MU, Ozdem C. Effect of blood transfusion on tumor recurrence and postoperative pharyngocutaneous fistula formation in patients subjected to total laryngectomy. Acta Otolaryngol (Stockholm) 1995; 115:566-568.

Cole RR, Robbins T, Cohen JI, Wolf PF. A predictive model for wound sepsis in oncologic surgery of the head and neck. Otolaryngol Head Neck Surg 1987; 96:165-171.

Girod DA, McCulloch TM, Tsue TT, Weymuller EA. Risk factors for complications in clean-contaminated head and neck surgical procedures. Head Neck 1995; 17:7-13.

Huang DT, Giovanna T, Wilson WR. Stomal seeding by percutaneous endoscopic gastrostomy in patients with head and neck cancer. Arch Otolaryngol Head Neck Surg 1992; 118:658-659.

Johnson J, Bloomer WD. Effect of prior radiotherapy on post surgical wound infection. Head Neck 1989; 11:132-136.

McCulloch TM, VanDaele DJ, Hillel A. Blood transfusion as a risk factor for death in stage III and IV operative laryngeal cancer. Arch Otolaryngol Head Neck Surg 1995; 121:1227-1235.

Peat BG, Boyd JB, Gullane PJ. Massive pharyngocutaneous fistulae: Salvage with two-layer flap closure. Ann Plast Surg 1992; 29:153-156.

Redleaf MI, Bauer CA. Topical antiseptic mouthwash in oncological surgery of the oral cavity and oropharynx. J Laryngol Otol 1994; 108:973-979.

Robbins KT, Favrot S, Hanna D, Cole R. Risk of wound infection in patients with head and neck cancer. Head Neck 1990; 12:143-148.

Velanovich V. A meta-analysis of prophylactic antibiotics in head and neck surgery. Plast Reconstr Surg 1991; 87:429-434.

Weber RS, Callender DL. Antibiotic prophylaxis in clean-contaminated head and neck oncologic surgery. Ann Otol Rhinol Laryngol 1992; 102:16-20.

Weber RS, Read I, Frankenthaler R, et al. Ampicillin-sulbactam vs clindamycin in head and neck oncologic surgery. Arch Otolaryngol Head Neck Surg 1992; 118:1159-1163.

Zbar RIS, Funk GF, McCulloch TM, et al. The pectoralis major myofascial flap: A valuable tool in contemporary head and neck reconstruction. Head Neck 1997.

FAR-ADVANCED HEAD AND NECK CANCER

The method of
David E. Schuller
by
David E. Schuller
Pramod K. Sharma

Contemporary treatment of far-advanced head and neck cancer continues to be challenging despite an improved understanding of the biologic behavior of the disease and the impact of multimodal treatment strategies. It is initially imperative to define certain terms about this disease category for purposes of describing recommended approaches. Treatment varies depending on the surgical resectability of the disease. However, there are certain components of treatment, such as pain relief and overall support issues, that apply to all categories. In this chapter, we define the term *far-advanced* as stages III or IV previously untreated resectable or unresectable, recurrent resectable or unresectable without distant metastases, or recurrent cancer with distant metastases.

■ PREVIOUSLY UNTREATED RESECTABLE DISEASE

This group of patients has been vigorously studied with clinical research over the past 20 years. The reason for this intense focus is because conventional treatment programs yield far from satisfactory results. Conventional therapy in the United States involves a combined therapy approach of surgery and radiotherapy, with the latter modality given in a postoperative sequence. However, results of clinical trials have demonstrated that the survival rates for squamous cell carcinoma arising from the four most common anatomic sites (larynx, oral cavity, oropharynx, and hypopharynx) in this category are approximately 38 percent disease-free, 4 year actuarial survival). Neoadjuvant or adjuvant chemotherapy regimens have been evaluated in a variety of combinations. The use of 5-fluorouracil (5-FU) in combination with cisplatin has become the "gold standard" of chemotherapy regimens because it has the greatest activity against squamous cell carcinoma arising in the upper aerodigestive tract. Concurrent chemoradiotherapy using cisplatin has also been employed in this patient population in combination with surgery.

The largest phase III trial for this patient population, which accrued 448 evaluable patients, was sponsored by the Head and Neck Cancer Intergroup and involved the member institutions of all of the existing cooperative groups in the United States. The experimental arm of that study consisted of a sequential regimen of surgical resection, followed by three cycles of cisplatin and 5-FU, and then followed by a course of radiotherapy (50 to 60 Gy). This study demonstrated, for the first time in head and neck cancer patients, that systemic chemotherapy statistically lowered the chances of developing distant metastases. However, there was no statistically significant difference in survival when compared with conventional therapy consisting of surgical resection with postoperative radiotherapy. This trial also continued to demonstrate frequent and unsatisfactory treatment failure rates at the primary site, neck nodal region, and distant sites.

Multiple pilot studies are currently under way to hopefully build on what has been learned from prior clinical trials for this patient population. We have been involved with evaluating a multimodal treatment program that was developed to intensify treatment for local, regional, and distant disease. This regimen includes preoperative accelerated fractionation radiotherapy administered concurrently with cisplatin for 3 days, followed immediately by surgery with intraoperative irradiation, and postoperative concurrent chemoradiotherapy. The preliminary results of this pilot experience have been published and demonstrate a high compliance rate with the schema in addition to strong locoregional control rates. However, distant metastases still occurred in this group, and currently are a focus of a subsequent clinical trial that incorporates three courses of paclitaxel postoperatively in addition to the postoperative chemoradiotherapy using cisplatin.

No matter what the treatment regimen, it is important for the clinician to recognize that this is a patient population that has a strong chance of treatment failure within the first 12 to 18 months. Accordingly, immediate reconstruction of the defect following surgical resection is an important quality-of-life consideration. These patients are often debilitated with comorbid conditions, including poor nutritional status. It is imperative that the head and neck oncologic surgeon have a full armamentarium of reconstructive capabilities, including the use of a multitude of musculocutaneous flaps as well as the availability of free tissue transfer using microvascular surgery.

■ PREVIOUSLY TREATED RESECTABLE DISEASE

Patients who have recurrent cancer that is believed to be resectable with no evidence of distant metastases represent special challenges. Comorbid conditions and the overall nutritional status play an important role in the patient's ability to tolerate further treatment. We have found that the involvement of a knowledgeable internist as a member of the head and neck oncologic team is invaluable. The optimal situation, in our opinion, includes an internist who repeatedly deals with this substance-abusing and noncompliant patient population and is familiar with the stresses created by head and neck oncologic surgery. It is obviously important for the internist to be involved with both the preoperative assessment to help determine treatment suitability and perioperative care, when requested.

In this patient population, it is important for the clinician to recognize that the prior treatment, whether it be surgery and/or radiotherapy, produces fibrosis in the area of disease that decreases the vascularity of the tumor bed and subsequently compromises the delivery of systemic chemotherapy and healing following additional surgery. It is imperative for these factors to be accurately communicated to the patient so that the patient and physician have a clear understanding of the realities of the situation. However, it is also important to recognize that a cure is still a possibility in this situation, and we recommend a vigorous and appropriately aggressive course of treatment when desired by the patient.

Protection of the carotid artery is of critical importance in all head and neck oncologic procedures that enter the oral cavity and/or pharynx. It is especially important in this group of patients with probable compromised healing capabilities. The muscular pedicle of a pectoralis musculocutaneous flap used in the reconstruction of a defect often provides effective coverage of the carotid artery. If that type of muscle coverage is not feasible, then a dermal graft should be strongly considered whenever the oral cavity or pharynx is entered.

Resection of the recurrent disease becomes more challenging because of the fibrosis created by the prior therapy. It is more difficult for the surgeon to clinically distinguish neoplasm from uninvolved tissue as a result of the fibrosis. Accordingly, it is usual to require wider margins of resection around the recurrent cancer. Once again, quality-of-life issues dictate reconstructive techniques that rehabilitate the patient as quickly as possible. It is important for the patient to understand that swallowing and speech rehabilitation occur slower in this group than in those patients undergoing similar treatment for previously untreated disease.

Adjunctive treatment before or after surgical resection is still considered investigational. There has been no demonstrated survival benefit in prior trials using neoadjuvant or adjuvant chemotherapy in this patient population. Intraoperative radiotherapy has been used extensively by the authors in this patient population with the hope that it would provide enhanced local control. Our Ohio State experience has demonstrated that this modality is certainly feasible and has acceptable toxicities. There is not sufficient experience yet to determine whether it provides a survival advantage.

In those patients who do not have cure as their goal or who have contraindications to additional surgery, systemic chemotherapy is an alternative. Response rates can be anticipated to be lower than in those with previously untreated disease, and this is presumed to be related to the fibrosis of the disease site compromising the vascularity. The combination of 5-FU with cisplatin continues to be the benchmark for comparison when investigational agents are being evaluated. There is interest and some reports of favorable activity using paclitaxel for this patient population. If radiotherapy was not administered as the initial treatment, that is another nonsurgical option that has potential for cure for small volume disease. Larger volume disease without prior radiotherapy is often treated with a combined approach using surgery and postoperative radiotherapy.

■ PREVIOUSLY UNTREATED UNRESECTABLE DISEASE

This patient population continues to be a major challenge. Of course, the determination of unresectability is critically important and should not be approached casually by the clinician. The definition of surgical unresectability differs among surgeons, and there is no single definition that is agreeable to all. There is no question that the relationship of the disease to surrounding structures, especially the carotid artery, cervical spine, and deep neck musculature, is often a part of this consideration. Surgical experience can also be a factor in the determination of surgical resectability. It is imperative for the treating surgeon to provide the patient with the opportunity for additional opinions if the surgeon thinks that his or her inexperience may be playing a disproportionately large role in the definition of surgical unresectability.

This previously untreated group of patients with unresectable disease has been studied in the past and is currently being evaluated. There is currently a trial open in the Southwest Oncology Group and Eastern Cooperative Oncology Group. This trial compares continuous course radiotherapy (35 fractions, 7,000 cGy), continuous course radiotherapy and concurrent chemotherapy (cisplatin), versus split-course radiotherapy with concurrent chemotherapy (cisplatin and 5-FU). Patients in the split-course radiotherapy arm receive 3,000 cGy with two courses of concurrent cisplatin and 5-FU. Following this, clinical evaluation identifies patients with a partial response, who are now candidates for surgical resection. These patients, upon recuperating from surgery, along with the patients who remained unresectable, receive a second course of radiotherapy and one course of concurrent cisplatin and 5-FU. All the patients in the various treatment arms are then evaluated, and surgical salvage is performed, if possible.

Overall, this is a group of patients who have a grave prognosis. It is imperative for the clinician to accurately communicate this matter to the patient at the onset. Obviously, quality-of-life issues, such as pain control and other supportive interventions, are critically important.

■ PREVIOUSLY TREATED UNRESECTABLE DISEASE

Treatment programs with curative potential are less common for this patient population compared with some of the other groups of patients that have been discussed. If the patients have not received radiotherapy, it is conceivable that some type of concurrent chemoradiotherapy program has curative potential. However, that is about the only possibility for cure, albeit small. The other options for treatment include chemotherapy regimens that are designed to provide protracted disease-free interval. Once again, the 5-FU–cisplatin regimen is the frame of reference for all other investigational agents, including paclitaxel and others. A cure for upper aerodigestive tract squamous cancer with chemotherapy alone has not yet been described.

■ PALLIATIVE SURGERY

There is no evidence of improved survival by following the strategy of partially resecting the disease and then adding adjunctive chemotherapy and/or radiotherapy. However, there are certain clinical situations in which surgery can improve the quality of life without having treatment survival outcome as the primary motivation. There are times when a bleeding mass of a far-advanced head and neck cancer in the neck can be surgically resected and improve the patient's quality of life. A bleeding maxillary sinus cancer can be resected with a chance for relatively little morbidity. There are other times when neck disease progression threatens the carotid artery system. A patient would certainly benefit from surgical attention to a carotid artery with a sentinel bleed before this becomes an emergent situation. Therefore, there are clinical situations in which disease can be surgically approached with the goals primarily linked to quality-of-life priorities rather than survival.

■ PAIN MANAGEMENT

Patients who have head and neck cancer may suffer from acute and chronic pain. Acute pain is generally associated with surgical procedures. The standard therapeutic intervention involves the use of opioid agents. It is important to note that there is great variation among patients in the dose of opioids needed to control pain of similar intensity. Additionally, opioids have an almost all-or-none effect. Clearly, if a patient has excruciating pain, a certain dose of opioids is needed to control the pain. Below that dose, the patient will obtain little pain relief. If the patient receives a dose that is higher than the amount needed, side effects such as nausea, vomiting, sedation, and respiratory depression (at higher doses) will develop. Therefore, the therapeutic window for an opioid in a particular patient with a particular intensity of pain is narrow. The use of patient-controlled analgesia allows better titration of the opioid dose than does an as-needed analgesia order. The computerized pump allows the physician to set specific parameters, including analgesia dose per bolus; time allowed between boluses; maximum amount of opioid for a given time period; and also continuous infusion, if indicated.

Most patients who have advanced head and neck cancer will experience disease-related pain. This is especially problematic in patients whose tumors are deemed unresectable and with disease progression. Chronic pain is caused by the effect of the cancer on surrounding structures. This pain may have somatic, visceral, or neuropathic components. Mild to moderate pain can be effectively controlled by relaxation and imaging techniques in addition to the use of nonsteroidal anti-inflammatory drugs (NSAIDs). Moderate to severe pain is best treated with appropriate dose opioids. Pain caused by bone metastases or an inflammatory component will be helped by adding an NSAID to the opioid therapy. Patients who have neuropathic pain may benefit from the addition of amitriptyline, carbamazepine, or neurontin. Patients who have intractable pain may benefit from the use of a cervical epidural catheter (short-term or permanent). Some patients may need sedatives (benzodiazepines) or other agents (ketamine). Patients who have difficulties tolerating oral medications are given transdermal fentanyl patches. This method is easy to use, long acting (currently every 72 hours), and may be less constipating and sedating.

Patients suffering from advanced head and neck cancer will require analgesia at some point in their care. Otolaryngologists–head and neck surgeons should be familiar and comfortable with the various methods of pain control. In addition, physicians specializing in pain therapy should be enlisted to help with pain management if the treating physician is unable to provide adequate pain control.

■ GENERAL SUPPORTIVE MEASURES

The majority of patients who have far-advanced cancer have been exposed to the usual tobacco and alcohol risk factors for an extended time. It is common for them to have the usual comorbid conditions associated with these agents, such as chronic obstructive pulmonary disease, hypertension, coronary artery disease, and peripheral vascular disease. The senior age grouping also increases the chances of other health problems, such as diabetes mellitus. In addition, this patient population usually has a poor nutritional status and thus requires nutritional support. The involvement of an internist knowledgeable about the head and neck cancer patient population is an invaluable asset in helping to develop a strategy for management.

The nutritional impact is usually related to difficulty with oral ingestion due to the anorexia commonly associated with advanced-stage cancers. Therefore, enteral hyperalimentation programs are important to begin as soon as possible. It is unrealistic to have the luxury of time that permits a dramatic impact on the nutritional deficit before beginning treatment. Unfortunately, the progression of disease mandates instituting treatment before the time when enteral hyperalimentation can produce a measurable improvement. The route of administration depends on the patient's ability to swallow and his or her preference for nasogastric or percutaneous endoscopic gastrostomy (PEG) tubes for administration. The PEG tube route provides increased patient comfort and has the aesthetic benefit of being concealed by clothing.

There are a variety of other considerations that can have a positive impact on quality of life, such as physical therapy, occupational therapy, and prosthetic support. Psychosocial support for the patient, families, and friends also needs to be an integral part of any comprehensive rehabilitation program. Head and neck cancer support groups provide an avenue for psychosocial support.

■ EFFECT OF MANAGED CARE

It would be inappropriate for a contemporary discussion of the management of far-advanced head and neck cancers to not include a discussion about the potential impact on this patient population of managed care insurance programs. There is no question that the treatment of this patient population is personnel and technology intensive, which translates into high cost. It is realistic to recognize that heavy utilization in a capitated environment will at times be challenged. The costs will be weighed against potential for patient benefit. When those costs are subtracted from a defined pool of funds, there is the potential that economics will certainly play an increasing, if not disproportionately prominent, role in decision making. It is critically important for the physician to assume a vigorous role as patient advocate in this type of potentially charged environment where economics and ethics may be opposing forces. It will be increasingly important for the clinician to be able to objectively defend treatment strategies. Treatment recommendations will have to be defended based on published results or involvement in an organized clinical trial that is attempting to develop a database to resolve unanswered questions. It will be difficult to defend treatment strategies based on physician opinion and bias.

■ PATIENT COUNSELING

This is a difficult patient population for many reasons. One reason is that often the treatment is difficult and the likelihood of cure or long-term disease control is not high. These patients demand clinician involvement based on expertise and experience, including the full spectrum of knowledge about the disease as well as the nonsurgical and surgical treatment options. Often, no one treatment strategy is clearly superior to another. In such cases, the clinician needs to individualize recommendations based on the patient's disease as well as on numerous other variables, including the patient's psychosocial status. It is also imperative that the clinician minimize his or her personal bias so that the decision is clearly that of the patient. However, that requires the physician's willingness to be a supportive partner. If the physician does not feel capable of being that type of partner, it is reasonable to involve another physician. The patient should be the decision maker after the physician has thoroughly informed the patient of the alternatives. Physician and patient can then work as a team to achieve mutually identified treatment and outcome goals.

Suggested Reading

Forastiere AA, Neuberg D, Taylor SG IV, et al. Phase II evaluation of taxol in advanced head and neck cancer: An Eastern Cooperative Oncology Group trial. J NCI Monogr 1993; 15:181-184.

Fu KK. Combined modality therapy for head and neck cancer. Oncology (in press).

Haller JR, Mountain RE, Schuller DE, Nag S. Mortality and morbidity with intraoperative radiotherapy for head and neck cancer. Am J Otolaryngol 1996; 17:308-310.

Laramore GE, Scott CB, Al-Sarraf M, et al. Adjuvant chemotherapy for resectable squamous cell carcinomas of the head and neck: Report on intergroup study 0034. J Radiat Oncol Biol Phys 1992; 23:705-711.

Schuller DE, Grecula JG, Gahbauer RA, et al. Intensified regimen for advanced head and neck squamous cell carcinomas. Arch Otolaryngol Head Neck Surg 1997; 123:139-144.

Vokes EE, Weichselbaum RR. Chemoradiotherapy for head and neck cancer. PPO Updates 1993; 7(6):1-12.

MALNUTRITION FROM CANCER

The method of
Barry L. Wenig
by
John D. Goldenberg
Barry L. Wenig

Squamous cell cancers of the upper aerodigestive tract have a devastating effect on the nutritional status of the afflicted individual These patients are often first seen with locally advanced disease, resulting in significant dysphagia and weight loss. Furthermore, years of alcohol and tobacco abuse predispose them to a nutritionally compromised state. Definitive intervention by way of chemotherapy, radiotherapy, and/or surgery exacerbates swallowing dysfunction and further compromises the patient's ability to maintain oral nutrition. In fact, 50 percent to 60 percent of all newly diagnosed head and neck cancer patients manifest some signs and symptoms of malnutrition. The negative impact of malnutrition on healing is well known, and many head and neck surgeons report increased recurrence and mortality rates in those patients who have depleted nutritional reserves. It has now been conclusively shown that early and aggressive enteral nutrition is linked to decreased morbidity and mortality rates in cancer patients, as well as in patients undergoing major surgical procedures. It is incumbent upon the head and neck surgeon to promptly identify malnutrition, establish its severity, and institute corrective measures.

■ EVALUATION

The nutritional evaluation of the head and neck cancer patient begins with the first office visit. The presumptive diagnosis of cancer is often obvious, and is rapidly confirmed with biopsy or fine needle aspiration. A detailed history of alcohol and tobacco use is taken, as well as the determination of other medical conditions that would predispose to a nutritionally compromised state, such as diabetes, cirrhosis, cardiac disease, or dental caries. Typically, patients who have small lesions of the oral tongue or floor of the mouth have minimal weight loss on presentation, whereas comparable lesions of the oropharynx or hypopharynx result in greater degrees of dysphagia and weight loss. Laryngeal lesions most often involve the glottis, and malnutrition is not a prominent feature in these cases. Advanced lesions (T_3, T_4) of any site in the upper aerodigestive tract, however, result in significant cachexia and malnutrition.

Anthropometrics

We find that the use of body weight is an excellent means to establish the presence of malnutrition and to follow up the progress of somatic repletion. Patients are weighed at every outpatient appointment and weekly while they are inpatients. Patients are asked about their predisease weight, and their ideal body weight (IBW) is calculated:

IBW males =

106 lb for 5 feet + 6 lb per inch over 5 feet

IBW females =

100 lb for 5 feet + 5 lb per inch over 5 feet

The percent of ideal body weight is then determined.

W = current weight/IBW 100

A reduction of 20 percent below IBW or a 15 percent loss of weight from the predisease state is considered evidence of malnutrition. We do not routinely measure triceps skinfold or midarm circumference as a means of establishing protein depletion.

Laboratory Studies

The most useful of the serum evaluations during the initial workup of nutritional status is the measurement of serum albumin. This protein has a half-life of approximately 20 days, which makes it a useful predictor of chronic protein stores, but a poor measure of short-term protein depletion. A normal range is 3.5 to 5.0 g per deciliter, and mild visceral protein depletion is present with a level of 3.0 to 3.5 g per deciliter. Moderate compromise is present with serum values of 2.5 to 2.9 g per deciliter, and less than 2.5 g per deciliter indicates severe malnutrition.

Serum transferrin is another protein that reflects nutritional status, but it is more sensitive to change because it has a half-life of 8 to 10 days. Therefore, we use this as our measure of nutritional depletion. Transferrin levels are measured weekly on an inpatient basis, and then monthly after the patient is discharged, until the weight stabilizes. The normal value of transferrin is 200 mg per deciliter, with 150 to 200 mg per deciliter indicating mild depletion, 100 to 150 mg per deciliter moderate depletion, and less than 100 mg per deciliter indicating severe protein depletion. Prealbumin is even more sensitive to rapid changes in protein stores, with a half-life of 2 to 3 days, but it is not routinely used at our institution. A complete blood count (CBC) is measured periodically to assess for anemia as well as to calculate the total lymphocyte count (TLC):

TLC (cells per cubic millimeter) =

white blood cell count % lymphocytes/100

The total lymphocyte count is similar to albumin in its ability to assess for evidence of chronic malnutrition. With a normal value greater than 2,000 cells per cubic millimeter, 1,500 to 2,000 cells per cubic millimeter indicates mild malnutrition, 1,200 to 1,500 cells per millimeter indicates moderate malnutrition, and fewer than 1,200 cells per cubic millimeter indicates severe malnutrition. Finally, the calculation of nitrogen balance is an excellent assessment of the adequacy of nutritional supplementation and is performed during an inpatient admission.

Nitrogen balance (g per day) =

Protein intake/6.25 − urine urea nitrogen + 3

The protein intake is calculated from the amount of enteral and oral feeds per 24 hours, and the urine urea nitrogen is determined from a 24 hour urine collection. In the normal nondiseased state, the nitrogen balance should be zero. A goal of a positive nitrogen balance of 4 to 6 g per day is used to confirm the adequacy of enteral protein repletion. However, the nitrogen balance may not be valid in the presence of a large-volume fistula because this can lead to abnormally high nitrogen losses.

Immune Status

We do not routinely apply an anergy panel (antigens such as mumps, *Candida,* or tuberculin) to confirm immunologic integrity as a measure of nutritional status. However, this technique is used at many institutions and is a valid criterion for the diagnosis of malnutrition.

MANAGEMENT

Once the degree of malnutrition is determined, efforts are made to correct the factors that have contributed to the compromised state. Head and neck cancer patients often have a life-style that contributes to malnutrition. Patients are instructed to discontinue alcohol and tobacco use, and are encouraged to begin nutritional oral supplementation with Ensure. Dental caries are often evident, and early intervention with a dentist familiar with cancer treatment patients is instituted. Prescriptions for folate, a multivitamin, and vitamin B_{12} are given. The cancer itself has a cachectic effect on the patient, irrespective of site or degree of dysphagia. These patients experience anorexia, weight loss, early satiety, and muscle wasting secondary to an increased basal metabolic rate created by the metabolism of the tumor. Obviously, treatment of the underlying disease process will ameliorate these effects.

Percutaneous Endoscopic Gastrostomy

Percutaneous placement of a feeding tube into the stomach via an endoscopic approach was first described in the early 1980s and has gained widespread acceptance. We have been routinely using percutaneous endoscopic gastrostomy (PEG) tubes preoperatively for all patients undergoing definitive resection of advanced (stages III and IV) carcinomas of the oral cavity, oropharynx, and hypopharynx, as well as for selected other scenarios. With the increasing use of chemotherapy and radiotherapy protocols for patients who have advanced lesions, placement of a PEG is a prerequisite for initiating therapy. All endoscopic gastrostomy tubes are placed using intravenous sedation and local anesthesia by the gastrointestinal service in a specially designed suite. Alternatively, for those patients undergoing pretherapy panendoscopy and tracheotomy, a PEG is placed at the same time. The patients are monitored for 24 hours, instructed on the care of the tube and the process of enteral feeding, and discharged home. In our recent review, the complication rate associated with PEG placement in the head and neck cancer patient was 5 percent and included superficial cellulitis at the puncture site only. This was less than the complication rate associated with nasogastric (NG) tube placement in a matched cohort. Furthermore, the hospitalization for those patients receiving preoperative PEGs was significantly shorter than for those patients using NG tubes. Bulky, friable lesions of the oropharynx or supraglottis were initially believed to be relative contraindications to PEG placement, but we have subsequently found this not to be the case. The number of surgical, open gastrostomy or jejunostomy tubes placed in our cancer patients is now exceedingly low.

Enteral Therapy

The goal of enteral therapy is to maintain or increase the weight of the patient during therapy while improving objective measures of visceral protein stores. Maintenance of fluid balance is also ensured by the use of the gastrostomy tube for free water requirements. We use 25 to 35 kilocalories (kcal) per kilogram weight as an estimate of the total daily caloric requirement. This number is then confirmed by calculation of the resting energy expenditure by the dietary service. Additionally, the protein requirement is calculated at 2 grams of protein per kilogram per day. For most of the standard enteral preparations we use (Table 1), 85 percent of the required free water is provided by the food. Therefore, 15 percent of the total delivered volume must be supplemented by way of free water (i.e., 2,000 cc of formula would require an additional 300 cc H_2O over 24 hours). In the absence of fever or abdominal tenderness, gastrostomy tube feedings are initiated after 24 hours at a continuous rate of 25 cc per hour full strength. This is increased by 25 cc per hour every 8 hours until the goal rate is met, if there is no abdominal distention or cramping. After 24 hours at the goal rate, the patient is converted to bolus feeds broken up four times per day.

SWALLOWING DISORDERS AFTER TREATMENT OF HEAD AND NECK CANCER

Although the patient's life-style, tumor, and resultant dysphagia all contribute to malnutrition, the effect of therapy can often be more dramatic with respect to the rapidity of nutritional decline. Therefore, we not only analyze the patient's pretreatment nutritional status, but we also attempt to predict the resultant dysfunction of definitive intervention.

Radiotherapy

For patients undergoing radiotherapy, the resultant mucositis, xerostomia, dysgeusia, and potential for esophageal stricture all have a significant negative effect on nutritional status. Early treatment with pilocarpine, 5 mg by mouth twice a day, has been shown to have a beneficial effect on radiation-induced xerostomia, and all patients begin pilocarpine use before the onset of the dry mouth symptoms (i.e., during the first week of irradiation). Patients are also instructed to increase water intake, use artificial saliva, and are prescribed an oral analgesic composed of viscous 2 percent lidocaine, Cepacol, and Maalox (ratio of 1:1:1). The adverse effects of irradiation on the ability to maintain oral nutrition are promulgated by the concurrent use of chemotherapy, with the additional symptoms of nausea, vomiting, and diarrhea. Prochlorperazine, 10 mg by mouth four times per day, and more recently ondansetron, 8 mg by mouth three times per day, have been very effective in relieving the nausea and vomiting associated with chemotherapy and radiotherapy treatment protocols.

Surgery of the Oral Cavity

Surgical resection of less than 50 percent of the oral tongue with primary closure or a wide local excision of a small floor of the mouth lesion with granulation results in transient dysarthria and dysphagia, and requires no long-term nutritional supplementation. However, resection of greater than 50 percent of the oral tongue with a portion of the floor of the mouth does require preoperative enteral access via a PEG secondary to increased risk of dysphagia and aspiration.

Table 1. Enteral Preparations Commonly Used at the University of Illinois, Department of Otolaryngology—Head and Neck Surgery

PRODUCT	KCAL/CC	OSMOL	PROTEIN	FAT	CHO	Na^+	K^+	NOTES
Ensure	1.06	470	37	37	145	798	38	Standard 1 kcal/cc, tube or oral
Ensure Plus	1.5	690	55	53	200	761	36	High calorie and protein
Resource	1.06	450	37	37	145	802	38	Standard 1 kcal/cc, tube or oral
Osmolite	1.06	300	37	38	145	599	24	Tube feed only
Osmolite HN	1.06	300	44	37	141	877	38	—
Jevity	1.1	310	44	37	152	877	38	Fiber containing
Sustacal	1.0	620	61	23	140	926	52	High protein

kcal, kilocalories; Osmol, osmolarity (mOsmol/kg H_2O); CHO, carbohydrate (g/l); Na+, sodium (mg/1,000 kcal); K+, potassium (mEq/1,000 kcal).

Recovery from this procedure is significantly delayed by the placement of a bulky, adynamic, pectoralis major myocutaneous flap for reconstruction, and our current approach to these defects is a sensate microvascular radial forearm free graft. Anterior mandibulectomy, if required, is rehabilitated with a fibula osseocutaneous free flap because of established functional benefits over placement of a reconstruction plate and axial soft-tissue flap. Tongue flaps are almost never used because of their tethering effects and disruption of the oral phase of swallowing.

Surgery of the Oropharynx

In general, resection of lesions of the base of the tongue, tonsil, and retromolar trigone region dramatically impairs swallowing. The faucial arches are the trigger zone for reflexive swallowing and the cornerstone of the pharyngeal phase of swallowing. Small (T_1) lesions, which are treated by a wide local excision or tonsillectomy, do not disrupt the tonsillar pillars, and are managed with an intraoperative nasogastric tube and early postoperative swallowing. All other lesions, including resections involving the mandible (composite), are managed with preoperative PEG placement and gradual swallowing rehabilitation with the speech pathology service. These defects often require reconstruction with an axial flap, further worsening the dysphagia secondary to pooling of secretions at the adynamic, epithelialized portion. Lateral mandibulectomy defects are not reconstructed with vascularized bone flaps, because functional improvement is found when compared to the traditional methods of reconstruction plating and soft-tissue coverage with a pectoralis flap or no reconstruction at all. Total glossectomy requires a total laryngectomy to manage the aspiration problem; however, this is rarely done as a primary treatment modality with the advent of nonsurgical, multimodality treatment options.

Surgery of the Hypopharynx

Surgery of the piriform sinus, exclusive of the larynx, is rare and isolated to small lesions of the lateral wall. Although limited in size and scope, these resections result in significant dysphagia and aspiration secondary to pooling of secretions at this level. Percutaneous gastrostomy tube placement is important in this scenario. It is more common that extensive lesions of the hypopharynx require a total laryngectomy and partial or complete pharyngectomy. In our department, complete pharyngectomy defects are reconstructed with a jejunal free flap in the vast majority of patients. Rarely, a gastric pull-up will be used if a total esophagectomy is required, or if the jejunum is not accessible. Mild dysphagia is common after a jejunal free flap secondary to poor peristalsis. However, the majority of patients will be able to maintain their weight via an oral route. Stenosis of an anastomosis may be a postoperative sequela in approximately 10 percent of patients.

Surgery of the Larynx

Small lesions (T_1 and some T_2) of the larynx are treated with primary radiotherapy and result in little swallowing dysfunction. A hemilaryngectomy is used for unilateral T_2 lesions or for the salvage of radiotherapy failures. These patients have a stent placed for 1 week and are fed via nasogastric tube. After stent removal, approximately 80 percent of patients recover swallowing in a few days through the aid of a speech pathologist, and they experience minimal dysphagia and aspiration. However, the remaining 20 percent may experience up to 6 months of aspiration during the pharyngeal phase of swallowing, and will require placement of a PEG postoperatively. Supraglottic laryngectomy results in a greater degree of dysphagia than a vertical hemilaryngectomy, which is secondary to the loss of sensation in the distribution of the superior laryngeal nerve and the loss of two of the three protective mechanisms of the airway (epiglottis-aryepiglottic folds and false vocal folds).

Extension of the procedure to involve the base of the tongue or an arytenoid greatly increases the degree of swallowing dysfunction. We have found that a cricopharyngeal myotomy is a useful adjuvant to decrease postoperative aspiration. Careful selection of patients who have adequate pulmonary reserve is vital for the success of this operation, and strong consideration to preoperative PEG placement should be given. For patients who have advanced laryngeal carcinoma, one of three treatment protocols is used. Patients undergoing therapy with chemotherapy and radiotherapy all have a pretreatment PEG placed for aggressive enteral nutrition. Selective patients undergoing a near-total laryngectomy such as a Pearson procedure or a supracricoid laryngectomy require semipermanent enteral access because of the potential for severe aspiration. For patients undergoing total laryngectomy, nutritional management consists of preoperative oral supplements, intraoperative placement of a nasogastric tube, and total enteral supplementation for 7 to 10 days. The longer interval is used for those patients who have had previous irradiation. The NG tube is removed provided there is no evidence of pharyngocutaneous fistula, and the patient resumes oral feeding with a nutritional supplement. A small percentage of total laryngectomy patients will develop a pharyngeal stenosis as a result of surgery and radiotherapy, and they are treated with serial dilation and continued oral feeding.

Suggested Reading

Conley J. Swallowing dysfunction associated with radical surgery of the head and neck. Arch Surg 1960; 80:602.

Gibson S, Wenig BL. Percutaneous endoscopic gastrostomy in the management of head and neck carcinoma. Laryngoscope 1992; 102:977-980.

Moore FA, Feliciano DV, Andrassy RJ, et al. Early enteral feeding, compared with parenteral, reduces postoperative septic complications: The results of a meta-analysis. Ann Surg 1992; 216:172-183.

Portugal LG, Wenig BL. Dysphagia after radical operations on the head and neck. In: Surgery of the esophagus, stomach, and small intestine. Boston: Little, Brown, 1995.

MANDIBULAR DEFECT

The method of
Neal D. Futran

Modern head and neck oncologic surgery is characterized by an emphasis on reconstruction and rehabilitation. Nowhere is this more apparent than when attempting to reestablish the oromandibular complex.

The mandible provides structural support for the mouth and lips, an essential element in lower facial structure and cosmetic appearance. It supports the tongue and floor of mouth musculature, permitting mastication, speech, deglutition, and saliva control.

Ideally, all mandibular defects should be reconstructed to preserve or restore lower facial contour, maintain mobility of the tongue, provide a denture-bearing surface, maintain or recreate occlusal relationships, and promote oral continence. The oral cavity is unique among sites in the head and neck in that several factors come into play when considering which techniques will be used to achieve these goals.

■ PREOPERATIVE DECISION MAKING

Mandibular involvement by carcinoma is primarily a clinical diagnosis and is likely when physical examination reveals complete fixation of the tumor to the mandible. Radiographic studies, particularly computed tomographic (CT) images of the mandible and a panorex radiograph, also aid in the assessment of the mandibular bone invasion. Magnetic resonance imaging (MRI) appears to be superior to CT for imaging the soft tissues of the oral cavity, but this is not necessarily used on a routine basis to determine bony invasion.

Once the decision is made that a segmental portion of the mandible must be resected, the choice of reconstruction depends on several factors. Patient age, associated medical problems, diet, performance status, individual motivation, and family dynamics all must be considered.

The extent of disease dictates the surgical resection. Anatomic variables to be considered for reconstruction are (1) location (anterior versus lateral) of the mandibular defect; (2) length of the mandibular defect; (3) size, location, and bulk of associated soft-tissue defects; (4) whether external skin is involved; and (5) concomitant loss of adjacent nerves, muscles, and vascular tissues.

In addition, the problem of salivary contamination must be addressed in almost every case, particularly when the patient has undergone previous radiotherapy or if this modality will follow surgical treatment. In the former case, the use of vascularized, nonirradiated tissue to reconstruct the defect promotes healing and decreases the rate of orocutaneous fistula formation. These same reconstructive techniques in the latter instance allow rapid wound healing, thus reducing the risk of delay in starting postoperative radiotherapy.

■ OPERATIVE DECISION MAKING

Controversy still exists concerning whether all mandibular defects require reconstruction (Fig. 1). Resection of the anterior mandibular arch produces the "Andy Gump" deformity, a debilitating functional and aesthetic problem. Oral competence suffers from the patient's inability to manage oral secretions, speak, eat, or swallow. This is, therefore, the most important mandibular defect to reconstruct primarily. The need for bone, intraoral soft tissue, and external skin coverage must be assessed carefully, with attention paid to the relative amounts of each tissue required. Reconstruction of this defect with an immediate microvascular, bone-containing free flap is the optimal method for achieving the best result. Additional absolute indications for this type of reconstruction include through-and-through mandibular defects requiring reconstruction of mucosa, bone, and external skin; failure of previous attempts at mandibular reconstruction; and severe osteoradionecrosis of the mandible.

When the posterior body, angle, or ascending ramus of the mandible is removed, the defect can be dealt with in a variety of ways, with equal restoration of form and function. Free flaps have no demonstrable superiority in the reconstruction of these defects. In fact, not all of these patients need to undergo reconstruction. Simple collapse of the segments often allows closure of the soft-tissue defect primarily. Although facial contour is slightly disturbed by shift of the anterior mandible to the affected side, these patients maintain adequate speech and swallowing. This technique is especially suited for the medically compromised patient and will minimize operative time. It may also be applicable to edentulous patients on soft diets preoperatively who do not expect prosthetic rehabilitation.

Intraoral tissue concerns are a higher priority for the aforementioned defects than immediate restoration of the mandibular bony continuity. The use of reconstruction plates in conjunction with soft-tissue free flaps or pedicled flaps allows an expedient method to obtain an excellent cosmetic and functional result with minimal donor site disability. This technique is best for lateral and posterior low-volume defects in the debilitated or elderly, and in those patients who have a poor prognosis. This method is no panacea. Reconstructive failure usually requires revision with a vascularized bone graft. Complications include fistulas, late plate extrusions, and plate fracture. Plate removals are significantly more frequent for reconstructions in irradiated fields. With proper selection of patients, however, this will rarely be necessary.

Restoration of coexistent temporomandibular joint (TMJ) and mandibular defects is challenging. Ideally, the TMJ joint is necessary for full mandibular range of motion. Realistically, immediate restoration of the articulation between the mandible and the glenoid fossa may not significantly contribute to cosmetic or functional improvement following radical ablative surgery.

Several approaches are available for synchronous reconstruction of the TMJ and other associated mandibular defects. Initially, intermaxillary fixation is applied to pre-

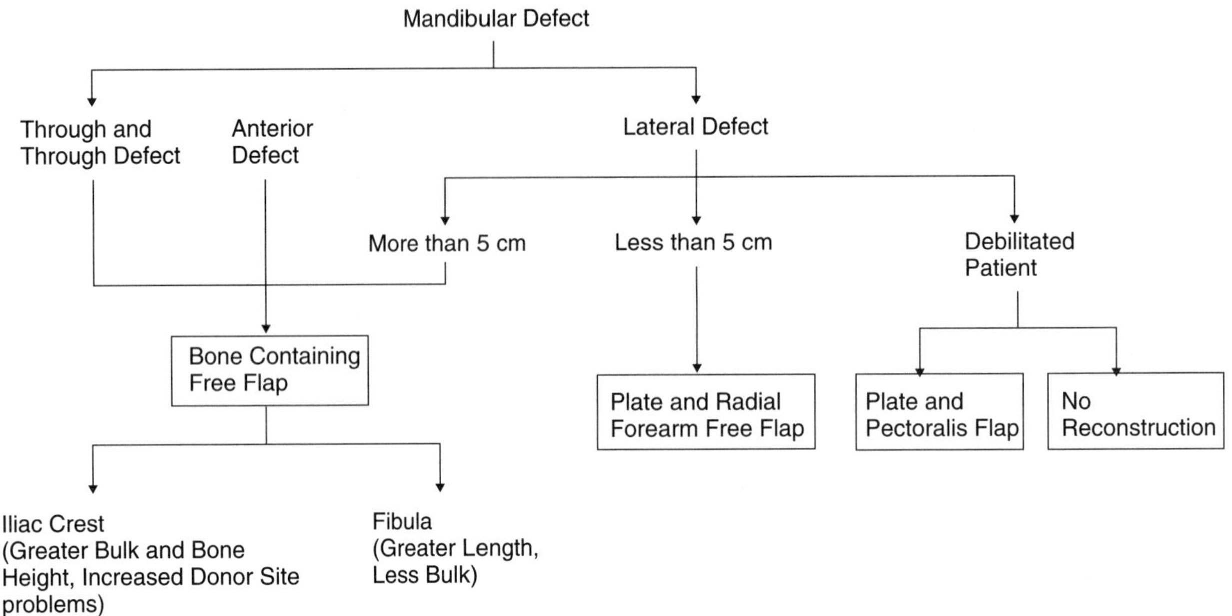

Figure 1.
Algorithm for the management of mandibular defects.

existing dentition to maintain occlusion. The use of reconstruction plates with a condylar head allows for a unilateral reconstruction in conjunction with skeletal fixation of a vascularized bone graft to residual mandible, or the resected condyle may be autotransplanted and fixated to the graft. Soft-tissue arthroplasty using temporalis tissue or other tissue during bone transfer has facilitated TMJ reconstruction, particularly in older patients. In younger patients, and especially children, costochondral grafts can be used along with the vascularized bone technique to maintain the vertical position of the mandibular ramus and allow for further growth. Any method used must recognize and address the risk to the facial nerve, both during the procedure and with subsequent mandibular function.

■ FLAP SELECTION AND TECHNIQUE

Although a variety of osseocutaneous free flaps have been described to reconstruct the mandible, the fibula and iliac crest are clearly preferred. Both flaps allow for two teams (extirpative and reconstructive) to operate simultaneously, which results in decreased operative time. Both flaps will support osseointegrated dental implants in all patients.

Free Fibula Flap

The free fibula flap is based on the peroneal vessels and provides the greatest length of bone. Up to 25 cm of bone is available to reconstruct a defect of any length. Its segmental periosteal blood supply safely permits multiple osteotomies so as to properly contour the mandibular reconstruction. Because it is primarily cortical bone, miter joints must be created to maintain bone-to-bone contact and promote primary healing. The skin paddle is reliably harvested when including a cuff of soleus muscle and is sufficient for many soft-tissue defects; however, the arc of rotation is limited due to the short, small caliber perforating cutaneous vessels. Sensate potential is achieved by incorporation of the lateral sural cutaneous nerve during flap harvest. In order to prevent vascular compromise to the donor leg and flap, preoperative noninvasive color flow Doppler ultrasonography provides reliable assessment of the lower extremity vasculature and can identify cutaneous perforating vessels to aid in flap design and harvest. The donor site can be closed primarily in most instances, and there is limited donor site morbidity. Postoperatively, the patient is placed in a lower leg splint for 4 days and then allowed to ambulate without restriction.

Iliac Crest Free Flap

The iliac crest free flap is based on the deep circumflex iliac vessels and provides an excellent stock of bone that is more "pliable" than the fibula in that it has a greater cancellous component. An average height of iliac bone as compared to the fibula (2.5 cm:1 cm) allows a more physiologic reconstruction of the anterior and anterolateral mandible in the dentate patient. Further, when the reconstructed segment and residual mandible are equal in height, less disruptive stresses are placed on the intraoral tissues and osseointegrated dental implants so as to simplify prosthetic rehabilitation. In addition, the iliac crest flap is usually harvested with a skin paddle and/or an internal oblique muscular paddle. The combined osseomusculocutaneous flap is excellent for through-and-through mandibular defects where the muscle reconstructs the mucosal defect and the skin paddle fills the cutaneous defect.

The primary disadvantages of the iliac crest flap are its inherent bulk and donor site morbidity. Even in the thinnest patient, secondary soft-tissue contouring is necessary to provide optimal intraoral soft-tissue contour and external cosmesis. The donor site must be closed meticulously to prevent the development of hernia or abdominal weakness. Additionally, significant gait disturbance is universally present for 3 to 4 weeks postoperatively and requires aggressive physical therapy.

Scapular Osseocutaneous Flap

The scapular osseocutaneous flap, based on the deep circumflex subscapular vessels, is the third choice in bony reconstruction of the mandible. Its major limitations are the inability to simultaneously harvest this flap while resecting the tumor, and relatively limited supply of bone when compared with the iliac crest or fibula. Its one major advantage is the ability to move the soft-tissue component of the flap along a wide arc of rotation independent of the bony segment without compromising flap viability. This can be advantageous in cases of small bony defects and complicated soft-tissue defects.

Radial Forearm Free Flap

Bony continuity, however, as mentioned previously, does not need to be re-established in every case. If the mandibular defect is near the angle, not tooth-bearing, and less than 5 cm, the soft-tissue reconstructive requirements far outweigh the bony requirements. In this setting, the radial forearm free flap is frequently used. It is thin, pliable, and has the potential to become sensate by incorporating the medial or lateral antebrachial cutaneous nerve. The flap is easily harvested, and donor site morbidity is minimal except for an unsightly scar. This flap is particularly well suited to reconstruct the tonsillar fossa, palatal defects, and those defects involving tongue tissue. I rarely incorporate radial bone with this flap because it possesses poor length and vertical height, risks debilitating radial bone fracture, and at least 6 weeks of donor site immobilization is required. The pectoralis major myocutaneous flap is readily available, reliable, and decreases operative time. However, it is nonsensate, bulky, and the effect of gravity is likely to increase the rate of wound dehiscence and plate exposure, especially in the irradiated patient. I have found that the incidence of plate exposure using the radial forearm free flap is negligible and is greatly preferred over pedicled tissue transfers if the medical condition of the patient permits its use.

Simultaneous double free flaps have been advocated by some authors to reconstruct extensive mandibular defects. In my experience, the need for two free flaps is a rare event, and virtually all defects can be restored with a single flap. The increased operative time, additional donor site morbidity, and potential for complications do not justify this approach. Moreover, there are no studies to support improved function and cosmesis of dual free flaps when compared with using a single flap.

Technical Considerations

When primarily reconstructing the mandible at the time of tumor extirpation, bony stabilization can be achieved before initial resection. In those cases in which the neoplasm has not penetrated through the buccal cortex of the mandible, a reconstruction plate may be adapted to the mandible before resection of the tumor. In most cases, a sufficient proximal condylar segment may be preserved without compromising the oncologic extirpation. A titanium hollow osseointegrated reconstruction plate is preferred because it is more rigid and has the potential for osseointegration of its screws. In addition, the use of the inner expansion screw within the osseointegrated screw head allows the applied plate to be anchored to the screw rather than being compressed to the underlying mandible. Theoretically, pressure necrosis of the underlying bone is reduced, thereby avoiding plate failure. At least three holes are drilled on either side of the anticipated defect. Screws are placed, and then the plate and screws are removed. An operative map greatly aids in the orientation and replacement of the plate and screws after tumor resection. Early fixation maintains essentially perfect contours. Tumor resection and recipient vessel identification then ensue. The surgical specimen is available as a visual reference for graft shaping as well as serving as a template for graft size and length. The plate is then reapplied to the mandible. Final harvest of the free tissue transfer is completed, and initial osteotomies are made to provide accurate contour of the neomandible and maximize bone-to-bone contact. Only the periosteum overlying the osteotomy should be elevated so as not to jeopardize the blood supply to the bony segments. The bone is then rigidly fixated in place. Although this is my preferred method, some cases dictate the use of miniplates to fixate the graft to the native mandible. A watertight, tension-free mucosal closure, especially in the floor of the mouth and gingivobuccal sulcus, is critical in preventing postoperative plate exposure and fistulas.

Microvascular anastomoses are then performed, and the transplanted tissues are assessed for viability. The advantages of primarily insetting the flap are the ability to work in a bloodless field, accurate creation of vascular pedicle geometry, and reduced risk of disruption of the vessel anastomoses. These composite flaps easily tolerate at least 4 hours of warm ischemia time.

Once the composite graft is revascularized, primary placement of osseointegrated implants allows more rapid dental rehabilitation They provide the most rigid form of stabilization to withstand the forces of mastication. In situations in which soft-tissue reconstruction or the height of the alveolar ridge is not sufficient for a tissue-borne denture, implants offer the most suitable alternative to restore masticatory and occlusal function. Four to 6 months after surgery, when the integration process has occurred and postoperative radiotherapy has been completed, the implants are unroofed, loaded, and ready for prosthetic placement. Primary implantation facilitates early dental rehabilitation and restoration of function.

When the neoplasm extends anteriorly through the mandibular buccal cortex and into the soft tissues, contouring the reconstruction plate to maintain ideal mandibular form is impossible before resecting the tumor. In order to maintain proper position of the condyles in the glenoid fossa, external fixation devices such as the Joe-Hall-Morris or Anderson biphasic splint may be applied. Alternatively, a universal reconstruction plate may be used to achieve the same result. Adequacy of anterior mandibular projection is determined by the surgeon's judgment as bone grafts are placed in relation to the anterior maxillary arch.

Success of free tissue transfer reconstruction relies on precise surgical technique, careful postoperative monitoring, and early integration of allied health personnel (particularly nursing staff and the speech-swallowing therapist) in the overall management of the patient. I have achieved a 99 percent rate of flap viability in more than 200 transfers, one-third of which were to reconstruct the mandible. Efforts must be increased, however, to optimize the functional success of these patients.

■ PRIMARY VERSUS SECONDARY RECONSTRUCTION

Whenever possible, immediate single-stage reconstruction is preferred over delayed reconstruction when the former can be achieved with acceptable success rates and low morbidity. This is especially important for patients who have advanced neoplasms, for whom prognosis is poor, and for whom early palliation is crucial to maintain quality of life over their limited life expectancy. Immediate restoration of the mandible prevents the development of muscle contracture and restores mandibular form with a template and surgical specimen as guides. It is also not in the patient's best interest to live with a devastating aesthetic and functional deformity after tumor extirpation without reconstruction, and also be subjected to two long operative procedures instead of one. Many patients who undergo delayed reconstruction will have had radiotherapy immediately after extirpative surgery. The resultant decreased tissue vascularity and fibrosis mandates the need for vascularized tissue transfer to achieve reconstructive goals.

The presence of scar contracture after tumor extirpation causes malalignment of the remaining mandibular segments if not initially maintained by a reconstruction plate or external fixation device. The proximal condylar segment is pulled upward and medially, and the distal segment shifts toward the side of the defect, distorting occlusion. Realignment and precise reconstruction of the defect become a more formidable task in this setting. As a result, graft shaping in secondary reconstruction is a mystery at best. Additionally, soft-tissue reconstruction becomes more challenging because the recipient tissues are fibrotic and have poor vascularity. Although restoration of mandibular continuity can be achieved, the sequential approach to reconstruction creates an inevitable delay in functional dental rehabilitation.

Reconstructive challenges are similar to those in delayed reconstruction when repairing oromandibular defects created by salvage surgery. Frequently, these patients have extensive scarring from previous procedures and/or are undergoing radiotherapy, which reduces the host tissue's ability to support alloplastic materials. Free vascularized tissue transfer is almost always necessary in this group of patients if definitive reconstruction is to be achieved.

■ MANAGED CARE CONSIDERATIONS

State-of-the-art oromandibular reconstruction incurs great costs in both the operative and rehabilitative phases. Clearly, the cost of procedures involving two teams of surgeons and increased operative time when using free tissue transfers is greater than procedures that use plate and/or pedicle flap techniques. Recent studies, however, reveal that overall hospital cost is greater in the latter group due to increased rate of postoperative complications, longer hospitalization, and increased need for home-based services.

In those patients for whom one goal is to achieve functional dental prosthetic rehabilitation, planning with the insurance carriers must be initiated before tumor treatment to ensure financial coverage. Most medical insurance carriers will not cover costs of the prosthetic restoration without a concerted lobbying effort by the reconstructive surgeon, oral surgeon, and prosthodontist at the time of initial treatment planning. It must be emphasized that the dental implants and/or prosthesis are an integral part of cancer care and a functional component of the patient's daily existence.

It is unclear at this time how managed care will influence the resources allocated to those patients who usually have advanced disease and marginal or poor prognoses. To what extent various parameters of the original disease, magnitude of resection, and properties of the reconstruction contribute to function in different anatomic circumstances is also not resolved in the current literature. Progressive functional assessment will benefit individual patients, enhance general quality of care, and critique reconstructive techniques. This approach may also isolate those key surgical properties underlying procedures for oral cavity reconstruction so that clear guiding principles for optimal results may be developed over time and justify the allocation of increasingly limited health care dollars to these reconstructive pursuits.

■ DISCUSSION

Oromandibular reconstruction continues to be one of the most challenging areas of head and neck reconstruction. Efforts to restore function and cosmesis impact patient speech, swallowing, nutrition, self-esteem, and quality of life. Advances in free tissue transfer offer optimum reconstruction of both primary and secondary defects in most patients. Primary restoration of the oromandibular complex offers the distinct advantage of recreating oral anatomy so that the patient is not forced to live with deformity. It is done in one operation, so additional hospitalizations are unnecessary. Multiple donor sites are available to choose the optimal flap for the soft-tissue and bony defects.

Each patient and the defect to be reconstructed must be evaluated and treated individually. The surgeon must use those techniques that best suit his or her abilities in order that reconstructive goals be achieved in a timely, efficient manner. Morbidity and patient hospitalization must be minimized to meet the demands of economic medicine while trying to restore the patient to a postoperative condition that more closely approximates the predisease state.

Suggested Reading

Hidalgo DA. Fibula free flap mandibular reconstruction. Clin Plast Surg 1994.

Klotch DW, Gump J, Kuhn L. Reconstruction of mandibular defects in irradiated patients. Am J Surg 1990; 160:396-398.

Sullivan M, et al. Free scapular osteocutaneous flap for mandibular reconstruction. Arch Otolaryngol Head Neck Surg 1986; 115:1334.

Urken ML, Weinberg H, Vickery C, Buchbinder D, Lawson W, Biller HF. The internal oblique-iliac crest free flap in composite defects of the oral cavity involving bone, skin, and mucosa. Laryngoscope 1991; 101:257.

REFRACTORY POSTERIOR EPISTAXIS

The method of
Fredrick A. Kuhn
by
Martin J. Citardi
Fredrick A. Kuhn

Epistaxis ranks among the most common of otolaryngologic emergencies. Despite its high prevalence, the management of epistaxis—especially profuse, posterior epistaxis—remains controversial. Today, the nasal telescope essentially permits total visualization of the intranasal cavity anatomy and affords the option of direct, minimally invasive epistaxis treatment.

■ ANATOMY

Each side of the nose receives dual blood supply from both internal and external carotid systems. The major blood supply is from the sphenopalatine artery (SPA), which is a terminal branch of the internal maxillary artery (IMA)— a direct branch of the external carotid artery. In addition, the anterior and posterior ethmoidal arteries, which are branches of the ophthalmic artery from the internal carotid artery, also contribute significantly to nasal blood flow (Fig. 1).

The sphenopalatine artery is one of the terminal branches of the IMA (Fig. 2). The SPA branches from the IMA in the pterygomaxillary fossa and enters the nose through the sphenopalatine formen, which is located on the lateral nasal wall, where the inferior portion of the middle turbinate basal lamella meets the medial orbital wall. After entering the nose, the SPA divides into the lateral nasal artery, which supplies the lateral nasal wall, and the posterior septal nasal artery, which supplies the corresponding portion of the septum.

After leaving the ophthalmic artery, the anterior and posterior ethmoidal arteries enter the superior nasal cavity through the anterior and posterior ethmoidal foramina, respectively (Fig. 1). The anterior ethmoidal artery is the major blood supply for the anterior third of both the lateral nasal wall and the septum. The posterior ethmoidal artery, which may be absent, supplies a small area on the superior concha and adjacent septum.

The labial artery, a branch of the facial or external maxillary artery, also sends twigs to the nasal vestibule. In addition, branches of the greater palatine arteries pass through the incisive foramen to supply the inferior anterior septum.

The network of vessels that is found in Little's area on the anterior septum is known as Kiesselbach's plexus. It has a rich blood supply from the anterior ethmoidal artery and the SPA. The naso-nasopharyngeal plexus, also known as Woodruff's plexus, is located at the posterior 1 cm of the nasal floor, inferior meatus, inferior turbinate, and middle meatus. This plexus also extends to the vertcal strip of mucosa anterior to the eustachian tube cartilage and the mucosa lateral and superior to the posterior choana covering the adjacent sphenoid rostrum.

■ CLASSIFICATION OF EPISTAXIS

Anterior epistaxis refers to bleeding from Little's area on the nasal septum. This type of epistaxis also may originate from the anterior lateral nasal wall, although this is much less common. From a practical standpoint, epistaxis that is controlled by anterior nasal packing is considered to be anterior epistaxis.

Posterior epistaxis occurs in the area of Woodruff's plexus. Any episode of epistaxis that fails routine anterior nasal packing may be operationally defined as posterior epistaxis.

Refractory posterior epistaxis is defined as continued hemorrhage that occurs with anteroposterior nasal packing in place or shortly after its removal.

■ POSTERIOR NASAL PACKING

The initial management of posterior epistaxis traditionally has involved the placement of an anteroposterior (AP) nasal pack. The details of this procedure are well described in various textbooks of otorhinolaryngology. Failure rates of nearly 20 percent to more than 25 percent have been reported.

Although this is a rather routine procedure, posterior nasal packing carries significant morbidity and mortality. Fairbanks divided the potential complications of posterior packs into those related to pack insertion (such as hypovolemic shock, nasal-vagal reflexes, topical anesthetic and vasoconstrictor reactions, and technical packing issues) and those related to maintaining the pack (such as hypoxia, hypoventilation, respiratory obstruction, local infection, bacteremia, toxic shock syndrome, and inadequate oral intake and/or malnutrition). Wang and Vogel published a retrospective review that noted a rate of major complications (i.e., hypoxia, sepsis, respiratory obstruction, cardiac arrhythmia and/or ischemia, aspiration pneumonia, transfusion reaction) of 19.7 percent among 31 patients who received posterior packs. These researchers also reported that the rate of minor complications (i.e., nasal necrosis, synechiae, sinusitis, incorrect pack placement, hemotympanum, hypesthesia, oroantral fistula) was 49.1 percent in their patient sample.

The respiratory morbidity from AP packs was commonly ascribed to a poorly defined "nasopulmonary reflex"; however, physiologic studies demonstrate no significant changes in lung volumes, flow, and alveolar gas exchange due to posterior packs. The pulmonary compromise in patients who have AP packs can probably be ascribed to pre-existing lung diseases, aspiration, and sedation. In addition, posterior packs may precipitate signs of obstructive sleep apnea, as indicated by an increased apnea index on polysomnography.

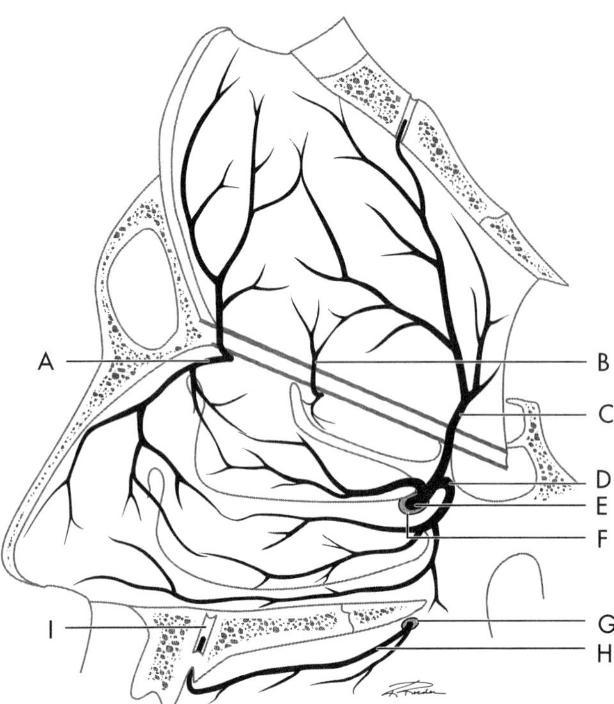

Figure 1.
Nasal blood supply. Major nasal blood vessels and their relative positions are depicted. Note that the nasal septum has been reflected superiorly. *A,* Anterior ethmoidal artery; *B,* Posterior ethmoidal artery; *C,* Posterior septal nasal artery; *D,* Lateral nasal artery; *E,* Sphenopalatine artery; *F,* Sphenopalatine foramen; *G,* Greater palatine foramen; *H,* Greater palatine artery; *I,* Incisive canal.

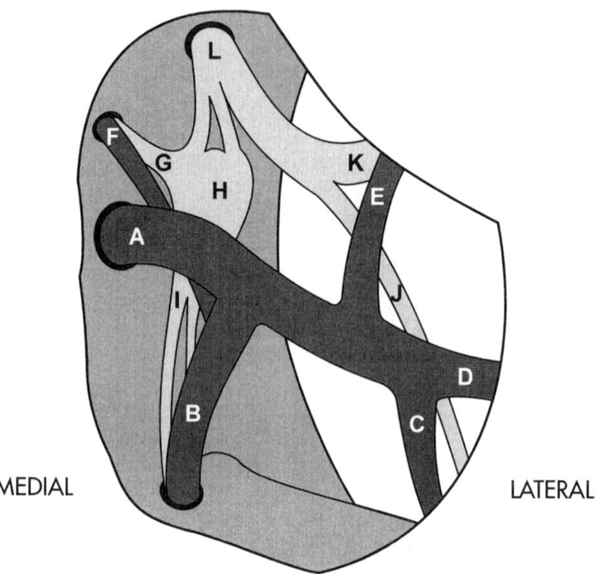

Figure 2.
Transantral view of the pterygomaxillary space. *A,* Sphenopalatine artery; *B,* Descending palatine artery; *C,* Superior alveolar artery; *D,* Internal maxillary artery; *E,* Infraorbital artery; *F,* Vidian artery; *G,* Vidian nerve; *H,* Sphenopalatine ganglion; *I,* Descending palatine nerve; *J,* Superior alveolar nerve; *K,* Infraorbital nerve; *L,* Maxillary nerve.

■ THERAPEUTIC INTERVENTIONS

Internal Maxillary Artery Ligation

The transantral approach to internal maxillary artery ligation is relatively straightforward. Preoperative radiographs should be obtained to ensure that the maxillary sinus is aerated. Under general anesthesia, a Caldwell-Luc maxillary antrotomy is performed. The soft tissues of the upper lip and face are retracted with a McCabe retractor or similar device. The remainder of the procedure is performed through the operating microscope (with a 300 mm focal length objective lens). The posterior maxillary sinus wall is identified, and a laterally based mucosal flap is made. The posterior bony sinus wall is removed, and the periosteum is opened via cruciate incision. The contents of the pterygomaxillary fossa are then carefully explored. Using a variety of blunt hooks, the IMA and its major branches are carefully dissected free of the fibrofatty tissue in this area. The neural structures are deep to the vessels and should not be disturbed. Vascular clips are then applied to the IMA as well as the SPA and the descending palatine artery (to prevent collateral flow). The mucosal flap is then replaced, and the Caldwell-Luc incision is closed in the usual fashion.

Transantral IMA ligation has many advantages. Overall, the procedure has a high success rate for an intractable problem, probably because the ligation occurs close to the bleeding point. The Caldwell-Luc approach and operating microscope are well known to all otolaryngologists who are comfortable with the procedure. Proponents of transantral IMA ligation also purport that this technique has minimal morbidity.

The complications of transantral IMA ligation are well recognized. The procedure carries all the morbidity associated with Caldwell-Luc antrotomies. Facial numbness, antral fistula, postoperative pain, cranial nerve palsies, and blindness are all potential sequelae. Ipsilateral total ophthalmoplegia due to transantral IMA ligation has also been described.

Transantral IMA ligation is widely reported in the literature, which reflects its acceptance in the field of otolaryngology. One review by Schaitkin and co-workers reported a failure rate of only 14 percent, and success rates of 90 percent are possible. Of note, Metson and Lane noted that half of all failures in their review were due to obvious technical errors in the procedure.

Anterior Ethmoidal Artery Ligation

Anterior ethmoidal artery ligation has a special role in the management of severe epistaxis. In the situation of refractory epistaxis after nasal fracture, laceration of the anterior ethmoidal artery is likely, and anterior ethmoidal artery ligation specifically targets this problem. Furthermore, this procedure is an important adjunct to procedures directed at the IMA or SPA. Singh noted that among 15 posterior epistaxis patients treated with IMA ligation alone, three patients rebled (failure rate of 20 percent), but that among 14 similar patients treated with IMA ligation and anterior ethmoidal artery ligation, no rebleeding occurred. If the blood flow from the anterior ethmoidal artery is not interrupted, it may rapidly reconstitute the entire nasal blood supply, even after IMA ligation.

The approach to the anterior ethmoidal artery is through a standard Lynch incision. The anterior ethmoidal foramen, through which the artery passes, is located at or just above the frontoethmoidal suture of the medial orbit, approximately 15 mm posterior to the maxillolacrimal suture. After the artery is identified, it may be secured with a hemoclip, or coagulated with the bipolar cautery.

Potential complications of this procedure include the sequelae of the Lynch approach (i.e., facial scarring, intraorbital or intracranial injury). Except in the situation of epistaxis after nasal fracture, anterior ethmoidal artery ligation should only be employed with procedures directed at the IMA and/or SPA.

Posterior ethmoidal artery ligation is not routinely recommended. Because the optic nerve is only 3 to 5 mm posterior to the posterior ethmoidal artery, inadvertent blindness is possible during this procedure (which is completed via a Lynch incision). In addition, this artery may be absent in many patients. Also, clinical experience indicates that therapy directed to the posterior ethmoidal artery is not necessary, because procedures aimed at only the IMA and/or SPA and anterior ethmoidal artery are very likely to be successful.

Embolization

The endovascular technique of embolization for epistaxis was first reported by Sokoloff and associates in 1974. Since then, numerous series and case reports have appeared in the literature.

The procedure is performed with only intravenous sedation in the angiography suite. Bilateral external carotid and internal carotid angiography is performed through a transfemoral catheterization. The initial arteriograms, which typically do not show active hemorrhage, guide the endovascular placement of a catheter within the IMA, and embolization with absorbable Gelfoam and/or polyvinyl alcohol particles is performed through that catheter. Both ipsilateral and bilateral embolizations have been used in the treatment of unilateral epistaxis.

Proponents of embolization outline the following advantages: (1) the procedure is safe and efficient, (2) the procedure is performed under local anesthesia, (3) hospital stays tend to be shorter in patients who have undergone embolization, (4) the procedure is easily repeatable if hemorrhage recurs, and (5) the morbidity of carotid arteriography is low.

Potential complications are not insignificant. After embolization, patients may have significant pain. Femoral catheterization is associated with local issues, including hematoma (both local and retroperitoneal) and pseudoaneurysm formation. Carotid arteriography carries a defined risk of cerebral thromoembolic events. Overaggressive embolization can produce soft-tissue necrosis (i.e., tonsillar ulceration). Facial atrophy can occur after endovascular embolization. Facial nerve palsy has also been reported.

IMA embolization ignores the importance of the anterior ethmoidal artery in epistaxis. Because of technical limitations, selective angiography cannot be performed through the internal carotid system and the ophthalmic artery for anterior ethmoidal artery embolization without entailing significant risks of cerebrovascular compromise or blindness.

Three recent papers illustrate the current status of embolization. In 1993, Siniluoto and co-workers reported that among 31 epistaxis patients undergoing embolization 20 patients (64.5 percent) had permanent control of the hemorrhage, two patients (6.5 percent) had delayed bleeding after initial success, and nine patients (29 percent) failed embolization therapy. Anterior ethmoidal artery ligation was needed in seven patients. In 1994, Elden and co-workers presented their retrospective review of 97 patients who were treated with endovascular therapy. In this series, permanent control of epistaxis was achieved in 80 patients (82 percent), and embolization was unsuccessful in 11 patients (11 percent) who underwent emergent embolization. In the 1995 series of Elahi and co-workers, angiography was abandoned in three patients (5 percent) due to atherosclerosis; 43 patients (75 percent) had long-term control of their hemorrhage; and six patients (11 percent) developed delayed, recurrent epistaxis (at a mean time of 8.6 months from embolization).

Endovascular embolization has a role in certain specific situations. In many institutions, it is employed for recurrent epistaxis after surgical intervention. Also, embolization may be used for intractable epistaxis in patients who have inoperable nasal tumors. Also a candidate for embolization is the patient whose general medical condition renders him or her at too great an anesthetic risk. In other situations, the use of embolization therapy is at the discretion of the otolaryngologist.

Nasal Endoscope–Guided Bipolar and Monopolar Cautery

The nasal endoscope has also been applied to the problem of epistaxis. Initially, the flexible nasopharyngoscope was used, but more recently, rigid telescopes have become the mainstay of this approach.

The technique is relatively simple. Under general or local anesthesia, nasal telescopic examination is completed, and the bleeding site is localized. Irrigation devices for the nasal telescopes are helpful. Cauterization is completed with a malleable monopolar suction cautery or bipolar cautery. It is important to cauterize feeding vessels in the vicinity of bleeding points to permanently control the epistaxis.

The main advantage of endoscopic cauterization is its simplicity. The bleeding site itself is controlled directly. Endoscopic nasal procedures tend to be well tolerated, with minimal morbidity. Nonetheless, nasal endoscope–guided cauterization has serious limitations. In the face of profuse hemorrhage, visualization is severely compromised and potentially impossible. Furthermore, many patients with posterior epistaxis have undergone nasal packing, and it can be very difficult to distinguish between the true bleeding point and the mucosal trauma associated with packing insertion and removal.

In the report by Wurman and colleagues, 12 of 18 patients were successfully treated with this technique. In McGarry's presentation, 10 of 12 patients treated with endoscopic cauterization tended to have shorter hospitalizations. In a smaller series, O'Leary-Stickney and co-workers reported success in five of 6 patients. Most recently, Silimy reported 27 successful endoscopic cauterizations in patients who had failed AP packing.

Transnasal Endoscopic Sphenopalatine Artery Ligation

Nasal endoscopy has also been applied to isolation and ligation of the SPA at the sphenopalatine foramen. Transnasal endoscopic SPA ligation (TESPAL) combines the advantages of endoscopic surgery with the direct approach of IMA ligation. Endoscopic approaches to epistaxis are clearly preferable, because they offer the advantages of minimally invasive surgery (equal or greater efficacy, minimal scarring, shortened hospitalization, and so forth). However, routine transnasal endoscopic cauterization has serious limitations. For practical reasons, most patients who have posterior epistaxis receive posterior packs, because nasal telescopes are not routinely available during the initial evaluation of these patients. Furthermore, profuse, potentially life-threatening epistaxis precludes the use of the telescopes. After packing is in place, it becomes virtually impossible to discern the original bleeding site from the trauma associated with packing placement and removal; in this situation, directed cauterization under endoscopic guidance becomes problematic. TESPAL overcomes these problems by targeting the SPA as it enters the nose.

Initially, TESPAL was performed only after endoscopic ethmoidectomy and maxillary antrostomy, procedures that were believed to provide anatomic information for the SPA localization. Now, ethmoidectomy and maxillary antrostomy are considered unnecessary. After decongestion of the nasal mucosa with topical cocaine or epinephrine, the lateral insertion of the middle turbinate on the medial orbital wall is identified. A Cottle elevator or similar instrument is used to lift a flap of mucosa off the lateral nasal wall and the middle turbinate basal lamella, revealing the SPA as it exits the sphenopalatine foramen (Fig. 3). With a ball-tipped seeker, the SPA is carefully isolated. A vascular clip is applied proximally. In addition, the visible distal SPA is cauterized with a bipolar microcautery. The mucosal flap is repositioned and held in place with a microfibrillar collagen slurry pack. Traditional anterior ethmoidal artery ligation through a Lynch incision can be performed as an adjunctive procedure. For reasons described previously, this increases the likelihood of epistaxis control after completion of procedures directed at the SPA.

TESPAL offers significant advantages over other approaches to refractory epistaxis: (1) the likelihood of success

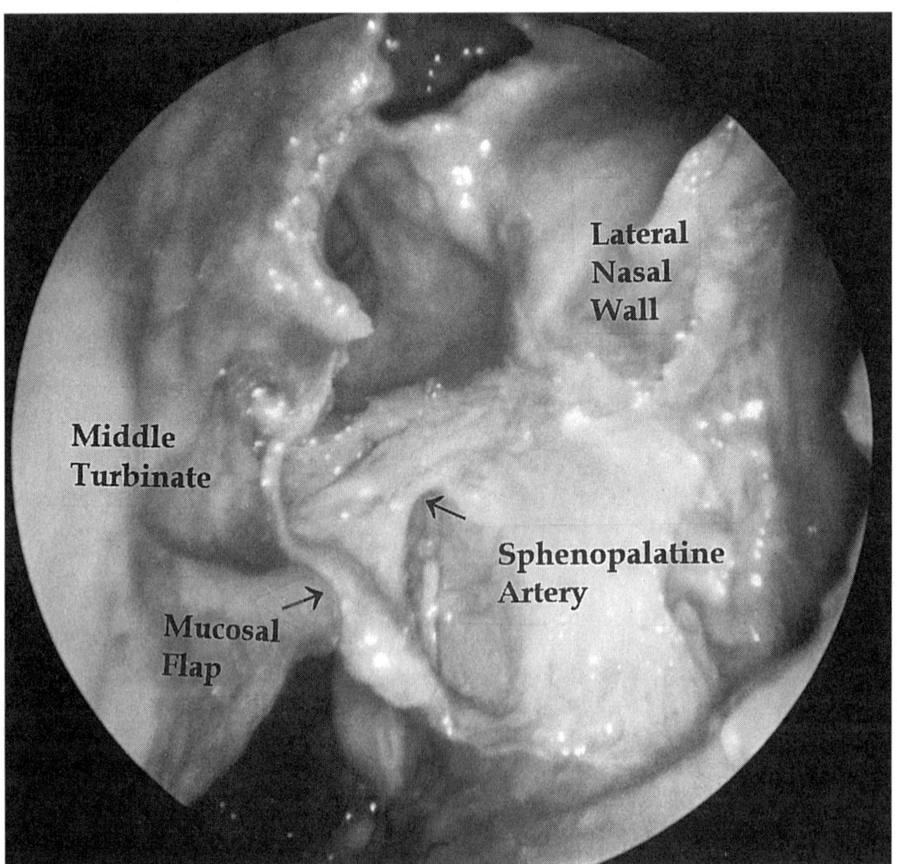

Figure 3.
Transnasal endoscopic sphenopalatine artery dissection (cadaver). Sphenopalatine artery is identified by raising a mucosal flap off the middle turbinate ground lamella, as demonstrated.

is high, (2) telescopic visualization is outstanding, (3) postoperative hospitalization is minimal, (4) patient acceptance is excellent, (5) instrument availability is very good, and (6) overall morbidity is low. Similar to any surgical procedure, TESPAL has potential disadvantages: (1) complications of ethmoidectomy may occur, (2) advanced endoscopic techniques are required, and (3) instrumentation for endoscopic surgery must be available.

In the initial series performed by Citardi and co-workers, TESPAL was successful in all five patients who underwent the procedure. Because this is a relatively new technique, overall experience is limited; nonetheless, early reports and anecdotal evidence demonstrate considerable promise for TESPAL.

■ INTEGRATED APPROACH

The otorhinolaryngologist may assess epistaxis in two possible scenarios. In the initial evaluation of epistaxis, it is relatively easy to perform nasal endoscopy and cauterization under local anesthesia in the office or even emergency room setting. These maneuvers may potentially arrest the bleeding, and nasal packing is avoided. If endoscopic cauterization is unsuccessful, or if the required equipment is unavailable, traditional nasal packing can be employed. Here, surgical management would be reserved for those patients who continued to hemorrhage 3 to 5 days after placement of AP packing.

The second scenario involves patients who have undergone nasal packing. In this situation, endoscopic cauterization is less likely to be successful for the control of persistent bleeding. Consequently, TESPAL may be employed. The potential morbidity associated with TESPAL is less than both transantral IMA ligation and transarterial embolization, and TESPAL is probably more likely to be successful.

■ DISCUSSION

Despite the technologic advantages of the past 2 decades, refractory posterior epistaxis continues to challenge otorhinolaryngologists. Nonetheless, certain conclusions may be offered:

1. At this time, traditional AP nasal packing remains the mainstay of posterior epistaxis management, and transantral IMA ligation is commonly reserved for the treatment of persistent hemorrhage.
2. The initial results of transarterial embolization are good, but are less impressive over time. Furthermore, this procedure carries significant risks that should not be overlooked.
3. Endoscopic cauterization offers directed therapy with minimal morbidity; however, in the setting of profuse epistaxis or previous nasal packing, this technique has much less utility.
4. The new technique of TESPAL combines the advantages of IMA ligation with those of minimally invasive surgery.
5. Routine use of nasal telescopes in the evaluation of epistaxis is advocated. Initial endoscopic cauterization may obviate the need for nasal packing. In the situation of refractory posterior epistaxis after attempted endoscopic cauterization and/or AP packing, TESPAL may serve as definitive therapy.

Suggested Reading

Beall J, Scholl P, Jafek B. Total ophthalmoplegia after internal maxillary artery ligation. Arch Otolaryngol Head Neck Surg 1985; 111:696-698.

Borgstein JA. Epistaxis and the flexible nasopharyngoscope. Clin Otolaryngol 1987; 12:49-51.

Budrovich R, Saetti R. Microscopic and endoscopic ligature of the sphenopalatine artery. Laryngoscope 1992; 102:1390-1394.

Citardi MJ, Vining E, Alberti PAA. Endoscopic transnasal sphenopalatine artery ligation for control of profuse epistaxis: A preliminary report. Presented at the American Rhinologic Society Spring Meeting, Palm Desert, Calif, May 1, 1995.

Elahi MM, Parnes LS, Fox AJ, et al. Therapeutic embolization in the treatment of intractable epistaxis. Arch Otolaryngol Head Neck Surg 1995; 121:65-69.

Elden L, Montanera W, Terbrugge K, et al. Angiographic embolization for the treatment of epistaxis: A review of 108 cases. Otolaryngol Head Neck Surg 1994; 111:44-50.

Fairbanks DNF. Complications of nasal packing. Otolaryngol Head Neck Surg 1986; 94:412-415.

Jacobs JR, Levine LA, Davies H, et al. Posterior packs and the nasopulmonary reflex. Laryngoscope 1981; 91:279-284.

Maceri DR. Epistaxis and nasal trauma. In: Cummings CW, ed. Otolaryngology—Head and neck surgery. St. Louis: Mosby–Year Book, 1993: 723.

Malcolmson KG. The surgical management of massive epistaxis. J Laryngol Otol 1963; 77:299-314.

McGarry GW. Nasal endoscope in posterior epistaxis: A preliminary evaluation. J Laryngol Otol 1991; 105:428-431.

Metson R, Hanson HG. Bilateral facial nerve paralysis following arterial embolization for epistaxis. Otolaryngol Head Neck Surg 1983; 91:299-303.

Metson R, Lane R. Internal maxillary artery ligation for epistaxis: An analysis of failures. Laryngoscope 1988; 98:760-764.

O'Leary-Stickney K, Makilski K, Weymuller E. Rigid endoscopy for control of epistaxis. Arch Otolaryngol Head Neck Surg 1992; 118:966-967.

Schaitkin B, Strauss M, Houck JR. Epistaxis: Medical versus surgical therapy: A comparison of efficacy, complications and economic considerations. Laryngoscope 1987; 97:1392-1396.

Silimy O. Endonasal endoscopy and posterior epistaxis. Rhinology 1993; 31:119-120.

Singh B. Combined internal maxillary and anterior ethmoidal artery occlusion: The treatment of choice in intractable epistaxis. J Otolaryngol Otol 1992; 106:507-510.

Siniluoto TMJ, Leinonen ASS, Karttunen AI, et al. Embolization for the treatment of posterior epistaxis: Analysis of 31 cases. Arch Otolaryngol Head Neck Surg 1993; 119:837-841.

Sokoloff J, Wickborn I, McDonald D, et al. Therapeutic percutaneous embolization in intractable epistaxis. Radiology 1974; 111:285-287.

Wang L, Vogel DH. Posterior epistaxis: Comparison of treatment. Otolaryngol Head Neck Surg 1981; 89:1001-1006.

Wetmore SJ, Scrima LS, Hiller FC. Sleep apnea in epistaxis patients with nasal packs. Otolaryngol Head Neck Surg 1988; 98:596-599.

Wurman LH, Sack JG, Flannery JV, Lipsman RA. The management of epistaxis. Am J Otolaryngol 1992; 13:193-209.

Wurman LH, Sack JG, Flannery JV, Paulson TO. Selective endoscopic electrocautery for posterior epistaxis. Laryngoscope 1988; 98:1348-1349.

CHRONIC NASAL OBSTRUCTION

The method of
Donald A. Leopold
by
Quoc A. Nguyen
Donald A. Leopold

Chronic nasal obstruction is one of the most common patient complaints in the field of otolaryngology at the present time. Despite the prevalence of the symptom, it is often overlooked and not adequately treated. Patients who have nasal obstruction frequently have associated complaints such as rhinorrhea, postnasal drip, headache, facial pain and/or pressure, and generalized irritability. More often than not, they have tried various combinations of over-the-counter and prescription medications. Some have even had surgery, most likely on their septums and inferior turbinates. Even so, most of these patients are still unhappy with their nasal status.

In treating nasal obstruction, it is important to give equal attention to the anatomy and physiology of this organ. Form and function go hand in hand, and successful treatment requires careful consideration of both.

Inspiratory airflow is distributed throughout the nose, with approximately 50 percent entering the middle meatus, 35 percent going through the nasal floor, and 15 percent passing into the olfactory cleft. The quantity and, even more important, the distribution of airflow determine the satisfactory sensation that a person receives from each respiration. The middle turbinates and meatuses with their rich innervation seem to be of particular significance in this regard. Not infrequently, patients will be initially seen with large airways along the nasal floors, but they still report obstruction. In these patients, the subjective complaint seems to be due to a lack of feedback from trigeminal receptors in the middle meatal regions. Another important location is the nasal valve area, because this is where the airway is at its narrowest and easily compromised. Finally, it should be remembered that systemic diseases can adversely affect the respiratory system and that a patient's overall state of health has an impact on his or her nasal well-being.

■ EVALUATION

There are three equally important components in the diagnosis and management of chronic nasal obstruction: history, physical examination with nasal endoscopy, and computed tomography (CT). Usually, but not always, they are in agreement with one another. All patients are initially managed with medical therapy. Surgery is considered only when two of the three components point toward failure of conservative treatment and there is a clearly defined anatomic problem.

History

It is important to ascertain exactly what a patient means by the complaint of "congestion." Is it a reduction of airflow through the nose, or is it a feeling of stuffiness? The latter symptom is sometimes associated with osteomeatal or anterior ethmoid disease.

The duration and character of the obstruction (unilateral versus bilateral, fixed versus alternating side, continuous versus intermittent) must be determined. The severity and any worsening or alleviating factors also need to be determined. Information regarding the patient's associated nasal symptoms, other medical problems, and current medications should also be included in the history. Any previous treatment, medical and surgical, that the patient has already had, and its result, also need to be determined. In addition, the patient's social history (work and home environments, recent changes of jobs, vacations, use of cigarettes and recreational drugs) and any seasonality in symptoms should be assessed.

Physical Examination

A complete head and neck examination with the nose saved for last is performed The nasal examination starts with an evaluation of its external appearance. The shape of the dorsum often influences the position of the nasal tip and the septum. The shape and strength of the columella, medial crural feet, and alae should be carefully evaluated. Particular attention should be paid to the presence of a ptotic tip and collapsible upper lateral cartilages. Anterior rhinoscopy using a nasal endoscope without touching the nose is performed next. The position of the caudal septum; the appearance of the inferior and at times middle turbinates; the color, thickness, and character of the mucosa; and the presence or absence of mucus and its viscosity and color should be noted. The status of the internal nasal valve is next examined, with particular attention paid to the presence of a high septal deflection and a narrow angle. This area is of interest in patients who have had rhinoplasty and who are seen with a complaint of nasal obstruction. Frequent findings in these patients include weak upper lateral cartilages and/or scarred angles. These patients often report relief with the Cottle's test (pushing malar skin laterally) or having the angles anesthetized with lidocaine soaked on a cotton swab.

In recent years, the advent of nasal endoscopy has revolutionized the diagnosis and treatment of nasal and sinus diseases. Either flexible or rigid nasoendoscopy can be performed, with each having its own advantages. It is often necessary to examine the nose both before and after the application of decongesting and anesthetic agents. Information regarding the patient's physiologic mucosal state can only be gathered before spraying, whereas visualization of posterior structures, especially of their bony details, is better after medicating. Flexible endoscopy is generally more available and allows examination of the entire upper respiratory tract. It, however, has lower image quality and does not permit procedures to be done concurrently with the examination. Rigid endoscopic equipment provides better optics and allows the physician a free hand to suction, biopsy, and so forth, but the technique is harder to learn initially. In our clinic, we perform rigid endoscopy the majority of the time, using either 4 mm or 30 degree endoscopes. Three passes are made into each nostril. The first pass is along the nasal floor going into the nasopharynx. The status of the inferior turbinate and the adenoid pad can be determined at this time. The second pass is used to look at the middle turbinate and its posterior insertion, the uncinate process, as well as the middle meatus. The anterior insertion of the middle turbinate and the olfactory cleft are examined during the last pass. The anterior middle turbinate needs to be examined closely, because subtle edema here often indicates middle meatal and frontal recess pathology. During all three passes, the shape of the septum; the status of the mucosa; and the presence of mucus, polyps, and any abnormal lesions should be noted.

Computed Tomography

The radiation exposure, scan time, and cost of a sinus CT scan have decreased in recent years as a result of better equipment and increased utilization. A full set of coronal CT scans offers better visualization of important landmarks than does a limited coronal CT. In addition, a complete coronal CT is needed for surgery; if a patient has only had limited CT, the study has to be repeated. For these reasons, we obtain a full set of coronal CT scans in all of our patients who need imaging studies of their paranasal sinuses.

■ TREATMENT

Medical Therapy

In most cases, patients are initially given a trial of medical treatment. This includes patients who have failed previous medical therapy by the referring physicians. Patients who have acute or chronic rhinosinusitis are prescribed a 6 week course of an oral antibiotic, a combination mucolytic-decongestant medication, and a topical nasal steroid spray. In addition, they are instructed to perform nasal irrigation using a commercially available WaterPik tip twice a day. Patients who have granulomatous diseases frequently have crusty, irritated mucosa. In these patients, diligent WaterPik irrigation three times a day, bihourly saline misting, application of petroleum jelly to the anterior nares, and use of a topical steroid spray may provide relief. It is also important for the patient to remember that their nasal pathology is only part of a systemic disease that should be adequately treated concurrently.

The mainstay of therapy for patients with allergic rhinosinusitis is avoidance. If this is not possible, a topical steroid spray, an oral antihistamine with or without decongestant, and at times nasal irrigation are given. Immunotherapy is considered in those patients who do not respond well to this standard regimen. Our experience with the newly introduced leukotriene receptor antagonists (e.g., zafirlukast) is too limited to make any definitive recommendation.

Increased parasympathetic tone is responsible for symptoms of vasomotor rhinitis. For these patients, we prescribe ipratropium and saline irrigation. An oral decongestant and a topical steroid spray are added to this therapy in patients who have recalcitrant symptoms.

In order to treat rhinitis medicamentosa, the first and most important step is eliminating the offending medication. Topical steroid spray, oral decongestant, saline misting, and a short course of oral steroid are often successful in relieving congestion in patients who have this disorder.

Patients who have pronounced concern regarding intermittent obstruction to airflow through one or both nostrils are frequently relieved when they are provided with an adequate explanation and caring assurance.

Surgical Therapy

Patients who do not improve with medical therapy go on to have a full set of coronal sinus CT scans. As indicated previously, they are considered for surgery only if at least two of the following three factors—history, physical examination, and CT—indicate failure of medical management and the presence of surgically correctable pathology.

External Nasal Pathology

Widened or deformed columellae are almost never responsible for nasal airway obstruction. Ptotic tips are rotated upward using standard rhinoplastic techniques or a "push-down" method. Collapsed upper lateral cartilages are corrected with cartilage graft and/or lateral scoring. Narrowed internal nasal valve apexes could be widened with spreader grafts. Care must be taken not to incise the nasal mucosa during this procedure; otherwise, webbing may form. Scars in this area should be excised and splinted with a piece of Gelfilm.

Intranasal Pathology

The aim of surgery in the nasal cavity is not simply to create a big airway but rather to establish physiologic airflow in the nose, especially through the important middle meatuses. Therapy is directed to specific anatomic abnormalities observed during physical examination and on CT that are related to the patient's symptoms. Conservative tissue removal and meticulous mucosal preservation are the rules.

Patients who have septal perforation need to have treatable causes ruled out. The size and site of the perforation often determine the degree of discomfort. The larger and more anteroinferior lesions tend to create more turbulence and crusting. Most patients get along fine with supportive measures such as saline misting and irrigation, petroleum jelly, and topical steroid spray. If surgery is needed, rotational mucosal flaps from the nasal floor and the superior septum could be used in patients who have dorsal prominence, and the size of the perforation could be reduced by downfracturing the bony septum before the mucosal flap closure (push-down technique).

Isolated obstructive lesions such as a large adenoid, discrete papillomas, or polyps could be easily removed. More frequently, however, patients have multiple pathologies, such as enlarged middle and/or inferior turbinates, septal deviation, mucosal edema, and polyposis. Over the years, we have gradually directed our attention away from the septum and toward the lateral nasal wall, specifically toward the middle meatus area.

Polyps

In the preoperative period, patients who have diffuse polyposis are given a 4 to 5 day course of oral steroid. The vast majority of our procedures are done under local anesthesia with intravenous sedation. Approximately 15 to 20 cc of 1 percent lidocaine with 1:100,000 epinephrine are given on each side. Injection is first administered through a sublabial approach into the areas surrounding the nasal spine and the piriform apertures using a 27 gauge needle. A 3 inch 25 gauge needle is then used to deliver the local solution to the sphenopalatine ganglion region, the posterior and anterior insertions of the middle turbinate, and the uncinate process. When administered properly, excellent anesthesia and vasoconstriction are obtainable. The keys to a successful operation are the patient's comfort and minimal bleeding.

We do not medialize the middle turbinate because it can become unstable and drift laterally after surgery. If the middle turbinate contains a concha bullosa, then its lateral half is removed. The remaining medial half is still covered with undisturbed mucosa and therefore has a low risk of forming synechiae with the lateral nasal wall. If there is minimal space around the anterior middle turbinate, then its anterior 2 to 3 mm border is removed with a large Tru-Cut forceps. This maneuver leads to an adequate opening for airflow in this region, allows sufficient working room, preserves the mucosa of the turbinate's lateral wall, and at the same time keeps the turbinate stable. After the uncinate process has been removed, a groove, the so-called "final common pathway," is often readily visible. Following this pathway anteriorly will lead to the maxillary ostium. If the ostium is otherwise not involved with disease, it is left undisturbed.

We use powered "microdebrider" instrumentation in all of our cases. This equipment allows precise removal of not only polyps but also targeted mucosa and bone. Normal mucosa is not disturbed to facilitate postoperative healing.

The Messerklinger technique is employed in most of our cases. In revision surgeries where landmarks are not readily identifiable, a posterior to anterior approach is preferred in order to allow the skull base to be visualized early. If there is a large amount of posterior ethmoid disease, then the partition between these air cells and the posterior maxillary sinus is taken down. The anterior face of the sphenoid sinus is usually removed when the posterior ethmoid or sphenoid sinuses are opacified. This procedure can be done quite efficiently with a powered instrument. The posterior ethmoid and branches of the sphenopalatine arteries should be avoided because they can be troublesome sources of bleeding in this area.

As a rule, we do not disturb the frontal recess except when there are large obstructing agger nasi cells. In this area, it is helpful to leave a small tag of the superior uncinate behind to prevent postoperative scarring.

Nasal Septum

A few words about the septum and the inferior turbinate. At the present time, we do not perform as many septal surgeries as we have in the past. In general, we would rather enlarge the airway along its preferred physiologic pathway, the middle meatus. During endoscopic sinus surgery in patients who have deviated septum, the more patent side is operated on first. The septum is then gently pushed to this side when the other nostril is worked on. We have found that this technique is satisfactory in the majority of patients. When this conservative approach fails, a limited septoplasty under endoscopic guidance is performed. Septal bone and cartilage are always put back once the deformity has been corrected. At the end of the surgery, we use magnetic septal splints and sometimes quilting sutures. In addition to holding the newly positioned septum in place and helping to prevent hematoma, these splints also serve as space keepers to prevent adhesion of the turbinates to the septal flaps No other intranasal packing is used because the splints are usually sufficient. The same conservative approach is also used in patients who only need septoplasty. Inferior septal spurs are usually left in place. We usually do not put any space keepers in the middle meatal area unless the middle turbinate has been destabilized. However, if magnetic splints are used, Merocel tampons are placed to prevent lateralization of the middle turbinates.

Inferior turbinate surgery is avoided. Creating a large space in this area not only reduces the more physiologic airflow to the middle meatus but also can cause nasal dryness and crusting. These patients frequently complain of congestion due to a lack of feedback from middle meatal nerve endings. In addition, the efficiency of their nose in warming, humidifying, and filtering air is reduced because proportionately more airflow is directed straight to the nasopharynx and the gland-rich turbinate tissue is removed.

Postoperative Care

Patients are started on saline irrigation, usually with a WaterPik, on postoperative Day 2. If nasal packings are used, they are usually removed on Day 5. Topical nasal steroid sprays are prescribed to patients who have polyposis or edematous mucosa. Patients who are receiving preoperative oral prednisone are tapered over 7 to 10 days. Meticulous cleaning during office visits is important. Patients are usually seen 1 week after surgery and 2 weeks thereafter until their surgical sites are healed. Successive visits can be stretched out beyond the 2 week intervals in patients who have minimal debris.

Suggested Reading

Hong SC, Leopold DA. Disorders of the nose and paranasal sinuses. In: Conn RB, Borer WZ, Snyder JW, eds. Current Diagnosis. 6th ed. Philadelphia: WB Saunders, 1997:275.

Schere PW, Hahn II, Mozell MM. The biophysics of nasal airflow. Otolaryngol 1989; 22:265.

NASAL SEPTAL PERFORATION

The method of
Thomas Romo III
Paul H. Toffel

Patients seek medical attention for perforations of the nasal septum when symptoms arise. These symptoms may include the following: whistling, epistaxis, crusting with obstruction, malodorous discharge, and paranasal pain. Concomitant paranasal sinusitis is found in some of these patients, and this condition should be evaluated with coronal computed tomographic (CT) scans. Whistling is associated with small perforations and arises from disruption of nasal laminar airflow. Most symptomatic perforations are large and involve the anterior cartilaginous portion of the septum. Posterior perforations tend to be less symptomatic because of the rapid humidification of inspired air by the nasal mucosal lining and turbinates.

Large septal perforations may be managed in suitable patients with surgery, but failure rates range from 60 percent for the methods used in older studies to 18 percent for the best of modern two-stage procedures in experienced hands. Therefore, a viable alternative to closure surgery, in this era of managed care and repeat cocaine abuse, is the use of a Silastic flanged septal prosthesis, with or without concomitant simple septoplasty.

When surgery is selected for management of septal perforations smaller than 2 cm, these are routinely corrected through a transnasal approach using the extended external rhinoplasty technique. This variation on the standard external rhinoplasty approach eliminates the need to dissect between the medial crura and membranous septal flaps, thereby allowing a direct exposure of the caudal nasal septum.

When septal perforations are greater than 2 cm or when additional endonasal mucosa is needed for perforation closure, a two-stage procedure is performed. The first consists of placement of small skin expanders under the bilateral nasal floor mucosa. The peripheral ports are placed on the face of the maxilla. Following long-term mucosal expansion, a midface degloving approach is used to remove the expanders and close the perforation with rotation of bilateral posterior, pedicled, expanded nasal mucosal flaps.

■ ORIGINS

Perforations of the septum are a well-recognized complication of septal surgery. Most postsurgical perforations follow the classic Killian submucous resection with a swivel knife. Other iatrogenic causes of perforation include cryosurgery, cautery for epistaxis, or nasotracheal intubation. Unrecognized or untreated septal hematoma may progress to abscess formation and perforation.

In recent years, substance abuse with drugs such as cocaine or methamphetamine accounts for an ever-increasing number of septal perforations. These perforations are usually large and progressive. They represent even more difficult surgical and medical challenges. The treating physician must aggressively treat both the nasal pathology and the patient's chemical addiction to ensure successful results.

■ PREPROCEDURE PREPARATION

Preprocedure evaluation and preparation is very important in the management of significant septal perforations. Few patients have clean, stable perforations. More frequently, there is significant crusting with malodorous discharge and low-grade infection. The mucosa is friable, bleeds easily, and is chronically inflamed. Sinusitis from chronic rhinitis and obstruction may be associated and should be evaluated and treated. If cocaine abuse is ongoing, surgery is absolutely contraindicated. The patient is told that postoperative substance abuse will result in reperforation. Prosthesis procedures are an alternative for patients who may not be reliable.

A regimen of intensive nasal care and hygiene is begun. The patient is instructed to use nasal irrigations two or three times per day with a Grossan nasal tip and a WaterPik. Emollients such as petroleum jelly or mupirocin may assist in lubricating the nose and lessening crusting. At times, a course of antibiotic therapy is prescribed in conjunction with the irrigations. The patient is seen weekly, if possible, for nasal suctioning and cleansing. Once the infection is eradicated and good hygiene is established with control of crusting, a course of intranasally administered topical steroid spray will decrease inflammation and help stabilize the mucosa. Prosthesis insertion or repair surgery is undertaken only when the mucosa has stabilized and inflammation and crusting are under control.

■ PROSTHESIS TECHNIQUE

In those patients selected for prosthesis procedures, insertion is simply performed by trimming the two septal button flanges to fit comfortably, without pressure, against the upper lateral cartilage–septum junction, and likewise, without pressure against the septal floor (Fig. 1). A key to success is that the portions of the septum anterior and posterior to the perforation must be relatively straight in order for the prosthesis to be tolerated by the patient. An intermediate procedure between simple prosthesis insertion and complete perforation closure surgery, therefore, is simple septoplasty anterior and posterior to the septal perforation in order to prepare the septum for successful prosthesis tolerance (Fig. 2). This does not require the time or risks involved with full septal perforation repair, and offers a cost-effective alternative that is nearly universally successful. Prosthesis insertion does commit the patient and physician to indefinite periodic follow-up and hygiene visits every few months for as long as the prosthesis remains. Our longest patient use has now been over 20 years.

SURGICAL TECHNIQUE

Small Perforation

The surgical technique used for closure of nasal septal perforations smaller than 2 cm consists of an extended external rhinoplasty approach, with elevation, rotation, and meticulous suture closure of the perforation, with bilateral posteriorly based unipedicled intranasal mucosal flaps. This is often done in conjunction with septoplasty on the remaining septum. An AlloDerm decellularized dermal matrix graft is inset as an interposition graft between the closed nasal mucosal perforation flaps. The denuded nasal floor is covered with a full-thickness postauricular skin graft.

All of these procedures are performed with the patient under general endotracheal anesthesia. The intranasal mucosa is topically treated with 0.25 percent phenylephrine hydrochloride by using Merocel sponges impregnated with 3 ml of solution. The nasal and paranasal soft tissues are injected with 1 percent lidocaine with 1:100,000 epinephrine.

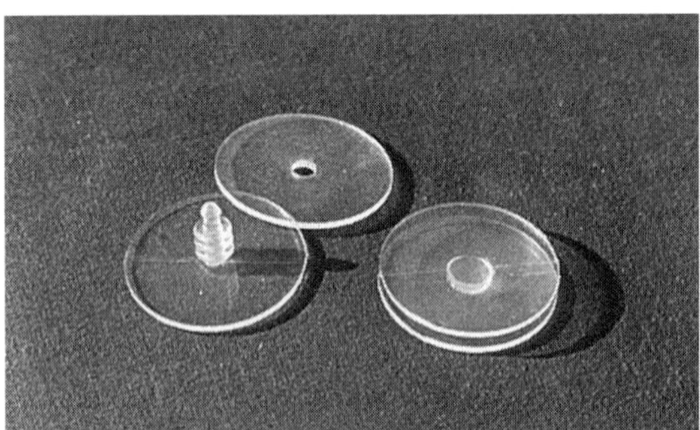

Figure 1.
Septal flanged prosthesis.

A transverse columella incision is made at the columella philtrum border (Fig. 3). This incision is carried vertically superior until the caudal septum is encountered. A full transfixion incision is performed through the membranous septum and carried over the septal angle. The columella and medial crural flap are elevated superiorly with a single hook directly exposing the caudal septum.

Next, the septal perforation is incised along its circumference with a No. 15 scalpel blade and an oval ear knife. Bilateral posterior tunnels over the remaining septum are carefully developed. Any deviated bone or septal cartilage is removed and straightened.

Elevation of the mucoperichondrium of the residual cartilaginous septum is accomplished with a calibrated Cottle elevator. This dissection is carried superiorly to the septal–upper lateral cartilage junction, anteriorly to the caudal septum and septal angle, and inferiorly to the maxillary crest (Fig. 4).

A transverse mucosal incision is now made from the posterior caudal septum across the anterior nasal sill, up onto the lateral piriform aperture, to the level of the insertion of the inferior turbinate.

A curved Cottle elevator is then used to elevate the nasal floor and inferior meatus mucoperiosteum back to the intersection of the hard and soft palates. Laterally, dissection continues to the insertion of the bony turbinate stalk and medially to the maxillary crest. Care is taken to incise the decussation fibers at the maxillary crest in an anterior to posterior manner. Sharp dissection with fine scissors and scalpel blades is usually required.

Next, the inferior turbinate is infractured and a through-and-through incision of the inferior meatus mucosa just inferior to the turbinate stalk is incised in a posterior to anterior manner. At the posterior portion of this incision, a back cut is made toward the nasal floor. This allows for

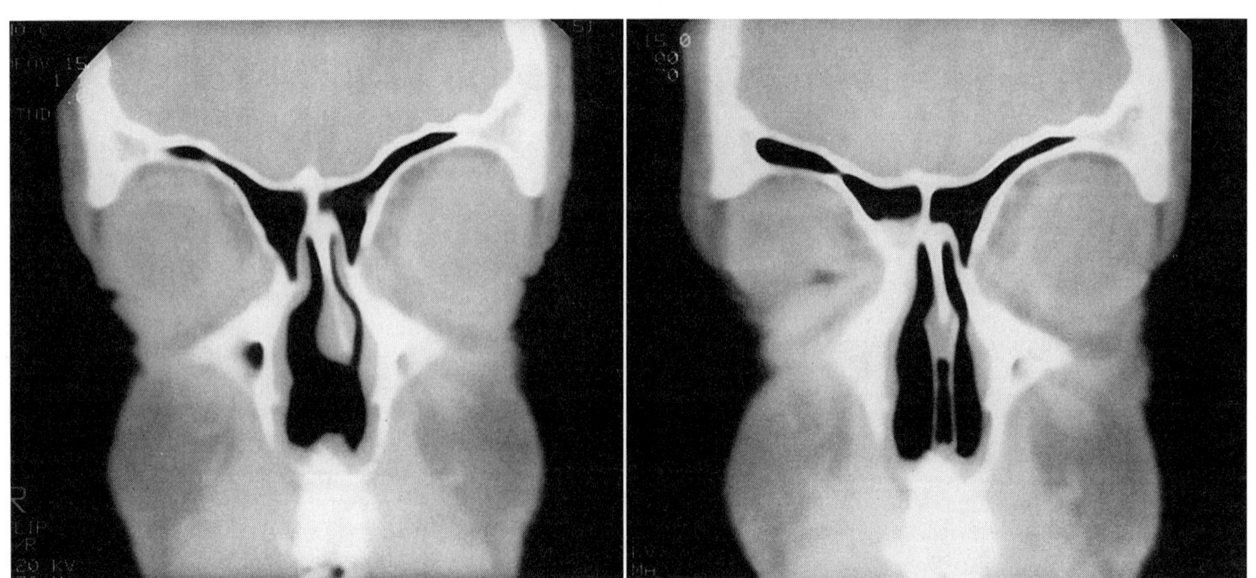

Figure 2.
Preoperative and postoperative coronal CT scans of a patient who underwent insertion of a septal prosthesis with simple septoplasty for straightening.

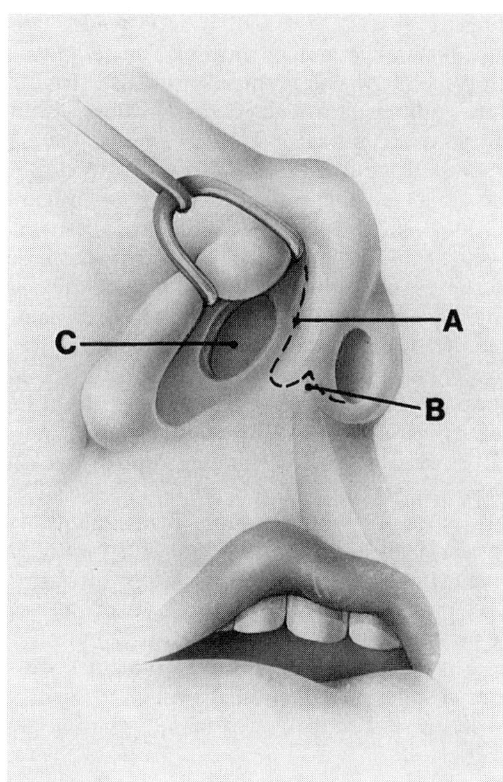

Figure 3.
A, Full transfixion incision; *B*, Transcolumella incision; *C*, Septal perforation.

unencumbered medialization of the posterior-based floor and inferior meatal nasal mucosal flap.

At this point, the intranasal mucosa is mobile from the upper lateral cartilages, across the nasal floor, and up to the inferior turbinate. The posterior-based mucosal flaps are medialized, with the inferior edge of the perforation being advanced to the superior edge of the perforation. These two mucosal edges are closed with interrupted 5–0 Vicryl sutures in a posterior to anterior manner. If excessive tension remains on the superior mucosal flap, an incision is made in the mucosa near the septal–upper lateral cartilage junction. This creates a bipedicle flap and allows inferior displacement of the superior flap, which reduces tension on the suture line.

An AlloDerm decellularized dermal matrix graft is then used as an interposition graft. This graft is secured to the septal cartilage with 5–0 Vicryl sutures superior to the perforation and allowed to drape over and totally cover the perforation on one side of the septal cartilage (Fig. 5). The repaired mucoperichondrial flaps are laid into position, and the denuded lateral nasal floor is covered with a previously harvested full-thickness postauricular skin graft. This graft is secured in place to both the nasal sill and medialized mucosal flap with interrupted 5–0 Vicryl sutures (Fig. 6).

Bilateral Silastic sheeting is fixated externally to the mucosal flaps with a 4–0 nylon suture. Finally, a Telfa pad is placed overlying a Merocel sponge to provide packing and intranasal support (Fig. 7).

Large Perforation

When perforations are greater than 2 cm in diameter or when closure requires additional endonasal mucosa, then a two-stage procedure is performed.

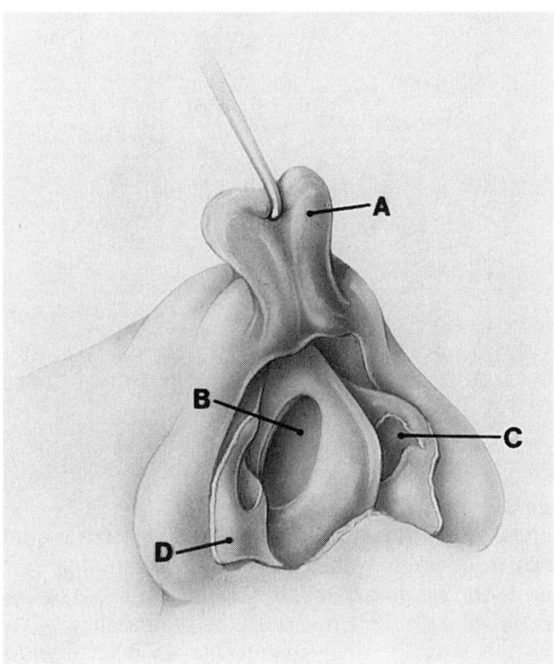

Figure 4.
A, Columella flap retracted; *B*, Cartilaginous perforation; *C*, Mucosal perforation; *D*, Mucosa elevated and reflected laterally.

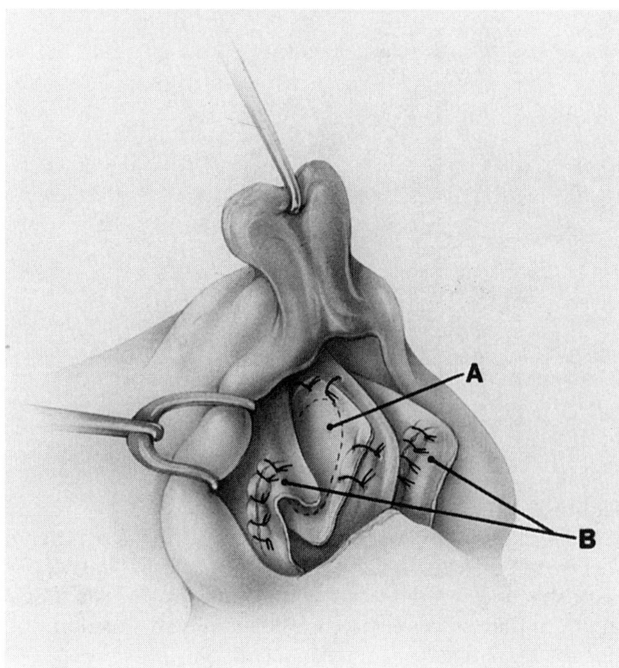

Figure 5.
A, AlloDerm decellularized dermal matrix covering septal perforation; *B*, Mucosal perforations closed with interrupted sutures.

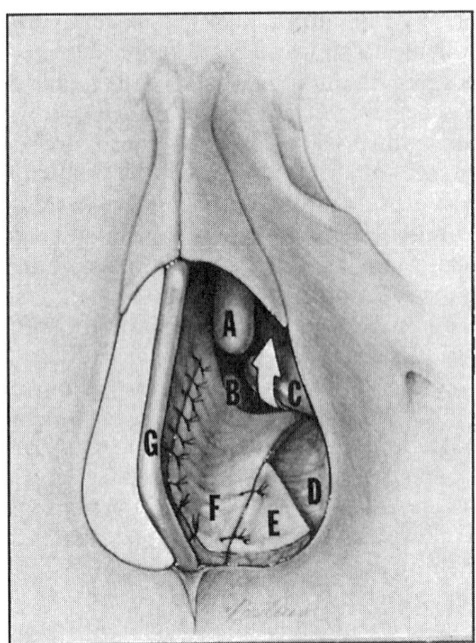

Figure 6.
Completion of flap elevation rotation, and repair of perforation. *A,* Indicated middle turbinate; *B,* Posterior nares; *C,* Inferior turbinate infractured; *D,* Raw surface area left by flap rotation; *E,* Full-thickness skin graft on floor of nose; *F,* Rotated flap; *G,* Septal angle. *(From Romo T, Foster CA, Korovin GS, Sachs ME. Repair of nasal septal perforation utilizing the midface degloving technique. Arch Otolaryngol Head Neck Surg 1988; 114:739–742; with permission.)*

During the first stage, small tissue expanders are inset under the bilateral nasal floor mucosa. The peripheral ports are then placed onto the premaxillary fossae (Fig. 8). This procedure is initiated through an incision along the anterior nasal sill mucosa, and carried lateral up onto the piriform aperture. Again, a curved Cottle elevator is used to elevate the nasal floor and inferior meatus mucoperiosteum. A 1 cm × 3 cm tissue expander is inset into the nasal floor pocket. Elevation of the premaxillary soft tissues is accomplished through the piriform mucosal incision. The peripheral port is placed onto the premaxillary fossae and connected to the expander via tubing and connecting rod. Care is taken not to kink or bend the tubing. A small amount (0.2 cc) of sterile saline dyed with methylene blue is instilled into the peripheral port to slightly expand the expander. The mucosal incision is closed with interrupted 4–0 chromic sutures, and no nasal packing is used.

Following a 2 week healing time, small aliquots of sterile saline are injected into the peripheral port through an intraoral approach. Each injection measures 0.5 cc to 1.0 cc, performed on a weekly protocol. A transcutaneous injection into the peripheral port may be performed, but this usually requires a preinjection infraorbital nerve block with local anesthesia. Total expansion time requires 6 to 8 weeks, with a total volume of 4 cc to 7 cc of saline being injected into the expander.

Once the desired amount of mucosal expansion is achieved, the second stage of the procedure is commenced. This consists of a midface degloving approach to fully expose the endonasal vault and septal perforation. The bilateral tissue expanders and peripheral ports are removed. Next, bilat-

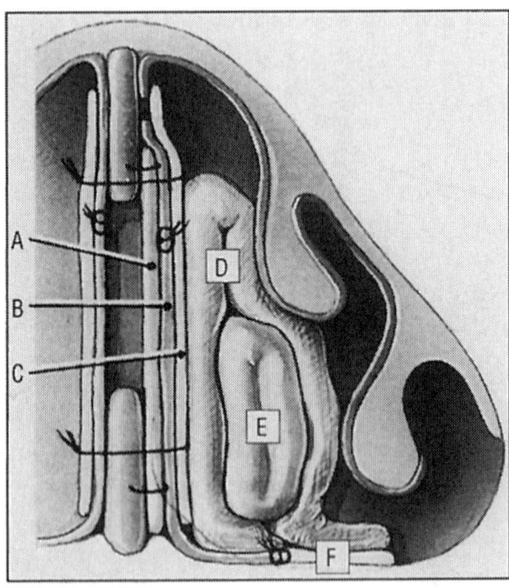

Figure 7.
Closure of perforation and nasal packing. *A,* AlloDerm dermal matrix graft; *B,* Rotated nasal floor mucosal flaps; *C,* Silastic sheeting secured to nasal mucosal flaps; *D,* Telfa dressing; *E,* Surgical sponge (Merocel); *F,* Skin graft covering donor site. *(From Romo T, Jablonski RD, Shapiro AL, McCormick SA. Long term nasal mucosal tissue expansion use in repair of large nasoseptal perforations. Arch Otolaryngol Head Neck Surg 1995; 121:327–331; with permission.)*

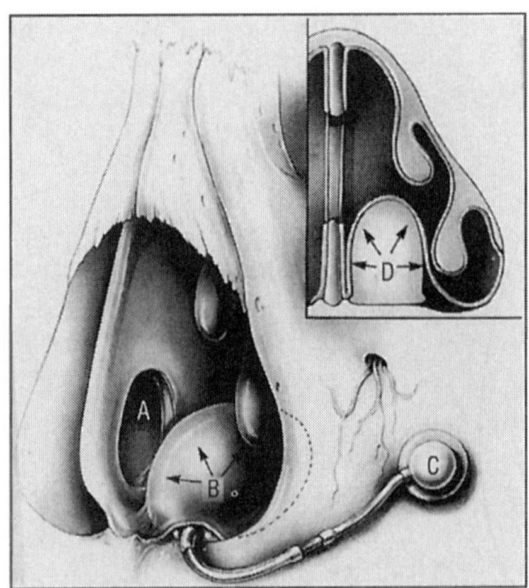

Figure 8.
A 1 cm × 3 cm tissue expander is inserted into a submucoperiosteal pocket on the nasal floor. *A,* Nasoseptal perforation; *B,* Long-term expanded nasal floor mucosa (arrows); *C,* Peripheral port implanted onto the premaxillary fossae (arrows); *D,* Inflated tissue expander in nasal floor submucoperiosteal pocket (arrows). *(From Romo T, Jablonski RD, Shapiro AL, McCormick SA. Long term nasal mucosal tissue expansion use in repair of large nasoseptal perforations. Arch Otolaryngol Head Neck Surg 1995; 121:327–331; with permission.)*

eral posterior-based expanded mucosal flaps are medialized, and the perforation is closed in the previously described manner over an AlloDerm decellularized dermal matrix graft. The midface degloving approach provides unparalleled exposure of the endonasal anatomy. This technique is initiated with the intranasal incisions being performed first (Fig. 9).

Bilateral intercartilaginous incisions are connected across the septal angle to a complete transfixion incision. The intercartilaginous incisions are carried laterally and inferiorly into the nasal floor and sill region, where they are connected to the complete transfixion incision.

Next, using cutting cautery, a complete gingivobuccal sulcus incision is performed from the region of one first molar across the midline to the other first molar.

The osteocartilaginous nose is then degloved over the upper lateral cartilages and nasal bones. The dissection is carried posteriorly and laterally over the nasal bones down onto the maxilla (Fig. 10). The intranasal incisions are then connected to the gingivobuccal incision from piriform apertures across the anterior nasal spine with a Stevens scissors.

The face of the maxilla is then stripped, with a periosteal elevator identifying the edges of the piriform apertures and the infraorbital nerves. This dissection is connected with the nasal degloving dissection. The tip structures and upper lip are retracted superiorly. The last remaining bridge of tissue lateral to the piriform aperture and upper lateral cartilages is carefully divided with the cutting cautery. The midface degloving is now complete, isolating the nasal fossae at the level of the piriform apertures, nasal valve, and septal angle. The tissues of the nasal tip, upper lip, and midface are retracted superiorly and secured with 0.5 inch Penrose drains (Fig. 11).

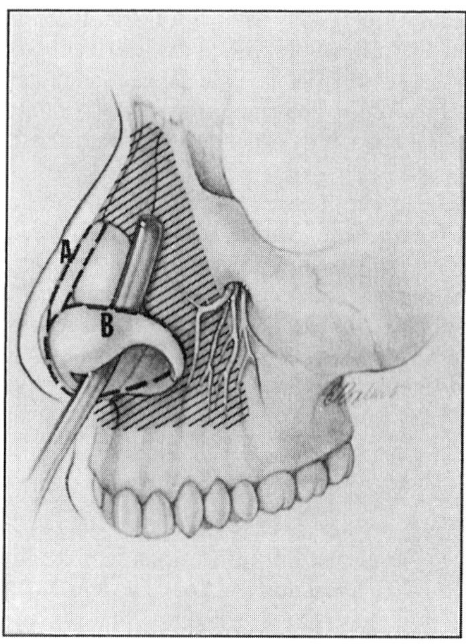

Figure 10.
Area of dissection for midface degloving. *A*, Indicated nasal dorsum and upper lateral cartilages; *B*, Lower lateral cartilages with elevator through intercartilaginous incision. *(From Romo T, Foster CA, Korovin GS, Sachs ME. Repair of nasal septal perforation utilizing the midface degloving technique. Arch Otolaryngol Head Neck Surg 1988; 114:739–742; with permission.)*

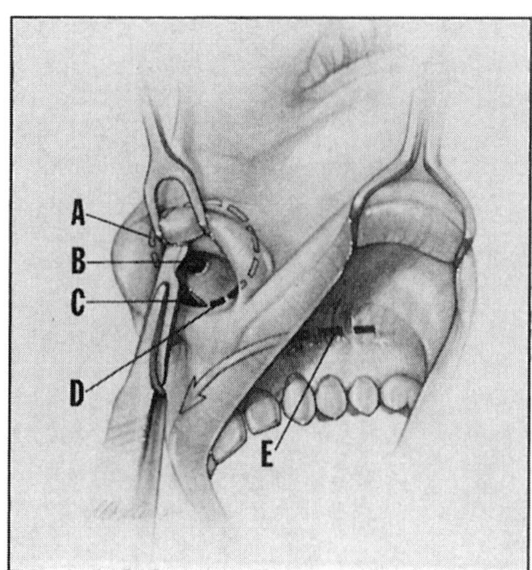

Figure 9.
Incisions used for midface degloving. *A*, Indicated intercartilaginous incision; *B*, Perforation; *C*, Complete transfixion incision; *D*, Nasal floor and sill incision; *E*, Buccal vestibule incision. *(From Romo T, Foster CA, Korovin GS, Sachs ME. Repair of nasal septal perforation utilizing the midface degloving technique. Arch Otolaryngol Head Neck Surg 1988; 114:739–742; with permission.)*

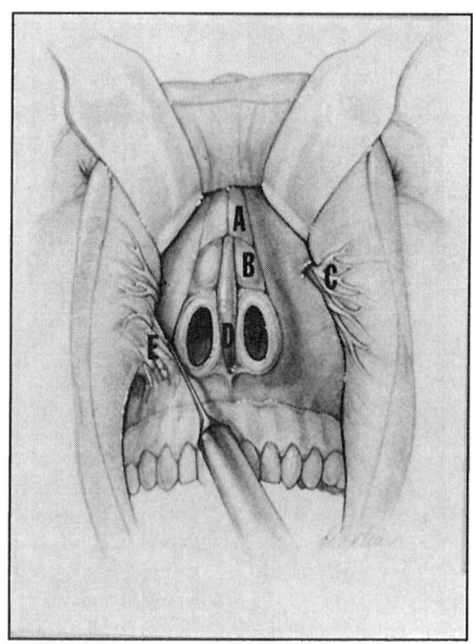

Figure 11.
Completing midface degloving. *A*, Indicated nasal bone; *B*, Upper lateral cartilages; *C*, Infraorbital nerve; *D*, Septal angle; *E*, Soft tissue lateral to piriform aperture being divided. *(From Romo T, Foster CA, Korovin GS, Sachs ME. Repair of nasal septal perforation utilizing the midface degloving technique. Arch Otolaryngol Head Neck Surg 1988; 114:739–742; with permission.)*

Next, elevation of the nasal floor and inferior meatus mucoperiosteum is accomplished as described earlier, with the additional removal of the tissue expander and peripheral ports. As previously described, the posterior-based intranasal mucosal flaps, now expanded, are medialized, and the perforation is closed.

The midface soft tissues are repositioned, and the intranasal incisions are closed with 4–0 and 5–0 chromic sutures. The intraoral incision is closed with 3–0 chromic sutures. The previously described nasal pack is placed, and all packing and external splints are removed on the seventh postoperative day. The internal nasal Silastic stent is removed at the fourth to sixth postoperative week.

■ RESULTS

Twenty-two patients at our institutions (University of California Medical Center and New York Eye and Ear Hospital) have undergone insertion of silicone septal prostheses with concomitant simple septoplasty for straightening and preparation of site. These devices have been maintained successfully for up to 21 years of follow-up without complication, except one patient who required retrievial of the prosthesis secondary to pressure complaints against the upper lateral cartilage–septal junction. Two prostheses were trimmed too small and were sneezed out by the patient; these required reinsertion with larger flanges. This technique has been a relatively simple and cost-effective management of septal perforations for appropriately selected patients.

Thirty-six patients underwent repair of their septal perforation with either of the two different surgical approaches, depending on the size of the perforation and the need for additional endonasal mucosal lining.

An extended external rhinoplasty approach was used in perforations smaller than 2 cm. Fourteen patients were included in this group, with total closure of the perforation noted in 13 patients. One (7.1 percent) had a small inferior septal perforation. Because of persistent whistling of this small perforation, the patient underwent a secondary closure procedure at 1 year postoperatively, and this perforation remains totally closed at 5 months after revision. Twenty-two patients underwent long-term mucosal expansion and the midface degloving technique for perforations greater than 2 cm. Eighteen of the 22 patients had total closure of their perforations at their 1 year postoperative office visit; four patients (18.1 percent) had reperforation at the posterior superior margin. These perforations have been relatively asymptomatic because of their location and improved humidification, and have not required subsequent revision closure procedures.

Aside from reperforation, we have not noted any significant complications—including vestibular stenosis, nasal deformity, or oronasal fistula—using our graduated technique for perforation closure.

Suggested Reading

Romo T, Foster CA, Korovin GS, Sachs ME. Repair of nasal septal perforation utilizing the midface degloving technique. Arch Otolaryngol Head Neck Surg 1988; 114:739.

Romo T, Jablonski RD, Shapiro AL, McCormick SA. Long term nasal mucosal tissue expansion use in repair of large nasoseptal perforations. Arch Otolaryngol Head Neck Surg 1995; 121:327.

Romo T, Leinhardt RR. Treatment of septal perforation. In: Rees TD, LaTrenta GS, eds. Aesthetic plastic surgery. 2nd ed. Philadelphia: WB Saunders, 1995:484.

GENERAL AND PEDIATRIC OTOLARYNGOLOGY

ALLERGIC RHINITIS

The method of
John R. Stram

Allergic rhinitis is a diagnosis that means different things to different practitioners of medicine. To the pediatrician and internist, it connotes sneezing, nasal discharge, and recurrent nasal or sinus infection. To the family physician and geriatrician, it means nasal obstruction and postnasal discharge. To the sinus surgeon, it may mean persistence of patient symptoms after surgery. Patients may be referred for symptoms as divergent as epistaxis, nasal dryness, headache, or nasal obstruction. Often, the most accurate referrals are made by satisfied past patients. The physician or surgeon who acts therapeutically without excluding allergy as the cause of the patient's complaints does so at the risk of professional reputation and patient trust. Acute allergic rhinitis causes rhinorrhea, sneezing, and epistaxis, symptoms all related to the mast cell release of preformed mediators of cell response. Chronic allergic rhinitis presents with obstruction, pain, and sinusitis, all related to newly formed mediators of cell response that result in cellular proliferation.

Progressive urban civilization has eliminated many human ills through habitat technology. This same technology, however, has exacerbated, if not created, many allergic disease entities. Petroleum combustion carbon residue present in ever-increasing amounts in our urban atmosphere acts as an adjuvant to inhalant allergic response to already present ambient levels of inhalant antigens, Pollens and mold spores have enhanced antigenicity in a polluted urban atmosphere. Tollbooth workers, traffic policemen, and taxicab drivers have their allergic responses augmented to clinically significant levels in a polluted urban atmosphere. Actors and singers are less tolerant of the mold and dust antigens in a theater atmosphere that contains dry cleaning and pesticide residue in costumes and theater draping. Efficiently heated indoor environments are rendered excessively moist by construction vapor barriers and, along with insulation that supports the growth of mold after becoming wet, combine to create an ever-larger mold spore contamination of the indoor work and living spaces. The outgasing of furniture and work surface finishes enhances inhalant allergy development. Personal items ranging from stuffed toys to insulated sports clothing are often manufactured outside of the U.S. government requirements for accurate identification of all components and preservatives, fire retardants, and pesticides contained in the product. Therefore, the down-filled jacket or quilt may contain animal products of unknown origin. The stuffed toy may be filled with the floor sweepings of the textile industry and treated with a pesticide to render it insect-free. After months in a crib or playpen, this toy becomes a major cause of dust mite exposure to its owner. Live animal companions add to the total allergen load of modern living. These life companions are often not reported by patients until they are specifically asked about pets in the history taking. Cats, birds, dogs, and rodents of many varieties add their saliva, dander, and waste droppings to the total allergic load. A rushed, nondirected, and abbreviated history taking will usually lead to a failed conservative therapy plan. I cannot quote a numeric incidence of population inhalant allergy, but the number of allergens and adjuvants continues to increase.

■ PATIENT MANAGEMENT

History

In that the definition of allergic rhinitis differs by referring specialty, the patient is often referred for symptoms or secondary disease management. The patient who has epistaxis, headache, nasal crusting, and nasal stuffiness with or without a computed tomographic (CT) scan in hand deserves a careful medical history review before being scheduled for radioallergosorbent testing (RAST), skin testing, or surgery. I have used mold culture plate technology to identify offending molds in the home, workplace, or automobile in order to plan conservative therapy or select antigens for testing. Ventilator or automobile source mold spores must be identified in order to establish environmental controls. In like manner, the side effects of medication for hypertension, glaucoma, hormone replacement, and contact lens management must be evaluated. All this is in addition to the usual questions about environmental flora and fauna and the diurnal variations of symptoms.

Examination

A competent rhinologist will be familiar with the intranasal findings of diseases and deformities capable of causing the patient's symptoms. Naclerio divides these findings into three groups: mechanical, infectious, and miscellaneous. In my experience, only cystic fibrosis can have a presentation that is difficult to diagnose without biopsy and molecular biologic tests for incomplete genetic trait penetrance. Until recently, many cystic fibrosis patients underwent failed surgery or ineffective immunotherapy for symptoms of nasal edema, tissue proliferation, and rhinorrhea.

At the time of the initial physical examination, I obtain a nasal smear for cytologic examination with Wright's stain or Hansel's stain. I also order blood drawn for a total immunoglobulin E (IgE) level and a RAST screen. If the IgE level is above 10 mg per 100 ml, and there are one or more positive findings from RAST screening antigen tests, a full RAST battery for the northeastern United States is done.

Initial Therapy

Initial therapy consists of instructions for twice daily nasal douching with buffered hypertonic saline solution (Table 1). This is followed by use of a topical nasal steroid spray, an antihistamine, and local control measures suggested by the medical history. In patients who have extremely acute symptoms and in those patients who are very troubled by their symptoms, I order a short course of oral steroids. I prescribe a broad-spectrum antibiotic if I suspect secondary infection. My first choice is a first- or second-generation cephalosporin. In approximately one-third of the patients I treat, I find signs and symptoms of gastroesophageal reflux. In these patients, I prescribe antireflux therapy. I have assigned "probably nonallergic" diagnoses to nearly one-third of the patients referred to me for "allergy shots." These diagnoses include anatomic disease requiring surgery, medical therapies that explain the symptoms, rhinitis medicamentosus after previous self-treatment of viral rhinitis, and hormonal and anatomic changes of aging causing symptom onset after age 60.

■ LABORATORY RESULTS AND ASSESSMENT OF PATIENT RESPONSE

At the time of the second visit, most patients express some positive response to therapy. Any patient who has an IgE level below 10 mg per 100 ml and no positive findings on RAST screen is not further evaluated for immunotherapy. Patients who have an IgE level over 1,500 mg per 100 ml are returned to the referring physician after first ordering a stool analysis for ova and parasites and electrophoresis. Diagnoses eventually made on these patients include multiple myeloma, schistosomiasis, and ascariasis. Patients who have an IgE level over 10 mg per 100 ml and at least one positive finding on the RAST screen have already had a full Northeast RAST panel run (Table 2). The exceptions to this panel are the elimination of dog epithelium if there is no contact by history. If there is associated asthma or cough, I test for both mite antigens and cockroach. It is important that the treating otolaryngologist be familiar with the molecular biology of cross-reacting pollens. Use of diagnostic and treatment panels based on this concept are efficient and effective in my experience. Only in the case of treatment failure or significant patient exposure would I order additional individual antigen tests within a biologic family of pollens.

At this time, the patient is re-examined, informed of the allergy test results, and given a collection of their individual allergen information and environmental control sheets selected and collated from our file. Patients who are doing well are instructed to continue on their regimen but without steroids. They are seen again in 6 weeks, and medication is adjusted down to the lowest dose that provides relief. Patients who are not adequately controlled are offered either three different additional antihistamines and topical preparations to try or immunotherapy. My own curiosity and the work of Corey prompted the first use of environmental culture plate exposure on a theater stage, a work station, and an automobile. Now I reserve ordering these tests for mold-sensitive patients who have failed to respond to immunotherapy.

Skin Testing

My practice includes free care as well as private and health maintenance organization patients. When insurance or financial limitations interdict RAST, I do serial endpoint skin testing (SET). Skin testing is the time-honored traditional procedure to identify abnormal sensitivity to inhalant antigens. Both otolaryngologic allergists and conventional allergists use commercially available stock bottles of antigen measured in weight by volume or protein nitrogen units. Most stock bottles are prepared in a 1:20 dilution. Conventional allergists dilute the stock bottles by a tenfold series to form

Table 1. Buffered Hypertonic Saline for Nasal Douching

1 qt tap water, temperature 90–100° F
2 tsp of kosher or canning salt
1 tsp of baking soda
Rubber bulb ear syringe

Table 2. Northeast Regional Inhalant Panels

Panel 1		
Johnson grass	Bermuda grass	June grass
English plantain	Short ragweed	Lamb's-quarter
White oak	Maple	Sycamore
	American elm	Mite F
Panel 2		
Cephalosporin	*Alternaria*	*Aspergillus*
Hormodendrum	Epiciccum	*Helminthosporium*
Penicillium	*Candida*	*Mucor*
	Cat epithelium	Dog epithelium

more diluted test and treatment sets (1:20, 1:200, 1:2,000, and so forth). Initial skin testing is done at 1:20 by a standard pinprick technique. Negative antigens are then tested by an intradermal injection of 0.03 cc of a 1:200 dilution. Otolaryngologic allergists use the same stock antigen but prepare a serial dilution in a fivefold manner. (1:20, 1:100, 1:500, 1:2,500, and so forth) The first dilution is referred to as a No. 1 dilution, the second as a No. 2 dilution, and so on. Skin testing is begun on a No. 6 dilution and proceeds toward a No. 1 dilution, with the additional testing stopping when the progressive skin wheal increases with progressively increasing solution concentration injections. A 0.03 cc injection is used, and the test is reported in numbers reflecting the wheal size (i.e., 3, 5, 7, 9, 11). The level of sensitivity is considered to be the level at which progressive increase in whealing size begins. I screen with the same panel used in RAST: rye grass, *Alternaria, Penicillium, Pteronyssinus* mite, ragweed, and maple comprise the screening panel. Instead of a full six-dilution test, I screen at dilutions No. 6 and No. 5. If nonreactive, I then test with a No. 1 dilution. This regimen does not subject the patient to any greater physical chemical exposure to antigen than the conventional allergy practice of prick testing at 1:20 followed by an intradermal test at 1:200. It preserves the option of completing the SET panel to identify a safe starting treatment dose. If the medical history strongly suggests mold allergy, patients evaluated by RAST and found to be mold negative are also screened by this modified skin test regimen. A full mold panel is used for the intradermal screen.

Patients who have normal IgE levels and negative RAST or SET panels are further worked up with limited CT sinus scan, serum antinuclear antibody titer determination, erythrocyte sedimentation rate determination, and nasal biopsy. Without further workup, some patients have been offered turbinate cautery, alternate-day steroid therapy, or intraturbinal steroid injection.

IMMUNOTHERAPY

Whether diagnosed by RAST or SET testing, all immunotherapy patients are treated by subcutaneous injection of commercially available antigen concentrate diluted in a fivefold manner as endorsed by the American Academy of Otolaryngic Allergy (AAOA) and the American Academy of Otolaryngology—Head and Neck Surgery (AAO–HNS). The injections are given weekly in increasing volume of dilute antigen by increments of 0.05 cc per week to a maximum volume of 0.50 cc. The starting antigen concentration is determined by the RAST or SET sensitivity levels, which are identical. For most antigens, the starting concentration is the RAST or SET sensitivity level plus one. This means that a patient who has an antigen sensitivity level of 1:500 (RAST class No. 2, SET No. 2 dilution) would begin therapy with a fivefold less concentrated antigen solution (1:2,500). Multiple antigens are mixed together in vials of similar strength. All class 4 and 5 antigens are mixed in one vial, and the lower sensitivity antigens are mixed in another. Each vial is skin tested on the patient before use with a 0.03 cc intradermal injection. If the resultant wheal is less than 16 mm at 5 minutes, the vial is deemed safe for use. Larger wheals result in a fivefold dilution of the treatment vial and a retest. I have seen patients with RAST class 5 sensitivity who required initial treatment vials mixed at a 1:1,560,000 dilution. All of these patients had asthma as a part of their allergic manifestation. By using single representative antigens of biologically cross-reacting pollens, the risk of systemic reactions from an enhanced shared antigenic stimulus is avoided.

Antigen vials are prepared in 5 cc amounts. Once the vial is used up in progressive weekly injections, a new vial fivefold more concentrated is made up, and the process is begun again at a 0.05 cc injection and progresses. This process continues until the patient can tolerate a 0.5 cc injection of a 5 cc vial prepared from concentrate antigen (0.2 cc concentrate in 5 cc total volume of diluent). The patient is then given weekly injections for 2 years. At that time, weaning to a 2 week injection interval is tried. If tolerated, the injection interval is lengthened to 3 and 4 weeks. If the patient remains asymptomatic through the duration of an allergy season while receiving monthly injections, cessation of therapy is tried.

Some patients get relief from symptoms at lower doses only to become symptomatic again at higher doses. These patients are treated long term with their symptom-relieving dose. Using this regimen, approximately 60 percent of my patients stop allergy therapy after 3 years. The remainder of my patients require either monthly injections or preseasonal therapy for selected antigens. Some mold-sensitive patients refuse to stop monthly therapy after 20 years.

SPECIAL PROBLEMS

Some antigens are more capable than others of inducing systemic responses during coseasonal therapy. Birch, ragweed, dust mites, and *Alternaria* are antigens that cause me to begin coseasonal therapy at an RAST or SET sensitivity level plus two. Some mold-sensitive patients complain of a delayed injection site induration or tenderness commencing 12 hours after injection. This complaint was eliminated by adding 0.2 cc of aqueous dexamethasone to each of the first two treatment vials. This same regimen was used successfully in a patient who had delayed asthma at one No. 7 dilution of the house dust mite *Pteronyssinus.* No steroid was used after the initial treatment vial.

Approximately 30 percent of my patients who are sensitive to ragweed and birch pollen require supplemental topical nasal spray and systemic antihistamines during coseasonal therapy.

No allergy therapy or skin testing is begun without a crash cart in the treatment area and an attendant office team who are familiar with the treatment of anaphylaxis.

FOOD ALLERGY

My experience with allergic and food allergy has been based on IgE levels that confirm food allergy suspected by history taking or review of a 2 week diet diary kept by the patient. Milk and fish have been the two most frequent offending

Table 3. Possible Cross-Reacting Pollens and Food During Pollen Season

Ragweed	Grasses
Watermelon	Buckwheat
Cantaloupe	Potato
Cucumber	Carrot
Honeydew melon	Apple
Zucchini	Mugwort
Banana	Celery
Birch	Melons
Apple	Apple
Carrot	
Potato	
Celery	
Orange	
Walnut	

foods for the patients in my practice. Treatment has consisted of complete avoidance of offending foods. Many inhalant allergy patients have rhinitis symptoms that are provoked by selected foods, which relate to their inhalant allergens (Table 3). Again, food allergy identification and avoidance are my treatment recommendations to patients.

Acknowledgment
My collaborator in the practice of allergy and preparation of this chapter is my allergy nurse, colleague, and wife, Jean C. Stram, R.N.

Suggested Reading

Ali M. Allergy diagnosis and management. Molecular Medicine, NJ, 1993.
Goldman JL. Principles and practice of rhinology. New York: John Wiley & Sons, 1987.
King HC. An otolaryngologist's guide to allergy. New York: Thieme Medical Publishers, 1990.
Mygind N, Naclerio RM. Allergic and non-allergic rhinitis: Clinical aspects. Copenhagen: Munksgaard, and Philadelphia: WB Saunders, 1993.
Roitt IM, Brostoff J, Male D. Immunology. 4th ed. St. Louis: Mosby–Year Book, 1996.

ACUTE SINUSITIS

The method of
William J. Richtsmeier

This chapter is intended to give a perspective of community-acquired acute infections that may be seen by the otolaryngologist–head and neck surgeon or primary care physician. There are many other dimensions to sinusitis. I do not discuss in any great detail the transition from acute to chronic sinusitis and reactivation or repeated acute infections.

■ RISKS

Organism Exposure

The primary reason that patients contract a sinus infection is that they are exposed to a virulent organism. Cultures have shown that infection is caused predominantly by aerobic bacterial pathogens, that is, *Streptococcus pneumoniae, Haemophilus influenzae, Branhamella catarrhalis,* and *Streptococcus pyogenes.* However, a variety of other organisms contribute, including viruses that may initiate an acute mucosal reaction, allowing subsequent growth of pathogens once the sinus is obstructed. The passage of organisms from hand to hand has been well documented for transmittance of the common cold. Sinusitis is probably transmitted in a similar fashion. Airborne infections produced by sneezing and coughing may contribute to a lesser extent.

Anatomic Predisposition

Some patients possess anatomic predispositions that allow a sinus to become obstructed with minimal mucosal change. Anatomic features may cause such changes, including septal deviation; middle turbinate variations such as concha bullosa or paradoxical (laterally deviated) turbinates; nasal polyps; or masses.

Mucosal Dysfunction

A variety of conditions can contribute to mucosal dysfunction. Allergy does so by producing a thin watery mucus that is not transported well out of the nose or sinus. Reactive mucosa, such as that seen in intrinsic asthma, allows swelling and noninfectious inflammation. Fundamental cilial abnormalities, such as those of cystic fibrosis, usually lead to chronic sinusitis, but the paralyzing activity of topical decongestants may secondarily lead to mucociliary transport abnormalities. The physician should keep this possibility in mind when treating patients who have recurrent acute sinusitis.

Immunosuppression

Acute sinusitis can appear in a variety of patients who have immunosuppression, including those with serologic abnormalities such as immunoglobulin A or selective immunoglobulin G deficiencies. Significant immunosuppressive states, such as human immunodeficiency virus infection, chronic steroid treatment, and immunosuppression due to transplantation or other medical conditions, can contribute to initiation of acute sinusitis. Pregnancy often provides an engorged nasal mucosa, and although not essentially an immunosuppressive state, is a transient condition that may also contribute to mucosal dysfunction and abnormalities.

■ DIAGNOSIS

The patient who has acute onset of purulent rhinorrhea, pain, fever, and physical examination findings that show an inflamed middle meatus with mucopurulent secretions from the sinus is easily diagnosed with acute sinusitis. Often, these patients have abnormal results from transillumination of the sinus, but transillumination as a diagnostic feature varies enough from patient to patient to be of limited value. Transillumination may be useful once the diagnosis is established radiologically to follow up on patients, particularly those in whom further radiologic evaluation is undesirable, such as pregnant women. Criteria for the diagnosis of sinusitis used in formal studies are rarely employed for the routine clinical condition. The physiologic impetus to provide therapy generally has to do with the amount of discomfort and length of time the patient has been ill. Patients who have myalgia, low-grade fever, and acute nasal obstruction for less than 48 hours can often be assumed to have a simple viral upper respiratory infection, unless localizing pain or physical findings indicate purulent pyogenic infection. Plain radiographs may be helpful but usually only serve to confirm clinical impressions. Radiographs are occasionally useful in patients who chronically complain about nasal obstruction. In most circumstances, if a radiologic evaluation is indicated, a noncontrast computed tomographic scan of the sinuses is most helpful. It identifies the specific sinuses involved as well as other abnormalities that may predispose the patient to prolonged recovery.

■ NATURAL HISTORY OF SINUSITIS

Evidence of humans living on this planet suggests a presence of more than 30,000 years. It is likely that sinusitis in one form or another has been occurring for at least that long. Only a limited amount of data regarding the natural history of sinusitis is published. Axelsson reported on 32 patients treated only with nasal decongestant in a study of acute maxillary sinusitis and found 23 (72 percent) patients restored or improved at 10 days and only nine patients unimproved or deteriorated. Similarly, Linbaek reported a control group of 44 patients of whom 25 (57 percent) had recovered or were much better. The mean response from these two studies would suggest that two-thirds of patients should be significantly improved at 10 days with no antibiotic therapy. For most patients, it is presumed that the acute immune response by leukocytes and the subsequent production of immunoglobulin against the offending organism is responsible for containment of the infection and eventual re-establishment of mucociliary transport, thus allowing the sinus to return to health. For certain organisms that cause excessive granulation and scarring, such as that commonly seen with some streptococcal infections, narrowing of the sinus os or adhesions between the uncinate and other structures within the osteomeatal complex may result in narrowing of the drainage pathways and lead to prolonged recovery or chronic sinusitis, even after the acute infection is contained. With most cases of acute sinusitis occurring in winter when the relative humidity is lower, the general physiology of the nose may come into play. Dry mucus exhibits increased viscosity and decreased mucociliary transport. Many patients who develop sinusitis experience eventual clearing when the weather improves. The exceptions are patients who have strong spring allergies whose nasal physiology may deteriorate as the year progresses.

■ MICROBIOLOGY

Pathophysiology

The primary pathogens involved in acute sinusitis are aerobic organisms. A number of studies have demonstrated anaerobic organisms in chronic maxillary sinusitis, but few studies, if any, have shown significant anaerobic organisms in acute ethmoid disease. Figure 1 demonstrates the difference in mucosal swelling between the ethmoid and the larger sinuses such as the maxillary, frontal, and sphenoid. In the ethmoid, the sinus itself is small enough so that when the mucosa swells, the air-containing space within the sinus can be completely obliterated by edematous mucosa. This swelling essentially leaves no space within the sinus that is not reached by blood and, hence, oxygen transport. In contrast, the larger sinuses, although they may have thickened mucosa, often have a central space that is not completely obliterated by the swollen mucosa. After the os is obstructed, the oxygen is removed from the sinus cavity in a relatively short period of time. The remaining nitrogen is slowly resorbed as fluid replaces the gas in the center of the sinus. In these sinuses, anaerobes can exist and proliferate, which accounts for the approximate 10 percent incidence of anaerobes. In the acute setting, there is not usually enough time for complete obstruction, removal of the oxygen, and proliferation of the anaerobes. After days of compete obstruction, there is a greater possibility of contribution by anaerobes to the infection.

The fluid space that exists in these larger sinuses also represents an important conceptual difference between infections that occur predominantly in the ethmoid as opposed to the other large sinuses because of antibiotic levels that exist in the center of the sinus, which must be carried there by serum exudate.

Pathogen Identification

As stated earlier, the primary organisms that cause sinusitis are well known and have been characterized for many years.

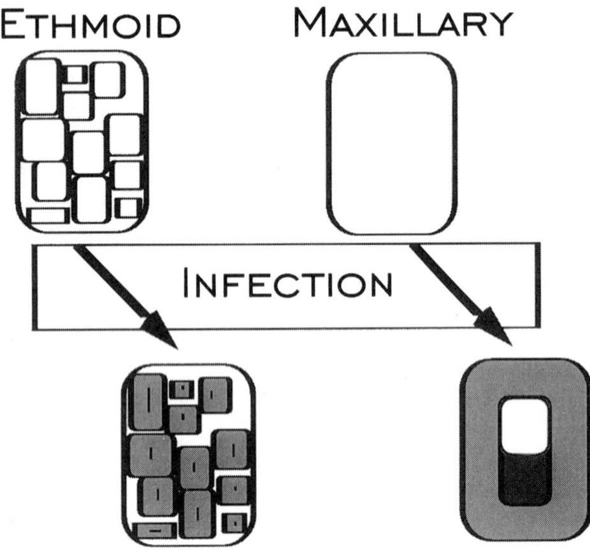

Figure 1.
Relative air space of the ethmoid and maxillary sinuses is contrasted. Infection causes swelling within the sinus mucosa and ethmoid that completely obliterates the internal air space. Oxygen is delivered to the interior of the ethmoid sinus through the blood supply to the engorged mucosa. By contrast, the swelling within the maxillary sinus leaves an internal space that can be filled with fluid and create an anaerobic environment.

Studies of sampling from normal sinuses for a variety of conditions have shown that aerobic pathogens are occasionally recovered from the sinus, but anaerobes are virtually never identified. Obstruction of the sinus by trauma or a viral inflammatory process can subsequently allow proliferation of such pathogens, which leads to acute pyogenic bacterial sinusitis. Whenever possible, it is best to culture the sinuses with the techniques that are available. Antral lavage is the most common method and should be combined with a Gram's stain to place culture findings in relative proportions, because many common nasal pathogens may also be cultured. Generally speaking, it is not useful to swab the nose because of the routine colonization of *Staphylococcus aureus* in the nares and nasal vestibule of many individuals. Techniques that allow selective suctioning of purulent secretions from the sinus ostia, particularly in conjunction with the Gram's stain that confirms the relative abundance of organisms, may be useful in identifying any specific microbial strategies for therapy.

The strategies that have been employed by organisms such as fungi and those determined by man predominantly use the differences between eukaryotes and prokaryotes, as demonstrated in Figure 2. As their name implies, prokaryotes are organisms that do not have organized chromosomes. This fundamental difference of having naked DNA within the bacterial cell is not regularly used as a strategy by which chemotherapeutic agents can selectively inhibit the activity of bacteria as opposed to the higher organisms, although the quinolones act on bacterial DNA. The presence of a cell wall and the effective disruption of its synthesis by penicillins and cephalosporins is a major distinction between bacteria and the higher organisms. Because the physiology for cell wall simply does not exist in higher organisms, a remarkable therapeutic advantage occurs. The penicillins and cephalosporin agents are particularly useful during pregnancy because of the minimal chance of affecting the fetus. The difference between the ribosomal system in eukaryotes and bacteria is an area where mother nature has evolved a strategy by demonstrated fungal organisms (i.e., *Streptomyces)* producing antibacterial substances. Many agents have been found that use this difference in protein synthesis machinery. Antibiotics acting on the bacterial ribosome include the tetracyclines, the macrolides, the streptomycin family, aminoglycosides, and others. The 55s ribosomal bacteria and the ribosomes contained within the mitochondria have been shown to be more similar than different, and in fact some antibiotics found in the tetracycline group have a profound antiprotein synthesis effect in mitochondria. Such antibiotics (oxytetracycline) are therefore not used in human therapeutic circumstances. The metabolic machinery of the bacteria finds another opportunity for selective toxicity, which would include activity of the sulfonamides and the quinolones.

Although acute fungal infections are not intended to be covered in this chapter, it should be noted that there is very little difference between fungi, which are eukaryotes, and other higher organisms like humans. Therefore, selective differences are much harder to find, and hence the agents that have therapeutic benefit often have significant toxicity, such as that seen with amphotericin B.

Resistance

Resistance of bacterial organisms to antibiotics can be caused by at least four processes: (1) the inability of the antibiotic to adequately penetrate the bacterial cell, (2) β-lactamase production, (3) penicillin-binding protein affinity, and (4) methicillin-resistance pattern. Cell penetration resistance can be conferred via a multiple drug–resistance genetic transfer. Thus far, it has not been a common problem for the usual organisms causing acute sinusitis. Nosocomial sinus infections with gram-negative organisms that have resistance to multiple antibiotics may be significant problems in the hospital setting and occasionally in hospital personnel such as critical care nurses. β-lactamase production by organisms was the first resistance to penicillins to occur. This problem was largely overcome by the production of β-lactamase–resistant penicillins (i.e., dicloxacillin). The cephalosporins, a group of antibiotics derived from fungi, have a different composition, but the active binding site is essentially the same as that of the penicillins. In general, this family of antibiotics is resistant to β-lactamase production. β-lactamase production, particularly by *H. influenzae,* has been extremely important clinically, and the β-lactamase produced by *B. catarrhalis* in mixed infections may provide a relative resistance when that organism is combined with other penicillin-sensitive infectious agents, such as pneumococcus. Penicillin-binding protein (PBP) affinity changes has been the mechanism by which *Pneumococcus* has evolved a resistance to the penicillins. In this circumstance, the enzymes that ordinarily link the cell wall chains decrease their affinity for penicillins as opposed to the normal building

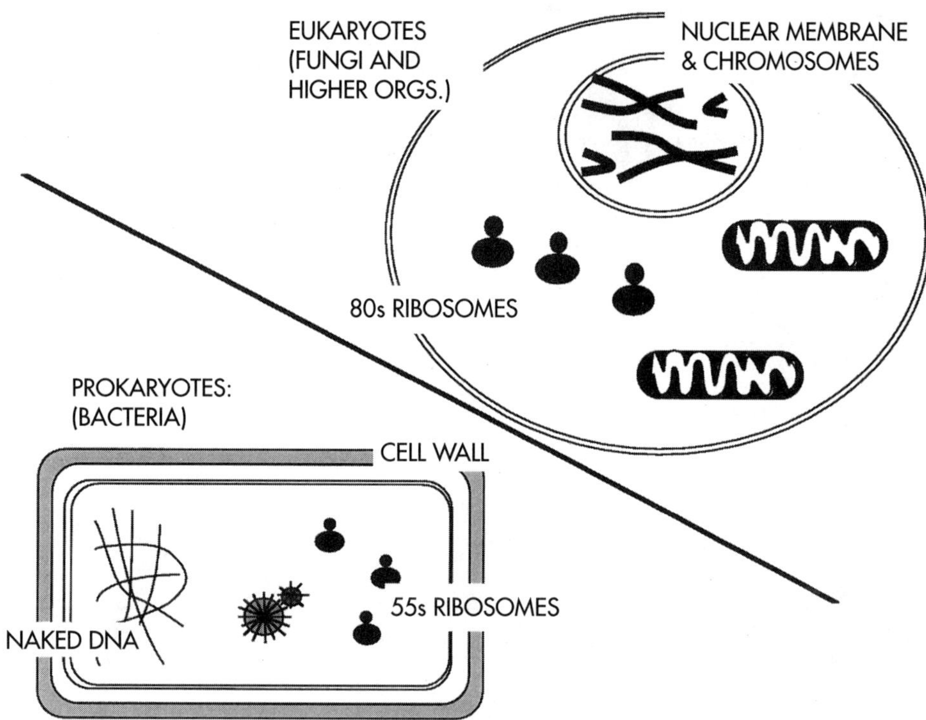

Figure 2.
Primary differences between the eukaryotes and prokaryotes are shown. The primary differences between these two classes of organisms allows for the antibiotics to affect prokaryotes and not eukaryotes. Antibiotics primarily affect the cell wall, ribosome, protein synthesis mechanism, and internal machinery of the bacterial cell.

blocks of the cell wall. In this circumstance, a relative resistance occurs proportional to the affinity of the organism's PBP. Often, this relative resistance can be overcome by increasing concentrations of the drug. Because this resistance does not involve chemical degradation of the β-lactam ring. It can extend to the cephalosporin group and to antibiotic combinations that employ irreversible lactamase inhibitors, such as clavulanic acid. The resistance for methicillin-resistant staphylococcus is not a common feature of acute sinusitis and is not further discussed here. Anaerobes provide their own antibiotic resistance patterns. In addition, if an anaerobe can live in a space, it means that blood is not getting there. Consequently, antibiotics delivered by serum or blood will be low in that space as well.

■ THERAPY

Antibiotics

Antibiotics provide the major armamentaria for treatment of acute sinusitis. Most antibiotics routinely employed for treating acute sinusitis have relatively good serum levels after intravenous or oral administration (Table 1). One oral antibiotic has a relatively unique pharmacology that is worth mention: the macrolide zithromycin. This antibiotic is rapidly bound in the intracellular space and never enjoys a significant peak serum level. Because the serum levels essentially predict what antibiotic concentration will enter into body fluids, such as that within the center of the major sinuses, it is unlikely that significant concentrations of zithromycin can be found in the fluid in the center of the maxillary sinus. Erythromycin is particularly useful for cellulitis or when intracellular killing is on course, such as infections with mycoplasma or in patients with defective leukemia. But in my opinion, zithromycin provides a significant disadvantage for therapy of acute maxillary sinusitis in which the central sinus fluid is to be treated. The pharmacology is quite different from that of azithromycin. Erythromycin or clarithromycin both enjoy relatively good serum levels. Clarithromycin has an extended spectrum to include significant activity against *H. influenzae,* by virtue of its active metabolites. The distribution of the penicillins, cephalosporins, sulfonamides, and quinolones all have reasonably good serum levels, which should penetrate sinus mucosa and sinus fluid contents adequately.

In picking an antibiotic and evaluating the response, it is important to keep in mind the natural history of sinusitis. No one knows how long patients need to be treated with antibiotics. A study of the length of time required to treat sinusitis used long (10 day) and short (3 day) trimethoprim-sulfamethoxazole oral therapy. In this study, slightly more than 60 percent of patients treated for 3 days no longer had sinusitis. Of patients treated with sulfonamides, only approximately 70 percent were improved at 10 days, which has led me to assume that sulfonamides are not a particularly good antibiotic for acute sinusitis, even when given for 10

Table 1. Clinical Activity of Oral Antibiotics Against Common Organisms Causing Adult Sinusitis

		SINUSITIS ORGANISMS					
		S. PNEUMONIAE	PEN RESISTANT *S. PNEUMO*	*S. PYOGENES*	*H. INFLUENZAE*	*B. CATARRHALIS*	*MYCOPLASMA PNEUMONIAE*
	Relative incidence	36%	Unknown	5–10%	27%	2–23%	Causes 1° URI
	Resistance		24% of pneumonia	rare	63% β-lactamase +	80% β-lactamase +	No cell wall
Penicillins	Amoxicillin	*****	**	*****	**	*	na
	Amoxicillin-clavulanate	*****	**	*****	*****	*****	na
	Cefaclor	*****	***	*****	***	****	na
Cephalosporins	Cefpodoxime	*****	****	*****	*****	*****	na
	Cefprozil	*****	ni	*****	*****	*****	na
	Cefuroxime axetil	*****	***	*****	****	*****	na
Macrolides	Clarithromycin	*****	****	*****	*****	*****	*****
	Erythromycin	****	ni	****	na	*	*****
	Zithromycin	***	***	Not 1st choice	**	***	*****
Quinolone	Ciprofloxacin	Not 1st choice	****	ni	*****	*****	ni
Sulfa	Trimethoprim-Sulfamethoxazole	**	ni	**	**	**	na

The relative activity of various oral antibiotics against organisms associated with sinusitis are shown. The information is based on combinations of personal clinical experience reported, indications and usage recommendations from the *Physicians' Desk Reference* (1997), reported clinical activity, and reported in vitro sensitivities. *Mycoplasma pneumoniae* is included as an agent that causes sinusitis in a manner similar to virus infection but whose clinical course can be affected by oral antibiotics. See text for further comments.
Na, no activity; ni, no information.

days. Short-term antibiotic therapy appeared to give the same results as that for untreated controls. Reports of other more active antibiotics, such as clarithromycin or the combination of amoxicillin and clavulanic acid, yield clinical Day 10 results in excess of 90 percent (and radiologic improvement for more than 80 percent of patients), which is the outcome I would expect for current oral antibiotic therapy. Pharmacokinetics of the newer quinolones reveal that essentially the same serum concentrations are reached after oral or intravenous administration, which is a remarkable achievement and potential cost savings (even in hospitalized patients) for infections requiring extended gram-negative coverage.

Few good studies have addressed the issue of how long the patient needs to be treated. Common sense dictates that a patient needs to be treated long enough to (1) reverse the sepsis or toxicosis; (2) allow resolution of the edema and hence the sinus ostia obstruction, especially in patients who have had severe squamous cell metaplasia occur within the sinus; and (3) re-establish mucociliary transport. This may occur in a few days for some patients; it may take 2 to 4 weeks for others. It is likely that this varies to some extent, depending on the organism. The community history of infections that are "going around" is very beneficial to the clinician in designing therapy for individuals.

Dose

For the two-thirds of patients who are going to get well anyway, the antibiotic dose is not important. I tend to think of sinusitis (particularly if the patient has a history of pressure) as an abscess, so I use doses recommended for serious illnesses.

Lavage

Maxillary sinus lavage enjoyed a more common role in the United States before the invention of antibiotics. It is still used more actively in other countries. This technique provides immediate relief of pressure from the maxillary sinus as well as removes a large amount of infected material (which can be cultured). The disadvantage is that it can only be applied to the maxillary sinus with any relative ease. Also, some discomfort is associated with the procedure. The Pretz type of sinus lavage, which is basically an aggressive nasal irrigation, may be of benefit to the patient by removing infected purulent secretions from the nose. Using saline irrigation may be beneficial, particularly for patients who have extremely thick secretions. In the setting of decreased humidity and dryness, lavage may substitute for increased humidification, which may not be realistic or possible in many clinical settings.

Decongestants

Oxymetazoline and other decongestants that minimize rebound congestion and maximize the opening into which the purulent secretions can be drained may significantly benefit patients. The paralysis of nasal cilia by oxymetazoline should be appreciated, and when this drug is used it should be limited to a maximum of 3 or 4 days of therapy.

Topical Steroids

Although not proved, many clinicians recommend topical steroids for their patients who have acute sinusitis. Although there are few data to support this use, it is commonly employed by many clinicians and for the most part not thought to be detrimental.

Analgesics

The discomfort from acute sinusitis should be treated adequately so that patients can rest, eat, and return to work when appropriate. Severe pain in the maxillary area can be treated with lavage.

Surgery

Surgery is seldom indicated for treating acute sinusitis except for patients who have (1) dehiscent bone, (2) symptoms of meningismus, or (3) primary sphenoid sinusitis. Because of the proximity of the sphenoid sinus to the central nervous system, and direct drainage into the cavernous sinus, sphenoid sinusitis presents a particular risk for patients who have acute infection. Patients who have pansinusitis for the most part are thought to be able to have their infections resolve with oral antibiotics, even when the sphenoid and frontal sinuses are involved. Patients who have questionable frontal dehiscence are considered candidates for surgical intervention. Unless some complication of acute sinusitis occurs, such as periorbital abscess or other signs of extension of the disease outside of the sinuses, surgical intervention is rarely required. When it is required, a conservative approach, decompressing the sinus to allow egress of fluids, which is similar in concept to incision and drainage of an abscess, should be used. This technique can usually be accomplished endoscopically. Once the acute infection is under control, further surgical intervention can be considered, if necessary, when visualization of normal structures is improved. This surgery also can usually be accomplished endoscopically.

Therapeutic Failures

Therapeutic failures have a variety of causes. The first is that the infection being treated is not a bacterial infection, and therefore it does not respond to conventional antibiotics. Usually, this type of infection is viral in origin or generally some other inflammatory symptomatology that mimics sinusitis. Very occasionally, fungal infection can have an acute sinusitis presentation. When the patient fails to respond to antibiotics within a few days, it is important to check cultures and consider the immunologic status of the patient. There are several reports in the literature of acute fungal infections in immunologically intact individuals; therefore, immunosuppression is not a prerequisite for fungal sinus infection, although these infections certainly are considered to be unusual.

The next most common reason for failure in my experience is infection by resistant organisms. If the patient is initially treated with an antibiotic, such as amoxicillin, for which numerous resistant organisms exist, switching to an antibiotic with a better resistance pattern is indicated. The second antibiotic should be β-lactamase–resistant, and it should encompass the usual organisms that cause sinusitis. Such antibiotics include the macrolide clarithromycin (erythromycin does not have good coverage of *H. influenzae)*, second-generation cephalosporins (such as cefoxitin and cefpodoxime), or combination antibiotics such as (amoxicillin and clavulanic acid). For pediatric patients, Pediazole, a combination of erythromycin and sulfisoxazole, extends the spectrum to cover the most common organisms. Most of the anaerobes involved in acute sinusitis are sensitive to amoxicillin. Occasionally employing metromidzate or clindamycin may tip the therapeutic balance in a stubborn infection.

Occasionally the patient fails to respond because of a foreign body in the maxillary sinus, such as dental material from a root canal, bone fragments from previous trauma, inspissated mucus, or other materials associated with surgical procedures. The patient should have a history compatible with such findings. Imaging patients with acute sinusitis who fail to respond to routine therapy may allow confirmation.

An obstructed os, particularly stenosis of the maxillary sinus ostia associated with acute pyogenic infection, may limit the egress of purulent secretions from the maxillary sinus and prolong the recovery period. This problem may ultimately result in chronic sinusitis and the need for surgical intervention.

Acute pyogenic sinusitis is likely to remain with us, and infections with resistant organisms may become an increasing problem. Fortunately, most individuals who have healthy immune systems and who lack anatomic problems in their noses and sinuses eventually recover on their own. This perspective is reassuring from a general public health standpoint, but may not be comforting to the individual who has acute discomfort or prolonged illness. Antibiotics remain the mainstay of therapy for acute purulent sinusitis, and choice of antibiotics is largely directed by the severity of the illness and the likelihood of infection with a resistant organism.

Suggested Reading

Anonymous. Clarithromycin and azithromycin. Med Lett Drug Ther 1992; 34:45-46.

Axelsson A, Chidekel N, Grebelius N, Jensen C. Treatment of acute maxillary sinusitis. Acta Otolaryngol 1970; 70:71-76.

Axelsson A, Brorson JE. The correlation between bacteriological findings in the nose and maxillary sinus in acute maxillary sinusitis. Laryngoscope 1973; 83:2003-2011.

Bauernfeind A, Jungwirth R, Eberlein E. Comparative pharmacodynamics of clarithromycin and azithromycin against respiratory pathogens. Infection 1995; 23:316-321.

Dubois J, Saint-Pierre C, Tremblay C. Efficacy of clarithromycin vs. amoxicillin/clavulanate in the treatment of acute maxillary sinusitis. ENT J 1993; 72:804-810.

Feldman C, Kallenbach JM, Miller SD, et al. Community-acquired pneumonia due to penicillin-resistant pneumococci. New Engl J Med 1985; 313:516-617.

Gungor A, Corey JP. Pediatric sinusitis: A literature review with emphasis on the role of allergy. Otolaryngol Head Neck Surg 1997; 15:4-15.

Hamory BH, Sande MA, Sydnor A Jr, et al. Etiology and antimicrobial therapy of acute maxillary sinusitis. J Infect Dis 1979; 139:197-202.

Lindback M, Hjortdahl P, Johnsen UL. Randomized doubleblind, placebo controlled trial of penicillin V and amoxycillin in treatment of acute sinusitis in adults. Br J Med 1996; 313:325-329.

Shapiro GG, Rachelefsky GS. Introduction and definition of sinusitis. Allergy Clin Immunol 1992; 90:417-418.

Van Cauwenberge P, Kluyskens P, van Renterghem L. The importance of the anaerobic bacteria in paranasal sinusitis. Rhinology 1975; 13: 141-145.

Wald ER. Antimicrobial therapy of pediatric patients with sinusitis. J Allergy Clin Immunol 1992; 90:469-473.

Wald ER, Reilly JS, Casselbrant M, et al. Treatment of acute maxillary sinusitis in childhood: A comparative study of amoxicillin and cefaclor. J Pediatr 1984; 104:297-302.

Wald ER, Chiponis D, Ledesma-Medina J. Comparative effectiveness of amoxicillin and amoxicillin-clavulanate potassium in acute paranasal sinus infections in children: A double-blind, placebo-controlled trial. Pediatrics 1986; 77:795-800.

Williams WJ Jr, Holleman DR Jr, Samsa GP, Simel DL. Randomized controlled trial of 3 vs 10 days of trimethoprim/sulfamethoxazole for acute maxillary sinusitis. JAMA 1995; 273:1015-1021.

SINUSITIS IN CHILDREN

The method of
Richard M. Rosenfeld

Recent improvements in functional endoscopic sinus surgery (FESS) have allowed children who have refractory sinusitis to experience symptomatic relief heretofore impossible with medical management alone. As with most surgical techniques, however, it is easier to learn *how* to cut, than *when* to cut, or—more important—when *not* to cut. Consequently, I deal primarily with decision making and not the nuances of surgical technique.

FESS is optimally viewed as the end point in a stepped management protocol, not as an isolated intervention. The steps in this protocol are (1) primary control through risk factor modification, (2) enlightened antibiotic therapy, (3) adenoidectomy, and (4) FESS. The protocol described herein is based on my background in public health and on the successful medical and surgical treatment of hundreds of children with refractory sinusitis.

■ DIAGNOSIS

Acute sinusitis has a presentation most often as cold symptoms that are unimproved after 10 days, including nasal discharge of any quality (clear, cloudy, or colored); daytime cough; and bad breath odor. Fever, if present, is usually low grade and transient. Less often, acute sinusitis has a presentation of more severe symptoms with high fever (greater than 39° C) and purulent nasal discharge, with or without eye swelling or headache. Preschool children, however, are less verbal and rarely report headache or facial pain. Instead, nonspecific symptoms such as fatigue, lethargy, irritability, or loss of appetite are observed.

Chronic sinusitis implies a symptom duration of 3 months or longer, and generally has a presentation of nasal congestion, cough, and foul breath. Nonspecific behavioral symptoms are often present; parents describe their children as not being themselves. In contrast to acute sinusitis, children who have chronic symptoms have few physical findings. Anterior rhinoscopy findings performed with an otoscope are frequently normal, and rhinorrhea may or may not be present. Thickened or purulent secretions may be seen in the posterior pharynx, with cobbling of the pharyngeal lymphoid follicles.

The particular sinus(es) involved depend on the age of the child. Children are born with well-developed ethmoid sinuses and small maxillary sinuses (approximately the size of the middle ear space). Development of the frontal sinuses begins at approximately age 4 to 5 years, whereas a small sphenoid sinus can be seen as early as 2 years of age. Clinically important sinusitis is less common in infants younger than 1 year of age; however, in older children ethmoid involvement associated with a viral upper respiratory infection (URI) is common and can develop into clinically apparent bacterial sinusitis.

Imaging studies are unnecessary for initial management of sinusitis, and should be reserved for children who are surgical candidates because of chronic symptoms or a complicated disease course. Computed tomography (CT) is the "gold standard" for sinus imaging, because it provides exquisite bony detail and a wealth of soft-tissue information. Axial images must be supplemented by coronal views to assess the ostiomeatal complex and skull base; intravenous contrast is unnecessary unless an abscess or other complication is suspected. Although plain sinus radiographs are readily available, they are not useful for surgical decision making because of limited bony resolution and poor visualization of the ethmoid sinuses.

■ NATURAL HISTORY

Approximately 50 percent to 60 percent of placebo-treated children in clinical trials have cure or improvement of acute sinusitis symptoms within 10 days. When antibiotics are administered, cure or improvement rates increase to 80 percent to 90 percent. Further, symptom relief occurs more rapidly with antibiotics than placebo. Although antibiotics have a favorable impact, the efficacy of placebo suggests that the host immune response is often sufficient for symptom relief. Consequently, observation alone may be appropriate for selected children (aged 2 years or older) who have *nonsevere* symptoms of *uncomplicated* acute sinusitis, provided that timely antibiotic therapy can be given at the earliest sign of any suppurative sequelae.

The natural history of untreated chronic or recurrent sinusitis is unknown, although most children observed in prospective studies improve gradually with time. Spontaneous resolution is most likely multifactorial, reflecting midface growth, steady immune maturation up to 8 years of age, and gradual involution of pharyngeal lymphoid tissue (adenoids). The time to resolution, however, can be quite lengthy, requiring up to several years of patient optimism by parents and suffering children. For example, approximately 90 percent of pediatric patients in a Netherlands study had spontaneous relief of refractory maxillary sinusitis at a mean age of 7 years. In contrast, the stepped treatment protocol that I outline in this chapter offers short-term resolution rates of 70 percent to 90 percent that remain stable after 1 year of follow-up.

■ STEPWISE APPROACH TO REFRACTORY SINUSITIS

The protocol that follows is intended only for the management of uncomplicated chronic or recurrent sinusitis; complicated cases require intravenous antibiotics and open surgical intervention and are not discussed further. The first step in management is to define *disease burden,* which is the global impact of sinusitis on the child and family, by discussing and recording the following:

- Major sinusitis symptoms (two or three), in order of parental importance.
- Minor or other symptoms considered attributable to sinusitis.
- Frequency, duration, and severity of symptoms (including seasonal variations).
- Frequency of physician visits for sinusitis and medication use.
- Baseline state of the child between episodes.
- Impact of symptoms on child behavior and school performance.

Information on disease burden is gleaned from discussions with the child, parents, and primary care practitioner (PCP). Communication with the PCP cannot be overemphasized; the specialist's impressions are incomplete without the global assessment of disease burden and family dynamics that only the generalist can provide. If an allergist or pulmonologist is also involved, they should be contacted as well.

Parental expectations concerning proposed therapy often become apparent once disease burden has been defined. But the family may have other expectations in mind—either realistic or unrealistic—about what can and cannot be accomplished. Therefore, the physician must ask parents to *specifically* define expectations at the start of treatment. A useful way of obtaining this information is to ask, "If I could wave a magic wand over your child's sinuses and make them better, what change(s) would you want to occur?" Common responses include the following: relieve general symptoms, reduce the need for antibiotics, improve the child's behavior and well-being, reduce relapses of infection, relieve specific sinonasal symptoms, improve baseline asthma, and reduce school absences.

Step 1: Primary Control

Primary control reduces disease burden by direct impact on causative factors (Table 1). Passive smoke exposure can be either eliminated completely or reduced by adequate ventilation and not smoking in closed spaces (e.g., while driving). Inhalant and food allergies should be evaluated by a pediatric allergist in light of a suggestive clinical history (watery rhinorrhea, ocular pruritus, repetitive sneezing) or physical findings (allergic shiners), nasal crease, facial or buttock rash). Optimal control of asthma, when present, is also mandatory.

Table 1. Primary Control of Sinusitis in Children

CONTRIBUTING FACTOR	INTERVENTION
Immature immune system	Patience; improves with growth and development
Passive smoke	Reduce or eliminate exposure; improve ventilation
Inhalant allergies	Environmental measures; immunotherapy
Food allergies	Dietary modifications; soy-based or elemental formulas
Large-group day care	Small group day care with six or fewer children
Gastroesophageal reflux	Optimize dietary and medical management

Approximately 5 percent to 10 percent of viral URIs in early childhood progress to acute sinusitis. The incidence of URIs can be reduced by eliminating passive smoke and considering day care alternatives; however, contact with an older sibling at home can negate the benefits of day care cessation. The size of the day care group—not day care per se—is responsible for an increased viral URI burden. When the group size is six children or fewer, risk is not increased. Consequently, small-group day care centers are preferable to large-group centers, whenever feasible.

Children, by definition, have a relative immunodeficiency because of a continued rise in plasma immunoglobulin G (IgG), immunoglobulin M (IgM), and immunoglobulin A (IgA) production until approximately 6 to 8 years of age. In particular, IgA undergoes a steady rise into later childhood. Although nothing can be done to accelerate immune development, "watchful waiting" may be effective in young children. Attainment of immunocompetence coincides with gradual involution of pharyngeal lymphoid tissue, including the adenoids. Bacteriologic and clinical studies show a direct correlation between sinonasal symptoms and the concentration of bacterial pathogens in the adenoid core. Adenoid involution reduces this local bacterial reservoir, and may affect sinusitis in a similar manner as for otitis media.

Step 2: Antibiotics

All children referred for treatment of refractory sinusitis should receive additional antibiotics beyond those administered by the child's primary care physicians (PCP), *regardless* of the duration of treatment. Sinusitis is caused by similar bacteria as for otitis media *(Streptococcus pneumoniae, Haemophilus influenzae,* and *Moraxella catarrhalis),* but unlike otitis media, sinusitis is often polymicrobial, with anaerobes and penicillin-resistant *Staphylococcus aureus* contributing to chronic infection. Therefore, treatment with several different antibiotics (Table 2), including those with adequate β-lactamase stability and anaerobe coverage, may be necessary to achieve a satisfactory response.

First-line sinusitis therapy begins with well-tolerated, inexpensive drugs such as amoxicillin or trimethoprim-sulfamethoxazole (TMP-SMX). Persistent symptoms require an extended-spectrum antibiotic, preferably one that the child has not previously received. Special use antibiotics are reserved for refractory cases. Clindamycin will destroy anaerobes and pneumococci that are resistant to penicillins or cephalosporins. The incidence of pseudomembranous enterocolitis with clindamycin is comparable to that of other antibiotics, including amoxicillin. Resistant *H. influenzae* should respond to cefixime. Finally, doxycycline offers superior penetration into respiratory secretions and may prove effective when other agents have failed.

Optimum duration of therapy is largely empiric, but 10 to 20 days appears prudent; longer courses of a single agent are unlikely to be of benefit. For severe acute sinusitis, antibiotics are continued for 1 week following symptom relief. Culture of rhinorrhea may guide therapy, although for many children who have chronic symptoms rhinorrhea is scant or absent. Treatment with intravenous antibiotics may help

Table 2. Recommended Antibiotics for Treating Sinusitis in Children

CATEGORY GENERIC (TRADE) NAMES	DOSING INTERVAL	COMMENTS
Prophylactic antibiotics		
amoxicillin (Amoxil)	qd	Must refrigerate; refill every 2 weeks
sulfisoxazole (Gantrisin)	qd	No refrigeration necessary
First-line antibiotics		
amoxicillin (Amoxil)	t.i.d.	Still the drug of choice for initial therapy
TMP-SMX (Bactrim; Septra)	b.i.d.	When child is penicillin-allergic
Extended-spectrum antibiotics		
amoxicillin-clavulanate (Augmentin)	b.i.d.	B.i.d. formulation reduces diarrhea
azithromycin (Zithromax)	qd	Suspension can be given without regard for food, but capsules cannot; useful if penicillin-allergic
clarithromycin (Biaxin)	b.i.d.	Well tolerated; useful if penicillin-allergic
cefpodoxime (Vantin)	b.i.d.	Broad-spectrum, but bitter taste
cefuroxime (Ceftin)	b.i.d.	Broad-spectrum, but bitter taste
Special use antibiotics		
clindamycin (Cleocin)	t.i.d.	Superb for anaerobes and pneumococcus
cefixime (Suprax)	qd	Superb for *H. influenzae*; 20 percent to 30 percent GI upset
doxycycline (Vibramycin)	b.i.d.	Superb sinus penetration; age 9 years and older

TMP-SMX, trimethoprim-sulfamethoxazole; GI, gastrointestinal.

refractory symptoms, but the duration of any carryover benefit is unknown.

Prophylactic antibiotics should be considered for children who have three or more recurrences over 6 months, or four or more episodes annually (same criteria as for otitis media). Amoxicillin or sulfisoxazole are administered nightly at one-half the usual daily dosage for 2 months or longer; extended-spectrum drugs may also be used, but their safety for long-term use is unconfirmed. Prophylaxis is *not recommended* for children in group day care because of an increased risk for multidrug-resistant *S. pneumoniae.* The efficacy of prophylaxis for recurrent sinusitis is at present unsupported by randomized, controlled trials.

Adjuvant medical therapy for sinusitis may promote symptom relief, but efficacy has not been shown in placebo controlled clinical trials. Consequently, I advise a minimalist approach in this area. Topical decongestants are used up to 3 days for acute intranasal edema, but decongestants should be given systemically if they are required for longer periods. Antihistamines are contraindicated because they thicken secretions and impair ciliary activity. In contrast, children who have concurrent allergic rhinitis may benefit from judicious use of antihistamines or topical nasal steroid sprays. Mucolytics offer unproved benefits and are not routinely prescribed. Saline sprays or steam inhalations may be used if the patient finds them beneficial.

Step 3: Adenoidectomy

Enlightened medical therapy will help some, but not all, children who have refractory sinusitis. Unfortunately, many children are either intolerant or allergic to more than a single class of antibiotic, and parents may be hesitant about the near-continuous use of medications to control symptoms. These children are candidates for step 3, adenoidectomy. Although there is no consensus on the timing of adenoidectomy in relation to endoscopic surgery, I recommend performing adenoidectomy before FESS for children who meet the criteria listed in Table 3.

The efficacy of adenoidectomy for refractory sinusitis is widely debated, but a relationship is probable. Longitudinal studies show a 70 percent cure or improvement of symptoms following surgery, with stable results for at least 12 months. The improvement seen after adenoidectomy most likely reflects a physiologic effect on the nasopharyngeal microflora, with a reduction in bacterial pathogens and an increase in commensal organisms. Adenoid vegetations provide a safe haven for pathogenic bacteria, which then have ready access to sinus ostia during periods of compromised mucociliary function (e.g., URI, flareups of allergic rhinitis or asthma). Presumably for sinusitis, as for otitis media, the adenoids do not have to be hyperplastic to adversely affect the paranasal sinuses.

The goals of adenoidectomy are to reduce bacterial reservoir by creating a smooth posterior nasopharyngeal wall, and to relieve choanal obstruction by precise removal of obstructing tissue and intranasal adenoid tags. To achieve these goals, the surgeon must visualize the nasopharynx and posterior choanae during surgery with either a mirror or an endoscope after initial curettage; digital palpation alone is insufficient. The St. Clair-Thompson adenoid forceps is an ideal instrument for directed removal of choanal or intranasal adenoid tissue. Any final remnants of tissue are cauterized using the monopolar suction cautery. I have not found any benefit to the carbon dioxide laser or powered microdebrider for routine adenoidectomy.

While the child is under anesthesia for adenoidectomy, sinus endoscopy may be performed to gain additional prognostic information in the event that FESS is eventually required. Particular attention is directed to the patency of the maxillary sinus natural ostium, and to the presence of any anatomic malformations that would predispose to ostiomeatal obstruction. When preoperative sinus imaging shows opacification of the maxillary sinus or an air-fluid level, antral lavage via inferior meatal puncture may be performed concurrently with adenoidectomy. Before attempted irrigation, however, a CT scan should be obtained to rule out antral hypoplasia as the source of opacification.

Step 4: Endoscopic Surgery

Approximately 20 percent of children who come to the otolaryngologist with refractory sinusitis may ultimately be candidates for endoscopic surgery. Indications for FESS are listed in Table 4. Note that the CT scan is performed *only* after 2 or more weeks of the use of an extended-spectrum antibiotic to minimize false-positive readings caused by edema or untreated acute infection. When a child comes for evaluation with a CT scan already in hand, the parents should be asked about treatment and symptoms at the time the scan was performed. If the child had incomplete antibiotic therapy or a URI, the scan should be repeated.

The goals of FESS are to (1) eliminate foci of residual disease that may cause reinfection or relapse; (2) relieve ostiomeatal complex obstruction; and (3) correct anatomic anomalies that may interfere with sinus drainage, such as an air cell within the middle turbinate (concha bullosa), or an enlarged infraorbital cell obstructing maxillary sinus drainage (Haller cell). Using the criteria for FESS in Table 4, I have observed an 85 percent to 90 percent chance of meeting or exceeding parental expectations and a 50 percent chance of exceeding them at 12 months postsurgical follow-up. All children I have treated with FESS experienced a reduction in their major sinusitis symptoms after FESS, but complete symptom relief was seen in only 33 percent. Therefore, FESS should be undertaken with caution when families define a successful outcome as complete resolution of all major symptoms.

Successful FESS in children requires conservatism, gentle tissue handling, and familiarity with the small confines of the pediatric ethmoid cavity. Ethmoid width increases in a roughly linear fashion from age 2 years to age 16 years, expanding anteriorly from 4 mm to 8 mm and posteriorly from 6 mm to 11 mm. During the same period, the ethmoid height also increases, but less dramatically. Septoplasty is rarely necessary for ethmoid access in children younger than 10 years of age, but may be necessary in older children or adolescents. An obstructing concha bullosa is treated by bivalving the turbinate and excising the lateral lamina.

FESS begins with uncinectomy performed from inferior to superior using a disposable myringotomy knife. The natural ostium of the maxillary sinus is identified with an angled telescope, and is enlarged, if stenotic, by incising the posterior fontanel; a backbiter is not used because of proximity to the nasolacrimal duct. Ethmoidectomy begins by removing the ethmoid bulla and its contents. The ground lamella is then penetrated, and the posterior ethmoid cells are examined. If no disease is encountered, the surgery ends at this point. Otherwise, the posterior skull base is identified, and ethmoidectomy is completed from posterior to anterior. Finally, the agger nasi cells are cleaned retrograde while the anterior skull base is visualized. Manipulation of the frontal recess or sphenoid sinus is generally not required. A rolled Gelfilm stent is placed in the ethmoid cavity, with care not to occlude the maxillary ostium.

After surgery an extended-spectrum antibiotic and saline spray are used for 3 weeks while the Gelfilm absorbs. I have not found any benefit to routine debridement under anesthesia after 2 weeks; I abandoned this technique several years ago, although it continues to remain popular. Intranasal manipulation in the office is limited to removing any large obstructing clots or debris from the vestibule or anterior nasal cavity. When the course of antibiotics has been completed, a topical nasal steroid spray is given for 3 additional weeks to resolve any mucosal edema.

Table 3. Indications for Adenoidectomy

1. Refractory symptoms despite primary control efforts, AND
2. Refractory symptoms despite use of therapeutic or prophylactic antibiotics, AND
3. Obstructive, hyperplastic, or infected adenoid vegetations seen on endoscopic examination, CT scan, or lateral radiograph, AND
4. No overt or submucous cleft palate, AND
5. Realistic parental expectations

Table 4. Indications for Functional Endoscopic Sinus Surgery

1. Refractory symptoms despite adenoidectomy if hyperplastic, obstructing, or infected adenoid vegetations were initially present, AND
2. CT evidence of chronic sinus disease, ostiomeatal complex obstruction, or anatomic malformations associated with sinusitis, AND
3. Discussion of proposed surgery with child's primary care practitioner, allergist, and pulmonologist, AND
4. Commitment by surgeon to follow up the child for at least 12 months after surgery, AND
5. Realistic parental expectations and understanding of potential complications

SINUSITIS IN SPECIAL CHILDREN

Children who have asthma are prone to sinusitis, and occult sinusitis should be suspected whenever the asthma becomes difficult to control. Although comparative studies are lacking, most parents report better control of their child's baseline asthma symptoms following appropriately indicated FESS. Inhalant allergies are generally present and must be managed concurrently.

Chronic sinusitis is highly prevalent in Down syndrome, but surgical results are disappointing. Sinonasal symptoms tend to persist because of nasal edema, chronic nasal secretions, and a shallow nasopharynx with minimal adenoid tissue. Therefore, adenoidectomy or FESS should be undertaken only with appropriately pessimistic parental expectations. Growth and development combined with gradual immune maturation are often more effective than surgery for long-term control.

Nasal polyps are rare in young children and should prompt a sweat test for cystic fibrosis. The presentation of cystic fibrosis includes characteristic CT findings of pansinusitis, with bilateral medial displacement of the lateral nasal wall and uncinate process demineralization. Conservative FESS is indicated for obstructive or expansile symptoms, but disease recurrence and revision surgery must be anticipated. Unilateral nasal polyps with a negative sweat test suggest an antral-choanal polyp or allergic fungal sinusitis.

Children with a hypoplastic maxillary sinus often have refractory symptoms. CT imaging shows reduced antral volume, with a hypoplastic or laterally displaced uncinate process. FESS is indicated, but may be technically challenging because of a concave lateral nasal wall. Care must be taken during uncinectomy so as not to inadvertently enter the inferior orbit. Success rates are also lower than for nonhypoplastic sinuses, so parental expectations should be tempered accordingly.

■ DISCUSSION

Management decisions in treating pediatric sinusitis must balance disease burden against the emotional concerns of children and their parents. Disease burden has been previously discussed, but emotional needs have not been mentioned. Considering that most parental decisions involve some degree of emotion, the practitioner who focuses solely on logic will be at a disadvantage. Most emotional concerns relate to the real or perceived complications of alternative interventions.

Sporadic use of antibiotics is safe and effective, but repetitive or prolonged use may result in gastric upset, drug allergies, or accelerated bacterial resistance. Multidrug-resistant pneumococcus is a global problem, related in part to antibiotic exposure and horizontal transmission of bacteria in group day care settings. Anesthesia is an emotional word, but nonetheless extremely safe; adverse outcomes occur in only 1:20,000 to 1:50,000 of uncomplicated cases. Access to dedicated pediatric anesthesia services can help minimize risk, particularly when young children are involved. Educational videotapes and presurgical hospital visits may reduce child anxiety about anesthesia or surgery.

Adenoidectomy is extremely safe and well tolerated, with significant bleeding observed in fewer than 1:500 cases. Regrowth of tissue is uncommon when remnants are removed under direct visualization as described previously. Despite widespread parental concerns about a detrimental impact of adenoidectomy on the immune system, longitudinal studies have never shown significant immunosuppression or an increased tendency to infection after the adenoids are removed. Parents must understand that adenoidectomy is not a cure-all for refractory sinusitis, and that 20 percent to 30 percent of children may have persistent symptoms despite surgery.

Endoscopic surgery is also a safe and well-tolerated intervention. In most reported series, the incidence of major complications (orbital injury or a cerebrospinal fluid leak) is 1 percent or less for primary surgery. Revision surgery carries additional risk, but is necessary in less than 5 percent of children. Risk, however, is always a comparative issue; sinusitis is a closed-space infection that may cause suppurative orbital or intracranial complications (including blindness) *without* surgical intervention. Surgical risk is minimized through appropriate training and experience. Surgeons must be honest with parents (and themselves) regarding their level of comfort when operating in the pediatric ethmoid cavity.

Suggested Reading

Lee D, Rosenfeld RM. Sinonasal symptoms and adenoid bacteriology. Otolaryngol Head Neck Surg 1997; 116:301-307.

Lindbaek M, Hjortdahl P, Johnsen ULH. Randomized, double blind, placebo controlled trial of penicillin C and amoxycillin in treatment of acute sinus infection in adults. Br Med J 1996; 313:325-329.

Lusk RP, ed. Pediatric sinusitis. New York: Raven Press, 1992.

Otten FWA, van Aarem A, Grote JJ. Long-term follow-up of chronic maxillary sinusitis in children. Intl J Pediatr Otorhinolaryngol 1991; 22:81-84.

Rosenfeld RM. Pilot study of outcomes in pediatric rhinosinusitis. Arch Otolaryngol Head Neck Surg 1995; 121:729-736.

Wald ER, Chiponis D, Ledesma-Medina J. Comparative effectiveness of amoxicillin and amoxicillin-clavulanate potassium in acute paranasal sinus infections in children: A double-blind placebo-controlled trial. Pediatrics 1986; 77:795-800.

ORBITAL CELLULITIS AND ABSCESS

The method of
Scott C. Manning

Periorbital inflammation is principally a pediatric problem: approximately 80 percent of cases occur in patients under age 20. The term *orbital cellulitis* describes a wide range of clinical conditions, and therefore no single treatment approach is sufficient to cover all patients.

The starting point for formulating a treatment plan is with an anatomic assessment of the location of the inflammation. The most common form of orbital inflammation is preseptal cellulitis or infection limited to the soft tissue anterior to the periorbita. By definition, these patients do not have orbital signs such as proptosis. Preseptal cellulitis is most common in young children with mean ages in reported series usually around 2.5 years. Before 1988, the most common cause of preseptal cellulitis was *Haemophilus influenzae* type b (HIB) septicemia, but this organism is now rarely cultured due to the success of the HIB vaccine. At present, a majority of patients with preseptal cellulitis have negative results from blood cultures, but when cultures are positive, *Streptococcus pneumoniae* has emerged as the most common organism. In addition to septicemia, other potential causes of preseptal cellulitis include cutaneous injury, blunt trauma, or conjunctivitis. In patients who have cutaneous injury, *Staphylococcus aureus* and beta-hemolytic streptococci are the most common organisms cultured (Table 1).

Inflammation behind the orbital septum is characterized by physical signs including chemosis, proptosis, and gaze restriction. Progression of disease can lead to loss of vision via ischemia due to either increased intraocular pressure or septic thrombophlebitis of orbital vessels. Postseptal inflammation can be divided into infection outside the muscle cone or orbital periosteum and infection inside the cone. The most common form of extraconal infection is medial subperiosteal phlegmon or abscess, which is caused by extension of bacteria from adjacent ethmoid sinusitis, either directly or along vascular channels. In reported series of subperiosteal orbital abscesses, adjacent sinusitis is present in 50 percent to 80 percent of patients. Dental infections can also ascend directly through the maxillary sinus to the orbital floor.

Intraconal or true orbital abscesses are caused by direct extension of subperiosteal disease, penetrating injury, or septic thromboemboli. These infections are the rarest and most severe forms of orbital inflammation and have significant rates of permanent visual loss. Cavernous sinus thrombosis can rarely result from further extension of infection along valveless orbital veins. Patients who have this condition exhibit massive proptosis and a fixed globe.

Table 1. Microbiology of Orbital Inflammation

Preseptal Cellulitis
- Septicemia: *Streptococcus pneumoniae*
  - *Haemophilus influenzae* type b (if unvaccinated)
- Cutaneous lesion or trauma: Staphylococci
  - Streptococci

Postseptal Inflammation: Age <9 yr
- Streptococci

Postseptal Inflammation: Age >9 yr
- Mixed polymicrobial infection
  - Aerobes: Streptococci—alpha- and beta-hemolytic
    - Staphylococci
    - *Haemophilus influenzae*
  - Anaerobes: *Bacteroides*
    - *Peptostreptococcus*
    - *Fusobacterium*
    - *Eikenella corrodens*
    - Microaerophilic streptococci

RADIOGRAPHIC AND OPHTHALMOLOGIC ASSESSMENT

Patients who have preseptal infection do not need imaging unless the disease progresses. Likewise, patients who have postseptal infection without advanced signs such as visual loss are generally not imaged unless their disease progresses despite systemic antibiotics. Patients who present with or progress to massive proptosis, significant visual loss, or severe discomfort should be imaged, and generally computed tomography (CT) is selected because of its ability to image both bone and soft tissue. Magnetic resonance imaging may have a role in the future in trying to distinguish between phlegmon and abscess, and currently this modality is superior for demonstrating intracranial complications such as cerebritis, subdural empyema or cavernous sinus thrombosis.

Unfortunately, CT is not very sensitive in determining the point of tissue liquefaction and abscess formation. Therefore, most surgical series report a significant false-negative rate of CT abscess diagnosis. Absence of a definite abscess on CT scan should not justify delaying a decision for surgical therapy in the face of deteriorating orbital signs. Gas within the mass effect indicates a definite abscess, but this is a relatively unusual finding. Central low density with surrounding enhancement is the most common finding associated with surgically proven abscesses, but pus may appear anywhere along a spectrum of low to high density with CT.

Because of the difficulty in positioning young patients, axial views are generally obtained first and are adequate for defining medial subperiosteal inflammation. Depending on the spacing between views, superior and inferior subperiosteal abscesses may be missed. Coronal views should be obtained whenever possible in any patient scheduled for surgical drainage in order to define the anatomy from the surgeon's perspective and image any inflammation that may have been missed on axial views. Sinus CT imaging is not adequate for ruling out intracranial complications; patients who have neurologic signs such as lethargy, severe headaches, seizures, or focal signs should undergo formal head imaging.

Every patient presenting with significant postseptal signs, including proptosis and gaze restriction, should have a complete ophthalmic assessment that includes visual acuity and a fundus examination. From a practical standpoint, it is extremely difficult, and at times impossible, to obtain an accurate visual acuity in ill children and to obtain a fundus examination in an awake child who has massive lid edema. This fact obviously may render moot the common adage of obtaining serial eye examinations every few hours in order to assess response to antibiotic therapy in patients who have severe disease. Therefore, some authors now recommend emergent CT imaging for patients who have severe periorbital edema when a fundus examination cannot be performed.

■ MEDICAL THERAPY

The management of orbital inflammation is presented in Figure 1.

Preseptal Cellulitis

Young patients who have no cutaneous lid lesions, conjunctivitis, or trauma history should be treated with antibiotics appropriate for streptococcal organisms. Staphylococcal coverage should be added for patients who have skin lesions or trauma history. Blood cultures are usually obtained, but lumbar puncture is generally reserved for high-risk patients, which is defined by (1) age less than 2 months, (2) meningeal or focal neurologic signs, or (3) clinical toxicity. Patients who have mild infection are sometimes managed as outpatients, usually with intramuscular antibiotics such as ceftriaxone.

According to retrospective series data, oral antibiotics do not change the course of serious infection. Preseptal cellulitis in a large majority of young patients will resolve rapidly with medical therapy. Failure to respond or progression to postseptal inflammation should prompt radiographic assessment for adjacent sinusitis and hospital admission.

Postseptal Inflammation: Age Under 9 Years

The ideal antibiotic regimen for postseptal orbital inflammation should cover streptococcal and staphylococcal aerobic organisms, as well as anaerobic organisms, including *Bacteroides* sp.; the antibiotic should also effectively cross the blood-brain barrier. In practice, initial antibiotic therapy can be focused according to the patient's age and clinical severity at presentation. Harris has shown that when results are positive, cultures in children under age 9 who have subperiosteal orbital abscesses generally yield a single aerobic organism, most commonly a streptococcus. This author recommends initial antibiotic therapy with ceftriaxone sodium (50 mg per kg per day given once daily intramuscularly or intravenously for children), which is a third-generation cephalosporin that has excellent penetration across the blood-brain barrier. Another single-drug regimen recommended by some authors is ampicillin-sulbactam, which should cover potentially resistant *Haemophilus influenzae, Moraxella catarrhalis, Staphylococcus aureus,* and *Bacteroides fragilis* organisms. In areas with a high incidence of penicillin-resistant *Streptococcus pneumoniae,* clindamycin should be added to initial therapy.

Postseptal Inflammation: Age 9 Years or Older

Harris's studies show that (1) the likelihood of culturing multiple organisms, including anaerobes, increases with increasing age, and (2) mixed infection is almost always the case in patients over age 15 years who have subperiosteal orbital abscesses. Polymicrobial infections with aerobes and anaerobes allow for synergy, because aerobes consume oxygen, which creates an environment conducive to anaerobic growth and anaerobes produce β-lactamase, which renders generalized resistance to many antibiotics. Mixed infections in older children and adults are therefore more difficult to treat and more likely to require surgical drainage. The risk of intracranial suppurative complications secondary to sinusitis is also greatest in teenagers. Initial antibiotic coverage must therefore encompass aerobes including alpha-hemolytic streptococci (with consideration of *S. pneumoniae* penicillin resistance); beta-hemolytic streptococci, including groups A, B, and D; staphylococci; and anaerobes, including *Bacteroides* sp., *Peptostreptococcus, Fusobacterium* sp., *Eikenella corrodens,* and microaerophilic streptococci. Whenever possible, antibiotics with superior blood-brain barrier penetration should be chosen.

One common treatment regimen for postseptal orbital inflammation in older patients consists of clindamycin plus ceftriaxone. Clindamycin adds coverage for most anaerobes and is excellent for staphylococci and resistant *S. pneumoniae.* Unfortunately, it does not cross the blood-brain barrier well. The ceftriaxone plus clindamycin regimen appears to be replacing the older chloramphenicol plus nafcillin or oxacillin regimen in many institutions because it offers excellent coverage without the concern for aplastic anemia that chloramphenicol poses. For initial therapy of orbital inflammation of suspected dental origin, some authors recommend penicillin plus metronidazole. Obviously, the ultimate antibiotic choice depends on culture and sensitivity and response to therapy.

Intraconal Inflammation and Cavernous Sinus Thrombosis

Emergent medical therapy for massive proptosis due to intraconal inflammation or cavernous sinus thrombosis may include medications to reduce intraocular pressure such as mannitol and β-adrenergic blockers. Cavernous sinus thrombosis classically manifests as progression of orbital inflammation to pronounced chemosis, ophthalmoplegia, and eventual involvement of the contralateral eye. In addition to broad-spectrum intravenous antibiotics that have good central nervous system penetration, some authors recommend anticoagulation therapy with heparin and also intravenous steroids, although the latter treatment remains controversial.

■ SURGICAL THERAPY

Preseptal Cellulitis

Surgery is not indicated for inflammation anterior to the orbital septum, with the rare exception of necrotizing infection requiring debridement of the eyelids. Necrotizing cellulitis is generally caused by mixed infections, including streptococcal organisms, and the risk is greatest in patients who

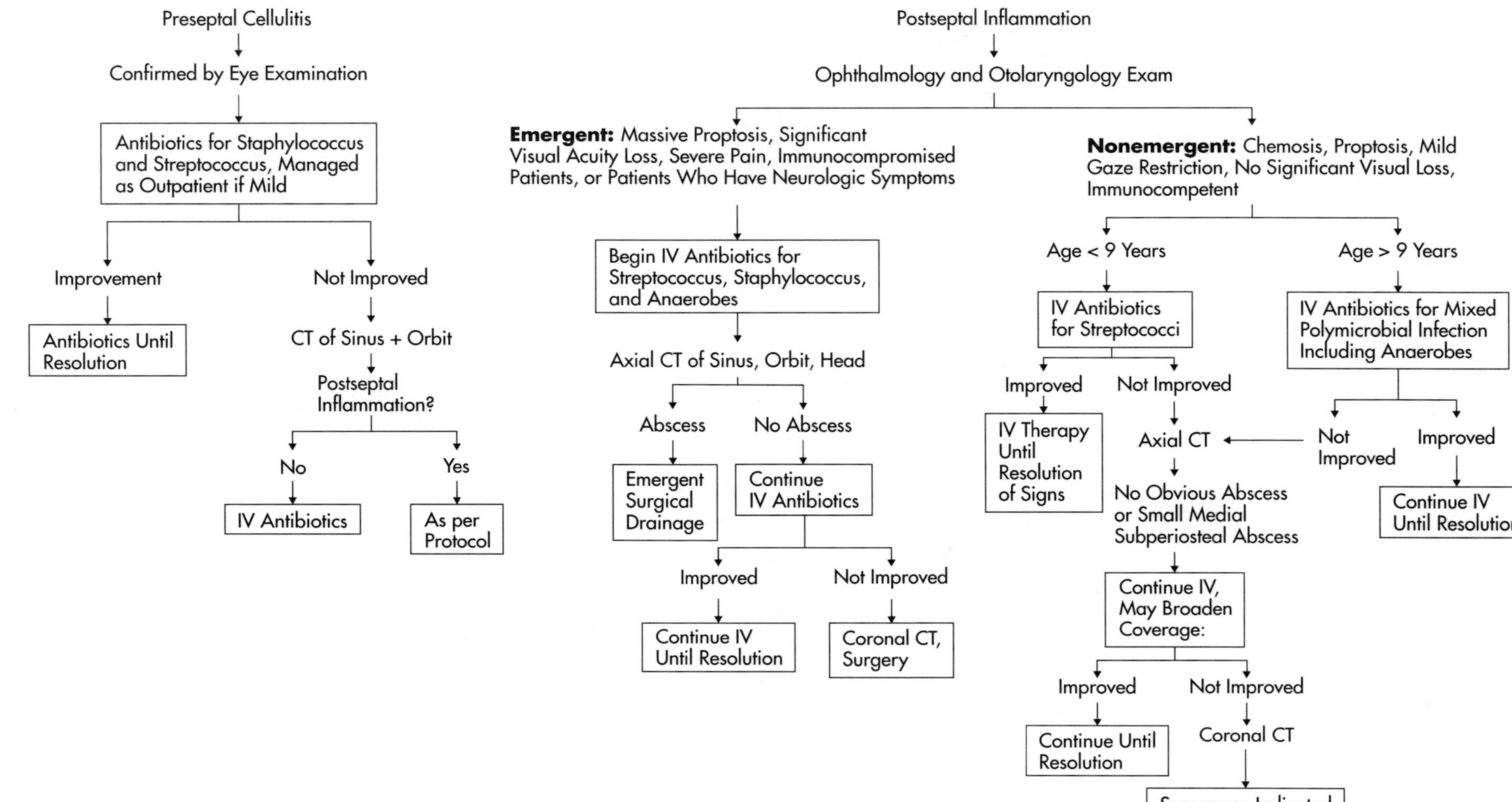

Figure 1.
Algorithm for management of orbital inflammation. CT, computed tomography; IV, intravenous.

have systemic diseases, including measles, diabetes, or alcoholism. Penicillin G remains the drug of choice for infections caused by group A beta-hemolytic streptococci.

Postseptal Inflammation: Age Less Than 9 Years

The large majority of young patients who present with orbital cellulitis with signs of proptosis and chemosis have normal or near-normal vision and minimal gaze restriction. These patients are initially treated with parenteral antibiotics; a decision for CT imaging is based on progression of signs or lack of improvement over 36 hours. For most of these patients, their disease will resolve with antibiotic therapy alone. A minority of patients will have a more severe clinical picture, and indications for emergent imaging include suspicion of intracranial inflammation based on neurologic symptoms, evidence of blindness or retinal ischemia, and severe discomfort, including deep-seated retro-orbital, vertex, or occipital headache. Indications for emergent surgery include CT evidence of an intraconal orbital abscess, massive proptosis with retinal or optic nerve ischemia and loss of vision (drainage of subperiosteal abscess and/or lateral canthotomy), and visual acuity of 20/60 or less in an immunocompromised patient (diabetes) who has a subperiosteal abscess.

When computed tomography demonstrates a probable subperiosteal abscess, most authors advocate immediate surgical drainage, including the adjacent sinus. However, a few series have reported resolution of disease with intravenous antibiotics alone (usually for 2 to 3 weeks) in patients who have small medial subperiosteal orbital abscesses. Harris reported that up to 25 percent of patients under age 9 years who had CT evidence of subperiosteal abscess can be adequately treated with antibiotics alone. Arguments in favor of medical treatment of small abscesses include the concern that surgery might potentially seed intracranial abscesses and the desire to avoid facial scars. The latter concern is potentially addressed by an endoscopic rather than an external ethmoidectomy approach to medial subperiosteal abscesses.

Postseptal Inflammation: Age Greater Than 9 Years

If CT obtained because of severe initial signs or progression of disease demonstrates a subperiosteal abscess, Harris has shown that the likelihood of resolution with a prolonged course of intravenous antibiotics decreases from approximately 10 percent in the 9- to 15-year-old age group to close to 0 percent in patients older than 15 years. One explanation for this finding, in addition to the high incidence of refractory polymicrobial infection in the older age group, might be the finding of some surgeons that the older patients often have significant ethmoid polyposis contributing to sinus obstruction.

The normal development of the maxillary sinus brings it in contact with maxillary molar tooth roots by age 12 years on average; therefore, dental infection becomes a significant predisposing factor for periorbital inflammation in this age group. A thorough dental examination should be a part of the initial evaluation of all patients, with appropriate dental radiographs as indicated. Drainage of the maxillary sinus with removal of the abscessed molar is necessary when treating severe orbital inflammation of dental origin.

Extraconal Subperiosteal Abscesses

The large majority of orbital abscesses are located in the medial orbital subperiosteal space adjacent to ethmoid sinusitis. The traditional approach to drainage of these abscesses has been via an external ethmoidectomy approach, but many authors are now reporting series of patients undergoing intranasal approaches. The endoscopic technique that I prefer offers the advantages of avoidance of facial scars and more rapid resolution of periorbital inflammation with shorter hospital stays. The principal disadvantage is the difficulty of performing endoscopic sinus surgery within the smaller confines of pediatric noses in the face of acute inflammation and increased potential for bleeding. Endoscopic drainage of medial subperiosteal abscesses should only be performed by surgeons who are experienced with endoscopic ethmoidectomy in pediatric patients.

The technique is that of a standard endoscopic ethmoidectomy, with the addition of removal of a portion of the lamina papyracea in order to ensure drainage of the medial subperiosteal space. Slow and deliberate technique, with frequent pauses to place oxymetazoline-soaked cottonoids, is necessary in order to maintain adequate visualization. Microdebrider power instruments can be extremely helpful in minimizing tissue trauma and bleeding from inflamed mucosa. Often, the only view of the abscess that the surgeon obtains is a glimpse of pus as the ethmoidectomy is completed. Once the lamina is well visualized, gentle pressure on the globe will demonstrate any cracks or natural dehiscences in the lamina. I remove a portion of the lamina at the site of the abscess with a blunt right-angled hook and then visualize white periorbita through the defect in order to confirm drainage of the subperiosteal space. All ipsilateral infected sinuses are also endoscopically drained at the time of abscess drainage.

When abscesses are successfully drained via this technique, patients usually experience dramatic improvement of their proptosis, chemosis, and lid edema within 12 hours. Failure to improve should prompt repeat imaging. Depending on the experience of the surgeon, medial inferior subperiosteal abscesses can also be successfully managed endoscopically. However, superior and lateral infection must be approached with open techniques.

Intraconal Orbital Abscesses

Intraconal orbital abscesses are ocular emergencies with a significant risk of permanent visual loss, even when managed aggressively. Lateral canthotomy surgery may be necessary in the face of massive proptosis with retinal ischemia. I enlist the help of an experienced ophthalmologist whenever draining the orbit inside the muscle cone; specific approaches depend on the location of the abscess. The orbit is approached via transconjunctival incisions, with endoscopic sinus techniques reserved for drainage of ipsilateral sinusitis.

Suggested Reading

Brook I, Frazier EH. Microbiology of subperiosteal orbital abscess and associated maxillary sinusitis. Laryngoscope 1996; 106:1010-1013.

Harris GJ. Subperiosteal abscess of the orbit. Ophthalmology 1994; 101: 585-595.

Patt BS, Manning SC. Blindness resulting from orbital complications of sinusitis. Otolaryngol Head Neck Surg 1991; 104:789-795.

CHRONIC ETHMOID SINUSITIS

The method of
Reuben C. Setliff III

Although the perception of the anatomy of the ethmoid bone is one of infinite complexity, the reality is that the basic components are in fact only four: the ethmoidal bulla, the agger nasi cell(s), the sinus lateralis, and the posterior ethmoid cells. The former two components represent the bulk of what is known as the anterior ethmoid complex. The sinus lateralis is not a cell, but a space of quite variable location and dimensions posterior to the bulla. It may be thought of as a pneumatized portion of the basal lamella, a lateral reflection of bone from the middle turbinate to the lamina papyracea and the bony reference used to divide anterior from posterior cells. The variation in the configuration of the basal lamella is largely a function of the location and extent of the sinus lateralis. The basal lamella may be pneumatized in any combination of the four quadrants of its vertical portion. The inferior horizontal portion of the basal lamella is not so pneumatized.

All of the aforementioned in conjunction with the uncinate process, lamina papyracea, middle turbinate, and portions of the skull base are, to the anatomist, one, and only one, bone: the ethmoid bone. The variations on the basic architecture of the ethmoid bone, as any experienced endoscopist will confirm, are almost legion and may be further altered by the disease process. Consequently, the surgical anatomy defies a predictable configuration, allowing only generalizations about surgical landmarks. However, the components of the surgical anatomy of the ethmoid bone are, although variable in configuration, constant enough that an anatomic dissection is both possible and desirable.

The variations in the sinus lateralis and basal lamella have been addressed. The ethmoidal bulla may be single or tiered. It may or may not have a back wall in addition to the basal lamella posteriorly. The agger nasi, the most anterior and superior cell of the basic architecture, may also be tiered, and, more important, it may pneumatize the frontal bone as well. Cells from either the anterior or posterior complex, if one considers the drainage pattern, may pneumatize the middle and/or superior turbinate. A variation of posterior ethmoid cellular development is a pneumatized extension beyond the face of and over the sphenoid sinus, the Onodi cell.

The boundaries of the anterior and posterior ethmoid complex are the lamina papyracea laterally, the skull base superiorly, and the middle turbinate medially. Absent the Onodi cell, the face of the sphenoid sinus is the posterior limit of the complex. If the skull base is dissected, neurovascular bundles, both anterior and posterior, may be seen traversing the skull base from medial to lateral. The drainage for the frontal sinus is frequently found immediately anterior to the anterior ethmoid bundle.

Spaces relating to the ethmoid are the middle meatus, the hiatus semilunaris, the infundibulum, the hiatus semilunaris posterior, the superior meatus, the sphenoethmoid recess, and the space into which the frontal sinus drains. The infundibulum is a three-dimensional space anterior to the ethmoidal bulla and bounded otherwise by the lamina papyracea laterally and the uncinate process medially. The hiatus semilunaris is a two-dimensional space defining the most medial extent of the infundibulum between the bulla and the posteromedial extent of the uncinate process.

The hiatus semilunaris posterior is bounded by the medial wall of the bulla, the lateral aspect of the middle turbinate, and the vertical portion of the basal lamella posteriorly. The superior meatus is a recess beneath and lateral to the superior turbinate. The sphenoethmoid recess is a space of varying dimensions at the most posterior extent of the interface between the middle turbinate and the nasal septum The most common drainage pattern for the sphenoid sinus is into the sphenoethmoid recess. Although the ultimate drainage for the frontal sinus is dictated by the insertion of the uncinate process superiorly, the most common pattern of egress from the frontal sinus is into the space posterior and medial to the agger nasi cell.

PATHOGENESIS

Even though honest observers may differ about the aforementioned designations and definitions, there is now little argument about the location of the initiating event in the pathogenesis of sinusitis. The location is anterior with respect to the ethmoid bone, and, as will be discussed, most likely in the infundibulum and/or the hiatus semilunaris posterior. The sinuses most often involved early in the disease process are, as expected, the anterior ethmoid and maxillary sinuses. Seldom do the posterior ethmoid or the sphenoid sinuses initiate difficulty and clinically seem to be reluctant participants in the disease process.

One possible explanation for the difference in susceptibility between the anterior and posterior sinuses is to be found in the marked difference in their respective drainage patterns. The posterior sinuses have the luxury of a direct entry into the nose, the posterior ethmoid via the superior meatus, and the sphenoid into the sphenoethmoid recess. By contrast, both the maxillary and ethmoidal bulla drain into transition spaces that subsequently empty into the nose. The transition space for the maxillary sinus is the infundibulum. For the ethmoidal bulla, drainage in most instances exits from a posterior and medial opening into the hiatus semilunaris posterior before it actually enters the nasal cavity.

Another way to underscore the significant difference in the entry of the anterior and posterior sinuses is that the openings for the sphenoid and posterior ethmoid sinuses may be visualized by simple endoscopy, which is in marked contrast to the hidden entry of their anterior neighbors. In the absence of a more plausible theory of the pathogenesis of sinusitis, the transition spaces of the anterior sinuses (the infundibulum and hiatus semilunaris posterior), and not the sinuses themselves or even their ostia, may well be the location of the initiating event and thus the cause of the difficulty. If an extension of this theory includes, in most instances, that the disease within the sinuses is not end-stage and thus not deserving of removal, surgery limited to the elimination of the transition spaces may well suffice, even in the presence of advanced pathology The anterior sinuses would then enjoy the direct entry of the less susceptible posterior sinuses. Removal of the posterior-medial wall of the agger nasi cell serves the same purpose for the frontal sinus.

PREOPERATIVE PREPARATION

Selecting the patient for sinus surgery is more a function of the art and not the science of medicine. Most otolaryngologists who formerly hoped that the information on the computed tomographic (CT) scan of the sinuses would make the decision an objective one now know that the information factored into the decision to operate or not must be ultimately obtained from the patient. Although many variables must be considered, two final determinations are decisive: (1) Is the patient miserable enough, or is the situation dire enough to justify operative intervention? (2) Are medical options no longer attractive, or have they been exhausted, or does the situation preclude resolution via conservative measures? Under this model, CT scan is essential for the actual surgical intervention, and it is considered a bonus if there is good correlation with the clinical findings.

The preparation of the patient before going to the operative suite is critical to both the patient's and the surgeon's experience. Inquiry regarding the ingestion of salicylates and/or nonsteroidal anti-inflammatories should be made enough in advance to allow a 10 to 14 day abstention.

Local Anesthesia and Hemostasis

I use serial 0.05 percent oxymetazoline sprays followed by serial sprays of a 10 percent cocaine and 1:1,000 (1:50,000 when delivered as spray to patient) epinephrine mix. The combination delivers both a profound vasoconstriction and topical anesthesia, and no significant systemic responses have been observed in either children or adults. The surgeon enjoys an immediate access to the nasal cavity under local or general anesthesia and can begin surgery without a "pack and wait" interval.

There appears to be no valid argument to support anything more than a theoretic advantage for operating in a sitting or a standing position. Neither is there a conclusive argument that operating off the monitor or through the endoscope is more beneficial for patient or surgeon. Better arguments obtain, particularly in ethmoid surgery, for implementing a variety of measures to minimize bleeding. They include both a hypotensive technique and a low end-tidal CO_2 when operating under general anesthesia.

Other measures apply to both local sedation and general anesthesia cases and include care not to traumatize the septum or lateral nasal wall when introducing the needle for injections. In most instances, leading with the needle in advance of the endoscope obviates this concern. Lateral wall injections of limited number and not along the path to the middle meatus are also helpful. Leaving mucous membrane at the limits of the dissection serves the dual purpose of reducing both bleeding and the healing burden for the patient. Where feasible in general anesthesia cases, early extubation will reduce immediate postoperative blood loss.

SURGICAL TECHNIQUE

The actual surgical technique delivered is the result of the combination of the surgeon's philosophy and the chosen instrumentation. Both will impact the degree of bleeding during the procedure. As mentioned, if mucous membrane of any degree of pathology is retained in lieu of the exposure of bare bone, both the amount of bleeding and the healing burden of the patient are reduced. Instrumentation, such as powered instrumentation, which delivers both precision and real-time suction brings advantages not available otherwise.

A precision cutting technique has obvious advantages over the traditional "grab and tear" approach coupled with the burden of removing all diseased tissue. I have no experience with the recently available "cutting" instruments.

Advances in both visualization and instrumentation have brought the issue of the necessary extent of sinus surgery to the forefront. The issue is especially applicable to intervention in the ethmoid complex. If ethmoid sinus disease begins in the hiatus semilunaris posterior, removal of the medial wall of the ethmoidal bulla eliminates the transition space of the bulla and provides direct entry into the nasal cavity. The removal must extend posteriorly to include marsupialization of the opening from the bulla into the hiatus semilunaris posterior. If the bulla is tiered, there may be an opening for each cell. Absent the cause of the disease, progressive improvement may then be expected without the necessity of removing all diseased tissue from the bulla. Surgery is therefore directed toward the cause of the disease rather than the disease itself.

Agger Nasi

Surgery for disease in the other component of the anterior cells, the consistently present agger nasi cell(s), is a function of removing the upper portion of the uncinate process to access the cell from below. The approach to the cell(s) is much more posterior than the location of the agger nasi would indicate by endoscopy or CT findings. The uncinate must be removed from posterior to anterior, working both superiorly and laterally. As with the maxillary sinus and ethmoidal bulla, neither the agger nasi cell nor its exit for egress may be seen at simple nasal endoscopy.

Upon entering the cell, both the opening from the cell and the space behind the posterior and medial wall can be visualized with a 30 degree endoscope. Surgery is limited to marsupialization of the cell and its outflow tract, leaving the mucous membrane intact and where indicated, removing the posterior-medial wall of the cell to open the transition space for the frontal sinus. An extended pneumatization from the agger nasi cell into the frontal bone is not unusual and may compromise frontal drainage, which dictates a more extensive removal of the posterior and medial wall.

Middle Turbinate

If the middle turbinate is pneumatized, the cell(s) are subject to the same disease processes as other ethmoid cells. In addition, nasal obstruction and compromise of drainage pathways when the turbinate is enlarged greatly are frequently present. The lateral aspect of the cell may closely contact the lateral nasal wall, uncinate process, and ethmoidal bulla. The precise removal of the lateral portion of the cell is possible without the necessity for sacrificing the bulk of the turbinate or removing the lining from the residual medial portion. The most common exit for the cell if it is completely enclosed is posterior and medial into the middle meatus or hiatus semilunaris posterior. In such cases, the marsupialization of the cell must include the opening of the outflow tract as well. However, the medial lip of the opening is retained.

Alternatively, the drainage for a pneumatized middle turbinate may be the superior meatus, in which case the lateral wall of the cell within the middle turbinate will reflect posteriorly and laterally to become the basal lamella, and the cell itself may be followed posteriorly as the most medial portion of the ethmoid complex, with egress into the superior meatus and extension posteriorly to the skull base, Surgery is thus limited to the marsupialization of the cell and retention of mucous membrane unless the basal lamella is taken down to address posterior disease.

Extensive intervention for both anterior and posterior ethmoid disease has been reported by many observers to be therapeutic. In most instances, all cells are marsupialized, all partitions are removed, and most, if not all, diseased tissue is removed. The middle turbinate is frequently sacrificed as part of the procedure, Currently, surgeons performing such extensive surgery are advising caution about extensive tissue removal with the exposure of bare bone, suggesting retention of mucous membrane along the lamina papyracea and at the base of the skull. As discussed next, an argument may be made that perhaps even less intervention than currently recommended would suffice, particularly with respect to the posterior ethmoid cells.

Posterior Cells

If the anterior cells are the first to participate in the disease process, the posterior cells are surely the last. Even in the face of extensive disease anteriorly, the posterior cells are frequently minimally diseased, if at all. The reason or reasons for the discrepancy are not clear, but the only significant difference other than the location within the skull is the direct entry of the posterior cells as opposed to the previously described entry of the anterior neighbors. The posterior cells are thus "last in" in terms of participating in the disease process. If they become involved secondarily, perhaps clearing of the disease anteriorly would reverse the process, allowing them to be "last out," thus obviating the need for surgical intervention at all. At most, intervention should be limited to the removal of secretions and/or polyps without the stripping of mucous membrane and exposure of bare bone. The limited number of cells and their relatively larger size are quite conducive to this surgical approach.

Ostia

With no evidence of a minimal threshold size for sinus openings into the nose and with abundant evidence that, in most instances, small holes function very well, respect for the ability of sinuses to function with a small outflow tract serves both patient and surgeon well. However, in the presence of fungal sinusitis, the requirement to remove all of the fungal debris, but not the underlying mucous membrane, dictates that adequate openings be made to accomplish that goal. The degree of surgery needed in such cases will vary from case to case and is a judgment decision for which no surgical guidelines exist. Secondary surgery for fungal sinusitis is the rule inasmuch as the marsupialization and removal of debris from every cell at the primary sitting is a goal seldom achieved.

Postoperative Care

The recommendations for postoperative care following surgery in the ethmoid complex are as diverse as the surgery itself. A full spectrum of postoperative management from skillful neglect with or without nasal irrigations or sprays to meticulous "clean-outs" have been reported to produce comparable results. Spacers of various types to no spacers of any kind are reported to produce equally favorable outcomes.

The minimally invasive surgical approach described in detail in prior studies (and briefly here) has been in continuous use for more than 1,500 consecutive patients since February 1993. Postoperative management consists of a Gelfilm roll in the middle meatus to be removed at 10 to 14 days. No nasal packing is used, even if a septoplasty with resection is done. Both intraoperative intravenous and postoperative intramuscular steroids are given. Irrigations with a hypertonic buffered saline solution at body temperature are begun in 24 hours in conjunction with the use of postirrigation nasal steroids. Noseblowing is allowed from the outset, and no restrictions are placed on diet or activity.

Outpatient surgery under monitored sedation is the rule when the surgery is limited as described previously. Further, most patients return to preoperative activity levels within 24 to 48 hours. There are no scheduled return visits until 10 to 14 days, which is in obvious disagreement with the early admonitions regarding the necessity for early postoperative crust removal. Early healing is to be expected and indeed occurs given the low healing burden associated with limited intervention and minimal bare bone in the surgical wound. Many patients are discharged on an as-needed status for the first postoperative visit. Apart from the presence of nasal polyposis in association with fungal disease, the necessity for secondary surgery has been reduced from 15 percent to 5 percent.

Suggested Reading

Setliff RC 3rd. The small-hole technique in endoscopic sinus surgery. Otolaryngol Clin North Am 1997; 30:341-354.

Setliff RC 3rd. Minimally invasive sinus surgery: The rationale and the technique. Otolaryngol Clin North Am 1996; 29:115-124.

NASAL POLYPOSIS

The method of
James A. Duncavage
by
James A. Duncavage
Jenny A. Van Duyne
John J. Murray

Patients who have nasal polyps present a challenge to otolaryngologists.

Nasal polyposis is a common disorder resulting in edema of mucous membranes, with swelling in the nasal and sinus cavities. The precise etiology remains unknown, although there are many proposed mechanisms. There are a number of systemic diseases with which nasal polyps are associated: cystic fibrosis, asthma, and ciliary motility disorders, to name a few.

Nasal polyps represent the most common benign intranasal tumor. They are seen in all ages, although various underlying causes or associated conditions differ with age. The male-female ratio for this condition is 2:1. Many patients undergo multiple operations for polyp removal; some patients undergo as many as 25 or more surgical procedures.

In this chapter, we present several theories of pathogenesis. We discuss making the diagnosis and evaluating the differential diagnosis. Medical and surgical treatment are outlined. Associated illnesses with their respective treatment considerations are then addressed.

HISTORICAL PERSPECTIVE

Writings about nasal polyps date back 3,000 years and can be found in the Indian scriptures of 1000 BC. Hippocrates (460–370 BC) wrote of polyps. Further accounts were subsequently contributed by prominent physicians of Arabia. One of the earliest references to a nasal speculum was made by As Sayzari circa 1193.

By the mid-nineteenth century, there was quite a difference of opinion about the pathology of nasal polyps. Physicians of the Middle Ages believed that polyps resulted from local infiltration of mucous membranes with serum. Some physicians followed this concept, whereas others (Billroth) considered polyps to be adenomatous swelling. Virchow referred to polyps as myxomata. Edward Wookes (1837–1912) was the first to suggest that polyps arose from chronic infection. He called polyps "necrotizing ethmoiditis," proposing that the ethmoids were the origin. Through the years beginning with the physicians of Arabia, snarelike instruments for polyp removal were developed. Physicians also developed hot irons for cauterization. A variety of odors, herbs, caustics, leaves, and vines were used to treat patients. The application of weak acids, such as chloracetic acid, gained popularity. The most popular treatment, made possible by the invention of electricity, was galvanic cautery.

Endoscopic surgery of the nasal sinuses is a range of procedures based on the use of endoscopes. The history of the procedure's development is short. Rigid-angled telescopes were used without the microscope beginning in 1981 by Buiter and Straatman. Messerklinger (1980, 1984) and Stammberger (1985, 1986) were the first authors to describe partial and total ethmoidectomy via endoscopic methods.

ETIOLOGY

There is an increased incidence of nasal polyposis in patients who have chronic rhinitis, chronic inflammation, and abnormal vasomotor response. There is often increased interstitial fluid pressure and edema. Dilated glands in the nasal mucous membrane obstruct blood flow in capillaries and superficial venules, which results in edema and distention of stroma, which eventually prolapse and form a polyp.

Nasal polyps can be self-perpetuating by interfering with sinus drainage. Subsequent sinusitis results in more venous stasis and mucosal edema, which leads to enlargement of polyps. Although nasal polyps were first described more than 3,000 years ago, a good many questions still exist with regard to incidence, causes, pathogenesis, and treatment. Pathogenesis is unknown. The histology pattern shows marked uniformity. However, in the presence of allergy, plasma cells are abundant; with infection, eosinophils dominate; and with cystic fibrosis, there are abundant polymorphonuclear leukocytes. Two main proposed theories of pathogenesis are allergic and infectious. The allergy theory is supported by elevated histamine and immunoglobulin E (IgE) in polyps, as well as degranulated mast cells and eosinophils. However, only 0.5 percent of atopic patients develop polyps. Also there is no increased incidence of allergies in patients who have polyposis.

DIAGNOSIS: HISTORY AND PHYSICAL EXAMINATION

The most common chief complaint is nasal obstruction. This obstruction may be described as a foreign body sensation or a valvelike flapping. Other symptoms include allergic complaints (watery rhinorrhea, sneezing, itchy eyes); decreased sense or change of taste; hyposmia; anosmia; and cough. Patients may complain of pain or discomfort between the eyes or over the nasal bridge. Usually, pain is a complaint only if acute infection exists. Patients who have recurrent and/or chronic sinusitis may also complain of posterior nasal drainage. Frequently, patients will have had previous nasal surgery. The physician should be aware that many patients may have rhinitis medicamentosus from having used a variety of topical vasoconstrictors.

On physical examination, the nasal bones may be widened, with polyps extruding from the nose. The polyps appear as smooth, gray, glossy lesions hanging from a narrow stalk. They are soft, mobile, and nontender to palpation. Polyps are nontender because they are devoid of nerves.

Some polyps may appear reddish in nature, which indicates chronicity. They are frequently multiple, bilateral, and vary in size. They can be seen projecting beyond the anterior nares or can descend posteriorly into the choana. If not extruding from the nose, polyps may be readily visible by speculum examination or may be seen with an endoscope. Recent introduction of topical steroid sprays has resulted in polyps sometimes only being found at the time of surgery when the middle turbinate is displaced medially.

The location and the attachments of the polyps should be noted. Nasal anatomic abnormalities such as septal deviations, concha bullosa cells, and so forth are noted. Previous nasosinus surgeries are examined closely to determine whether alteration in ciliary flow is occurring, that is, circular flow in a maxillary sinus. If there is concern about neoplasm, a biopsy should be considered.

■ HISTOLOGY

Histologically, the polyp surface is comprised of respiratory epithelium that exhibits squamous metaplasia, with non-neoplastic collections of inflammatory mucosal tissue that originate from the sinus mucosa. This mucosa is chiefly filled with edema fluid, sparse fibrous cells, and few mucous glands.

The cellular infiltrate is composed of plasma cells, lymphocytes, a moderate number of mast cells and plasma cells, and an often striking eosinophilia. There are data to suggest that the more eosinophils, the more likely infection is present; however, the more plasma cells, the more atopy. If the ratio of eosinophils to plasma cells is greater than 5, infection is likely. If neutrophils are present, there should be a strong index of suspicion for other conditions, including cystic fibrosis. The polyps contain concentrated immunoglobulin A (IgA), immunoglobulin E (IgE), immunoglobulin G (IgG), and immunoglobulin M (IgM). There is more histamine in the mucosa of patients who have nasal polyps than in nasal mucosa of normal patients. However, there is less histamine in patients who have aspirin sensitivity and those patients who have asthma. Ultrastructure analysis reveals ciliated respiratory epithelium with branching microvilli. Mast cell degranulation indicative of a hypersensitivity reaction is revealed as well.

■ SPECIAL STUDIES

Investigations should include a basic immunologic workup, pulmonary function testing, computed tomography (CT), and biopsy for ultrastructural analysis when ciliary dysfunction is suspected.

Immunologic assessment may consist of skin testing (after stopping antihistamines for at least 48 hours or longer). Blood testing for specific IgE may be necessary in some cases. Pulmonary function testing may detect asthma. Children who have polyps require a sweat chloride test to detect cystic fibrosis. CT scan examination can elicit retention cysts and air-fluid levels. Bony expansion or destruction when seen on CT scan may be an indicator of a malignant process, but this finding is usually a result of the polyps.

The use of CT scan for evaluation of the paranasal sinus is mandatory. A coronal CT scan with bone windows is the standard type of x-ray study obtained. An axial scan may be obtained to complement the coronal view or in cases when patient positioning in the scanner limits the use of the coronal scan. The review of the CT scan is done in a systematic manner. The anatomy is recorded with attention to the nasal septum, the middle turbinates, and the bony sinus walls. It is not unusual for bony erosion to occur with nasal polyposis. Air-fluid levels within any sinuses are noted and recorded. Completely opacified sinuses are noted and recorded. The densities of the opacification are noted. Any irregularities in the densities are recorded. Any expansion of bony sinus walls is noted.

When polyps are present on physical examination but the CT scan examination shows polyps without evidence of infection, the polyps may be of an allergic nature. When irregular densities are seen in opacified sinuses, allergic fungal sinusitis should be considered. Soft-tissue windows are more diagnostic of allergic fungal sinusitis than are bone windows. The deposition of calcium salts by the fungus accounts for the CT appearance of irregular density.

■ THERAPY

Medical

The planning of treatment combines the history, endonasal examination, and CT scans. For routine polyposis, polypectomy is not the treatment of choice. The initial approach is medical. However, a combined medical and surgical approach is frequently required for the long-term management of the disease. Unfortunately, despite appropriate medical and surgical management, polyposis does recur. Initial medical therapy can be in the form of topical nasal steroids for mild disease. However, after a trial of 1 to 3 months of topical treatment without reduction in the size of the polyps or upon initial assessment that there is extensive mucosal and polyp swelling to prevent the entrance of the drug, oral steroids are indicated. The dose of steroids should be started at 40 to 60 mg of prednisone per day (or 6 to 8 mg of dexamethasone), which should be given in a slow taper over a period of 2 to 4 weeks. Because topical steroids may provide some additional therapeutic benefits in addition to oral administration, this treatment should be continued concurrently. Antibiotic treatment can also be added if it is warranted based on symptoms and physical examination. Given the chronic nature of the disease, a long course of treatment using polymicrobial coverage, including that for anaerobic organisms, is appropriate. These drugs would include amoxicillin-clavulanic acid, trimethoprim-sulfamethoxazole, clindamycin, or metronidazole. *Pseudomonas* treatment (e.g., in cystic fibrosis patients) may require an agent like ciprofloxacin. Further antibiotic coverage can be dictated by culture results obtained as a routine part of the endoscopic examination. At the end of the treatment intervention period, the response should be reassessed by endoscopy and CT scan, and a decision should be made as to whether an additional oral steroid and/or antibiotic course should be given. Topical steroid treatment should be continued indefinitely.

Certainly when severe nasal obstruction and anosmia are present and are unresponsive to medical therapy, polypectomy is indicated. Direct injection of polyps with steroids is too risky to suggest for a routine treatment option.

Surgical

Before surgical intervention, all attempts should be made to control the underlying reactive airway disease to prevent significant surgical complications. This concern about safety of surgical removal causing an exacerbation of the underlying asthma is particularly important in aspirin-sensitive individuals. After surgery, close follow-up with endoscopy should be routine in individuals who require surgical intervention, because intensive medical treatment and minor surgical debridement can reduce recurrence. Individuals who have undergone surgical treatment or who have significant disease requiring frequent medical treatment should be placed on regular topical steroids forever as mandated by the high recurrence rate. In an atopic individual, allergy desensitization can be considered an additional option because this will prevent recurrences but may not shrink existing polyps. The use of antihistamines and decongestants (both topical and oral) provides symptomatic relief but does not reverse or prevent polyposis. Cromolyn appears to be of little benefit.

In the treatment of nasal polyposis, we must consider two populations: those who do not have sinusitis and those who have sinusitis. The presence of nasal polyps in the absence of CT scan evidence of sinusitis is an uncommon finding in our experience. The absence of CT scan evidence of sinusitis allows the surgeon to offer removal of the polyps to improve nasal obstruction. Cases of an isolated polyp, polypoid changes to the middle turbinates, and small polyps easily viewed can be considered for removal in the office. The office removal of the polyps is done with a topical anesthetic and the infiltration of 1 percent lidocaine with 1:100,000 epinephrine into the polyps and surrounding tissue. The patient is instructed to avoid aspirin products and nonsteroidal anti-inflammatories for 2 weeks before the office procedure. The use of endonasal sinus telescopes and microdebriders allows for the precise removal of the polyps. Our experience with removal of polyps in patients without CT scan evidence of sinusitis has been gratifying in that this group of patients has not shown recurrent polyposis when they are maintained on medical treatment.

Patients who have polyps and CT scan evidence of sinusitis are managed differently from patients who have polyps only. The association of sinus infection with the development of nasal polyps determines our approach to the removal of the polyps. The removal of the polyps without surgical drainage of the infected sinuses will result in recurrence of the nasal polyps. Therefore, the patient who has nasal polyps and CT scan evidence of sinusitis is managed with the endonasal telescopes and endoscopic techniques not only to remove the polyps but also to drain the involved sinuses.

Polyps are removed in the operating room (OR) under general anesthetia using the sinus telescopes. The monitoring of blood pressure and keeping the systolic pressure under 140 mm Hg is helpful with bleeding. The patient is placed in reverse Trendelenburg's position and topically decongested with oxymetazoline in OR holding and topical cocaine in the OR, and then infiltrated with lidocaine with epinephrine. A greater palatine foramen block is also used. Large polyps are then individually infiltrated and removed. The removal of the polyps can be done with a polyp snare, grasping forceps, or microdebrider. The polyps should be sent for histologic examination.

After removal of the polyps, the infected sinuses are approached. All of the infected sinuses are opened endoscopically, and all pus is removed.

Maxillary Sinuses

The presence of polyps in the maxillary sinuses may present the surgeon with a problem. If the polyps are not removed, they may herniate from the maxillary sinus out through the maxillary antrostomy and obstruct the nasal cavity. The endoscopic frontal sinus instruments provide the ability to reach and remove most maxillary sinus polyps. If the surgeon cannot reach the polyps, a decision must be made to either leave the remaining polyps or remove the polyps via a Caldwell-Luc approach. We have been able to remove the polyps endoscopically but always obtain permission for a Caldwell-Luc when the maxillary sinus is completely opacifed on CT scan before surgery, should this procedure become necessary.

The ethmoid sinuses in our experience are believed to be the site of the infection that leads to most polyp formation. The presence of polyps with ethmoid changes on CT scan consistent with infection is an indication to do an endoscopic ethmoidectomy. Polyp recurrence is likely when only a polypectomy is done. All the ethmoid sinuses are opened endoscopically. A microdebrider has been helpful in removing the polyps when the polyps are protruding from the ethmoid sinuses.

Sphenoid Sinuses

The sphenoid sinuses become infected by blockage secondary to polyps in the sphenoethmoidal recess. The endoscopic removal of the polyps when the polyps are attached around the sphenoid ostium may result in ostial stenosis. We enlarge the sphenoid ostium when a concern for stenosis is present. The presence of polyps in the sphenoid sinus may increase the risk of surgical injury to the optic nerve and internal carotid artery because of increased bone erosion. The CT scan should be examined carefully to determine if any evidence of bony dehiscence is present. The removal of the polyps is done using blunt instruments. A No. 12 Frazier suction and the round, olive tip 90 degree suction instruments are helpful for the polyp removal. We do not use a grasping instrument in the depths of the sphenoid.

Frontal Sinuses

The treatment of polyps at the frontal recess presents the greatest challenge to the surgeon. If the frontal sinus is completely opacified on CT, the surgeon does not know whether the sinus is filled with polyps, has only an edematous lining, or is filled with pus. The frontal sinus that is filled with polyps may not be infected. Recurrent infection in the frontal sinus once the frontal recess polyps are removed may cause recurrent polyps. We believe that sinus infection in patients who are predisposed to polyp formation will lead to the formation of new polyps. If the polyps recur at the frontal recess, then the patient's frontal sinus infection will persist due to sinus ostium obstruction. The concern for recurrent sinus infection and polyps is greater in patients who have asthma. The frontal sinusitis will exacerbate the asthma, causing the asthma to become difficult to manage. In addition, the purulent material, when it drains out of the frontal sinus, will infect the maxillary and sphenoid sinuses and will also lead to polyp formation along the roof of the ethmoid or in the ethmoid area if the ethmoids have not been surgically opened. The evaluation of the CT scan of the frontals is very helpful in making a surgical decision as to what type of surgical procedure to employ. The CT scan may reveal a small anteroposterior diameter of the frontal sinus or may show intrasinus septations within the frontal sinus, which make it difficult to treat the frontal sinus endoscopically. We believe that the osteoplastic frontal obliteration is a low morbidity operation with a 94 percent success rate in arresting frontal sinus disease. It is used as a last resort, but is considered in our experience to offer the best chance for definitive cure of chronic frontal sinusitis with nasal polyps.

In addition, if previous CT scans of the frontal sinuses are available for review, a correlation with treatment can be done. When the frontal sinus over months to years despite medical treatment (even sometimes including systemic steroids) never shows aeration, we advise the patient to consider an osteoplastic frontal sinusotomy with obliteration.

When frontal sinus disease shows improvement with medical treatment but the CT scan shows supraorbital ethmoid or bullar cells obstructing the frontal recess, it is reasonable to correct these anatomic abnormalities as a first surgical procedure via an endoscopic frontal sinusotomy.

Also, if the patient has only mild asthma (based on physical examination and pulmonary function tests) or no asthma, it is reasonable to consider an endoscopic approach. The endoscopic frontal sinusotomy is much less invasive than the osteoplastic flap.

■ ASSOCIATED CONDITIONS

Patients with cystic fibrosis have polyps 20 percent of the time and greater than 30 percent of the time if asthma is a comorbid condition. Thirty percent of patients with nasal polyps have allergic rhinitis, whereas 70 percent of patients with nasal polyps have asthma. Most patients who have polyps are over 40 years old. Males with polyps outnumber females three to one, but there are more women with polyps who are asthmatic. Of the subpopulation of asthmatics who are sensitive to aspirin, one-half have polyps, and one-third have evidence of sinusitis. Kartagener's syndrome (immotile cilia syndrome); cystic fibrosis; chronic sinusitis; asthma (nonallergic and allergic); aspirin intolerance; Sampter's triad (nasal polyposis, nonallergic asthma, and aspirin sensitivity); Churg-Strauss syndrome (vasculitis); and Young's syndrome (sinopulmonary disease, azoospermia, nasal polyps) are all associated with nasal polyposis and should be kept in mind.

■ DIFFERENTIAL DIAGNOSIS

Benign polyps may look like a number of childhood nasal masses. Meningoceles or meningomyeloceles may project out the nose through a defect in the cribriform plate. Under the age of 2 years, a defect in the anterior cranial fossa most likely represents a neoplasm or dermoid cyst. Hemangiomas and other benign neoplasms or malignancies such as rhabdomyosarcoma can appear in children, with a presentation that mimics polyposis. Preadolescent males may present with a juvenile nasopharyngeal angiofibroma (JNA). JNAs frequently arise from the nasopharynx but can originate within the nose. Tumors and neoplasms including squamous cell carcinoma, sarcoma, angiofibroma, encephalocele, and inverting papilloma can present features similar to nasal polyposis. However, neoplasms are often unilateral, friable, firm, and bleed spontaneously.

The antrochoanal polyp may occur in all ages. The polyp originates from antral mucosa, projects through the middle meatus, and proceeds toward the posterior choana, often into the nasopharynx. It is a benign, unilateral lesion.

Suggested Reading

Anonymous. Endoscopic sinus surgery: Sinonasal polyposis and allergy. Ear Nose Throat J 1993; 72:544-554.

Calenoff E, McMahan JT, Herzon GD, et al. Bacterial allergy in nasal polyposis: A new method for quantifying specific IgE. Arch Otolaryngol Head Neck Surg 1993; 119:830-836.

Cowart BJ, Flynn-Rodden K, McGeady SJ, Lowry LD. Hyposmia in allergic rhinitis. J Allergy Clin Immunol 1993; 91:747-751.

Drake-Lee AB. Medical treatment of nasal polyps (review). Rhinology 1994; 32:1-4.

Jankowski R, Moneret-Vautrin DA, Goetz R, Wayoff M. Incidence of medico-surgical treatment for nasal polyps on the development of associated asthma. Rhinology 1992; 30:249-258.

Massegur H, Adema JM, Lluansi J, et al. Endoscopic sinus surgery in sinusitis. Rhinology 1995; 33:89-92.

Nishioka GJ, Cook PR, Davis WE, McKinsey JP. Immunotherapy in patients undergoing functional endoscopic sinus surgery. Otolaryngol Head Neck Surg 1994; 110:406-412.

Ogino S, Abe Y, Irifune M, et al. Histamine metabolism in nasal polyps. Ann Otol Rhinol Laryngol 1993; 102:152-156.

Settipane GA, Lund VJ, Bernstein J, Tos M. Nasal polyps: Epidemiology, pathogenesis and treatment. Internal book on nasal polyps—1997.

Stoop AE, van der Heijden HA, Biewenga J, van der Baan S. Eosinophils in nasal polyps and nasal mucosa: An immunohistochemical study. J Allergy Clin Immunol 1993; 91:616-622.

PROPTOSIS

The method of
Richard E. Gliklich

Dysthyroid orbitopathy is the term used to describe the ocular manifestations of Graves' disease. It implies orbital congestion secondary to enlargement of both extraocular muscles and fat, which leads to exophthalmos, corneal exposure, lid retraction, and optic neuropathy in severe cases. Clinically, dysthyroid orbitopathy is independent of changes in or treatments of the thyroid gland. It is a gradual, insidious process. The typical progression of signs and symptoms has been described by the acronym NOSPECS (Table 1). Graves' orbitopathy is typically bilateral (80 percent to 90 percent).

There are two distinct phases of the process. First, an acute phase is associated with inflammation of orbital contents, which leads to an increase in soft-tissue volume and intraorbital pressure. This typically results in anterior displacement of the globe. As a result of this, lid closure is poor and exposure keratitis may threaten the visual axis. At the same time, stretching of the optic nerve and posterior pressure may result in optic neuropathy. This phase may last from 6 to 18 months. Initial treatment usually consists of corticosteroids that control inflammation but do not affect proptosis, retraction, or myopathy. Low-dose radiotherapy (20 to 35 Gy) is another option that can effectively limit the lymphocytic infiltrates in many patients.

A more stable chronic period is reached from 18 to 36 months after onset of the orbital findings. Enlargement of the intraorbital contents becomes permanent. It is in this stage that surgery is most often used to treat this disease. There are three elements to surgical management: orbital decompression, strabismus surgery, and eyelid surgery. Orbital decompression, which involves removal of part of one to four walls of the orbital cavity, is used to decrease exophthalmos and its consequences, which include exposure keratopathy and optic neuropathy. Following a period of stabilization, strabismus surgery is performed to treat the diplopia that may arise from the congestive process and is often worsened by the decompression. Therefore, strabismus surgery is always performed after decompression. Lid retraction and excess eyelid fat are subsequently addressed.

Table 1. Classification of Dysthyroid Orbitopathy*

CLASS	DESCRIPTION
0	No signs or symptoms
1	Only signs (eyelid retraction, lid lag, edema)
2	Soft-tissue signs and symptoms (e.g., resistance to retropulsion, injection)
3	Proptosis (mild, 21 to 23 mm; moderate, 24 to 27 mm; severe, >28 mm)
4	Extraocular muscle involvement (minimal to frozen globe)
5	Corneal involvement (superficial to necrosis and perforation)
6	Sight loss by optic neuropathy (visual field defects, color vision, acuity)

* Adapted from descriptions by Werner SC. Modification of the classification of eye changes of Graves' disease. *Am J Ophthalmol* 1977; 83:725.

SURGICAL CONSIDERATIONS

Surgical procedures are ideally performed in a stable orbit. The goal is to enlarge the confining space of the orbit. This is achieved through removal of one to four walls of the bony orbit and incision of the periosteum to allow the orbital soft tissues to prolapse into the adjacent spaces. Theoretically, up to 15 mm of decompression can be achieved by removing all four walls of the orbit. However, in general, surgery achieves 3 to 7 mm of posterior displacement. Significant complications, including intractable strabismus and hypoglobus, may result from excessive decompression.

INDICATIONS

Indications for surgical decompression are severe exophthalmos, globe prolapse anterior to the lids, exposure keratitis, and optic neuropathy (Table 2). Cosmesis is a relative indication that should be balanced against potential complications. Patients who have exophthalmos in excess of 24 mm are more common candidates for decompression. Those patients who have less proptosis may benefit from eyelid procedures alone.

APPROACHES

Multiple surgical approaches to orbital decompression have been popularized. Each technique involves one or more bony walls (Table 3). The sinus cavities provide the largest

Table 2. Indications for Orbital Decompression

Optic neuropathy
Severe proptosis
Exposure keratopathy
? Cosmesis

Table 3. Approaches to Surgical Decompression

ORBITAL WALL(S) REMOVED	ASSOCIATED NAMES
Lateral	Kronlein
Inferior	Hirsch/Urbanek
Superior	Naffziger (transcranial)
Medial	Sewall
Medial/inferior	Ogura (transantral)
Medial/inferior (medial aspect)	Endoscopic (transethmoid)

potential volume for decompression, whereas the temporal fossa and orbital roof provide the least. The most commonly performed decompressive procedures involve the orbital floor and medial wall. Walsh and Ogura described a transantral approach with removal of the orbital floor (preserving the infraorbital nerve) and medial orbital wall and ethmoid. Modifications of this procedure have attempted to leave bone lateral to the infraorbital nerve canal to prevent vertical subluxation. Although this procedure may be performed without an external incision, the procedure has the same morbidity as that of a Caldwell-Luc procedure and provides limited visualization of the optic nerve near the orbital apex. Lateral decompression allows for decompression into the temporal fossa. In the Kronlein orbitotomy, removal of the lateral orbital rim with a saw and rongeur and incision of periosteum allows prolapse up to the temporalis fascia. Another approach to lateral decompression is excavation of the lateral orbital wall to the temporal fossa from the orbital side, which is performed with a cutting bur. Access is obtained through a standard upper eyelid orbitotomy incision.

Decompression in the horizontal plane theoretically reduces the risk of vertical dystopia. Such an approach can be achieved through a medial decompression combined with a lateral or Kronlein procedure. The portion of the orbital floor medial to the infraorbital nerve can also be removed without significant change of the globe in the vertical plane. Five millimeters or more of decompression, similar to that reported for the Walsh-Ogura technique, can be achieved by combining a medial orbital decompression, including the orbital floor medial to the infraorbital nerve, and a lateral decompression, when necessary. Medial decompression via a transethmoid approach provides on average more than 3 mm of decompression alone while giving excellent access to the orbital apex in cases of optic neuropathy.

The nasal-sinus endoscope provides unsurpassed visualization of the medial orbital wall to the orbital apex. The endoscopic transethmoid approach avoids an external incision, has limited morbidity, provides excellent access to the optic nerve at the orbital apex, and may even be performed under local anesthesia. For these reasons, endoscopic transethmoid orbital decompression, combined when necessary with lateral decompression, is the approach of choice in our institution.

■ PREOPERATIVE EVALUATION

Preoperative evaluation includes a full ophthalmologic examination with Hertel exophthalmometry to assess the degree of proptosis. Visual acuity, visual fields, and color saturation are assessed to rule out optic neuropathy. Nasal endoscopy is performed to diagnose nasal and sinus problems, such as septal deviation, nasal polyps, or infection, which may complicate surgical management. Axial and coronal computed tomographic scans are obtained and reviewed.

■ ENDOSCOPIC TECHNIQUE

The patient is placed on the operating table in a slight reverse Trendelenburg's position. Oxymetazoline spray is used for initial decongestion. Both eyes are left uncovered in the surgical field, with scleral shells used for corneal protection if lid closure is poor. Pledgets soaked in 4 mL of 4 percent cocaine solution are placed in the nasal cavity. If the patient is under general anesthesia, submucosal injections of 1 percent lidocaine with epinephrine 1 : 100,000 are begun along the lateral nasal wall and along the middle turbinate.

A standard uncinectomy is performed with a sickle knife just posterior to the maxillary line, a bony prominence that extends from the anterior attachment of the middle turbinate to the root of the inferior turbinate. A large maxillary ostium is created, and a 30 degree telescope is used to identify the position of the infraorbital nerve bundle in the roof of the maxillary sinus. A total ethmoidectomy is completed, and the sphenoid ostium is identified and enlarged. The lamina papyracea is skeletonized. The position of the anterior and posterior ethmoidal arteries is noted. The middle turbinate is resected before exposure of the periorbita. This facilitates exposure as well as postoperative cleaning. A spoon curet is used to crack the lamina in its thin midportion. A Cottle elevator is used to bluntly elevate bone away from the periosteum. Care is taken to preserve the periosteum so that orbital fat does not herniate into the field and obstruct the view. Bone fragments are meticulously removed. Bone is removed superiorly to the roof of the ethmoid (Fig. 1, *A*), which is confirmed by the position of the ethmoidal arteries. Posteriorly, bone is removed to the face of the sphenoid. Inferiorly, bone is removed to the maxillary ostium and anteriorly to the maxillary line. The last portion of bone to be removed is the orbital floor medial to the infraorbital nerve. Downward pressure on the remaining bony rim of the maxillary ostium with a large spoon curet accomplishes this maneuver (Fig. 1, *B*). The bone will typically fracture along the cleavage plane of the infraorbital canal.

A sharp sickle knife is used to incise the periorbita (Fig. 1, *C*). This is begun posteriorly to avoid fat prolapse obscuring visualization. The tip of the knife must be kept superficial to avoid injury to the extraocular muscles, which are enlarged in Graves' disease. Multiple cuts through the periosteum, or its removal, allow for herniation of orbital fat into the ethmoid and maxillary sinuses (Fig. 1, *D*).

Local Anesthesia

In some cases, local anesthesia may be preferred to general anesthesia. These situations include patients who have an only-seeing eye, those patients who have significant medical comorbidities, or those who have a strong preference for local anesthesia. Ideal sedation is achieved with an intravenous bolus of propofol at 0.4 to 0.8 mg per kilogram before local injection, followed by a maintenance infusion of 95 to 75 μg per kilogram during the procedure. Supplemental midazolam may be used to achieve an appropriate level of sedation. Submucosal infiltration of 1 percent lidocaine with epinephrine 1 : 100,000 is performed exactly as for the procedure that uses general anesthesia. Regional blocks are usually not necessary. Patients may report discomfort during removal of the lamina papyracea, and this may require a small additional infiltration of anesthetic solution into the periorbita.

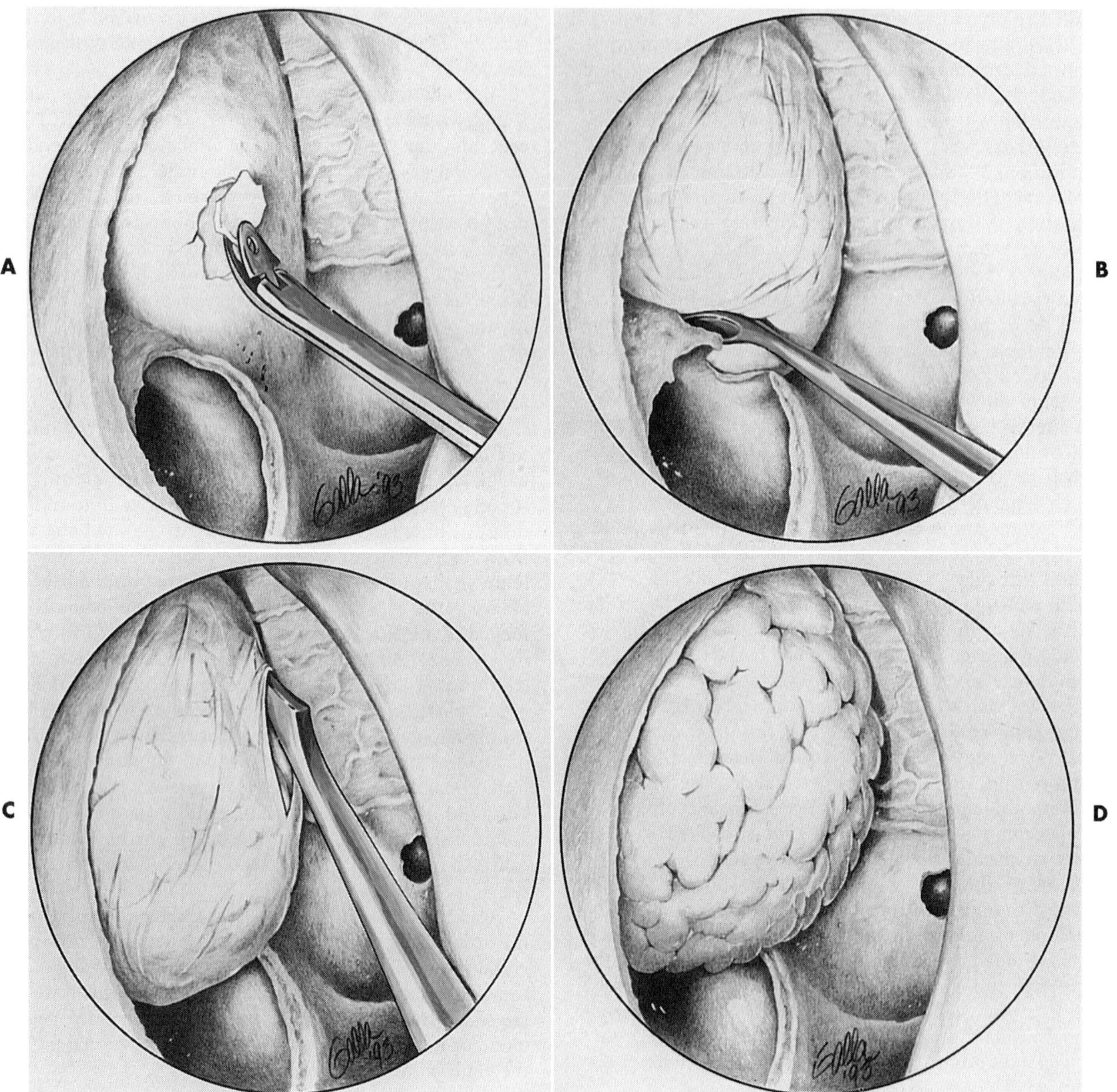

Figure 1.
After completion of a total sphenoethmoidectomy, removal of the middle turbinate, and skeletonization of the lamina papyracea, the thin bone of the medial orbital wall is removed *(A)*. A large spoon curet is used to downfracture the orbital floor medial to the infraorbital nerve *(B)*. Once the bone has been removed as far posteriorly as the face of the sphenoid, the periorbital fascia is incised with a sickle knife *(C)*. At the end of the procedure, herniated fat bulges freely into the ethmoid and maxillary sinuses *(D)*. *(From Metson R, Dallow RL, Shore JW. Endoscopic orbital decompression. Laryngoscope 1994; 104: 950–957; with permission.)*

Lateral Decompression

Lateral decompression, either through a standard Kronlein orbitotomy or via an upper eyelid crease incision, is performed after medial decompression. This allows for retraction of the orbital contents in a medial direction, which provides excellent exposure for the lateral bony wall to be excavated or removed. To approach the lateral orbit through the upper lid, the skin is marked as for upper blepharoplasty. The incision is carried laterally enough to gain exposure of the rim. Infiltration is performed with lidocaine 1 percent with epinephrine 1 : 100,000. The lateral rim is exposed from the reflection of the zygomatic arch to the frontozygomatic suture. A deep subperiosteal dissection is created into the orbit to expose the lateral wall, roof, and floor. The canthus is left intact. A high-speed cutting bur is used to excavate the lateral orbital wall while a malleable retractor protects the orbital fat. Bone is removed to the level of the lateral periosteum, the fascia of the temporalis muscle, and the dura superiorly while leaving the orbital rim intact. Excess orbital fat may be trimmed via this incision as well.

Results

Endoscopic medial decompression results in an average reduction in proptosis of 3.5 mm, whereas combining endoscopic medial and external lateral decompression yields an average reduction of 5.4 mm.

■ POSTOPERATIVE COURSE

When surgery is completed, visual acuity and extraocular movements are assessed. Nasal packing is avoided. Patients may be discharged in less than 24 hours on oral antibiotics and nasal irrigations with saline. Postoperative cleaning is performed under endoscopic visualization as would occur in routine sinus surgery. In general, bilateral orbital decompressions are performed as a staged procedure at an interval of 1 week.

■ COMPLICATIONS

There are many potential complications of orbital decompression; fortunately, most are rare. Visual loss can occur from hemorrhage or direct optic nerve injury. Poor visualization may lead to infraorbital nerve injury or direct muscle injury. Transient intraorbital nerve paresthesias may follow aggressive downfracture of the medial orbital floor. It is common for strabismus to worsen after any orbital decompression procedure. However, it is difficult to correct secondary enophthalmos from excessive decompression, and this should be avoided. The risks of postoperative epistaxis or cerebrospinal fluid leak are the same as those for standard endoscopic sinus procedures. Delayed sinusitis may occur in patients in whom an extensive decompression is required. Creating a large maxillary antrostomy, particularly in its inferior aspect, and sparing bone in the lateral frontal recess may help avoid these difficult problems.

■ DISCUSSION

Endoscopic medial orbital decompression with or without lateral decompression is a safe and effective technique for managing Graves' orbitopathy when surgical intervention is warranted. In addition to providing excellent visualization of the medial orbital wall and the orbital apex, the procedure can be performed under general or local anesthesia, and it can be customized to the needs of the individual patient.

Suggested Reading

Dallow RL, Netland PA. Management of thyroid ophthalmolopathy (Graves' disease). In: Albert DM, Jacobiec FA, eds. The principles and practice of ophthalmology. Philadelphia: WB Saunders, 1974:1905.

Kennedy DW, Goodstein ML, Miller NR, et al. Endoscopic transnasal orbital decompression. Arch Otolaryngol Head Neck Surg 1990: 116:275-282.

Metson R, Dallow RL, Shore JW. Endoscopic orbital decompression. Laryngoscope 1994; 104:950-957.

Metson R, Shore JW, Gliklich RE, Dallow RL. Endoscopic orbital decompression under local anesthesia. Otolaryngol Head Neck Surg 1995; 113:661-667.

Walsh TE, Oqura JH. Transantral orbital decompression for malignant exophthalmos. Laryngoscope 1957; 65:544.

Wilson WB, Manke WF. Orbital decompression in Graves' disease. The predictability of reduction of proptosis. Arch Ophthalmol 1991; 109: 343-345.

ANOSMIA

The method of
Louis D. Lowry
by
Louis D. Lowry
Beverly J. Cowart

Olfaction may be the most important primitive sense and is certainly the most poorly understood. The sense of smell depends on odorants reaching the olfactory mucosa and penetrating the mucous layer to stimulate the olfactory neurons. In conjunction with cranial nerves V, IX, and X (mostly V), the complex signals are processed and identified.

Because various authors use the same words with different meanings, the terminology for our chapter is defined as follows:

- Anosmia: absence of the sense of smell.
- Specific anosmia: inability to smell a specific compound or class of compounds with intact general olfactory abilities.
- Hyposmia: diminished smell sensitivity (threshold similar to change in threshold for pure tones in hearing testing).
- Dysosmia: odor quality distortion (like poor discrimination with testing of hearing).
- Phantosmia: perception of an odor without any external stimulation (perhaps this could be equated to tinnitus).

■ ETIOLOGY

We present some general considerations from our experience at the Monell/Jefferson Taste and Smell Center, Philadelphia, PA, combined with literature review from the University of Connecticut and the University of Pennsylvania, before looking at some specifics.

Approximately two of three persons coming to the Monell/Jefferson Center complain of taste loss (savor, flavor, and bouquet), but just under 9 percent have taste changes identified with our tests. However, 67 percent do have objective changes in the sense of smell.

Trauma

Trauma accounts for 10 percent to 19 percent of persons reporting a loss of smell. In general, the amount of loss correlates with the severity of trauma. Phantosmia and dysosmia are greater than that with nasal sinus disease (NSD), but less than that with upper respiratory infection (URI).

Upper Respiratory Infection

Numbers vary from 14 percent to 26 percent. Viral URI followed by secondary bacterial infection is a common history. This etiology is more common in persons over 40 than under 40 years of age. Women are more commonly affected than men. Less anosmia is found with URI than with NSD. At Monell/Jefferson Center, odor quality distortions were greater than in NSD; dysosmia was reported in 27 percent of URI and 3 percent of NSD patients. We believe that this may represent a decreased number of neurons that regrew or abnormal regrowth of neurons.

Nasal Sinus Disease

NSD, including allergic rhinitis, generally accounts for 20 percent to 30 percent of diagnoses. Phantosmia is reported by just over 10 percent and quality distortion by approximately 6 percent. Olfactory sensitivity does not correlate with nasal patency, which suggests that obstruction is not the only mechanism causing loss of smell. When steroids produce a rapid recovery, this generally indicates a good prognosis.

Idiopathic Disorders

Ten to 24 percent of patients have no known cause of their anosmia. This percentage will decrease as we become more astute in identifying causes.

Miscellaneous Causes

Various causes such as age, inhalation of vapors, genetic or congenital etiology, and medications have been identified in small numbers of patients.

■ DIAGNOSTIC AND TREATMENT PROTOCOL

A careful history will be of greatest benefit, and routine otolaryngologic nasal examination is mandatory before any decisions are made about further testing or medications. Our approach for NSD, URI, and head trauma are outlined in the following paragraphs, followed by a brief discussion of the large group of remaining patients.

Head Trauma

There is a history of head trauma followed by loss of smell. Often, trauma is to the occiput, but almost any head trauma with or without loss of consciousness may be associated with loss of smell.

The first step in diagnosis is to order magnetic resonance imaging (MRI) with contrast and a computed tomographic (CT) scan of the sinuses. If sinus disease is found, follow the steps described under the later section "Nasal Sinus Disease." If no sinus disease is found and there are no fractures or changes visible on MRI, proceed with formal smell testing. When smell testing results are normal, no treatment is necessary. You will need to explain this finding to the patient. With anosmia or hyposmia that has been present for less than 2 years, there is a good possibility that some function will return. If either of these conditions has been present longer than 2 years, permanent impairment is likely, and the patient should be informed of this probability. Dysosmia is rare in patients who have experienced head trauma. In such a case, redo the history to determine whether URI is the actual cause.

Upper Respiratory Infection

When there is a history of URI with acute loss of smell, CT scanning of the sinuses is appropriate. If findings are abnormal, follow the protocol outlined under "Nasal Sinus Disease" (see subsequent section). If CT findings are normal, proceed with formal smell testing. Normal smell testing results mean that no treatment is indicated. With a finding of hyposmia or anosmia, return of function is possible if the condition has been present less than 2 years. If present longer than 2 years, the condition is probably permanent. Patients who have dysosmia will likely have further return of function.

Nasal Sinus Disease

If the patient reports a history of NSD and/or allergic rhinitis, treat with methylprednisolone, sulfamethoxazole-trimethoprim, one tablet twice daily for 30 days, plus nasal steroids. At the end of this time, order a CT scan without contrast for review. If CT findings are normal, no treatment is needed. If there has been a transient return of smell during the treatment period and CT findings are normal, functional endoscopic sinus surgery (FESS) may be helpful, or treatment with antibiotics and steroids may be continued. If, however, the patient remains anosmic, it is difficult to justify any surgical intervention.

If the CT scan shows abnormalities, one of several courses may be followed. For the asymptomatic patient whose sense of smell has returned to normal, give antibiotics for recurrent acute sinus attacks and continue on nasal steroids. If there are symptoms (e.g., pain, pus, anosmia, congestion), FESS is appropriate, with close follow-up care, including antibiotics as needed and nasal douches of saline solution and steroids. The anosmic or hyposmic patient should be treated with oral steroids (for less than 1 week), antibiotics, and nasal douches of saline solution and steroids for 1 month. Re-evaluate the patient's sense of smell at that time. Dysosmia is rarely related to NSD, but sinus signs and symptoms should be treated before assigning the patient to another category.

Idiopathic Disorders

When the history and physical examination are not helpful in directing our attention toward a particular diagnosis, we come to the very large category of idiopathic etiology. At the Monell/Jefferson Center, this category includes approximately one-fourth of all patients. CT scanning is ordered. Patients who have normal CT findings are treated with methylprednisolone and steroid nasal spray. Those patients who have abnormalities on CT scan are removed from the idiopathic category.

Miscellaneous Causes

We include in the miscellaneous group congenital and genetic conditions and loss of smell related to vapors, medications, stroke, or previous nasal surgery, because of the small number of each types of these cases that we have seen. To date, we have found only one brain tumor (a meningioma) after testing more than 1,500 patients.

■ TESTING PROCEDURE

Two charts from a set of patients tested in our center give some insight into the complexity of the problem, even with thorough testing procedures. Table 1 compares our patients' "diagnoses" of the etiology of their loss of smell with our diagnosis after smell testing. Table 2 illustrates our categorization of etiology after patients have undergone a complete history, physical examination, and smell testing.

Formal smell testing at the Monell/Jefferson Center consists of a 20 item identification task and taste testing. Pyridine and phenylethyl alcohol are used in undiluted strengths. The latter is a pure olfactory stimulant; the former produces trigeminal stimulation at undiluted strength, and thus is useful in cases of possible malingering.

Our odor identification task consists of 20 different odors in various strengths in polypropylene bottles. We use a forced-choice alternative method of testing. We have found that our results correlate well with those of other centers.

Office-Based Testing Suggestions

Olfacto Laboratories (P.O. Box 757, El Cerrito, California 94530; contact John Amoore; phone, 510-235-0203; fax 510-235-1635) markets premade threshold tests in polypropylene bottles, as well as premade kits for threshold and identification tests. A manual is provided. Testing kits range in price from $175 to $975. Each kit has a shelf-life of 2 years and can be used to test up to 100 patients.

Table 1. Etiology of Patients' Presenting Complaints Versus Our Diagnosis (After Testing)

PATIENT'S "DIAGNOSIS"	NORMAL	HYPOSMIC	ANOSMIC	DYSOSMIC	PHANTOM ONLY	TOTAL
Head trauma	20	19	57	1	13	110
URI	34	57	25	37	7	160
NSD	12	25	42	1	5	85
Congenital	0	0	7	0	0	7
Toxin exposure or medication	6	12	6	3	0	27
Miscellaneous						
Stroke/surgery	9	10	21	3	4	47
Idiopathic	38	50	85	15	15	203
NSD & URI	8	16	9	3	3	39
NSD & toxin exposure	2	2	9	0	0	13
NSD & surgery	0	4	5	1	0	10

URI, upper respiratory infection; NSD, nasal sinus disease.

Table 2. Diagnosis of Patients Tested for Smell Problems

ETIOLOGY	NORMAL	ANOSMIC	DYSOSMIC	PHANTOM ONLY	TOTAL
Head trauma	18	54	14	0	86
URI	68	30	40	8	146
NSD	51	89	5	6	151
Congenital	2	27	0	0	29
Toxin exposure or medication	2	0	0	0	2
Miscellaneous					
Stroke, surgery	22	25	6	5	58
Idiopathic (includes aging)	44	43	13	16	116

URI, upper respiratory infection; NSD, nasal sinus disease.

A Smell Identification Test is manufactured by Sensonics, Haddonfield, N.J. (phone, 609-428-1161; fax, 609-547-5665). The price is $24.95 per test, with a minimum order of six tests. The manual describing administration of the test costs $15. Tests have a shelf-life of approximately 2 years.

■ RESULTS

A complaint of change of taste or smell deserves a workup. Because only patients who have nasal sinus disease can be helped medically, it is important to document the problem. Thorough testing and categorization may give a prognosis (such as dysosmia documented shortly after a viral URI). A short course of oral steroids with nasal steroid supplement leading to return of smell is an excellent prognostic sign. Follow-up interviews with 268 patients at Monell/Jefferson Center show that just over 60 percent of dysosmics (44 patients) can expect improvement in their sense of smell, compared with approximately 20 percent of hyposmics (109 patients) and approximately 35 percent of anosmics (115 patients).

INVERTING PAPILLOMA

The method of
Thomas C. Calcaterra

Inverting papilloma of the nose and paranasal sinuses is a histologically benign tumor with an unusual propensity for recurrence after surgical removal. Using conventional transnasal and Caldwell-Luc approaches, the recurrence rate often exceeds 50 percent. Another challenge facing clinicians is the risk of malignant conversion, which ranges from 5 percent to 15 percent in most large series.

The mechanism for recurrence or even the cause of the tumor remains unknown. Recent evidence suggests that human papillomavirus may play a role in the pathogenesis of this tumor, and certain virus types may be associated with malignant transformation. There is not much correlation between tumor aggressiveness and propensity for recurrence with histologic grading. Very histologically benign-appearing tumors are capable of eroding bone and extending throughout all of the paranasal sinuses, eustachian tube, and nasopharynx, eroding into the anterior cranial fossa.

One of the reasons attributed to tumor recurrence is the finding of metaplastic respiratory mucosal cells adjacent to the tumor bed. Although all visible tumor may be removed, adjacent metaplastic mucosa may eventually evolve into new tumor formation. Multicentric tumor is also seen; it is not rare to find tumor concurrently arising on more than one site within the nasal cavity and paranasal sinuses.

■ PATIENT EVALUATION

The majority of patients have unilateral nasal airway obstruction. Less frequently, there is epistaxis or maxillary pressure or pain. On rhinoscopy, it is often difficult to precisely distinguish inflammatory nasal polyps from inverting papilloma. In many instances, both types of pathologic tissue are present within the nasal cavity. Whereas polypoid inflammatory sinus disease is usually bilateral, inverting papilloma is almost always unilateral. When bilateral inverting papilloma is found, it is usually the result of extension of tumor through septal erosion.

If inverting papilloma is suspected, biopsy under local anesthesia is preferable before planning definitive treatment. Removing and sampling as much tissue as possible is important to determine the presence of inverting papilloma, because there are often copious inflammatory polyps associated with papilloma. Furthermore, foci of malignant mucosal degeneration may be identified.

To assess the anatomic extent of disease, a complete computed tomographic (CT) scan with axial and coronal views is essential. It is not uncommon to find concurrent obstructive sinusitis, particularly involving the frontal or sphenoid sinuses. If differentiation between obstructive mucus retention and direct tumor extension is difficult to determine by CT scanning, a magnetic resonance imaging (MRI) scan can usually distinguish each disease process. An MRI scan is also very helpful if there is suspicion of intracranial extension because this study is more accurate in defining intracranial anatomy.

■ SURGICAL THERAPY

Surgical excision is considered the optimal treatment for inverting papilloma. Because of its tendency for recurrence, multicentricity, and malignant transformation, excision with wide margins has been traditionally advocated. With the advent of endoscopic techniques, some surgeons have employed transnasal excision in more limited tumors.

Transnasal Approach

For limited tumors arising from the septum and inferior and middle turbinates, a transnasal endoscopic technique can be employed. Using this method, a complete amputation of the middle turbinate and most of the inferior turbinate along with a complete ethmoidectomy and sphenoidotomy can be accomplished. Biopsies of mucosal margins using frozen section analysis can be performed to determine clearance of tumor.

Midface Degloving Technique

For lower tumors not involving the upper or anterior ethmoid, the degloving approach is very satisfactory because it avoids an external facial incision. This operation provides reasonably ample exposure and permits an en bloc resection of the medial wall of the maxilla. The primary limitation is poor exposure of the anterior skull base, anterior medial orbit, and lacrimal sac. Because considerable retraction of the infraorbital nerve is often required, long-term or permanent numbness of the face may result.

Lateral Rhinotomy with Medial Maxillectomy

When tumors extend into the ethmoid complex, particularly around the upper lacrimal system, ethmoid roof, or frontal sinus, lateral rhinotomy is the optimal approach because of its versatility, direct access, and maximum exposure. Its only shortcoming is potential facial scarring, but this is usually not a problem or is substantially minimized when certain surgical adjuncts are incorporated.

■ SURGICAL HIGHLIGHTS: MEDIAL MAXILLECTOMY

The upper end of the incision begins at the medial inferior edge of the eyebrow and passes inferiorward halfway between the nasal dorsum and the medial canthus. The lower part of the incision passes through the alar crease into the nasal vestibule. Throughout the entire orbital portion, the incision is modified by multiple small W-plasty incisions to minimize any webbing and produce a less conspicuous postoperative scar line. The upper lip is almost never divided.

The lateral osteotomy is placed incorporating a portion of the premaxilla. The upper portion of the osteotomy is placed as high as possible into the frontal process. A medial osteotomy through the frontal process facilitates fracture rotation of the lateral bony complex. Preservation of this large bone fragment with the soft tissues of the nose usually eliminates any asymmetry of the nasal skeleton after surgery.

The lamina papyracea is exposed, and a small vascular clip is usually placed on the anterior ethmoidal artery before division of the artery. The lacrimal duct is exposed by removing the anterior maxillary buttress with a curved sharp osteotome. The sac is sharply divided obliquely with a scalpel just below the orbital rim. Sufficient anterior maxillary wall is removed to provide adequate exposure of the maxillary sinus, and all abnormal-appearing mucosa within the sinus is dissected toward the medial wall. An osteotomy is carried out between the floor of the nose and the maxillary sinus as far back as the posterior wall of the maxillary sinus.

The upper resection margin depends on the superior extent of the disease. If tumor fills the ethmoid sinus, it is usually necessary to remove most of the lamina papyracea and transect the ethmoid complex at the level of the cribriform plate and ethmoid roof, where all mucosa is removed. If tumor has eroded through the cribriform plate and/or ethmoid roof and extended to the aura, a craniofacial resection is the optimal treatment. The posterior cut of the en bloc resection can be accomplished satisfactorily with heavy right-angled scissors. The anterior wall of the sphenoid sinus is taken down, and all mucosa is stripped from the sinus if there is any evidence of mucosal disease.

A thin margin of infraorbital rim can usually be preserved in most cases. It is desirable to avoid any tears of the orbital periosteum to prevent late enophthalmos. To avoid delayed frontal sinus obstruction with mucocele formation, the floor of the frontal sinus is widely opened. If there is any evidence of a cerebrospinal leak at the cribriform plate, the area can be repaired with a mucoperiosteal graft from the septum and secured with Surgicel or Gelfoam.

If the lacrimal sac has been transected cleanly and obliquely with an adequate lumen, it is unnecessary to stent the sac with plastic tubing. A single suture is employed to evert the anterior cut margin of the sac. The lateral nasal bone complex is restored to its former position against the premaxilla; this is usually done without wiring. The medial canthal ligament can be wired to the nasal bone, but careful suture alignment of the medial canthus to the deep incision edge will also avoid any lateralization of the medial canthus. Meticulous closure of the W-plasty incision with fine suture is important to minimize scarring. If there is any question about the stability of the lateral nasal bone complex, an external nasal splint can be maintained for approximately 1 week. Light packing is placed and is usually removed by postoperative Day 3. Facial sutures can be removed on postoperative Day 4 or 5. Rubber bulb irrigation of warm tap water mixed with a small amount of salt is started a few days after pack removal and continued daily for 2 to 3 months.

■ POSTOPERATIVE OBSERVATION

Patients are advised to return twice yearly for approximately 5 years for an office endoscopic examination of the nasal and sinus cavities. Because it is not uncommon for recurrence to develop after 5 years, subsequent annual examinations are recommended. If a small recurrence is documented by biopsy, excision can usually be accomplished endonasally by employing an endoscope or operating microscope, because the altered sinus and nasal anatomy allows much better visualization and access.

Cancer arising in inverting papilloma must be treated aggressively by full maxillectomy and possible orbital exenteration, followed by postoperative radiotherapy.

Although endoscopic excision of inverting papilloma has recently engendered considerable interest, it must be remembered that this is either a potentially debilitating disease if multiple recurrences develop or a fatal disease if carcinoma is missed. At least a 5 year follow-up is required before judging the merit of any operative method. Until the success of more limited approaches can be confirmed, the lateral rhinotomy with medial maxillectomy should be the treatment of choice for most patients who have inverting papilloma. Using appropriate surgical techniques, facial scarring is almost always very inconspicuous and of little concern to the patient.

Suggested Reading

Bielamowicz S, Calcaterra TC, Watson D. Inverting papilloma of the head and neck: The UCLA update. Otolaryngol Head Neck Surg 1993; 109:71-76.

Calcaterra TC, Thompson JW, Paglia DE. Inverting papilloma of the nose and paranasal sinuses. Laryngoscope 1980; 90:53-60.

Lawson W, Ho BT, Shaari CM, Biller HF. Inverting papilloma: A report of 112 cases. Laryngoscope 1990; 100:481-490.

Stankiewicz JA, Girgis SJ. Endoscopic surgical treatment of nasal and paranasal sinus inverted papilloma. Otolaryngol Head Neck Surg 1993; 109:988-995.

Vrabac DB. The inverted schneiderian papilloma: A 25 year study. Laryngoscope 1994; 104:582-605.

WEGENER'S GRANULOMATOSIS

The method of
Ronald G. Amedee
by
Ronald G. Amedee
Mark A. Jabor

In 1931, Heinz Klinger, a German medical student, described the first reported case of a systemic vasculitis that involved the upper and lower respiratory tracts and kidneys. Five years later, Dr. Friedrich Wegener, a pathologist, provided detailed information about patients who had illness similar to that seen by Klinger. Some time later, this disease entity became known as Wegener's granulomatosis (WG). WG is still regarded as vasculitis of unknown etiology that primarily affects the respiratory tracts and kidneys, but the treatment and prognosis of this disease has greatly improved.

Wegener's granulomatosis affects both sexes equally, occurs in patients of all ages (mean age, 41 years), and is more commonly seen in whites. Patients can generally be divided by site of disease into locoregional involvement (isolated to the upper or lower respiratory tracts) and systemic involvement (kidneys plus upper and/or lower respiratory tracts). Untreated WG usually runs a rapidly fatal course, with a mean survival of approximately 5 months; 82 percent of patients are dead within 1 year, and 90 percent are dead within 2 years. Due to this fact, it is important that the correct diagnosis and treatment begin immediately.

■ CLINICAL PRESENTATION AND DIAGNOSIS

Symptoms and Signs

It is essential for the otolaryngologist to be able to recognize the patient who has WG because more than 70 percent of presenting features are related to the ear, nose, and throat (Table 1). Symptoms develop insidiously, with sinusitis being the most common presenting problem; *Staphylococcus aureus* is the most predominant organism. Nasal disease is a prominent presenting feature in approximately one-third of WG patients. Symptoms and signs include nasal congestion, crusted nasal ulcers and septal perforations, serosanguineous discharge, epistaxis, and rarely saddle nose deformity. Serous otitis media is the most common otologic manifestation. Laryngotracheal disease may range from hoarseness to stridor and life-threatening upper airway ob-

Table 1. Otolaryngologic Manifestations of Wegener's Granulomatosis

MANIFESTATION	PRESENTING FEATURE (%)	FREQUENCY (%)
Sinusitis	52–67	85
Epistaxis	11	32
Saddle nose deformity	<1	9–29
Otalgia	10	14
Hearing loss (conductive > sensorineural)	6–15	12–14
Otitis media (serous > suppurative)	25	44
Oral lesions (ulcers, gingivitis)	2–6	6–13
Subglottic stenosis	1	16
Combined otolaryngologic manifestations	73	92–94

struction. The most common lesion affecting the airway is subglottic stenosis, which occurs in 16 percent of all WG patients but is much more frequently seen in the pediatric and adolescent populations (48 percent). Pulmonary involvement is one of the cardinal features of WG. Forty-five percent of patients are affected at presentation, and 87 percent develop pulmonary involvement during the course of the disease. The most common radiologic findings are pulmonary infiltrates and nodules that are usually multiple, bilateral, and cavitate. Renal involvement distinguishes between generalized and limited WG and is also the most frequent cause of death. However, the exact frequency of renal disease is difficult to determine. Microscopic urinalysis is the primary tool for assessing active glomerulonephritis, and red blood cell casts are also highly suggestive of this process. Ocular, cutaneous, musculoskeletal, neurologic, gastrointestinal, genitourinary, and cardiac system involvement may also be seen.

Clinical Evaluation

Every patient suspected of having WG should undergo a minimal set of laboratory and radiologic tests consisting of a complete blood cell count, erythrocyte sedimentation rate, rheumatoid factor, serum creatinine level, chest radiograph, and CT scan of the sinuses. Yet none of these tests will have findings pathognomonic for WG. Assessment of antineutrophilic cytoplasmic antibodies (ANCA) in serum is subdivided into cytoplasmic staining (c-ANCA) and perinuclear staining (p-ANCA). Perinuclear staining has not proved useful in the evaluation of WG. The sensitivity of c-ANCA is approximately 90 percent in active WG and 40 percent when the disease is limited or in remission. The specificity of c-ANCA in the diagnosis of WG is also approximately 90 percent. Positive c-ANCA is rarely found in other forms of vascular diseases (relapsing polychondritis, classic polyarteritis nodosa, and granulomatous diseases of infectious or noninfectious nature) or in patients who have systemic necrotizing small-vessel vasculitis. The c-ANCA should never be used as a sole source for diagnosis and should not replace a biopsy in the evaluation of a patient suspected of having WG. Baseline levels of c-ANCA may be useful in the long-term follow-up of WG patients. There is some correlation between a rise in c-ANCA in stable patients and exacerbation of disease, although the absolute level of c-ANCA has limited usefulness. This may help differentiate intercurrent infections from exacerbations. It is important to realize that no clinical or laboratory marker can distinguish which patients will continue to have limited, indolent, nonrenal forms of the disease versus those who will rapidly progress to fulminant renal involvement.

Histology

Wegener's granulomatosis initially begins as a granulomatous lesion that then evolves into a vasculitis. Inflammatory lesions of WG classically include a triad of granulomatous changes, vasculitis of small and medium-sized arteries and veins, and necrosis. Intranasal biopsies are the simplest and most common form of tissue analyzed. Unfortunately, the small amount of tissue obtained from the nasal mucosa usually makes it difficult to distinguish the classic triad of pathologic features that are seen in only 3 percent to 16 percent of biopsies. Regardless, nasal biopsies are considered diagnostic in more than half of patients who have WG. When reviewing the nasal biopsies, the presence of palisading granulomas appears to be the single most important observation leading to the diagnosis of WG. The diagnostic yield of lung biopsies typically reflects sample size. Transbronchial biopsies have very low yield, and open lung biopsies show a triad of pathologic features in 90 percent of cases. Renal biopsy is usually characterized by the presence of segmental glomerulonephritis.

Biopsy

After careful history and physical examination, a patient who is suspected of having WG should undergo intranasal biopsy; a generous piece of viable nasal mucosa should be obtained. Biopsies are taken from the turbinates, lateral nasal wall, or nasal septum and should include samples larger than 5 mm in greatest dimension. The biopsy can be performed under general or preferably local anesthesia with intravenous sedation. Neosynepherine or 4 percent cocaine-impregnated packs for vasoconstriction should be placed 10 minutes before biopsy, and specimens should be sent to pathology fixed in formalin. Biopsies should not be sent for frozen section because freezing the tissue can interfere with recognition of vasculitis. Biopsy specimens should also be sent for both routine and fungal culture and sensitivity as well as staining for acid-fast organisms. After obtaining hemostasis, antibiotic-impregnated nasal packs are inserted and left in place for approximately 1 to 2 hours.

Differential Diagnosis

In its typical presentation, WG is usually fairly easy to characterize and diagnose. Nonetheless, if all of the typical features are not present, it needs to be differentiated from other diseases, including lymphomatoid granulomatosis (polymorphic reticulosis); idiopathic midline granuloma; Churg-Strauss syndrome (systemic necrotizing vasculitis associated with a history of atopy, asthma, eosinophilia, and sometimes nasal polyps); Goodpasture's syndrome; lymphoma; sarcoidosis; tuberculosis; rhinoscleroma; fungal infections; and relapsing polychondritis. Of particular note is differentiation of lymphomatoid granulomatosis and idiopathic midline granuloma. Lymphomatoid granulomatosis is characterized by lung, skin, central nervous system, and kidney involvement. Histologically, it displays lymphocytoid and plasmacytoid cell infiltrates that have an angioinvasive manner, which are not typical of a classic inflammatory vasculitis. Approximately 50 percent of these patients will develop lymphoma. Idiopathic midline granuloma frequently erodes through the skin of the face, which is a feature never seen in WG.

■ THERAPY

Medical Therapy

Whenever the diagnosis of WG is being entertained, the otolaryngologist should refer the patient to an internist (preferably a rheumatologist), who should be the coordinator of all treatment. Although many different combinations of drugs have been used to treat WG, the "gold standard" remains cyclophosphamide (CY) and glucocorticoids (GC) (Table 2). This combination has proved extremely successful in long-term follow-up of patients and has drastically changed the lethal prognosis of patients afflicted with WG. The actual therapy administered usually depends on the disease extent and toxic effects of the drugs. Cyclophosphamide therapy is instituted at doses of 2 mg per kilogram daily, but in an acute life-threatening situation (pulmonary hemorrhage or rapidly progressive glomerulonephritis), doses may be increased to 3 to 5 mg per kilogram daily for 3 to 4 days and then reduced to conventional levels. The leukocyte count is used to guide subsequent dosage adjustments; tapering of CY usually lags behind the tapering and discontinuation of GC. Cyclophosphamide is continued for at least 1 year after the patient achieves complete remission and is then tapered by 25 mg increments every 2 to 3 months until discontinuation or until disease recurrence requires an increase in the dose. Serious side effects caused by CY include bone marrow suppression causing leukopenia, hemorrhagic cystitis, bladder fibrosis, and bladder cancer. Patients receiving daily CY require regular leukocyte count and lifelong surveillance for bladder cancer. Cyclophosphamide is also teratogenic and should be avoided during pregnancy.

Glucocorticoids are generally initiated in combination with CY at high doses. Prednisone given at 1 mg per kilogram daily is most commonly used and maintained until all major manifestations of WG have ceased. After the major manifestations of the disease are under control, GC therapy is slowly tapered. Most studies have tapered GC in an alternate-day fashion so that if a patient is without relapse or exacerbation, a dose of 1 mg per kilogram every other day is achieved in 2 to 3 months. During the next several months, GC can be further tapered until discontinuation is reached. Pulse intravenous methylprednisolone of 1 g daily for 3 days has also been used in life-threatening disease. Although palliation of limited indolent disease may be achieved by GC alone, there should never be the expectation that in generalized WG remission can be achieved with single therapy using GC.

Side effects are dose related, and patients are much more tolerable of alternate-day therapy than daily dosing. Pneumonia is the most prevalent life-threatening infection and usually occurs most commonly when daily GC are given with CY. Other side effects include hyperglycemia, hypertension, electrolyte imbalance, peptic ulcer disease, cataracts, myopathy, and osteoporosis. Glucocorticoids alone have modestly increased mean survival time to 12 months. Recent clinical studies have shown that adding CY resulted in 75 percent of patients achieving complete remission, but induction of remission may take up to 5 years. Disease relapse occurs in 50 percent of patients; 86 percent suffer permanent morbidity from the disease; and a 13 percent mortality rate is attributable to the disease. Permanent morbidity as a result of concurrent drug therapy occurs in 42 percent of patients.

Methotrexate (MTX), 0.05 to 0.3 mg per kilogram weekly, has been used in combination with daily GC therapy in patients who do not have life-threatening disease. Results are promising, but long-term follow-up is lacking. A clinical role for MTX will probably develop in the treatment of selected WG patients, such as those patients who do not have life-threatening disease and/or those patients who are refractory to or have suffered serious toxicity from CY.

Trimethoprim-sulfamethoxazole (TMP-SMX), 800/160 mg twice daily, has been used with success in treating WG patients who have upper airway involvement as the main clinical finding. However, TMP-SMX is not advocated as a single-treatment modality for WG patients. The use of TMP-SMX, 800/160 mg twice daily, over a 24 month period in combination with CY and GC has resulted in a reduction in the number of relapses and a decrease in the number of respiratory and nonrespiratory infections.

Isolated sinus disease may be treated with topical cortico-

Table 2. Recommended Medical Treatment for Wegener's Granulomatosis

SYSTEMIC DISEASE OR RAPIDLY PROGRESSIVE DISEASE
Not acutely life-threatening
CY 2 mg/kg/day (begin to taper 1 year after complete remission)
Prednisone 1 mg/kg/day (begin to taper 2 to 3 months after complete remission)
? TMP-SMX 800/160 mg b.i.d. (continue for 24 months?)
Acutely life-threatening*
CY 3 to 5 mg/kg/day for 3 to 4 days and then decrease to 2 mg/kg/day
Methylprednisolone 1 g IV for 3 days and then decrease to prednisone 1 mg/kg/day
NONSYSTEMIC LOCALIZED INDOLENT DISEASE
Upper airway
Nasal steroids
Saline irrigations
Antibiotics for superimposed bacterial infection
Lower airway
? TMP-SMX 800/160 mg b.i.d.
? Prednisone 1 mg/kg/day

* Pulmonary hemorrhage or rapidly progressive glomerulonephritis.

CY, cyclophosphamide; TMP-SMX, trimethoprim-sulfamethoxazole; IV, intravenous; ?, no generally accepted time frame or dosing of drugs.

steroid sprays, daily saline nasal irrigations, and empiric treatment with appropriate antibiotics when bacterial superinfection is suspected. Refractory isolated sinus disease may also respond to low-dose (10 to 20 mg per day) prednisone. Nasal obstruction and crusting are chronic nagging problems in WG patients. Patients should be scheduled for regular appointments to remove nasal crusting; judicious use of saline irrigations and cool mist humidification at night should be advocated to decrease the amount of crusting.

Surgical Therapy

The need for surgical intervention in WG is limited; intranasal biopsies are usually the only procedure indicated. Occasionally, other surgical procedures are needed for the following conditions: maxillary antrostomies and Caldwell-Luc operation for acute or chronically infected sinus disease refractory to medical treatment; myringotomy and placement of ventilation tubes for persistent or recurrent otitis media with effusion; dacryocystorhinostomy for nasolacrimal sac or duct obstruction; and orbital decompression for pseudotumors with proptosis. Saddle nose deformities can be corrected in various ways if remission has occurred for 1 year or longer.

Subglottic stenosis (SGS), which is much more prevalent in the pediatric population, requires individualized multidisciplinary intervention. It is important to determine whether the stenosis is secondary to scarring, active inflammation, or both. When present, the active inflammatory process should always be suppressed concurrent with or before surgical intervention. Severe SGS may require immediate tracheotomy, and manual dilation of minimally noninflamed lesions may be adequate. Definitive treatment of significant SGS may require laryngotracheoplasty with microvascular free flap.

Renal transplantation is an option for patients who have end-stage renal disease; patients who are in sustained remission are good candidates. Unfortunately, there has been occasional documentation of recurring glomerulonephritis in WG patients who have transplanted kidneys. WG patients who are good candidates for transplantation are subjected to the same protocol that other patients who have end-stage renal disease undergo.

Suggested Reading

Duna GF, Galperin C. Hoffman GS. Wegener's granulomatosis. Rheum Dis Clin North Am 1995; 21:949-986.

Fauci AS, Haynes BF, Katz P, et al. Wegener's granulomatosis: Prospective clinical and therapeutic experience with 85 patients for 21 years. Ann Intern Med 1983; 98:76-85.

Hoffman GS, Kerr SG, Leavitt RY, et al. Wegener's granulomatosis: An analysis of 158 patients. Ann Intern Med 1992; 116:488-498.

Kallenberg CG. Treatment of Wegener's granulomatosis: New horizons? Clin Exp Rheumatol 1996; 14:9-16.

Lebovics RS, Hoffman GS, Leavitt RY, et al. The management of subglottic stenosis in patients with Wegener's granulomatosis. Laryngoscope 1992; 102:1341-1345.

Sneller CM, Hoffman GS, Williams-Talar C, Kerr GS. An analysis of forty-two Wegener's granulomatosis patients treated with methotrexate and prednisone. Arthritis Rheum 1995; 38:608-613.

CEREBROSPINAL FLUID RHINORRHEA

The method of
Anthony J. Yonkers
by
Gary F. Moore
Anthony J. Yonkers

Cerebrospinal fluid (CSF) drainage from a dural defect rarely occurs, but its consequences may be catastrophic. Dural fistulas are due to a defect or "tear" in the pia-arachnoid that allows CSF to leak from the subarachnoid space into an extradural area. CSF rhinorrhea accounts for approximately 90 percent of all CSF fistulas. The flow of CSF into the nasal cavity may take place across the frontal sinus, the cribriform plate of the ethmoid, the sphenoid sinus, the sella, or via the temporal bone into the middle ear through the eustachian tube (Fig. 1). Leaks are usually the result of trauma or are iatrogenically induced by surgical or invasive therapy. Less frequently, leaks can be congenital or idiopathic in origin.

Many CSF fistulas heal with conservative management and without the development of complications. However, pneumocephalus, meningitis, and hydrocephalus are potentially life-threatening complications that can arise secondary to CSF leakage and require medical and/or surgical treatment. Due to the widespread use of nasal endoscopy for rhinologic procedures and an increase in extensive skull base neurotologic surgical procedures, the practicing otolaryngologist needs to have a thorough understanding of the anatomy and potential problems that can be created by these techniques and also how the same techniques can be used to correct the underlying anatomic problem causing the CSF drainage. We discuss the laboratory, radiographic, and clinical technique used in our practice to help identify the pres-

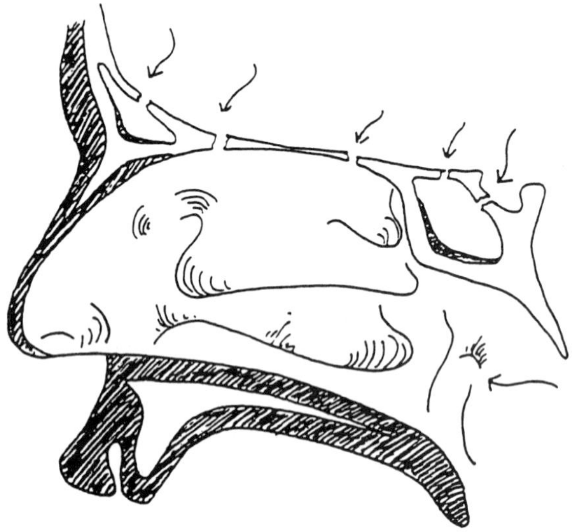

Figure 1.
Potential routes of cerebrospinal fluid leakage into the nose.

ence and site of fistulas as well as their medical and surgical treatment.

■ PATHOGENESIS OF SPONTANEOUS (ATRAUMATIC) RHINORRHEA

Spontaneous CSF rhinorrhea is divided into normal-pressure and high-pressure leaks (Table 1). The initial leak is frequently precipitated by coughing, sneezing, or straining. The large majority are precipitated by slow-growing tumors, most commonly from the pituitary gland. In these cases, by the time the tumor produces a large enough increase in intracranial pressure to precipitate a leak, there are generally other neurologic signs and abnormalities identifiable by radiography.

Normal-pressure CSF leaks account for approximately one-half of spontaneous leaks and are due to the slow erosion of the skull base secondary to fluctuations in the intracranial pressure, which leads to focal bony erosion and CSF rhinorrhea. The large majority of leaks originate from congenital or potential pathways, such as a persistent craniopharyngeal canal or nasal encephalocele. Other potential pathways include the olfactory nerve, stalk of the hypophysis, or an empty sella syndrome. A few are due to direct erosion of the skull base by tumor or infections. Examples include osteomas of the frontal ethmoids, nasal pharyngeal angiofibromas, and osteolytic erosion secondary to sinusitis.

In contrast to normal-pressure CSF leaks, high-pressure CSF rhinorrhea is not due to direct invasion of the skull base but from intrinsic conditions that cause abnormalities within the CSF pressure.

■ DIAGNOSIS

Clinical and Laboratory Tests

The diagnosis of CSF rhinorrhea involves (1) determining that fluid is draining from the nose, (2) ascertaining that this fluid is CSF, and (3) attempting to identify the portal of entry into the nose or nasal chamber. The most reliable means of clinically examining a patient with suspected CSF rhinorrhea is to lean the patient forward while he or she is seated. This position should be maintained until clear liquid drainage is identified, which often requires several minutes. Small amounts of fluid can often be collected in a test tube for laboratory assay.

Nasal discharge exhibiting a clear "halo" surrounding a central blood stain after trauma is thought of as a clinical diagnosis for CSF rhinorrhea. Although this "handkerchief" test is a classic example given as a means of identifying CSF, it is only a gross test and produces false-positive results if saliva or tears are mixed with the fluid obtained from the nose.

Another test that has been historically used to identify the presence of CSF uses a glucose oxidase paper or dextrose sticks. Unfortunately, this test is also unreliable and should not be counted on to give reliable results

Beta-2 transferrin (tau transferrin) analysis has been described as a technique that identifies nasal fluid as being of CSF origin. This protein is highly specific for human CSF and is not present in other body fluids. One advantage of this test includes the small sample size required, that is, less than 1 cc, and the fact that no special handling or refrigeration is required. The samples can be analyzed by immunochromatographic assay or gas chromatography. Because samples of fluid can be mailed to reference laboratories, this technique is not limited by the presence of a laboratory in your hospital. Because we currently do not have this laboratory test at our hospital, we do not use it primarily. However, if other means of identifying CSF rhinorrhea fail, this test is a resource that we have used for helping to make the diagnosis.

Table 1. Etiologies of Cerebrospinal Fluid Rhinorrhea

TRAUMATIC: 90%	ATRAUMATIC: 10%
Iatrogenic	High-pressure
Rhinologic surgery	Intracranial tumor
Craniotomy	Hydrocephalus
Skull base tumors	Normal-pressure
Nonsurgical	Facial bony erosions
Blunt trauma	Tumor
Missile trauma	Infection
	Congenital defect
	Idiopathic

Radiographic Examination

Computed tomographic (CT) scans are the study of choice in diagnosing temporal bone or basilar skull fractures, particularly when a history of trauma is present. Thin-cut CT scans are particularly helpful to identify bony abnormalities within the sinuses and skull base. These scans have the ability to delineate the exact fracture site as well as the presence of tumors, abscesses, bony erosions, or hydrocephalus. The thin-cut CT scans with and without intrathecal tracer studies are the present workhorses for identifying and delineating

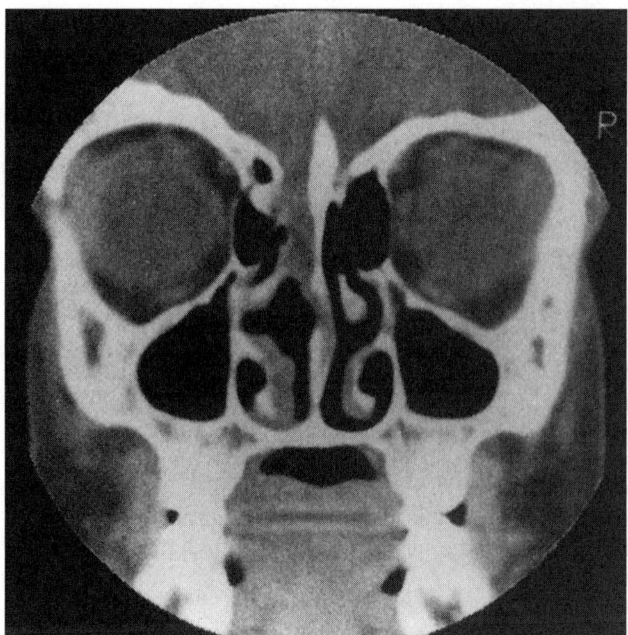

Figure 2.
Computed tomographic scan through cribriform plate demonstrating bony defect.

CSF leaks at our institution (Fig. 2). Magnetic resonance imaging (MRI) has only been occasionally helpful in identifying or diagnosing the location of CSF leaks, usually in conjunction with a nasal mass or brain tumors. A new technique, magnetic resonance cisternography, has been reported but is not currently used at our institution.

Intrathecal Tracers

A single reliable diagnostic protocol to identify CSF leaks has not been generally accepted. During the past 50 years, several types of intrathecal tracer studies designed to locate the site of the CSF leak have been used, reported, and abandoned, primarily because they produced neurologic symptoms, such as seizures, and accomplished poor localization of the leak. Dyes such as indigo carmine and methylene blue were originally used. Fluorescein has been reported at many institutions as being diagnostically useful; however, we do not use it because of transient neurologic complications that we have seen, even when the patients were pretreated with diazepam.

Intrathecal metrizamide, a water-soluble contrast material, in conjunction with thin-cut CT scans was used frequently in the past at our institution to help identify and localize CSF leaks. However, metrizamide still bears the risk of neurotoxicity, and for that reason it is not used by us.

We currently use radionuclide scans to assess for the presence of CSF rhinorrhea. Specifically, 500 mg diethylene-5-triamine penta-acetic acid (DTPA) is injected intrathecally into the lumbar space. DTPA stays within the CSF space as it rises to the basal cistern. It flows to the parasagittal area, where it is transferred unmetabolized by the arachnoid villi to the vascular component. There are no medial contraindications to its use, although in some patients a lumbar puncture may require fluoroscopy for placement of the catheter. Preceding the intrathecal installation of DTPA, the nasal cavity is sprayed with a 4 percent solution of cocaine to anesthetize and shrink the mucous membranes. Cotton pledgets are carefully placed within the nasal cavity, one superiorly near the cribriform plate and ostium of the sphenoid, one under the middle turbinate near the ostium of the frontal sinus, and one inferiorly near the orifice of the eustachian tube. Careful technique is important during any scan involving nasal pledgets to avoid contamination of neighboring cotton pledgets. Our current recommendations include using three pledgets in each nasal passage to identify all possible routes of leakage that are indicated in Figure 1. The cotton pledgets are scanned immediately at 1 and 2 hours after injection to identify the presence of DTPA. The nasal pledgets are also weighed dry and wet to help detect the presence of CSF accumulation. Thin-cut CT scans looking for bony defects are also obtained, with special emphasis on the cribriform plate and temporal bone areas.

■ THERAPY

Medical Therapy

Conservative medical management is advocated to allow the body's reparative process a reasonable chance to heal itself without the possible detrimental effects of surgical exploration. Our protocol includes keeping the head of the bed at 30 degrees while the patient is at bed rest. Coughing, sneezing, noseblowing, and straining are to be avoided. Laxatives are given, and fluids are restricted. We do not use acetazolamide, dexamethsaone, or furosemide or other diuretic agents. Conservative management of CSF leaks attempts to reduce the CSF pressure to allow the dura to approximate and subsequently heal. This approach is recommended for up to 2 weeks in a patient who has a leak immediately following head trauma, depending somewhat on the patient's other symptoms. However, repair of facial fractures should not be delayed during a trial of conservative management for a CSF fistula because realignment of the body fragments will often speed the healing of dural tears.

Although the prophylactic use of antibiotics is controversial, we have been giving broad-spectrum antibiotics to patients whose CSF rhinorrhea is traumatic in origin. This is based on the premise that the traumatic wound is contaminated by CSF exposure to potentially pathogenic organisms. Thus, technically, antibiotics used in this fashion are not prophylactic but are given for treatment of this contamination. We are currently not using broad-spectrum antibiotic coverage in those patients whose CSF rhinorrhea has a spontaneous or nontraumatic etiology. Ceftriaxone, 1 mg twice daily given intravenously, is the antibiotic that we primarily have used due to its spectrum and ability to cross the blood-brain barrier.

As an adjunct to both surgical and conservative management, we have found a large-bore Cordis lumbar subarachnoid catheter to be an effective, reliable treatment to decrease the intracranial pressure, thus allowing the dura a better chance to heal. The catheter system is made up of implant-grade Silastic and can be left in place for several days. We have chosen the closed drainage system over repeat lumbar taps to decrease the discomfort to the patient and decrease the risk of infection by contamination. Recently, we have begun using AVI pump connected to the Cordis catheter, which runs through the IMED into a closed sterile collecting bag. This setup essentially runs an infusion pump in reverse, placing it between the patient and the collecting bag, which allows us to obtain a constant flow rate of approximately 75 to 100 cc per shift. The major advantages of this system are that it is flow-regulated and the amount of CSF drained is not affected by changes in the patient's head position or the level of the closed CSF chamber or reservoir. Care must be taken to ensure that no medications are inadvertently injected into the system.

■ POTENTIAL COMPLICATIONS

CSF drainage from a dural tear created iatrogenically secondary to traumatic or nontraumatic etiology may have catastrophic consequences. The potential complications include meningitis, pneumocephalus, and hydrocephalus, as well as the continuing CSF leak.

Meningitis

CSF leak may be responsible for bacterial meningitis. The incidence of meningitis secondary to CSF leak is approximately 5 percent. Pending culture and sensitivity testing, patients who have clinical signs of meningitis should be started on penicillin and chloramphenicol. The antibiotics can then be adjusted for specific culture and sensitivity results.

Pneumocephalus

The presence of pneumocephalus after a surgical procedure in which the dura is not intentionally entered is of clinical significance. By far, the most common cause of pneumocephalus is trauma. Tumors, infections, and iatrogenic or idiopathic cases account for the remainder. The situation gives rise to pneumocephalus when there is a communication between the intracranial and extracranial spaces. Creation of a pneumocephalus secondary to a dural tear during mastoidectomy or sinus surgery is theorized as being the combination of two processes: the ball-valve effect and the "coke bottle" effect.

The ball-valve effect is a reflux of air up the eustachian tube or nose and through the dural tear into the subarachnoid potential space when the patient coughs, strains, or swallows. After the pressure wave has forced itself through the dural tear, the defect is tamponaded by the downward pressure of the brain. Repeated instances of the pressure wave continue to cause increasing intracranial pressure. In the "coke bottle" effect, as the CSF leak occurs, a slight negative intracranial pressure is compensated for by the inflow of air into the subarachnoid space, much like the inflow of air into a soda bottle as liquid is poured from the container. After sufficient CSF has escaped, a negative intracranial pressure exists, and air enters via the same channel as the CSF leaves (Fig. 3). Pneumocephalus formation via middle cranial fossa defect is facilitated by the dura and arachnoid being closely adherent.

Hydrocephalus

Hydrocephalus is by definition a dilatation of the cerebroventricular system caused by an imbalance in production and adsorption of CSF. The pathogenesis of hydrocephalus is obscure. Obstruction of the CSF in its course through the subarachnoid space is the only proven cause. Normal-pressure hydrocephalus is a well-recognized but poorly understood syndrome whose symptoms include decreased mentation, occasional incontinence, and gait difficulties. CT

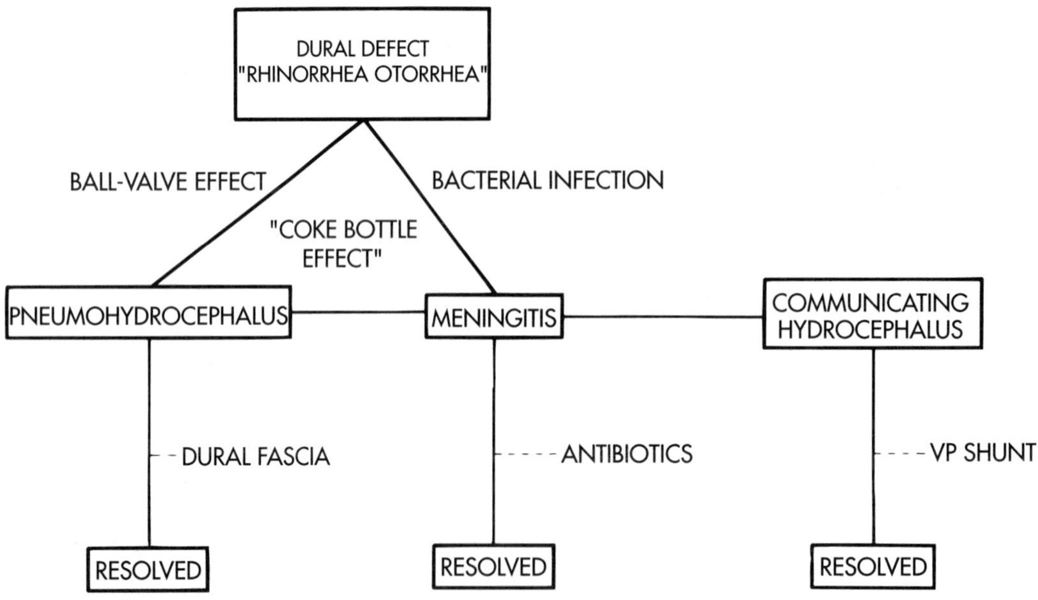

Figure 3.
Mechanisms of complications secondary to cerebrospinal fluid leaks and their treatment.

scan shows a very enlarged lateral ventricle that appears to be due to the obstruction of CSF flow due to blockage in the subarachnoid pathways, which can follow meningitis or subarachnoid hemorrhage. When normal-pressure hydrocephalus is secondary to meningitis, the symptoms may not appear for weeks or months after the meningitis has occurred. The treatment for a patient who has normal-pressure hydrocephalus is either a ventriculovenous or ventriculoperitoneal shunt to divert the excess CSF from the cerebral ventricles to the venous pathways. These are neurosurgical procedures that are necessary to allow the patient's neurologic status and gait to return to normal. The inter-relationship between complications of unrecognized CSF leak and their management are shown in Figure 3.

■ SURGICAL REPAIR

Extracranial Ethmoid–Cribriform Plate Repair

The ethmoid roof and cribriform plate region is the area most often involved in cases of leakage associated with trauma. It is also susceptible to iatrogenic insults during intracranial, nasal, and orbital surgery. Spontaneous leaks are also common in this area. Repairing the ethmoid area is classically approached by an external ethmoidectomy, with the development of mucoperiosteal flaps using either the septum or turbinate as the donor area. We currently prefer to use rigid intranasal endoscopy to repair ethmoid defects when possible due to the decreased morbidity. However, it is important to be able to do an extracranial repair, because some leaks from the ethmoid have failed intranasal repair.

Once the complete ethmoidectomy is performed through the nasal orbital incision, the dural defect is exposed. A mucoperiosteal flap is then constructed, using either nasal septum, middle turbinate, or lateral wall as the donor area. Septal flaps anteriorly or posteriorly based, depending on the defect site, are used to provide coverage of both the ethmoid roof and the cribriform plate (Fig. 4). Once the flap is rotated into position, we reinforce it with the placement of a free fascial graft taken from either the temporalis fascia or the fascia lata. This is secured in place by packing the nose with antibiotic-impregnated gauze. The packing is removed 6 to 10 days postoperatively. Failure of an extracranial ethmoidectomy approach has not burned any bridges behind, and the surgeon can still follow this procedure with a neurosurgical intracranial repair if this approach fails.

Extracranial Frontal Sinus Repair

CSF leak from the frontal sinus is best approached with an osteoplastic flap technique. An eyebrow or coronal incision is used, depending on the patient's sex and family preponderance for male-pattern baldness. After the sinuses are entered and the mucosa is removed, the bony defect in the posterior wall is identified. Lowering the head of the bed, and a Valsalva's maneuver by the anesthesiologist may help define the area of leakage. Removal of bone in the posterior wall will reveal the dural tear. Direct repair of the dural defect can be accomplished by using interrupted sutures of 4–0 to 6–0 silk. If the defect is large, we repair it using fascia lata graft or homograft dura tucked medial to the bony defect and then held in place with silk sutures. The frontal sinuses are then obliterated with fat harvested from the left lower quadrant of the abdomen, and the frontal sinus anterior bone flap is replaced. The bone flap is secured into position with miniplates.

Rigid Intranasal Endoscopic Repair

With the advent of functional endoscopic sinus surgery, traditional repair of CSF leaks occurring from the sphenoid, ethmoid, and occasionally the frontal sinuses has changed. There has been an evolution in our practice toward using the rigid transnasal endoscope due to the enhanced angle of visualization and improved illumination as well as magnification. We have occasionally been able to use the rigid endoscope not only to help repair a CSF leak but also to

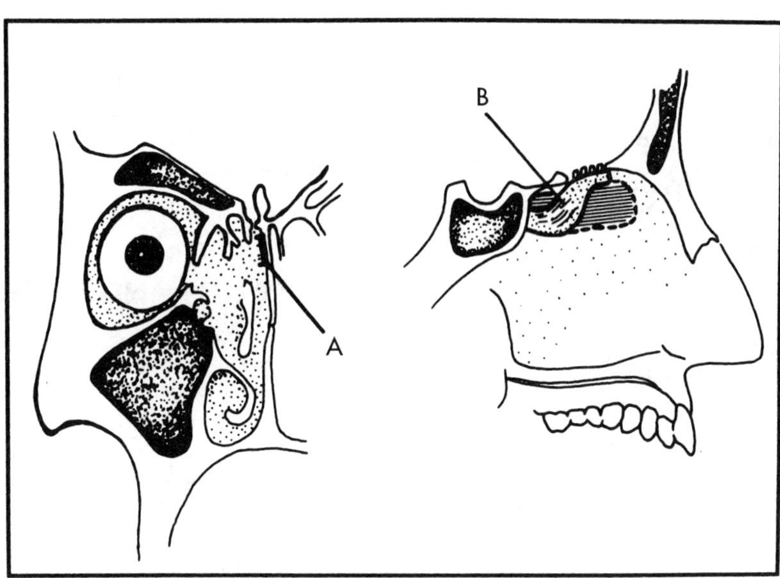

Figure 4.
External ethmoidectomy approach using septal flap (*A*) reconstruction of dural defect (*B*).

help define the location of the leak originating from a paranasal sinus.

Sphenoid Sinus Repair

Our first choice of repair for sphenoid sinus leaks is using intranasal endosocpy. During the repair of a trans-sphenoidal defect, we use the neurosurgical nasal speculum placed onto the anterior wall of the sphenoid cavity. Using the 0 degree 4 mm rigid endoscope, careful visualization of the area of the sphenoid cavity is obtained after routine vasoconstriction. If direct visualization cannot document CSF leak, a 30 degree or 70 degree 2.7 mm nasal endoscope is introduced to look into the lateral and superior recesses. While inspection is going on, Valsalva's maneuvers by the anesthesiologist may actually increase the ability to see a CSF leak directly. To repair the defect, we use fascia placed directly onto the defect and held in place with abdominal fat strips. Once the nasal speculum is removed, the nasal vaults are packed with Neosporin-impregnated 0.5 inch gauze strips left in place for 48 hours. An indwelling Cordis subarachnoid catheter allows the margins of a dural tear to approximate each other and increases the chance of healing by primary intention.

Intranasal sinus repairs are currently our first choice of repair of ethmoid sinus leaks, using the same techniques of direct visualization and repair outlined for sphenoid sinus repair. The frontal sinus is still primarily repaired by extracranial techniques, but intranasal endoscopy has been helpful in aiding the location of a leak from the frontal sinus.

Therefore, functional transnasal endoscopic sinus surgery not only can be useful in making a diagnosis of a CSF leak as well as helping to identify the location, but also can be used to repair the defect, thus eliminating the need for a craniotomy or extracranial surgery and reducing operating time, bleeding, and postoperative morbidity.

Suggested Reading

Moore GF, Nissen AJ, Yonkers AJ. Potential complications of unrecognized cerebrospinal fluid leaks secondary to mastoid surgery. Am J Otol 1984; 5:317-323.

Swanson SE, Chandler WF, Kocan MJ, Bogdasarian RS. Flow-regulated continuous spinal drainage in the management of cerebrospinal fluid fistulas. Laryngoscope 1995; VOL:104-106.

Yokoyama K, Hasegawa M, Shiba KS, et al. Diagnosis of CSF rhinorrhea: Detection of tau-transferrin in nasal discharge. Otolaryngol Head Neck Surg 1988; 98:328-332.

INVASIVE FUNGAL RHINOSINUSITIS

The method of
Robert W. Seibert
by
Robert W. Seibert
Charles M. Bower

Invasive fungal sinusitis is recognized as an important cause of morbidity and mortality in a number of clinical scenarios. These include immunocompromise (most common), poorly controlled diabetes with ketoacidosis, and other conditions resulting in metabolic acidosis, such as severe diarrhea and renal failure. Prolonged neutropenia of any cause and overuse of broad-spectrum antibiotics and steroids may be contributing factors in this disease. The immunocompromised group includes patients undergoing treatment for hematologic malignancies, especially bone marrow transplantation, as well as those patients who have head and neck solid tumors who are treated with irradiation. Kavanagh and co-workers reported the incidence of fungal infections in children who were dying from leukemia as from 22 percent to 28 percent. In another series, Berlinger reported that 93 percent of patients with fungal sinusitis had aplastic anemia, leukemia, or primary immunodeficiency, and nearly 50 percent of patients who had fungal sinusitis were bone marrow transplantation recipients.

Increasingly, fungal sinusitis has been found in the later stages of disease associated with the human immunodeficiency virus (HIV). Nosocomial factors have also been implicated with outbreaks of the disease, such as a reported association with hospital construction.

■ ETIOLOGY AND PATHOGENESIS

Numerous fungal agents have been reported to cause invasive disease in isolated cases. *Aspergillus* species causes the majority of cases of invasive fungal sinusitis. *Candida* is the second most commonly found organism, followed by *Mucor* and *Rhizopus* species. These organisms are found as saprophytes in the environment (soil, decaying matter) and as nonpathogens in the upper respiratory and gastrointestinal tracts of normal individuals. *Aspergillus fumigatus* is the most common species implicated in paranasal sinus disease in the United States. Histologically, *Aspergillus* is identified as septate hyphae with dichotomous branching at 45 degrees.

Four distinct clinical variants of aspergillus sinusitis are recognized: (1) allergic aspergillus sinusitis; (2) aspergilloma [both 1 and 2 are benign saprophytic infections]; (3) indolent invasive aspergillosis, a slowly progressive but destructive infection; and (4) fulminant (invasive) aspergillosis, which is a rapidly progressive disease associated with a high mortality rate that usually affects immunocompromised patients. Fulminant invasive aspergillosis was first recognized by McGill in 1980 in a neutropenic patient who had a hematologic malignancy. Similarly, mucormycosis is an opportunistic infection caused by fungi of the family Mucoraceae. Infected patients are usually immunocompromised and/or have metabolic ketoacidosis. Rhinocerebral mucormycosis was first reported by Paultauf in 1885. *Rhizopus oryzae* accounts for more than 90 percent of cases of mucormycoses. Histologic findings characteristic of mucormycosis include tissue necrosis and angioinvasion by organisms with nonseptate hyphae.

Loss of normal immune competency results in fungal invasion of mucosa with a predilection for vascular, especially arterial, invasion. Ischemia and necrosis result from thrombosis. This produces further propagation of fungus along blood vessels. Bone and skin involvement occur rapidly. Major arterial and brain invasion herald advanced disease and poor prognosis.

■ DIAGNOSIS

Successful outcome of these highly fatal infections depends on early diagnosis and prompt aggressive treatment. A high index of suspicion based on knowledge of the usual clinical setting is crucial. Early symptoms are nonspecific (fever [in 100 percent of patients], nasal congestion, rhinorrhea, facial pain), occurring often in the presence of common bacterial sinus infections. A new onset of facial pain and edema in an immunocompromised patient who has fever is an important symptom of invasive fungal sinusitis. There may be lethargy and decreased mentation out of proportion to the appearance of illness severity. With orbital involvement occur retro-orbital pain, diplopia, and decreased vision. Contralateral eye findings are ominous signs of central nervous system disease. Signs of invasive disease include serosanguineous nasal discharge and necrotic-appearing crusting or ulceration of the septum and turbinates. The nasal mucosa may vary in appearance from pale ischemia to black necrosis. Septal perforations may be present. Orbital signs include chemosis, proptosis, and ophthalmoplegia. Ischemic and necrotic changes may also occur on the skin and palate. Central nervous system invasion results in lethargy, coma, brain infarction, and death. Anterior rhinoscopy may be inadequate to identify mucosal change consistent with invasive fungal sinusitis.

Nasopharyngoscopy after adequate vasoconstriction may reveal a pale or granular middle turbinate, which suggests the need for biopsy, and should be performed in all suspicious cases. Imaging studies are helpful in demonstrating bony destruction, which is usually a late sign. Extent of disease is demonstrated by computed tomographic scanning of the sinuses. Magnetic resonance imaging is useful in demonstrating invasion of major arteries, cavernous sinus, and the brain. The identification of maxillary sinus involvement with contiguous nasal fossa involvement and extension into the facial or orbital soft tissue suggests fungal sinusitis, especially if bony necrosis is evident. Unfortunately, these findings overlap enough with bacterial infection to preclude making a definitive diagnosis by imaging.

Definitive diagnosis is made by histologic identification of fungal organisms in biopsy tissue. Potassium hydroxide preparation of crushed tissue may result in rapid identification of fungal elements. Staining of biopsy material with hematoxylin and eosin, periodic acid-Schiff, and silver methenamine should lead to the correct identification of the organisms. Cultures may be necessary for ultimate identification, but they have no bearing on the onset of treatment. Surveillance cultures of the nose are found to be unreliable because they cannot rule out invasive disease. Histologically, invasive sinusitis exhibits hemorrhagic thrombosis, infarction, and tissue necrosis. Septate hyphae with dichotomous branching at 45 degrees *(Aspergillus)* or broad nonseptate hyphae *(Mucor)* can usually be identified. Care must be taken on frozen section diagnosis because certain gram-negative bacteria such as *Pseudomonas* can cause vasculitic lesions similar to those of fungal sinusitis.

■ TREATMENT AND PROGNOSIS

Treatment of invasive fungal sinusitis is directed by several principles.

1. Reversal or correction of the underlying disease process, if possible. This is the most important factor in determining ultimate outcome. Correction of ketoacidosis in the diabetic patient and neutropenia in the immunosuppressed patient is essential. This correction may consist of administration of granulocyte transfusion, granulocyte colony–stimulating factor, or bone marrow transplantation. There is, however, limited evidence of the effectiveness of such treatment when there are complications, such as in the case of pulmonary infiltrates during the course of granulocyte transfusions.
2. Surgical treatment. Surgical debridement of all infected nonviable soft tissue and bone to bleeding margins is essential in the management of invasive fungal sinusitis. Such radical excision removes fungus growing in necrotic, thrombosed tissue and facilitates penetration of antifungal agents (see principle number 3). The extent of excision, for example, whether to exenterate an invaded orbit, depends on consideration of overall prognosis in individual patients. Thrombocytopenia requires correction by platelet transfusion before surgery.

   Sinus drainage procedures may be indicated; however, radical debridement appears to offer increased survival rate. Because the maxillary sinus seems to be the most commonly involved sinus, medial maxillectomy via an external approach (lateral rhizotomy) may be indicated. Endoscopic resection is adequate for more limited disease and as a means of assessing recurrences. Endoscopic surgery may be adequate if isolated turbinate involvement is found, because this procedure allows complete resection of diseased tissue. If irrigation of the nose and sinuses with topical antifungal agents is planned, an indwelling catheter can be placed at the same time as resection (see principle number 3). Invasion of overlying soft tissue, as evidenced by black necrotic skin, requires excision of these areas to healthy margins, with possible secondary closure once the disease is under control. Progression of necrosis after initial debridement is common, and repeated excisions may be necessary as often as every few days.

3. Antifungal agents. Amphotericin B, although only fungistatic, is nevertheless the mainstay in limiting progression of invasive fungal sinusitis. Given intravenously at doses of 0.8 to 1.5 mg per kilogram per day depending on disease severity and patient tolerance, this drug is continued for weeks or months. Side effects, such as nausea and vomiting, a flulike syndrome, hyperkalemia, and especially nephrotoxicity, are common and severe. Severe renal damage is dose dependent and occurs in approximately 15 percent of patients if the total dose of amphotericin is less than 2 g but in 80 percent of patients if the dose exceeds 5 g. Frequent monitoring of renal status by serum creatinine levels or creatinine clearance should be performed. Recently, less toxic amphotericin B preparations such as amphotericin B colloidal dispersion and liposomal amphotericin B have been reported to show increased efficacy and fewer side effects. Topical administration of amphotericin B in the maxillary sinus via catheter may be considered adjunctive treatment. Fifty milligrams of amphotericin B in a liter of water is irrigated, 20 ml four times a day. Such irrigation also helps control nasal crusting in the postoperative patient.

PROGNOSIS

Combined aggressive surgical and medical therapy has been shown by Zieske and co-workers to improve survival in patients who have fungal sinusitis. Unfortunately, mortality rates remain high. Only two of 11 patients responded completely to therapy in one series by Drakos and associates. Fifty percent survival has been noted in other studies. In a study by Kavanagh and co-workers, an 80 percent survival rate was found in patients who were in remission, but there were no survivors in relapse.

FUNGAL SINUSITIS AND HIV

Fungal sinusitis occurs late in the course of HIV disease, generally when CD4+ lymphocyte counts are less than 50 per cubic millimeter. Recognition of fungus in the nose or sinuses in these patients indicates a need for treatment without confirming the presence of invasive disease. Treatment is based on the same principles as in the non–HIV patient: surgical drainage and/or excision of infected tissue and antifungal agents administered as early as possible. Prognosis is guarded with combined therapy, which offers the best possibility of cure or suppression of these infections.

Suggested Reading

Berlinger N. Sinusitis in immunodeficient and immunosuppressed patients. Laryngoscope 1985; 95:29-35.

Blitzer A, Lawson W. Fungal infections of the nose and paranasal sinuses. Otolaryngol Clin North Am 1993; 26:1007-1035.

Drakos PE, Nagler A, Or R, et al. Invasive fungal sinusitis in patients undergoing bone marrow transplantation. Bone Marrow Transplant 1993; 12:203-208.

Forman SJ, Robinson SV, Wolf JL, et al. Pulmonary reactions associated with amphotericin B and leukocyte transfusions. New Engl J Med 1981; 305:584-585.

Kavanagh KT, Parham DM, Hughes WT, Chanin LR. Fungal sinusitis in immunocompromised children with neoplasms. Ann Otol Rhinol Laryngol 1991; 100:331-336.

Leopairut J, et al. Fungal sinusitis: The important role of the histopathology in the clinical management. J Med Assoc Thai 1992; 75 (Suppl 1): 60-70.

McGill D, et al. Fulminant aspergillosis of the nose and paranasal sinuses: A new clinical entity. Laryngoscope 1980; 90:748-754.

Morpeth JF, Rupp NT, Dolen WK, et al. Fungal sinusitis: An update. Ann Allergy Asthma Immunol 1996; 76:128-140.

Paultauf A. Mycosis mucorina. Virchows [A] 1885; 102:543-564.

Polacheck I, Nayler A, Okon E, et al. Aspergillus quadrilineatus, a new causative agent of fungal sinusitis. J Clin Microbiol 1992; 30:3290-3293.

Shugar MA. Mycotic infections of the nose and paranasal sinuses. In: Goldmon JL, eds. The principles and practice of rhinology. New York: John Wiley & Sons, 1987:717.

Sholer HJ. Mucorales. In: Howard DH, ed. Fungi pathogenic for humans and animals. New York: Marcel Dekker, 1983:9.

Venezio FR, Tucker PC. Zygomycosis. Elsevier Science Publishers, 1988: 467.

Yousem DM. Imaging of sinonasal inflammatory disease. Radiology 1993; 88:303-314.

Zieske LA, Kopke RD, Hamill R. Dematiaceous fungal sinusitis. Otolaryngol Head Neck Surg 1991; 105:567-577.

CHOANAL ATRESIA

The method of
Harlan R. Muntz

The infant is an obligate nasal breather. The unique anatomy of the newborn requires a patent nasal airway to continue normal respiratory function, which is likely due to the position of the tongue related to the palate. The infant also has an obstructed oral airway during suckling, which makes nasal breathing vital for feeding. Even a partially obstructed nose will cause difficulty in this vital task.

The child with choanal atresia has the classic case of neonatal airway obstruction. The cessation of dissolution of the oronasal membranes during fetal development leaves the infant with an obstruction of the airway that often is life threatening. Unilateral atresia and stenoses may also be problematic.

Airway obstruction noted during feeding but relieved by crying demonstrates that the oral airway is intact while the nasal airway is obstructed. Although the degree of obstruction and the degree of symptoms may vary, cyanosis and respiratory collapse may occur. Feeding difficulties may also lead to failure to thrive. Any infant who has significant breathing or feeding difficulties must be evaluated for choanal atresia, and repair should be considered based on the severity of the problem.

A unilateral obstruction from choanal atresia may be undiagnosed for some time. These children are frequently seen with thick mucoid nasal drainage, which is often interpreted as chronic sinusitis. Because the contralateral nose is patent, there is minimal complaint of nasal airway obstruction. The social ramifications of the nasal drainage are frequently the parental main issue. Obstruction on the contralateral side from infection, adenoid enlargement, or nasal septal deviation may precipitate increased airway symptoms and prompt medical evaluation. The treatment goal is to improve the overall airway status and allow normal mucus flow.

■ EVALUATION

Prompt evaluation of airway obstruction is a necessity. At the initial encounter, one must evaluate the severity of the obstruction. If the child is in extreme distress, urgent endotracheal intubation or tracheotomy allows safe, controlled evaluation and care. If the child has a moderate or mild obstruction, additional evaluation may take place before intervention. Close monitoring is essential to document and act on any worsening of airway status.

Nasal Airflow

Frequently, the site of airway obstruction can be determined by a detailed history. Nasal airway obstruction from bilateral choanal atresia is usually demonstrated immediately after delivery. Suckling or a mouth-closed posture will precipitate a crisis.

Airway distress is less common in unilateral choanal atresia because the patent contralateral airway may only intermittently become obstructed. The severity of distress is predicated on the degree of nasal obstruction and the age of the patient, because at some point the child will change from an obligate nasal breather to one who tolerates nasal obstruction. Feeding difficulties may lessen, as does the frequency of episodic obstruction.

Airflow through the nose may be seen by using a small cotton whisp placed beneath the nose when the mouth is closed or during feeding. Movement of the whisp signifies air motion. Similarly, a laryngeal mirror placed beneath the nose will fog with airflow. The documentation of the airflow rules out an atresia, but does not preclude a stenosis. This documentation does not suggest normal airway resistance but only that a passage exists.

Dye Study

If it has been determined that a total obstruction is present on one side but uncertainty exists about the other side, the physician can place a drop of methylene blue in the anterior nares of the side in question. If the blue dye appears in the oral cavity, a patent system is confirmed. Nasal airway resistance may still be quite high, and the nose could be functionally occluded, but atresia is ruled out.

Catheter Passage

The classic evaluation is to attempt the passage of a small catheter through the nose. If the catheter is seen in the oral cavity or pharynx, a nasal airway is present. The catheter may, however, roll in the nasal vault, giving the false impression that the nasal airway has been traversed. The high tongue position and the level of the palate in the neonate may make the observation of the catheter in the pharynx very difficult. Unfortunately, the attempt to pass a catheter through a patent but attenuated airway may cause edema and/or bleeding, making a partial obstruction complete. The resultant airway crisis could have been prevented by other means of evaluation.

Endoscopy

The preferable evaluation is with the use of a flexible fiberoptic endoscope to inspect the nasal airway. Although the differential diagnosis of nasal airway obstruction includes choanal atresia, it is certainly not the most common or only diagnosis entertained. Through the use of an endoscope, the physician can both assess nasal patency and evaluate the anatomy, including the nasal vestibule, nasal septum, and lateral nasal wall. Congenital nasal septal deviation may cause significant distress in the neonate, as can piriform aperture stenosis, encephalocele, nasal lacrimal duct cysts, nasal dermoid, or glioma. Diagnosis and treatment planning may start at the bedside with flexible endoscopy. Less trauma should result with the flexible endoscope than with a catheter because the airway can be navigated under direct vision. Nasal mucus should be suctioned before the endoscopy to allow better visualization.

Radiographic Imaging

If the diagnosis of choanal atresia or stenosis is established, radiographic imaging will allow the surgeon to plan the appropriate procedure to resolve the airway compromise. Lateral soft-tissue films with contrast in the nose will show the presence of the atretic plate, but will not define its nature. An axial computed tomographic scan will define the thickness of the atresia as well as the bony and membranous nature. Nasal septal pathology is also defined. The atresia most often involves a widening of the posterior septum and a dense bony thickening of the lateral buttress. The nature of the atresia and the thickness of the plate will be delineated and thus will allow for better surgical planning.

■ SURGICAL INTERVENTION

Tracheotomy

If the respiratory distress is severe and an airway cannot be established by endotracheal intubation, an emergency tracheotomy should be performed. This will stabilize the airway until further evaluation and treatment can be instituted. Some children may have choanal atresia as part of a syndrome, for example, CHARGE syndrome, or accompanying many other congenital deformities. In these cases, it may be far safer to establish a secure airway with a tracheotomy until the child is older and the bulk of the other deformities are corrected. Early surgical correction of the atresia may lead to a false sense of security about the airway and result in more problems for the child.

Surgical Repair

Repair of the choanal atresia has taken many forms. Early descriptions relate that the transnasal trochar tearing of an opening in the posterior choana is associated with much bleeding and an occasional success. Three major approaches are commonly in use: the transpalatal, the transnasal and the trans-septal. Each approach has certain advantages and potential difficulties.

Transpalatal

Although the transpalatal approach may be considered the standard, many surgeons today have not done this type of repair. This approach to the choana allows for preservation of mucosal flaps, with the hope that there will be less postoperative scarring in the area of the atresia. This is most often used for difficult bony atresia.

After induction of general anesthesia and endotracheal intubation, the palate is exposed with a Dingman mouth gag. One of two different incisions can be used. A large U-shaped palatal flap can be raised off the hard palate, which preserves both greater palatine neurovascular bundles. I prefer the alternative, a midline incision through the proximal soft palate and hard palate mucoperiosteum. Lateral elevation will expose the posterior hard palate. The posterior hard palate and bony septum are drilled away using a microdrill and operating microscope. Care is taken to preserve the mucosa. The mucosa is opened, and nasal stents are placed through the choana into the posterior pharynx. The palatal incision is closed.

This route should preserve the mucosa and allow removal of the bone plates causing the atresia, but as in most of the other techniques, stenting is still required. Dilation is planned after the stent removal. As high as a 50 percent incidence of midface retrusion is expected with this approach. This retrusion rate as well as the difficulty in execution of the technique have led many to seek alternative approaches.

Transnasal

The transnasal route has become far more sophisticated than the early attempts with a trochar. If there is only a thin membranous web, the method of removal may matter little, but the use of a stent to prevent restenosis is often required. Frequently, the atretic plate will have both a membranous and a bony component, and both components will need to be treated if a good nasal airway is to result.

CO_2 laser resection of the atretic plate offers some advantages. Bleeding is controlled as the tissue is resected. On low wattage, there is little adjacent soft-tissue trauma. A membranous atretic plate without much bone can be managed occasionally without the use of a stent, but still may require dilation. Resection of bone is possible, but only at higher wattage with an increase in the heat produced and a concurrent increase in the adjacent soft-tissue injury. The need for a direct line of sight may limit the resection in children who have a high arched palate, nasal septal deviation, or craniofacial deformities. The use of other wavelengths may allow the use of fiber delivery, but access still may be limited, and removal of bone is difficult. CO_2 laser can also be used to resect granulation at the time of subsequent dilations.

Many surgeons who operate on the nose have used microscopic techniques similar to those used in the ear. Development of stellate mucosal flaps followed by drilling away the atretic plate allows opening. The very tight space and the same limitations discussed with laser excision make for a challenging procedure. Stenting is still required, and dilations are necessary.

Since the development of equipment for pediatric endoscopic sinus surgery, a greater ability has been afforded to approach the choana from the anterior nose. The use of endoscopes and especially angled endoscopes often allows greater visualization. Mucosa may be removed with Tru-Cut instruments or powered microdebriders. Some bone can be removed with the bone cutting forceps, although these are often not sufficient to remove the dense bone at the lateral buttress. After flaps have been raised, the bone may be removed with a powered drill. Greater precision seems to be afforded with these techniques. In the case of totally membranous atresia, the surgeon may believe that a stent is not necessary. Further work with this technique will give us greater insight into its overall utility and success.

Trans-septal

Although the trans-septal route has typically been reserved for unilateral atresia in an older child, I have found it successful even in the small child or infant who has bilateral atresia. The anatomy of atresia is most frequently not really a "plate," but a narrowing from both the septum and the lateral buttress. Because the transpalatal route relies heavily on the removal of this abnormal area of the posterior septum, the transnasal approach similarly will open the nasopharynx by removal of the posterior aspect of the septum. Unlike the transnasal route that leaves two small lateral ports, the trans-septal route allows for creation of a single larger central port.

The Cottle septal approach creates anterior, bilateral posterior, and inferior tunnels. The mucosal flaps are maintained. The mucosa may be elevated off the atretic plate, which exposes the bone and/or fibrous tissue. If the infant's nose is too small to allow the introduction of the instruments, a sublabial incision is used to assist access. The use of telescopes, as used in endoscopic sinus surgery, assists visualization. Minimal bleeding is present because the mucosa has still not been traversed.

The posterior septum can be removed with any one of many bone forceps or chisels. As the dissection moves laterally across the atretic plate toward the lateral buttress, the bone may be removed with a drill or Spurling neurosurgical bone forceps. Incision first through the nasopharyngeal mucosa and then through the nasal mucosa opens the atresia. Minimal damage is incurred to the mucosa. Resection is well controlled. The use of well-developed mucosal flaps should prevent circumferential scarring.

To date, I have still used stents in this procedure. A nonrolled Silastic sheet can be extended from the anterior nasal septum through the repair side and secured to the septum with a single trans-septal stitch. This will not allow an adequate airway in bilateral atresia. A tubular stent is needed to allow both adequate airway and stenting of the mucosal flaps.

■ POSTSURGICAL CONSIDERATIONS

Stents

To prevent restenosis of the choana, a stent, usually made of an appropriately sized endotracheal tube, is used. This stent acts to maintain the position of mucosal flaps and establish an airway. Stents are fashioned to follow the curve of the nasal vault into the nasopharynx. Airway through these stents must be maintained, except in the case of a unilateral repair without significant airway compromise. The stent may be secured to the nasal septum and left within the nasal vestibule to reduce the risk of damage to the nasal ala.

Airway Maintenance

Because this is frequently the child's only airway, the caretaker in the postoperative period must be aware that obstruction of the airway stents will precipitate airway compromise. Aggressive saline lavage and suctioning at frequent intervals will reduce the risk of obstruction. Constant monitoring of the child for oxygen saturation and heart rate will alert the parent or nurse to any difficulty.

Dilations

The wounds are expected to be well healed by 4 to 6 weeks postoperatively. The stents are maintained until such time as the surgeon believes that the repair is healed. In some cases of trans-septal or transnasal repair, success has been seen with minimal duration stenting. Some restenosis usually occurs after the removal of the stent. Dilation helps break up the forming scar band and eventually leads to better patency. Three to four dilations at 2 week intervals are often required to maintain a good airway.

Under general anesthesia, increasingly larger diameter male ureteral sounds are lubricated and gently passed through the nose into the nasopharynx. Laser excision of granulation tissue has been used as an alternative, although there are no data showing this procedure to be more effective.

■ RESULTS

All of the previously described procedures work. Because no one surgeon who operates for choanal atresia has an enormous case volume, prospective randomized controlled studies have not been done. These studies would need to stratify for some of the more obvious vagaries of the population, including the membrane-bone ratio and thickness of the bone plate. The required population size for such a study would require multi-institutional cooperation. Success must be defined with follow-up endoscopy. Restenosis frequently occurs, but in the absence of symptoms, it is most often not investigated. Close observation and frequent follow-up is a necessity regardless of the technique.

Suggested Reading

Benjamin B. Evaluation of choanal atresia. Ann Otol Rhinol Laryngol 1985, 94:429-432.

Caldarelli DD, Friedberg SA. Transnasal microsurgical correction of choanal atresia. Laryngoscope 1977; 87:2023-2030.

Carpenter RJ, Neel HB. Correction of congenital choanal atresia in children and adults. Laryngoscope 1977; 87:1304-1311.

Connelly JP, Montgomery WW, Robinson JC. Choanal atresia. Part I: Medical aspects of a serious anomaly. Clin Pediatr 1965; 4:65-70.

Healy GB, McGill T, Jako GJ, et al. Management of choanal atresia with the carbon dioxide laser. Ann Otol Rhinol Laryngol 1978; 87:658-662.

Krespi YP, Husain S, Levine TM, Reede DL. Sublabial transseptal repair of choanal atresia or stenosis. Laryngoscope 1987; 97:1402-1406.

Leclerc JE, Fearon B. Choanal atresia and associated anomalies. Int J Pediatr Otorhinolaryngol 1987; 13:265-272.

Montgomery WW, Connelly JP, Robinson JC. Choanal atresia. Part II: Surgical management. Clin Pediatr 1965; 4:71-76.

Stankiewicz JA. The endoscopic repair of choanal atresia. Otolaryngol Head Neck Surg 1990; 103:931-937.

SUBMUCOUS CLEFT PALATE

The method of
William H. Lindsey

The word *velopharyngeal* is derived from the Latin word for *veil (velum)*, a sail-like structure resembling a curtain. The term *velum palatinum*, or *velopharyngeal*, thus refers to the interaction of the veil-like soft palate and the posterior pharyngeal wall. Together the velopharyngeal mechanism can be thought of as a complex sphincter made up of the soft palate and uvula; lateral pharyngeal walls and their constrictor muscles; posterior pharyngeal wall, including the Passavant's ridge; and, when applicable, the adenoid pad and tonsils (Fig. 1).

Velopharyngeal insufficiency (VPI) refers to insufficient or dysfunctional tissue in this region. This can result in poor closure of the palatal sphincter and a consequent poor separation of the nasopharynx from the oropharynx. Although this condition is commonly seen in patients who have clefts of the palate and thereby diagnosed in early evaluations, VPI can be overlooked in patients who have secondary or submucous clefts. In this latter population, the diagnosis can be delayed until a child enters the educational system, at which time faulty speech is detected by skilled personnel. History (reported by parents), physical examination, speech analysis, and fiberoptic nasopharyngoscopy can then confirm the diagnosis.

Symptoms and signs range from a mild alteration of speech patterns to gross reflux of food matter into the nasal cavities. In VPI of this magnitude, correspondent otitis and sinusitis sequelae have been demonstrated. The much more common manifestations of VPI center on the production of speech with a nasal quality. In addition, persistent VPI after primary cleft repair can affect up to 38 percent of patients.

■ DIAGNOSIS

The evaluation of suspect patients begins with a thorough history and physical examination. I often first have the parents relate in their own words the problems a child is having. This provides information about speech and may also shed light on recurrent otitis and sinusitis problems. I ask parents to describe the patient's swallowing ability for liquids, semisolids, and solids from birth to present. A review of past medical events should center on oral cavity procedures. If a tonsillectomy and/or adenoidectomy has been performed, what time relationship did the symptoms have to this procedure? A family history should determine whether other relatives have similar symptoms or have had clefts of the palate. Be attentive to the parent's dialect because on at least one occasion, the parents' speech during this history has led to the diagnosis of a submucous cleft in both the parent and the child.

Next, I begin the physical examination by having the patient elaborate upon any symptoms the parent may have mentioned. This elaboration is, of course, age dependent, but it can often give clues to the presence of VPI and its severity. A complete head and neck inspection includes evaluation for repaired or unrepaired cleft lip and/or palate disorders. The symmetry, shape, and length of the soft palate and uvula are ascertained and followed by digital palpation of these structures. If tonsils are present, determine whether their size inhibits the normal up and back movement of the soft palate during speech and swallowing.

Next, I perform a minispeech analysis on patients who are old enough to cooperate. This usually includes at least some investigation of other domains of communication such as hearing and language development skills. An articulation battery that surveys several phonemes is read, and the patient is asked to repeat each word (Table 1). This simple test includes nasal and non-nasal phonemes; fricative, affricative, and plosive phonemes; and vowel sounds that are often phoneme-specific difficulties secondary to VPI. When functioning properly, the velopharyngeal sphincter separates the resonating column of air in the oropharynx from the nasopharynx in all phonemes except /m/, /n/, and /ng/. VPI results in distortion of speech when this separation is inadequate. Resonance disorders, specifically hypernasality and nasal emission, are the hallmarks of VPI.

Hypernasality refers to an increase in the nasal resonance of sounds that are not in the /m/, /n/, and /ng/ phonemes, whereas nasal emission describes the escape of air from the nose during phonation. Compensatory articulation occurs during the attempt to enunciate fricative and plosive sounds by stopping, starting, or otherwise manipulating the speech air column at a point lower in the airway, such as at the glottis or hypopharynx.

Transoral and transnasal examination of the palate during phonation is performed in the office. With the mouth open, the patient is is asked to say "k" repeatedly as the soft palate and uvula are inspected. Attention should be focused on the detecting posterior and superior movement of the palate and its approximating the position of that movement to the posterior pharyngeal wall. Topical anesthesia is then applied to the nasal mucosa, and a small fiberoptic scope is inserted to the posterior nasal choanae. I repeat the simple

Table 1. Simple Therapy Test Words and Phrases Helpful in the Diagnosis of VPI

NASAL VS. NON-NASAL	PLOSIVE AND FRICATIVE	COMBINATION SENTENCES THAT ALSO TEST AIRFLOW
Nancy	Airplane	Papa puts paper in his pipe
Mama	Function	Sassy cats raced across the ice
Running	Ping-pong	
Global	Papa	
Boatload	Seesaw	
	Sister	
	Mississippi	
	Kick-the-can	
	Sixty-six	

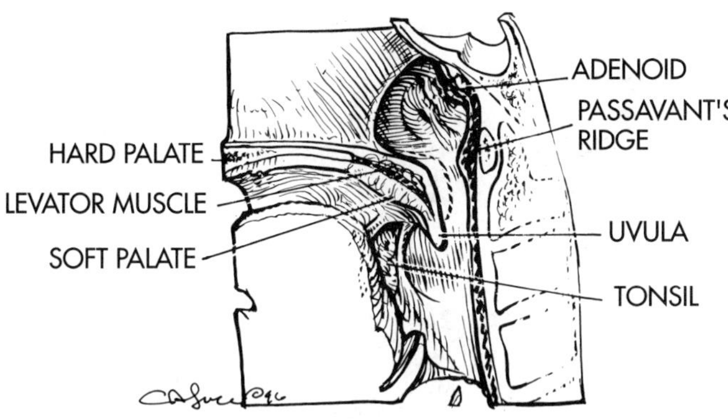

Figure 1.
Anatomy of normal nasopharynx.

speech analysis list and carefully inspect the nasopharynx for motion. First, the posterior and superior movement of the soft palate is observed. Next, any anterior motion of the posterior pharyngeal wall and the presence and size of a Passavant's ridge is quantified. Then, any medial motion of the lateral pharyngeal walls during constrictor contraction is measured. Finally, the scope is passed into the nasopharynx, and visualization of the palate and tonsils is achieved, with attention being given to any limitation in palate movement by the tonsils themselves. When complete, this examination should provide insight into the degree of contact between the soft palate and posterior pharyngeal walls during speech. If there is no contact, an approximation of the velopharyngeal gap is obtained, which allows therapeutic planning. Additionally, any specific wall motion abnormalities are noted. *In summary, patients with VPI have a velopharyngeal gap. Where is it, how big is it, and what needs to be augmented to fix this gap?*

Other diagnostic tests have been described. Videofluoroscopy with radiographic imaging of the nasopharynx has been used by many authors. I do not find that this adds information, and thus I do not expose patients to the radiation dose. Nasomanometry is a new approach to measuring nasal airflow and therefore has the potential to detect nasal emission. I have not used this approach yet, but I look forward to the literature reports concerning this technique. Two additional and important tests are always performed in my practice. First, I ask all patients to try to blow up a balloon before (and after) intervention. This baseline gives insight into the degree of seal that any velopharyngeal procedure achieves. Second, a competent speech pathologist who has clinical expertise in phonatory disorders examines my patients; coupled with the instrumental findings already noted, the speech pathologist's findings yield invaluable pre- and postinterventional diagnostic and therapeutic information. The role of the speech pathologist can not be underestimated.

■ THERAPEUTIC OPTIONS

The goal in treating VPI is to restore a functional seal between the nasopharynx and the oropharynx so that a more normal production of speech and deglutition occurs. It is also important to achieve these results while maintaining normal midface growth. Several options are available. Prosthetic speech appliances can be classified as speech bulbs and palatal lift prostheses. They artificially lengthen the soft palate and can be used in unrepaired or failed repairs of clefts and when surgery is either not desired or contraindicated. Posterior pharyngeal wall augmentation has been used for small velopharyngeal gaps.

Augmentation materials have ranged from Teflon and Silastic to autologous cartilage. Advantages of posterior wall augmentation include its relative simplicity and the fact that it does not alter the nasal airway. Sphincter pharyngoplasty creates a dynamic muscular sphincter by rotating the palatopharyngeus muscles transversely into the velopharynx. Theoretic advantages of this procedure are its dynamic nature and the fact that it does not obstruct the nasal airway. However, it has not been reported in large enough numbers for complete evaluation.

Pharyngeal flap surgery is a commonly performed procedure that creates a nonanatomic structure statically separating the nasopharynx and oropharynx. Drawbacks include a high rate of postoperative problems related to nasal airway obstruction by the flap itself. This obstruction of the airway can lead to hyponasal speech, mouth breathing, severe snoring, and obstructive sleep apnea. In addition, if the flap is not large enough, VPI may persist. Palate-lengthening procedures, including the Wardill V-Y pushback procedure and Dorrance incision, have been used. Lengthening the palate at the time of initial cleft repair is controversial. The use of these procedures for management of VPI without clefts has not been established and may alter hard palate growth by the elevation of large amounts of periosteum.

The Furlow palatoplasty offers an alternative to conventional palate-lengthening procedures. Performed by Leonard Furlow since 1976, this procedure as initially described simultaneously repairs clefts of the palate and lengthens the soft palate and velum. Other researchers who have noted the success of this procedure with VPI have used the Furlow palatoplasty after primary cleft repair and with submucous cleft palates. Patients selected for surgical intervention undergo a double-opposing Z-plasty, as described by Furlow. Briefly, a soft palate Z-plasty is designed and incised (Fig. 2). On one side only, palatal mucosa and submucosa are elevated as an anteriorly based flap. On the opposite side, a posteriorly based mucosal and levator–palatopharyngeus muscle flap is elevated. Next, a mirror image of the Z-plasty is developed on the nasal side, with the posteriorly based flap containing the remaining muscle. The flaps are transposed and inset, and the incisions are closed. Patients are given nothing by mouth for 24 hours and are gradually advanced to a soft diet over 2 weeks. A 5 day course of antibiotic therapy is prescribed to control oral flora. Postoperative evaluation, including speech analysis and flexible nasopharyngoscopy, allows assessment of surgical results.

■ DECISION MAKING

A thoughtful approach to therapeutic interventions for VPI allows for some flexibility. Together with the patient and

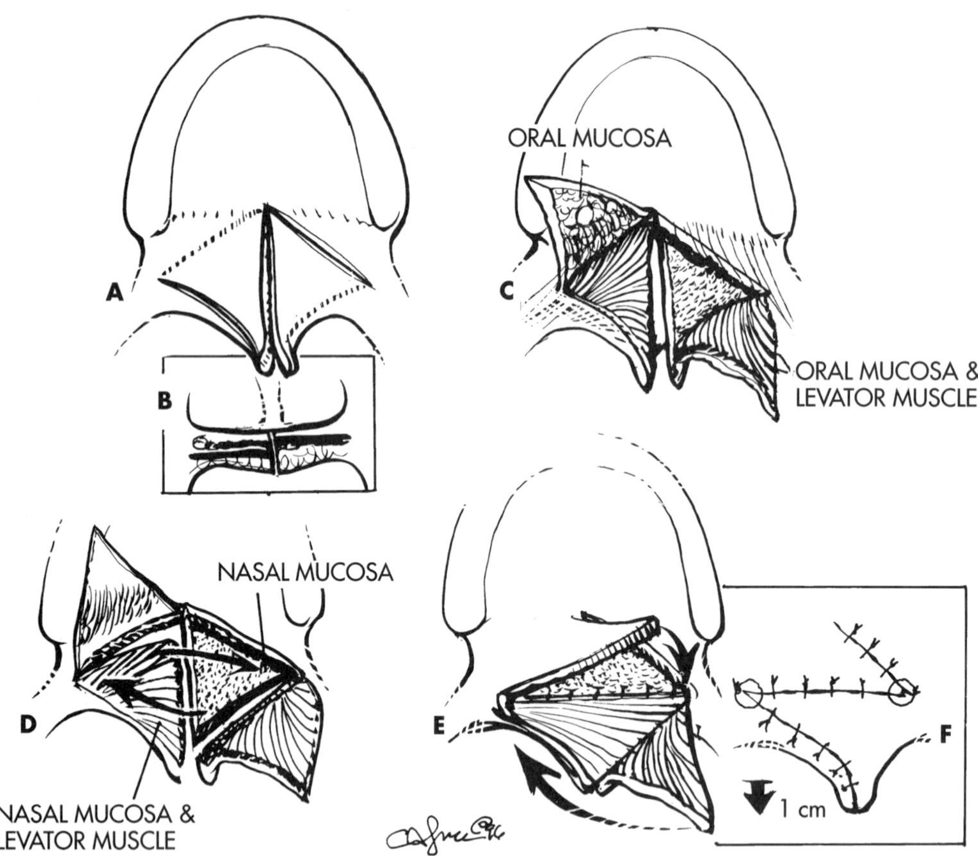

Figure 2.
Technique of the Furlow palatoplasty (see text).

parents, the speech pathologist and I discuss options and reasonable expectations. Much of the decision is influenced by the velopharyngeal gap size and location. For gaps of 0 to 2 mm either before or after surgical intervention, prolonged speech therapy and balloon exercises are often a successful and conservative modality. For limited posterior wall gaps associated with a small or absent Passavant's ridge and yet with a reasonable palate length, local augmentation with cartilage is used. In patients who have gaps of 3 to 8 mm, I prefer the Furlow palatoplasty. The procedure is not difficult to perform and is accomplished in roughly the same time frame as are other palatal procedures. The Furlow palatoplasty has several unique physiologic advantages over other methods of treating VPI.

The use of double-opposing Z-plasty lengthens the velum, just as a Z-plasty for scar revision lengthens the central limb of the scar. Furthermore, the nonlinear design of the incision allows less scar contracture in an anterior to posterior direction than do the linear incisions of some other procedures. More important, the levator sling in patients who have cleft palate and other types of VPI is misdirected anteriorly, which potentially increases the palatal gap with contraction. The Furlow palatoplasty both redirects and suspends the levator sling in a more transverse fashion (Fig. 2). In the muscle dissection itself, the mucosal covering is elevated on one side only. Thus, myomucosal flaps rather than isolated muscle flaps (as are used in other techniques) are transposed. When used to correct VPI rather than to repair hard palate clefts, the Furlow palatoplasty involves no periosteal elevation. Periosteal elevation has been correlated with hard palate scarring and altered growth. Push-back procedures for VPI have been shown to produce maxillary deformities and cross-bite malocclusion. Finally, unlike other procedures, the Furlow palatoplasty does not interfere with the dynamic muscular contractility of the rest of the pharynx, nor does it obstruct the nasal airway as a route for respiration.

For patients who have velopharyngeal gaps of greater than 8 mm or failures from other techniques, a pharyngeal flap procedure is chosen. Postoperative speech therapy is emphasized for all VPI patients.

Traditional articulation exercises are beneficial to remediate compensatory articulation patterns. The efficacy of exercises or drills to improve VPI is somewhat controversial. Currently, interventions with biofeedback, including endoscopy and nasomanometry, appear advantageous. The role of continuous positive airway pressure warrants further investigation in the treatment of VPI.

Suggested Reading

Furlow LT Jr. Cleft palate repair by double opposing Z-plasty. Plast Reconstr Surg 1986; 78:724-736.

Furlow LT Jr. Correction of secondary velopharyngeal insufficiency in cleft palate patients with the Furlow palatoplasty. Plast Reconstr Surg 1994; 94:942-943.

Grobbelaar AO, Hudson DA, Fernandes DB, Lentin R. Speech results after repair of the cleft soft palate. Plast Reconstr Surg 1995; 95:1150-1154.

Hudson DA, Grobbelaar AO, Fernandes DB, Lentin R. Treatment of velopharyngeal incompetence by Furlow Z-plasty. Ann Plast Surg 1995; 34:23-26.

Lindsey WH, Davis PT. Correction of velopharyngeal insufficiency with Furlow palatoplasty. Arch Otolaryngol Head Neck Surg 1996; 122:881-884.

Witt PD, D'Antonio LL. Velopharyngeal insufficiency and secondary palatal management; a new look at an old problem. Clin Plast Surg 1993; 20:707-721.

UNILATERAL CLEFT LIP AND PALATE

The method of
Craig W. Senders

The surgical correction of cleft lip and palate has been challenging surgeons since the first recorded repair in 300 AD during the Tien dynasty in China. In general, surgeons today are able to achieve excellent results regarding both function and aesthetics. However, the unilateral cleft nasal deformity continues to be an area where additional innovations will benefit all of us.

Approximately 1 in 1,000 neonates in the United States has a cleft lip. Two-thirds of these patients have an associated cleft palate. Although more than 250 syndromes are associated with cleft lip and palate, most of these patients develop their deformity from multifactorial inheritance, in which genes from both the mother and the father as well as environmental factors contribute to the expression of the cleft deformity.

Patients who have cleft lip and palate require treatment from many disciplines, including audiology, facial plastic surgery, genetics, orthodontics, oral surgery, otolaryngology, social services, and speech pathology. Because the treatment plans are complex and involve multiple disciplines, care should be coordinated by a cleft team.

■ FEEDING

Infants who have a cleft palate are unable to generate a normal sucking reflex and therefore have difficulties with feeding. Although a child who has a cleft lip alone may breast-feed, all children who have a cleft palate require specialized feeding techniques. The MeadJohnson cleft palate nurser accomplishes this by using a larger than normal nipple with an enlarged opening. In addition, the bottle is plastic, and the parent is able to squeeze the bottle in coordination with the infant's sucking reflex to allow a more efficient egress of formula.

Children should be seen weekly until consistent weight gain is demonstrated. All infants are expected to have a 10 percent weight loss in their first week of life, but thereafter they should gain 20 to 30 g per day. Persistent failure to gain at least 15 g daily requires admission to the hospital for intensive feeding instruction and/or nasogastric feedings. Children who require nasogastric feedings despite appropriate feeding techniques should be evaluated by a geneticist. The incidence of syndromes in this population is much higher.

■ PREOPERATIVE ASSESSMENT

Most surgeons follow the "rule of tens" in determining surgical eligibility, which states that the infant has achieved 10 weeks of age, a weight of 10 pounds, and a hemoglobin level greater than 10 g/dL. In recent years, consideration of the preoperative hemoglobin level has become optional.

Many surgeons use the pinch test to determine whether an infant will require presurgical orthopedics before the definitive lip repair. The surgeon pinches the cleft together to determine how much tension the repair will be under. If the surgeon is unable to make the edges of the cleft approximate, the child definitely requires presurgical orthopedics. If the cleft's edges easily approximate, presurgical orthopedics are not necessary. With experience, the surgeon will determine at what level of tension presurgical orthopedics will benefit a patient.

An easy and inexpensive method for presurgical orthopedics is the "tape technique," in which 1/2 inch paper tape is applied from cheek to cheek to exert pressure across a cleft. In applying the tape, the cheeks should be pinched together with one hand. The placement of successive layers of tape allows each subsequent piece of tape to exert slightly more pressure. The use of an extra-thin stoma adhesive on the cheeks will prevent skin irritation and allow frequent changing when the tape becomes soiled. For the University of California at Davis Cleft and Craniofacial Team, the use of the tape technique has always been successful, and a lip adhesion has not been used in a unilateral cleft lip and palate patient. Please see the suggested reading section for additional information on presurgical orthopedics.

■ TIMING OF SURGERY

The cleft lip repair is performed when the infant is between 10 and 14 weeks of age. If the cleft nasal deformity is significant, a primary cleft rhinoplasty is performed at the same setting. Additionally, short-acting middle ear ventilating tubes are placed in patients who have otitis media with effusion.

The cleft palate is repaired when the infant is between 10 and 14 months of age. At the same surgery, the short-acting middle ear ventilation tubes are replaced with long-acting T-tubes.

■ ROTATION ADVANCEMENT UNILATERAL CLEFT LIP REPAIR (MILLARD REPAIR)

Patients typically receive a prophylactic antibiotic of penicillin or a cephalosporin even though there are no definitive studies that demonstrate this to be necessary. A local anesthetic of 1 percent lidocaine with 1:100,000 epinephrine can be injected before making the markings for the rotation advancement repair as long as the anesthetic is used in moderation and the injections are away from the sites of the intended incisions. Local anesthetic can therefore be injected at the superior margin of the oral commissure to vasoconstrict the superior labial arteries at the bases of both ala and at the base of the columella of the nose. If a primary rhinoplasty is anticipated, the nasal tip is injected as well.

The marking points are indicated in Figure 1. The location of the medial peak of Cupid's bow on the cleft side (point 3) is determined. This point is the same distance from the low point of Cupid's bow (point 2) to the high point of Cupid's bow on the normal side (point 1). Next, the lateral peak of Cupid's bow on the cleft side (point 8) is identified. The distance from point 6 to point 1 should equal the distance from point 7 to point 8. Alternatively, this point can be determined as the point where the white roll disappears. The distance from point 8 to point 9 should equal the distance from point 3 to point 5 to point X. If the distance from point 8 to point 9 will be inadequate, point 9 can be moved further internasally or, conversely, point 8 can be moved more laterally.

The intended incisions are marked as indicated in Figure 2. There is a tendency to make the incision from point 3 to point 5 overly curved. The more curved this incision is, the smaller the c-flap will be. Also, the approximation of the advancement flap (point 8 to point 9), which is relatively straight with a highly curved rotation flap, is more difficult.

Point 3 and point 8 are tattooed with a 27 gauge siliconized needle (a nonsiliconized needle is not necessary).

■ INCISIONS

Beginning with the advancement segment, the vertical vermilion border incision is made with a No. 11 blade from the intended peak of Cupid's bow (point 8) outward. The cutaneous incisions are made with a No. 15C blade. The mucosal incisions are then made with a No. 15 blade. The l-flap is then elevated. A mucosal incision is made in the buccal-alveolar sulcus.

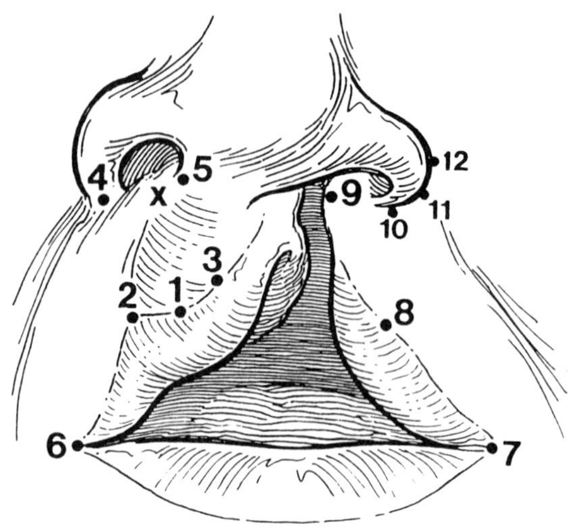

Figure 1.
Marking points for rotation advancement repair: (1) Low point of Cupid's bow; (2) Peak of Cupid's bow, noncleft side (NCS); (3) Medial peak of Cupid's bow, cleft side (CS); (4) Ala base (NCS); (5) Columella base; (X), Back-cut point; (6) Commissure (NCS); (7) Commissure (CS); (8) Lateral peak of Cupid's bow (CS); (9) Medial tip of advancement flap; (10) Midpoint of alar base; (11) Lateral alar base; (12) Maximum extent of alar incision. *(From Ness JA, Sykes JM. Basics of the Millard rotation advancement technique for repair of the unilateral cleft lip deformity. In: Facial plastic surgery. New York: Thieme, 1993:176; with permission.)*

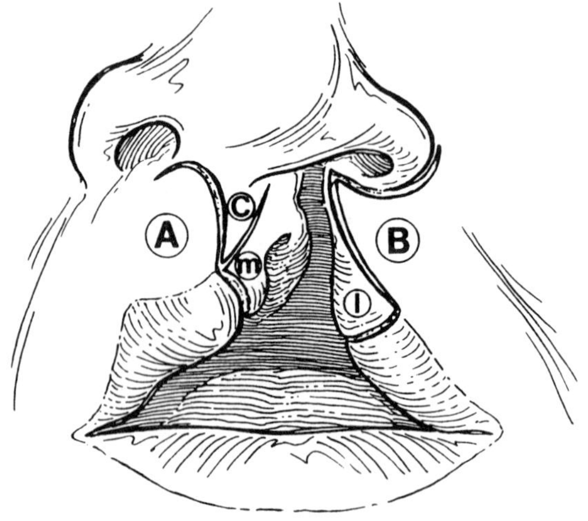

Figure 2.
Incisions and flaps for rotation advancement repair. *(From Ness JA, Sykes JM. Basics of the Millard rotation advancement technique for repair of the unilateral cleft lip deformity. In: Facial plastic surgery. New York: Thieme, 1993:176; with permission.)*

The lip release is accomplished by connecting the alar incision (point 9 to point 11) to the buccal-alveolar incision. The muscle fibers are sharply separated from the base of the ala. Scissors are used to separate the lip from the face of the maxilla. Care is taken not to injure the inferior orbital nerve. In some clefts. it is necessary to extend the alar incision (point 9 to point 11) to point 12.

The nasal release is accomplished by connecting the intranasal incision to the alar incision (point 9 to point 11). In designing the intranasal incisions, care is taken to preserve all the cutaneous tissue possible for reconstruction of the nasal floor. It is often necessary to sharply separate the ala from the piriform aperture. At this point, both the nose and the lip should be completely free and mobile, and they should easily reach their intended closing positions. With a No. 15 blade, the epithelium is undermined 2 mm. The vermilion border is undermined 3 mm. It is normally not necessary to undermine the mucosa.

A similar procedure is performed on the rotation segment. Here, the m-flap and the c-flap are elevated before the lip release. The lip release connects the rotation incision with the buccal-alveolar sulcus incision. Again, scissors are used to separate the malinserted muscle fibers from the base of the columella. A No. 11 blade is used to make the back-cut from point X to point 5. The back-cut is extended until adequate rotation is achieved. Undermining of the rotation segment is similar to that of the advancement segment, except the undermining near the columella is only 1 mm.

A primary rhinoplasty can be performed through the advancement and/or rotation incisions. Please see the suggested reading section for additional details on primary rhinoplasty.

■ SUTURING

The nasal floor is closed first with 4–0 chromic suture. Closure of the nasal floor can determine the superior and inferior position of the alar base as well as the lateral position. The mucosal incisions are closed next with interrupted 4–0 chromic suture. The m-flap and l-flap can be used to close the floor of the nose, but they are often discarded. The mucosal incisions within approximately 15 mm of Cupid's bow are left unapproximated at this time. A temporary 6–0 nylon suture is placed at the vermilion cutaneous junction to aid in alignment of the muscles. The muscles are then closed with 4–0 PDS suture from superior to inferior. The temporary vermilion cutaneous junction suture is removed to allow careful approximation inferiorly.

A 6–0 nylon suture is replaced at the vermilion cutaneous junction, and another suture is placed where the advancement flap fits into the rotational flap defect. The remainder of the cutaneous skin sutures are closed with 6–0 fast-absorbing catgut. The c-flap is generally closed on itself for one or two sutures and then is used to help recreate the floor of the nose. Any redundant C-flap is excised. The vermilion is now closed with 5–0 chromic suture. Any redundant vermilion tissue is excised (Fig. 3). Bacitracin ointment is placed over the suture line.

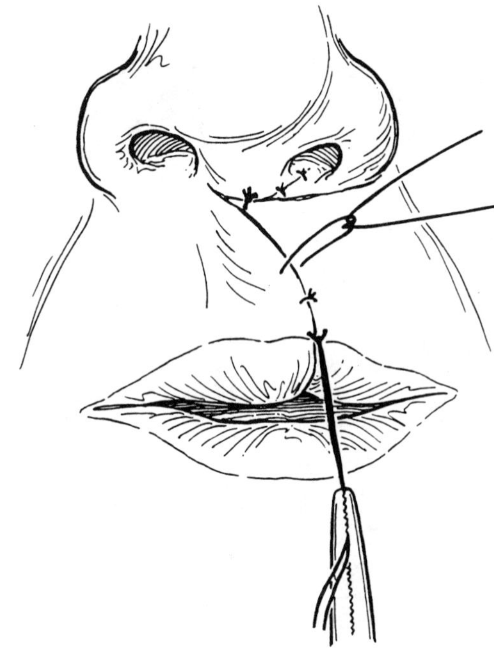

Figure 3.
Final suturing. *(From Ness JA, Sykes JM. Basics of the Millard rotation advancement technique for repair of the unilateral cleft lip deformity. In: Facial plastic surgery. New York: Thieme, 1993:176; with permission.)*

■ POSTOPERATIVE CARE

All patients are kept in arm restraints and are fed with syringe feedings for approximately 3 weeks. The external incisions are cleansed with half-strength hydrogen peroxide, followed by bacitracin ointment four times a day for the first 7 to 10 days. The two permanent nylon sutures are removed between 5 and 7 days postoperatively. Two weeks following surgery parents are encouraged to massage the suture line for 5 minutes twice a day.

■ TWO-FLAP PALATOPLASTY

All patients receive prophylactic penicillin (20,000 U per kilogram) before surgery and for 24 hours after surgery. Additionally, patients receive dexamethasone (0.25 mg per kilogram) before surgery and for 24 hours postoperatively. The palate is injected with 1 percent lidocaine with 1 : 100000 epinephrine to aid with hemostasis.

The incisions are marked as indicated in Figure 4. The hard palate incision is made slightly on the oral surface of the hard palate. On the soft palate, the incision is midway between the oral and nasal surface of the cleft. Using scissors and a forceps, the medial one-quarter to one-third of the uvula is resected bilaterally. Failure to perform this maneuver often results in a dehiscence of the uvula. A No. 15 blade is used to carry the incision anteriorly from the uvula, splitting the soft palate approximately 3 mm. As this incision reaches the hard palate, the blade is angled slightly to ensure

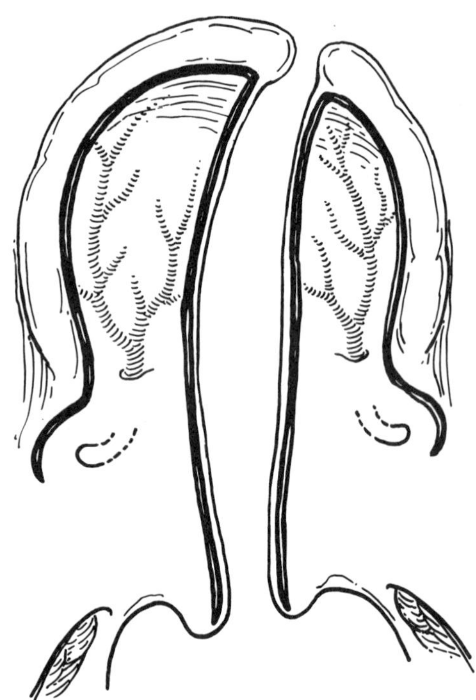

Figure 4.
Markings for two-flap palatoplasty. *(From Senders CW, Sykes JM. Advances in palatoplasty. Arch Otolaryngol 1993; 119: 375–377; with permission.)*

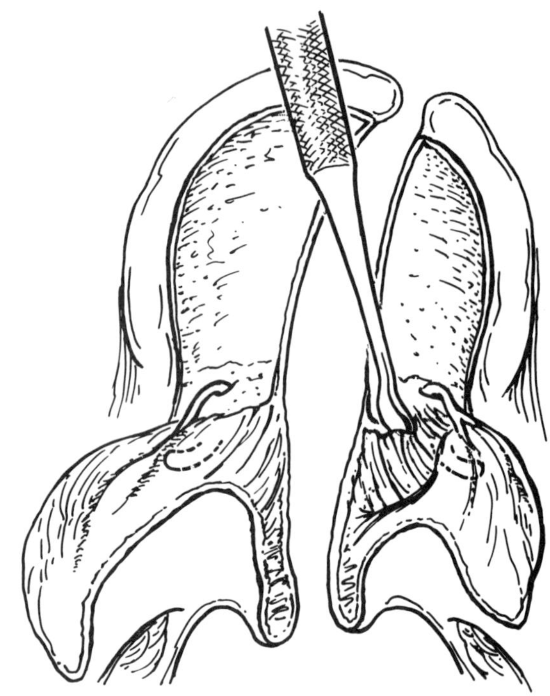

Figure 5.
Elevation of flaps allows direct dissection of the greater palatine vessels. *(From Senders CW, Sykes JM. Advances in palatoplasty. Arch Otolaryngol 1993; 119:375–377; with permission.)*

that the knife strikes the bone of the palate. Laterally, the incision is made through mucosa behind the alveolar process and passes around the alveolar process. On the patient's right side, the surgeon's left hand is used to ensure that the blade angles away from the greater palatine vessels. This incision is then carried just onto the palatal aspect of the alveolar ridge until it meets the midline cleft incision.

The palatal flaps are elevated with the use of a Woodson elevator. Care is taken not to damage the greater palatine vessels. Once this flap is elevated, bleeding points are cauterized. A Paget elevator is used to separate the muscle attachments from the bony palate posteriorly. This can then be followed anteriorly to elevate the nasal mucosa from the palatine shelf. Care should be taken not to fenestrate the nasal mucosa, which is quite thin.

A similar procedure is done on the opposite side. Using a tooth forceps in each hand, the surgeon approximates the oral mucosa at the bony soft palate junction. The palatal mucosa should approximate without significant tension. If there is still tension, care is taken to further dissect the greater palatine vessels and occasionally separate the aponeurosis of the velum palatinum muscle after it wraps around the hamulus (Fig. 5).

■ CLOSURE

The palate is closed in three layers. The nasal layer is closed with 4–0 chromic suture from anterior to posterior. Next, the muscle layer is approximated with 3–0 or 4–0 polyglactin

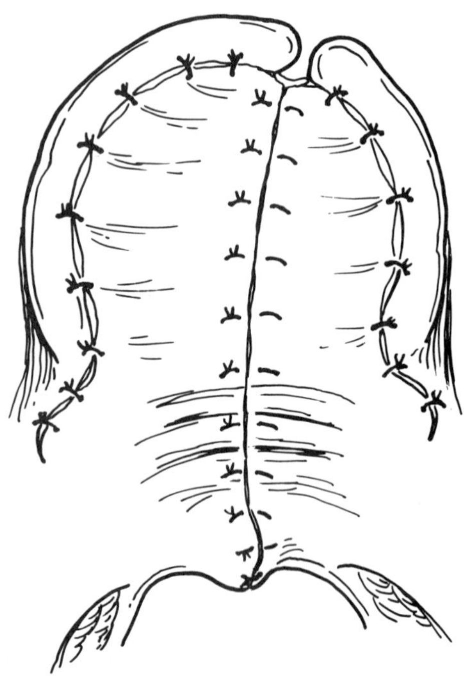

Figure 6.
Final suturing result. *(From Senders CW, Sykes JM. Advances in palatoplasty. Arch Otolaryngol 1993; 119:375–377; with permission.)*

910. Last, the oral layer is closed with 4–0 or 3–0 polyglactin 910 suture using interrupted vertical mattress sutures. In two sutures the deep loop of the vertical mattress sutures should pass through the nasal mucosa in the hard palate region to ensure elimination of dead space. Typically, one or two simple sutures are placed anteriorly. Closure in this manner will typically leave some small areas of exposed bone laterally. The lateral incision is closed where practical. One or two sutures are usually placed laterally near the posterior alveolus (Fig. 6).

■ POSTOPERATIVE CARE

The child is kept in a mist tent until he or she begins to take oral fluids. The child should also be kept in arm restraints and on oral fluids for 2 weeks postoperatively. Children are kept in the hospital until they demonstrate good oral fluid intake.

■ COMPLICATIONS

Five to 10 percent of palatoplasties will result in a fistula formation. Roughly 25 percent of patients who undergo a palatoplasty will have difficulty with velopharyngeal dysfunction. Therefore, these patients should be carefully monitored by a speech pathologist yearly until good speech is demonstrated. Surgery for velopharyngeal dysfunction should be accomplished between the ages of 4 and 5 years. Waiting until the child is older can make catch-up speech more difficult.

Suggested Reading

Millard DR Jr. Cleft craft: The evolution of its surgery. Vols. 1 and 2. Boston: Little, Brown, 1976.

Ness JA, Sykes JM. Basics of the Millard rotation advancement technique for repair of the unilateral cleft lip deformity. In: Facial plastic surgery. New York: Thieme, 1993:176.

Senders CW. Presurgical orthopedics. Surgery of the cleft lip and palate deformities. Facial Plast Surg Clin North Am 1996; 4:333-342.

Senders CW, Sykes JM. Advances in palatoplasty. Arch Otolaryngol 1993; 119:375-377.

Senders CW, Sykes JM. Cleft palate. In: Smith JD, Bumsted R, eds. Pediatric facial plastic reconstructive surgery. New York: Raven Press, 1993:159.

Senders CW, Sykes JM. Surgical treatment of the unilateral cleft nasal deformity at the time of lip repair. Facial Plast Surg Clin North Am 1995; 3:69-77.

VELOPHARYNGEAL INSUFFICIENCY

The method of
Howard W. Smith
Joseph Haddad, Jr.

Velopharyngeal insufficiency (VPI) is a functional defect in the pharynx whereby oral speech is diverted in varying degrees through the nasal passage. The cause of the defect may be in the pharyngeal muscles, the palatal muscles, or the osseous pharyngeal cavity. This area modifies sounds created by the vibrating vocal cords or creates sounds with air passing through a nonvibrating larynx.

Defective speech with nasal emission is easy to recognize when it is severe but requires sophisticated analysis by a speech pathologist if it is minimal. Depending on the degree of insufficiency, the individual may suffer social and financial problems. Inability to properly speak can be an embarrassment not only from the speech itself but also from facial distortions due to abnormal jaw and tongue movements during efforts to close off the nasal escape of air and attempts to shift the production of speech posteriorly into the pharynx.

Patients who have a history of cleft lip and palate repair, craniofacial syndromes, and neurologic disorders often exhibit nasal regurgitation of liquids, snoring, and sleep apnea. The examining physician needs a discriminating ear to detect the lesser degrees of insufficiency, especially those evident only on connected speech. Concerned parties in the diagnosis and management of VPI include the family physician or pediatrician, speech pathologist, radiologist, orthodontist, plastic surgeon, and otolaryngologist.

■ EVALUATION

Minimal VPI requires more sophisticated assessment. The more obvious cases of hyponasality developing or persisting after closure of a palatal cleft suggest a scarred, thickened, shortened palate or even a palatal fistula (Fig. 1). Regardless of the cause, all patients deserve a competent workup to arrive at a diagnosis on which a reliable treatment plan can be established.

A complete assessment includes an intraoral examination, voice recording with speech analysis, cephalometric radiographs, videofluoroscopy, nasal endoscopy, and possibly airflow studies.

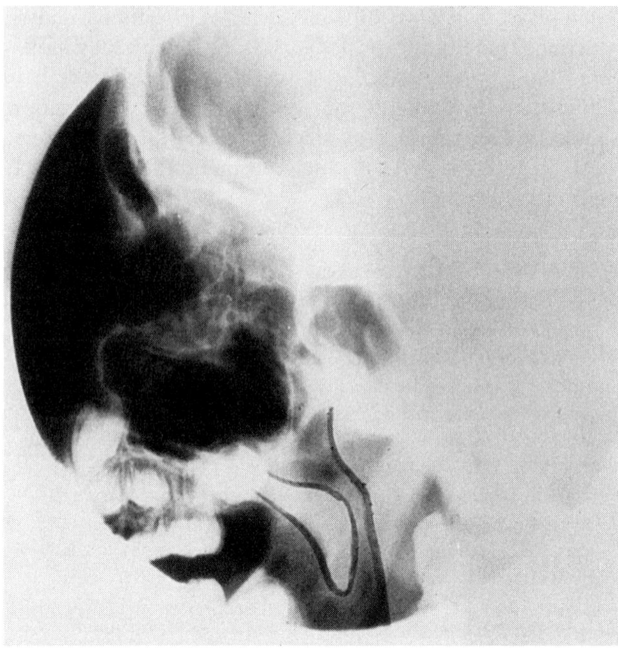

Figure 1.
Radiograph of patient with velopharyngeal insufficiency taken during phonation showing thick and stiff soft palate after cleft palate closure.

Intraoral Examination

Much can be gained by evaluating the patient's ability to open and close the mouth quickly. The lips provide an anterior movable muscular curtain and are a valuable aid in articulating speech. Defects in dentition such as missing teeth and a high, narrow palatal arch can affect articulation. The length and movement of the soft palate, as well as lateral pharyngeal muscle movement, can be evaluated by provoking the gag reflex. This upward movement of the palate in a patient who has a submucous cleft will demonstrate a midline separation of the muscles and the presence of a short, stubby uvula with a hint of bifurcation (Fig. 2). Palpation of the posterior border of the hard palate will reveal a cleft in the bone. Often, the anterior-posterior depth of the nasopharynx can be visualized with the palate at rest, but it is best evaluated by phonating cephalometric radiographs (Figs. 3 and 4). Large tonsils should be considered for removal, especially if the treatment plan calls for a pharyngeal flap.

Cephalometric Radiographs

Lateral cephalometric radiographs taken both at rest and on phonation provide valuable information on the length, shape, and movement of the soft palate and movement of the posterior pharyngeal wall (Fig. 5). The size of the nasopharyngeal cavity and the size of the adenoids are clearly seen. The anterior-posterior phonating cephalometric radiograph will show medial movement of the lateral pharyngeal walls.

Video Nasopharyngeal Endoscopy

This procedure is possible in all children. Even though a child may not cooperate, important information on the dimensions and dynamics of the nasopharynx can be obtained, as well as palate and pharyngeal muscle movement. Older children can cooperate more easily by phonating. A videorecording with voice provides a direct view of the soft palate muscles and the superior constrictor muscles in action. The recorded test can be reviewed at leisure with the speech pathologist to correlate sounds with muscular action and efficiency of the sphincteric closure.

Speech Analysis

The specialist in speech pathology and speech therapy is a great help to the physician examiner. Most physicians can recognize severe hypernasality and possibly distinguish it from hyponasality. In true VPI, articulated speech needs to be analyzed for degrees of hypernasality, nasal air emissions, weak pressure consonants, and compensating articulation.

The surgeon planning the surgical correction of VPI should at least have a basic knowledge of articulation, phonation, resonance, and compensatory articulation in order to have a meaningful conference with the speech pathologist.

- Articulation is achieved by the lips, mandible, palate, tongue, and pharynx to achieve speech.
- Phonation is of two types: that produced by the vibrating vocal cords and that produced by air passing through the larynx; in both instances the sound is modified by articulated speech.
- Resonance occurs in the entire vocal tract above the larynx as a response to sound. Resonance may be hypernasal, hyponasal, or mixed.
- Compensatory articulation is an attempt to achieve articulation in the presence of VPI. These attempts are recognized by the speech pathologist, but are not meaningful to the average surgeon.

■ THERAPY

Nonsurgical

Speech therapy may be considered in patients who have minimal or intermittent VPI. The operating surgeon must rely on the speech therapist for identifying these patients. Training may be effective in cases in which compensatory movements have been discovered. In general, speech therapy does not correct true VPI but should be considered in borderline cases. Biofeedback has been suggested as a treatment for minimal VPI.

If surgery is contraindicated for health reasons, a prosthetic appliance may be considered (Fig. 6). These devices were in common use many years ago, but are infrequently constructed today with the advent of controlled anesthesia and new surgical techniques, primarily pharyngeal flaps.

Surgical Prevention

In recent years, progress has been made to avoid the occurrence of VPI following surgical closure of the cleft palate. There is no consensus on the correct time to perform cleft palate surgery. Most surgeons perform cleft palate repair on patients between the ages of 6 and 18 months. The need for pharyngeal flaps has reportedly been reduced by using a two-flap technique versus the V-Y or Van Langenbech tech-

A

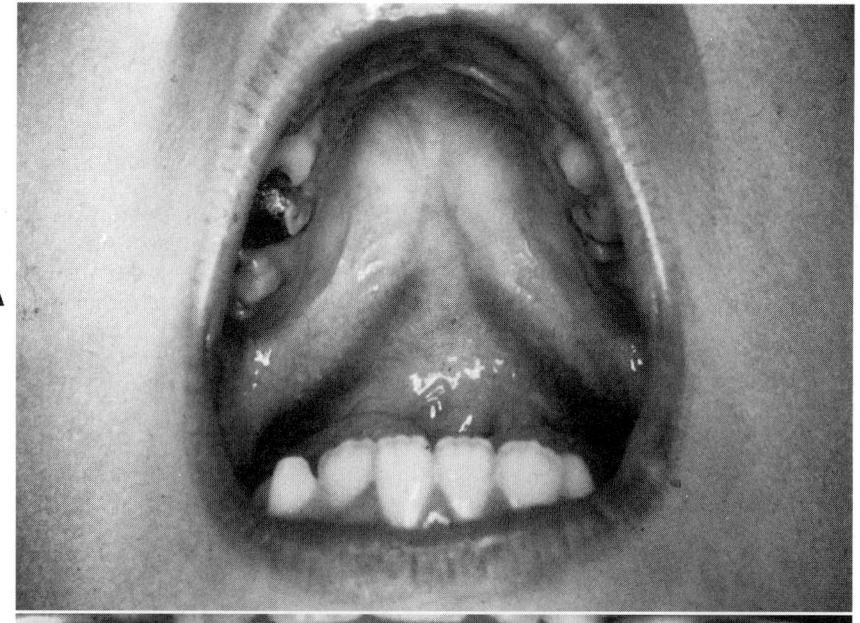

B

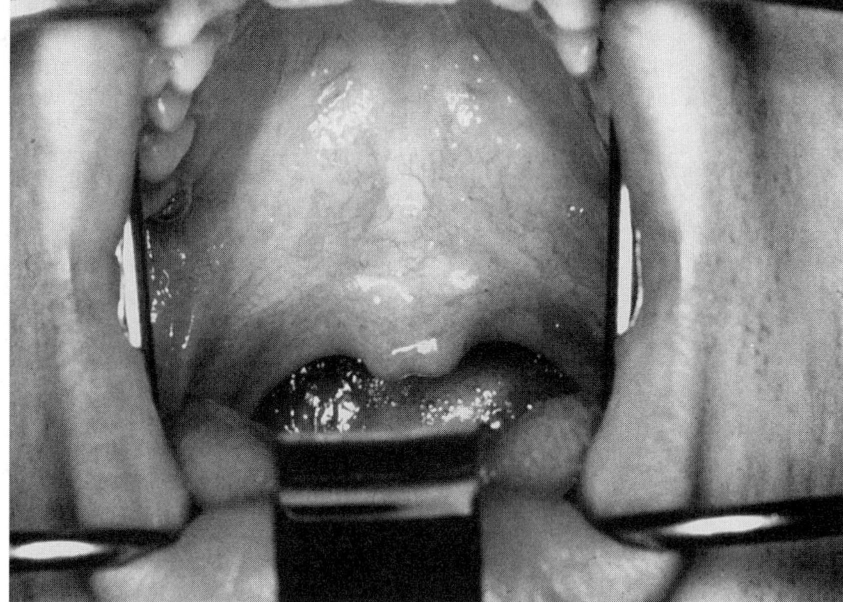

Figure 2.
Submucous cleft palate. *A,* Deficient hard palate bone; *B,* Short, stubby uvula with a hint of bifurcation.

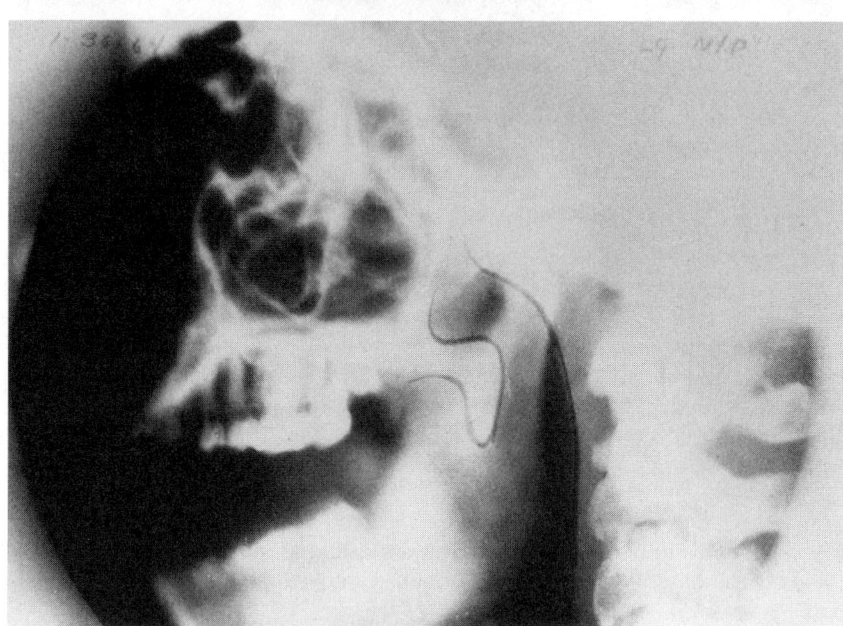

Figure 3.
Radiograph of patient with velopharyngeal insufficiency showing a short soft palate.

niques, in part because a two-layer closure can be achieved in the hard palate area, and a three-layer closure can be achieved in the soft palate.

In the Perko technique, the periosteum is left on the hard palate, and a Z-plasty is placed at the anterior border of the soft palate. In the Furlow technique, two opposing Z-plasties are performed in the soft palate.

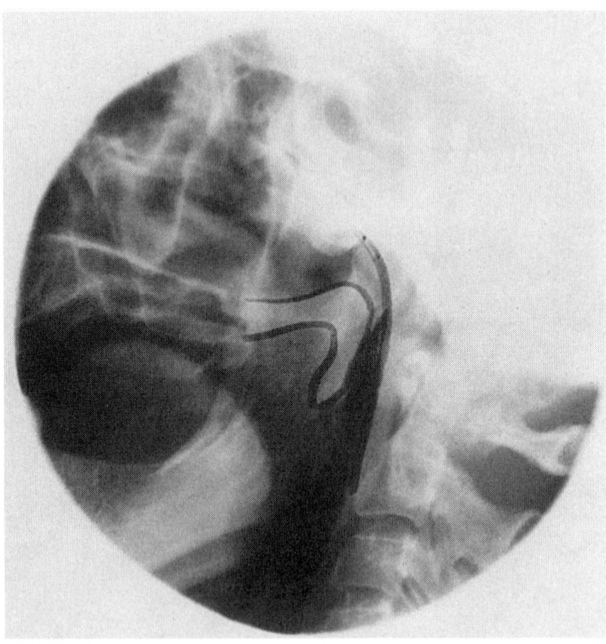

Figure 4.
Radiograph of patient with velopharyngeal insufficiency showing a long soft palate and a deep nasopharynx.

Corrective Surgery

The goal of surgical treatment of VPI in general should be to correct the deficit with the least amount of surgery. Because there are varying degrees of deficiency, multiple surgical techniques have been developed. Evaluation of each of these methods requires a large series of cases over a number of years. Some techniques have stood the test of time, whereas others have been discarded.

The goal in all cases is to achieve an effective functional sphincter in the pharynx to monitor the degree of airflow through the nasal airway during speech and normal breathing. Too much air through the nose creates hypernasality. No air through the nose during speech causes hyponasality.

Surgery is directed toward either lengthening the soft palate or changing the position and action of the superior constrictor muscle. Timing of the surgery is very important because the surgery itself has long-term effects on facial growth. Palatal lengthening using mucoperiosteum from the hard palate can cause severe scar formation in some but not all patients, which results in malocclusion and narrowing of the dental arch (Fig. 7). Delaying palate-lengthening procedures until the 6 year molars have erupted makes it possible to initiate preventive orthodontia.

The soft palate problem may be one of insufficient length, stiff scar tissue, submucous cleft, cervical spine defect, or a neurologic defect. The pharyngeal musculature may lack a Passavant's ridge or insufficient lateral function to effect a closure in combination with the soft palate. The pharyngeal deficiency may result from adenoid resorption, removal of adenoids, a deep nasopharynx, or a neurologic defect.

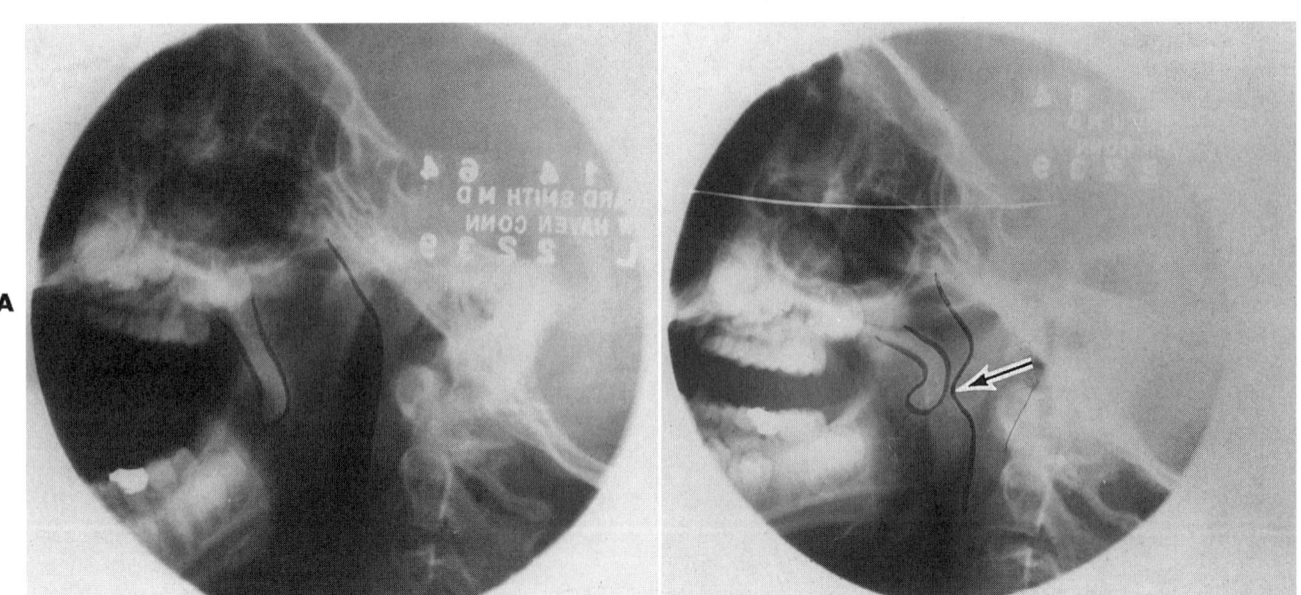

Figure 5.
A, Radiograph of pharynx in a patient with normal speech showing a deep nasopharynx and a long soft palate; *B,* Radiograph of same patient showing forward movement of Passavant's ridge on phonation.

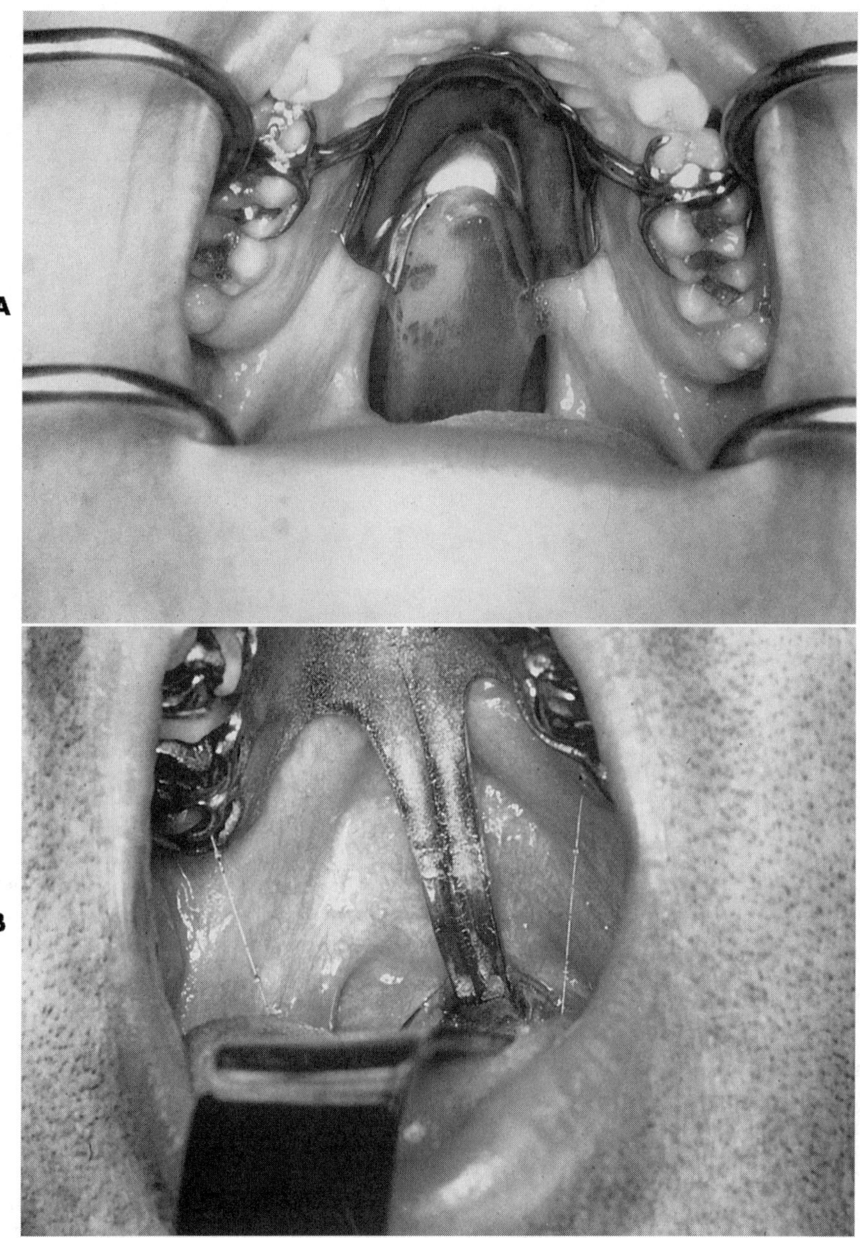

Figure 6.
A, Patient with repaired soft palate wearing dental appliances with nasopharyngeal bulb to correct velopharyngeal insufficiency; *B,* Patient with an unrepaired cleft palate wearing a dental appliance.

Regardless of the cause, the degree of deficiency must be assessed and the surgical procedure tailored to provide "just enough" correction.

A wide variety of surgical procedures has been developed. Some are directed toward the soft palate alone, others toward the superior constrictor alone, and others combine soft palate and superior constrictor procedures.

Summary of Techniques

Soft Palate Lengthening Alone Using Tissue from the Hard Palate

1. V-Y palatal pushback
2. Dorrance palatal pushback
3. V-Y or Dorrance pushback plus a Cronin nasal flap
4. V-Y or Dorrance pushback combined with an island flap

Superior Constrictor Procedures Alone

1. Hynes pharyngoplasty
2. Orticochea sphincteric pharyngoplasty
3. Smith superior constrictor pulldown

Combined

1. Inferiorly based pharyngeal flap inserted into the soft palate musculature
2. Superiorly based pharyngeal flap inserted into the soft palate musculature
3. V-Y or Dorrance palatal pushback with superiorly based pharyngeal flap grafted onto the raw area created in the nasal area by the pushback
4. V-Y or Dorrance palatal pushback combined with a nasopharyngeal pushback using a superiorly based pha-

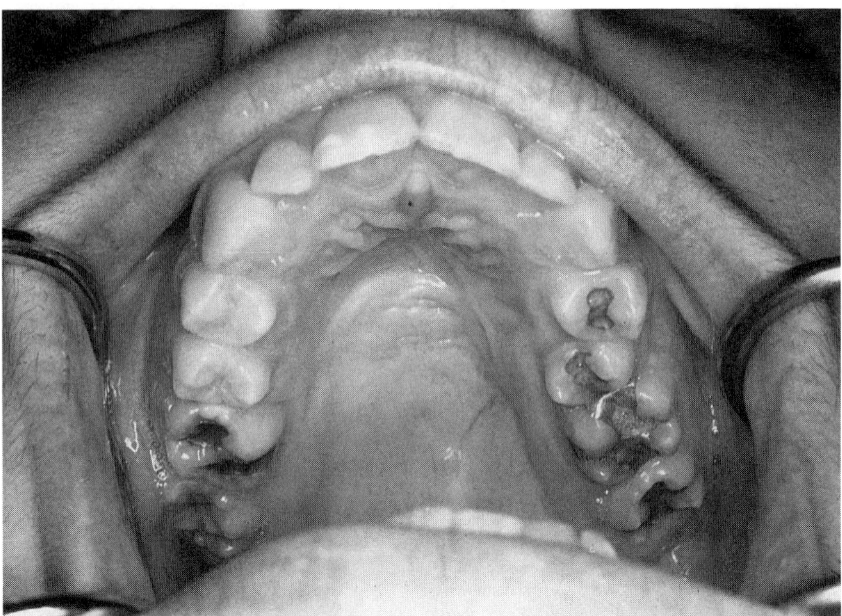

Figure 7.
Maxillary dental arch showing malocclusion caused by palatal scar tissue (island flap donor site).

ryngeal flap to graft the raw area on the nasal layer of the soft palate

5. Double palatal pushback
   a. First operation: V-Y or Dorrance combined with a Cronin nasal flap
   b. Second operation: Repeat V-Y or Dorrance palatal pushback combined with superiorly based pharyngeal flap
6. Superiorly based pharyngeal flap: Hogan's variation

Description of Techniques

Wardill V-Y or Dorrance Palatal Pushback

This technique alone achieves only a limited lengthening because the raw area created in the nasal layer of the retropositioned soft palate heals with scar tissue and forward contracture.

Wardill V-Y or Dorrance Pushback with Cronin Nasal Flap

This very ingenious technique uses the mucosa from the floor of the nose to graft the raw area created by the pushback. We like this procedure for treating a minor degree of VPI (Fig. 8).

Wardill V-Y or Dorrance Pushback with an Island Flap

An island of oral mucoperiosteum is dissected with its attached greater palatine artery, and then sutured into the nasal mucosal defect created by the pushback. We have found this flap to be too hard and stiff, and it reduces flexibility of the soft palate (Fig. 9).

Hynes Pharyngoplasty

Two superiorly based posterior pharyngeal wall flaps are raised and sutured into a horizontal incision at the level of the Passavant's ridge. This is intended for minor degrees of insufficiency in an attempt to recreate a Passavant's pad. We found this technique to fail because the tissue tended to flatten with time. Jackson added the medial edge of the tonsil pillar to the procedure.

Orticochea Sphincter Pharyngoplasty

An inferiorly based pharyngeal flap is raised. Bilateral superiorly based flaps from the posterior tonsillar pillar are raised and sutured to the inferiorly based flap. We have no experience with this flap; however, moderate success is reported by Bardach.

Jackson's modification of the Orticochea procedure is essentially a Hynes pharyngoplasty plus the addition of the two palatopharyngeus muscles sutured into the same area. This creates a Passavant's pad and reinforces it with the crossed palatopharyngeus muscle.

Smith Superior Constrictor Pulldown

This technique was used with success in adult patients who had almost no soft palate—only a thick mass of mobile scar tissue. Access to the nasopharynx was obtained through a semilunar incision above the level of the mid–hard palate. The superior constrictor muscle was freed from the posterior pharyngeal wall and pulled down, and sutured on itself in the midline. This was used on adults for correction of hypernasality. The usual problems of snoring, difficulty clearing mucus, and established vocal substitutions persisted, although these improved with speech therapy.

Inferiorly Based Pharyngeal Flap Inserted into Soft Palate Musculature

We have not seen good results with this procedure. It has some merit for the paralyzed palate by acting as a shield to divert air away from the nasal cavity.

Superiorly Based Pharyngeal Flap Inserted into Soft Palate Musculature

In our experience, the superiorly based pharyngeal flap is a superior technique; however, we believe that it is more effec-

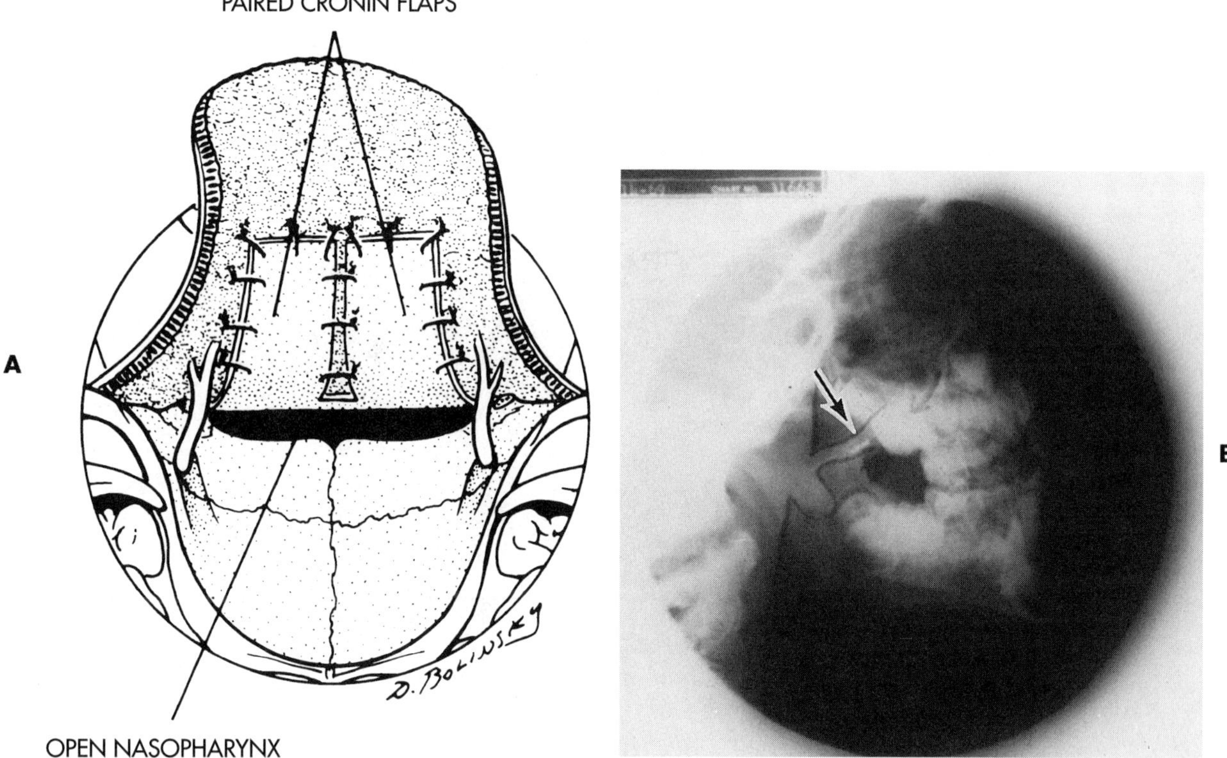

Figure 8.
A, Cronin nasal flap, sutured to soft palate; *B,* Radiograph showing lengthened and flexible soft palate following Cronin nasal flap procedure (arrow).

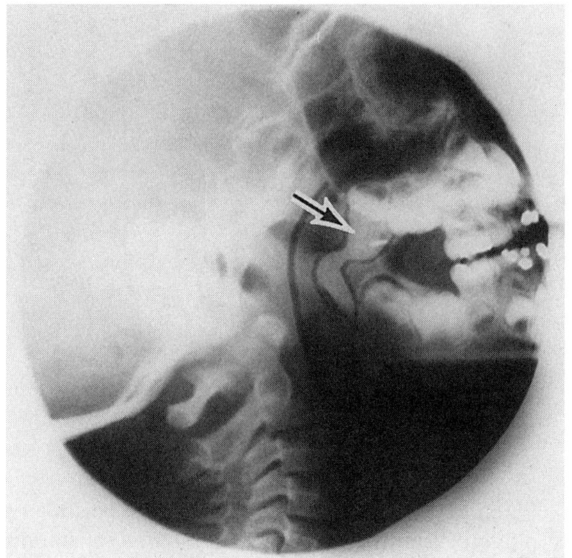

Figure 9.
Radiograph of palate following palatal pushback and island flap techniques. Note thick graft hindering soft palate flexibility. (arrow).

tive when attached to the raw area created by a palatal pushback, which allows the musculature of the soft palate to remain flexible. (Fig. 10).

V-Y or Dorrance Palatal Pushback

This technique, with an incision in the nasal mucosa from one hamular process to the other along the free border of the hard palate, creates a raw area of approximately 2 cm. The superiorly based pharyngeal flap is sutured into the defect (Fig. 10). The width of the superiorly based pharyngeal flap is tailored to the degree of VPI. It is our opinion that this is the most effective area to attach the flap because the soft palate is free to function as before, but more effectively and with added length and a more posterior position (Fig. 11).

V-Y or Dorrance Palatal Pushback Combined with a Nasopharyngeal Pushback and a Superiorly Based Pharyngeal Flap

In cases of gross nasopharyngeal insufficiency and yet a flexible soft palate, added palatal pushback can be achieved by extending the incision in the nasal mucosa from the hamular process of the medial pterygoid plate up the medial surface of the plate and through the attached superior constrictor muscle to the apex of the nasopharynx below the eustachian tube orifices. This allows the soft palate to retroposition another 2 cm. The superiorly based pharyngeal flap is at-

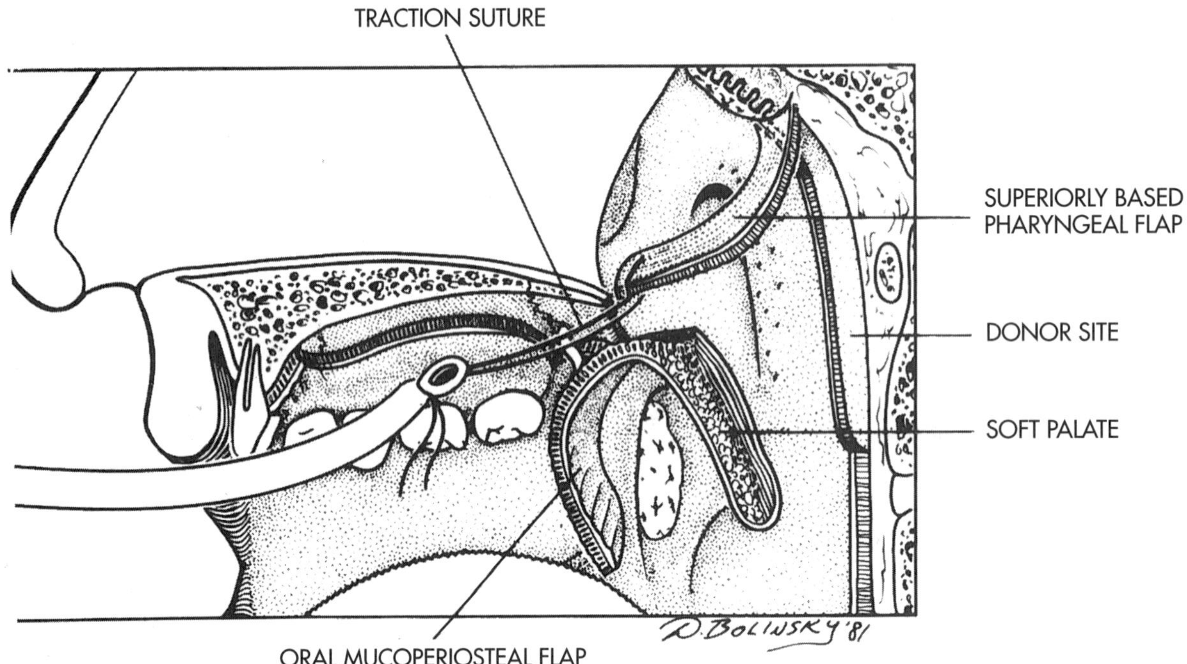

Figure 10.
Superiorly based pharyngeal flap.

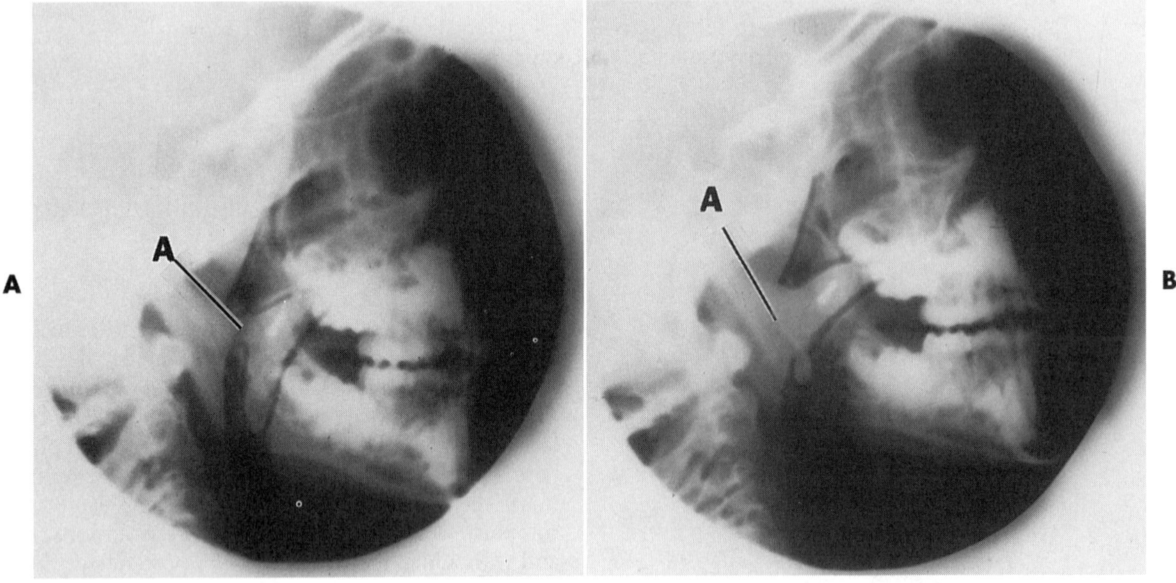

Figure 11.
Radiographs of palatal pushback and superiorly based pharyngeal flap. *A*, At rest; *B*, Phonating.

tached to the raw area. This incision does not influence soft palate movement.

Double Palatal Pushback

When it appears that a superiorly based pharyngeal flap will not be sufficient to correct VPI, a two-stage operation can be performed provided that the soft palate is flexible. The first operation consists of a V-Y or Dorrance palatal pushback plus a Cronin nasal flap. The second operation 6 months later is a repeat V-Y or Dorrance palatal pushback and a superiorly based pharyngeal flap. To get added length, the nasopharyngeal pushback can be added. This two-stage operation can also be used when a Cronin flap is selected and later found to be insufficient.

In our experience, this is a very workable combination. It is helpful to have a broad, flat hard palate arch. Orthodontic treatment is anticipated to prevent scar contractions and subsequent malocclusion (Fig. 12).

Hogan's Modification of Superiorly Based Pharyngeal Flap

The soft palate is split in the midline. The superiorly based pharyngeal flap consists of the posterior wall of the nasopharynx down to the prevertebral fascia, with approximately 5 mm of posterior pharyngeal wall left on each side of the flap. The flap is raised, transected inferiorly, and sutured to the nasal surface of the split soft palate. The donor site is closed. Lateral ports are thereby created, and the oral portion of the soft palate is sutured over the flap, thus covering the raw surface. This technique is designed so that the flap can be tailored to the degree of VPI; however, variables in healing can alter the lateral port size. Although this technique has attained considerable support, its attachment discourages action of the soft palate almost in the same way as does an inferiorly based pharyngeal flap.

■ COMPLICATIONS

Surgical results do not always meet the surgeon's expectations and render the patient free of VPI. Perhaps the most frequent complication is snoring, and if it is severe enough this complication may result in obstructive sleep apnea. Mucus may accumulate in the upper surface of the soft palate and require irrigations for removal. Oral breathing may give patients a sense of suffocation and cause fatigue on exercise. With shrinkage of the pharyngeal flap, some degree of VPI may return. With proper care and prevention of infection, flap loss is not a common problem. With palatal pushback surgery, fistulas may occur in the hard palate. Most patients need follow-up speech therapy in an attempt to correct some of the preoperative speech substitutions.

Many patients who have had repair of cleft lip and cleft palate experience retarded growth of the maxilla. These patients may require orthognathic surgery for good occlusion and facial harmony. Patients should be advised that such surgery may compromise their corrected velopharyngeal insufficiency, so they should not enter into the surgery without careful consultation and evaluation.

■ DISCUSSION

1. Surgeons should become familiar with both the Perko and the Furlow techniques of cleft palate closure.
2. In all instances, the V-Y or Dorrance types of oral mucoperiosteal pushback flaps must be anchored to the hard palate, and there must be no space left between the layers of the palate. Adequate fixation of these flaps can be achieved by drilling the palate bone through to the nasal passage and using mattress sutures. Additional protection of these flaps can be provided by stenting.
3. Either palatal or superior constrictor muscle function should be preserved whenever possible rather than having static blockage of the posterior nasal passages.
4. Extending the nasal mucosal incision beyond the hamular process of the medial pterygoid plates to the skull base does not affect soft palate movement.
5. Attaching the superiorly based pharyngeal flap to the raw area created by a pushback allows for a more flexible and functional soft palate.
6. Repositioning of the palatopharyngeus muscle (Or-

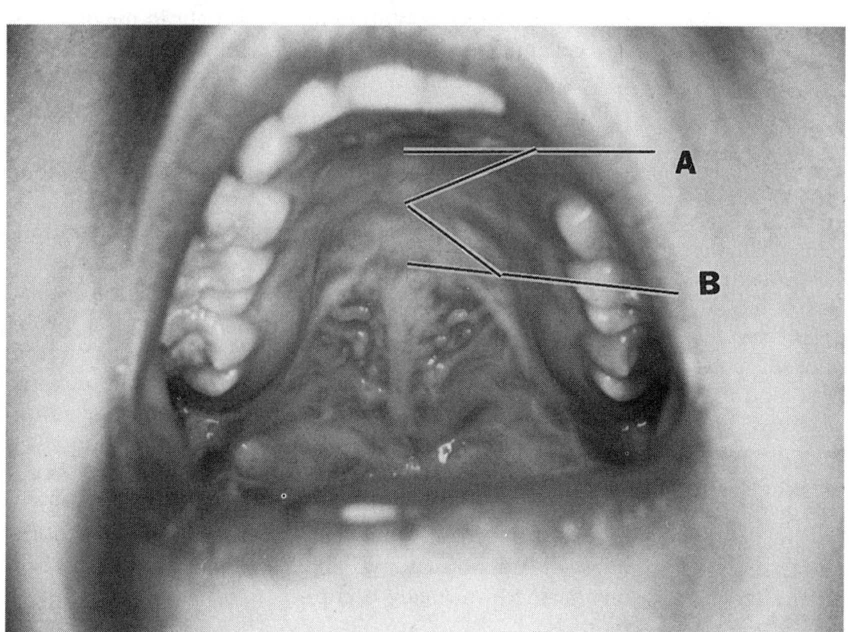

Figure 12.
Photograph of palate showing donor sites for double palatal pushbacks without disturbance of dental arch. *A*, Dorrance palatal pushback No. 1; *B*, Dorrance palatal pushback No. 2.

ticochea technique with Jackson's modification) should be more widely used.

7. Pharyngeal flaps—whether inferiorly based or superiorly based— that are sutured into the soft palate musculature tend to lessen soft palate flexibility.
8. Surgical procedures designed to attempt the "impossible" should be discouraged because of complications. The art of obturator construction and use should be reintroduced to treat some cases of velopharyngeal insufficiency.

Suggested Reading

Bardach J, Salyer KE. Surgical techniques in cleft lip and palate. ed 2. St. Louis: Mosby–Year Book, 1991.

Cronin TD. Method of preventing raw area on nasal surface of soft palate in pushback surgery. Plast Reconstr Surg 1957; 20:474.

Dorrance GM. Lengthening of soft palate in cleft palate operations. Ann Surg 1925; 82:208.

Furlow LT Jr. Cleft palate repair by double opposing Z-plasty. Plast Reconstr Surg 1986; 78:724-738.

Hogan VM. A clarification of the surgical goals in cleft palate speech and the introduction of the lateral port control (LPC) pharyngeal flap. Cleft Palate J 1973; 10:331-345.

Hynes W. Pharyngoplasty by muscle transplantation. Br J Plast Surg 1950; 3:128.

Jackson I, Silverton JS. The sphincter pharyngoplasty as a secondary procedure in cleft palates. Plast Reconstr Surg 1977; 59:518-524.

Millard DF Jr. The island flap in cleft palate surgery. Surg Gynecol Obstet 1963; 116:297.

Orticochea M. Construction of a dynamic muscle sphincter in cleft palate. Plast Reconstr Surg 1968; 41:323.

Perko MA. Two-stage closure of cleft palate. J Maxillofacial Surg 1979; 7:46-80.

Rosenthal W. Zur frage der gaumenplastik. Zentralbl Chir 1925; 82:208.

Sanvanero-Russelli. Divisione platina e sua chirugico. Lau Cong INT. Stomatol 1935; 36:391.

Smith HW. Superior constrictor muscle pulldown. In: Atlas of cleft lip and cleft palate. New York: Grune & Stratton, 1983:93.

Smith HW, Hughes M, Rosnagle RS. Double palatal pushback: A technique for correction of severe velopharyngeal insufficiency. Arch Otolaryngol 1972; 95:33-41.

Wardill WEM. The technique of operation for cleft palate. Br J Surg 1937; 25:117.

OROANTRAL FISTULA

The method of
William Lawson
Anthony J. Reino

Oroantral fistulas (OAF) occasionally occur during extraction of the postcanine teeth in the maxilla because of the close relationship between the apex of those teeth and the floor of the maxillary antrum. OAF may occur when the bone that separates the teeth from the maxillary antrum is thin or has been resorbed. Von Bonsdorf studied 84 human skulls and found that roots of the second molar have the most intimate relationship to the floor of the maxillary antrum, followed by the first molar, third molar, second premolar, first premolar, and the canine, respectively. This study confirmed that the roots of posterior teeth in the maxilla are in close proximity to the floor of the sinus, especially the first and second molars; therefore, the risk of OAF is increased when these teeth need to be extracted. An analysis of 250 cases of oroantral fistula by Killey and Kay showed that more than 50 percent of the cases occurred after the removal of the first molar, and approximately 25 percent of the cases were associated with extraction of the second molar.

Chronic oroantral fistulas are much less common than one would suspect considering the compromising anatomy, the high incidence of upper respiratory infections frequently involving the maxillary sinus, and the relative insouciance with which posterior maxillary teeth are extracted.

Maxillary sinusitis, on the other hand, is a common clinical occurrence. Its symptoms may be localized to the posterior teeth, and its resolution may be sought in the dentist's office. Pain in the posterior maxilla, along with pressure and tenderness in the lateral tuberosity area, can and often does lead to the unfortunate extraction of the suspected tooth. Although tooth extraction under these circumstances may result in the formation of an oroantral fistula, it seldom occurs.

Excluding obvious communications that follow trauma or neoplastic surgery, it appears that certain circumstances predispose to the formation of a chronic oroantral fistula. These circumstances include (1) immediate surgical penetration of the antral membrane, which is the most common etiology; (2) periapical, granulomatous, or cystic disease, which on radiographs appears contiguous with the sinus; (3) a retained root tip located near the antral floor; (4) an impacted tooth—generally a third molar; (5) advanced periodontal disease; (6) maxillary tuberosities requiring reduction for dental prostheses; and (7) large cysts that have distorted anatomy and have grossly encroached on the space normally occupied by the antrum of Highmore.

CLASSIFICATION OF OROANTRAL FISTULAS

Table 1 describes the three categories of oroantral fistulas. Category I is most common. The etiology is the extraction of a maxillary molar or second premolar, with accidental penetration into the underlying maxillary sinus. The involved maxillary sinus is free of infection and well aerated. Category II is the second most common. The etiology is the same (dental extraction), but the maxillary sinus is acutely or chronically infected. Category III is the least common and usually results from the surgical removal of a neoplasm or cystic lesion of the maxilla, which may leave a large communication from the oral cavity to the maxillary sinus. On rare occasions, this opening may extend to the floor of the nasal cavity. Other possible etiologies for category III lesions are tissue breakdown from radiotherapy, osteomyelitis, and traumatic loss of portions of the maxilla.

The therapeutic approach to each of the three categories is usually different (Table 2). Category I lesions are rarely seen by the otolaryngologist because they almost always heal spontaneously, with or without minor local procedures by the general dentist or oral surgeon. If these lesions fail to heal, they may be treated as category II fistulas.

Category III fistulas are usually best managed by a dental prosthesis. The general dentist or prosthodontist may cover the defect with a portion of the base plate required by the patient for the tooth loss that accompanies these fistulas. When these fistulas are small and the surrounding tissues are healthy, they may be repaired as category II lesions.

Category II fistulas are by far the most commonly encountered in the practice of general otolaryngology. Often, these patients have undergone a number of failed procedures performed by a general dentist or oral surgeon. The most common site for these fistulas is the socket of the maxillary first molar. These first molars erupt at approximately age 6 years, and are often neglected as "baby teeth." Therefore, they are the most frequent permanent tooth involved with advanced dental caries.

Table 1. Classification of Oroantral Fistula

CATEGORY	DESCRIPTION	SIZE
I	Cause: dental extraction Maxillary sinus: healthy	1 to 5 mm
II	Cause: dental extraction Maxillary sinus: signs of acute or chronic disease	6 mm to 1.9 cm
III	Large fistula secondary to extirpative surgery and/or trauma; may include oronasal fistula	>2 cm

Table 2. Treatment of Oroantral Fistulas by Category

CATEGORY	TREATMENT
I	Spontaneous healing is the rule; if they become chronic, may be treated as category II.
II	Sinus disease must be eradicated; may be managed by local flaps, with or without insertion of autogenous or alloplastic material.
III	Dental prosthesis is treatment of choice; smaller defects with healthy surrounding tissue may be treated with local flaps.

In category II lesions, the entered sinus is either secondarily infected by the diseased tooth or involved with chronic sinusitis of a nondental etiology. When presented with a chronic oroantral fistula, the otolaryngologist's first step is to assess the health of the paranasal sinuses. This is best done with a computed tomographic (CT) scan. Attempts to repair these fistulas without adequately treating any concomitant sinus disease will result in failure.

MANAGEMENT OF CHRONIC OROANTRAL FISTULA

A chronic oroantral fistula differs considerably from the acute one and likewise must be free of concurrent sinus disease before closure is attempted. An accurate history and physical examination should also be performed to rule out other possible contributing factors, that is, previous sinus disease, nasal obstruction, benign or malignant neoplasms, or osteomyelitis. A CT scan of the paranasal sinuses should be performed to determine the presence of sinonasal pathology. In cases with displaced teeth, exposed roots, root canal material, packs, severe periodontal disease, or questionable OAF, a dental CT scan may be obtained. These scans have been used successfully to determine both the size and the existence of OAF.

The efficacy of drainage is ascertained. Too small an aperture or one located off the alveolar crest and blocked by the folding buccal tissues will not permit adequate drainage and will thus prolong the healing process. Both apertures can be enlarged by removing the surface bone without the necessity of making a classic flap.

When infection of the communicated sinus is present, the patient should be placed on oral antibiotics, and antral irrigations should be performed through the oral aperture. This treatment should continue until the scheduled date of surgery. A large-gauge, blunt, spinal needle attached to a cannula, which in turn is fitted to a syringe, may be used. When the fistula is too large and the sterile water solution refluxes into the mouth, dental compound may be used to obliterate the space around the needle. The patient is asked to lower the head below the level of the fistula and hold a kidney basin under the nose. Gentle plunger pressure will fill the sinus and bring the return through the nasal ostium. The return is observed for purulence. Repeating this procedure three or four times a week for approximately 14 days or less should clear the uncomplicated sinus infection. Irrigating through the nasal ostium is equally effective. Generally, surgery may be performed after clear nasal effluent is observed on 3 consecutive days. It is essential here to note that failure to clear the sinus strongly suggests the possibility of other factors, that is, nasal blockage due to polyps, turbinate hypertrophy, and/or chronic sinusitis.

Sinus Exploration and Curettage

If no cause for the cloudy return is identified, exploration of the sinus is indicated. The procedure can be performed through the fistula, or through an anterior sublabial incision, with or without the use of a sinus endoscope. The oral side of the fistula should be opened first, and all granulations as well as the epithelialized tract should be removed. A small anterior maxillary antrostomy will allow inspection of the upper side of the fistula. Identification and removal of persistent granulation tissue, infection, or bony sequestrum should be performed during this procedure. An attempt at closing the fistula at this time is contraindicated.

Flap Selection

The buccal mucoperiosteal advancement flap as described by Berger is the simplest and most effective way of closing an established fistula. A review of 75 such operated cases revealed three failures, which were successfully closed 3 months later.

Advantages of the Buccal Flap

The buccal flap is a familiar one and is routinely used in oral and maxillofacial surgery. The labial and buccal tissues are more elastic than are the palatal mucosa. The buccal flap can be lengthened and modified as needed during surgery. It permits wide opening into the sinus and thus replaces the Caldwell-Luc approach for the required curettage. This flap does not leave raw surfaces to heal by secondary intention. Partial denture prostheses may be used in many cases.

Disadvantages of the Buccal Flap

A decrease in the depth of the mucobuccal fold is an immediate postoperative consequence, which to a large extent is normalized by function in 5 to 6 months. It is important, however, to borrow tissue laterally from the cheek and not infraorbitally.

■ TECHNIQUE

Local anesthesia with intravenous sedation is the anesthesia of choice. Complete excision of the fistula is mandatory. Should the root of a tooth adjacent to the fistula constitute any part of the fistulous tract, it must be extracted. This extraction is generally done at the time of surgery. Inspection and curettage of necrotic or polypoid antral mucosa is considered to be an integral part of the operation. Antral bleeding is controlled by a gauze pack, which may be left in place until the suturing phase. A nasal antrostomy is advisable. Sharp edges of bone under the flap are rongeured and filed. Abrupt bony margins that cause undue pressure and folding of the flap are reduced and contoured. The length and width of the flap are increased conventionally by lengthening the anterior and posterior incisions. Advancement of the flap over the defect requires division of the periosteum so that tissue may be mobilized from the buccal mucosa.

The wound is closed without tension in one layer using 3–0 silk sutures. If there is a possibility of the lower teeth contacting the operated site, either inadvertently or during sleep, a previously fabricated bite block should be inserted. Sutures are removed in approximately 10 days. Antibiotics and decongestants are routinely administered for approximately 2 weeks.

■ POSTOPERATIVE CARE

The patient should have nothing by mouth for approximately 6 hours. For the first 24 hours, the head should be elevated when the patient is in the supine position. Increased antral pressure should be avoided; this is aided by not blowing the nose and opening the mouth to sneeze. A full liquid diet (not using a straw) is taken until sutures are removed. Subsequent to this, the patient may advance gradually to a mechanical soft diet. There should be no smoking until sutures are removed, and the patient is advised to avoid strenuous physical activity until closure is assured.

■ ALTERNATIVE METHODS OF CLOSURE

The palatal rotation flap has been a very popular choice for closure of OAF. Aside from the inherent anatomic deficits suggested earlier, it has other disadvantages. An additional buccal flap is required, and once designed, this flap permits little room for error. Preparation of a template on a model, as recommended by Williams, can be useful.

Metal foil and gold plate became popular approximately 40 years ago because closure could be accomplished with minimal surgery and without the loss of sulcus depth. Their neutrality to tissues and easy malleability allow easy placement onto the margins of the aperture. A small mucoperiosteal flap is raised on the buccal aspect, and an accompanying release of the palatal mucosa is made to expose the entire bony margin of the fistula. The flaps are mobilized sufficiently to secure the burnished margins of the plate beneath them. These margins are not approximated; they are simply held down by sutures. In 2 to 4 weeks, granulation tissue forms under the plate and closes the fistula. When motion of the plate is noted, it is removed, and epithelialization is left to heal by secondary intention. This procedure is recommended by many investigators for the immediate perforation. However, for the chronic fistula, some in the field prefer the plate to be completely covered by the flaps and left in place indefinitely. Crolius and others believe that a metal plate closure always should be tried before resorting to other procedures.

Smaller lesions (1 to 5 mm) can be closed by using the interseptal alveolotomy. This procedure incorporates autogenous alveolar bone through the performance of proximal and distal vertical osteotomies, which allows infracturing of the buccal cortex to close the fistula. The wound is then closed primarily.

Larger defects can be closed by a variety of methods, which include pedicled or free buccal fat pad interposition (up to 6 × 5 cm); anteriorly based buccinator myomucosal island flap (up to 7 × 5 cm); and/or temporoparietal fascia flaps.

■ COMPLICATIONS

Wound breakdown and flap necrosis are the most common complications of oroantral fistula repair. Careful preservation of the flap's blood supply and tension-free wound closure are the keys to avoiding these complications. If associated paranasal sinus disease has been adequately treated, there is reasonable hope of the fistula closing by secondary intention. Any plans for a secondary procedure should allow adequate time for this healing to occur.

When a small fistula redevelops around a healthy flap, the sinus disease has not been eradicated, and treatment should be directed appropriately. This fistula should close shortly after the sinus becomes healthy.

Suggested Reading

Berger A. Oroantral openings and their surgical closure. Arch Otolaryngol 1939; 30:400.

Budge CT. Closure of an antraoral opening by use of tantalum plate. J Oral Surg 1952; 19:32.

Crolius WE. The use of gold plate for the closure of oroantral fistula. Oral Surg Oral Med Oral Pathol 1956; 836.

Killey HC, Kay. An analysis of 250 cases of oroantral fistulae treated by the buccal flap operation. Oral Surg 1967; 24:726.

McClung EJ, Chipps JE. Tantalum foil use in closing antral-oral fistulas. US Armed Forces Med J 1951; 2:1183.

Williams PE. Diseases of the maxillary sinus of dental origin. In: Kruger CO, ed. Textbook of oral and maxillofacial surgery. 5th ed. St. Louis: CV Mosby, 1979.

DROOLING

The method of
Mark A. Richardson

Drooling or sialorrhea is a significant problem in children who have oral motor dysfunction; it is a significant care issue because these children are integrated into school, play with other children, and eventually work. A variety of approaches have been used to control drooling, including physiotherapy, drug treatment, and surgical methods. If physiotherapy is unsuccessful and drug side effects are unacceptable, my surgical approach is rerouting of the submandibular ducts with the addition of parotid duct ligation as a staged procedure if submandibular duct rerouting alone is unsuccessful in controlling the sialorrhea.

Drooling is a manifestation of a neurogenic disturbance in the complex movements of the muscles of the mouth, pharynx, and esophagus that occurs during swallowing. A variety of neurogenic deficits, both central and peripheral, may contribute to drooling. Sialorrhea, however, is generally not due to hypersecretion but to an inability to move normal secretions from the anterior oral cavity to the pharynx, where in most cases a normal swallow reflex is present and will eliminate the saliva from the upper portion of the digestive tract.

Saliva is secreted by the three large groups of paired salivary glands, the parotid, submandibular, and sublingual, as well as numerous smaller minor glands located on the palate, buccal mucosa, and tongue. The overwhelming majority of saliva is produced by the large paired glands, with approximately 70 percent of resting salivary flow coming from the submandibular and sublingual groups. Food ingestion causes stimulation of the parotid glands as well as further secretion of saliva from the submaxillary and minor salivary glands, which then more actively aid in the digestion of food and deglutition.

Secretion of saliva from the large salivary glands is under the control of the parasympathetic nervous system. The parasympathetic innervation of the parotid begins as fibers leave the inferior salivary nucleus traveling with a glossopharyngeal nerve. These fibers leave the glossopharyngeal nerve as its tympanic branch (Jacobson's nerve) enters the middle ear inferiorly. Here it receives a branch from the carotid plexus (the sympathetic portion of the nerve) and proceeds anteriorly, crosses the promontory where it begins to branch off to the round and oval windows, the middle ear mucosa, and the region of the eustachian tube. On the promontory, the tympanic plexus may lie in a bony canal or a bony semicanal, or it may simply be covered by mucosa. The tympanic nerve exits the middle ear as the lesser superficial petrosal nerve and travels to the otic ganglion near the foramen ovale. Postganglionic fibers leave the otic ganglion and ultimately reach the parotid gland. Parasympathetic innervation to the sublingual and submandibular glands begins in the superior salivary nucleus. Fibers join with the nervus intermedius and travel with the facial nerve into the mastoid. The chorda tympani nerve, which carries the parasympathetic fibers. emerges from the facial nerve in its descending portion and passes through the middle ear, exiting through the petrotympanic fissure and traveling along the lingual nerve to the submandibular ganglion. Postganglionic fibers are then distributed to the sublingual and submandibular glands.

Saliva facilitates chewing, transport, and breakdown of food and speech articulation and also protects the teeth and the oral cavity mucosa. Any method for control of sialorrhea should be based on maintaining normal function and physiology, if possible.

■ PATIENT SELECTION

Objective measurements of sialorrhea are difficult and may or may not correlate well with the magnitude of the problem as perceived by the patient, parents, and/or nursing staff. The history is generally sufficient to evaluate the problem. The number of bibs and shirts soiled daily; whether salivation is worse at a particular time of day, such as with stress or feeding; the amount of voluntary control that can be exerted; and psychosocial factors, such as being teased by playmates or poor family reactions to the drooling, should all be assessed and determined. Generally, I consider that soaking three shirts or bibs during the day is evidence of a significant problem.

Physical examination is performed, with particular attention to tongue control, evidence of dental problems or caries, sores on the lips or chin, and swallowing ability. Any factors contributing to nasal obstruction are carefully evaluated. Adenoidectomy, diathermy to the turbinates, or treatment of vasomotor or allergic rhinitis can improve swallowing by improving normal breathing patterns. Hypertrophic tonsils causing an open-mouth posture or otherwise contributing to swallowing ability difficulties might also be removed and could facilitate control of oral secretions.

Usually by the time a surgical consultation is requested, the patient has had months or years of physical therapy. If not, certainly in younger patients, a consultation with a physical therapist is obtained to evaluate the possible benefit of physiotherapy for control of sialorrhea. Any indication of chronic aspiration, esophageal stricture, or other esophageal motility disorders might affect what type of procedure would be indicated in any individual patient.

■ NONSURGICAL TREATMENT

Nonsurgical therapy includes physiotherapy to facilitate oral motor control. This is certainly the most logical procedure to attempt first because oral motor control is the primary defect in the development of drooling. Unfortunately, the results even with intensive therapy have been mixed, and to be effective, this therapy must be started at an early age. The availability of videofluoroscopic swallow examinations has resulted in all of my patients being referred for radiographic evaluations before surgical treatment.

Drugs have been used and continue to be used for the control of drooling. Because salivary secretion is primarily under parasympathetic control, anticholinergic drugs have been used to inhibit this. Side effects may result from drug treatment. Constipation, urinary retention, xerostomia, blurred vision, and restlessness all have accompanied the use of either glycopyrrolate or scopolamine. The lack of availability of transdermal scopolamine has limited its use. Currently, however, Robinul given orally does have a moderate success rate in patients who are able to tolerate the mode of drug administration.

■ SURGICAL METHODS

The lack of consensus on surgical management means that no one procedure is ideal for any patient; all surgical treatment must be individualized to a certain extent. Surgical approaches can be divided into the following categories: (1) direct reduction of salivary flow; (2) redirection of salivary secretions; and (3) elimination of the parasympathetic supply to the glands, thereby diminishing secretion.

Gland excision is an obvious solution to the problem of sialorrhea. Submandibular gland excision is a simple procedure that head and neck surgeons are quite familiar with and has a high success rate in controlling sialorrhea. Surgical removal of the parotid glands would have a significantly higher morbidity rate related to the potential for facial nerve injury, a longer surgical procedure, and accompanying side effects to this surgery, such as Frey's syndrome.

Denervation procedures usually consist of bilateral tympanic neurectomy or bilateral chorda tympani nerve section, or both. These procedures are technically simple to perform and relatively free of complications. To achieve an adequate success rate, tympanic neurectomy and chorda tympani nerve section must be performed. Disadvantages include loss of taste in the anterior two-thirds of the tongue, production of a somewhat thicker salivary consistency, and a late failure rate due to denervation hypersensitivity.

Duct ligation is simple to perform but may be associated with minor discomfort secondary to swelling of the gland and may be followed by recurrent infection. It also eliminates saliva. Duct rerouting does require intraoral dissection and may cause transient tongue swelling and edema in the floor of the mouth. Ranula formation has been associated with submandibular duct rerouting. In the case of parotid duct rerouting, the procedure is technically difficult and may be associated with fistula formation along the rerouting tract. Rerouting does, however, retain the normal amount of saliva and places it in an area of the oral cavity where it more easily passes into the hypopharynx and esophagus.

■ SURGERY

Once the patient has been evaluated and selected for a potential surgical procedure, the exact nature of the surgical procedure to be performed can be chosen from the list of available processes. In general, for those patients who are highly motivated and have milder neurologic problems that are more limited to the oral motor area, submandibular duct rerouting has been my method of choice for the control of sialorrhea. For patients who have more complicated neurologic problems, I begin with submandibular duct rerouting, but I approach the patient and problem as a potentially staged procedure that may later involve the ligation of the parotid duct as a separate and secondary procedure. This would be done after a 5 to 6 month interval with a continual objective assessment of the drooling problem. If the parents and other caretakers are unsatisfied with the results, the parotid duct ligation can be performed as an outpatient procedure, with the only side effect being occasional transitory swelling in the parotid area that usually resolves after 48 to 72 hours. For those significantly impaired individuals who are nonintegrated into school or work, it may be more appropriate to consider submandibular gland excision and parotid duct ligation as a single stage, especially if swallowing difficulties or aspiration accompany that patient's neurologic deficit. It must also be noted that patients may continue to improve throughout their early childhood; early intervention before 5 years of age is contraindicated. Most patients we deal with are between the ages of 8 and 15 years.

Goals and objectives of the surgery, which should be to reduce the saliva but not eliminate it, are discussed with the parents ahead of time, as well as the potential need for second-stage procedures if indicated. If chorda tympani nerve section is to be performed, the possible effect on taste and enjoyment of food should be an important part of the preoperative discussion.

■ TECHNIQUE

Prophylactic antibiotics of the cephalosporin type are administered parenterally approximately 1 hour before surgery and for 3 days postoperatively. General anesthesia is delivered through a nasotracheal tube. A side mouth gag is used to open the mouth, and a pharyngeal pack is placed. A heavy tongue suture of zero silk is placed on the ventral surface of the tip of the tongue to retract the tongue and expose the sublingual papilla. The punctum is then cannulated with a lacrimal probe, and an elliptical incision is made to form a 3 mm or greater cuff of mucosa surrounding it. The mucosal cuff is marked medially and laterally with 4–0 polyglactin 910 sutures of different colors. The submandibular duct with the lacrimal probe still in place is bluntly dissected from the surrounding tissues for a distance of 3 to 4 cm; any adjoining sublingual ducts are ligated. This dissection may be performed without the necessity of the lacrimal probe once experience is gained with the procedure. A suture of zero silk is then placed laterally on the tongue, and a submucosal tunnel is created with a curved tonsil hemostat from the furthest point of the dissection to a point just posterior to the anterior tonsillar pillar at the base of the tongue. The polyglactin 910 sutures are then passed through the tunnel to maintain their proper spatial relationships by first passing a zero silk suture through the tunnel created, tying the polyglactin 910 sutures to the silk and gently advancing the duct and sutures through the created tunnel, maintaining the spatial orientation so no kinking of the duct will occur. The cuff of mucosa is then tacked to the tongue mucosa using the polyglactin 910 stitches and a free needle. A similar procedure is performed on the opposite side. The resulting wound in the floor of the mouth is closed using an absorbable suture. As additional skill is gained in the performance of the procedure, swelling in the tongue and the floor mouth area is minimal, and the hospital stay is shortened.

The patient generally remains in the hospital for 24 to 48 hours following surgery. The limitation on discharge relates to the intake of fluids orally. Initially, there may be an increase in the amount of drooling due to the discomfort in the oral cavity from the surgery, but usually by 6 weeks the final result has been obtained, and the effectiveness of the procedure can be judged.

■ COMPLICATIONS

Complications have been primarily related to initial postoperative edema and swelling, infection in the floor mouth, and ranula formation. Ranulas are uncommon but remain a complication encountered in 2 percent to 3 percent of all patients. Approximately 20 percent of patients selected for submandibular duct rerouting require additional procedures to help control their drooling, which in my hands has consisted of parotid duct ligation. In these patients, control of drooling has been quite effective; other than the temporary swelling of the parotid gland immediately after the procedure, no complications have been encountered. With the addition of the parotid duct ligation, however, the development of thicker oral secretions has been the result, although drooling has been controlled.

Suggested Reading

Cotton RT, Richardson MA. The effect of submandibular duct rerouting in the treatment of sialorrhea in children. Otolaryngol Head Neck Surg 1981; 89:535-541.

Gross CW, Linden BS. Drooling. In: Gates GA, ed. Current therapy in otolaryngology—Head and neck surgery. 4th ed. Philadelphia: Mosby–Year Book, 1990:327.

Kaplan I. Results of the Wilkie operation to stop drooling in cerebral palsy. Plast Reconstr Surg 1977; 59:646-648.

Michel RG, Johnson KA, Patterson CN. Parasympathetic nerve section for control of sialorrhea. Arch Otolaryngol Head Neck Surg 1977; 103: 94-97.

Parisier SC, Blitzer A, Binder WJ, et al. Tympanic neurectomy and chorda tympanectomy for the control of drooling. Arch Otolaryngol Head Neck Surg 1978; 104:273-277.

Rogawski MA. Transdermal scopolamine and sialorrhea (letter). Arch Neurol 1984; 41:25.

Sochaniwskyj AE, Koheil RM, Bablich K, et al. Oral motor functioning, frequency of swallowing and drooling in normal children and children with cerebral palsy. Arch Phys Med Rehabil 1986; 67:866-874.

Talmi YP, Finkelstein Y, Zohar Y, Laurian N. Reduction of salivary flow with Seopoderm TTS. Ann Otol Rhinol Laryngol 1988; 97:128-130.

Wilkie TF. On the bad effects of nerve sections for the control of drooling. Plast Reconstr Surg 1977; 60:439-440.

Wilkie TF, Brody GS. The surgical treatment of drooling—A ten year review. Plast Reconstr Surg 1977; 59:791-797.

TONSIL AND ADENOID DISORDERS

The method of
Linda Brodsky

Diseases in the tonsils and adenoids are among the most common disorders seen by the otolaryngologist. Recent advances in the understanding of these diseases has led to medical therapy as an alternative to tonsillectomy and/or adenoidectomy in appropriately selected patients.

A standardized classification of adenotonsillar disease has not yet emerged; this places the practicing otolaryngologist at a disadvantage when treatment plans are considered. Recurrent or persistent (chronic) infection and/or obstructive hyperplasia are the most commonly encountered problems. Peritonsillar abscess, unilateral tonsillar hyperplasia, and infectious mononucleosis are discussed separately.

Tonsillectomy and adenoidectomy (T & A) are the most common major surgical procedures performed in children in the United States today. Even so, the variability of use of surgical technique, preoperative evaluation processes, and postoperative care instructions is astounding. I describe in this chapter the rationale and procedure for certain aspects of pre-, intra-, and postoperative care of T & A patients.

The management of adenotonsillar disease is made most difficult by the many variables that must be considered and are not always readily quantifiable. The wide variation in diagnostic criteria, the failure of primary care physicians to recognize "noninfectious" disease, and the inherent suspicion within the medical community against previous practices of the seemingly ubiquitous need for T & A, all challenge the otolaryngologist to be most thoughtful in offering therapy options to patients and their families. Furthermore, the tendency to consider the tonsils and adenoids as one entity must be resisted, because they manifest disease differently and should always be considered separately.

The key to developing an evaluation and treatment plan begins with assessing the perception of the effect of the illness upon the family and the child. Even when a patient meets criteria for surgery (as described next), the severity of each illness (i.e., whether the child has a slight sore throat or spends 4 days in bed with a high fever); the impact on chronic medical conditions (such as asthma and congenital heart disease); *or* the possible risk of chronic medical conditions (such as hematologic disorders or immunodeficiencies) should all be weighed against the risk of surgery. Previous therapies, household illness, and child or parental anxieties are other salient features to be considered.

INFECTIONS OF THE TONSILS AND ADENOIDS

Recurrent Acute Tonsillitis

Recurrent tonsil infections are characterized by (1) changing bacterial flora (with greater presence of β-lactamase–producing micro-organisms), and (2) the presence of chronic cryptitis with crypt obstruction on pathologic examination of these tonsils. Consequently, in select cases, antibiotic therapy may be useful, although its application should be weighed against the individual patient's situation and the environmental pressures for increasing bacterial resistance to antibiotics.

In children who have been affected for only one season and in whom chronic changes in the tonsils (peritonsillar erythema, loss of surface crypts, and dilated surface blood vessels) are not apparent, I offer a prolonged course (30 days) of full-dose antibiotic therapy with either clindamycin (if halitosis is a prominent feature) or amoxicillin-clavulanate. Alternatively, using the same antibiotics as prophylaxis for 4 to 6 months at a low dose (one-third to one-half the therapeutic dose), is often effective in "breaking" the cycle.

Indications for surgery in patients who have recurrent acute tonsillitis are five to seven (or more) episodes of acute tonsillitis occurring in 1 calendar year. Five episodes per year for 2 consecutive years or three episodes per year for 3 consecutive years are also useful guidelines. A single episode of acute tonsillitis is characterized by sore throat; odynophagia; fever; exudative, erythematous tonsils; and tender cervical lymph nodes. The absence of a positive finding on culture for group A β-hemolytic streptococcus does not exclude the presence of acute bacterial tonsillitis. Symptoms clear between episodes.

Persistent Chronic Tonsillitis

A prolonged course (30 days) of antibiotics with either clindamycin or amoxicillin-clavulanate may be helpful. Chronic cryptitis is particular troublesome in persistent tonsillitis. Irrigation of the tonsillar crypts and/or antibacterial mouth rinses have also been advocated by some otolaryngologists.

Surgery for persistent tonsillitis is indicated when a chronic sore throat is present for more than 12 weeks and is associated with enlarged cervical nodes, halitosis, and often otalgia and odynophagia. The tonsils almost always exhibit cheesy exudate (which in its most extreme form presents as tonsillolithiasis), erythema of the tonsils and peritonsillar area, and occasionally dilated surface blood vessels. The tonsils themselves may or may not be enlarged.

RECURRENT ACUTE NASOPHARYNGITIS (ADENOIDITIS)

Recurrent infection in the adenoid is an ill-defined entity primarily because it is often confused with or accompanied by acute rhinosinusitis, both viral and bacterial. Purulent rhinorrhea, nasal obstruction, postnasal drip, fever, and often otitis are harbingers of infection in the adenoids. Four or more episodes of acute nasopharyngitis in 1 year, particularly associated with otitis and/or sinusitis, warrants adenoidectomy.

Substantial benefit in the elimination of chronic adenoid infection and/or inflammation can be gained from assessing the role of environmental irritants. Eliminating smoke, woodburning stoves, dust, and animal dander—*even in the nonallergic child*—may prove to be sufficient. A very effective nasal hygiene program should be implemented, which includes nasal saline containing antibiotics dissolved within the solution followed by use of topical nasal steroids. The use of a broad-spectrum antibiotic (effective against β-lactamase–producing micro-organisms) either at full dose for 30 days or at a prophylactic (one-third to one-half dose) for 3 to 6 months may be undertaken cautiously, with consideration of bacterial resistance patterns in the particular geographic area, severity of disease, and likelihood of resolution based on patient age, duration of symptoms, and season of the year.

Chronic Nasopharyngitis (Adenoiditis)

Persistent infection in the adenoids as manifested by chronic nasal discharge and congestion is also difficult to differentiate from chronic rhinosinusitis. Nonsurgical management is the same as for recurrent acute adenoiditis (see preceding text). For chronic nasal discharge of longer than 3 months' duration not attributable to other causes such as foreign body or allergy, adenoidectomy may be considered.

■ OBSTRUCTION IN THE TONSILS AND ADENOIDS

Obstructive Tonsillar Hyperplasia

General Considerations

Enlarged obstructing tonsils can be present even in the absence of a history of infection. Conversely, enlarged tonsils that have no clinically apparent manifestations, such as dysphagia, snoring with sleep disturbances, or speech abnormalities attributable to tonsil enlargement, may be observed over time for the emergence of symptoms.

Indications for Surgery

Tremendous controversy exists as to how to document obstruction caused by the tonsils. Clinically, sleep disturbances such as loud snoring with snorting, choking or pauses (apneas), restless sleep, morning headaches, lethargy, and growth disturbances may all be more or less prominent. Although the diagnostic usefulness of multichannel polysomnography (PSG) has been well worked out for adults, standardization and meaningful parameters to determine the effects of apnea and hypopnea (duration and frequency) have yet to emerge from the pediatric literature. Furthermore, dysphagia and speech disturbances are not addressed by PSG. The use of audiotape or videotape may be helpful if the findings are strongly positive, but a tape with negative findings has no diagnostic usefulness. Thus, it is most important in these situations to determine the effect of any of these disturbances on the quality of sleep and life for that child. Duration of symptoms is important only in relationship to severity of disease. A long duration of less severe symptoms may be as important as a very severe obstruction of short duration. Precise indications are difficult to establish given the multifactorial nature of the manifestations.

Alternatives to Tonsillectomy

Both idiopathic tonsillar hyperplasia and recurrent tonsillitis with persistent hyperplasia harbor excessive numbers of potential pathogens, particularly *Haemophilus influenzae*, which often produces β-lactamase. Thus, the use of 4 to 6 weeks of a broad-spectrum antibiotic such as amoxicillin-clavulanate is effective in reducing the size of the tonsils for at least 1 year in approximately 15 percent of children. Unilateral tonsillectomy has been recommended by some otolaryngologists when a noninfectious etiology is present.

Obstructive Adenoid Hyperplasia

Indications for Surgery

Obstruction from the adenoids is more readily established. The triad of mouth-breathing, snoring, and hyponasal speech in the presence of a normal intranasal examination is indicative of enlarged obstructing adenoids. Often, otitis, orofacial dental abnormalities, and speech articulation disturbances are present. Adenoidectomy is indicated when these symptoms are present for more than 4 to 6 months despite medical therapy. However, these guidelines may be altered for severe manifestations of disease.

Alternatives to Adenoidectomy

The pathogenesis of obstructive adenoid hyperplasia most likely results from persistent nasal secretions with antigenic stimulators that sit on the adenoids and cause the loss of ciliated columnar epithelium, which is replaced with antigen-presenting squamous epithelium. Antigenic stimulation of the adenoids results in enlargement and obstruction. Thus, several nonsurgical treatment strategies are available. First is environmental control—lessening smoke exposure, irritants from woodburning stoves, animal dander, and dust. A consistent program of nasal hygiene with nasal irrigants (saline-antibiotic preparations, natural irrigants) followed by the use of intranasal steroids to reduce inflammation and the possible effects of immunoglobulin E–mediated allergic stimulations to the nose and nasopharynx are quite helpful.

■ SPECIAL SITUATIONS IN THE TONSILS

Peritonsillar Abscess

Peritonsillar abscess results from a collection of pus lateral to the tonsillar capsule. Hydration, analgesia, and antibiotics (usually parenteral) effective against *Staphylococcus aureus* and oral anaerobes are useful. Immediate tonsillectomy is recommended when the patient presents with a recurrent peritonsillar abscess and/or clear-cut history of recurrent acute or chronic tonsillitis.

For a first occurrence of a peritonsillar abscess, needle aspiration is an effective treatment. An 18 gauge needle on a syringe of 10 mL may be inserted at the superior aspect of the tonsil on the soft palate at the point of maximum bulge or fullness. If after the aspiration, the patient can tolerate fluids orally, a dose of intravenous antibiotics and a fluid bolus are given in the office or emergency department. Close outpatient follow-up is recommended over the next several days until complete resolution is ensured. If there is poor oral intake, impending airway obstruction, systemic toxicity, severe trismus, and/or a very large abscess, admission to the hospital for close observation, vigorous hydration, and administration of parenteral antibiotics is advised.

Unilateral Tonsillar Hyperplasia

Significant variation in size between the two tonsils is unusual. Sometimes one will be more deeply placed in the fossa, but this can usually be ascertained on physical examination alone. However, if one tonsil is larger than another, particularly if the tonsillar architecture is abnormal or ipsilateral cervical nodes are more prominent, tonsillectomy is warranted. Specimen processing is of the utmost importance and should include a full set of cultures and a fresh tonsil specimen for pathologic evaluation to assess for lymphoma. Stains for mycobacterial infection as well as culture are in order. Prior consultation with the pathologist is helpful.

Infectious Mononucleosis

Infectious mononucleosis is not an uncommon cause of acute airway obstruction in children. Characteristic filmy white tonsillar exudate, severe odynophagia, and generalized lymphadenopathy should alert the practitioner to this possibility. Acute bacterial tonsillitis and rarely, peritonsillar abscess may further complicate the picture. Initial treatment includes securing the airway with a nasopharyngeal tube, antibiotics, hydration, and the use of systemic steroids. (Amoxicillin should be avoided because a rash may result; erythromycin has potential for hepatic toxicity.) Orotracheal intubation and immediate tonsillectomy are reserved for those patients who are not managed by the previously described initial treatment measures or in whom hemorrhagic complications are encountered. Experienced anesthesiologists and pediatric intensive care specialists are often consulted; postoperative care must include vigilance in monitoring the patient for pulmonary complications such as pneumonia and postobstructive pulmonary edema.

Postobstructive pulmonary edema may be encountered after relief of either an acute upper airway obstruction or a long-standing chronic upper airway obstruction. Hypoxia (in the face of adequate oxygen delivery and ventilation) may be an early sign; frothy secretions through the endotracheal tube are sometimes seen. Prompt recognition is the key to effective treatment. Positive pressure ventilation for up to 48 hours, diuretics, and morphine may be required.

■ TONSILLECTOMY AND ADENOIDECTOMY

Preoperative Evaluation

Tonsillectomy and adenoidectomy continue to be the mainstays of treatment for chronic tonsillar and adenoid disease despite advances in medical therapy. Many physicians regard T & A as a minor procedure because it is so commonly performed. Taking time for the preoperative preparation of the family and child will help decrease unrealistic postoperative expectations and perhaps complications. The risks of postoperative hemorrhage, emesis resulting in dehydration, and general malaise and throat pain should be discussed in detail with the parents and older child.

A careful medical history includes evaluation of a bleeding history in the family and child. Screening for coagulopathy should include determination of bleeding time and partial thromboplastin time. Malignant hyperthermia is also sought in the family history to screen for adverse reactions to anesthesia. Cervical spine films (extension and flexion) are recommended in the child who has Down syndrome to check for C1-2 subluxation so as to avoid hyperextension of the neck during surgery. (Even in the absence of definable C1-2 instability, I prefer to perform T & A in Down syndrome children in a neutral, nonextended head position.) Other underlying medical problems such as seizures, asthma, and cardiac abnormalities should also be thoroughly evaluated and stabilized before surgery in the elective situation.

Adenoidectomy

Principles of adenoidectomy include mirror visualization of the nasopharynx and removal of the tissue using a sharp curet, adenotome, or suction cautery. Complete removal of the adenoids is rarely necessary, especially in the peritubal Rosenmüller's fossa. I prefer to do an *almost* complete adenoidectomy using a curved curet, leaving the area of the eustachian tube relatively untouched so as to avoid postoperative scarring and possible permanent eustachian tube dysfunction. Rarely does the residual tissue around the eustachian tube orifice undergo hyperplasia to cause late nasopharyngeal obstruction. Great care should also be taken at the posterior choanae to prevent stenosis in that region as well. Direct visualization of the nasopharynx minimizes the chance that this problem will occur. Hemostasis is usually accomplished with packing, suction, or electrocoagulation of the adenoid bed.

Before surgery, a thorough evaluation of the palate is necessary to identify occult clefts or palatal hypotonia. Palatal clefting and velopharyngeal insufficiency are relative contraindications to adenoidectomy. However, if significant nasal obstruction with apnea is documented by PSG, a carefully done lateral or superior adenoidectomy may suffice to relieve the obstruction while having little impact on speech.

Nasopharyngeal stenosis, bleeding, torticollis, and rarely C1-2 subluxation from hyperextension during surgery are additional complications. The most common side effect is malodorous breath that lasts for up to 1 to 2 weeks after the surgery; this side effect is more troublesome to the parents than to the child.

Tonsillectomy

Many techniques are described for tonsillectomy. The principles of careful dissection in the subcapsular plane and meticulous hemostasis underlie all techniques. Variations in technique usually revolve around the method of dissection (cold knife versus hot knife and cautery) and the method for hemostasis (cautery, chemical, or suture). I believe that the lasers that are presently available for tonsillectomy add undue additional risk and cost, and therefore are not justifiable. Complications from laser therapy are as common, and healing is usually delayed.

I prefer the following technique:

- The patient is placed in Rose's position with a shoulder roll in place. A McGiver mouth gag with a slotted tongue depressor is gently placed in the mouth, with an untaped endotracheal tube in the slot. Cooperation with the anesthesia team is necessary. The mouth gag is suspended from the Mayo stand upon which are placed the tonsillectomy instruments.
- Retraction of the soft palate is accomplished using one or two red rubber catheters placed through one or both

Table 1. Postoperative Complications of Tonsillectomy

COMPLICATION	PRESENTATION	MANAGEMENT OPTIONS
Hemorrhage post-tonsillectomy	Bleeding from mouth/nose Frequent swallowing	Local control (cautery or vasoconstriction) Control in OR Evaluate for coagulopathy in selected cases
Post–T & A airway obstruction	Occurs in first 4–24 hours Palatal swelling Hypopharyngeal secretions	Nasopharyngeal airway Suction gently Steroids (IV)
Dehydration post–T & A	Poor oral intake Dry mucous membranes Lethargy	Control emesis if present IV hydration Parental education Pain control p.r.n.
Persistent VPI after adenoidectomy	Hypernasal speech (lasting beyond 2 months post surgery) Nasal regurgitation of fluids	Speech therapy Palate surgery

T & A, tonsillectomy and adenoidectomy; VPI, velopharyngeal insufficiency; OR, operating room; IV, intravenous; p.r.n., as necessary.

nares and secured with a clamp at the nasal tip. A microscope is brought into the field; adenoidectomy is performed as described previously, when indicated.

- Using the operating microscope, a curved Alyss clamp is applied to the superior pole of the tonsil. A blunt-tipped bipolar bayonet cautery (set at 10 W) is used to incise the mucosa of the anterior tonsillar pillar to expose the underlying capsule of the tonsil. The incision, made close to the anterior fold, is extended to the base of the tonsil.
- A subcapsular plane of dissection is developed by alternating cauterizing the blood vessels that are encountered and dissecting the muscle and fascia.
- The bipolar cautery is used to cut across the base of the tonsil, taking care not to invade the lingual tonsil.
- Little bleeding occurs, and little char is present. Packing the fossa is rarely needed. Irrigation of the naso- and oropharynx will clear debris and reveal residual bleeding points that may then be cauterized (bipolar bayonet cautery in tonsil bed, monopolar suction cautery in adenoid bed).

Postoperative Management

Airway protection is most important during extubation to prevent blood and secretions from causing reflex laryngospasm. For children who present little or no increased surgical risk and do not require a longer post–T & A in-hospital observation time, we have implemented procedures for early discharge. These include intraoperative administration of an antiemetic, antibiotic, analgesic, and fluid replacement for the 24 hours after surgery. The use of local analgesia and/or intravenous steroids varies by surgeon. When the child is alert enough for discharge, he or she can leave the same-day surgery unit. Establishing oral intake of any kind is not encouraged. Same-day surgery nurses call the family that evening and the following morning to inquire about eating, breathing, pain management, bleeding, and overall recovery. The child may return to normal activity and diet as tolerated, and whenever desired. Most patients complete a 10 day course of amoxicillin to help reduce the pain and malodorous breath often encountered after T & A. Pain control is accomplished by using acetaminophen with codeine early in the postoperative course, acetaminophen alone after that time. No aspirin or ibuprofen is allowed because bleeding may be a side effect of the platelet dysfunction associated with these analgesics. This information needs to be stated **boldly** on the postoperative instructions.

Stringent criteria should be applied for same-day discharge to ensure that children at greatest risk immediately after surgery are not sent home too early. Children who should be kept for a longer period of observation are those who (1) are younger than 3 years of age, (2) live more than 45 to 60 minutes from the hospital, (3) experience vomiting or hemorrhage, (4) have poor oral intake, (5) live in an environment in which inadvertent neglect may lead to complications, or (6) have other medical problems such as obstructive sleep apnea, Down syndrome, asthma, seizures, or unstable cardiac disease.

The most common complications after tonsillectomy are emesis, dehydration, hemorrhage, and airway obstruction. The presentation and management of these complications is found in Table 1.

Suggested Reading

Brodsky L. Modern assessment of the tonsils and adenoids. Pediatr Clin North Am 1989; 36.

Brodsky L. Tonsillitis, tonsillectomy, and adenoidectomy. In: Bailey BJ, ed. Otolaryngology—head and neck surgery. Philadelphia: JB Lippincott, 1993.

Pizzuto M, Brodsky L. Tonsillectomy and adenoidectomy. Pediatr Otolaryngol General Otolarynologist. Igaku-Shoin, 1996:3.

PERITONSILLAR ABSCESS

The method of
Fred S. Herzon

Peritonsillar abscess (PTA) is the most common head and neck fascial space abscess treated by otolaryngologists. It accounts for 70 percent to 80 percent of all fascial space abscesses of the head and neck. Although PTA occurs in all age groups, patients in their late teens to mid-thirties experience the highest incidence. In American otolaryngology patients who are 5 to 50 years old, PTA has an incidence of approximately 30 per 100,000 person-years. This accounts for approximately 45,000 PTAs per year. There are probably an additional several thousand cases of PTA treated annually in the United States by emergency room physicians or other generalists.

The treatment of an acute PTA is relatively straightforward. Once a diagnosis is made, the abscess cavity should be drained, antibiotics and pain medication should be prescribed, and attention should be directed to fluid intake. However, several variables in the management of PTA have significant impact on the comfort of the patient, the cost of treating the disease, and the long-term incidence of recurrent PTA or tonsillitis. These variables include, among others, the particular surgical procedure used for initial drainage of the abscess and the type of antibiotic used for medical management of the patient. The challenge in managing PTA in the present economic environment is to provide a cost-effective treatment that resolves the abscess quickly with low morbidity while decreasing the risk of recurrent PTA and tonsillitis.

Although it is commonly presumed that an antecedent pharyngeal infection causes PTA, the exact etiology of the disease is unclear. In the United States, there are more than 15 million ambulatory patient visits for sore throat each year and between 0.5 and 1 million tonsillectomies each year. Because there are only 45,000 to 55,000 cases of PTA annually, there may be other clinical variables that predispose a relatively small number of patients who have pharyngeal infections to develop PTA.

DIAGNOSIS

A diagnosis of PTA is indicated by a 2 to 4 day history of sore throat associated with the physical findings of trismus, unilateral tonsillar erythema, uvular deviation, and peritonsillar bulging. Peritonsillitis without abscess formation is the most common entity that must be differentiated from PTA. The simplest way to determine if an abscess is present is to aspirate the tonsil, a procedure that simultaneously confirms the diagnosis and drains the abscess. If the patient refuses aspiration because of age or anxiety, ultrasonic imaging of the tonsil may permit a definitive diagnosis. Occasionally, a patient will not allow any instrument to be placed in the pharynx. Under these circumstances, CT tomographic (CT) imaging may be helpful in making the diagnosis. If there is a high probability that the patient has a PTA, the patient can be taken to the operating room, examined, and treated at that time.

Treatment with parenteral antibiotics for 24 to 48 hours is an alternative to CT or surgery. In a study of a pediatric population, the variables of fever, sore throat, trismus, and tonsillar bulge were evaluated after 1 or 2 days of antibiotic treatment. An improvement in one of these clinical variables predicted peritonsillitis. No improvement after antibiotic treatment predicted the occurrence of PTA.

ACUTE SURGICAL MANAGEMENT

Once it is established that the patient has a PTA, the most important initial treatment is drainage of the fluid in the abscess cavity. This may be successfully accomplished with either needle aspiration, classic incision and drainage, or abscess tonsillectomy. Survey data indicate that 54 percent of otolaryngologists in the United States who treat PTA use incision and drainage, 14 percent drain the fluid with an abscess tonsillectomy, and 32 percent use needle aspiration. Although each procedure is effective in draining the abscess contents, they differ significantly in their morbidity, cost, and skills needed to do the procedure.

INTRAORAL INCISION AND DRAINAGE

Intraoral incision and drainage has been the accepted approach to draining PTAs for decades. Unfortunately, the procedure is tolerated poorly by patients of all ages, and repetition of the procedure may be required to achieve resolution of the PTA. Intraoral incision and drainage requires the services of an otolaryngologist, and there is a finite possibility that the patient may aspirate the contents of the abscess.

ABSCESS TONSILLECTOMY

Abscess tonsillectomy was initially popularized in Europe and was then adopted for the treatment of PTA in the United States approximately 30 years ago. Advocates of this technique maintain that abscess tonsillectomy is the only way to drain a PTA completely. Because PTA is such a strong indication for a tonsillectomy, it may be cost effective to drain the abscess and do the tonsillectomy at one time.

There are several problems with using abscess tonsillectomy as the initial approach to draining a PTA. Abscess tonsillectomy is the most expensive method for the initial treatment of this disease because it requires considerable personnel and equipment resources. There is often a delay of several hours between diagnosis and treatment while the resources are assembled to perform the procedure. In addition, there is no compelling evidence that all patients with a PTA should have a tonsillectomy.

NEEDLE ASPIRATION

The use of needle aspiration for the initial surgical drainage of PTA was first reported nationally approximately 20 years ago. Since that time, many well-controlled studies have confirmed the effectiveness of needle aspiration for the initial surgical drainage of PTA, either alone or in combination with intraoral incision and drainage. Several reports have demonstrated that a single aspiration will resolve a PTA in approximately 85 percent of patients and repeat aspiration, when necessary, brings the success rate to approximately 93 percent (Table 1).

The procedure consists of using an 18 gauge needle on a 10 mL syringe to aspirate the tonsillar apex approximately halfway between the base of the uvula and the maxillary alveolar ridge. Topical and infiltration of local anesthesia can be helpful, but the initial injection of local anesthetic is quite painful. If severe trismus prevents access to the abscess, a standard 1.5 inch, 18 gauge spinal needle can be used to aspirate the abscess cavity. The narrow diameter and length of the spinal needle permits easier access to the tonsil. Patients frequently have significant relief of their odynophagia within hours of the initial needle aspiration, and they should be markedly improved within 24 hours.

MEDICAL THERAPY

Antibiotics, Pain Relief, and Hydration

Basic medical treatment for PTA entails pain relief, hydration, and antibiotic therapy. Each patient should receive whatever pain medication is necessary for comfort. Fluid intake should be monitored, and if necessary parenteral fluids should be given. There is controversy over which antibiotic, if any, should be given to patients who have PTA. Several studies reported in the medical literature have examined the antibiotic sensitivities of the micro-organisms found in the fluid contents of PTAs. The results of these studies are contradictory. Approximately half of the studies concluded that the majority of micro-organisms identified in fluid aspirated from PTAs are sensitive to penicillin, whereas the remaining half reported that most micro-organisms identified in the fluid from PTAs are resistant to penicillin. Consequently, it is difficult to make a specific recommendation about which type of antibiotic is most effective in the treatment of PTA based on this evidence. The choice of an antibiotic to treat PTA should actually be guided by outcome studies that examine the use of different antibiotics to treat the disease rather than studies that examine only the antibiotic sensitivities of micro-organisms in abscess contents. However, outcome studies of this kind have not been reported to date.

In one of the largest series reported on the management of PTA, 96 percent of all PTA patients who were treated with penicillin experienced resolution of the abscess without having to change their antibiotic regimens. Penicillin is also necessary to treat the approximately 30 percent of β-hemolytic group A streptococcus *(Streptococcus pyogenes)* found in the fluid contents of PTAs.

Finally, there is anecdotal information that steroids may be used in conjunction with antibiotics to treat PTA more effectively. No scientific evidence is available in support of this approach to the medical management of PTA.

Table 1. Success Rate of Needle Aspiration for Initial Drainage of Peritonsillar Abscess

STUDY	ABSCESSES TREATED	ABSCESSES RESOLVED	SUCCESS RATE (%)
King	39	38	97
Strome	20	20	100
Herzon & Aldridge	23	19	82
Schechter et al. (1982)	52	48	92
Herzon	41	37	90
Spires et al.	41	39	95
Ophir et al.	75	64	85
Maharaj et al.	30	26	87
Weinberg et al.	31	29	94
Savolainen et al.	98	98	100
Wolf et al.	86	78	90
Herzon (1995)	130	125	96
Totals	666	621	93

OTHER CONSIDERATIONS

Culture of Fluid Contents

The first step in the treatment of most infectious diseases is the identification of the micro-organism responsible for the disease. This does not seem to be the case with PTA. Although some studies of PTA have questioned the value of identifying micro-organisms in the fluid contents of PTAs, it was not until recently that a study examined the effect of micro-organism identification on the outcome of the disease. The results of this recent work suggest that there is no merit in culturing abscess contents in an otherwise normal patient because the identification of micro-organisms in the abscess has little or no bearing on surgical management of the disease.

Site of Treatment

Most patients who have PTAs can be managed as outpatients. Numerous studies support this recommendation. A minority of patients will need to be admitted for hydration and pain relief.

Pediatric PTA

Up to one-third of patients who have PTA are children. Although most studies of PTA include children, there have only been a small number of reports that have examined pediatric patients exclusively. Perhaps the biggest possible difference in treating PTA in a child is the child's ability to tolerate drainage of the abscess without a general anesthetic. Although there is a report that over 90 percent of children will allow a physician to aspirate their PTA without a general anesthetic, one should be prepared to provide whatever sedation or anesthetic is necessary to permit drainage of the fluid from a PTA.

The incidence of a recurrent PTA and prior tonsillitis

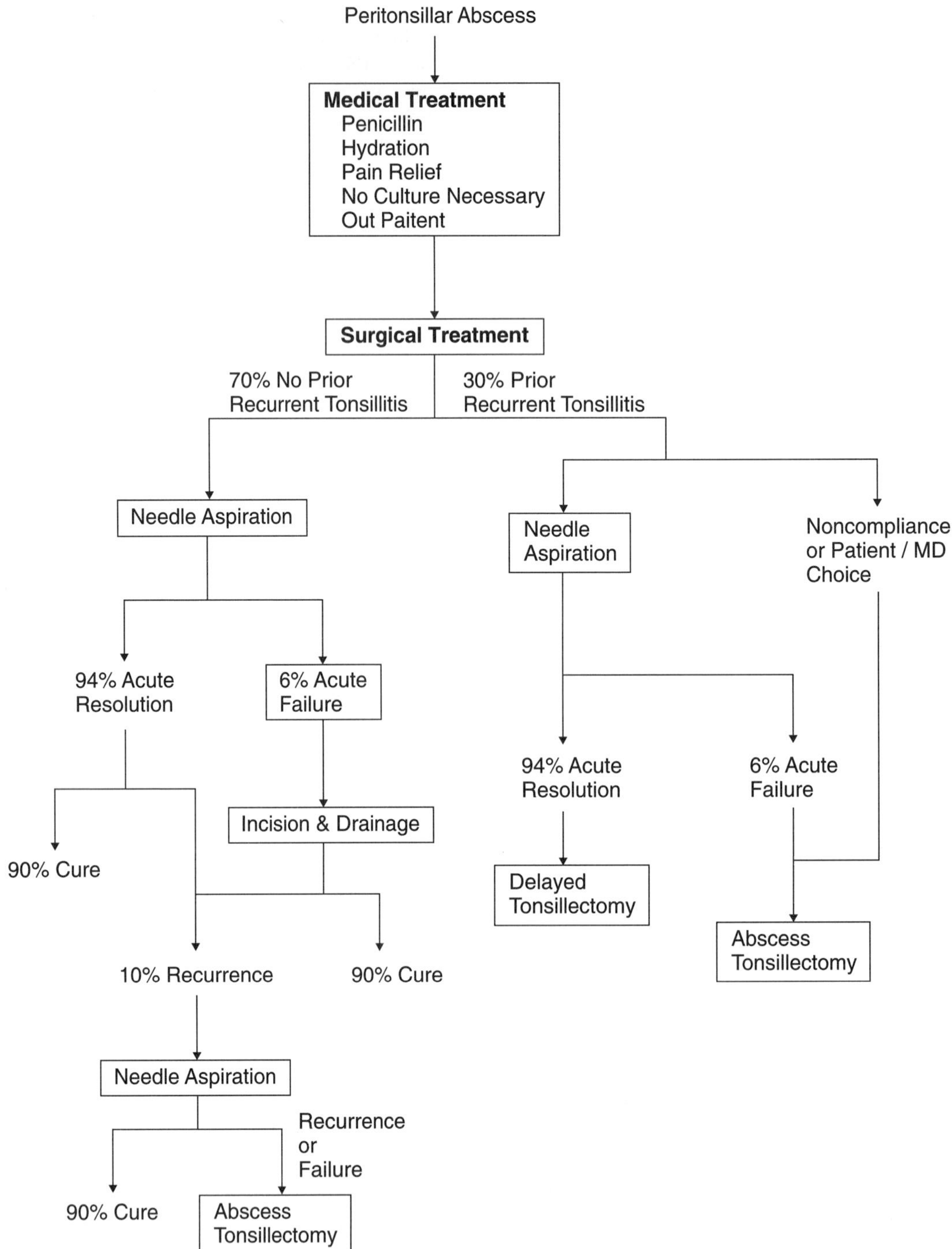

Figure 1.
Management guidelines for peritonsillar abscess. The surgical treatment of PTA should consist of drainage of the abscess with needle aspiration. Needle aspiration will result in a 94 percent resolution rate of the abscess. Patients treated with needle aspiration who have a history of recurrent tonsillitis or recurrent PTA should have a delayed tonsillectomy. If the patient is noncompliant and has a history of prior recurrent tonsillitis, an abscess tonsillectomy may be necessary. An abscess tonsillectomy should also be considered in patients who have multiple recurrent PTA or when needle aspiration or intraoral incision and drainage fail to resolve the abscess.

appear to be lower in children than in adults. Since these data influence the decision to perform a tonsillectomy either immediately or later in a patient who has PTA, available data would suggest that few children who develop PTA should have either an immediate or a delayed tonsillectomy.

Tonsillectomy and PTA

More than 90 percent of otolaryngologists in the United States consider PTA to be either an absolute or a relative indication for tonsillectomy. The major reasons for this appear to be the common beliefs that there is a high incidence of recurrent PTA and that all patients who have experienced PTA will have continued problems with recurrent tonsillitis. Therefore, tonsillectomy would be the logical therapy because it is the only way to drain a PTA completely. However, data on the recurrence of PTA and other related evidence do not support the use of tonsillectomy in most patients who have PTA. Although the recurrence rate for PTA has been reported to vary from 0 percent to 30 percent, a detailed review of the studies of PTA recurrence found that up to 90 percent of patients who have PTA do not suffer a recurrence. Additionally, there is no evidence that PTA alone is a predictor of recurrent tonsillitis. Therefore, the incidence of recurrent PTA or recurrent tonsillitis does not justify a tonsillectomy after a patient has had one episode of PTA.

Proponents of abscess tonsillectomy contend that the procedure is necessary for complete drainage of a PTA. Although it may be true that a tonsillectomy will drain a PTA completely, the success rate for needle aspiration is 93 percent. This strongly suggests that an acute tonsillectomy, with its higher cost and risk, is not necessary to manage PTA.

A substantial portion of patients who experience PTA would probably benefit from a tonsillectomy. Prior recurrent tonsillitis seems to be the best indication for recurrent PTA, but the results of studies that have examined this variable are not consistent. The best interpretation of the data from these studies suggests that any patient who has had two to three episodes of tonsillitis before their initial PTA will have an increased risk of recurrent abscess and tonsillitis and would likely benefit from either an immediate or a delayed tonsillectomy. Approximately 30 percent of patients who have PTA will have experienced recurrent tonsillitis before their PTA and would likely benefit from a tonsillectomy.

■ GUIDELINES FOR MANAGEMENT OF PTA

Once a presumptive diagnosis of PTA has been made, the abscess should be drained using needle aspiration as the initial surgical technique. Topical anesthesia is somewhat helpful, but injection of local anesthetic may be as painful as the therapeutic drainage. A single aspiration will be sufficient for drainage in 80 percent to 85 percent of patients. The patient can be treated in a outpatient setting with penicillin and medication for adequate pain control. Attention should also be paid to the fluid needs of the patient. There is no need to culture the fluid contents unless the patient is immunocompromised. Significant relief of symptoms should occur within hours of the aspiration. A call to the patient at the end of the day or the morning after the treatment will allow the health care provider to determine when the patient should be seen again. If there has not been symptomatic improvement in 24 to 48 hours, a repeat aspiration is indicated. This should bring the resolution rate to approximately 93 percent. Once the abscess is resolved, a delayed elective tonsillectomy should be scheduled for those patients who have a history of prior recurrent tonsillitis or prior PTA.

This acute management approach for PTA will be unsuccessful in approximately 7 percent of all patients. If there is no resolution of the abscess after the second aspiration, an alternative method should be used.

There are two approaches to managing a patient whose PTA is not resolved using needle aspiration as the initial drainage technique. The physician can perform a classic intraoral incision and drainage of the abscess, which should resolve the infection. An alternative is to perform an abscess tonsillectomy. A tonsillectomy may be indicated if the patient has a history of recurrent tonsillitis or if the patient refuses to allow incision and drainage without a general anesthetic. If a general anesthetic and operating room are required to manage the abscess, a tonsillectomy should be considered because this procedure successfully resolves 100 percent of PTAs (Fig. 1).

■ MANAGED CARE AND PTA

Management guidelines are becoming a major tool that health care organizations use to provide quality care to their patient population at a relatively predictable cost. This treatment approach manages effectively both the short-term and the long-term problems of patients who develop PTA at significant savings when compared with the costs of the procedures currently in use by members of the American Academy of Otolaryngology—Head and Neck Surgery who treat this disease.

Suggested Reading

Herzon F, Nicklaus P. Pediatric peritonsillar abscess: Management guidelines. Curr Prob Pediatr 1996; 26:270-278.

Herzon FS. Peritonsillar abscess: Incidence, current management practices, and a proposal for treatment guidelines. Laryngoscope 1995; 105 (Suppl 74):8.

Schechter GL, Sly DE, Roper AL, Jackson RT. Changing face of treatment of peritonsillar abscess. Laryngoscope 1982; 92:657-659.

Stringer SP, Schaefer SD, Close LG. A randomized trial for outpatient management of peritonsillar abscess. Arch Otolaryngol Head Neck Surg 1988; 114:296-298.

OBSTRUCTIVE SLEEP APNEA

The method of
Jonas T. Johnson

Interest among surgeons in the diagnosis of and therapy for sleep disordered breathing is a relatively new phenomenon. Both the medical and the lay literature contain numerous references to snoring, various sleep disorders, and even the pickwickian syndrome described centuries ago. Nevertheless, it has only been in the last 15 years that the potential for surgical intervention whetted the enthusiasm of surgeons for a better understanding of these entities.

Obstructive sleep apnea describes the syndrome in which temporary airway obstruction occurs during sleep. The site of obstruction may vary between individuals and, in fact, some individuals probably have obstructions in more than one site. With the advent of sophisticated polysomnography, we have come to recognize that some individuals may suffer from subtotal obstruction hypopnea, whereas others may have sleep disordered breathing manifested by increased upper airway resistance.

Snoring seems to be the common denominator among these various obstructive sleep syndromes. Snoring that is occasional or positional may be less likely to be associated with apnea. It is estimated that approximately 25 percent of men between the ages of 30 and 60 years snore. The incidence of snoring increases with age. Only approximately 10 percent of women report snoring. About one-half of snorers have apnea as determined by even the most stringent criteria for the diagnosis of sleep apnea. With the consideration of 10 or more obstructive apnea events per hour as a criterion, the prevalence of sleep apnea drops.

■ OTOLARYNGOLOGIC EVALUATION

As a health care provider, the otolaryngologist should be knowledgeable about the stigmata commonly attributed to obstructive sleep apnea (OSA). A history of snoring or perhaps even the recognition of excessive oropharyngeal soft tissue (draping soft palate, elongated and enlarged uvula, bulky tonsils, and relative macroglossia) might lead the surgeon to query the patient about observed respiratory pauses, daytime somnolence, hypertension, obesity, and family history.

There is general agreement that history and physical examination do not correlate closely with objective findings on polysomnography (PSG). Accordingly, patients suspected of having OSA should be referred for further evaluation. This is ideally undertaken in a certified sleep laboratory. The sleep laboratory staff should be prepared to objectively record sleep efficiency and submit a report quantitating obstructive events per hour, observed blood oxygen desaturation, associated cardiac arrhythmias, and sleep architecture.

The otolaryngologist should evaluate the upper aerodigestive tract in patients suspected or known to have OSA. Evidence of a discrete area of obstruction may lend itself to therapeutic intervention. I would caution, however, against intervening for OSA before establishing the diagnosis. Surgical procedures performed on patients who have OSA may be complicated by respiratory distress and sudden death in the immediate postoperative period. Narcotics and general anesthetics should be administered with all caution to patients who have OSA. Elective surgeries should probably be delayed until a PSG has been performed and intervention, if indicated, has been initiated.

A history of nasal obstruction or prior tonsillectomy may be helpful in formulating a treatment plan for patients who have OSA. If severe nasal obstruction is present, it is unlikely that a ventilator mask such as nasal continuous positive airway pressure (CPAP) or bilevel positive airway pressure (BiPAP) can be effectively administered. Our experience has been that patients who had prior tonsillectomy are less likely to benefit from procedures directed at the oropharynx such as uvulopalatopharyngoplasty or laser-assisted uvulopalatoplasty.

The examination of the upper aerodigestive tract with a flexible laryngoscope may help the surgeon appreciate the dynamics of the upper airway. Unfortunately, Müller's maneuver has not been generally acknowledged to be useful in predicting response to surgical therapy. It is estimated that among patients with OSA, more than 90 percent have obstruction at the level of the oropharynx (soft palate, tonsils, and uvula), but more than 80 percent have obstruction at the level of the hypopharynx (tongue base). These numbers indicate that the majority of patients have two sites of obstruction. This observation probably explains the low efficacy of surgery directed at one site alone. This can be appreciated during flexible endoscopy in many patients.

I have personally seen OSA secondary to midface deformity, laryngeal stenosis, and supraglottic edema secondary to radiotherapy. All of these cases have responded to appropriate intervention.

■ THERAPY

A variety of interventions are available for patients who have symptomatic OSA. Positive airway pressure during sleep delivered through a nasal or face mask, such as nasal CPAP or BiPAP, should probably be offered to all candidates. These techniques are effective in 75 percent or 80 percent of patients; however, compliance is low and only 40 percent of patients will consistently use the face mask for 4 or more hours per night.

A great deal of interest has developed around the potential to use a variety of oral devices for the management of snoring and OSA. These devices seek to either reposition the tongue and mandible, lift the soft palate, or stimulate soft-tissue proprioception during sleep. Large-scale, well-documented clinical trials are not available; however, anecdotal evidence suggests that these appliances are useful to some patients

Surgical therapy for OSA is well within the province of most otolaryngologists. Tracheotomy should relieve all symptoms in patients who are accurately diagnosed inasmuch as it effectively bypasses the obstruction. My tracheotomy patients wear the trach plugged during waking hours and open it at night to sleep. This provides remarkable relief of symptoms and is highly effective. Needless to say, the stigmata of tracheotomy make this an intervention that is rarely used.

Uvulopalatopharyngoplasty

Uvulopalatopharyngoplasty (UPPP) has been widely applied to the management of OSA. The procedure includes removal of the tonsils (when present), the anterior tonsillar pillar, and the posterior 1.0 to 1.5 cm of soft palate (including the uvula). I attempt to preserve the posterior pillars in their entirety to obviate the potential for nasopharyngeal stenosis. If the posterior pharyngeal wall and posterior pillars are injured during surgery, the surgeon has created a circumferential wound that with scar contracture may lead to nasopharyngeal stenosis. In my experience, this is the *worst* complication of UPPP and *must* be avoided at all costs.

In connecting the vertical incision from the anterior tonsillar pillar with the horizontal incisions for the soft palate resection, I attempt to make a 90 degree angle between these two incisions. This affords a broad velopharyngeal opening and avoids a Gothic arch effect. Following establishment of adequate hemostasis, I advance the posterior pillar to the cut edge of the mucosa anteriorly. This maneuver effectively smooths out and stretches redundant posterior pharyngeal wall mucosa and again tends to "fish mouth" the velopharyngeal opening. Attempts to recreate the uvula seem frivolous to me. Suture repair of the tonsillar fossa is unnecessary, but the corner stitch between the posterior pillar and the palate as well as closing of the palate seems to potentiate rapid healing. I use polyglycolic acid because reabsorbable suture seems inadequate for the task.

My experience with UPPP parallels that reported by others. Only 50 percent of patients have relief of apnea (fewer than 10 episodes per hour). In the subset of patients who have had prior tonsillectomy, fewer than 10 percent get complete relief of apnea. Overall, patients who have limited apnea (fewer than 20 events per hour) are more likely to have a cure. Accordingly, UPPP should probably not be offered to patients with significant apnea who have had prior tonsillectomy unless some further intervention is anticipated. Conversely, 80 percent of patients with tonsils experience at least an improvement after UPPP, as measured by a reduction of the apnea index by 50 percent. It is apparent, however, that patients who have an apnea index over 40 events per hour may still have symptomatic apnea after UPPP if they only get a 50 percent reduction in events per hour in their respiratory disturbance index

UPPP has been highly effective in the elimination of snoring. Approximately 50 percent of patients report absolute elimination of snoring, whereas another 35 percent to 40 percent report that snoring is vastly improved. For some reason that I do not understand, a small patient subset reports no change in their snoring. Additionally, 10 percent to 15 percent of patients may report recurrence of snoring months to years later.

The postoperative report of the efficacy of surgical intervention correlates poorly with objective PSG, because snoring may be relieved while apnea persists. Accordingly, I recommend that all patients who have symptomatic apnea be restudied with PSG following surgical intervention to document relief of apnea. Failure to do so puts the patient at risk for progression of cardiopulmonary disease secondary to unrecognized OSA.

Laser-Assisted Uvulopalatoplasty

Laser-assisted uvulopalatoplasty (LAUP) and other office-based procedures directed at limited palatal and uvula resection are less effective than is UPPP. Accordingly, the practitioner and the patient should be forewarned that these office-based procedures are perhaps best suited for management of simple snoring and very limited apnea and should not be offered to patients who have symptomatic OSA. I use LAUP for the outpatient management of individuals who have unacceptable snoring but no evidence of apnea. This is especially appropriate in the situation in which the patient's insurance will not cover in-hospital intervention for snoring because office surgical intervention for snoring is considerably less expensive than even an outpatient procedure done in a surgicenter.

Mandibular Advancement

At the other end of the spectrum are patients who have failed UPPP, patients with significant apnea who have had prior tonsillectomy, and patients who have respiratory disturbance greater than 20 or 25 events per hour. Under these circumstances, further intervention is required. Efforts to improve the hypopharyngeal airway have been successful in a high percentage of these individuals. The procedure I currently advocate is a horizontal mandibulotomy that allows advancement of the mentum 12 to 15 mm anteriorly. This procedure effectively reshapes the hypopharyngeal airway because the suprahyoid musculature has been repositioned. Excessive mental projection can be handled by trimming the mandible. Suspension of the hyoid to the mandible is currently employed in an effort to relieve the tension on the suprahyoid musculature during the convalescent phase. I suspect, however, that efforts at long-term suspension with wire, Gore-Tex, or suture eventually result in fatigue and failure with time.

Nasal Surgery

I believe that nasal surgery rarely has a material effect on snoring or OSA. I am impressed by what appears to be a rather remarkably high incidence of chronic nasal obstruction in the population of patients with snoring and sleep apnea. Certainly, efforts at relief of allergic rhinitis, reduction of excessive turbinates, and repair of septal deviation may afford the patient improved comfort and must facilitate the use of nasal CPAP. In view of this, I am an advocate of aggressive management of nasal obstruction for this population of patients. It must be stressed, however, that I have rarely encountered patients who report relief of snoring, apnea, and its associated stigmata (hypertension, hypersomnolence, and so forth) following nasal surgery. Fairbanks suggests a trial of night-time oxymetazoline in an effort to identify the occasional patients who may experience relief of snoring with intranasal surgery. This seems a reasonable approach to me.

Suggested Reading

Johnson JT. Uvulopalatopharyngoplasty. In: Myers EN, Carrau RL, Cass SP, eds. Operative otolaryngology head and neck surgery. Philadelphia: WB Saunders, 1997:208.

McGuirt WF, Johnson JT, Sanders MH. Previous tonsillectomy as prognostic indicator for success of uvulopalatopharyngoplasty. Laryngoscope 1995; 105:1253-1255.

Riley RW, Powell NB, Guilleminault C. Inferior sagittal osteotomy of the mandible with hyoid myotomy-suspension: a new procedure for obstructive sleep apnea. Otolaryngol Head Neck Surg 1996; 94:589-593.

Riley RW, Powell NB, Guilleminault C. Maxillary, mandibular, and hyoid advancement for treatment of obstructive sleep apnea: a review of 40 patients. J Oral Maxillofac Surg 1990; 48:20-26.

Waite PD, Wooten V, Lachner J, Guyette RF. Maxillomandibular advancement surgery in 23 patients with obstructive sleep apnea syndrome. J Oral Maxillofac Surg 1989; 47:1255-1256.

INFLAMMATORY LARYNGEAL DISEASE IN CHILDREN

The method of
Sylvan E. Stool

Inflammatory disease of the larynx is frequently encountered in pediatric practice; most episodes are self-limited and of viral origin. The management depends on the etiology, which is not necessarily apparent upon presentation of the patient. The patients encountered by the otolaryngologist are those whose course is unusual and for whom there is often concern regarding the possibility of sudden or complete airway obstruction.

When the otolaryngologist evaluates a patient, he or she must consider the entire spectrum of diseases and be aware of the significant symptoms and signs. A brief history is necessary to gather information about pertinent developmental milestones and prenatal conditions, such as prematurity, intubation, and previous episodes of respiratory distress. The course of the present illness, time and rapidity of onset, and progression alert the otolaryngologist to the severity. Since the advent of immunization for *Haemophilus influenzae* B, supraglottitis has become very rare.

Three major conditions must be considered in the child who has inflammatory laryngeal disease: croup, supraglottitis, and bacterial tracheitis. Less frequent but important considerations include foreign body and laryngeal papilloma. These may be distinguished on the basis of the characteristics listed in Table 1.

MANAGEMENT

At Children's Hospital of Denver, we have established a protocol for management that I summarize in the following paragraphs.

Emergency Department

The emergency department team includes the otolaryngologist, pediatric senior resident, anesthesiologist, and intensive care unit staff. They are notified when advance notice is received or promptly in case of an unannounced arrival of a child in respiratory distress.

Assessment

The triage nurse and emergency resident rapidly assess the child and assemble the emergency kit, which includes a

Table 1. Distinguishing Characteristics of Croup, Bacterial Tracheitis, and Supraglottis

FEATURE	CROUP	BACTERIAL TRACHEITIS	SUPRAGLOTTITIS
Age	>2 years	Any age	3–5 years
Organism	Respiratory syncytial virus, parainfluenza	*Staphylococcus aureus*	*Haemophilus influenzae*
Site of involvmeent	Subglottis	Trachea	Supraglottis
Stridor	Biphasic	Expiratory	Inspiratory
Voice	Barking cough	Hoarseness	Unaffected
Position	Not characteristic	Not characteristic	Erect, chin jutting forward
Swallowing	Unaffected	Unaffected	Drooling
Treatment	Humidity, epinephrine, steroids?	Bronchoscopy, suctioning, intravenous antibiotics, monitoring in intensive care unit	Artificial airway, intravenous antibiotics, humidity

mask, laryngoscope, endotracheal tube, and drugs for intubation and resuscitation.

Disposition

The disposition depends on the degree of severity (Table 2).

Mild. These children usually have a slowly progressive illness, are alert, are not cyanotic, have a pulse rate under 100, and have an occasional cough. The pharynx may be examined, and treatment may involve cool mist.

Moderate. The progression is fairly rapid. The child is alert but anxious and is hoarse. Radiographs may show a steeple sign. Treatment with racemic epinephrine and steroids may be instituted. These children may be admitted for careful observation.

Severe or Extreme. The child who is deemed to have supraglottic disease should be transferred to the operating room (OR) promptly. The parent may accompany the patient to the OR. During transport all emergency equipment is carried. Visualization of the pharynx should not be attempted. If the patient cannot be moved, positive pressure with a bag and mask should be applied.

Operating Room

The parent or a surrogate holds the child on the lap. All endoscopic equipment is available. The child is preoxygenated, an inhalation anesthetic is started, and the parent is excused. Usually ventilation can be maintained as the child relaxes, and after adequate level of anesthesia is achieved an intravenous line is established. Examination is performed using the endoscope to establish the diagnosis. If the diagnosis is supraglottic disease, an endotracheal tube may be inserted, and cultures are obtained. If the diagnosis is laryngotracheal bronchitis or bacterial tracheitis, a decision is made regarding intubation or tracheotomy, depending on the extent of the laryngeal involvement and character of the secretions. The decision for intubation or tracheotomy is multifactorial and depends on the expertise available for patient care. If the hospital has an experienced intensive care unit (ICU) with personnel available for reintubation, this procedure is appropriate. Obviously, if this is not the situation, tracheotomy may be preferable. If there is evidence of laryngeal damage or thick secretions, a tracheotomy is preferred.

Tracheotomy is preferably performed after an airway is established with a bronchoscope or endotracheal tube, and the patient is stabilized. In very small infants (especially those who have a fat neck), the bronchoscope has some advantages.

The surgeon should position the patient so that the shoulders are elevated. The neck is palpated to ascertain the position of the larynx and trachea. The stomach may be aspirated, but an orogastric tube should not be inserted. Minimal draping should be used, because the position of the head and face should be monitored. Turning the head displaces the trachea. The anesthesiologist holds the chin to hyperextend the neck.

I usually prefer a horizontal incision, one finger breadth above the sternal notch. The dissection is performed in the midline, with each fascial layer being identified. Much of the dissection is accomplished by palpation. When the trachea is identified, stay sutures are applied 1 to 2 mm to the right and left of the midline. These are of value if there is an accidental decannulation. They should be taped to the chest and identified left and right.

The vertical incision into the trachea is made with a knife and enlarged with scissors. The tracheotomy tube is inserted through the tracheotomy incision. In acute inflammatory disease, the child usually is not ventilated so a large tube is not necessary. The tracheal secretions can be aspirated and sent for culture. A postoperative chest radiograph is ordered.

The duration of intubation depends on the resolution of the disease. Because most patients requiring tracheotomy have severe tracheitis, resolution is often slow, and it may be necessary to perform an endoscopic examination before decannulation. When the resolution is rapid, the tube can be removed without downsizing; if it exceeds 1 to 2 weeks, insertion of progressively smaller tubes may be necessary.

Occasionally, the diagnosis of viral laryngotracheal bronchitis is made, in which case intravenous steroids can be administered and an artificial airway need not be provided.

Intensive Care Unit

The intubated child is usually sedated and restrained to prevent accidental extubation. The choice of antibiotics depends on the results of blood and throat culture and what treatment has been most effective in the community.

■ EXTUBATION

The otolaryngologist and ICU fellow examine the larynx every 24 hours, observing structure and presence of a leak around the tube. Extubation is performed when the swelling has subsided and the child is alert. Postextubation racemic

Table 2. Characterization of Severity of Respiratory Distress

FEATURE	MILD (DAYS)	MODERATE (HOURS)	SEVERE (MINUTES)	EXTREME (IMMEDIATE)
Tussive (cough)	Occasional	Hoarse	Bark	Bark or depressed
Retractions	Absent	Suprasternal	Supra- and infrasternal	All accessory muscles
Anxiety	Calm	Anxious when disturbed	Restless	Agitated or stuporous
Cyanosis	0	0	In room air	In 40% oxygen
Heart rate	<120	<140	>140	>140
Stridor	Occasional	Inspiratory and expiratory	Inspiratory and expiratory	Marked or diminished

epinephrine can be used if the child has a croupy cough without obstruction.

■ DISCUSSION

There are few conditions in which proper planning and expeditious management can be as satisfying as the management of inflammatory disease of the larynx in children; conversely, there are few conditions that are as treacherous. The principles of adequate oxygenation and not increasing work of breathing without providing an adequate airway cannot be overemphasized.

Suggested Reading

Ledwith C, Shea L, Maauro R. Safety and efficacy of nebulized racemic epinephrine in conjunction with oral dexamethasone and mist in the outpatient treatment of croup. Ann Emergency Med 1995; 25:3.

Witmore R. Tracheotomy. In: Bluestone CD, Stool SE, Kenna MA, eds. Pediatric otolaryngology. 3rd ed. Vol. 2. Philadelphia: WB Saunders, 1996:1425.

RESPIRATORY PAPILLOMATOSIS

The method of
Brian J. Wiatrak

Respiratory papilloma (RP) is the most common benign tumor of the larynx in children. There is evidence that the incidence of this often debilitating disease has recently been increasing. Although RP is also prevalent in the adult population, it seems to have a particular preponderance toward aggressive recurrences in children, with statistically devastating developmental, social, and familial consequences. Currently, there is no cure for recurrent RP. Disease management is focused on endoscopic surgical extirpation of disease, often combined with adjuvant medical therapy, to bring the disease process under control until a period of long-term and possibly permanent quiescence is reached. There is no absolute consensus among otolaryngologists as to the ideal management approach. It should be emphasized, however, that this disease should be managed as a team effort, involving the physician, appropriate nursing staff, operating room personnel, and most important, the patient's family.

■ ETIOLOGY

Respiratory papillomatosis is a disease of viral origin representing infection by human papillomavirus (HPV) types 6 and 11 in the vast majority of cases. However, premalignant viral subtypes, that is, types 16 and 18, have also been implicated. It is presumed that children who have RP obtain the virus from infected mothers who have vaginal HPV disease, although this has not been clearly substantiated. There are reported pediatric cases of patients with RP who have obtained the disease after birth by cesarean section. Although the majority of patients in my practice have mothers with evidence of HPV disease (vaginal condyloma or cervical dysplasia), this is not a universal finding.

Once the respiratory tract has been infected with HPV, the viral DNA establishes itself in the basal layer of the mucosal epithelium, stimulating viral protein production and also stimulating rapid epithelial growth, which results in papilloma formation. The actual viral capsids are formed in the more superficial and mature layers of the epithelium. Viral DNA has been identified in areas of clinically normal mucosa in the airways of infected patients and in the airways of patients who have undergone remission. The implication is that even in patients who have inactivated disease, this viral DNA presence may be representative of a period of quiescence, with reactivation of the disease process possible in the future.

The vast majority of involved sites in the pediatric airway include the glottic and supraglottic larynx, although other sites that might become involved include the subglottis, trachea, bronchi, pulmonary parenchyma, esophagus, pharynx, and palate. The most common sites of predilection have been demonstrated to be transition zones between different types of epithelium, that is, the junction between squamous and ciliated epithelium. It has also been demonstrated that patients who have serious disease warranting tracheotomy may have a higher incidence of tracheal involvement by papillomatosis.

■ INITIAL MANAGEMENT

The vast majority of pediatric patients who have RP are first seen within the first 3 years of life, typically with aphonia or hoarseness as the primary presenting symptom. Although airway obstruction is a component of the presentation, it is the unusual patient who is initially seen with severe airway obstruction. Over the past 5 years, three of 40 patients have initially been seen by me after undergoing emergent tracheotomy at other institutions. It must be remembered that, although papillomas may contribute to significant obstruction of the laryngotracheal airway, they result in a soft, fairly dynamic stenosis, and there may be significant compromise of the airway before significant respiratory distress develops, unlike a case of firm stenosis, such as subglottic stenosis, in which airway symptoms may be quite severe.

Although the true diagnosis cannot be made until histologic confirmation is obtained in the operating room, the initial diagnosis in most cases is made using flexible laryngoscopy in the office setting. Videolaryngoscopy equipment is used, so that video and photographic documentation can be obtained for the patient's record and for patient education purposes. Once the diagnosis of RP has been made, surgery is scheduled according to the severity of the patient's symptoms. Obviously, patients who have evidence of significant airway compromise need urgent surgical intervention, whereas others who have less severe airway compromise can be scheduled at the surgeon's discretion.

At this point in the management of the patient, family counseling plays an extremely important role. In the majority of cases, the parents of a child diagnosed with RP are completely lacking in knowledge of this disease process. The family should be educated immediately about laryngeal papillomas and about the possible implications of their child's potential long-term chronic illness. The true impact of this disease on patients and their families may not be realized immediately. However, the process of education should start at the first suspicion of this diagnosis. It is very helpful to show the parents the appropriate anatomy on the flexible laryngoscopy videotape and possibly use models or diagrams that demonstrate the affected anatomy of their child. Although not always the case, a significant number of patients with RP are from families of lower socioeconomic means and may be poorly educated and will require extensive educational sessions. The importance of close follow-up should be stressed, and both the patient and the family should be clearly made aware of who to contact when significant respiratory symptoms develop. It is also important to educate the family's primary caregiver about the patient's diagnosis, its implications, and the need for close medical supervision over a potentially long period. If medical insurance is a problem for the family, these issues should be worked out early on in the management process to alleviate this source of significant stress and anxiety on the family before they feel overwhelmed, as is often the case in families of patients who have RP.

■ SURGICAL PLANNING

When performing endoscopy on a patient who has a compromised airway, anesthetic management is extremely important. It is crucial to communicate ahead of time with the anesthesiologist regarding the extent of disease in that particular patient and agreement about the type of anesthetic that will be used. No anesthetic should be delivered until the primary surgeon has also confirmed that all necessary equipment is available in the operating room and functioning appropriately. Once anesthesia has been administered to a patient who has a severely compromised airway, urgent airway intervention may be necessary if the anesthesiologist is not able to continue oxygenating the patient adequately. Fortunately, in cases of laryngeal papillomatosis, the soft stenosis allows adequate mask ventilation of the patient with positive pressure. If the degree of airway obstruction is unclear, it is not wise to administer any muscle relaxant until the larynx has been examined initially and the amount of obstruction has been assessed. Administering muscle relaxants to a patient who has a severely compromised airway could potentially have catastrophic results.

Various anesthetic techniques have been used for the surgical management of recurrent RP. However, at the Children's Hospital of Alabama at Birmingham, the intermittent apnea technique has been found to be ideal. This technique allows a clear, unobstructed view of the entire larynx, especially the posterior larynx, which otherwise would be hidden by the presence of an endotracheal tube. Other techniques that may be used include the Sanders-Venturi ventilation technique or spontaneous respiration with halothane, possibly combined with propofol.

■ SURGICAL TECHNIQUE

The intermittent apnea technique is used for the majority of my patients who have RP. The general anesthesia is initially induced with inhalation agents, most commonly halothane. At this point, intravenous access is established, and laryngoscopy is performed using a Parson's laryngoscope (Fig. 1) and Storz-Hopkins rod lens telescope. Topical lidocaine is applied to the larynx under direct visualization before the endoscope is introduced. Using the rod lens telescope, the larynx and trachea are assessed, as well as the proximal right and left mainstem bronchi. At this point in the procedure, spontaneous respiration technique is used. However, when the airway has been assessed and determined to be safe, neuromuscular relaxants can be given for the remainder of the case.

At this point, after the appropriate photograph and video documentation has been obtained, the patient is intubated

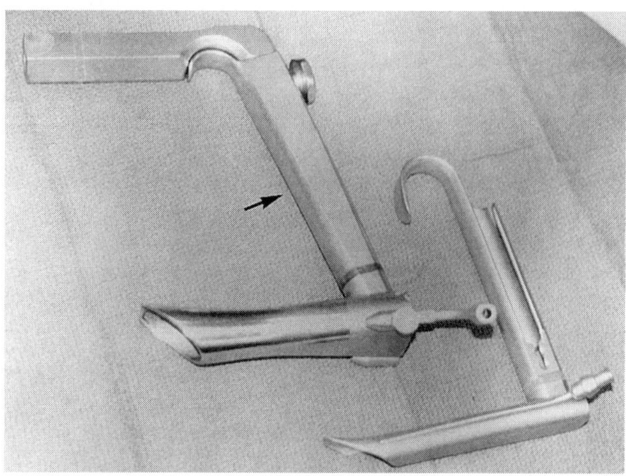

Figure 1.
Lindholm (arrow) and Parson's laryngoscopes.

with an appropriate-sized endotracheal tube, and the larynx is suspended with a Lindholm laryngoscope (Fig. 1). If the larynx is particularly anterior or if the anterior commissure is particularly difficult to visualize, another laryngoscope, that is, Dedo, may be required for more appropriate visualization during the case. We prefer the Lindholm laryngoscope because of the wide distal opening of this instrument, which allows a wide field of visualization during the microlaryngoscopy and also allows for less frequent repositioning of the laryngoscope during the procedure.

Suspension laryngoscopy is performed using a suspension platform that fits over the patient directly on the operating table (Fig. 2). This allows manipulation of the bed frequently during the case without the need for repositioning a Mayo stand. Microlaryngoscopy is then performed using an operating microscope. Biopsies are obtained using straight and angled forceps from appropriate locations within the larynx. The specimens are obtained for histopathology to demonstrate any potential areas of dysplasia or malignant degeneration; specimens are also sent to research laboratories for basic science research. At this point, the CO_2 laser is connected to the microscope. Moist eye patches are placed on the eye; moist towels are applied to the head, neck, and upper chest; and the laser is set on a relatively low wattage (3 to 5 W). All operating room personnel should be wearing protective glasses to shield from potential injury from the CO_2 laser beam. All personnel coming in contact with the patient during the procedure should be wearing masks, gowns, and gloves to protect themselves from potential viral contamination. Although there are no reported cases of health care personnel becoming infected with HPV while performing or assisting with endoscopy in RP patients, these precautions should be maintained. The laser used at my institution is the Coherent ultrapulse laser, which allows high-frequency ultrapulse delivery of the CO_2 laser, with cooling between pulses and, secondarily, less charring during the endoscopy. A highly focused beam is used. However, defocusing the beam may help with hemostasis when needed. Bleeding can also be controlled with cottonoids soaked in phenylephrine hydrochloride applied directly to the bleeding point.

As was mentioned earlier, the intermittent apnea technique is used. The endotracheal tube is removed, and laser excision is performed. When oxygen desaturation begins to occur, as reported by the anesthesiologist monitoring the case, the endotracheal tube is placed back directly through the laryngoscope.

Excision of tracheal papillomas is more difficult due to the more distal location in the airway. Different options exist for the management of tracheal papillomas. One option is to place the rod lens telescope directly through the Lindholm laryngoscope into the trachea, simultaneously placing an appropriate cup forceps (straight or angled) alongside the telescope. Under direct endoscopic visualization, the tracheal papillomas can be debrided (Fig. 3). This works very well at my institution for cases of tracheal papillomas. Another option is to use the KTP laser. This laser can be delivered through a flexible optical fiber that can be threaded through the suction port of a rigid bronchoscope that has been placed into the trachea (Fig. 4). This allows ventilation during the case while laser excision is being performed. Another option is to use a CO_2 laser bronchoscope, which currently is not used at my institution. Finally, the papillomas may be excised using optical foreign body forceps, which may be

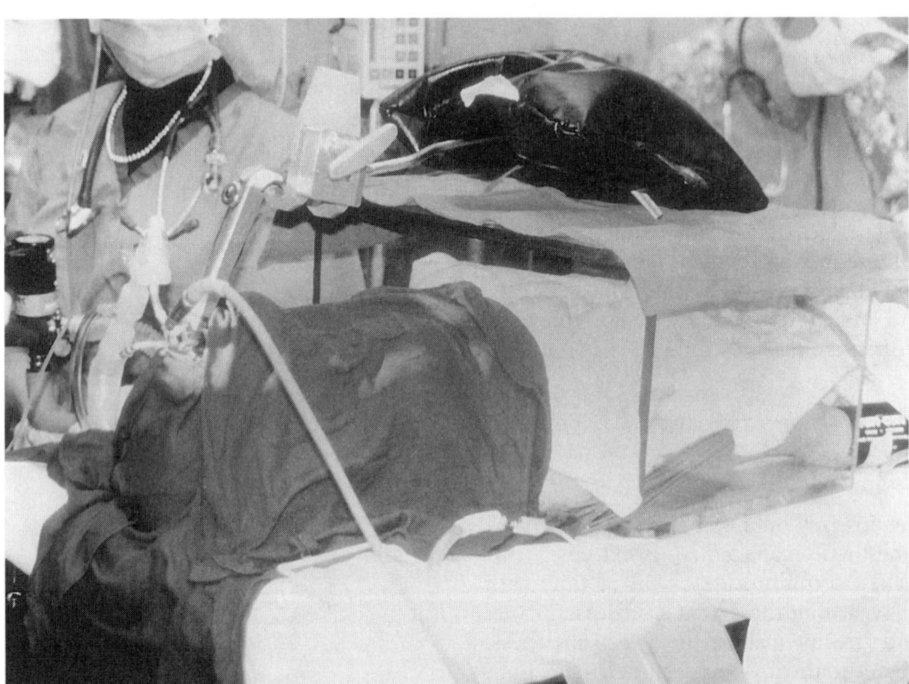

Figure 2.
Patient undergoing suspension laryngoscopy with Lindholm laryngoscope and CO_2 laser. Note suspension table overlying the patient.

passed directly through a ventilating bronchoscope into the trachea.

When excision of papillomas is complete and hemostasis has been obtained, the laryngoscope is removed. To maintain a safe airway during this process, the endotracheal tube adapter is removed from the endotracheal tube. The endotracheal tube is then grasped with a large straight alligator forceps, and the laryngoscope is completely removed from the oral cavity, leaving the endotracheal tube in the endotracheal airway. The adapter is then replaced on the endotracheal tube so that ventilation can be maintained for the remainder of the procedure.

During the procedure, the extent of disease is staged using a staging sheet we have created at the Children's Hospital of Alabama (Fig. 5).

■ MEDICAL MANAGEMENT OF PATIENTS WHO HAVE RECURRENT RP

Many medical therapeutic options have been attempted for the treatment of severe cases of recurrent RP. Few of these options have been well studied, and some are currently under investigation and show promise. No clear national standards exist at this time as to when to begin a patient on medical therapy for recurrent RP. At my institution, a patient who has severe papillomatosis requiring frequent laser procedures in the operating room (> 6 weeks between laser procedures) is a candidate for medical therapy.

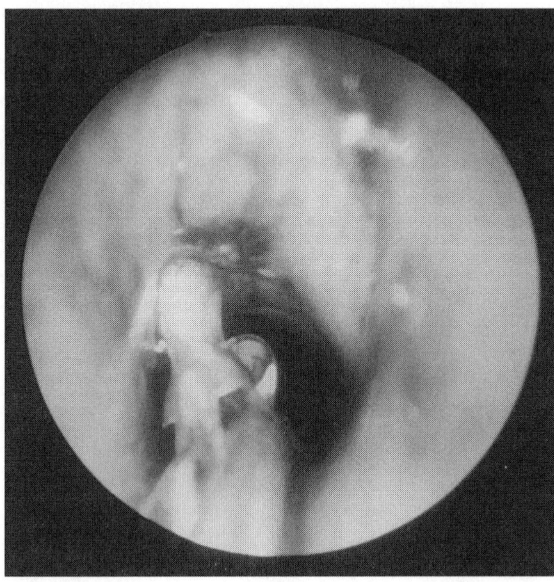

Figure 3.
Cup forceps in trachea visualized with 0 degree rod lens telescope for excision of tracheal papillomas.

Interferon

Numerous medical options have been suggested for patients who have RP. The best known is the use of interferon alpha-2a. This glycoprotein has been well studied in numerous prospective blinded clinical trials and has demonstrated clinical efficacy. Although there are some significant side effects, in general treatment with interferon is well tolerated.

The current interferon protocol that is used at my institution is an initial dose of 1 million U per square meter per day for 3 days, followed by 2 million U per square meter for 3 days, then 3 million U per square meter for 3 days, and finally 4 million U per square meter for 3 days. After this, the patient is maintained on 5 million U per square meter per day for 30 days and subsequently decreased to three doses per week of 5 million U per day. A patient who has not been placed on interferon before has the initial dose monitored in the hospital. Patients younger than 2 years old are usually admitted to the hospital for observation. Patients older than this are observed as outpatients for 4 to 6 hours after the first dose for any side effects. Initial studies obtained include a chest radiograph, complete blood count (CBC) with differential, platelet count, prothrombin time, partial thromboplastin time, fibrinogen, fibrin split products, aspartate aminotransferase, alanine aminotransferase, alkaline phosphatase, total and direct bilirubin, electrolytes, blood urea nitrogen, creatine, calcium, uric acid, serum iron, iron binding capacity, and urinalysis. These studies are obtained based on prior scientific literature regarding interferon and in conjunction with consultation with the pediatric hematology department. Parents are educated about the potential side effects of interferon. Follow-up monitoring includes CBC with differential on Day 14, and a repeat of the complete metabolic workup on Day 28. These laboratory tests are then repeated on Day 60 and Day 90. After 90 days, a CBC with differential is obtained monthly, and the full metabolic workup is obtained quarterly.

Side effects of interferon are flulike symptoms, including fever that may be quite high at times; muscle aches and joint aches; fatigue; headaches; chills; and tachycardia. These side effects, which may be quite common within the first week of treatment, subside significantly after 10 to 14 days of

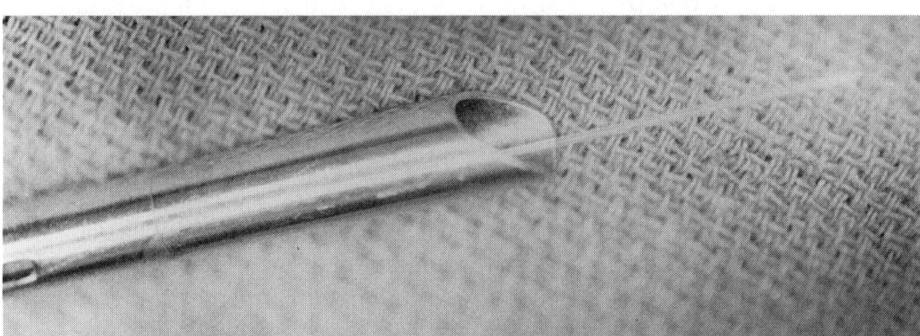

Figure 4.
KTP laser fiber protruding from suction port in distal end of bronchoscope.

DATE OF SURGERY ___________
ADJUVANT THERAPY __________
INITIATION DATE __________

NAME
M.R. #

SEVERITY RATING
0 NONE PRESENT
1+ MINIMAL
2+ MODERATE
3+ SEVERE

LARYNX
EPIGLOTTIS _____
LINGUAL SURFACE _____
LARYNGEAL SURFACE _____
ARY-EPIGLOTTIC FOLDS LEFT_____ RIGHT_____
FALSE VOCAL CORDS LEFT_____ RIGHT _____
TRUE VOCAL CORDS LEFT_____ RIGHT _____
ANTERIOR COMMISSURE _____
POSTERIOR GLOTTIS _____
SUBGLOTTIS _____
OTHER _____

TRACHEA
UPPER 1/3 ANTERIOR _____ POSTERIOR _____
MIDDLE 1/3 ANTERIOR _____ POSTERIOR _____
LOWER 1/3 ANTERIOR _____ POSTERIOR _____
BRONCHI RIGHT _____ LEFT _____
TRACHEOSTOMY STOMA _____

OTHER
NOSE _____ ESOPHAGUS _____
PALATE _____ LUNGS RIGHT _____ LEFT _____
PHARYNX _____ OTHER _____

TOTAL SCORE _____

Figure 5.
Disease staging sheet for respiratory papillomatosis.

therapy. Other reported side effects may include nasal congestion; urinary urgency; dizziness; and gastrointestinal symptoms, including loss of appetite, vomiting, diarrhea, weight loss, and dysgeusia. There may be associated elevation of liver enzymes as indicated by liver function tests. Circulatory hypotension may occur, with occasional fainting in rare cases. Hematologic effects include decreases in the white blood cell count, red blood cell count, and platelet count. Approximately 15 percent to 20 percent of patients who receive interferon develop mild protein spilling in the urine, and skin rashes may occur.

Interferon is delivered as a subcutaneous injection that requires significant parental education. The costs of interferon obtained at my institution is approximately $50.00 for 3 million U.

13-*Cis*-Retinoic Acid

Another medical option that has been well described in the literature and that has resulted in significant success at my institution is retinoic acid. Although a large prospective randomized trial using retinoic acid for treating RP has not been performed, significant responses to this drug have been reported in the literature. Retinoic acid works as a potential regulator of epithelial differentiation and as such has been shown to affect synthesis of keratins, response to certain growth factors, cornified envelope formation, and cell-to-cell adhesion. In ciliated and secretory cells derived from tracheal and bronchial epithelium, retinoids have been shown to regulate proliferation and maintenance of the differentiated structure and function inherent to respiratory epithelium.

In my institution, a significant number of patients who have received retinoic acid have had a profound, long-lasting remission. Based on this experience, it appears that patients will have either a significant profound response or no response whatsoever.

The dosage for retinoic acid is 1 to 2 mg per kilogram orally on a daily basis. The therapy is maintained for 6 months or until significant side effects develop that are not tolerated by the patient. Monitoring includes baseline liver function tests, and triglyceride levels followed by biweekly liver function testing and monthly triglyceride testing. Restrictions include no supplemental vitamin A and limiting exposure to the sun, because retinoic acid causes severe skin sensitization to sunlight. Patients should not be placed on any tetracycline, limit the amount of fat in their diets, and have no alcohol intake (this restriction applies to older patients during treatment). Female patients of childbearing age should have a negative serum pregnancy test and use effective birth control for 1 month before starting retinoic acid. The drug should be started on the second or third day of a menstrual cycle.

Side effects from retinoic acid include dry skin and lips, skin irritation, headaches, nausea, vomiting, blurred vision, changes in mood, severe abdominal pain, diarrhea, rectal bleeding, persistent dryness of the eyes, jaundice, or dark urine. In my experience, patients who have had a clinical response to retinoic acid with respect to their laryngotracheal papillomas also have had significant side effects. The patients who had no clinical effect had no significant side effects from the drug. Apparently, there is a subgroup of patients who have profound sensitivity to retinoic acid, which on the one hand allows a significant clinical response, but on the other hand allows for development of side effects.

The cost of retinoic acid for patients at my institution is $6.00 for one 40 mg capsule.

Other Potential Medical Therapies

Indole-3-carbinol is a metabolite of estrogen metabolism and has been shown to have some potential clinical effect in treating conditions such as breast cancer and laryngeal papillomatosis. Prospective studies are only in their early stages at this point. However, anecdotal evidence exists indicating that there may be benefit from dietary supplementation using indole-3-carbinol as an adjunctive therapy in the treatment of RP. Indole-3-carbinol is considered a dietary supplement and may be found in cruciferous vegetables, that is, cabbages, or it may be obtained as a purified dietary supplement at a relatively low cost. As of yet, the staff at my institution has not detected a significant response in our patients to supplementation with indole-3-carbinol. This medical option has been offered at my institution to newly diagnosed patients as an early, easily tolerated, relatively inexpensive adjuvant therapy. Further research is warranted in this area before global recommendations can be made. Numerous other adjuvant medical therapies have been recommended, that is, acyclovir, methotrexate, ribavirin, and, most recently, cidofovir, which has recently been approved for treatment of cytomegalovirus retinitis in acquired immunodeficiency syndrome patients. More research is necessary before the efficacy of these medications can be truly elucidated. At this point, the staff of my institution is not recommending any of these adjuvant medical therapies to our patients.

■ DISCUSSION

Although new adjuvant medical therapies have been recently proposed, the treatment of children who have RP remains unchanged over the last 15 years: surgical excision with adjuvant medical therapy in selected severely recurrent cases. Further research is required on a national, or possibly, international, scale to determine (1) why certain patients are susceptible to RP when infected with HPV, whereas others are not; (2) standards for requirement of adjuvant medical therapy; (3) which medical therapy or therapies, either alone or in combination, are required to best manage this disease. With recent advances in molecular biology, it is very likely that many of these issues will be elucidated, hopefully over the next 10 to 15 years.

Suggested Reading

Avidano MA, Singleton GT. Adjuvant drug strategies in the treatment of recurrent respiratory papillomatosis. Ann Otol Rhinol Laryngol 1995; 112:197-202.

Bell R, Hong WK, Itri LM, et al. The use of cis-retinoic acid in recurrent respiratory papillomatosis of the larynx: A randomized pilot study. Am J Otolaryngol 1988; 9:161-164.

Crockett DM, McCabe BF, Lusk RP, Mixon JH. Side effects and toxicity of interferon in the treatment of recurrent respiratory papillomatosis. Ann Otol Rhinol Laryngol 1987; 96:600-607.

Derkay CS. Task force on recurrent respiratory papillomatosis. Arch Otolaryngol Head Neck Surg 1995; 121:1386-1391.

Healy GB, Gelber RD, Trowbridge AL, et al. Treatment of recurrent respiratory papillomatosis with human leukocyte interferon. N Engl J Med 1988; 319:401-407.

Kashima H, Mounts P, Leventhal B, Hruban RH. Sites of predilection in recurrent respiratory papillomatosis. Ann Otol Rhinol Laryngol 1993; 102:580-583.

Leventhal BG, Kashima HK, Weck PW, et al. Randomized surgical adjuvant trial of interferon alfa-n1 in recurrent papillomatosis. Arch Otolaryngol Head Neck Surg 1988; 114:1163-1169.

Pignatari S, Smith EM, Gray SD, et al. Detection of human papillomavirus infection in diseased and nondiseased sites of the respiratory tract in recurrent respiratory papillomatosis patients by DNA hybridization. Ann Otol Rhinol Laryngol 1992; 101:408-412.

PEDIATRIC TRACHEOTOMY AND LONG-TERM MANAGEMENT

The method of
Audie L. Woolley

Tracheotomy in children is a surgical procedure that may not only be technically difficult, but may also often present a dilemma for the surgeon concerning postoperative management and discharge planning. The literature on pediatric tracheotomies includes complication rates as high as 46 percent and tracheotomy deaths ranging from 1 percent to 8.7 percent. The classic indications for tracheotomy are to (1) alleviate upper airway obstruction, (2) facilitate artificial ventilation, and (3) access the airway for suctioning and improved tracheobronchial toilet.

A recent survey of members of the American Society of Pediatric Otolaryngology found that in their practices, 40 percent of all pediatric tracheotomies were performed for ventilator dependency, 30 percent for extrathoracic obstruction, 20 percent for neurologic dysfunction, and 10 percent for intrathoracic obstruction. These figures represent a significant change in the indications for tracheotomies in children over the past 2 decades. Tracheotomies once performed for acute inflammatory conditions have now been replaced by nasal or orotracheal intubations. Tracheotomy today is performed most often for chronic conditions such as ventilator dependency and neurologic problems that often result in long-term tracheotomies. Parental and home care is continuing to increase, which makes the role of parent and family education extremely important.

The use of a tracheotomy management team for preoperative teaching and postoperative tracheotomy care greatly facilitates home care. The team consists of the otolaryngologist; clinical nurse specialists; and a variety of other specialists, including occupational therapists and social workers. Once the decision has been made to proceed with tracheotomy in a child, the tracheotomy management team spends a significant amount of time preoperatively counseling the family about the need for tracheotomy, the advantages of tracheotomy, the estimated length of time the child will need the tracheotomy, and, if the child is to be discharged home with the tracheotomy tube, the care of the tracheotomy. This helps relieve the inevitable anxiety when parents are confronted with the need for tracheotomy in their child.

■ OPERATIVE TECHNIQUE AND POSTOPERATIVE CARE

In performing the tracheotomy, the airway is first secured with either an endotracheal tube or a bronchoscope. A straight vertical tracheotomy incision is used in children, with placement of retention sutures lateral to the tracheal incision to help retract open the stoma intraoperatively, and to help reguide the tracheotomy tube into the trachea during the first postoperative week in case of accidental dislodgement. I routinely mature the tracheotomy stoma by plicating the strap muscles to the dermis of the skin. This technique is helpful in the event of accidental dislodgement in the early postoperative period.

All patients are sent to a monitored unit for the first 72 hours until the first tracheotomy change is performed. The nurses in these units are trained in tracheotomy care, and in these units there is a high nurse-patient ratio, sophisticated oxygen saturation monitors, and electrocardiographic monitors. After the first tube change, the children are sent to a floor with nurses trained in tracheotomy care, but the children are not kept on monitors unless the monitors are needed for other reasons (respiratory or neurologic problems).

■ DECANNULATION PROTOCOL

Adherence to a few basic guidelines can facilitate a successful routine decannulation. First, the underlying pathologic condition and resolution of this condition largely determine the appropriate time for removal of the tube. In cases of supraglottic infection, edema usually resolves quickly with treatment of the underlying disorder, and decannulation can be attempted in a few days. In a tracheotomy performed for a pulmonary condition, neurologic condition, or congenital anomaly, decannulation must be carefully approached, with every effort made to ensure that the problem necessitating the tracheotomy has resolved. Any suggestion of aspiration or pulmonary dysfunction should receive further intense evaluation before decannulation. Evidence of aspiration, atelectasis, bronchiectasis, or infections are all contraindications for decannulation. Likewise, any patient who needs supplemental oxygen or frequent pulmonary toilet through the tracheotomy tube is probably not a candidate for decannulation. If additional future surgical procedures will be required, it is often desirable for these to be completed before decannulation.

A physical examination must include a thorough head and neck and pulmonary evaluation. In children, particular attention should be directed toward the nose, nasopharynx, and oral cavity. If upper airway obstruction is present after tracheotomy tube removal, the patient may experience obstructive sleep apnea. If there is any concern, a sleep study should be carried out before decannulation with the tracheotomy tube plugged. It may be necessary to perform tonsillectomy and adenoidectomy before decannulation in children who have tonsillar adenoid hypertrophy. Evidence of proper craniofacial growth or adequate maturation of previous obstructive craniofacial deformities must be determined in children who have craniofacial abnormalities. In a child who has micrognathia, the mandible must have grown sufficiently as to allow good visualization of the larynx for safe intubation in case of failed decannulation.

Patients who have had a long-standing tracheotomy may have associated supraglottic or glottic pathology that will preclude a successful decannulation. A wide variety of anatomic or functional findings can be identified. I believe that an evaluation of the airway by endoscopy is mandatory just before decannulation in children who have had their tracheotomy tubes for a prolonged period. This is helpful to evaluate the original pathologic condition and also to ascertain whether complications have arisen secondary to the presence of the tracheotomy. The examination begins with flexible endoscopy of the nasopharynx, oropharynx, and supraglottic area. Flexible endoscopy will identify potential sites of upper airway obstruction before decannulation and will allow assessment of glottic and supraglottic dynamics.

Once flexible endoscopy has been performed, direct laryngoscopy with bronchoscopy under general anesthesia is carried out. It is again essential that the dynamics of the supraglottis and larynx be evaluated during the bronchoscopy, because dynamic conditions that may prevent decannulation will be missed if the patient is paralyzed during bronchoscopy. Inhalation agents such as halothane can be given through the tracheotomy tube, allowing the patient to breathe spontaneously. Topical 1 percent lidocaine can be applied to the vocal folds, which prevents laryngospasm as the bronchoscope is introduced. Intravenous propofol may also be used as a supplement to the halothane. I use a 4 mm 0 degree telescope to initially view the subglottis and trachea. This telescope provides excellent visualization and photo documentation of the airway. For neonates or children who have subglottic stenosis, smaller telescopes are available (2.7 and 1.9 mm rigid telescopes). The telescopes are small enough that they do not dilate the airway when inserted, and thus malacic segments of the airway are not masked by the endoscope.

Once endoscopy has confirmed that the airway is normal and that the underlying condition requiring the tracheotomy has resolved, the decannulation is safely performed in an intensive care setting by the use of progressively smaller diameter tubes. Once the smallest caliber tube is in place, the tracheotomy tube can be plugged for 24 hours. Decannulation in children may be met with anxiety from both the parents and the patient. When the tracheotomy tube is removed, an increase of 300 percent in airway resistance will be added to the work of breathing, and dead space will be doubled. This may be quite frightening to a child, particularly one who has been tracheotomy dependent for a long time. Periodic occlusion of the tube by corking the tube may allow the patient to become adjusted to laryngeal breathing before final decannulation. These children are placed on appropriate cardiorespiratory monitors during the period when the tracheotomy tube is plugged. If the patient has no difficulty with the tube plugged while awake and asleep during a 24 hour period, the tracheotomy tube is removed.

Decannulation should take place during the day, in a place that is not frightening to the patient and with resuscitation equipment nearby. The child will be hospitalized for another 24 hours with the tracheotomy tube and will be monitored by pulse oximetry. Once the patient tolerates this, he or she may be discharged home. In infants and small children, tracheotomy tube plugging cannot be carried out because the size of the tube frequently occludes the airway. In these children, once endoscopy confirms that the airway is adequate for decannulation, the tube is simply removed.

Another technique that is helpful in small children is to fenestrate the tracheotomy tube. The placement of the fenestration is confirmed endoscopically. Once the tube is fenestrated and the child has adjusted to the fenestrated tube, the tube is plugged, allowing the child to breathe through the fenestration. If the child can tolerate this for 48 hours, the tube is removed. It has been my experience that most of the difficulty with decannulation in children is mechanical and not psychological. With endoscopic techniques, precise diagnosis can be made and appropriate therapy can be instituted. In children who have chronic airway edema seen on physical examination for which decannulation is not successful, attention should be focused on gastroesophageal reflux disease, and pH probe placement is indicated.

If there is any doubt that the underlying pathology that precipitated tracheotomy placement may recur, the child will be sent home for a period of time, with plugging of the tube only while the child is awake. This period of time may range from weeks to months.

The Passy-Muir one-way speaking valve can be used as a step in decannulation. I use this in children who will not experience respiratory difficulty once the Passy-Muir has been placed and in those children in whom adequate phonation is possible. Contraindications to the use of the Passy-Muir valve include abnormal supraglottic or subglottic airway, neurologic dysfunctions, and age less than 1 year. If the voice quality is poor and there is no evidence of aspiration, the tube can be fenestrated or downsized. Fenestration should not be performed in a child who is actively aspirating.

■ CAUSES OF FAILED DECANNULATION

Stomal Granulation or Keloid Formation

The formation of granulation tissue along the upper margin of the tracheal stoma is a frequent, if not universal, finding in children who have tracheotomies. This granulation tissue should be expected to some degree as a normal sequela. The amount of tissue can vary from insignificant to a large amount that must be removed before decannulation. Successful removal of tracheal granulomas has been reported by endoscopic means with biopsy forceps, the resectoscope, and/or CO_2 laser. It is very important to judge the size and length of the lesion because this will determine the type of resection needed to successfully remove the granuloma. Most tracheal granulomas in children can be removed through the stoma by the use of a small single hook and dissecting scissors. This technique is accomplished by passing a bronchoscope beyond the granuloma and using the bronchoscope to help push the granulation tissue into the stoma. Under endoscopic vision with the use of the bronchoscope, the tracheal granuloma can be grasped with a single hook and withdrawn through the stoma to the external surface, where it can be cauterized at the base with bipolar electric cautery and then trimmed sharply. I have successfully used the resectoscope to remove small tracheal granulomas, but care must be taken to prevent inadvertent burning of the tracheal lumen with the resectoscope.

If the granuloma is very large and sessile, endoscopic removal may not be possible. In these cases, an open approach in which the granuloma and involved anterior tracheal wall to which it is attached are resected in continuity, and the resected cartilage is replaced with auricular cartilage or rib, depending on the length of cartilage excised. Most of the time, auricular cartilage works very well because the amount of cartilage that needs to be resected is small.

Laryngomalacia

Examination for laryngomalacia cannot be done on the paralyzed patient. A dynamic mobile airway is needed for this pathology to be appreciated. Flexible endoscopy or rigid endoscopy with spontaneous ventilation technique can be used. Mild laryngomalacia alone should not prevent decannulation, but significant laryngomalacia confirmed on endoscopy may require a supraglottoplasty in order to decannulate the patient successfully.

Suprastomal Collapse

Isolated tracheal collapse above the stoma is a problem that is usually a direct result of the tracheotomy itself. The etiology is believed to be related to either chondritis of the tracheal wall or mechanical stress from the pressure of the tracheotomy tube, which weakens the tracheal arches. This is easily appreciated in a dynamic situation in which the suprastomal collapse may be significant enough to cause complete collapse of the suprastomal airway. If the area of collapse is small, the malacic segment can be excised and allowed to heal by secondary intention, with the tracheotomy tube left in place during the healing phase. If a large segment of cartilage requires excision, this area can be replaced with auricular cartilage in a single-stage procedure, in which the patient is intubated for a short time to allow the graft to heal, as with an anterior cartilage graft laryngotracheoplasty.

Tracheomalacia and Bronchomalacia

Acquired malacia of the trachea and bronchi may be seen in patients who have been on ventilator support with high pressures; this condition is caused by either the tracheotomy itself or inflammatory processes that produce severe tracheobronchitis. Mair and Parsons have called this major airway collapse type 3. In these patients, the trachea has a characteristic endoscopic appearance, with flattening of the cartilaginous anterior arch and widening of the posterior membranous wall. The collapse may extend below the tracheotomy tube and involve the mainstem bronchi. The tracheotomy tube may bypass the malacic segment, which alleviates the problem, but once the tube is removed, tracheal collapse is apparent. If the collapse extends to involve the distal trachea and bronchi, this is a very difficult problem to manage. Aortopexy with suspension of the anterior tracheal wall, resection of the malacic segment with reanastomosis or reconstruction, and endoscopic placement of expandable splints have all been reported in the literature. If there is significant malacia of the distal airway and bronchi, successful decannulation is unlikely.

Vascular Compression of the Trachea

This is a rare entity and can easily be overlooked by the inexperienced endoscopist. A common mistake is to keep the tracheal wall taut during insertion of the bronchoscope such that vascular compression of the trachea can be missed. The most common pediatric vascular anomaly that may lead to difficulty in decannulation is late takeoff of the innominate artery. Innominate artery compression may be diagnosed by a pulsatile mass compressing the anterior wall of the trachea. This diagnosis can be confirmed if the right radial pulse is obliterated by lifting the tip of the bronchoscope against the collapsed, pulsating anterior tracheal wall. Although rare, other pediatric vascular anomalies that may cause tracheal compression include the double aortic arch and right atrial dilation.

Vocal Cord Dislocation and Fixation

Cricoarytenoid joint dislocation is a recognized, but rare, complication of laryngeal trauma. In children, it may occur as part of a complex injury or an isolated lesion. The classic symptoms of hoarseness and odynophagia in adults will be missed or disregarded in the premature infant who has undergone prolonged intubation for weeks or months, repeated instrumentation, and subsequent tracheotomy for failed extubation. Prolonged dislocation results in a fibrous ankylosis of the joint, and this may occur in as little time as a few weeks. Dynamic evaluation of the larynx is again important to confirm the position of the vocal cords. At the time of rigid endoscopy, palpation of the cricoarytenoid joint should be carried out. In children who have a fixed vocal cord that impedes decannulation, laser arytenoidectomy and partial cordectomy can be carried out to achieve successful decannulation. This must be thought out very carefully, and the family must be intimately involved in this decision. The voice will be sacrificed with these types of procedures, and it is important that the family realizes the compromise of voice for the gain of tracheal decannulation in their child.

Subglottic Anomalies

Although these lesions are unusual, subglottic cysts, hemangiomas, or other benign lesions of the subglottis must be recognized and treated before attempts at decannulation.

Adhesions, Webs, and Strictures

Varying degrees of laryngeal scarring constitute the most common of postintubation disorders; scarring is almost always assumed to be present in cases of difficult decannulation. Subglottic stenosis must be ruled out and corrected before attempted decannulation. In cases of moderate to severe stenosis, laryngotracheal reconstruction will need to be carried out before attempts at decannulation.

Neurologic Conditions

Neurologic conditions account for many of the tracheotomies performed in children today. This may range from diverse central nervous system (CNS) diseases, to traumatic CNS injury, to isolated peripheral cranial nerve disorders. These patients may have many problems that contribute to difficulty with decannulation, including gastroesophageal reflux, aspiration, neuromuscular disorders, and cranial nerve injuries with resultant aspiration and vocal cord paralysis. In children who have cerebral palsy, mixed sleep apnea may be found in which not only glossoptosis and palatal and/or pharyngeal collapse contributes to the apnea, but also a component of central apnea may exist. In these patients, it is extremely important to ascertain whether the condition necessitating the tracheotomy has now completely resolved. Adjuvant studies include the use of a modified barium swallow to rule out aspiration, esophageal pH probe to rule out significant gastroesophageal reflux, speech and/or occupational therapy to assess dysphagia, and a sleep study with the tracheotomy tube plugged to assess the presence of sleep apnea.

Mediastinal Lesions

Mediastinal lesions may easily be overlooked until decannulation because the presence of the tracheotomy tube will mask the obstruction. Once the tube is removed, the airway is compressed. Any significant mass in the mediastinum can cause tracheal compression. Neurogenic tumors, bronchogenic cysts, teratomas, cystic hygromas, pectus excavatum, thyroid goiter, and thymus enlargement have all been reported to cause tracheal obstruction.

■ HOME CARE

In children in whom decannulation is not possible, suitable provisions must be made for prolonged tracheotomy care. The most skilled emphasis should be placed on properly training the parents because they are the primary care providers. Home care may not be feasible for every patient who must endure a prolonged period of tracheotomy use.

Before discharge of the patient, the parents must be trained in the use of equipment; tracheotomy care; and early detection of complications and emergency techniques, including cardiopulmonary resuscitation. The facilities of the home must be arranged with the necessary equipment. Family responsibility should be assigned, and instruction of the parents should be organized. At the Children's Hospital of Alabama, the tracheotomy nurse and physician become both teachers and counselors for these parents, promoting total patient management, instilling knowledge and confidence, and providing support for difficult adjustments. Visiting nurses are used during the initial weeks after discharge. They are very helpful in providing counseling, giving parents relief and extra training, and reporting back to the physician about the family and the patient's progress. It is extremely important that both parents participate in the hospital training; in the case of a single parent, an extended family member should also participate. It is unsatisfactory for one parent to receive training and then train the other parent after the child returns home. We have both parents spend the night with the child 24 hours before discharge. During this time, they have complete charge of their child. We also make every opportunity to introduce the parents of a child who has a tracheotomy to other parents of tracheotomized children who have been in a home care program. This is probably one of the most helpful services we provide. The interactive parent group becomes a valuable source of information and dispersion of experience.

Discharge equipment includes a suction machine with necessary accessories. The suction machine should have an adapter so that it can be easily connected to household current.

■ POSTOPERATIVE CARE

Patients with long-term tracheotomies have regular endoscopic examinations every 3 to 6 months. Early intervention by speech-language pathologists is extremely important to prevent delays in oral-vocal speech and voice production in those children who will need their tracheotomies for an extended period of time. The Passy-Muir speaking valve is used at my institution in those children who clinically can use a speaking valve in order to prevent the loss of speech skill.

Suggested Reading

Benjamin B, Curley JWA. Infant tracheotomy-endoscopy and decannulation. Int J Pediatr Otolaryngol 1990; 20:113-121.

Friedberg J, Giberson W. Failed tracheotomy decannulation in children. J Otolaryngol 1992; 21:404-408.

Mair EA, Parsons DS. Pediatric tracheobronchomalacia and major airway collapse. Ann Otol Rhinol Laryngol 1992; 101:300-309.

Wetmore RF, Handler SD, Potsic WP. Pediatric tracheostomy: Experience during the past decade. Ann Otol Rhinol Laryngol 1982; 91:628-632.

Wiatrak BJ, Myer CM III, Cotton RT. Atypical tracheobronchial vascular compression. Am J Otolaryngol 1991; 12:347-356.

Woolley AL, Muntz HR, Prateri D. Physician's survey on the care of children with tracheotomies. Am J Otol 1996; 17:50-53.

SPASMODIC DYSPHONIA

The method of
Gayle E. Woodson

Currently, botulinum toxin is considered to be the treatment of choice for spasmodic dysphonia (SD). Laryngeal injections of this substance vastly improve the voice, yet do not completely restore normal function. Voice therapy can enhance results and prolong the therapeutic response. In my experience, the outcome of botulinum toxin treatment is critically dependent on identification of the optimal dose, which varies greatly among patients. Systematic clinical evaluation is required to identify the proper treatment protocol. Treatment is highly effective for adductor SD. However, botulinum toxin treatment is less successful in patients who have abductor SD, some of whom require adjunctive surgery.

■ THERAPEUTIC ALTERNATIVES

For many years, spasmodic dysphonia was generally considered a hopeless disorder, probably psychological in origin. Psychotherapy and speech therapy were rarely effective, and no effective surgical procedures were available. Then, in the late 1970s, section of the recurrent laryngeal nerve (RLN) was reported to be dramatically effective in nearly all SD patients. However, many patients had a breathy, weak voice, and spasmodic symptoms recurred within 3 years in approximately two-thirds of patients. Vocal breathiness is due to inadequate glottal closure and is most common in patients whose presenting symptoms are less severe. Experimental results and clinical experience indicate that recurrent spasms are due to regeneration of the RLN, even when the cut ends of the nerve had been securely ligated. Despite its shortcomings, RLN surgery is a viable option for some patients who have severe spasm, particularly when frequent injections of botulinum toxin are required for control. When, for whatever reason, the patient prefers a permanent surgical solution, RLN avulsion is preferred to RLN section. As described by Netterville, RLN avulsion carries a lower incidence of recurrent spasm.

An implantable RLN stimulator has been investigated as a possible treatment for SD. Initial experience with five patients was encouraging, but long-term outcome is not known, and safety is not known. Some indication of long-term safety may be extrapolated from the reported clinical experience with vagus nerve stimulators implanted for the treatment of epilepsy. No significant complications have been encountered in a large number of these patients.

Resection of a portion of the thyroarytenoid (TA) muscle has been proposed as a potential permanent alternative to the temporary chemodenervation achieved by botulinum toxin in patients who have adductor SD. Experiments in rabbits indicate that the muscle can be easily approached via a window in the thyroid cartilage, and that the muscle does not regenerate. After 3 months, the defect is replaced by loose fibroareolar tissue, with no impairment of the vibratory edge of the vocal fold. Currently, use in humans has not been studied.

Laryngeal framework surgery has been reported as a treatment for adductor SD. Anterior commissure retrusion has been used in an attempt to relax the vocal fold. However, this procedure is not recommended due to unsatisfactory results and the extreme difficulty encountered in attempts to surgically reverse this procedure.

To administer botulinum toxin to the larynx, I prefer percutaneous electromyographic (EMG)–guided injection. This technique causes minimal patient discomfort and provides objective confirmation that the injector needle is in active muscle tissue. Several alternative approaches have been reported. Injection can be accomplished transorally, using a long, curved needle and visualizing the larynx with a mirror or endoscope. A flexible needle through the working channel of a fiberoptic endoscope has also been used. Most patients find internal manipulations to be significantly uncomfortable, and such methods require time-consuming local anesthesia of the mouth, throat, and larynx. Further, the endoscopic injection requires two clinicians, an endoscopist, and an injector (e.g., a nurse or another doctor). Additionally, the long catheter contains a considerable volume of dead space so that dose delivery is less accurate and the toxin required to fill this space is wasted. Another alternative is termed the *point-touch* technique, which also requires both an endoscopist and an injector and does not employ EMG guidance. Injection is percutaneous and transcartilaginous, with endoscopic confirmation of needle position.

■ PREFERRED APPROACH

Diagnostic criteria for SD are not clearly defined. Recognition of these patients becomes easier with increasing clinical experience, relying on the sound of the voice, the patient's history, physical examination of the larynx, and careful neurologic examination. A characteristic strained or strangled voice in a patient who has a morphologically normal larynx is highly suggestive of adductor SD. A continuously breathy voice or the occurrence of breathy voice breaks are observed in patients who have abductor SD. The onset of the disorder is usually gradually progressive, and symptoms vary with the speaking situation. Most patients note an increase in symptoms when they are under stress or use the telephone.

It is crucial to listen carefully to the patient in order to characterize the specific speech disorder. Laryngeal injection of botulinum toxin is indicated for laryngeal spasms that disrupt *phonation,* but is not an effective treatment for *dysarthria.* It is also essential to determine whether the patient has adductor, abductor, or mixed SD. The severity level must also be assessed because this is important in determining the dose needed. Patients who have severe and constant spasm require larger doses than do patients who have mild or intermittent problems. Although SD often fluctuates in severity, extreme variability in the nature of the vocal symptoms suggests a psychogenic problem, which generally does not respond well to botulinum toxin therapy.

The larynx should be observed with a flexible laryngoscope during connected speech, sustained phonation, and respiratory activities. Positive physical signs that support the diagnosis of SD are the findings of tremor in the larynx and/or palate and pharynx, or observable spasms of the larynx during speech and/or breathing. Tremor of the palate is most easily detected during sustained phonation of the vowel "i." Although spasms are pathognomonic of SD, tremor is not present in all patients. The status of the thyroarytenoid muscle should also be assessed, because patients who have atrophy experience greater side effects with lower doses of botulinum toxin. Abductor spasms are most apparent during specific tasks when the patient switches suddenly from an unvoiced, plosive consonant to a vowel. For example, when the patient says, "pay Paul a penny," the arytenoids tend to "hang up" laterally just after articulation of the "p's," delaying the onset of the voiced portions of the words.

A neurologic examination is essential to seek possible focal lesions and to rule out other neurologic disorders that can result in speech that sounds much like adductor SD. These include parkinsonism, myoclonus, pseudobulbar palsy, tardive dyskinesia, cerebellar disorders, multiple sclerosis, and amyotrophic lateral sclerosis. Although some of these patients may be candidates for botulinum toxin therapy, the underlying disease process must be identified to permit general medical treatment and patient counseling. Botulinum toxin is of benefit to some patients who have parkinsonism, myoclonus, and cerebellar disorders, but only when the primary speech problem is adductor laryngeal spasm. It is not effective for hypokinetic parkinsonism or, as mentioned previously, for dysarthria.

Imaging studies, such as magnetic resonance imaging or computed tomography, have a very low diagnostic yield in isolated spasmodic dysphonia and are only indicated if the neurologic examination detects focal signs.

Diagnostic EMG is not useful in managing most patients who have SD. Although sophisticated analysis of EMG signals can document inappropriate levels of muscle activity in most SD patients, routine quantitative or qualitative analysis does not reveal any characteristic patterns that are diagnostic of SD. However, in those patients in whom botulinum toxin is ineffective or is losing its efficacy, EMG can be helpful in elucidating the problem. There may be a failure of botulinum toxin to adequately denervate the muscle, due to misplacement, inadequate dose, a "bad" batch of botulinum toxin, or resistance to the toxin. Another possibility is an atypical muscle activation pattern during phonation such that the TA is suppressed, and the excessive adduction is being affected by the lateral cricoarytenoid or interarytenoid muscle. EMG can identify the atypical activity and guide the selection of an alternate injection site.

Temporary RLN blockade is not recommended in the routine pretreatment evaluation of candidates for botulinum toxin therapy. The results could be misleading, because the effects of focal denervation and global unilateral paralysis are quite different. However, blockade can be useful in evaluating patients who do not respond to botulinum toxin. Vocal function testing is important, not to diagnose the disorder, but to quantify severity, to aid in determining whether injection should be bilateral or unilateral, and to establish the optimal dose. To accomplish this, patients should be assessed before and at 1 week and 1 month after injection. Muscle weakness and its related side effects of breathiness and dysphagia are maximal in the first 3 to 14 days. By 1 month, function has usually stabilized at a level that will persist for 3 to 4 months. The primary parameters useful in documenting these effects are voice break factor, phonatory airflow, and the rate of voice breaks. This assessment schedule should be adhered to for all injections until the optimal dose and schedule have been determined. The patient can then be treated based on symptoms, without the need for routine endoscopy or vocal function testing.

A sudden silence or decrease in amplitude of a voice recording indicates laryngeal spasm and is termed a *voice break.* Voice breaks are rare in normal voices but occur as often as once per second in patients who have SD. They are most reliably measured during sustained phonation. A major sign of successful botulinum toxin is the elimination or drastic reduction of voice breaks, and this can be used as an end point for therapy. This does not mean that more toxin is indicated for a patient who is satisfied with his voice despite some persistent voice breaks. But the elimination of voice breaks indicates that any persistent vocal dysfunction will not improve with additional botulinum toxin.

Phonatory airflow can also be used to guide therapy. It is important to calibrate equipment regularly. Normative data should be established for each voice laboratory, using the identical equipment and protocol used in clinical testing, rather than referring to control values in the literature. In adductor SD, mean airflow rates have been shown to range from normal to extremely low, and adductor spasms correlate with sudden drops in airflow, which correspond to voice breaks. With successful botulinum treatment, the airflow is normal or slightly elevated, and sudden drops are eliminated. However, increased airflow correlates with the side effect of breathiness, and therefore, when airflow rises much above normal, the effects of botulinum toxin become counterproductive.

In abductor spasmodic dysphonia, mean phonatory airflow is generally above normal, with bursts of increased airflow. Successful botulinum toxin treatment reduces and stabilizes phonatory airflow. Measurement of phonatory airflow may identify a component of abductor SD in a patient who has predominantly adductor symptoms. In such patients with mixed adductor and abductor spasms, a more conservative initial dose is prudent.

■ ADDUCTOR SPASMODIC DYSPHONIA

The major clinical question in managing patients who have adductor SD is not whether botulinum toxin is likely to work, but how much toxin should be used, and whether injection should be unilateral or bilateral. Both unilateral and bilateral injection can eliminate voice breaks, but there are significant differences. Bilateral injection requires a smaller total dose to achieve the same clinical effect. Using the American preparation of toxin (Botox), injection of 1.25 U into each TA muscle is therapeutically equivalent to a unilateral injection of 10 to 15 U. However, bilateral injection is generally associated with more pronounced side effects of breathiness and swallowing problems, particularly in the first 2 weeks after injection. Injection of 1.25 U is the lowest dose that can be reliably delivered, and therefore the lowest bilateral injection totals 2.5 U. Unilateral injection permits the use of a wider therapeutic range, so that unilateral injections of 1.25 to 10 to 15 U may be used in patients who cannot tolerate the side effects of bilateral injection of 1.25 U. The reason for the difference in effects of unilateral and bilateral injection is not known. However, it is clear that bilateral injections are not simply additive, but are synergistic.

Botulinum toxin type A is marketed in the United States as Botox and in the United Kingdom as Dysport. The two preparations differ significantly in potency. Although both are ostensibly dispensed according to the same international unit of botulinum toxin activity (LD_{50} for Swiss mice), approximately 2.5 times more units of Botox are required to achieve the same degree of muscle weakness produced by a given dose of Dysport. Therefore, when referring to the literature for treatment recommendations, it is important to note which preparation is used. Treating with Dysport according to guidelines established for Botox could result in serious overtreatment.

Clinical evaluation usually permits selection of a dose and site of injection that is effective, but sometimes the dose needs to be adjusted. If side effects are excessive, the next injection, when the patient returns with recurrent symptoms, should be reduced. If the injection is not sufficiently effective, a "booster" dose can be given. Ideally, this should be given as near in time as possible to the first injection, so that the prediction of the optimal dose in the future is valid. If the injection has been accurately placed in the appropriate muscle, the results at 1 day after injection are an excellent indicator of function during the stable period, which is 1 to 4 or more months after injection. Therefore, if at 1 day after injection, the dose appears to be inadequate, a booster can be given. However, caution must be used, because if the toxin was not accurately placed and must diffuse even a tiny distance, the therapeutic effect will be delayed. Therefore, a booster at 24 hours could result in overtreatment with unacceptable side effects.

The dose to be used should be determined by severity and constancy of symptoms. For mild or intermittent symptoms, unilateral injection of 1.25 to 2.5 U should be used initially, increasing the dose if needed. For moderate symptoms, unilateral injection of 5 to 10 U is usually required. Patients who have significant or severe SD require bilateral treatment of 1.25 to 2.5 U. The dose should be conservatively estimated in patients who have atrophy of the vocalis muscle.

As mentioned previously, my preferred injection technique is percutaneous and EMG–guided. Patients should be comfortable, preferably reclining in an examination chair. To minimize discomfort, the skin over the cricoid is very superficially infiltrated with 1 percent plain lidocaine. The cricothyroid space is palpated. If the space is very narrow, the cricothyroid muscle is in spasm, generally due to patient anxiety. Steps should then be taken to relax this muscle, such as mental imagery, patient encouragement, or even sedation. In the presence of active cricothyroid muscle contraction, it is difficult and painful to pass the needle between these cartilages. In some patients, particularly smokers, the sensation of the needle in the larynx stimulates a brisk cough reflex, requiring premedication with codeine or dextromethorphan. However, if the needle is introduced 1 to 2 cm off the midline, the injection can be accomplished without entering the lumen, so that there is no mucosal stimulation. The needle enters the skin over the cricoid, to one side of the midline, and is advanced upward and medially, passing between the cricoid and thyroid cartilages. To ensure location in an adductor muscle, the patient is asked to phonate. The TA muscle is maximally activated by modal phonation, while the cricothyroid is activated at a higher pitch. The patient should also be asked to flex the neck to rule out inadvertent position in a strap muscle. Excessive 60 cycle interference noise, despite adequate grounding, usually indicates that the tip of the needle is not only not in a muscle, but also not even in tissue, resting instead in the air space of the larynx.

The optimal response is no voice breaks, normal airflow, and at least 16 weeks of therapeutic benefit. If the patient becomes aphonic, or if breathiness and swallowing discomfort persist for 4 weeks or more, the dose should be reduced for the next injection. If results are either unsatisfactory, produce only a brief improvement, or have persistent breaks or low airflow, the dose should be increased. If the dose is determined to be inadequate within 1 or 2 weeks, a booster injection can be given. But if a longer interval has elapsed, it is best to wait 12 weeks, allowing the toxin to wear off completely, so that an accurate assessment of the dose can be accomplished.

Treatment should be repeated when symptoms reappear, usually within 12 to 16 weeks. Patients rarely return to the pretreatment level of severity, but usually require reinjection of the same dose. The duration of effect often increases with sequential injections. Voice therapy improves the voice and prolongs the duration of benefits. Some patients may require less toxin with repeated injections, and rarely are escalated doses needed. If the dose requirement increases, the possibility of antibody formation to the toxin, although not reported for treatment of SD, must be considered. Most patients settle into a schedule of a stable dose at regular intervals, often scheduling repeat injections before symptoms recur. The schedule may be modified by patient needs or preferences. For example, patients may not want an injection immediately before some important event, because the voice is frequently unstable for the first 2 weeks after injection.

■ ABDUCTOR SPASMODIC DYSPHONIA

Results of botulinum toxin therapy for abductor SD are disappointing when compared with the results achieved for adductor SD. Slightly more than half of the patients who have abductor SD respond significantly to botulinum toxin. The duration of benefit is shorter, and the magnitude of improvement is less impressive. In part, these differences can be attributed to dose limitation incurred by the side effects of injecting an abductor muscle (the posterior cricoarytenoid muscle). Paresis sufficient to control abductor spasms can compromise laryngeal motion with respiration, resulting in airway obstruction. But it also appears that the pathophysiology of abductor SD is more complex than that of adductor SD. Not only do patients have abductor muscle spasm, but also there is insufficient activation of the TA muscle with phonation. Thus, even when abductor spasms are eliminated, there may still be glottal insufficiency and a breathy voice, because the vocal folds are not actively closed. Some patients also have spasms of the diaphragm and cricothyroid muscles. Injection of the diaphragm has not been attempted, but would seem ill-advised because of the size and vital function of this muscle. Cricothyroid muscle injection has been reported, with variable success.

Botulinum toxin may be injected into the posterior cricoarytenoid (PCA) muscles in an effort to suppress abductor spasm and increase phonatory airflow. This generally requires bilateral, asymmetric injection. In almost all abductor SD patients, a dominant side can be identified that has a larger amplitude of abductor spasm. The nondominant PCA is injected with 1.25 U. The dominant PCA muscle is injected with from 5 to 20 U of botulinum toxin, beginning with 5 U and titrating upward, until a satisfactory voice is attained or until the airway is impaired.

Several methods have been described for injecting the PCA muscle, including endoscopic and percutaneous approaches. I prefer the percutaneous EMG–guided approach, manually rotating the larynx to move the PCA of interest closer to the skin. I palpate the cricothyroid joint and pass the needle through the skin 1 to 2 cm lateral and inferior to this landmark, aiming the needle to pass just behind the cricothyroid joint and just over the surface of the cricoid. During insertion, I continuously monitor the position of the carotid artery. The patient is asked to sniff to activate the PCA, so that position can be confirmed by EMG. If possible, the patient should be asked to speak, so that abductor spasms can be confirmed. Then the toxin is injected and the needle is withdrawn.

When botulinum toxin is ineffective for abductor SD, surgical procedures to medialize the vocal fold should be considered. Arytenoid adduction is not recommended, because the goal is to facilitate approximation of the membranous vocal folds, not to close the respiratory glottis. Either type I thyroplasty or fat injection can be used, but thyroplasty is more precise and results in a more reliable long-term solution. Before any permanent medialization, a trial of Gelfoam injection is recommended to determine the likelihood of success.

■ VOICE THERAPY

Speech therapy has been used to treat SD for many years. Although a few authors have encountered success, most have reported frustration with voice therapy alone. However, voice therapy is a very effective adjunct to botulinum toxin therapy. The duration of beneficial effect from botulinum toxin is significantly longer in patients who also receive voice therapy aimed at regulating breath support and avoiding excessive glottal adduction.

■ PROS AND CONS OF TREATMENT

Botulinum toxin is a minimally invasive treatment that provides dramatic relief of symptoms in most patients who have SD, without serious side effects. In the uncommon situation in which the response to therapy is unfavorable, the problem is temporary, because the effects of the toxin will wear off in 3 to 4 months.

The major limitation of botulinum toxin therapy is that it only mitigates the symptoms of SD and does not treat the underlying cause. Even when the voice is dramatically improved, normal function is never completely achieved. Frequently, some abnormal activation persists. And suppression of spasm is always accompanied by some loss of vocal power. The side effects of breathiness and swallowing problems, although usually mild and transient, can be severe and occasionally last for several weeks. Pronounced side effects may preclude therapy in some patients, particularly those who have abductor SD.

Suggested Reading

Blitzer A, Brin MF, Stewart C, et al. Abductor laryngeal dysphonia: A series treated with botulinum toxin. Laryngoscope 1992; 102:163-167.

Friedman M, Toriumi DM, Grybauskas VT, Applebaum EL. Implantation of a recurrent laryngeal nerve stimulator for the treatment of spastic dysphonia. Ann Otol Rhinol Laryngol 1989; 98:130-134.

Maloney AP, Morrison MD. A comparison of the efficacy of unilateral versus bilateral botulinum toxin injections in the treatment of adductor spasmodic dysphonia. J Otolaryngol 1994; 23:160-164.

Murry T, Woodson GE. Combined modality treatment of adductor spasmodic dysphonia with botulinum toxin and voice therapy. J Voice 1995; 9:460-465.

Rodriguez AA, Ford CN, Bless DM, Harmon RL. Electromyographic assessment of spasmodic dysphonia patients prior to botulinum toxin injection. Electromyogr Clin Neurophysiol 1994; 34:403-407.

Van Pelt F, Ludlow CL, Smith PH. Comparison of muscle activation patterns in adductor and abductor spasmodic dysphonia. Ann Otol Rhinol Laryngol 1994; 103:192-200.

Weed DT, Jewett BS, Rainey C, et al. Long-term follow-up of recurrent laryngeal nerve avulsion for the treatment of spastic dysphonia. Ann Otol Rhinol Laryngol 1996; 105:592-601.

Woo P, Colton R, Casper J, Brewer D. Analysis of spasmodic dysphonia by aerodynamic and laryngostroboscopic measurements. J Voice 1992; 6:344-351.

Woodson GE, Allegretti J. Spasmodic dysphonia. Curr Opin Otolaryngol HNS 1996; 4:121-125.

Zwirner P, Murry T, Woodson GE. A comparison of bilateral and unilateral botulinum toxin treatments for spasmodic dysphonia. Euro Arch Otorhinolaryngol 1993; 250:271-276.

VOCAL PROBLEMS OF SINGERS

The method of
Robert W. Bastian

In order to diagnose, manage, and document the voice disorders of singers, proper tools are required. Depending on the particular clinicians involved and other local circumstances, these tools may be mastered by one individual who is responsible for the entire diagnostic process, or they may be divided among, for example, the laryngologist, speech pathologist, and singing teacher. (In either case, a team representing each of these professions will enable comprehensive management on an individualized basis for singers in distress.) The tools are:

1. A sophisticated voice history
2. Assessment of the voice's capabilities and limitations through a series of vocal task elicitations and skillful auditory perceptual interpretation (special examiner skills required here)
3. A high-quality laryngeal examination, often including videostroboscopy

Unfortunately, "objective" measures of phonatory function such as acoustic analysis and airflow measurement have not yet earned a place in the diagnostic arena as tool number 4, although these methodologies continue to be interesting for voice science purposes.

Prerequisites for tool number 2 in particular include a detailed understanding of normal or adequate vocal capabilities for each voice type (soprano, mezzo-soprano, contralto, tenor, baritone, bass, and their subtypes) as well as the vocal demands and performance circumstances of various genres of singing. Also required is the ability to elicit vocal tasks—particularly very high-frequency, low-intensity vocal tasks that reliably detect mucosal swelling—and to judge the presence or absence, nature, and degree of impairment. Equipped with this sort of background understanding and mastery of the three "tools," virtually all of the problems of singers can be diagnosed and managed efficiently and effectively.

In one sense, each performer in vocal distress brings to the clinical encounter a unique set of circumstances. This is because of the variety of disorders combined with the following factors: acuteness, severity, degree of vocal training, importance of the performance, patient temperament, beliefs about voice, underlying medical conditions, and so forth. The laryngologist serving this population will, however, encounter certain circumstances that tend to be more common than others. Some of these are addressed next.

■ VOCAL OVERDOER SYNDROME

To define the "vocal overdoer," it is helpful to consider both the innate drive to talk ("push from within") and external demands or commitments ("pull from without"). As one way to assess the former, patients can be asked the following: "On a 7 point scale, where 1 represents a shy, untalkative introvert, and 7 an unusually expressive, sociable, talkative individual, 4 being moderately talkative, and so forth, where would you put yourself? This is your innate, lifelong, average degree of talkativeness." The overdoer syndrome is generally seen in persons who rate themselves as "6" or "7." The answer to this simple question correlates better by far with the vocal fold mucosal injury than with any other issue, with the exception of those who indulge in extreme use of voice (singers of aggressive rock music, for example). Questions about occupation, rehearsal and performance schedule, childcare responsibilities, church, community, and social activities give an appreciation of the "pull from without."

Many vocal overdoers have recurrent bouts of hoarseness from acute vocal fold mucosal edema—often incorrectly attributed by singers to phlegm, reflux, allergy, and so forth—or singers may also refer to this state as, "my voice is tired." Another group of overdoers has an established mucosal or submucosal injury such as nodules, polyps, epidermoid cysts, or capillary ectasia.

Treatment for patients both with and without mucosal injury begins with the simplest part of a comprehensive plan for rehabilitation: optimization of medical issues (acid reflux, insufficient hydration, and so forth). These factors are virtually always secondary to the primary issue of behavioral management. It is helpful to focus on the "management of 7-ness," not an attempt to change that personality profile. Said another way, the emphasis is on additional skills of personality and social life management, not on crash "vocal diets." In brief summary, behavioral management is administered by the speech pathologist and voice teacher and consists of the following:

1. Vocal hygiene—reduce caffeine and alcohol use, hydrate, attend to dietary management of acid reflux (see next section), and so forth
2. "Management of 7-ness"—for example, preplanning social life for quiet rather than noisy venues, learning to optimize occupational use of voice, increasing vocal personality awareness
3. Work on voice production for both speaking and singing, to make it as "inexpensive" as possible

Often, this sort of behavioral management alone will suffice to eliminate bouts of mucosal edema or hoarseness or to resolve a chronic mucosal injury. On the other hand, when mucosal injuries are proved to be chronic, and when the disturbance to voice is unacceptable to the patient, surgery can be considered.

■ VOCAL UNDERDOER SYNDROME

Those who answer "1 or 2" on the 7 point talkativeness scale generally fit the profile of the vocal underdoer. Paradoxically, a common symptom is vocal fatigue. This is not hoarseness, but rather a tendency for the voice to fade with use as well as anterior neck discomfort and difficulty being heard in noisy places. The correlated examination findings are often, but not always, vocal fold bowing and atrophy, even in young persons.

Because vocal underdoers often self-select to vocally undemanding occupations, this personality is less common among active solo performers, but occasionally a short-term "underdoer syndrome" is seen in the performer who is otherwise a "4, 5, 6, or 7." The performer may have, for example, gone through several weeks or months of relative vocal disuse. This may have occurred because of illness; a break from singing during an extended holiday; convalescence from a surgical procedure; or an unsophisticated diagnosis of "vocal nodules," which has caused the singer to rest the voice extensively. The singer in this circumstance presents weeks or months later with the belief that the voice remains weak and impaired because of the illness, surgical scarring from the tonsillectomy, the nodules, and so forth. In a high percentage of such patients, the problem is actually that the voice has become deconditioned. Even the singer with nodules functions much better when the vocal apparatus is conditioned!

In each of these cases, barring a specific diagnosis to the contrary, the advice should be to systematically recondition the voice. The laryngologist might suggest three 10 minute practice sessions for 3 days; three 15 minute sessions for 3 days; and so forth until a total of at least an hour a day of practice is reached. Especially initially, the emphasis is on "putting in the time" and not on what the voice will not yet do. It is surprising how frequently this approach brings the voice back to its previous level of functioning. In the case of the singer who has nodules, that level may include some impairment that is easily detected by the clinician but is considered normal and acceptable by the singer.

■ ACUTE VOCAL DYSFUNCTION

Obviously, whether the dysfunction results from vocal fold mucosal edema due to overuse or upper respiratory infection, the greatest consideration is given to the patient's vocal safety. Also of great importance are the voice's ability to "get through" the performance, and the risk of doing the next performance but having to cancel future ones as a result. With these primary issues in mind, the laryngologist will, however, want to help the singer continue when possible. This is because considerable harm can also be done by canceling: to the patient's sense of professionalism, finances, and even career. Thus, aside from (1) acute infectious laryngitis, (2) mucosal edema of overuse or abuse so great as to preclude performance even with the assistance of steroids, and (3) hemorrhage, most often the performer can be helped through the event(s). There are various forms this assistance might take:

1. Basic information about vocal anatomy and function, often taught from the singer's videotaped examination
2. General medical teaching or advice concerning hydration; environmental humidification and steaming; cessation of the use of tobacco, alcohol, nonessential aspirin, nonsteroidal anti-inflammatory drugs (NSAIDs), inhalers, and drying medications
3. Individualized medical assistance in the form of (as appropriate) short-term, high-dose tapering steroids; antibiotics; mucolytics; nondrying antihistamines; acid reflux medications; nasal inhalers; and so forth
4. Formulation of overall strategy: when to rest the voice; changes to the performance (musical keys, miking, cuts); which, if any, of a run of shows the understudy will be called upon to perform; warm-up considerations; who, if anyone, will need to be telephoned, and exactly what will be said

It is surprising how frequently the laryngologist may see a singer with significant mucosal edema of overuse and considerable impairment who can later the same day perform to public accolade, if not to his or her own complete satisfaction. Again, primary issues that necessitate cancellation include acute hemorrhage, infectious laryngitis, and edema so great that even with steroid treatment and careful preperformance warm-up the voice simply cannot fulfill the task at hand. It is also surprising how often a singer may describe acute difficulties when it is later agreed by all parties that he or she actually had an exacerbation of a long-standing mucosal injury, such as vocal nodules.

■ ACID REFLUX LARYNGITIS (GASTROESOPHAGEAL REFLUX)

A surprising percentage of singers may experience nocturnal acid reflux to the level of the larynx due to dysfunction of the lower esophageal sphincter. Some patients may have obvious daytime symptoms such as heartburn or acid eructations to suggest the diagnosis. Many, however, are unaware that they have acid reflux. They may have only vague, indirect symptoms such as (1) chronic, mild, raw sore throat, generally worse in the morning and improving as the day continues; (2) excessive morning phlegm, halitosis; (3) a chronic irritative cough or need to continually clear the throat; or (4) a particularly low or husky morning voice requiring prolonged warm-up.

When severe, laryngeal findings can be dramatic: redness of the arytenoid apices, interarytenoid pachyderma, hazy leukoplakia, increased mucus production. In mild cases there may be little seen on laryngeal examination to suggest the diagnosis. There is debate about the need to work up every individual who may have this problem. To procure one or more of the following—a barium esophagram, 24 hour pH monitoring, or esophagogastroduodenoscopy—for every individual suspected of the diagnosis would add enormously to the nation's health costs! Thus, for persons who have obvious symptoms in particular, it may be justified to prescribe an empiric trial of the following treatment measures:

1. After noon, avoid caffeine, alcohol, spicy foods, chocolate, mint, and citrus fruits, all of which may increase stomach acidity and/or make the lower esophageal sphincter function poorly.
2. Eat the last meal or snack of the day 3 or more hours before going to sleep. The "back pressure" of a full stomach may facilitate reflux.
3. Put 4 to 6 inch blocks between the floor and headposts

of the bed to place the entire bed on a slight downward slant from head to foot. This allows gravity to assist in keeping stomach acid in the stomach.

4. Use one of a variety of medical approaches. They are, from most to least effective:
   a. Omeprazole or lansoprazole. These are powerful proton pump drugs that inhibit the formation of stomach acid. They are most appropriately taken an hour before the evening meal.
   b. An H2-receptor blocker such as ranitidine, nizatidine, famotidine, or cimetidine. One of these is best taken approximately an hour before retiring.
   c. An antacid such as Gaviscon, taken at bedtime.

■ ALLERGY

A mild degree of skepticism is appropriate when singers believe their problems are the result of allergy. This is because the following scenario is so common: the singer, a "7" who is also dramatically overcommitted vocally, has vocal nodules. Despite the obvious "vocal overdoer" explanation for the vocal nodules, the singer believes the source of difficulty to be "allergy." She is using antihistamines, a nasal inhaler, and herbal remedies. In fact, review of allergy symptoms and even the results of skin testing throw doubt on the significance of allergies as compared with the overdoer history. All the same, when addressing allergy in singers, consider the following:

1. Help the singer see the relative importance of allergy to his or her vocal problem accurately.
2. Rely when possible on nondrying, nonsedating antihistamines such as fexofenadine.
3. When allergy does indeed seem to be present and a significant problem, refer the patient for expert evaluation and management by an allergist who is sensitive to singers.

■ ACUTE VOCAL FOLD HEMORRHAGE

This condition can occur as a "vocal accident" when a strenuous high note, yell, or even loud sneeze causes a capillary to rupture. Sometimes, the exact moment of the hemorrhage can be pinpointed because of the abruptness of the vocal deterioration. Upon presentation, the singer's speaking voice quality may be anywhere from mildly husky to severely hoarse. The upper voice is generally markedly impaired. Physical findings are variable. One may see a thin suffusion of blood in Reinke's space (superficial layer of lamina propria), with little, if any, effect on vocal fold margin contour. Under strobe light, the mucosa may even oscillate rather well. In this case, the voice will be affected relatively little.

On the other hand, the otolaryngologist may see a pocket hemorrhage with the appearance of a "blood blister" (hemorrhagic polyp). In this case, the voice will be dramatically impaired. Many months can be required for resolution, and there is a significant chance that the patient will be left with a unilateral fleshy polyp, which, although less vocally impairing than the acute turgid hemorrhagic polyp, remains a source of considerable limitation.

Acute management generally includes an initial period of complete voice rest (there are exceptions to every rule). Unnecessary aspirin and NSAID use is discontinued. The patient is questioned about such prior hemorrhages or bruises and whether he or she fits the "vocal overdoer" profile (see previous section on this subject). In the case of thin-suffusion hemorrhage and depending on the nature of the performance, judicious return to voice use is sometimes possible within a week or so—after mucosal oscillation normalizes but before all signs of hemorrhage have disappeared.

There is room for debate when the "hemorrhagic polyp" variant is first seen. When this polyp is very small, complete resolution may occur, although even in this case months may be required. With larger hemorrhagic polyps, it is quite likely that surgery will eventually be required if the goal is complete voice restoration. Thus, there is some reason to consider early intervention: after administering a brief general anesthetic, a tiny incision is made, and the blood or clot is evacuated from the polyp. With the larger, long-term hemorrhagic or nonhemorrhagic polyp, surgery (see next section) becomes a strong option after an appropriate trial of voice therapy.

■ CHRONIC MUCOSAL INJURY LEADING TO VOCAL FOLD MICROSURGERY

On occasion, singers will have vocal impairment caused by proven irreversible mucosal lesions. Typically, "surgical" lesions of this sort include large polyps; persistent capillary ectasia responsible for recurrent hemorrhage, polyp formation, or reduced vocal endurance; epidermoid and mucus retention cysts; glottic sulcus; and nodules that have persisted with unacceptable symptoms or limitations after an appropriate trial of voice therapy. In these cases, the option of vocal fold microsurgery may be gently introduced.

Until very recently, surgery was virtually condemned to treat singers. Some in the field, including "expert" laryngologists, said that surgery always left a scar, and was therefore unsafe in this patient population. This prevailing belief did keep many singers safe from the risk of poorly performed surgery, which can have disastrous consequences to the voice. On the other hand, it left some singers struggling to continue to perform despite a considerable vocal handicap. In some cases, vocal impairment forced a change in career. In other cases, singers coped as best they could but experienced frustrating symptoms such as (1) reduced vocal endurance, (2) day-to-day variability of vocal capabilities, (3) loss of high soft singing, (4) delayed phonatory onsets, and (5) upper voice hoarseness and air escape.

Fortunately, surgery has now been shown to be safe and highly effective (although not entirely without risk), provided each of the following conditions is met:

1. The lesion must be amenable to surgery and proved to be chronic or unresponsive to behavioral and medical management.
2. The singer must be highly informed about procedural details, risks, potential benefits, and postoperative care.

3. The surgeon must be well versed in vocal fold layer structure (microarchitecture) and mucosal vibratory physiology.
4. There must be pre- and postoperative documentation of both the vocal capability battery and videostroboscopy, which the patient of course reviews with the surgeon.
5. The surgeon must have both training and experience in vocal fold microsurgery.

Those clinicians who cannot supply all of the aforementioned prerequisites should not perform surgery in this patient population, because the stakes are so high and because of the heightened potential for disaster when these prerequisites are not met.

Concerning the risks of surgery, singers are told about the remote risks of general anesthesia, and that there is also a very small risk of a chipped, scratched, broken, or dislodged tooth. Finally, the singer must know that the precise vocal outcome cannot be known in advance. The routine expectation is for marked improvement, but whether this means the voice will be normal, near-normal, or only partially back to normal is the question. The possibility that the voice will be worse is mentioned, although this possibility is put into perspective as being very small. It is helpful for patients to hear before and after excerpts from videotapes of others who have undergone surgery and have consented to let their tapes be used in this fashion. Sometimes, a postsurgical singer will also agree to speak by telephone to another singer who is contemplating surgery.

Surgical details are to be found in a wide body of the literature. Based on knowledge of the layer structure of the folds along with vibratory physiology, the surgeon must focus on highly controlled, precise, and superficial removal of the offending lesion. If possible, nonlaser techniques are preferred. The goal is to remove the abnormality, and nothing more! For submucosal lesions (cysts, sulci), the technical demands on the surgeon are great.

Instructions about postsurgical voice use may vary according to the lesion and the singer involved. Generally, only a few days of voice rest are suggested, followed by gradual increase in the amount of talking and singing on a week-by-week basis. Early postoperative singing through the entire expected range of the voice is helpful for dynamic healing. Vocal recovery is expected to be very rapid after superficial trimming of nodules and polyps. The voice should show marked improvement within 2 weeks of surgery, and the "final result" can be seen as early as 4 weeks postoperatively, thus permitting the singer judicious return to public performance. On the other hand, when disturbance to the fold is greater, as after cyst and sulcus surgery, improvement can still be seen quite early, but the final result may take many months to achieve.

Suggested Reading

Bastian RW. Benign mucosal and saccular disorders: benign laryngeal tumors. In: Cummings CW, Fredrickson JM, eds. Otolaryngology—head and neck surgery. 2nd ed. St. Louis: CV Mosby, 1993:897.

Bastian RW. Vocal fold microsurgery in singers. J Voice 1996; 10:389-404.

Bastian RW, Keidar A, Verdolini-Marston K. Simple vocal tasks for detecting vocal fold swelling. J Voice 1990; 4:272-283.

Cornut G, Bouchayer M. Phonosurgery for singers. J Voice 1989; 3:269-276.

Hirano M, Kurita S, Nakashima T. The structure of the vocal folds. In: Stevens KN, Hirano M, eds. Vocal fold physiology. Tokyo: University of Tokyo, 1981:33.

Sataloff RT. Professional singers: the science and art of clinical care. Am J Otolaryngol 1981; 2:51-66.

CONTACT ULCERS AND GRANULOMAS OF THE LARYNX

The method of
Robert Thayer Sataloff

Contact ulcers and granulomas of the larynx usually occur on the posterior aspect of the vocal folds, often in or above the cartilaginous portion. They may be bilateral or unilateral; and it is common to see a sizable granuloma on one side and a contact ulcer on the other. Patients who have ulcers or granulomas may complain of pain (laryngeal or referred otalgia), a globus (lump in the throat) sensation, hoarseness, painful phonation, and occasionally hemoptysis. It is surprising that even large granulomas are often asymptomatic. These benign lesions usually contain fibroblasts, collagenous fibers, proliferated capillaries, leukocysts, and sometimes ulceration. However, granulomas and ulcers may be mimicked by more serious lesions, such as carcinoma, tuberculosis, and granular cell tumor. Consequently, the clinical diagnosis of laryngeal granuloma must always be made with caution and must be considered tentative at least until the patient has been followed up over time, and a good response to treatment has been observed.

Understanding the etiology of laryngeal ulcers and granulomas is essential to clinical evaluation and treatment. Traditionally, ulcers and granulomas in the region of the vocal processes have been associated with trauma, especially intubation injury. However, they are also seen in young, apparently healthy patients who have no history of intubation or obvious laryngeal injury. In fact, the vast majority of granulomas and ulcerations (probably even those from intubation) are caused or aggravated by laryngopharyngeal reflux disease. In some patients, muscular tension dysphonia producing forceful vocal process contact may be contributory or causal, especially in patients whose adduction patterns are determined by lateral cricoarytenoid activity (LCA).

■ PATIENT ASSESSMENT

History

Evaluation of patients who have laryngeal ulcers or granulomas begins with a comprehensive history. In addition to elucidating specific voice complaints and their importance to the individual patient's life and profession, the history is designed to reveal otolaryngologic and systemic abnormalities that may have caused dysphonia. Special attention is paid to symptoms of laryngopharyngeal reflux. It must be remembered that reflux laryngitis is commonly not accompanied by pyrosis or dyspepsia. Common symptoms of reflux laryngitis include morning hoarseness; prolonged vocal warm-up time (greater than 20 to 30 minutes); halitosis; excessive phlegm; frequent throat clearing; globus; dry mouth; coated tongue; throat tickle; dysphagia; chronic sore throat; nocturnal, chronic, or recurrent cough; difficulty breathing (especially at night), laryngospasm; regurgitation of food; poorly controlled asthma (which also contributes to dysphonia by interfering with the support mechanism); pneumonia; and only occasionally dyspepsia or pyrosis. Symptoms suggesting voice abuse include voice fatigue; voice deterioration during the course of a business day or week; improvement in laryngeal symptoms following quiet vacations or weekends away from work; a family history or personal history of previous vocal nodules; occupational or social history, including extensive voice use, especially over background noise; and throat discomfort or pain associated with phonation. The history also specifically seeks symptoms consistent with asthma, including voice fatigue following extensive use. Exercise-induced asthma can be provoked by the exercise of voice use, and even mild reactive airway disease undermines the power source of the voice and may lead to compensatory muscular tension dysphonia and consequent laryngeal granuloma or ulcer. Also, systemic investigations are made of all body systems for evidence of other diseases that may present initially as a laryngeal mass. It is important to include a psychological assessment. Excessive stress may lead to increased acid production and symptomatic reflux, and to muscular tension dysphonia. In such cases, it is important to identify and treat the underlying stressor as well as the symptomatic expressions of the stress.

Physical Examination

Physical examination begins with an assessment of the patient's general health. Specific attention is directed toward the patient's speaking voice. The laryngologist should note the range, ease, quality, breathing patterns and coordination; an excessive number of harsh glottal attacks; frequent throat clearing; and head and neck muscle tension associated with phonation. Indirect laryngoscopy is included during every examination; it provides excellent information on the color of the laryngeal mucosa, reveals most sizable masses, and provides information on the severity of the patient's gag reflex. Symmetry of gag response should be tested routinely. I routinely test the gag reflex with the handle of the laryngeal mirror following indirect laryngoscopy on every patient. Laryngopharyngeal reflux classically produces arytenoid erythema and edema; erythema of the cartilaginous portion of the vocal folds and mucosa in the region of the vocal processes; and often edema of the false vocal folds, which may partially obscure the ventricles. The most prominent erythema is typically on the apices and posterior aspects of the arytenoids. Marked muscular tension dysphonia more commonly produces erythema on the anterior aspects of the arytenoids, the petiolus, and often the aryepiglottic folds. It is not unusual for the conditions to coexist.

Strobovideolaryngoscopy

Mirror examination usually reveals the presence of a granuloma or ulcer, but more sophisticated evaluation is invaluable. In the presence of suspected laryngeal granuloma or ulcer, I routinely perform strobovideolaryngoscopy using both flexible and rigid endoscopes. Flexible examination reveals patterns of phonation and is extremely helpful in identifying muscular tension dysphonia and determining phonatory behaviors associated with forceful adduction. Rigid laryngeal telescopic examination provides magnified, detailed information on the lesions under slow-motion light, allowing analysis of their composition (solid granulomas versus fluid-filled cysts) and their effects on phonation. This examination also permits assessment of other areas of the vocal folds to rule out separate lesions (such as vocal fold scar) that may be the real cause of the patient's voice complaints.

Evaluation also includes at the least formal assessment by a speech-language pathologist who is skilled in voice evaluation and care. In my practice, an objective voice analysis and a vocal stress assessment with a singing voice specialist (even with nonsingers) are also included. The information provided by these evaluations helps establish the degree to which voice abuse or misuse is present, and it guides the design of an individualized therapy plan.

Reflux Studies

Reflux must be suspected in virtually all cases of granuloma. It can be evaluated by 24 hour pH monitor, barium swallow with water siphonage (routine barium swallows are not satisfactory for diagnosing reflux), and/or therapeutic trial of medical management. If there is historical evidence of prolonged reflux symptoms, formal gastroenterologic evaluation to rule out Barrett's esophagus is often advisable. If a therapeutic trial without confirmatory tests is elected, marked improvement in symptoms and signs should occur within 1 month. If this is not the case, gastroenterologic assessment, generally with 24 hour pH monitor studies, is generally recommended.

TREATMENT

Medical

Treatment for laryngopharyngeal reflux should be aggressive. The condition requires high doses of medication for prolonged periods (often a lifetime). I generally start with 20 mg of omeprazole twice daily, a liquid antacid for most patients in addition to the proton pump inhibitor, avoidance of eating for a few hours before going to sleep, diet modification to avoid substances that aggravate reflux (e.g., spices, caffeine, alcohol, etc.), and avoidance of caffeine or alcohol. A more individualized regimen can be designed following 24 hour pH monitor studies. For example, some singers experience reflux severely whenever they sing, but do not experience reflux at other times, even when they are supine. Consequently, life-style modifications may be individualized. The efficacy of oral steroids for treating laryngeal granulomas and ulcers has not been proved, but these drugs are used commonly on the basis of anecdotal evidence, especially for granulomas and ulcers that appear acutely inflamed. For these conditions, low doses are usually given for longer periods, such as triamcinolone acetonide 4 mg twice a day for 3 weeks. Steroid inhalers are not recommended. They may lead to laryngitis or laryngeal candidal infections, and prolonged use may cause vocal fold atrophy.

Surgery

At the end of 1 month of therapy that includes antireflux measures, voice therapy, and possibly steroids, substantial improvement in the appearance of the larynx should be seen. Ulcers should be healed, and granulomas should be substantially smaller. Consistent strobovideolaryngoscopy examination technique allows comparison of lesion size over time. If such improvements are noted, aggressive therapy and close follow-up can be continued until the mass lesion disappears or stabilizes. If the mass does not disappear, or if response to the first month of aggressive therapy produces no substantial improvement, biopsy should be performed to rule out carcinoma and other possible causes. If the surgeon is reasonably certain that the lesion is a granuloma, injection of an aqueous steroid preparation into the base of the lesion at the time of surgery may be helpful. As long as a good specimen is obtained, the laser may be used for resection of suspected granulomas, because the lesions are usually not on the vibratory margin, and they are often friable. However, I usually use traditional instruments, wishing to avoid the third-degree burn caused by the laser (even with a microspot) in the treatment of this chronic, irritative condition.

It is essential that causative factors, especially reflux and voice abuse, be controlled strictly after surgery. The patient is kept on optimal doses of a proton pump inhibitor before surgery and for at least 6 weeks after surgery. Surgeons should not hesitate to use omeprazole 20 mg as frequently as four times a day under these circumstances. After surgery, absolute voice rest (writing pad) is prescribed until the surgical area has remucosalized. This period is usually approximately 1 week and virtually never longer than 10 to 14 days. There are no indications for prolonged absolute voice rest. Voice therapy is reinstituted on the day when phonation is resumed, and frequent short therapy sessions and close monitoring are maintained throughout the healing period.

Recurrent Granuloma

In some patients, granulomas recur. In all such cases, aggressive re-evaluation of reflux with 24 hour pH monitor studies is warranted. Often, endoscopy and biopsy of esophageal and postcricoid mucosa is appropriate. Twenty-four hour monitor studies should be conduted not only with the patient off all medications, but also with the patient on either a proton pump inhibitor or an H2-receptor blocker Some patients are resistant to omeprazole treatment and will have normal acid secretions despite receiving 80 mg of omeprazole per day. In such patients, the use of H2-receptor blockers is preferable. When medical management is insufficient, laparoscopic fundoplication should be considered before repeated granuloma excisions. Voice use must also be optimized with the help of the speech-language pathologist and voice team, and the laryngologist must be sure that good vocal technique is carried over outside the medical office into the patient's daily life.

Occasionally, patients develop multiply recurrent granulomas that may develop even after excellent reflux control (including fundoplication), surgical removal including steroid injection into the base of the granulomas, and voice therapy. Medical causes other than reflux and muscular tension dysphonia must be ruled out, particularly granulomatous diseases (sarcoidosis and tuberculosis) and neoplasm. Pathology slides from previous surgical procedures should be reviewed. When it has been established that the recurrent lesions are typical granulomas occurring in the absence of laryngopharyngeal reflux, the cause is almost always phonatory trauma. When voice therapy has been insufficient to permit adequate healing, some of these uncommonly difficult patient problems can be solved by temporary paresis using botulinum toxin. I favor injecting the botulinum toxin into the LCA rather than the thyroarytenoid in these patients. Although this treatment approach has been effective in a small number of patients, it is not recommended as initial therapy and is appropriate only for selected recalcitrant cases.

Suggested Reading

Bough ID, Sataloff RT, Castell DO, et al. Gastroesophageal reflux disease resistant to omeprazole. J Voice 1995; 9:205-211.

Koufman JA. Gastroesophageal reflux and voice disorders. In: Rubin J, Sataloff RT, Korovin G, Gould WJ, eds. The diagnosis and treatment of voice disorders. New York: Igaku-Shoin, 1995:161.

Sataloff RT. Professional voice: The science and art of clinical care. 2nd ed. San Diego: Singular Publishing Group, 1996.

Sataloff RT, Castell DO, Sataloff DM, et al. Reflux and other gastroenterologic conditions that may affect the voice. In: Sataloff RT, ed. Professional voice: The science and art of clinical care. 2nd ed. San Diego: Singular Publishing Group, 1997:319.

LARYNGEAL PARALYSIS

The method of
Henry T. Hoffman
by
Henry T. Hoffman
Timothy M. McCulloch
Luis Victoria

Management of vocal fold paralysis includes a diagnostic plan to identify the cause of the paralysis and a treatment plan to address voice and swallowing problems. Compromised breathing rarely accompanies unilateral paralysis but is a critical concern for most patients who have bilateral vocal fold paralysis. Intervention is prioritized for both processes to urgently address the life-threatening consequences of laryngeal dysfunction, such as airway obstruction and aspiration pneumonia.

Patients who have unilateral laryngeal paralysis most commonly complain of dysphonia that is characterized by a rough and breathy voice produced with effort and readily fatigable. Although voice problems are not life threatening, impaired verbal communication does threaten the quality of life. Recent studies by Smith and colleagues have identified that patients who have voice disorders suffer substantial disability and limitations in their work. Among 57 patients with unilateral laryngeal paralysis evaluated through the University of Iowa Voice Clinic, 46 percent identified a negative impact of their voice problems on their current job performance. A moderately to extremely adverse effect of their voice disorder on future career options was perceived by 65 percent of these patients.

This chapter addresses our management of laryngeal paralysis. Alternative methods are presented primarily to highlight the rationale for our approach.

UNILATERAL LARYNGEAL PARALYSIS

History and Physical Examination

The duration and quality of the breathing, swallowing, and voice problems should be determined. Further evaluation is focused on determining the cause of the paralysis, which is aided by knowledge of the most common etiologies. Trauma, which is most often surgical, is the most common cause of laryngeal paralysis at many institutions and rarely poses a diagnostic problem. Paralysis associated with infectious or neurologic disease usually presents with associated symptoms that are readily identified and help to direct further evaluation. Greater difficulty may exist in identifying the cause of the paralysis associated with neoplastic disease. The presenting signs and symptoms of thyroid cancer, lung cancer, and esophageal cancer may be limited to those resulting from laryngeal paralysis. Both benign and malignant skull base tumors as well as mediastinal lesions may have similar presentations with a paucity of other localizing signs. It is important to discriminate between these processes and idiopathic laryngeal paralysis in order that treatment be appropriately initiated.

A history of a viral infection at the onset of voicing difficulties should be solicited. Patients with "idiopathic" laryngeal paralysis may actually have a self-limited viral neuritis that can develop either with or without associated symptoms of an upper respiratory infection. A history of past laryngeal manipulation should be solicited to identify injury resulting in vocal fold fixation from direct trauma or paralysis from nerve injury. The evaluation should also attend to cardiopulmonary signs and symptoms. Nonmalignant chest disease such as cardiac enlargement with traction on the recurrent laryngeal nerve (Ortner's syndrome) is one of several benign processes associated with laryngeal paralysis. Careful palpation of the neck is necessary not only to address potential malignant disease, but also to identify benign lesions that have been reported to occasionally induce paralysis from pressure neurapraxia.

Abnormalities of the neuromotor system should be recorded, with specific attention to the lower cranial nerves. Nasal regurgitation of food and hypernasal speech resulting from impaired movement of the ipsilateral palate support the diagnosis of a high vagal lesion that affects not only the recurrent laryngeal nerve, but also the pharyngeal branches to the palate. Function of the hypoglossal and spinal accessory nerves should be evaluated by testing for tongue motion and shoulder weakness.

Sensory function of the supraglottic laryngeal nerve can be tested to help identify whether the immobile vocal cord results from an isolated recurrent laryngeal paralysis or a combined recurrent and superior laryngeal paralysis. Loss of sensation of the ipsilateral supraglottic larynx suggests a combined paralysis. The flexible fiberoptic laryngoscope may identify intact sensation by touching the supraglottic larynx, thus demonstrating a functioning superior laryngeal nerve. Although we have not found the routine use of this test to be useful, advances in instrumentation may improve the reliability of this type of evaluation.

The laryngeal configuration has been used in the past to determine whether a combined paralysis involving the superior and recurrent laryngeal nerves or an isolated recurrent nerve paralysis was present. This clinical assessment was based on the Wagner-Grossman theory, which states that an intact superior laryngeal nerve innervating the cricothyroid muscle results in median positioning of a vocal fold paralyzed by isolated recurrent laryngeal nerve injury. Most investigators currently believe that assessment of vocal fold position is not useful diagnostically to identify the site of injury. Although unilateral loss of cricothyroid muscle action may impair the degree to which the vocal folds may be lengthened, superior laryngeal nerve paralysis does not have a consistent effect on position of the paralyzed vocal fold during phonation. Partial reinnervation, scar contracture, muscle atrophy, and other unknown factors are important in determining position of the paralyzed vocal cord.

Laryngeal Imaging

Inspection of the larynx is needed to support the diagnosis of laryngeal paralysis. In most cases, an immobile vocal fold, which most commonly reflects laryngeal paralysis, is readily identified with indirect mirror or flexible fiberoptic transnasal laryngoscopy. The diagnosis of paralysis is not conclusively established by identification of an immobile vocal fold. Consideration should be given to other processes that impair vocal fold mobility, such as posterior glottic scarring and cricoarytenoid arthritis.

Identification of an immobile vocal fold may be difficult in pediatric patients as well as those who have abnormal anatomy or a vigorous gag reflex. Additionally, supraglottic movement due to function of extrinsic laryngeal muscles (i.e., strap muscles) may result in passive movement of the arytenoids that may be misinterpreted as vocal fold motion. The additional time and expense of videorecording endoscopic examination is justified when more than one observer is needed to interpret subtle findings and demonstrate to patients their altered laryngeal function. These demonstrations improve patients' understanding of their vocal disorders and allow for their greater participation in treatment choices. Interval comparisons of sequential recordings are also useful to evaluate the evolution of the paralysis and the patient's adaptation to it. These assessments are particularly helpful to assess responses to treatment and direct further intervention.

Stroboscopic evaluation of the paralyzed larynx provides the best dynamic imaging of vocal fold configuration during the glottic cycle. Despite apparently adequate glottic closure, differences in tension and stiffness between the two vocal folds commonly cause asymmetric vocal fold vibration that often correlates with vocal roughness. Although stroboscopy is the most effective way to assess this asymmetry, laryngeal paralysis may cause vocal fold vibration that is sufficiently chaotic as to preclude a stroboscopic evaluation. Stroboscopy requires that periodicity be present in the glottic cycle to permit imaging of progressive separate segments of the glottic cycle through asynchronous but periodic flashes of light. Electroglottography is commonly performed synchronously with videostroboscopy examinations and may be useful in assessing type and degree of glottic closure during phonation.

Radiographic Evaluation

The history and physical examination determine the need for radiographic imaging. A patient who has the new onset of a breathy dysphonia immediately after a pneumonectomy, thyroidectomy, or carotid endarterectomy may be assumed to have injury to the vagus or recurrent laryngeal nerve without need for further evaluation. A patient who has the onset of unilateral laryngeal paralysis coincident with an upper respiratory infection may be considered to have a viral (idiopathic) neuropathy without the need for advanced imaging at the initial evaluation. A chest x-ray radiograph should be included in the preliminary evaluation of almost all patients who have unexplained unilateral laryngeal paralysis. A chest radiograph is inexpensive and useful in excluding an intrathoracic malignancy that may require urgent attention. After evaluation that includes a normal chest radiograph, the patient who has presumed viral (idiopathic) laryngeal paralysis may be appropriately treated with the expectation that vocal fold mobility will spontaneously recover. Re-evaluation should be arranged to obtain a computed tomography (CT) or magnetic resonance imaging (MRI) if mobility is not restored within 2 to 3 months. Patients without a clear etiology for laryngeal paralysis and without localizing signs or symptoms should be evaluated for occult neoplastic processes by imaging the vagus and recurrent laryngeal nerves from their origin in the brain stem to their termination in the larynx.

Before MRI and CT imaging became readily available, radiographic imaging with a barium esophagram was considered important to assess for occult hypopharyngeal or esophageal neoplasms. Although these considerations are still valid and may warrant a diagnostic barium esophagram in selected patients, we generally restrict our use of barium contrast studies to assess the swallowing impairment that may accompany laryngeal paralysis. The modified barium swallow or "oropharyngeal motility study" (OPMS) is useful in selected patients to assess the risk of aspiration.

Electromyography

Laryngeal electromyography (EMG) is helpful in assessing the chance for return of vocal fold motion. Patients should be appropriately counseled, however, that EMG evaluation does not definitively determine prognosis. EMG should be performed within 6 months of the onset of paralysis because electrical activity in the paralyzed vocal fold after 6 months is difficult to interpret. It may result from reinnervation without topographic organization, which results in synkinesis and lack of vocal fold motion.

Judgment is needed to determine which patients will benefit from EMG analysis. Electromyography is most valuable to help determine the timing and type of therapeutic intervention (Fig. 1). Those patients whose recurrent laryngeal nerve has clearly been transected or is involved with cancer have such a poor chance for return of function that EMG analysis is generally not worthwhile. A definitive procedure may be offered to those patients without waiting for spontaneous return of function. In those patients without such a clear prognosis, EMG may be helpful in guiding the patient to choose between the options of observation; temporary medialization with Gelfoam injection; and a permanent medialization laryngoplasty by way of fat injection, thyroplasty, or arytenoid adduction.

Operative Direct Laryngoscopy

Rigid endoscopy is rarely needed as a diagnostic tool now that evaluation with transnasal fiberoptic laryngoscopy permits adequate visualization of most aspects of the larynx and hypopharynx. An occult hypopharyngeal cancer may escape detection despite use of maneuvers such as anterior traction on the larynx or performance of a modified Valsalva's maneuver, which are designed to expose the piriform sinuses during fiberoptic endoscopy. A hypopharyngeal or esophageal cancer that is sufficiently advanced to cause laryngeal paralysis is unlikely to escape detection by physical examination and MRI or CT scan. We therefore do not believe that we can justify the routine use of diagnostic esophagoscopy and direct laryngoscopy in patients who have idiopathic laryngeal paralysis in the absence of signs or symptoms suggestive of esophageal or hypopharyngeal neoplasms.

Many authors have advocated that direct laryngoscopy be performed in patients who have an immobile vocal cord

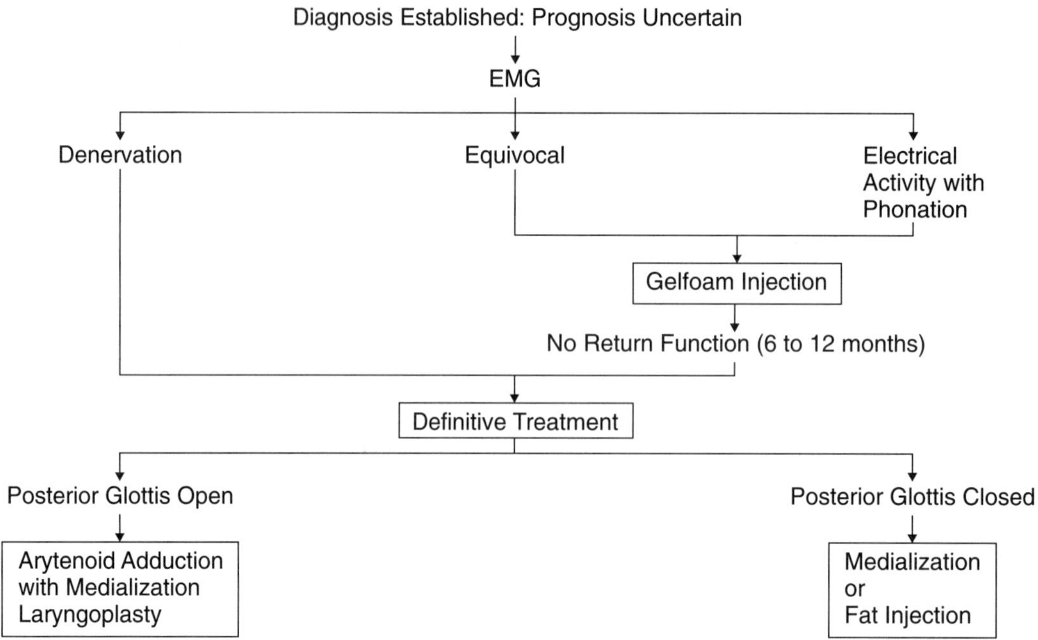

Figure 1.
Use of laryngeal electromyography to help determine choice of treatment for symptomatic unilateral laryngeal paralysis.

and recent neck injury or laryngeal manipulation in order to discriminate between laryngeal paralysis and injury to the cricoarytenoid joint. Arytenoid dislocation, which refers to complete separation between the arytenoid and cricoid, is not likely to occur without significant laryngeal injury and its associated mucosal and ligamentous disruption. Arytenoid subluxation refers to distortion of the usual cricoarytenoid relationship, with the arytenoid still partially in contact with the joint. The lack of muscle tone associated with paralysis of the laryngeal muscles may result in a partial subluxation through loss of adjacent muscular support. Although EMG and CT imaging have been reported as helpful in discriminating between these disorders, controversy still persists regarding the pathophysiology of arytenoid subluxation.

The finding of an immobile vocal cord in a patient following use of a general anesthetic may create a diagnostic dilemma. It may be difficult to discriminate intubation injury resulting in arytenoid subluxation from laryngeal paralysis developing from a pressure neurapraxia exerted by the endotracheal tube cuff on the recurrent laryngeal nerve. Intervention may be appropriately devised to treat both disorders through direct laryngoscopy with Gelfoam injection. Direct laryngoscopy permits palpation of the arytenoid, which may help support the diagnosis of subluxation. Whether or not the findings support the diagnosis of arytenoid subluxation, Gelfoam may be injected to improve glottic closure. If paralysis is responsible for the glottic insufficiency (and possibly the "subluxed" position of the arytenoid), Gelfoam will improve glottic closure. If a true subluxation (in the absence of paralysis) is present, the Gelfoam will help maintain the appropriate position of the arytenoid.

Other Studies

A battery of other studies, including glucose tolerance tests, serology, thyroid scans, and cine barium swallows, have been used to screen patients who have laryngeal paralysis. Although signs and symptoms may appropriately direct evaluation to include thyroid scans or barium esophagrams, we do not find these studies useful in screening for occult disease now that MRI and CT scans are available.

■ NONSURGICAL THERAPY

The role of voice therapy in the treatment of laryngeal paralysis is controversial. It is generally accepted that evaluation by a speech pathologist is useful to document the degree of the voice disorder and to address abnormalities that are either compensatory adaptations or separate unrelated behavioral voice abnormalities. Additionally, a speech pathologist who is trained in swallowing disorders may counsel the patient about strategies to improve swallowing technique. Controversy exists regarding the role of voice therapy as an alternative to surgery. We generally employ voice therapy as an adjunct to surgical treatment of laryngeal paralysis once the glottic configuration has been optimized. Those patients with glottic insufficiency who are not surgical candidates may benefit from voice therapy to maximize compensatory strategies.

■ SURGICAL THERAPY

Laryngeal Reinnervation

Reinnervation of a paralyzed larynx by repair of an injured vagus or recurrent laryngeal nerve is, in theory, the most appealing way to restore function. It is widely accepted, however, that this repair does not restore normal vocal cord mobility. Although it is likely that in many cases neural impulses are communicated to the larynx through the repaired nerve, the benefit from this reinnervation appears primarily to be limited to the atrophy that accompanies denervation. Crumley has proposed that this reinnervation, which is without topographic organization, results in mass movement or synkinesis of the laryngeal muscles without vocal fold mobility. Even without intentional neural repair, some degree of reinnervation commonly occurs.

Reinnervation procedures have not found general acceptance in the treatment of laryngeal paralysis. Although Tucker and Crumley have reported success with reinnervation procedures, other investigators have not replicated these authors' results. We have found that the omohyoid nerve muscle pedicle reinnervation is readily performed at the time of medialization laryngoplasty with a minimal amount of additional dissection. We have abandoned its use, however, because this reinnervation procedure requires sacrificing the function of an intact muscle to achieve a dubious benefit. Because static procedures designed to position the paralyzed vocal cord in the phonatory position are successful, we do not currently include reinnervation procedures among those offered to patients who have symptomatic unilateral laryngeal paralysis.

■ INJECTION LARYNGOPLASTY

Until recently, Teflon injection was widely accepted as the standard approach to restore glottic competence by adding bulk to an immobile cord. Problems with unpredictable foreign body reaction as well as induction of fibrosis with diffusion of Teflon through the injected cord have limited our treatment to rare cases. We do, however, continue to use injection laryngoplasty for selected patients, with either fat or Gelfoam to improve glottic closure by augmenting the paralyzed vocal fold.

Gelfoam Injection

Gelfoam injection is used to treat laryngeal paralysis when the prognosis for return of function is uncertain. We initially performed this procedure with the patient under local anesthesia in order to monitor vocal results as Gelfoam is added incrementally. Through this process, the patient's voice is generally at its best immediately after injection, with the expected deterioration in quality occurring over the ensuing 2 months as the Gelfoam is resorbed. Over the past 4 years, we have more commonly injected Gelfoam under general anesthesia both in deference to patient comfort and to permit the more accurate positioning and manipulation of the Gelfoam bolus. A slight overinjection is performed in anticipation of gradual resorption, with the understanding that a pressed voice is expected during the first weeks after injection and improvement is expected as the Gelfoam gradually resorbs.

General anesthesia is administered through a small (5.5 or 6) endotracheal tube, with the patient treated with short-acting paralysis. One gram of Gelfoam powder is made into paste by mixing it with 4 cc of injectable saline. It is then loaded into a Bruening syringe with a 22 gauge needle attached. The glottis is exposed through direct laryngoscopy, with care taken to avoid distortion of the vocal folds by positioning the end of the laryngoscope approximately 2 mm above the level of the vocal folds. The Gelfoam bolus is then injected into the vocal fold at the point of maximum vocal cord concavity. Two to four "clicks" are delivered through the syringe deep to the mucosa and laterally into the muscle of the vocal cord. Depending on the glottic configuration, a second injection may be added and is usually positioned posterior to the first injection, immediately lateral to the vocal process. Manipulation of the bolus within the substance of the vocal cord can be effected employing either a spatula or another blunt endoscopic instrument. We prefer using the end of a large upbiting biopsy forceps. With the tips closed, the end of the biopsy forceps is used to manipulate the bolus by pressing from superior and medial directions to mold a straight edge to the vocal cord at the expected level of contact opposite the contralateral fold.

Fat Injection

The technical features of fat injection that differ from Gelfoam injection relate primarily to harvesting and processing the fat. The key to successful transplantation is preservation of fat viability. To limit the trauma to the fat and permit delivery through the Bruening syringe, a large-bore (18 or 19 gauge) needle is used. Puncture of the vocal fold epithelium with a needle this size may create a sufficiently large opening that some of the injected fat may extrude. This extrusion is generally not problematic in that an adequate amount of fat usually persists in the substance of the vocal cord. An alternative approach to avoid this extrusion is to place the fat into the vocal cord through a percutaneous route. Placement of an 18 or 19 gauge short spinal needle percutaneous through the cricothyroid membrane into the vocal cord permits injection through a submucosal route in a manner similar to botulinum toxin injection without entering the airway. Accurate placement of an adequate fat bolus through this technique may be difficult. As a result, we prepare patients for an alternative injection through direct laryngoscopy if the planned percutaneous approach fails.

Methods to harvest and prepare fat before injection have been designed to emphasize different strategies to maximize survival of the transplant. We have successfully transferred fat by abdominal liposuction but prefer direct surgical excision in order to minimize trauma. Through a periumbilical incision in order to retrieve the fat without a visible scar, sharp dissection is employed to obtain fat superficial to the rectus abdominis fascia. The fat is then sharply dissected into 1 to 2 mm "pearls" and washed with saline to remove blood and fascia. The pearls are then loaded into the barrel of the Bruening syringe if transoral injection is planned or into a 1 cc syringe if percutaneous injection is to be done through a spinal needle.

Overinjection of the vocal fold by 50 percent is recommended because loss of bulk over the ensuing weeks is expected. Despite histologic studies demonstrating survival of injected fat for 5 or 6 months, it is still not clear that fat can be expected to persist for longer periods. Despite these concerns, fat injection still appears to have a role in the treatment of glottic incompetence. Those patients who refuse use of alloplastic implants are particularly suited to use of autogenous fat. Patients who have mobile vocal folds and glottic incompetence are also candidates for this procedure.

■ LARYNGEAL FRAMEWORK SURGERY

Although a critical comparative analysis is still lacking to define the best surgical approach for treating laryngeal paralysis, it is our impression that the best long-term results come from medialization laryngoplasty, often coupled with arytenoid adduction. Arytenoid adduction, when performed without an ancillary procedure to medialize the membranous vocal cord, does not consistently provide adequate glottic closure. It is best suited to position the vocal process in the phonatory position but does not always result in adequate medial positioning of the membranous vocal cord. A significant portion of the patients we have treated with arytenoid adduction alone have subsequently needed further treatment of the anterior glottis with either a fat injection or medialization laryngoplasty. As a result, most of the patients we now treat with arytenoid adduction receive a concomitant medialization laryngoplasty.

Those patients suitable for permanent vocal fold medialization are counseled about alternatives and generally treated with laryngeal framework surgery. Preoperative assessment of the vocal fold position permits an estimate to be made as to whether medialization laryngoplasty will be performed alone or in combination with arytenoid adduction. Regardless of the result of this assessment, we prepare patients for both procedures in the event that the medialization laryngoplasty alone is found to be inadequate at the time of surgery. Arytenoid adduction is then readily accomplished through the same incision, with only a few extra instruments required.

A variety of different types of implant materials can be used to help secure the vocal fold in the phonatory position during medialization laryngoplasty. Although Silastic (hardened silicone) is widely used as an implant material, we now use expanded polytetrafluoroethylene (EPTFE, or Gore-Tex) in the majority of medialization thyroplasties.

Technique

Intravenous sedation is begun along with the administration of antibiotics and steroids. The patient may be heavily sedated during the beginning of the procedure, but should be sufficiently awake toward the end to respond to verbal commands to permit assessment of the voice. The patient is positioned supine, with a small shoulder roll employed to slightly extend the neck. Oxygen by nasal cannula with attached CO_2 monitor is delivered to the nostrils, which are topically decongested and anesthetized. Transnasal flexible fiberoptic laryngoscopy is performed to confirm the laterality of the paralysis and identify changes that may have occurred in the interval from the time of the last evaluation. The flexible fiberoptic laryngoscope is coupled to a television monitor to permit all members of the operating team to view the appearance of the larynx. The patient is then prepped and draped from the lower lip to below the clavicles to permit intermittent nasal insertion of the fiberoptic laryngoscope during the procedure in order to assess vocal fold position as it is adjusted during the procedure.

After injection of local anesthetic, a 4 to 5 cm incision along a relaxed skin tension line is centered over the ipsilateral thyroid ala and extended slightly past midline. Subplatysmal flaps are elevated, and the strap muscles are separated in the midline and retracted laterally. The local anesthetic is reinjected as the dissection is deepened. The perichondrium is elevated in a medial to lateral direction over the ipsilateral thyroid lamina. This dissection plane permits bloodless elevation of the musculature from the oblique line and inferior tubercle. If an arytenoid adduction is to be done, the dissection is carried around the posterior edge of the thyroid lamina. Medialization laryngoplasty alone can be accomplished without dissecting around the posterior lamina, but this procedure is best done with wide exposure in order to permit assessment of the full extent of the external cartilaginous anatomy. Placement of a tracheotomy hook or heavy suture through the laryngeal prominence permits medial retraction and rotation of the larynx to improve exposure.

Medialization Laryngoplasty

As with other medialization techniques, a window is created in the thyroid cartilage lateral to the membranous vocal fold to permit its medial displacement. A rotating bur is employed to remove a 12 × 7 mm segment of thyroid cartilage positioned 1 cm posterior to the midline and 3 mm above the inferior border of the thyroid cartilage.

The inner perichondrium is bluntly elevated circumferentially from the undersurface of the thyroid cartilage. The inferior elevation allows direct communication between the window and the cricothyroid space as an elevator is passed underneath the inferior cartilage strut. The inner perichondrium is judiciously incised to permit accurate vocal fold medialization without lateral tethering. Temporary medialization is effected by depressing the vocal fold medially with a blunt instrument placed into the window. The voice is assessed, and vocal fold position is re-evaluated by flexible fiberoptic laryngeal examination during this trial, which helps indicate the correct location for implant placement.

The implant is fashioned as a 1 cm continuous strip (or ribbon) of EPTFE fashioned from a 0.6 mm thick cardiac patch graft. The implant is soaked in antibiotic solution before placement. In order to ensure adequate implant stabilization and maximize medialization at the appropriate inferior level, the EPTFE ribbon is wrapped once around the inferior strut of cartilage. The "tail" of the ribbon is then incrementally placed in the window as vocal fold position and voice are continuously assessed. This ribbon of EPTFE is partially secured by tucking it under the thyroid cartilage, which forms the edges of the window. Definitive fixation of the implant is effected through a 4–0 monofilament suture placed through the Gore-Tex circumferentially around the inferior strut and then tied on itself. The upper aspect of the implant is secured by two separate 4–0 monofilament sutures placed through the EPTFE and the unossified thyroid cartilage above the window. A final endoscopic examination is then done to confirm accurate medialization and an adequate airway. The wound is irrigated and closed over a Penrose drain. The patient is observed overnight and discharged the next day after the drain is removed.

This approach offers several advantages over other described techniques of medialization laryngoplasty. Use of a malleable ribbon as an implant permits incremental placement or removal as the voice and vocal cord position are dynamically assessed. Unlike preformed prostheses and segments of Silastic that require modification through carving, this EPTFE implant is positioned without the need to modify or change the prosthesis size. Degree of medialization is readily altered by adding or removing a portion of the continuous ribbon. Accurate positioning of the EPTFE ribbon is not dependent on precise placement of the window in the thyroid cartilage. Most other techniques of medialization laryngoplasty are critically dependent on accurate location of the window directly over the segment of the vocal fold to be medialized. This technique employing a ribbon of EPTFE as an implant is more flexible. Regardless of the position of the window, the implant may be placed anywhere in the paraglottic space and can be positioned into regions that do not immediately underlie the window.

As with all medialization laryngoplasties, some edema is expected from manipulation of the vocal fold. We have found it best to medialize the vocal fold slightly past midline in anticipation that approximately 2 to 3 mm will relapse over the ensuing months as the edema subsides.

Arytenoid Adduction

Arytenoid adduction is designed to permanently position the vocal process in the phonatory position. It is effected by placement of a suture through the muscular process of the arytenoid which, with anterior pull, rotates the arytenoid to place the vocal process in an inferomedial position. A critical component of the procedure is adequate exposure of the posterior cricoarytenoid (PCA) muscle and muscular process.

The procedure is accomplished through posterior extension of the dissection initiated by medialization laryngoplasty. An elevator is used to remove the soft-tissue attachments from the posterior aspect of the thyroid lamina, with care to avoid entry into the piriform sinus. Kerrison rongeurs are employed to remove a segment of the cartilage approximately 2 cm in width from just above the midportion of the posterior lamina to the cricothyroid articulation. Although earlier reports suggested that separation of the cricothyroid joint is useful to improve exposure of the muscular process, we have not found this separation to be routinely needed when an adequate amount of cartilage is removed from the posterior thyroid lamina.

The fibers of the PCA muscle are then exposed as the piriform sinus is pushed superiorly. The PCA muscle fibers converge in a "V" shape from a broad base on the cricoid cartilage to an apex inserting on the muscular process. The muscular process is identified by tracing these fibers from the base to the apex.

A 4–0 monofilament suture is placed through either the cartilaginous muscular process or the insertion of the PCA muscle. Two passes of the needle into the muscular process (figure eight) ensures that the suture will remain secure. The window created by medialization laryngoplasty facilitates passing the arytenoid adduction suture anteriorly from its position deep to the posterior aspect of the thyroid ala. Before passing the suture forward, an elevator is used to connect the posterior aspect of the window with the lateral aspect of the PCA muscle through medial displacement of the inner perichondrium of the thyroid cartilage. Both ends of the suture are brought forward. One end is placed through a small hole drilled 0.5 cm posterior to the midline and 0.5 cm above the inferior aspect of the thyroid cartilage. The second end of the suture is attached to a French-eye curved needle and drawn forward under the inferior strut of the thyroid cartilage through the cricothyroid membrane. The two ends of the suture are drawn forward with minimal tension and secured by tying one to the other as the larynx is inspected with the fiberoptic laryngoscope. When arytenoid adduction is done with medialization laryngoplasty, the sutures are placed but not tied before the EPTFE implant is secured. The sutures, which are superficial to the thyroarytenoid muscle but deep to the implant, are tied after the implant is placed.

The wound is then treated in a manner similar to that of medialization laryngoplasty with irrigation, placement of a drain, and overnight observation in the hospital before discharge the following morning.

Postoperative Considerations

Oral feedings are usually begun either the evening of surgery or the following morning. Judgment is required to determine the need for and timing of a barium oropharyngeal motility study (cookie swallow) in patients who have aspiration identified preoperatively. Sutures are removed at postoperative Days 6 or 7, and a repeat videoendoscopy is done at 6 weeks and then at 3 months postoperatively. Yearly evaluations are subsequently performed. Follow-up evaluations are needed to ensure adequate healing; identify speech, swallowing, or airway problems that may potentially require revision surgery; and identify the need for postoperative voice therapy.

■ BILATERAL VOCAL CORD PARALYSIS

Diagnosis

Identification of the etiology of bilateral vocal fold paralysis is usually not as difficult as for unilateral paralysis. Surgical trauma (thyroidectomy) is the most common cause. Rare cases of metabolic, toxic, or infectious disorders can cause a bilateral neuropathy that may be more difficult to identify. A common diagnostic problem in evaluating patients who have bilaterally immobile vocal folds is to discriminate between fixation and paralysis.

Posterior glottic scarring may cause symptoms that are indistinguishable from bilateral paralysis. Airway compromise usually dominates the clinical picture for both processes. The voice is commonly normal in patients who have posterior glottic scarring because the vocal folds are usually fixed in median positions. Variable voice quality in cases of bilateral paralysis is dependent on the position the vocal folds assume. Swallowing disorders are more common among patients who have bilateral paralysis. High vagal lesions causing paralysis with loss of sensation to the supraglottic larynx are frequently associated with swallowing difficulties. Those patients who have an open glottic configuration and immobile vocal folds from bilateral paralysis may have an adequate airway but often aspirate due to failure of glottic closure despite intact superior laryngeal nerve function. In contrast, patients who have posterior glottic scarring rarely have trouble swallowing but nearly uniformly have some degree of airway obstruction.

Videoendoscopic examination may help discriminate between these process by identifying subtle movement in the membranous portion of the vocal fold that is not apparent in cases of bilateral vocal fold paralysis. Fiberoptic examination of the undersurface of the vocal folds through a tracheotomy site usually makes this distinction more apparent. The definitive evaluation to discriminate between these processes is direct laryngoscopy with palpation of the arytenoids and vocal folds. It is usually not necessary to perform direct laryngoscopy as a separate procedure in that the diagnostic assessment can be performed under the same anesthesia as the definitive treatment. Full passive mobility should be present upon palpation of vocal folds and arytenoids in patients who have bilateral laryngeal paralysis. Posterior glottic scarring may affect only the soft tissue without causing cricoarytenoid fixation. In these patients, palpation of one arytenoid in a lateral direction will cause the other arytenoid to move in the same direction. Cricoarytenoid fixation is apparent through immobility of the arytenoid.

Although some similarities in surgical management are apparent for these two disorders, the following discussion focuses on the treatment of bilateral laryngeal paralysis.

Surgical Therapy

Compromises are generally required in the effort to restore function to the complex and dynamic glottic valve that is rendered incapable of motion through bilateral paralysis. A good voice without dysphagia can generally be preserved at the expense of treating airway obstruction with a tracheotomy. Removal of the tracheotomy to restore a laryngeal airway is generally associated with some diminution in vocal quality and some risk of developing aspiration with swallowing.

As with unilateral laryngeal paralysis, theoretically the most satisfying treatment is through reinnervation of the paralyzed larynx. Although a few investigators have reported success in maintaining an adequate voice and airway without a tracheotomy through this approach, reinnervation has not yet found wide acceptance. As a result, we limit our treatment to the options of (1) tracheotomy; (2) enlarging the posterior glottic aperture, usually through an endoscopic laser approach; and (3) observation without surgical intervention.

The surgical treatment of bilateral laryngeal paralysis usually includes tracheotomy either as the definitive procedure or as a means to secure the airway during the healing process following another intervention. Permanent tracheotomy is a valuable treatment for many patients, especially those who require use of their voice. Modifications to the tracheotomy by way of a valve to permit inspiration through the tube with expiration directed around the tube permit voicing without the need for digital occlusion of the tracheotomy tube.

Endoscopic laser resection of a portion of the posterior larynx is our preferred treatment for patients who desire removal of their tracheotomy. The larynx conceptually may be divided into an anterior "phonatory glottis" comprised of the region between the membranous vocal folds. This area is responsible for the majority of vibrator activity during phonation, which can be near normal despite air escape through the posterior "respirator glottis." The respirator glottis at the base of the glottic triangle has a much larger surface area than does the anterior glottis. Many of the procedures used to treat bilateral laryngeal paralysis are designed to exploit the perceived differences in function between the anterior and posterior glottis. In general, effort is made to enlarge the respiratory glottis to improve the airway posteriorly, with efforts made to preserve the proximity of the vocal folds anteriorly in the phonatory segment of the glottis.

A spectrum of endoscopic laser procedures to improve the airway have been reported and range from complete arytenoidectomy to partial arytenoidectomy to removal of variable portions of the vocal process, vocal fold, or the muscles around the arytenoid. We generally employ a conservative endoscopic laser resection of tissue at the junction of the posterior membranous vocal fold and vocal process through a "lateral cordotomy," as popularized by Kashima. An initial conservative approach is advocated to afford the greatest chance for voice preservation. Revision procedures to remove more tissue are much easier to accomplish than are procedures to restore bulk to the posterior glottis if an excessive amount of dissection results in an unacceptable voice. Some diminution in voice quality is expected with this approach.

The presence of bilateral vocal fold paralysis does not mandate surgical treatment. The desires of an informed patient are critical to appropriate management. Vocal fold position generally determines the symptoms, which can range from life-threatening airway obstruction with the vocal folds medially positioned to limitations in exercise, with a breathy voice if the vocal folds are more laterally positioned. Observation with counseling regarding the risk of airway obstruction may be sufficient treatment for the latter group.

Suggested Reading

Bigenzahn W, Hoefler H. Minimally invasive laser surgery for the treatment of basilateral vocal cord paralysis. Laryngoscope 1996; 106:791-793.

Crumley RL. Endoscopic laser medial arytenoidectomy for airway management in bilateral laryngeal paralysis. Ann Otol Rhinol Laryngol 1993; 102:81-84.

Crumley RL. Laryngeal synkinesis: Its significance to the laryngologist. Ann Otol Rhinol Laryngol 1989; 98:87-92.

Dennis DP, Kashima H. Carbon dioxide laser posterior cordectomy for treatment of bilateral vocal cord paralysis. Ann Otol Rhinol Laryngol 1989; 98:930-934.

Eckel HE, Thumfart M, Vossing M, et al. Cordectomy versus arytenoidectomy in the management of bilateral vocal cord paralysis. Ann Otol Rhinol Otolaryngol 1994; 103:852-857.

Hirano M, Bless DM. Videostroboscopic examination of the larynx. San Diego: Singular Publishing Group, 1993:120.

Hirano M, Yukizane K, Kurtia S, Hibi S. Asymmetry of the laryngeal framework: A morphologic study of cadaver larynges. Ann Otol Rhinol Laryngol 1989; 98:135-140.

Hoffman HT, Brunberg JA, Sullivan MJ, et al. Arytenoid subluxation: Diagnosis and treatment. Ann Otol Rhinol Laryngol 1991; 100:1-9.

Kashima HK. CO_2 laser arytenoidectomy and transverse cordotomy. In: Johns ME, ed. Atlas of head and neck surgery. Vol. 1. Philadelphia: BC Decker, 1990:44.

Meiteles LZ, Lin P, Wenk EJ. An anatomic study of the external laryngeal framework with surgical implications. Otolaryngol Head Neck Surg 1992; 106:235-240.

Ossoff RH, Duncavage JA, Krespi PY, et al. Endoscopic laser arytenoidectomy revisited. Ann Otol Rhinol Laryngol 1990; 99:764-771.

Remacle M, Mayne A, Lawson G, Jamart J. Subtotal carbon dioxide laser arytenoidectomy by endoscopic approach for treatment of bilateral cord immobility in adduction. Ann Otol Rhinol Laryngol 1996; 105: 438-445.

Smith E, Verdolini K, Gray S, et al. Effect of voice disorders on quality of life. J Med Speech-Language Pathol 1920; 4:223-244.

Tucker H. Long-term results of nerve-muscle pedicle reinnervation for laryngeal paralysis. Ann Otol Rhinol Laryngol 1989; 98:674-676.

ASPIRATION

The method of
Marshall Strome

The sequelae of aspiration of food or secretions can run the gamut from insidious to catastrophic. Management should be based on the etiology of the physiologic aberrations, and perhaps what is more important, on the short-term and long-term prognoses. Not only are the volume and origin of the aspirate important, but also its content and pH.

EVALUATION

History

For the cerebrally intact patient, a history of aspiration may involve intermittent hoarseness, coughing, a wet voice, dyspepsia, and substernal burning. A chronic cough may be the only symptom of intermittent aspiration of gastric contents. The associated hoarseness is caused by chronic irritation, with documentable changes being prevalent primarily in the posterior aspect of the larynx. The severity can be further assessed by investigating weight loss, dietary change, bolus consistency, the duration and frequency of meals, as well as special posturing of the head and neck musculature that may be used to facilitate deglutition. Because the etiology is multifactorial, considerations must include myopathies, neuropathies, cerebrovascular accidents, and carcinoma.

Physical Examination

The comprehensive head and neck examination must include a complete cranial nerve evaluation, with nerves IX, X, and XII being particularly relevant. Fiberoptic endoscopy as part of the initial evaluation gives detailed information regarding the tongue base, vocal cord mobility, laryngeal elevation and closure, as well as pharyngeal and upper esophageal synchrony. It is essential that no topical anesthesia be used when performing examination of the latter areas. In addition, the procedure enables an evaluation of the epiglottis, defining whether its length and width are adequate to be used in a closure procedure.

Fluoroscopy

Three techniques—cinefluoroscopy, videofluoroscopy, and esophageal manometry—are of value in assisting the surgeon in the management of aspiration. Cinefluoroscopy, frequently designated as a modified barium swallow, involves swallowing small aliquots of varying consistencies: cookie, paste, and liquid. The technique provides stop-frame analysis of deglutition. Simultaneous voice recording is attainable with videofluoroscopy, and frame analysis is similarly feasible. Although the standard barium swallow does not provide adequate detail of oropharyngeal and hypopharyngeal motility, it does enable the clinician to make a reasonably precise assessment of pharyngoesophageal structural lesions (i.e., neoplasms and aberrations of the lower esophagus). Its major disadvantage rests with the fact that a large volume of barium is necessary to complete the study in patients who are being evaluated for aspiration. One can anticipate that the two fluoroscopic techniques will assess transit time, laryngeal elevation, timing of aspiration, and, most important, the patient's ability to handle aspirated material (i.e., clear it with an effective cough or have a substantial amount enter the tracheal or bronchial tree). Further synchrony of the pharynx and upper esophageal sphincter as well as residue in the piriform sinuses can also be assessed.

Manometry

Manometry is not a test for aspiration per se, but it can give useful functional information by identifying pressure variances in the upper esophageal sphincter (UES). Simultaneous measurements can be recorded in the UES, pharynx, and esophagus. Combining videofluoroscopy with manometry, McConnel has further refined our ability to detect specific areas of malfunction.

Sensory Testing

A recently described laryngopharyngeal sensory test can provide additional data in the assessment of aspiration. The supraglottis and both sides of the pharynx are evaluated using a special Pentax fiberoptic laryngoscope. A puff of air, controlled for pressure and duration, is used to define the sensory pressure threshold.

THERAPY

Any treatment regimen considered must be relevant to the magnitude of the problem and the patient's prognosis as related to the etiology. The occasional aspiration that not infrequently accompanies the aging process needs no management. The aspiration of gastric contents that occurs with recumbency, particularly if associated with irritative change in the posterior larynx, can usually be managed with the well-known antireflux regimens. But life-threatening aspiration, as evidenced by recurrent pneumonia (which often occurs in the elderly), may be best managed by early surgical intervention. However, a decision to separate the laryngotracheal complex from the gullet should be reached only after intensive medical management and conservative surgery have failed.

Swallowing Measures

If diagnostic studies suggest that maintaining alimentation without system overload is feasible, it is essential that the physician educate the patient at the bedside on how this can be accomplished. When the cords are functioning properly, I instruct the patient on closure maneuvers, such as Valsalva's maneuver during deglutition, and stress that after the bolus has entered the esophagus, a clearing cough can itself prevent incapacitating aspiration from occurring in selected instances. Similarly, a lateral, semirecumbent position in which the neck is partially flexed can enable feeding to take place for some patients.

Gastrostomy

Parenteral feedings are initiated when oropharyngeal secretions are not problematic but larger boluses are associated with aspiration. Before considering gastrostomy, gavage feeding should be taught; it is relatively easily mastered. Later, if indicated, a pediatric feeding tube, used as a conduit for a continuous drip proprietary formula, can provide caloric intake and minimize gastric dilatation and reflux. However, a gastrostomy is preferable for long-term nutritional support and can have a protective function as well. Many patients can tolerate small amounts of saliva entering the upper airway, but not the large bolus introduced by active deglutition. Esophagostomy and piriformostomy are techniques available to all head and neck surgeons, yet are not indicated in this setting. In this instance, the further away from the laryngoesophageal region the nutritional port remains, the better.

Tracheotomy

When problematic aspiration persists after a gastrostomy, a tracheotomy should be considered, particularly if the etiology is determined to be short-lived. Irrespective of the theory of and known physiologic considerations surrounding tracheotomy and its contribution to aspiration and dysphagia, it is a requisite for all closure procedures. As such, recognizing its potential effect as an independent, therapeutic entity in selected circumstances is germane. Tracheotomy does not prevent all aspiration, but with a low-pressure cuff inflated it can eliminate most soilage and provide access for effective trachea and pulmonary toilet. The combination of a tracheotomy with an inflated low-pressure cuff and gastrostomy for nutritional support can provide a meaningful short-term solution. Acknowledging that small amounts of aspirate are the result of imperfect cuff seals, with expert nursing care, this is usually not problematic. Infrequent large aspirates become less of an issue with the availability of tracheal suctioning. Removing oropharyngeal secretions before cuff deflation can decrease or eliminate pulmonary contamination. Tracheotomy is not a long-term solution to the problem of aspiration, but as a temporizing measure it can provide humidification, airway access, and significant airway protection.

Cricopharyngeal Myotomy

When a modified barium swallow defines cricopharyngeal dysfunction related to primary cricopharyngeal achalasia or following major ablative head and neck surgery, a cricopharyngeal myotomy may be beneficial. It may, in selected instances, be useful for myopathies, for example, inclusion body myositis. Most patients who have cricopharyngeal achalasia do not require surgical intervention. Only those who have significant dysphagia and/or aspiration warrant myotomy. Technically, introducing a flexible cuffed endotracheal tube into the esophagus and inflating the balloon makes it far easier to cut all of the requisite muscle fibers. To be effective, the myotomy must include the cricopharyngeus plus an additional 3 cm of both pharyngeal and esophageal musculature. Postoperative swallowing studies are not essential in a capitated environment if swallowing symptomatically is improved.

Vocal Cord Augmentation

Aspiration that is associated with a unilateral vocal cord paralysis can usually be managed with medialization of the cord. Injection of an absorbable material, Gelfoam, can provide closure for several months and is the procedure of choice if there is any possibility of spontaneous recovery. Teflon paste will effect a long-term result when chronicity is anticipated. Thyroplasty type I has been gaining support. Although removal of a Silastic implant is possible, if mobility returns, function following implant removal is not normal. Because patients who have aspiration are frequently debilitated, the simplest technique is always the most prudent.

Closure Procedures

Whenever aspiration becomes life threatening and the aforementioned considerations are neither germane nor efficacious, closure procedures are frequently essential. The choice of the technique will depend in part on the surgeon's background and technical skills as well as on the patient's short- and long-term prognosis and vocal requisites. In choosing a procedure, there are several parameters to evaluate, the reliability of the procedure in controlling aspiration being foremost. Other issues include technical difficulty, ease of reversal of the procedure chosen, and the potential for and quality of voicing after reversal.

Laryngectomy

Total laryngectomy is the definitive procedure for aspiration and was widely espoused in the 1970s. However, in the 1990s, with many more elegant procedures available, its consideration should be limited to the permanently disabled, institutionalized patient, preferably an individual who has limited environmental awareness. Laryngectomy in mentally alert patients fosters depression, eliminates hope, and as such potentially hastens demise. Patients will almost uniformly (M. Strome, personal survey) choose voicing over oral alimentation if they are allowed to participate in the decision-making process.

Stents

To date, laryngeal stents have not been widely acknowledged as being successful in the management of chronic aspiration. Newer iterations should change current opinion. When tracheotomy with a low-pressure cuff is not sufficient and/or concern arises about the duration of cuff inflation, modern stents are the next logical step in management. Stenting is the simplest closure technique. Whereas solid stents did not afford vocalization, the most recent variation of the Eliachar stent does. It is made of soft silicone that is introduced through the tracheotomy site and is easily secured via an external silicone tongue. Most important, this stent is vented. It has been used satisfactorily for as long as 9 months. Disadvantages include potential soilage with improper sizing, granulation tissue formation, webs, and/or stenoses. The judicious use of antibiotics in patients who have acute or chronic airway infection can decrease the potential for delayed complications. I personally find the newer stents to be a very worthwhile step in managing aspiration.

Open Surgical Procedures

Three basic techniques have provided the foundation for most of the modifications that have been reported in the literature in recent years. These techniques include the epiglottic oversew, laryngotracheal separation with a proximal tracheoesophageal diversion and distal tracheostomy, and open endolaryngeal procedures, the most acknowledged of which is thyrotomy with vocal fold oversew.

Vocal Fold Closure

Vocal fold oversew is performed via a midline laryngofissure. The vocal cords are denuded, as are the ventricles and posterior commissure. The classic procedure has been an intricate suturing technique that approximates the true vocal folds; the false vocal cords can be included. This procedure has been later modified by interposing a superiorly based sternohyoid muscle flap, which is affixed to the interarytenoid area. Although the latter procedure enhanced closure, it also made potential reversal far more difficult. Reversal of these glottic and supraglottic stenoses were always at best technically demanding, and normal phonation could not realistically be expected. In my opinion, vocal cord suturing has always been the most efficacious technique for managing chronic and progressive aspiration when recovery from the underlying disease is guarded and all conservative measures have been exhausted. Botulinum toxin injected into both vocal folds before closure has further simplified this technique. Without cordal motion, after denuding the cover, simple suturing is adequate. The additional use of Gelfoam injected laterally approximates the cords, thus eliminating all tension on the sutures. The latter adjuncts eliminate the need for false cord apposition and/or external pedicled muscle. Also, postoperative failure is virtually eliminated. Reversal is now potentially much easier—laser lysis with keel insertion. As such, the utility of other endolaryngeal procedures is questionable (i.e., subperichondrial cricoidectomy and partial cricoidectomy, which are essentially not reversible).

Tracheal Separation

The tracheal separation technique has been updated and reported in the literature on multiple occasions. It has the advantages of both direct and indirect laryngeal assessment, which allow recovery to be monitored. Although technically challenging, this technique can be reversed, and an excellent quality of voice after reversal has been reported. The procedure necessitates interruption of the trachea at the third or fourth ring, with an associated distal trachea stoma and a proximal end-to-side tracheoesophageal anastomosis. Reversal requires resection of a tracheal ring and end-to-end tracheal anastomosis. The esophagotomy is closed with a conventional two-layer repair. A variation of the technique, designed for accommodating the high tracheotomy, includes oversewing the proximal tracheal stump. Removing an anterior wedge from the last upper tracheal ring can in some patients enhance formation of the blind proximal pouch. Rerouting the proximal segment through the sternocleidomastoid muscle and suturing the upper trachea to the skin has been described, but the potential for incontinence makes it little more than a historical consideration. The potential complications of this procedure are more serious than those of other procedures detailed. These complications include fistulization at the tracheoesophageal junction, with the danger of associated mediastinitis, leakage from the proximal pouch (if created), vocal cord paralysis, and laryngeal irritation that can occur when the larynx serves as a conduit for secretions. However, other than the technical demands of this procedure or its reversal, there can be no criticism of it. Based on the parameters detailed, the tracheal separation technique is an efficacious procedure.

Epiglottic Flap

The epiglottic flap was described by its originator as being successful in four of six patients reported. In one patient, a reversal was subsequently performed. After attempting several procedures as originally described, I modified the original technique, and this modification remains the technique that I prefer (an epiglottis that maintains its infantile characteristics, that is, is furled or stubby, precludes the use of this technique). Before considering surgery, I perform endoscopy because it is critical to determine the length, width, and anterior-posterior dimensions of the epiglottis. At endoscopy, I grasp the epiglottic tip and pull it over the arytenoids, thereby ensuring that closure is feasible. I now prefer an infrahyoid pharyngotomy through a transverse incision. Cutting the hyoepiglottic and thyroepiglottic ligaments is important to posterior positioning. The intrinsic spring of the cartilage can be reduced by linear striations made with either a scalpel or a laser, removal of wedges, and/or morselization; a thick epiglottis may need a combination of all three.

When the epiglottis falls posteriorly of its own accord and covers most of the inlet, preparation for suturing can commence. Mucosal surfaces of the aryepiglottic folds, arytenoids, and rim of the epiglottis are removed. I prefer a permanent, braided, synthetic suture (Ethibond) for closure. A two-layer closure is essential. Not infrequently after surgery, there may be a pinhole beneath the overhanging epiglottic rim that acts as a one-way valve for phonation, yet precludes aspiration.

My additional contribution to the technique was the consideration of sequential opening. The reversal is performed endoscopically with the laser. A probe is introduced through the tracheotomy site and passed in a retrograde fashion through the vocal cords until it is visible, elevating the epiglottis. With the use of a hand-held laser scope KTP fiber, any size fenestration can be created. Thus, beginning with a very small window, this technique offers a progressive functional assessment of improvement in the pathologic state. During separate procedures, the fenestra can be sequentially and conservatively enlarged. Increasing the diameter of the fenestra decreases the effort of phonation. If the technique is adhered to as described, failures should be few. The epiglottic flap technique is not for all patients. A lack of manual dexterity will in most instances preclude closure of the tracheotomy, thus limiting phonation potential. Severe arthritis and debilitating parkinsonism, among other disease states, could perhaps dictate the choice of a procedure for which closure, and not reversal, is the preeminent consideration. Similarly, patients who have expressive phonatory disorders would not necessarily have the potential for reversal as a prerequisite for treatment.

The major complication of this technique is basically the failure to achieve closure. However, if the surgeon pays attention to the details described in this chapter and defines suitable candidates, success is almost uniformly assured. Of the techniques currently available, the epiglottic procedure is the only one that offers the potential for immediate postoperative vocalization. This technique is not as technically demanding as some and is the one procedure that can be reversed in a graduated manner.

Severe aspiration that requires separation of the airway from the pharyngoesophagus is a rare entity. Therefore, the exposure to this condition that any one physician receives and thus the opportunity to assess the varied techniques available are limited. Nonetheless, one should not necessarily be wedded to a given procedure. The surgeon must integrate the patient's wishes, the etiology, and the prognosis in the decision-making process. There are ample techniques available to meet almost any contingency. In the future, vocal cord pacing could play a greater role. Miniaturization of a pacing device is in progress at The Cleveland Clinic Foundation, and synchronous pacing with the upper esophageal sphincter seems feasible. As such, the future seems to hold hope for significant progress in the management of aspiration.

ACUTE LARYNGEAL TRAUMA

The method of
Steven D. Schaefer

Early and proper management of the injured larynx is essential to preserve the patient's life, airway, and voice. Each case of external laryngeal trauma presents a unique set of problems, but despite the diversity of injuries, specific management guidelines can be applied to each situation.

Blunt trauma to the larynx may result in crushing of the laryngeal skeleton between the impinging object and the cervical spine. In such injuries, the momentum of the vocal folds causes a shearing effect between the vocalis muscle, the internal perichondrium, and the laryngeal ligaments. Arytenoid cartilage subluxation or dislocation may result in a fixed vocal fold. Unilateral recurrent laryngeal nerve injury is often associated with cricoarytenoid joint injuries due to the close proximity of the recurrent laryngeal nerve and the cricoid.

Penetrating trauma from knife and gunshot wounds causes injuries that may vary from minor lacerations to severe disruption of the cartilage, mucosa, soft tissue, nerves, and adjacent structures. The amount of energy absorbed by the cervical tissues secondary to a gunshot wound, and therefore the degree of injury, is directly related to the velocity and mass of the wounding missile. Knife wounds cause less peripheral soft-tissue damage and hence are cleaner, but it is difficult to determine the depth of penetration. Injuries to deep structures such as the thoracic duct, cervical nerves, great vessels, and viscera may occur well away from the entrance wound.

■ DIAGNOSIS AND EVALUATION

History and Physical Examination

Any patient who has anterior neck trauma should be considered to have an upper airway injury. The classic symptoms associated with laryngeal trauma include hoarseness, laryngeal pain, dyspnea, and dysphagia My experience suggests that no one symptom seems to correlate well with the severity of the injury. However, important clues about the potential consequence of the trauma can be learned from the history. For example, when patients are seen immediately after massive blunt trauma to the neck to have a normal-appearing larynx, the injury may not have fully evolved. Such patients may lose their airway several hours later to edema or hemorrhage.

The classic signs of external laryngeal trauma include stridor, hemoptysis, subcutaneous emphysema, and tenderness or deformity of the laryngeal skeleton. Along with a careful examination of the head and neck, direct fiberoptic laryngoscopy is essential to the evaluation of the upper airway. The larynx should be examined for vocal fold mobility, hematomas, lacerations, and airway patency.

Radiographic Evaluation

Computed tomography (CT) has replaced soft-tissue radiographs, xerograms, polytomography, and laryngograms as the examination of choice when evaluating laryngeal trauma. Such imaging should only be employed when the results will influence treatment rather than to document an obvious injury.

THERAPY

Figure 1 shows my management protocol for acute injuries of the larynx. There are two primary goals in such management: (1) preservation of life by maintaining the airway, and (2) restoration of lack of tracheotomy dependence and voice quality.

Emergency Care

The initial evaluation and treatment of the trauma patient consists of airway preservation, cardiac resuscitation, control of hemorrhage, stabilization of neural and spinal injuries, and a systematic investigation for injuries to other organ systems. If the airway is precarious, endotracheal intubation in this setting is potentially hazardous because the moderately traumatized larynx may be further injured during attempted intubation or may result in the loss of an already precarious airway. If orotracheal intubation is to be employed, it should be limited to those injuries in which the endolarynx is intact; the intubation should be performed under direct visualization by highly experienced personnel who use a small endotracheal tube. Because these conditions are often difficult to fulfill, I recommend tracheotomy under local anesthesia rather than endotracheal intubation in victims of laryngeal trauma who require an alternative airway.

Observation Versus Surgery

Once the airway has been stabilized, management is divided into observation versus surgical treatment, based on the extent of injury as determined by the physical examination and CT imaging. The decision to observe or surgically manage such injuries is determined by the likelihood that the injury will resolve without surgical intervention. At the University of Texas Southwestern Medical Center, Dallas, I studied 139 laryngeal trauma patients who were treated within 24 hours of injury, and found that observation alone achieved a satisfactory outcome for the following conditions: edema, small hematomas with intact mucosal coverage, small glottic or supraglottic lacerations without exposed cartilage, and single nondisplaced thyroid cartilage fractures in a stable larynx. The goal of observation or medical therapy is to eliminate further injury and promote rapid healing. Because the clinical course after significant blunt trauma to the neck is uncertain, hospitalization for the first 24 hours after injury is necessary. This time allows the physician to observe for signs of progressive airway compromise and to take steps to maximize a successful outcome. Bed rest with elevation of the head of the bed for several days promotes resolution of laryngeal edema. A period of voice rest may minimize further edema or reduce the progression of a hematoma or subcutaneous emphysema. The use of cool humidified room air helps prevent crust formation in the presence of mucosal damage and transient ciliary paralysis. Additional oxygen is not required (unless indicated by arterial blood gases) and may even be harmful, especially in older patients who are prone to carbon dioxide retention. Although the value of systemic corticosteroids in general for treating laryngeal trauma is questionable, they may be useful in the immediate postinjury setting to accelerate the resolution of edema in the aforementioned minimal injuries.

During this initial observation period, those patients who have significant endolaryngeal edema or hematomas may need to be restricted to a clear liquid diet, with intravenous supplementation as required by any additional injuries. Nasogastric tubes are best avoided because they are often unnecessary, may worsen the injury during their passage, and promote gastroesophageal reflux. The results of the treatment of patients who had the aforementioned injuries are shown in Table 1; these groups are referred to as types 1 and 2 management groups. Patients in the type 2 management group differ from patients in the type 1 group in that they required tracheotomy to stabilize their airway. Once the airway was stabilized, these patients underwent further evaluation via direct laryngoscopy and esophagoscopy, and were thereafter observed. An exception to the aforementioned recommendations are those patients who have single nondisplaced angulated fractures of the thyroid cartilage. Experimental evidence suggests that these patients should undergo open reduction and internal fixation to prevent subtle vocal changes.

In the same patient population, I found that injuries that would benefit from surgical treatment via open laryngeal exploration and repair include lacerations involving the free margin of the vocal fold, large mucosal lacerations, exposed cartilage, multiple and displaced cartilage fractures, avulsed or dislocated arytenoids, and vocal fold immobility. Injuries likely to require open exploration, primary repair, and endolaryngeal stenting include disruption of the anterior commissure, multiple and displaced cartilage fractures, and multiple and severe endolaryngeal lacerations. Stenting is indicated in the aforementioned injuries to prevent loss of the normal scaphoid shape of the anterior commissure, stabilize severely comminuted fractures or lacerations, and prevent endolaryngeal stenosis. In general, penetrating trauma is more likely to require open exploration than is blunt trauma. Olson believes that waiting several days after trauma allows the edema to resolve so that endolaryngeal lacerations

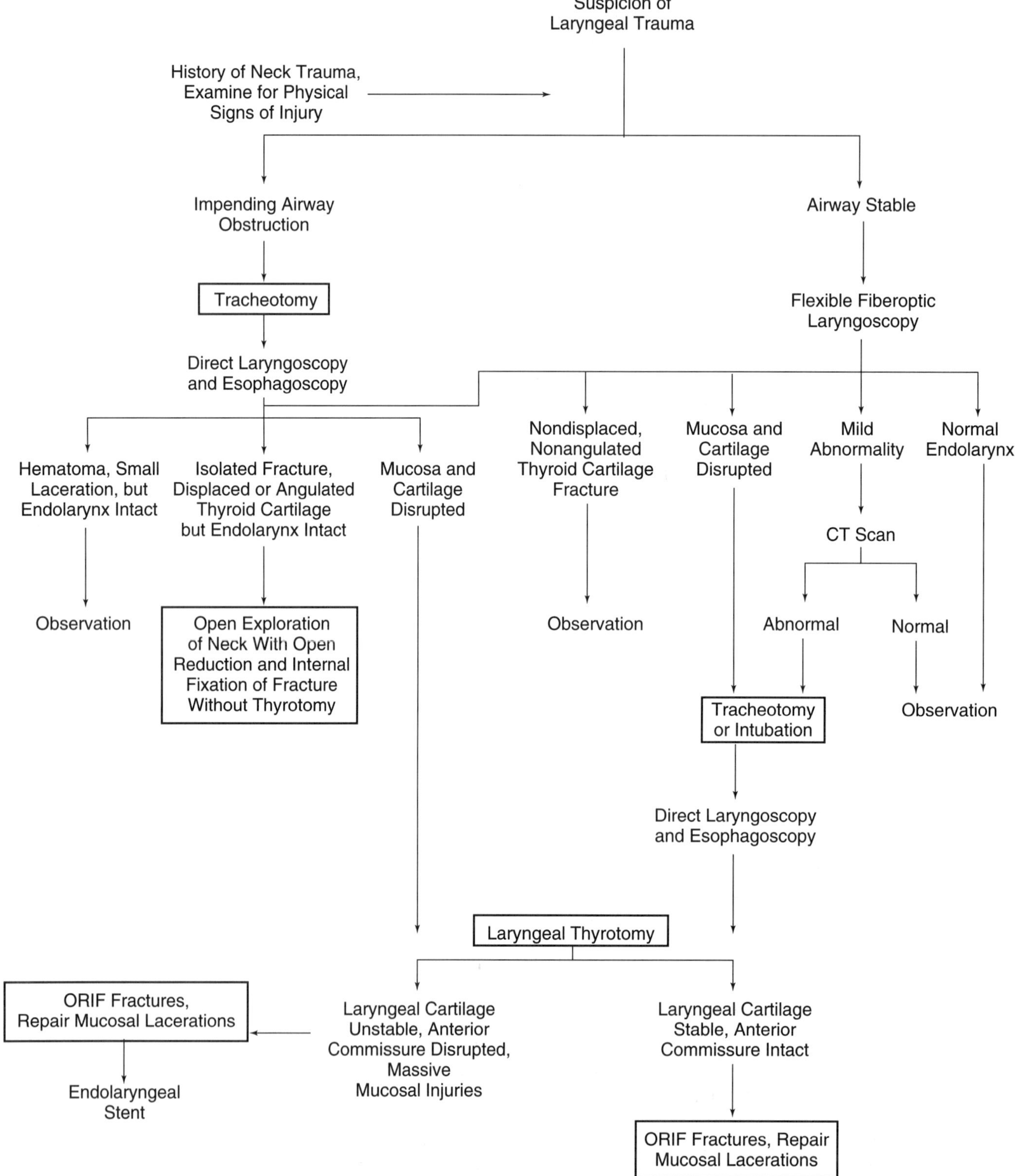

Figure 1.
Management protocol for the acutely injured larynx. ORIF, open reduction internal fixation. *(From Schaefer SD. The acute management of external laryngeal trauma. A 27 year experience. Arch Otolaryngol Head Neck Surg 1992; 118:598; with permission.)*

Table 1. Voice and Airway Results of Evaluable Patients by Management Groups*

GROUP	VOICE			AIRWAY			TOTAL
	GOOD	FAIR	POOR	GOOD	FAIR	POOR	(N = 115)
I	20	0	0	20	0	0	20
II	38	3	0	40	1	0	41
III	18	3	0	21	0	0	21
IV	23	10	0	31	0	2	33

* Group I patients had no airway compromise and were judged to have reversible injuries. They were managed by observation only. Group II patients had airway compromise and were considered to have reversible injuries. They were managed by tracheotomy, direct laryngoscopy, esophagoscopy, and observation. Group III patients were judged to have irreversible laryngeal fractures and/or lacerations that required management by open reduction and fixation of disrupted cartilage and/or mucous membrane. Group IV patients had more severe injuries as discussed in the text and management differed from group III in that endolaryngeal stents were used. (From Schaefer SD. The acute management of external laryngeal trauma. A 27 year experience. Arch Otolaryngol Head Neck Surg 1992;118:598–604; with permission.)

may be better identified and approximated. In contrast, I strongly believe that early surgical treatment offers the opportunity for a complete assessment of the injury, which potentially results in a lower postoperative infection rate, quicker healing, less granulation tissue, and subsequently less scarring. The results of such a management protocol are noted in Table 1. Such treatment begins with endoscopy to determine the full extent of laryngeal and adjacent aerodigestive tract injury.

■ OPERATIVE TECHNIQUE

Laryngeal exploration is done through a horizontal incision in a skin crease at the level of the cricothyroid membrane. Subplatysmal flaps are elevated superiorly to the level of the hyoid bone and inferiorly to just below the cricoid. The incision can be extended to explore and repair any associated neural, vascular, or visceral injuries. The infrahyoid strap muscles are separated in the midline and retracted laterally to expose the laryngeal skeleton and any fractures. The thyroid cartilage is incised at the midline, and the endolarynx is entered through the cricothyroid membrane. Under direct visualization, the incision is extended superiorly through the anterior commissure to the thyrohyoid membrane. The entire endolarynx is examined to identify the full extent of the injury. The arytenoids are palpated to assess their position and mobility.

All mucous membrane, muscle, and cartilage with a viable blood supply should be preserved and restored to their original position. Because exposed cartilage is the primary factor responsible for the formation of granulation tissue and subsequent fibrosis, it must be covered primarily. Failure to do so results in the need for grafting and healing by secondary intention. Lacerations are meticulously approximated with 5–0 or 6–0 absorbable suture material. Mucosal advancement flaps may be needed to relieve tension on suture lines and achieve complete cartilage coverage.

Cartilaginous fractures are fixated with wire, nonabsorbable suture, or miniplates. Small fragments of cartilage with no intact perichondrium are removed to prevent subsequent chondritis. The anterior margin of each true vocal fold is sutured to the thyroid cartilage or its external perichondrium at the thyrotomy site to reconstitute the anterior commissure. Finally, the thyrotomy is closed with wire, nonabsorbable suture, or miniplates. If part of the anterior cricoid ring is lost, suturing the infrahyoid strap muscles into the defect may help maintain the airway and voice.

Adhering to the principles of conservation of normal anatomy and immediate operative management makes the need for a graft rare. Mucous membrane or skin grafts have been used to cover areas of exposed cartilage that cannot be closed primarily. However, these wounds must heal by secondary intention, which leads to greater scar formation than with primary closure. In the rare situation in which a graft is required, mucous membrane, dermis, and split-thickness skin are suitable. Mucous membrane most closely resembles the normal endolaryngeal epithelium but has variable donor-site morbidity and requires entering the oral cavity. Grafting should never be considered a substitute for the careful closure of all significant laryngeal lacerations.

Laryngeal stents are reserved for injuries that include disruption of the anterior commissure, severely comminuted fractures, or massive endolaryngeal lacerations. Employing stents in lesser injuries invites potential infection and granulation tissue. Stents alone should not be considered a substitute for primary closure of mucosal lacerations and careful reduction and internal fixation of fractures. When a stent is used, it should be fixed in the larynx in such a fashion that it moves with the larynx during swallowing. In addition, the stent should be consistently and easily recoverable by endoscopy alone. A useful method is to pass a heavy synthetic nonabsorbable suture through the stent and the larynx at the level of the laryngeal ventricle and another at the cricothyroid membrane. These are then tied over buttons on the skin. Although superior and inferior sutures may be brought out through the nose and the tracheotomy site for additional safety, I have not employed this technique in more than 15 years.

There are various reports as to how long to leave a stent in place. The desired laryngeal stabilization must be achieved, and scar formation should be prevented, but the potential for infection and wound necrosis associated with prolonged stenting should be considered. If all wounds have been carefully closed and the fractures have been effectively stabilized, clinical experience suggests that 14 days is a reasonable compromise and yields good results.

The stent is removed via direct laryngoscopy, and the

operative result is assessed. Any granulation tissue can be removed with the conservative use of a CO_2 laser. The need for additional endoscopic manipulation should be determined by serial fiberoptic laryngeal examinations. Decannulation is best deferred until the patient can tolerate prolonged plugging of the tracheotomy tube.

Cricotracheal Separation

When managing cricotracheal separation, several factors unique to this injury must be considered, including a precarious airway, loss of cricoid support, a high incidence of recurrent laryngeal nerve injury, and the late development of subglottic stenosis. When a patient sustains lower cervical trauma, this injury must be considered and recognized so that the tenuous airway can be preserved. The airway is best controlled by performing a tracheotomy under local anesthesia. An alternative form of intubation is to use a ventilating bronchoscope, followed by repair of the injury and tracheotomy as needed. If the cricoid cartilage is found to be intact, direct mucous membrane repair is done with absorbable suture. To distribute the tension on the wound away from the cricotracheal anastomosis, nonabsorbable sutures are placed from the superior aspect of the cricoid to the inferior aspect of the second tracheal ring. In the presence of a fractured cricoid, the effectiveness of the repair is limited by the stability of the cricoid cartilage after internal fixation. Reconstitution of the severely injured cricoid cartilage, with the assistance of internal fixation and stenting, is preferable to significant resection of the cricoid with thyrotracheal anastomosis because of the likelihood of immobility of the vocal folds.

Transection of the Recurrent Laryngeal Nerve

The management of the severed recurrent laryngeal nerve continues to be a surgical dilemma. Even with careful microscopic repair of the transected nerve, vocal fold mobility is not regained due to the mixture of abductor and adductor fibers in the nerve. However, nerve regeneration may prevent muscle atrophy, which maintains some strength of the voice. Acute anastomosis of the phrenic nerve to the distal stump of the recurrent laryngeal nerve, or direct implantation of the phrenic nerve into the posterior cricoarytenoid muscle have not proved to be more efficacious than simple anastomosis of the severed nerve. Therefore, it appears at present that the best acute-phase management is to immediately reapproximate the nerve under the operating microscope.

■ OUTCOME

In my series of 115 evaluable of 139 patients with laryngeal trauma who were managed by the previously discussed protocol at the University of Texas Southwestern Medical Center at Dallas, only two patients were left with a poor airway, as defined by the inability to decannulate (Table 1). Time to decannulation in those patients undergoing tracheotomy along with exploration ranged from 14 to 35 days, whereas those patients who had stents (usually reserved for more severe injuries) needed 35 to 100 days to decannulation. All but 16 of the 115 evaluable patients achieved a good voice; these 16 patients were classified as having a fair voice.

Despite strict adherence to proper principles of management of laryngeal trauma, fibrosis and subsequent stenosis may occur. Therapeutic measures used in the treatment of stenosis depend, to some extent, on the level of the stenosis. Supraglottic stenosis may often be corrected by simply excising the scar tissue, then using local advancement flaps for wound coverage. Sometimes, this requires removing a significant portion of the epiglottis or aryepiglottic fold; rarely, a supraglottic laryngectomy is needed. A keel or stent may be used as needed to maintain the repair.

The rehabilitation of glottic stenosis depends on the extent of the lesion. Thin anterior glottic webs can be simply lysed, and then a keel can be placed to prevent recurrence. Posterior glottic webs or interarytenoid scarring can be excised along with an arytenoidectomy and resurfaced with local mucosal advancement flaps. Extensive glottic stenosis often requires a laryngofissure with direct excision of the stenotic area, followed by placement of a tissue graft with a stent to promote re-epithelialization.

Subglottic stenosis continues to be difficult to treat, no matter what the etiology. Less extensive lesions can be treated with repeated dilatation or conservative noncircumferential laser excision of the scar tissue. More significant stenosis may require anterior or posterior cricoid splits with cartilage grafting to increase the size of the subglottic lumen. Stenting is usually required, as well as multiple endoscopic procedures to excise granulation tissue after removal of the stent. Significant tracheal stenosis in a short segment is managed by resecting the stenotic area with end-to-end tracheal anastomosis. Lesions up to 4 cm can be resected with laryngeal release techniques.

After blunt trauma, a persistently immobile vocal fold may be due to either recurrent laryngeal nerve injury or cricoarytenoid joint fixation. Differentiating these causes is essential in selecting the proper form of therapy. This is best accomplished by observing the vocal fold for any sign of movement with either fiberoptic laryngoscopy or direct laryngoscopy under light anesthesia, followed by direct palpation of the arytenoid to assess its mobility. Laryngeal electromyography is also useful in determining the cause of immobility and the likelihood of reinnervation. Patients who have significant morbidity from sustained unilateral immobility and electromyography-documented reinnervation at 6 months are appropriately treated by thyroplasty.

Suggested Reading

Crumley RL. Phrenic nerve graft for bilateral vocal cord paralysis. Laryngoscope 1983; 93:444-448.

Gordon JH, McCabe BF. The effect of accurate neurorrhaphy on reinnervation and return of laryngeal function. Laryngoscope 1968; 78:236-240.

Olson NR. Surgical treatment of acute blunt laryngeal injuries. Ann Otol Rhinol Laryngol 1978; 87:716-721.

Schaefer SD. The acute management of external laryngeal trauma. A 27 year experience. Arch Otolaryngol Head Neck Surg 1992; 118:598-605.

Schaefer SD. The treatment of acute external laryngeal injures. Arch Otolaryngol Head Neck Surg 1991; 117:35-40.

Schaefer SD, Brown OE. Selective application of CT in the management of laryngeal trauma. Laryngoscope 1983; 93:1473-1477.

Stanley RB, Cooper DS, Florman SH. Phonatory effects of thyroid cartilage fractures. Ann Otol Rhinol Laryngol 1987; 96:493-496.

POSTLARYNGECTOMY APHONIA

The method of
Mark I. Singer
Carla DeLassus Gress

Laryngectomy results in a number of altered functions, of which aphonia is the most devastating. Traditional methods of alaryngeal speech include esophageal voice and the use of artificial devices, powered electronically or pneumatically, to provide a voicing source. Many laryngectomees achieve effective and efficient communication using these methods.

Tracheoesophageal puncture (TEP) has gained worldwide acceptance as the preferred method of speech restoration since its introduction by Singer and Blom in 1980. In this technique, communication between the trachea and esophagus is re-established endoscopically by creating a small puncture in the common wall at a location inferior to the cricopharyngeus and pharyngeal constrictor muscles. This permits the use of the pulmonary air supply to achieve esophageal vibration, which provides a voicing source for speech production. The tract is bridged by a silicone prosthesis that prevents the tract from closing and incorporates a one-way valve to eliminate aspiration of esophageal contents (Fig. 1). The success of this procedure is due to its simplicity, low cost, infrequent complications, lack of interference with cancer control, and superior voice characteristics in the majority of patients.

■ PATIENT ASSESSMENT

The voice restoration technique was originally developed as a secondary procedure to be performed at any point postlaryngectomy, allowing a few weeks for sufficient tissue healing. Candidacy for secondary tracheoesophageal puncture is determined with a concern for the relative importance of a number of factors, including the patient's general health, motivation, initial disease extent, operative technique, quality of peristomal tissue healing, radiotherapy, and reconstructive method. Dementia, significant respiratory compromise, reduced vision, and limited manual dexterity are relevant considerations in the evaluation. Microstomas should be dilated and stented with a laryngectomy tube or revised by Z-plasty technique to ensure easy manipulation of the prosthesis into the puncture tract after the voice restoration procedure. Reconstruction of the pharyngoesophagus through the use of radial forearm or jejunal free flaps, gastric pullup, or other myocutaneous flaps does not preclude tracheoesophageal voice restoration. However, in some cases, the reconstructed segment will have reduced vibratory capability that results in suboptimal vocal quality.

Esophageal Insufflation

Preoperative esophageal insufflation of the laryngectomized patient can provide important information regarding the potential of the vibrating segment. Using a catheter placed transnasally a distance of 25 cm into the upper esophagus, air is introduced by an external source or by a special connector fixed to the tracheostoma. As air passes across the pharyngoesophageal segment and the patient attempts to vocalize, vibration of the tissue should occur and result in a sustained vocal tone. The ability to prolong phonation for 10 to 15 seconds and count fluently from 1 to 15, without extreme effort or straining, suggests that the vibrating segment will be sufficiently supple for efficient vocal production following the restoration procedure.

In contrast, the patient who produces little or no sound, has a strained vocal quality, or complains of gastric filling and retrosternal pressure may be experiencing pharyngeal constrictor spasm. After ascertaining that the catheter is correctly placed in the esophagus, further assessment is performed by combining fluoroscopic imaging (lateral view) of the voicing dynamics with pharyngeal plexus nerve block using 150 to 200 mg of 2 percent lidocaine without epinephrine. Marked improvement in fluency accompanied by a reduction in esophageal distention and a decrease in the mass of the constrictor muscles is suggestive of pharyngeal constrictor spasm, thus identifying the patient as being at risk for voice failure following the restoration procedure. Other causes of failed insufflation include postirradiation edema, stricture, or the presence of recurrent disease.

■ SECONDARY TRACHEOESOPHAGEAL PUNCTURE

Puncture Technique

The operative procedure involves the introduction of a rigid esophagoscope through the laryngectomized pharynx and upper thoracic esophagus under general anesthesia. At the tracheostoma, the esophagoscope is rotated 180 degrees so that the longer side of the bevel is apposed to the posterior trachea. The membranous trachea is palpated through the stoma to ascertain that the esophagoscope is against the posterior trachea. A puncture location 5 mm from the superior trachea is identified, and the window of the esophagoscope is aligned with this point. A 14 gauge needle is curved and introduced through the wall of the trachea, which corresponds with the window, by using direct vision through the esophagoscope to guide the needle into the lumen of the endoscope.

With the needle in place, a 16 gauge intravenous catheter is threaded through until it is retrieved at the mouth. The needle is withdrawn, and the puncture is dilated carefully with a small hemostat while the catheter is used as a guide. Next, a urethral catheter (14 Fr, filiform, or other gradually tapered device) is attached to the intravenous catheter. With continuous traction at the mouth, the intravenous catheter/dilating catheter is pulled retrograde through the esophagus and hypopharynx into the oral cavity. The intravenous catheter is released, and in the absence of significant bleeding, the esophagoscope is reinserted. The integrity of the anterior esophageal wall is examined at the site of the puncture, and

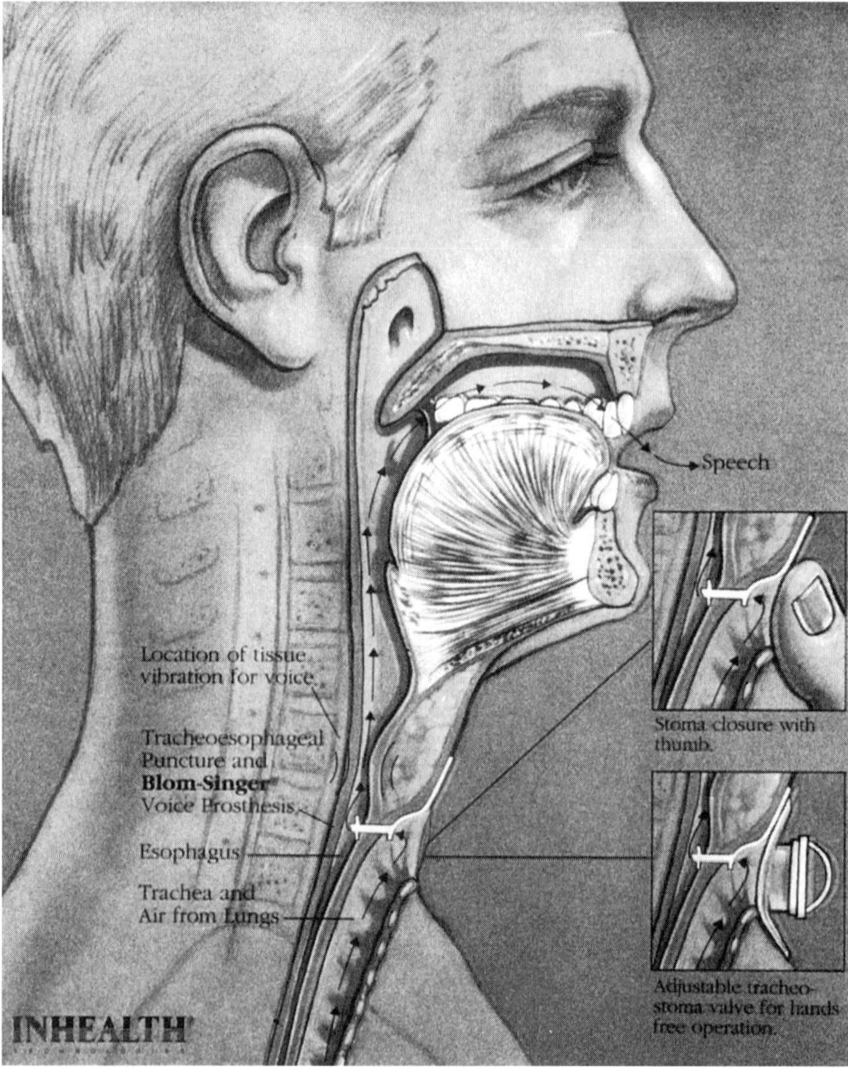

Figure 1.
Tracheoesophageal voice prosthesis. *(From International Healthcare Technologies, a division of Helix Medical, Inc. Blom-Singer is a registered trademark of Hansa Medical Products, Inc., Carpinteria, CA; with permission.)*

the tip of the endoscope is used to carefully direct the dilating catheter into the distal esophagus. The dilating catheter is tied in place with a suture at the lateral tracheostoma. The patient is released on an ambulatory basis with a 48 hour course of prophylactic antibiotics and can resume a normal diet.

Pharyngeal Constrictor Relaxation Techniques

There are several choices available if preoperative assessment has determined the need for a pharyngeal constrictor relaxation procedure. A pharyngeal constrictor myotomy can be performed at the time of tracheoesophageal puncture by using a dilator (French No. 36) in a manner similar to cricopharyngeal myotomy for dysphagia in patients who have an intact larynx.

A secondary unilateral pharyngeal plexus neurectomy, performed contralateral to radical neck dissection in a method similar to pharyngeal constrictor myotomy, represents an alternative approach. In this technique, the pharynx is distended with a mercury-filled dilator, and the parapharyngeal tissues are dissected to the level of the prevertebral fascia. The carotid sheath is reflected laterally, and the pharynx is rotated away from the sheath, which exposes the posterolateral wall of the pharyngoesophagus.

The fascia overlying the constrictor muscles is carefully dissected superiorly to the base of the tongue. The middle pharyngeal constrictor, which is bulkier than the inferior constrictor and represents less than 20 percent of the vertical length of the upper esophageal sphincter, serves as a key landmark; at its junction with the corresponding inferior pharyngeal constrictor, the main branches of the pharyngeal plexus course before dividing and innervating the underlying constrictor muscle fibers.

After identifying the pharyngeal plexus, which represents one to three nerve branches at this level, the fibers are electrocoagulated and divided. The wound is drained away from the stoma and closed. Moderate soft-tissue edema may result, especially in irradiated patients, or there may be tracheitis from intubation. The patient may resume a normal diet postoperatively and is usually discharged in 24 hours.

A third option for management of pharyngoesophageal spasm is the use of botulinum toxin injections. Although repeated injections are required approximately every 6 months, the procedure can be performed in the office and eliminates the need for additional surgery beyond the tracheoesophageal puncture.

Prosthesis Fitting Technique

Placement of the voice prosthesis can be initiated 48 hours after puncture, assuming there is adequate healing at the operative site. The dilating catheter placed at the time of puncture is removed, and the puncture is serially dilated using catheters to 18 Fr to ease placement of the measuring device and the prosthesis. The patient is instructed not to swallow while the puncture is unstented, because aspiration of pharyngeal secretions may occur and induce coughing. The horizontal distance from the membranous trachea to the anterior surface of the esophagus is determined using a measuring device.

Voicing is initially assessed "open tract" (in the absence of a prosthesis or stent) by covering the tracheostoma after inhalation and asking the patient to attempt phonation of a gentle "ah." Most patients will phonate easily, and connected speech may be attempted for a brief period. Usually the open tract voice represents the best possible vocal tone, because air will flow freely through the puncture without the resistance of a prosthesis. Absence of fluent phonation during the open tract test, in the presence of an adequately occluded stoma, suggests that the vibrating segment is not a viable sound-producing mechanism.

Following successful open tract voicing, the prosthesis is attached to its inserter and introduced into the puncture. As the prosthesis is advanced, its flexible retention collar will fold, which allows the prosthesis shaft to enter the puncture tract. When fully inserted, the retention collar unfolds in the esophagus and offers slight resistance to gentle retraction attempts. While still attached to the inserter, 360 degree rotation of the prosthesis confirms placement fully into the lumen of the esophagus. The inserter is withdrawn, and the silicone strap is affixed vertically above the tracheostoma with paper adhesive tape. Assessment of proper functioning of the prosthesis valve for prevention of aspiration can be accomplished by observing the absence of leakage as the patient sips water.

Initial voice production attempts commence with instruction in careful stoma occlusion for efficient airflow and proper breath control for easy voicing. Usually under the direction of a speech pathologist, the patient learns correct hygiene practices, prosthesis cleaning, and the replacement technique, in addition to the guidelines for emergency situations. Long-term success requires that the patient fully comprehend the importance of maintaining the puncture at all times through proper placement of a prosthesis, dilating stent, or catheter, and of diligently observing the prosthesis for signs of failure.

The early experience with the duckbill voice prosthesis demonstrated the need for development of additional prosthesis types designed to meet individualized patient requirements for aerodynamic characteristics, length of wear, and ease of insertion. Low-pressure devices feature lowered prosthesis resistance to airflow and usually result in less effortful voicing. Increased airflow, with associated louder vocal production, can be attained with the use of larger diameter (20 Fr) devices. Current trends include the development of long-wearing (approximately 4 to 6 months) devices with improved retention ability, which reduce the patient's responsibility for removal and reinsertion. These devices are cleaned externally while positioned in the puncture tract. Candidiasis can result in premature failure of the prosthesis (usually valve degradation with aspiration through the prosthesis), but can be managed effectively with nystatin oral suspension.

Tracheostoma Valve

Patients initially learn to cover the tracheostoma manually, but hygiene concerns and the associated social handicaps render this practice less than ideal. The preferred method of occlusion is using a tracheostoma valve attached to either the peritracheal skin or a silicone tube (similar to a laryngectomy tube) that is inserted into the tracheostoma. The device consists of a curled valve diaphragm that closes against a housing as a result of high-speech airflows, but remains open for normal respiration when flows decrease. Successful use of the "hands-free" valve requires adequate respiratory function and a meticulous technique if an adhesive attachment is used to ensure a long-lasting seal. It is estimated that approximately 25 percent to 30 percent of laryngectomized speakers are successful in using the tracheostoma valve for hands-free speech.

■ PRIMARY TRACHEOESOPHAGEAL PUNCTURE

The voice restoration procedure can also be performed at the time of laryngectomy without compromise of the oncologic technique. The tracheoesophageal puncture is placed after the stoma is constructed and before closure of the pharynx. The upper tracheal rings are fixed anteriorly and inferiorly to the skin flap rather than through a concentric skin defect. After the tracheostoma is stabilized, a right-angled hemostat is placed against the membranous trachea by way of the open pharynx. The membranous trachea is incised transversely 3 to 4 mm to allow protrusion of the hemostat into the tracheostoma. The tracheostoma common wall should be closed to prevent leakage of saliva into this space if it has become separated. A 16 Fr Foley catheter is directed downward into the esophagus using the tip of the hemostat and will serve to stent the TEP in addition to its use as a feeding tube.

Pharyngeal constrictor relaxation is accomplished by constrictor myotomy in the posterior midline raphe, or by a unilateral pharyngeal plexus neurectomy. For primary TEP, neurectomy is the preferred method, because it effectively reduces the tendency toward sphincter spasm while maintaining the vascularity and elasticity of the constrictor muscles, which theoretically produces a more pliable pharynx for the alteration of pitch.

The pharyngeal plexus is identified by rotating the intact larynx to midline after neck dissection and before blocking the specimen for resection. The main branches of the pharyngeal plexus travel through a muscular hiatus at the junction of the middle and inferior constrictor muscles through a space created by the cornu of the thyroid cartilage and the greater cornu of the hyoid bone. The neurectomy is completed by verifying the nerves through electrostimulation, followed by electrocoagulation and division.

■ COMPLICATIONS

The most common urgent complication occurs when the prosthesis is too short or improperly inserted and fails to bridge the entire length of the tracheoesophageal common wall. The initial complaint will be of increased effort in speaking, and in some cases the prosthesis will begin to extrude, as the TEP tract begins to close from the esophagus externally. Access to the lumen will be lost within 24 to 48 hours unless proper stenting is employed. Timely management involves serial dilation of the tract with plastic catheters ranging from 10 to 18 Fr done with as little resistance as possible to prevent separation of the tracheoesophageal common wall, followed by stenting with a flexible dilator for several hours to re-establish an adequate lumen.

Aspiration of the voice prosthesis occurs infrequently, usually when the prosthesis is unsecured in the tract as the patient attempts its replacement. The most common location for device impaction is at the level of the upper right mainstem bronchus and carina. Uncomfortable dyspnea and tracheal aspiration of saliva through the unstented puncture result. Detailed instruction in emergency measures provided at the time of initial prosthesis fitting will prevent this complication. The patient should first stent the puncture, then bend over as far as possible and attempt to cough out the prosthesis, avoiding deep inhalations that could result in deeper penetration of the prosthesis into the airway. If this fails, the patient should go to an emergency medical facility where retrieval can be accomplished using topical anesthesia and a rigid open bronchoscope with grasping forceps.

The presence of the TEP in the superior tracheostoma may induce an inflammatory process that has been linked to a low incidence of tracheostomal stenosis. Tracheal granulations (treated by cautery or laser), prolapse of esophageal mucosa through the puncture, and puncture tract dilation are other complications that occur in a small number of patients. Current estimates of successful tracheoesophageal voice restoration range from 85 percent to 95 percent. With primary TEP, successful speech is obtained in a relatively short period of time—an average of 22 days postoperatively. Measurements of intensity, fundamental frequency, and speaking rate have confirmed that tracheoesophageal speech is more acoustically similar to normal speech than is standard esophageal speech, as well as more acceptable and intelligible. The surgical technique of tracheoesophageal puncture is relatively simple, and complications are minimal. Thus, tracheoesophageal voice restoration represents the most effective and efficient means of postlaryngectomy voice rehabilitation.

Suggested Reading

Blom ED, Singer MI, Hamaker RC. An improved esophageal insufflation test. Arch Otolaryngol Head Neck Surg 1985; 111:211-212.

Blom ED, Singer MI, Hamaker RC. Tracheostoma valve for post-laryngectomy voice rehabilitation. Ann Otol Rhinol Laryngol 1982; 91:576-578.

Deschler DG, Doherty ET, Reed CO, et al. Tracheoesophageal voice following tubed free radial forearm flap reconstruction of the neopharynx. Ann Otol Rhinol Laryngol 1994; 103:929-936.

Kelly KE, Anthony JP, Singer MI Pharyngoesophageal reconstruction using the radial forearm fasciocutaneous flap: Preliminary results. Otolaryngol Head Neck Surg 1994; 111:16-24.

Robbins J, Fisher HB, Blom ED, Singer MI. Selected acoustic features of tracheoesophageal, esophageal, and laryngeal speech. Arch Otolaryngol 1984; 110:670-672.

Singer MI, Blom ED. An endoscopic technique for voice restoration after total laryngectomy. Ann Otol Rhinol Laryngol 1980; 89:529-533.

Singer MI, Blom ED. A selective myotomy for voice restoration after total laryngectomy. Arch Otolaryngol 1981; 107:670-673.

Singer MI, Blom ED, Hamaker RC. Further experience with voice restoration after total laryngectomy. Ann Otol Rhinol Laryngol 1981; 90: 498-502.

Singer MI, Blom ED, Hamaker RC. Pharyngeal plexus neurectomy for alaryngeal speech rehabilitation. Laryngoscope 1986; 96:50-53.

Singer MI, Blom ED, Hamaker RC, Yoshida GA. Applications of the voice prosthesis during laryngectomy. Ann Otol Rhinol Laryngol 1989; 98:921-925.

SUBGLOTTIC STENOSIS IN CHILDREN

The method of
Robin T. Cotton

The evaluation and management of pediatric laryngotracheal stenosis (PLTS) is complex and technically challenging. Teamwork is essential in caring for such infants and children, and their care should be restricted to institutions that have all the appropriate instrumentation and personnel. Medical support personnel are required with expertise in the following pediatric disciplines: anesthesia, surgery, pulmonology, gastroenterology, intensive care management, medicine, and genetics. Furthermore, nursing, speech therapy, and social service expertise is required for patient and parent teaching, counseling, rehabilitation, social assessment, tracheotomy care instruction, and home care assessment. These children have complex medical issues, and appropriate care of children with PLTS requires a high level of integration of the services, which is led by the otolaryngologist.

It is essential to develop a good rapport between the physician, nurse, patient, and family, because the relationship is often a lengthy one.

EVALUATION

Definition and Classification

There is no generally accepted definition of congenital or acquired PLTS. It occurs separately or in combination in the three anatomic areas of the larynx and often extends into the upper trachea. If the child already has a tracheotomy, therapy must include attention to the common suprastomal sequelae of tracheotomy in children, mainly suprastomal collapse, granulation tissue, or fibroma. The subglottis is almost universally involved in children who have acquired PLTS, which occurs most commonly secondary to prolonged intubation but may be congenital or secondary to extrinsic traumatic forces (Table 1). I use a grading system that divides the stenosis into four grades; this is useful in planning therapy and in discussing outcomes with the parents (Fig. 1). A useful classification of congenital pediatric subglottic stenosis is outlined in Table 2.

Most of the children who come for evaluation of PLTS are in one of three categories: (1) intubated in the neonatal intensive care unit (NICU); (2) have a tracheotomy in place with an established diagnosis of PLTS; (3) have not required an artificial airway but have a history suggestive of PLTS.

Patients Failing Extubation in the NICU (Group 1)

The intubated patient in the NICU has multiple extubation failures. Careful evaluation of the patient's history and medical problems is essential, and close dialogue with a neonatologist is mandatory. Expectations and outcomes of therapy for the patient need to be frankly discussed between the neonatologist and the otolaryngologist. Close attention should be paid to the patient's medical condition, with emphasis on cardiopulmonary status, ventilation status, oxygen requirements, and the details of previous extubation failures. Assuming that steroids and racemic epinephrine have been used appropriately, the duration of extubation before reintubation is an important determinant of the need for consideration of tracheotomy; the shorter the interval, measured in hours, the more likely that a tracheotomy is necessary. Patients requiring peak airway pressures above 35 mm Hg are poor candidates for any therapy, including tracheotomy. Under these circumstances, the endotracheal tube provides a better seal, and further airway management is best delayed until peak pressures can be reduced.

Flexible nasopharyngolaryngoscopy gives marginal information about the intubated patient. Nasopharyngolaryngoscopy and bronchoscopy in the operating room is by far the most important part of evaluation. This is best accomplished, if at all possible, under spontaneous ventilation so that dynamic as well as fixed obstruction can be diagnosed.

Important concomitant airway diagnoses need to be individually looked for because they affect treatment and outcomes of PLTS. Options at this point in time include reintubation, possibly with a smaller tube; proceed with anterior cricoid split (ACS) or laryngotracheal reconstruction (LTR); or tracheotomy. Controversial procedures that I do not find of value include repeated dilation or excision with a resecto-

Table 1. Etiology of Pediatric Laryngotracheal Stenosis

Congenital
Acquired
Intubation
External trauma
High tracheotomy
Infection/inflammation
Burn
Thermal
Chemical
Tumor
Dystrophic cartilage

Table 2. Classification of Congenital Subglottic Stenosis

SOFT-TISSUE STENOSIS	CARTILAGINOUS STENOSIS
Granulation tissue	Cricoid cartilage deformity
Submucosal fibrosis	Normal shape
Submucosal gland hyperplasia	Small for infant's size
	Abnormal shape
	Large anterior lamina
	Large posterior lamina
	Generalized thickening
	Elliptical submucous cleft
	Submucous cleft
	Other congenital cricoid stenosis
	Trapped first tracheal ring

scope; however, when isolated granulation tissue originating from the posterior larynx is present, the use of a CO_2 laser with a micromanipulator can be helpful.

Careful evaluation of the larynx for the sites and degree of injury helps with the decision making; pathology limited to the subglottis is more likely to have a good outcome with ACS than if there is considerable glottic involvement or eventration of the ventricles and considerable edema.

Patients Who Still Have Tracheotomy for PLTS (Group 2)

As in the assessment of the neonate, a thorough history and consideration of the total medical situation of the patient is required, but a microlaryngoscopy and bronchoscopy, supplemented by a flexible nasopharyngolaryngoscopy, provide the most important aspects of evaluation. Additional assessments are variously important, depending on the age of the patient.

Flexible nasopharyngolaryngoscopy, although of limited use in intubated patients, becomes very important in nonintubated patients, because it offers visualization of dynamic problems throughout the laryngotracheobronchial tree, but in particular at the vocal cord level. Abnormalities of glottic mobility due to neurologic problems, scarring of the glottis, or involvement of the cricoarytenoid joints complicate surgical therapy.

Roentgenographic evaluation of the airway itself is of limited use. Plain anteroposterior and lateral airway radiographs can give some information on the length of the stenosis. In my experience, computed tomographic (CT) scans give little additional information directly on laryngotracheal stenosis. I do not routinely obtain a CT scan unless I am looking for specific information on extrinsic lesions that could be affecting the airway. If a coincidental vascular compression is suspected, magnetic resonance imaging (MRI) is indicated. An MRI should also be considered in those cases of tracheobronchomalacia in which the etiology of the malacia is not clear. Radiologic studies for gastroesophageal reflux disease and aspiration are appropriate for some patients.

Gastroesophageal reflux, which is common in children, should be carefully evaluated by history and needs to be evaluated and managed if reflux is considered to be a possible aggravating factor in PLTS. I prefer the 24 hour double-lumen pH probe study and esophageal biopsies (both low and high in the esophagus) to help in the diagnosis of significant reflux that may be affecting the larynx.

Evaluation of the swallowing function of the larynx is necessary in children who have a history of swallowing problems or aspiration, or in those who have neurologic problems. This can be accomplished by a combination of contrast barium swallow and fiberendoscopic endoscopic swallow (FEES) study. Both studies are useful in certain circumstances, and while each gives specific information, they are also complementary to each other (Table 3).

Those children who have significant pulmonary disease need a consultation and appropriate investigation with a pediatric pulmonologist, especially if single-stage laryngotracheal reconstruction (SSLTR) is contemplated. In general, it is inadvisable to perform LTR in children who have an oxygen requirement, although in selected cases continued oxygen administration may be possible by nasal prongs after decannulation. SSLTR requires lung function adequate enough to withstand not only the surgery but also the postoperative course in the ICU and subsequent extubation.

Direct microlaryngoscopy and bronchoscopy under spontaneous ventilation anesthesia provides the most essential information on laryngeal pathology. Microlaryngoscopy is performed using a laryngoscope. A selection of instruments should be available because no one style of laryngoscope is applicable to all cases. Included in the assessment is the evaluation of passive arytenoid mobility. Glottic pathology may include anterior or posterior glottic webs, intra-arytenoid adhesions, and fixation or paralysis of one or both vocal cords. The subglottis, if patent, is best evaluated using

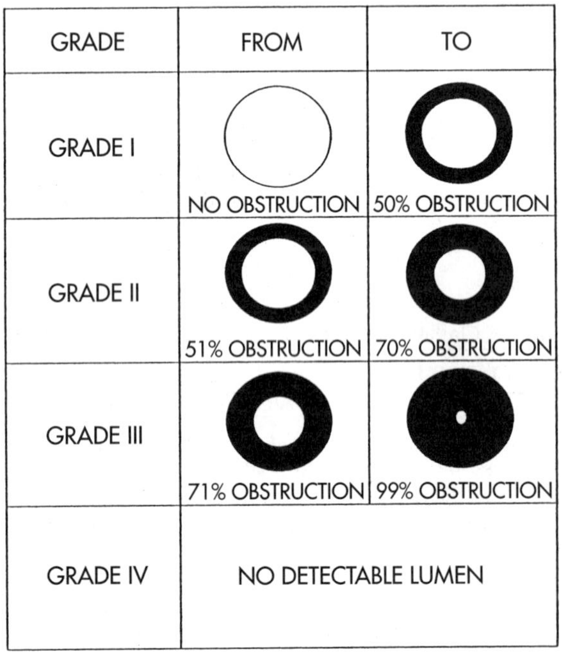

GRADE	FROM	TO
GRADE I	NO OBSTRUCTION	50% OBSTRUCTION
GRADE II	51% OBSTRUCTION	70% OBSTRUCTION
GRADE III	71% OBSTRUCTION	99% OBSTRUCTION
GRADE IV	NO DETECTABLE LUMEN	

Figure 1.
Stenosis grading system.

Table 3. Comparison of Methods for Evaluation of Swallowing Function

FEATURE	VSS	FEES
Oral preparatory phase	+ +	−
Premature spillage	+	+ +
Laryngeal penetration	+ +	+ +
Aspiration	+ +	+
Residue in hypopharynx	+	+ +
Esophageal motility	+	−
Gastroesophageal reflux to the pharynx	+	+
Hypopharyngeal pooling of oral secretions	−	+ +
Anatomic abnormality impacting swallow	+	+ +
Hypopharyngeal sensation	−	+

VSS, videofluoroscopic swallow study; FEES, fiberendoscopic swallow study.

a Hopkins rod lens telescope of appropriate size, with the determination of the site (anterior, posterior, circumferential); maturity; length; and consistency of the pathology. If the telescope passes through the subglottic stenosis, the suprastomal area is carefully assessed with attention to factors such as suprastomal collapse, granuloma, or fibrous tissue that could interfere with decannulation. The remainder of the laryngotracheobronchial tree is studied with the telescope either placed through the subglottis or, if the telescope is unable to be passed through the subglottis, through the tracheal stoma. If there is an available lumen, it is most important to size the airway with an endotracheal tube of known size and to measure at what pressure a leak (if any) occurs. In this way, knowing the airway size that the child should have establishes goals for reconstructive surgery. When assessing vocal cord function, it is important to realize that laryngeal neuromuscular function changes with growth. Very young infants may exhibit laryngeal dyskinesias, transient unexplained vocal cord paralysis, paradoxical vocal cord motion, aspiration, gastroesophageal reflux, and simple central apnea—all without definable etiology.

Patients Without Tracheotomy But With History Suggestive of PLTS (Group 3)

The assessment of this group of patients is identical to that of the previously described group, along with some additional special considerations. First, I always expect the airway to be very small; I am consistently amazed at how tiny an airway children are able to breathe through. Therefore, I have the smallest instruments and endotracheal tubes available before beginning the endoscopic evaluation. Induction of general anesthesia in these patients is potentially dangerous for the airway, and it is essential to have a game plan worked out with the pediatric anesthesiologist and operating room personnel before the induction of anesthesia. Fixed subglottic stenosis—no matter how small—does not normally cause obstruction during the induction of anesthesia, whereas significant supraglottic obstructions may cause inability of adequate ventilation during induction of anesthesia. Second, I use perioperative steroids to minimize edema of the airway that could further compromise the child's ability to breathe. Third, subglottic stenosis must be differentiated from subglottic cysts, which are relatively common sequelae of neonatal intubation.

■ THERAPY

Treatment is generally recommended for subglottic stenosis in children. In group 1 patients, the end point is either treatment to enable the endotracheal tube to be removed or eventually tracheotomy, because the patient cannot remain intubated past several months of life. In group 2 patients, unless there are significant mitigating issues, treatment designed to remove the tracheotomy tube is recommended because of the morbidity and mortality associated with a tracheotomy. The younger the patient and the more obstructive the lesion above the level of the tracheotomy tube, the higher the mortality. Other medical conditions, however, may preclude surgical reconstruction at that time. Such factors include age, weight, oxygen-dependent pulmonary disease, neurologic disease with significant potential for aspiration, and certain craniofacial anomalies.

In group 3 patients, surgery should be recommended in a young child if the airway is marginal or in an older child if exercise tolerance is markedly limited. For patients in this group who have a relatively mild stenosis, there is a place for "wait and see" management to determine whether the stenotic lumen grows and enlarges with the patient's growth.

Surgical intervention for PLTS is divided into endoscopic management, ACS in the infant, and open LTR techniques.

Endoscopic Management

Endoscopic management is most often performed with the CO_2 laser, but traditional endoscopic instruments work well in many cases. I do all CO_2 laser work in children of any age under spontaneous ventilation using microlaryngoscopes with anesthetic adapters. Using this technique, I have found it unnecessary to use endotracheal tubes, which are a potential fire hazard and also occupy valuable space. I do not use the apneic technique because this prevents adequate working time. The CO_2 laser should be used on short-pulsed duration with small spot size to minimize thermal damage. Newer micromanipulators with a spot size as small as 0.27 mm and 400 mm focal length are currently the instruments of choice. I use the CO_2 laser as a primary form of therapy for isolated supraglottic, glottic, or subglottic pathology of a relatively minor nature. Much more common in my practice is to use the CO_2 laser as a secondary adjunct to LTR procedures; the most common use of the CO_2 laser in such work is in partial removal of supraglottic arytenoid mucosa that may be infolding into the airway or in partial posterior vocal cordectomy in cases of vocal cord medialization secondary to paralysis or scar fixation. I do not use the CO_2 laser for anterior or posterior webs, and I have not found that the techniques of micro-trapdoor flaps are as useful in the pediatric larynx as they are in the older child, adolescent, or adult larynx.

Anterior Cricoid Split

ACS and LTR are started generally in the same manner. The patient is positioned with a shoulder roll for maximum exposure of the neck, as for a tracheotomy. The patient is draped so that an intraoperative endoscopy can be performed, if required, without contaminating the field, by using a 1000 3M Steridrape over the chin to isolate the mouth from the neck wound. A horizontal incision at the level of the cricoid is identified and injected with 1 percent lidocaine with 1:100,000 epinephrine. Standard dissection is used to expose the thyroid, cricoid, and upper tracheal cartilages. The incision into the airway starts at the cricoid; hemostasis is secured with a needle point electrocautery under very low power. Incision is enlarged superiorly through the level of the anterior commissure but stops short just inferior to the thyroid notch. The incision is enlarged inferiorly to the first and very often the second tracheal ring. A 4–0 Prolene suture is placed into each side of the cricoid to act as a traction suture, and the patient is reintubated, if necessary, with a tube of appropriate size (Table 4). The incision is approximated very loosely, and a small drain is always placed. The Prolene sutures are labeled and taped to the sides of the chest. If this incision is closed, the patient

Table 4. Guidelines for Stenting of Airway After Anterior Cricoid Split Procedures

Tube size (inside diameter)
3.0 mm for weight 1,500–1,199 g
3.5 mm for weight 2,000–2,499 g
4.0 mm for weight 2,500–3,000 g
Duration of stenting
14 days for weight <2,500 g
7 days for weight >2,500 g

may develop significant subcutaneous emphysema. In employing the ACS, I do not generally advise using cartilage, although I have no objection to the use of auricular cartilage under these circumstances. Strict criteria should be observed before performing an ACS.

Laryngotracheal Reconstruction

Anterior Costal Cartilage Graft

This operation was originally conceived for isolated, predominantly anterior, subglottic stenosis without glottic involvement. Of the several varieties of LTR, anterior cricoid cartilage grafting is the most appealing because (if there is a tracheotomy tube present) no stenting of the laryngeal lumen is necessary, and decannulation follows soon after re-epithelialization of the cartilage graft. The patient is anesthetized through the existing tracheotomy using a shortened RAE tube. The patient is placed in the typical tracheotomy position, and the neck and right hemithorax are prepped and then draped as separate wounds. For access to the mouth for intraoperative endoscopy, a 1000 3M Steridrape is placed over the chin to isolate the mouth from the neck wound. The airway is entered through a midline fissure that extends from just below the vocal cords through the cricoid to just above the tracheotomy stoma. The airway is sized with an endotracheal tube of appropriate size, and a decision is made whether an anterior graft alone will be adequate to enlarge the lumen or whether a posterior graft may be necessary as well.

Once this has been determined, sufficient costal cartilage graft material is removed to perform the reconstruction. The cartilage graft is placed in a wet saline sponge for use in the airway and, after ensuring that there is no pleural leak, the chest wound is closed in layers. The graft is carefully fashioned into an ellipse in such a way that the perichondrium will lie internally. The edges of the cartilages are beveled so that the widest part of the graft is seated externally. A mattress suture is performed between the cut edges of the laryngofissure and the costal cartilage graft, using 4–0 Prolene sutures on a PC1 needle. Approximately eight sutures are necessary, one at each apex and three on each side, thus securing the graft. Fibrin glue made from the patient's own blood is generally applied around the suture line between the cartilage and the airway to minimize postoperative airway leaks. The wound is closed in layers with adequate drainage.

The patient is discharged from the hospital within a few days of the surgery and returns at approximately 6 weeks for endoscopic evaluation to determine the adequacy of the airway and readiness for decannulation.

Posterior Costal Cartilage Graft

This procedure is used when there is primarily posterior subglottic scar tissue with or without posterior commissure scar. Similar to the procedure just described, the horizontal skin incision is made in the neck, the airway is exposed, and the airway is entered from the second tracheal ring through the anterior commissure and generally up to the thyroid notch. A tattoo mark is put on each side of the cartilage to help in accurate reapproximation. The posterior plate of the cricoid is now divided with a Beaver blade that is kept strictly in the midline. The interarytenoid muscles superiorly may need to be partially divided, and inferiorly the incision should extend below the inferior cricoid margin for approximately 1 cm. The airway is now sized with an age-appropriate endotracheal tube, and assessment is made for whether a posterior graft alone will be sufficient or whether an anterior graft should also be placed.

The costal cartilage graft is then removed and shaped appropriately into an ellipse of a size that will fill the space between the cut ends of the cricoid. This is sewn in place with 4–0 Vicryl on a P2 needle in a subcartilaginous plane such that the knots are buried. Stenting with an endotracheal tube or with a Cotton-Lorenz stent (see later section on stenting) is necessary when placing a posterior graft. The airway is carefully reapproximated, and the wound is closed in layers with a drain.

Anteroposterior Graft

A combination of the techniques previously outlined is required for severe PLTS. Often, the judgment to perform posterior cartilage graft or anterior or posterior cartilage graft is made at the time of surgery.

Cricotracheal Resection

Partial cricotracheal resection (CTR) with cricothyrotracheal anastomosis is an attractive alternative to expansion cricoid surgery, especially in patients who have severe subglottic stenosis without associated glottic pathology and at least a few millimeters of margin of normal airway beneath the vocal cords and the most significant part of the stenosis.

Exposure for CTR is similar to the procedures outlined previously, except that the exposure inferiorly below the tracheotomy stoma is greater; at least two rings below the stoma need to be identified. The scar tissue is sharply dissected off the cartilage of the thyroid and cricoid until the cricothyroid joint is identified. The airway is entered with a Beaver blade in the vertical midline at the level of the cricoid, and the incision is carried superiorly to the inferior margin of the thyroid cartilage. Endoscopy performed simultaneously can help identify the superior extent of the stenosis. A horizontal cut is made just above the superior extent of the stenosis from anterior to posterior, stopping at the level of the cricothyroid joint, and thus avoiding injury to the recurrent laryngeal nerves. Lateral cuts are then made anterior to the cricothyroid joints and continued inferiorly through the lateral aspects of the cricoid cartilage, thus exposing the posterior cricoid plate.

Dissection is now focused to the inferior aspect of the stenosis, generally at the level of the tracheotomy stoma. The trachea is incised just below the inferior aspect of the stenosis through the anterior and lateral wall. Dissection occurs in the subperichondral plane to avoid injury to the recurrent laryngeal nerves. The posterior membranous trachea is incised carefully to identify the party wall between the trachea and the esophagus. Often the placement of a bougie in the esophagus will aid in this dissection. The lateral and posterior tracheal incisions are then connected, and the stenotic segment of the anterolateral cricoid and upper trachea is removed, leaving the exposed posterior cricoid plate. Scar from the posterior cricoid plate is removed using an electric drill and bur until a thin, flat surface is present.

A suprahyoid release is performed, and adequate mobility of the distal trachea is obtained. Interrupted 4–0 Vicryl sutures are used for the posterior mucosal anastomosis, at which time the shoulder roll is removed and the sutures are tied. Now the airway is intubated nasotracheally if a single-stage procedure is planned, or with a Montgomery T-tube, and the anterior and lateral anastomosis is completed with 3–0 Prolene sutures between the thyroid cartilage and the uppermost tracheal ring. Two additional tension-releasing 2–0 Prolene sutures are placed between the thyroid ala and the tracheal rings below the anastomosis, At the end of the procedure, the neck is maintained in a flexed position with three cutaneous 0–0 Prolene sutures placed from the chin to the chest to prohibit the child from extending the neck for 10 days postoperatively.

Stenting

Use of Stents

The decisions to be made with respect to stenting include whether or not to use a stent, the type of stent, and the length of stenting. Ideally, no stent should be used, because most often the initial insult was from an artificial airway. The original description of the anterior costal cartilage graft LTR was performed without a stent, which is still recommended for this procedure.

The stents that I use include the Montgomery laryngeal keel for anterior webs; the Cotton-Lorenz Teflon stent, modeled after the Aboulker stent (itself modeled on a stent described by Chevalier Jackson); the Montgomery T-tube; and, for single-stage reconstruction, an endotracheal tube.

For isolated anterior costal cartilage grafts with a tracheotomy in place, no stenting is required under most circumstances. If there is some accompanying posterior pathology requiring manipulation (e.g., scar band revision), a short stent for a few days is acceptable. If the decision has been made to remove the tracheotomy site at the same time and perform an SSLTR, stenting is required for a variable time from 1 to 10 days, depending on the age of the patient. The younger the patient, the longer the period of intubation. Two factors need to be considered. First, the perichondrium swells for a few days and intrudes in the airway; the smaller the airway, the greater the intrusion. Second, the younger the child, and particularly if he or she is a graduate of the neonatal nursery and still has some residual lung disease, the greater the problem of removal of pulmonary secretions. In general, a 2-year-old child who has an isolated anterior costal cartilage graft is intubated for approximately 8 to 10 days, whereas an adolescent is intubated for a shorter time.

If posterior costal cartilage grafting has been performed, stenting is mandatory. The choices are a Cotton-Lorenz above-stoma stent for 4 weeks or proceeding with an SSLTR, in which case I recommend that the endotracheal tube be left in for 14 days. It is very important in these reconstructions to place age-appropriate endotracheal tubes.

For SSLTR patients, nursing and medical care occurs in an ICU setting. I do not advise paralyzing the patient unless the patient has pulmonary conditions requiring this for a brief period after the surgery. Careful selection of patients for SSLTR will minimize the number of patients who require prolonged paralysis after surgery. I do not heavily sedate these patients unless circumstances make this mandatory. Most patients over the age of 2 years can be managed appropriately in the ICU with minimal sedation. The older the child, the more likely they are to tolerate a normal diet during this phase of healing. The day before planned extubation, the patient is returned to the operating room, and under general anesthesia the patient is extubated, and the airway is examined for adequacy and patency. The patient is generally reintubated with a half size smaller endotracheal tube and is returned to the ICU for extubation the following morning. If there is still significant swelling or edema, reintubation with a one size smaller tube is recommended, and re-evaluation occurs within a few days. If there is continued airway granulation tissue at that time, retracheotomy may be necessary. This outcome can be minimized by carefully selecting the patients for SSLTR.

The Montgomery T-tube is useful in the management of post-cricotracheal resection patients. Its use is not advocated in very small children or in those children for whom meticulous care at home is not possible. I only use a T-tube in a patient after I have deemed that it is the most advisable stent to use and have had a thorough discussion with the parents regarding its care and potential dangers, thus making this a shared decision and responsibility. CTR (if not performed as a single-stage procedure) requires a Montgomery T-tube to be in place for approximately 6 weeks, and the T-tube limb is placed high in the supraglottis, with the anterior lip being longer than the posterior lip, which is left at the interarytenoid level. Most children tolerate the T-tube in this position without significant aspiration, although some require nasogastric feedings during the time the Montgomery T-tube is left in place.

Montgomery Keel

Acquired subglottic stenosis is often associated with significant anterior glottic webbing. I have found that after dividing the web, a Montgomery keel is the most effective means of preventing re-formation of the web. This keel can be used either in isolation or in combination with a Cotton-Lorenz stent, if appropriate indications for a Cotton-Lorenz stent are present.

Decannulation

The decannulation process may begin once the findings of microlaryngoscopy and bronchoscopy indicate that there is an adequate airway, including adequate vocal cord movement. The first step in the process of decannulation is a reduction in size of the tracheotomy tube in a controlled environment, followed by plugging of the tracheotomy tube in a monitored setting. The tube is plugged initially while the patient is awake. The tracheotomy tube remains plugged as long as the child shows no clinical evidence of respiratory distress or oxygen desaturation. If the child tolerates plugging while awake, night-time plugging of the tracheotomy tube is appropriate in a monitored setting that includes pulse oximetry.

Decannulation itself is carried out in a monitored setting (for at least 48 hours) to evaluate any significant oxygen desaturations for at least 48 hours. The actual removal of the tracheotomy tube should take place in the morning after the patient has had nothing by mouth (NPO) for a period of time, and the patient should remain at NPO status for a few hours following decannulation in case an emergency procedure becomes necessary.

If a child fails plugging at some point during this process, several possibilities should be considered, including supraglottic collapse, inadequate vocal cord movement, residual laryngeal stenosis, suprastomal collapse, and tracheobronchomalacia. If there is any question about the airway, plugging the tracheotomy tube for 3 months is advisable, during which time the child should be able to tolerate an upper respiratory infection without unplugging.

Following decannulation, a child should be evaluated either endoscopically or with radiographs for possible recurrent stomal granulation tissue.

FOREIGN BODIES OF THE AIRWAY AND ESOPHAGUS

The method of
Lauren D. Holinger

Most victims of foreign body aspiration are older infants and toddlers. Children under 5 years of age account for approximately 84 percent, and children under 3 years of age account for 73 percent of cases. The high incidence in this age group reflects the tendency of these children to explore their world using their mouths. In addition, these children have not yet developed a full posterior dentition, and the neuromuscular mechanisms for swallowing and airway protection may not be fully mature.

Vegetable matter is uniformly the most common foreign body found in the pediatric airway. Nuts, particularly peanuts, account for approximately 34 percent of foreign bodies. The offending objects range from nuts to pieces of raw carrot, apple, dried beans, popcorn, sunflower seeds, and watermelon seeds.

The types of foreign bodies ingested evolve slowly over time. Metallic objects, especially safety pins, have decreased in incidence with the era of disposable diapers. Plastic foreign bodies have risen in frequency due to the use of plastic parts in toys. These objects are inert and often contain no radiopaque substances. Because of their nonirritating and radiolucent qualities, plastic parts may remain in the tracheobronchial tree for prolonged periods.

Coins and discs are most commonly found in the esophagus. Less common are hardware and metal objects, which include tacks, nails, screws, staples, rivets, ball bearings, pen parts, and straight pins. Glass, which usually originates from a broken food container, may be visible radiographically and is often associated with perforation and mediastinal emphysema. Esophageal foreign bodies typically lodge immediately below the cricopharyngeus muscle. If they lodge lower, there may be an underlying condition (such as a congenital or acquired esophageal stricture); follow-up barium esophagram is ordered 2 to 3 weeks later to detect the underlying pathology.

MANAGEMENT PRINCIPLES

A Foreign Body Generally Is Not an Acute Emergency

In general, the treatment of choice for foreign bodies in the airway or esophagus is reasonably prompt endoscopic removal under conditions of maximum safety and minimum trauma. Most patients with foreign bodies who come to the endoscopic surgeon have already passed the acute phase. When there is no urgent danger to the patient's life, the problem is approached with complete and thoughtful consideration of the physiologic and mechanical factors involved. However, untoward delay of bronchoscopic removal of a foreign body in the airway is potentially harmful because the foreign body may become dislodged from the bronchus and impact in the larynx, causing asphyxiation.

Endoscopy is therefore deferred only until preoperative studies have been obtained and the patient has been prepared for surgery by adequate hydration, emptying of the stomach, and so forth. Foreign bodies in the larynx or tracheobronchial tree are generally removed the same day the diagnosis is first considered.

Urgent Situations

There are four situations in which a foreign body does constitute an acute emergency.

Actual or Potential Airway Obstruction

The most serious complication of foreign body aspiration is complete obstruction of the airway. Globular food objects, such as hot dogs, grapes, nuts, and candies, are the most frequent offenders, whereas rubber balloons and other toys are common among nonfood objects. Suspected objects in the larynx, trachea, or bronchi are considered actual or potential causes of airway obstruction. Large or multiple esophageal foreign bodies can compress the airway from behind, causing airway obstruction. These patients are taken to the operating room within the first 24 hours after the diagnosis is suspected.

Dried Beans or Peas

When a main bronchus is obstructed for more than 24 hours, absorbed moisture may burst the capsule, and asphyxia develops as the bean swells to occlude the airway. If the child does not asphyxiate, the swelling of the bean will at least obliterate forceps space, making the technical aspects of bronchial foreign body extraction extremely difficult. The sooner such a child is bronchoscoped, the greater the likelihood for successful endoscopic retrieval of the object.

Disc Battery Ingestion with Esophageal Lodgment

Prompt removal of disc batteries lodged in the esophagus is critical. Data show that mucosal damage occurs after 1 hour in the esophagus; erosion into the muscular layers occurs within 2 to 4 hours; and perforation of the esophagus occurs within 8 to 12 hours.

Disc batteries contain sodium hydroxide, potassium hydroxide, and mercury, which leak through the grommet seal of the battery and produce esophageal injury. This may lead to complications of esophageal stricture, perforation, tracheoesophageal fistula, mediastinitis, and death.

The following protocol offers a rational plan of management for disc battery ingestions:

1. Initial radiograph to locate the battery.
2. Urgent endoscopic retrieval if the battery is lodged in the esophagus.
3. Identification of the battery diameter and chemical system. This is done by determining the imprint code of a duplicate.
4. If the battery has passed beyond the esophagus, the patient may be discharged and observed for fever, pain, and hematochezia. Minor symptoms (vomiting, stool discoloration) should not prompt retrieval effort. A follow-up radiograph is obtained 4 to 7 days after ingestion.
5. In the asymptomatic patient when the battery has passed beyond the esophagus, the parents are instructed to check the stools regularly for the battery. A radiograph can be done after several days to confirm passage, which will alleviate parental concern and allow them to discontinue patient monitoring. For batteries of 15 mm or greater diameter, in a child under the age of 6 years, a radiograph is taken after 48 hours. Any such battery remaining in the stomach after 2 days is removed endoscopically.
6. Prompt operative intervention is carried out if signs or symptoms of bowel perforation develop at any time.

Esophageal Perforation

Any patient exhibiting signs and symptoms of esophageal perforation undergoes prompt confirmatory diagnostic studies, followed by retrieval of the foreign body and appropriate medical-surgical management of the perforation.

Complications of Nonendoscopic Means of Foreign Body Extraction

If the patient's airway is not completely obstructed, back slaps, the Heimlich maneuver, or other attempts at removal may unintentionally exacerbate the patient's symptoms. The child is taken immediately to a facility that has the equipment and personnel to manage the problem properly. When the proper laryngoscopes, bronchoscopes, forceps, tracheostomy set, and personnel (including anesthesia) are available in the operating room, the attempt is made to remove the foreign body.

Postural drainage (chest physical therapy) and bronchodilators have been suggested as an alternative to bronchoscopic removal of foreign bodies in the airway. This ill-advised and poorly conceived technique has led to respiratory arrest in at least four patients, one of whom also experienced transient cortical blindness. This throwback to the nineteenth century does no more than serve as a makeshift alternative for those who are unskilled in modern bronchoscopic techniques.

The use of papain, such as Adolph's meat tenderizer, to dissolve meat impaction in the esophagus is another nonendoscopic means of foreign body management that is also contraindicated. Its use has resulted in fatalities due to necrosis of the esophagus and rupture of a major blood vessel.

Balloon catheter extraction of radiopaque foreign bodies from the cervical esophagus has been recommended for discs such as coins that have had a brief sojourn. There are reports of complications such as mucosal laceration and esophageal perforation, aspiration of the object or other associated nonradiopaque foreign bodies, epistaxis, and laryngospasm. The psychological trauma is not to be disregarded either. Forceful restraint and invasion of an awake child, when more humane alternatives exist, is a backward step in the care of the pediatric patient.

■ EVALUATION

History

Positive findings from the history must never be ignored. Negative findings from the history may be misleading. Choking or coughing episodes accompanied by wheezing are highly suggestive of foreign body aspiration. A history of gagging or the statement by a young patient that he or she has swallowed something is taken seriously.

There are three stages of symptoms due to aspiration of an object into the airway

Initial Event

Violent paroxysms of coughing, choking, gagging, and possibly airway obstruction occur immediately when the foreign body is aspirated or swallowed. Such a history can be elicited in most cases, but unfortunately many parents tend to trivialize the significance of such an episode or do not recall the incident. Some parents engage in wishful thinking and minimize the symptoms, hoping that nothing is wrong and that no surgical intervention will be required. Older children are often reluctant to admit to such an episode for fear of being punished.

Asymptomatic Interval

During the second stage, the foreign body becomes lodged, reflexes fatigue, and the immediate irritating symptoms subside. This stage is most treacherous and accounts for a large percentage of delayed diagnoses and overlooked foreign bodies. It is during this second stage that the physician is inclined to minimize the possibility of a foreign body accident, being reassured by the absence of symptoms that no foreign body is present.

Complications

In the third stage, obstruction, erosion, or infection develop to again direct attention to the presence of a foreign body. Complications of airway foreign bodies include fever and malaise, cough, and hemoptysis. Pneumonia, atelectasis, and lung abscess may develop. Complications of esophageal foreign bodies are manifested by dysphagia, failure to thrive, mediastinal abscess, or even massive exsanguinating hemorrhage with erosion of a sharp point through the wall of the esophagus, which can penetrate a major blood vessel or even the heart.

Symptoms

Esophageal Foreign Bodies

Complete esophageal obstruction will cause secretions to overflow into the larynx, producing symptoms of laryngeal obstruction. These patients have a sensation of something being stuck as well as odynophagia. When the obstruction is not complete, odynophagia and dysphagia occur. Small infants may take little or nothing by mouth and present with failure to thrive. Older children may be reluctant to admit something is stuck and quietly eliminate solid foods from their diet.

Bronchial Foreign Bodies

In most cases, airway foreign bodies find their way into one of the main bronchi, more frequently the right main bronchus as compared with the left. This is due to the slightly greater diameter of the right main bronchus, its smaller angle of divergence from the tracheal axis, the greater airflow through to the right lung, and the position of the carina to the left of the midline. There is decreased air entry to the obstructed side, but symptoms may be constantly changing with movement of the foreign body, development of edema, or infection.

Laryngeal Foreign Bodies

Complete obstruction will asphyxiate the child unless promptly relieved with the Heimlich maneuver. Objects that are only partially obstructive are usually flat and thin and lodge between the vocal folds in the sagittal plane. Such objects commonly cause symptoms of croup, hoarseness, cough, stridor, and varying degrees of dyspnea, all of which increase as edema and inflammation progress. Odynophagia may also occur.

Tracheal Foreign Bodies

Choking and aspiration is present in 90 percent of patients who have tracheal foreign bodies. Stridor is present in 60 percent, wheezing in 50 percent, and cough in 40 percent.

Radiologic Evaluation

Posteroanterior (PA) and lateral chest radiographs are standard in the assessment of infants and children suspected of having aspirated or swallowed a foreign object. The abdomen is included.

Barium is not used to localize nonradiopaque esophageal foreign bodies for several reasons: (1) it complicates the subsequent attempt at endoscopic removal; (2) it can be aspirated during the study; and (3) it will delay the endoscopic removal for 6 hours because the child's status is no longer NPO once barium has been ingested. However, when the index of suspicion of an esophageal foreign body is quite low, a small sip of barium may be given to rule out esophageal lodgment of a nonradiopaque object.

With suspected bronchial foreign bodies, a good expiratory PA chest radiograph is most helpful. In the infant who is tachypneic and uncooperative, lateral decubitus chest radiographs or fluoroscopy may provide the same information. During expiration, the bronchial foreign body obstructs exit of air from the obstructed lung and produces obstructive emphysema—air trapping —with persistent inflation of the obstructed lung and shift of the mediastinum toward the opposite side. Air trapping is an immediate complication in contrast to atelectasis, which is a late finding.

If the parents have an idea of what the foreign body may be, they are asked to return home to obtain a duplicate. If this is not practical, they are asked to draw the object as accurately as possible. They are carefully questioned about the size of the object, its color, and its texture. When a duplicate object can be obtained, preoperative testing is undertaken to see which instruments work best for the particular mechanical problem.

■ OPERATIVE TECHNIQUE

Anesthesia

General anesthesia is used for endoscopic extraction of foreign bodies. A pulse oximeter is routinely used. Complete cooperation between the endoscopist and the anesthesiologist is of paramount importance and improves dramatically with experience and mutual trust. The details of the procedure as well as potential complications are reviewed before induction of general anesthesia. Endotracheal intubation is accomplished for all patients who have esophageal foreign bodies. For patients who have airway foreign bodies, spontaneous respiration is maintained. This is somewhat safer than apneic techniques in which the patient is completely paralyzed and cannot move any air should the airway be temporarily lost. Positive pressure ventilation (bagging) is avoided, because this tends to drive the foreign body further peripherally. As anesthesia lightens, an occasional cough may actually help move the foreign body toward the bronchoscope. An inhalation anesthetic, typically halothane, is delivered through the closed system of a rigid bronchoscope. The larynx and trachea are sprayed with topical lidocaine before introduction of the bronchoscope.

Instrumentation

Rigid bronchoscopes and esophagoscopes are the instruments of choice for foreign body extraction. The major drawback of flexible instruments is that they lack control of the foreign body and provide inadequate control of the airway. The rigid instruments offer a greater range of size and variety of forceps, allow better exposure of the foreign body, and permit sheathing of sharp parts within the tube during extraction.

Passive action forceps offer a wide range of blades for the various types of mechanical problems. There are four types: (1) forward grasping, (2) rotation, (3) ball bearing (globular object), and (4) hollow object forceps. Positive action (center action) forceps have the advantage of a narrower shaft and the capacity to dilate a bronchus. A magnified view may be obtained with a rod lens telescope or the optical forceps.

Recommendations

The Doesel-Huzly bronchoscopes with rod lens telescopes (Karl Storz, Tuttlingen, Germany) are most commonly used for bronchial foreign body extraction. A size of 3.75 × 30 cm (Storz) is most often used for bronchial foreign bodies. Two laryngoscopes and two bronchoscopes are lighted and prepared; should a light fail or forceps become jammed in one scope, a backup is available immediately.

Technique

Forceps are selected and tried with a duplicate object before surgery. The forceps are adjusted and lubricated so that they are smooth in operation. At least two forceps are selected preoperatively because unexpected circumstances arising after the procedure is under way may require an alternative.

The endoscopist resists the impulse to seize the foreign body as soon as it is discovered. A careful study is made to determine the size, shape, position, probable location of unseen parts, and relationship to surrounding structures before making any attempt at extraction. The forceps is advanced until it lightly touches the foreign body, and the endoscope is withdrawn a short distance to permit the blades of the forceps to be opened. The forceps blades are advanced so that the tips pass the equator of the object. The tip of the endoscope is advanced against the foreign body, which is held against the tube mouth. The grasp of the forceps is firmly maintained by the fingers of the right hand while all traction for withdrawal is made by the left hand. The thumb of the left hand firmly clamps the forceps to maintain the relationship between the forceps and the endoscope during the extraction so that the three units are extracted as one. The endoscope keeps the vocal folds apart until the foreign body has exited the glottis. The foreign body is rotated to the largest diameter of the lumen for extraction: in the esophagus, the coronal plane; in the larynx, the sagittal plane.

Pointed, Sharp, and Cutting Objects

Pointed objects pose a special problem. The first priority during the extraction procedure is to localize the point. The point is released and sheathed within the endoscope. It is often necessary to accomplish this by first moving the object distally to disengage the point, then advancing the endoscope over the object (rather than pulling the object into the tube).

Fluoroscopy

Fluoroscopic assistance is used for upper lobe foreign bodies, common pins in the lung periphery, sharp or irregular foreign bodies (such as dental bridgework), and gastric foreign bodies.

"Stripping Off"

As a foreign body is brought out through the larynx, the lateral pressure of the vocal folds may strip it from the grasp of the forceps. The airway is re-established immediately, either by removing the object or by pushing it down into the bronchus in which it had been lodged, which allows ventilation of the good lung. The faulty technique is corrected, and the object is relocated.

A foreign body lost in the trachea will most likely be carried into the normal bronchus. This occurs because the previously obstructed lung or lobe moves little air and is edematous or narrowed by granulation tissue. This creates an immediate and critical emergency, because the child's only normal lung is completely obstructed. The object must be immediately removed or relocated to the other bronchus.

Complications

Laryngeal, Tracheal, and Bronchial Foreign Bodies

Immediate complications of endoscopic extraction include pneumomediastinum, impaction and complete obstruction, and failure to recover the object, which necessitates thoracotomy or tracheotomy. Obstructive emphysema is an immediate finding, whereas atelectasis is a late finding. Longer term complications include pneumonia, atelectasis, and granuloma or stricture formation along with their resulting problems.

Traumatic laryngitis and laryngeal edema are treated with humidity, racemic epinephrine, and high-dose steroids (1 to 1.5 milligrams per kilogram of dexamethasone up to 30 mg intravenously as a bolus). The head of the bed is elevated.

Esophageal Foreign Bodies

Perforation or tear of the esophagus is the most feared complication. With very large objects there is a potential danger of uncontrolled traumatic laceration. External esophagotomy with careful repair may be used to avoid this problem. Long-standing esophageal foreign bodies may lead to abscess or stricture formation. Rarely, a long-standing foreign body will work its way through the wall of the esophagus to assume an extraluminal location between the trachea and the esophagus. Over time, this foreign body may be virtually asymptomatic. Barium esophagram will precisely define the extraluminal location in relationship to the esophagus.

Postesophageal Foreign Bodies

Most objects, even large or pointed objects, that pass into the stomach will traverse the entire gastrointestinal tract without complications. The patient is given a regular diet. The position and progress of pointed objects are checked radiographically every 3 or 4 days until the object passes. For smooth objects, the parents are instructed merely to check the stools. Foreign bodies that remain loose in the stomach for a long time are generally of little concern unless they are unusually large. A radiograph of the abdomen is obtained in 2 or 3 weeks if the object does not pass. If the foreign body remains in one position for more than 1 week, removal may be considered.

Lengthy objects that enter the stomach easily on their long access have difficulty passing through the duodenum in children who are under 2 years of age. Because these objects may cause perforation, they are removed endoscopically before they leave the stomach. Gastrotomy is not delayed if endoscopic retrieval is unsuccessful. Needles are removed as soon as the diagnosis is confirmed by radiograph.

Follow-up

Antibiotics or steroids are not used after routine endoscopic foreign body extraction. One exception is the child who has a bronchial foreign body and pneumonia; antibiotics are continued if the child has already been receiving antibiotic therapy. Postoperative chest physical therapy is employed in cases of pneumonia, purulent bronchitis, and atelectasis.

Patients are discharged the day following the procedure if the lungs sound clear and the patient is afebrile. A chest radiograph is taken if pulmonary symptoms have not improved or if the patient remains febrile. In cases of sharp contaminated objects, tetanus immunization history is reviewed and updated.

Suggested Reading

Berdon WE. Editorial comment. Pediatr Radiol 1983; 13:119

Darrow DH, Holinger LD. Foreign bodies of the larynx, trachea, and bronchi. In: Bluestone CD, Stool SE, Kenna MA, eds. Pediatric otolaryngology. 3rd ed. Philadelphia: WB Saunders, 1996.

Holinger LD. Management of sharp and penetrating foreign bodies of the upper aerodigestive tract. Ann Otol Rhinol Laryngol 1990; 99:684-687.

Jackson C, Jackson CL. Diseases of the air and food passage of foreign body origin. Philadelphia: WB Saunders, 1936.

Litovitz T, Schmitz B. Ingestion of cylindrical and button batteries: 2382 cases. Pediatrics 1992; 85:747-772

Maves MD, Carithers JS, Birck HG. Esophageal burns secondary to disc battery ingestion. Ann Otol Rhinol Laryngol 1984; 93:364.

CAUSTIC INGESTION

The method of
James W. Forsen, Jr.

Despite improvements in medical technology, federal legislation, and heightened public awareness, caustic ingestion continues to be a common and controversial problem facing the otolaryngologist. The modern era in the management of caustic ingestion began in the first quarter of this century with the efforts of Chevalier Jackson. In response to a significant number of severe esophageal burns due to lye ingestion, he developed the end-lighted esophagoscope and also lobbied for passage of the Federal Caustic Act of 1927. The Federal Hazardous Substance Labeling Act was passed in 1960 and was followed by the Safe Packaging Act of 1970. Nonetheless, the incidence of caustic ingestion remains high. Poison control centers in the United States estimate that 26,000 caustic ingestions occur per year. There is a bimodal distribution, with a large group of ingestions occurring in children and a second large group occurring in adults. The majority of this latter group consists of suicidal gestures and suicide attempts.

■ AGENTS

Caustic agents are substances that can burn the mucosa of the aerodigestive tract. Alkaline agents are the most common offenders and are responsible for the majority of severe oropharyngeal and esophageal burns. Alkalis cause tissue damage by way of liquefactive necrosis, which allows the agent to cause rapid and deep burns. Even short exposure to an agent with a pH of 12.5 may result in a significant burn. The alkali will continue to cause damage as long as it is in contact with soft tissue. Common alkaline agents include lyes (sodium hydroxide, potassium hydroxide), miniature or disc batteries, hair relaxers, ammonia, and Clinitest tablets. Acids comprise the second largest group of caustic agents. Acids cause a coagulation necrosis upon exposure to mucosa, whereby a coagulum forms at the interface between agent and mucosa that can act to reduce further penetration of the agent into the muscle layers. Acids are less likely than alkalis to cause severe esophageal burns. The most significant complications involving acids usually occur in the gastroduodenal region. Bleaches are substances that contain chlorides such as sodium chlorite; these substances rarely cause significant esophageal injury unless ingested at very high concentrations.

■ THERAPY

Emergency Management

Initial management of the caustic ingestion patient follows emergency room routine (Fig. 1). Securing an airway and

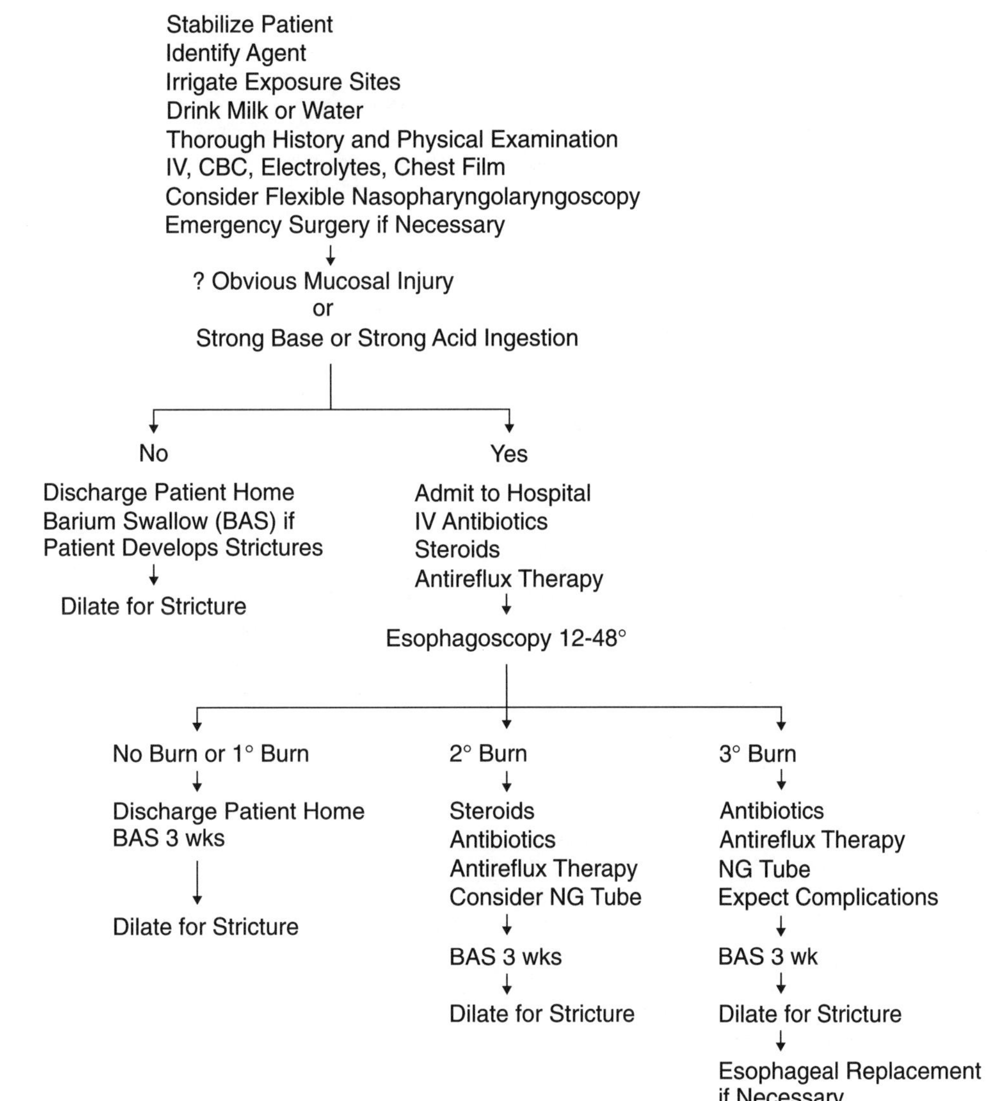

Figure 1.
Algorithm for management of caustic ingestion. CBC, complete blood count; NG, nasogastric.

cardiovascular support are priorities, although rarely necessary. An intravenous line should always be started, and blood samples for complete blood count and electrolytes should be sent, including a blood gas, if indicated. A concerted effort should be made to determine the type and amount of agent ingested. If possible, it is helpful to have a family member bring in any remaining agent and the original container. The pH, as well as other pertinent information, can be obtained by contacting a poison control center. Interviewing witnesses to the ingestion may help determine the amount ingested and whether the patient suffered aspiration, emesis, or respiratory distress.

After obtaining vital signs, a complete physical examination is performed, with particular attention paid to the upper aerodigestive tract mucosa. It is important to examine the patient's entire body to check for any skin burns due to agent spilled onto clothing. Any obvious skin or oral cavity burns should be washed with a copious amount of water. Flexible fiberoptic nasopharyngolaryngoscopy is most helpful in determining the presence of upper airway injury. A chest radiograph is routine, and abdominal radiographs are ordered, if indicated.

Water or milk can be administered to dilute or neutralize the agent, unless immediate surgery is planned. Giving an acid to neutralize an ingested base is not recommended. Gastric lavage, charcoal, and emetics are contraindicated. The passage of a nasogastric tube is controversial and is usually not recommended.

Children commonly have burns of the hands, lips, and oral cavity. Drooling and refusal to take liquids by mouth usually indicate some degree of mucosal injury. However, it is extremely important to remember that the presence or absence of burns in the oral cavity is not predictive of injury to the esophagus. It is estimated that 10 percent to 20 percent of significant esophageal burns occur without any evidence of injury to oral cavity mucosa. Hoarseness and stridor are signs of possible damage to the pharynx, larynx, or trachea. Rapid evaluation is necessary, and treatment may require tracheostomy. A patient who has acute chest or abdominal pain should be evaluated for possible viscus perforation. This is rare and usually occurs in an adult who has ingested a large amount of a strong acid or base in an effort to commit suicide. Emergent laparotomy with possible esophagogastrectomy is occasionally necessary.

Ingestion of miniature or disc batteries requires emergent management. These devices contain strong bases and can leak caustic agent from around the seals. If the battery is lodged in the esophagus, the patient should be taken directly to the operating room for esophagoscopy and removal, because esophageal perforation can occur in hours. If the radiograph demonstrates the battery to be in the stomach, it can be allowed to pass. If not detected in the stool within 4 days, a repeat radiograph should be performed. Retrieval is rarely necessary, although occasionally a large battery will not progress through the pylorus. As long as a battery is continuing to progress through the gastrointestinal tract, no intervention is necessary.

Because bleach ingestions are rarely associated with significant esophageal injury, many of these patients are sent home directly from the emergency room. Most bleaches used in the United States are less than 4 percent in concentration, and a large volume must be swallowed before esophageal erosion occurs. This is unlikely in cases of accidental ingestion. If there are oral cavity burns, however, these patients are investigated further. Bleach concentrations may be higher in Europe and other countries and are, therefore, more likely to cause esophageal injury in those geographic locations.

Caustic ingestion in the pediatric age group is often evidence of stress and discord within the patient's home. This sort of environment puts the child and siblings at risk for a repeat ingestion, as well as possible neglect or even abuse. Treating physicians should have a low threshold for involving social services in the care of these patients and their families. Obviously, any patient who has attempted suicide with a caustic agent requires urgent psychiatric consultation and suicide precautions.

■ INTERMEDIATE CARE

Any patient who is symptomatic or has ingested a strong acid or base should be admitted for overnight hospital observation. After life-threatening issues have been addressed, attention is directed toward evaluating and managing injury to the upper aerodigestive tract, particularly the esophagus. Traditionally, burns have been graded first-degree, erythema and/or edema of the mucosa; second-degree, full-thickness injury to the mucosa, including bleb formation, sloughing, or ulceration; and third-degree, full-thickness esophageal injury, with perforation into or through the muscular layer.

Early medical management of caustic ingestion using steroids is primarily concerned with the prevention of esophageal stricture formation; this approach remains controversial. General clinical consensus seems to maintain that first-degree injuries require no treatment because there is little or no risk of stricture. On the other hand, third-degree burns are likely to cause scar and stricture regardless of medical treatment and, therefore, steroids are not recommended. Disagreement continues as to the efficacy of steroid use in the management of second-degree burns. Because there may be some benefit in reducing the early local inflammatory response and there is little risk with short-term use, I routinely begin steroids for patients in whom I suspect more than first-degree burn. I do not wait until esophagoscopy to determine whether I will start steroids, because there is evidence that these drugs are more effective if given soon after the ingestion. Steroids are contraindicated in cases of esophageal or gastric perforation. There is no consensus on the appropriate dosing. I initially give a single dose of dexamethasone, 1 milligram per kilogram daily IV up to 25 mg, and determine the need for further steroid administration at the time of esophagoscopy. In these same patients, I begin broad-spectrum intravenous antibiotics (ampicillin, 100 milligrams per kilogram daily every 6 hours, or clindamycin, 40 milligrams per kilogram daily every 6 hours). The antibiotics act to decrease local bacterial colonization and formation of granulation tissue at sites of mucosal injury. Granulation tissue predisposes to fibrosis and possible stricture. Gastroesophageal reflux is common after caustic ingestion, and the acidic irritation can act to worsen ulceration. This problem is, therefore, treated with an H_2-receptor blocker such as ranitidine (4 milligrams per kilogram daily every 12 hours).

■ ESOPHAGOSCOPY

Definitive evaluation of the esophagus should be performed 12 to 48 hours after the injury. Earlier evaluation may lead to underdiagnosis because the full extent of mucosal damage may not yet be evident. Barium swallow is not as sensitive as esophagoscopy in the diagnosis of less dramatic, but potentially clinically relevant, esophageal burns. Therefore, the procedure of choice is esophagoscopy. The timing of esophagoscopy after the ingestion remains controversial. Although many clinicians advocate waiting at least 24 hours, it is unlikely that a significant burn will be missed if the procedure is performed only 12 hours after the ingestion. This interval also eliminates unnecessary hospital admission for the majority of patients who will fortunately have no significant esophageal injury. Essentially every patient who has ingested a strong acid or strong base other than bleach should undergo esophagoscopy. Esophagoscopy is a low-risk and inexpensive procedure that is very sensitive in detecting esophageal injury.

There is also controversy regarding rigid versus flexible endoscopic techniques. Traditionally, the latter has been more widely used by gastroenterologists and has the advantage of allowing for gastroduodenoscopy. Rigid esophagoscopy has been preferred by otorhinolaryngologists and, in experienced hands, the risk of perforation does not seem to be significantly higher than with the flexible endoscopes. After the patient is intubated, direct pharyngolaryngoscopy should always be performed. This may be followed by tracheobronchoscopy, if indicated. Esophagoscopy should be performed cautiously and not distal to a visualized full-thickness burn. If this is encountered, a nasogastric tube (soft Silastic) or esophageal stent (Reyes) is passed into the stomach and maneuvered to exit the nose. Flexible gastroduodenoscopy should always follow rigid esophagoscopy if there is any concern or possibility of gastric injury. If no esophageal burn is found at esophagoscopy, or if only minor first-degree burns are noted, the patient is discharged home. A barium esophagram is performed at 3 weeks after ingestion.

Corticosteroids

Patients who have second-degree esophageal burns are kept in the hospital for several days to 2 weeks. Prednisone is given at a dose of 1 milligram per kilogram twice daily for 2 weeks and then tapered over 4 more weeks. The long course of steroids is thought to decrease collagen deposition with subsequent fibrosis that occurs during healing. Antibiotics (ampicillin or clindamycin) are continued orally at the usual dosages for 2 weeks. Ranitidine is given for 2 to 4 weeks. These patients should all have a barium esophagram performed at 3 weeks after ingestion because this is when strictures first become evident. Dilations begin immediately for strictures.

For circumferential second-degree and all third-degree burns, a nasogastric tube or esophageal stent is left in place for 6 weeks. Antibiotics, along with ranitidine and a prokinetic agent such as cisapride, are used. Severely burned patients may remain in the hospital for an extended period due to the risk of late massive hemorrhage, which can result after esophagogastric necrosis. If stricture becomes evident, serial dilations are started.

Dilation

When esophageal stricture occurs, serial dilations are performed under general anesthesia. The procedure is initially performed several times per week, and later the frequency is determined by symptoms of dysphagia. In adults, dilations can later be performed in the office or at home. There are several different types of esophageal dilators; at our institution we use mercury-filled Maloney bougies. Acute complications of dilation include esophageal perforation and mediastinitis; therefore, a dilator is never forced through a stricture. Some patients can be managed for years with infrequent and effective dilations. Efficacy of the treatment is in large part determined by the degree of esophageal wall thickening.

If the stricture progresses or becomes difficult to dilate using the anterograde method, Tucker retrograde bougienage is an option. This form of dilation is performed through a gastrostomy with a continuous string in the esophagus that offers several advantages. The esophagus is often dilated above a stricture and funnel-shaped below it. In addition, strictures may be multiple, and lumina can be eccentrically placed. Anterograde dilation, therefore, runs the risk of creating a false passage with perforation. Retrograde bougies are safer and easier to advance in more severe or complicated strictures. Although usually done under general anesthesia, the technique can be performed outside of the operating room. In reality, the procedure is rarely used today.

It must be remembered that patients who have esophageal injury secondary to caustic ingestion are at significantly higher risk of developing squamous cell carcinoma of the esophagus. Chronic dilations may actually increase this risk. Therefore, these patients must be followed for many years. Late dysphagia can be due to stricture, tumor, or both.

■ ESOPHAGEAL REPLACEMENT

If esophageal stricture progresses or becomes complete, dilation attempts must be halted, and more definitive treatment should be sought. Several options are available for reconstruction or replacement of the esophagus. Jejunal free grafts have been used for high esophageal lesions. Colonic interposition is the procedure of choice for complete esophageal replacement, although gastric tubing or gastric pullup procedures may be considered. If there is at least some lumen remaining within the esophagus to allow for emptying into the stomach, the esophagus may be left in situ. If this is not the case, the esophagus is removed. Although esophageal replacement is usually successful, there is a relatively high incidence of complications, including stricture at anastomoses, fistulization, and dysphagia.

Suggested Reading

Adam JS, Birck HG. Pediatric caustic ingestion. Ann Otol Rhinol Laryngol 1982; 91:656-658.

Anderson KD, Rouse TM, Randolph JG. A controlled trial of corticosteroids in children with corrosive injury of the esophagus. N Engl J Med 1990; 323:637-640.

Gaudreault P, Parent M, McGuigan MA, et al. Predictability of esophageal injury from signs and symptoms: A study of caustic ingestion in 378 children. Pediatrics 1983; 71:767-770.

Hawkins DB, Demeter MJ, Barnett TE. Caustic ingestion: Controversies in management. A review of 214 cases. Laryngoscope 1980; 90:98-109.

Lovejoy FH Jr. Corrosive injury of the esophagus in children. N Engl J Med 1990; 323:668-669.

Maves MD. Esophageal burns secondary to disc battery ingestion. Ann Otol 1984; 93:364-368.

Moore WR. Caustic ingestions: Pathophysiology, diagnosis and treatment. Clin Pediatr 1986; 25:192-196.

Reyes HM, Hill JL. Modification of the experimental stent technique for esophageal burns. J Surg Res 1976; 20:65-70.

Schild JA. Caustic ingestion in adult patients. Laryngoscope 1985; 95:1199-1201.

DYSPHAGIA

The method of
Gary L. Schechter

Dysphagia, that is, difficulty in swallowing, is a common complaint in the otolaryngologist–head and neck surgeon's office. The swallowing mechanism is complex: it involves the actions of 26 muscles and five cranial nerves. Therefore, it is no surprise that disorders of this function occur frequently. In the United States, an estimated 10,000 deaths each year are attributed to choking. The incidence of dysphagia is higher in older age groups. Approximately 50 percent of nursing home residents suffer from some form of swallowing disorder. With the increasing numbers of older persons in this country, physicians are seeing more of this complaint and must know more about its diagnosis and treatment. The basis of this knowledge must start with an understanding of the normal anatomy and physiology of the swallowing process.

ANATOMY AND PHYSIOLOGY OF SWALLOWING

Swallowing, or deglutition, begins with actions of the lips and oral cavity. Competence of the orbicularis oris sphincter mechanism depends on a functioning facial nerve and is necessary for the transport and maintenance of food into the oral cavity. It assists the oral cavity to act as a suction or negative pressure pump. Once in the oral cavity, the combined actions of both the intrinsic and the extrinsic tongue muscles, the buccinators, and the muscles of mastication are required for the oral phase of deglutition (Fig. 1). It is in this phase that the basic food bolus is formed and brought to a consistency that is appropriate for passage into the pharynx, the positive pressure pump of the oral cavity.

Transferring the food bolus from the oral cavity to the pharynx is initiated by its contact with the anterior tonsillar pillars and soft palate. The sensory portion of this reflex is via the trigeminal nerve. Movement of the bolus into the pharynx triggers one of the most complex muscular interactions in the body, the pharyngeal phase of deglutition. The action to sweep the bolus back into the pharynx begins with a posterior and superior movement of the tongue. Simultaneously, the elevators of the palate, the levator veli palatini muscles, close off the nasopharyngeal isthmus to prevent nasal regurgitation.

While the tongue is moving the food bolus into the pharynx (Fig. 2), there are actions taking place to protect the laryngeal introitus and prevent aspiration. As the food bolus enters the pharynx, the geniohyoid muscles begin to contract along with the anterior bellies of the digastric muscles, which results in anterior and superior movement of the larynx. This, along with the posterior movement of the tongue, produces a posterior tilt of the epiglottis.

The combined effects of gravity and the pharyngeal constrictor muscles move the bolus inferiorly into the hypopharynx, where a complex reflex involving the vagus nerves begins. The sensory component is via fibers from the superior laryngeal branches of the vagus. The motor component is via branches of the superior laryngeal and parasympathetic nerve fibers of the vagus. The latter nerves stimulate relaxation of the cricopharyngeus muscle, whereas the former stimulate adduction of the vocal cords. At this time, there is simultaneous cessation of diaphragmatic muscle activity and further anterior and superior laryngeal movement under the tilting epiglottis. The net result is passage of the food bolus into the cervical esophagus without aspiration (Fig. 3). Residual food in the pharynx is stripped into the esophagus by sequential contractions of the pharyngeal constrictor muscles. A combination of laryngeal and hypopharyngeal movements produce a suction pump that pulls the bolus through the pharynx. Relaxation of the cricopharyngeal muscle ends this portion of the pharyngeal phase.

The entire interaction between oral and pharyngeal phases requires interplay between muscles innervated by the fifth, ninth, tenth, and twelfth cranial nerves. Coordination of these actions occurs in the swallowing center, which is located in the pons and medulla. This interaction is both voluntary and involuntary. The voluntary component moves the bolus, or liquid, into the pharynx and subsequently the esophagus, and the involuntary component strips any residual material downward. When involuntary or reflex swallowing occurs prematurely, aspiration or laryngeal obstruction may develop, that is, the "cafe coronary," in which food that has not been masticated adequately moves too far posteriorly in the oral cavity, touches the faucial arch, triggers the swallowing reflex prematurely, and then, because of the abnormal bulk of the bolus, lodges in the laryngeal introitus.

Once the bolus is in the esophagus, and the esophageal phase of deglutition is in effect, gravity plays a major role in its transit toward the lower esophageal sphincter and the stomach (Fig. 4). Passage of the bolus inferiorly requires coordinated contraction and relaxation of both the skeletal muscle in the cervical esophagus and the smooth muscle of the thoracic esophagus. These muscles, and those of the lower esophageal sphincter, are entirely under the influence of the autonomic nervous system, with the vagus nerve and associated sympathetic nerves acting in concert. The vagus nerves synapse with intramural ganglia, whereas those of the sympathetic system are in paraspinal locations. Neuromuscular activity in the esophagus is under the influence of both the central nervous system, via the swallowing center, and local reflexes stimulated by esophageal distention.

It is easy to appreciate the vulnerability of the deglutition process when it depends on such complex interactions between so many distinct neural and muscular components and functioning mandibular, temporomandibular, and salivary structures. Dysfunction may result from loss of any one or combination of factors. Thus, establishing a diagnosis in a patient who complains of dysphagia is a major challenge.

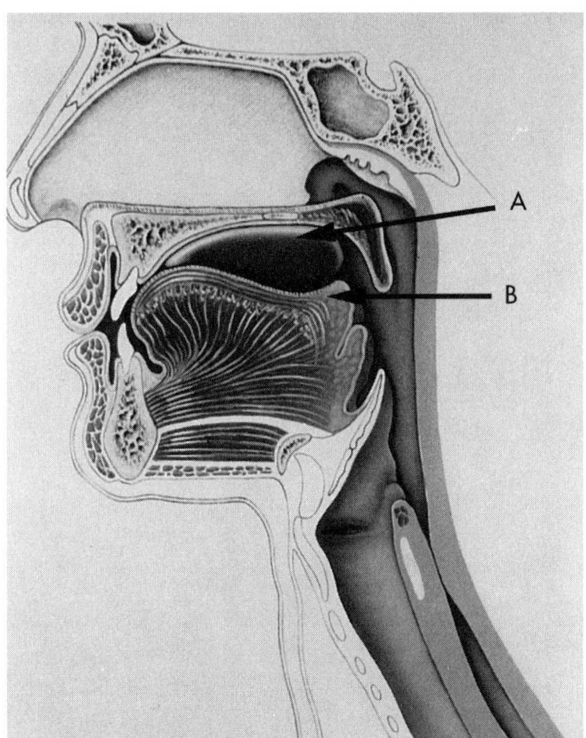

Figure 1.
The bolus *(A)* on the dorsum of the tongue during the *oral phase* of deglutition. Note the posterior elevation of the tongue *(B)* to prevent posterior movement of the bolus and the normal position of the larynx. *(From Schechter GL. When your patient complains "Doctor, I can't swallow." J Respir Dis 1985; 6:45–48; with permission.)*

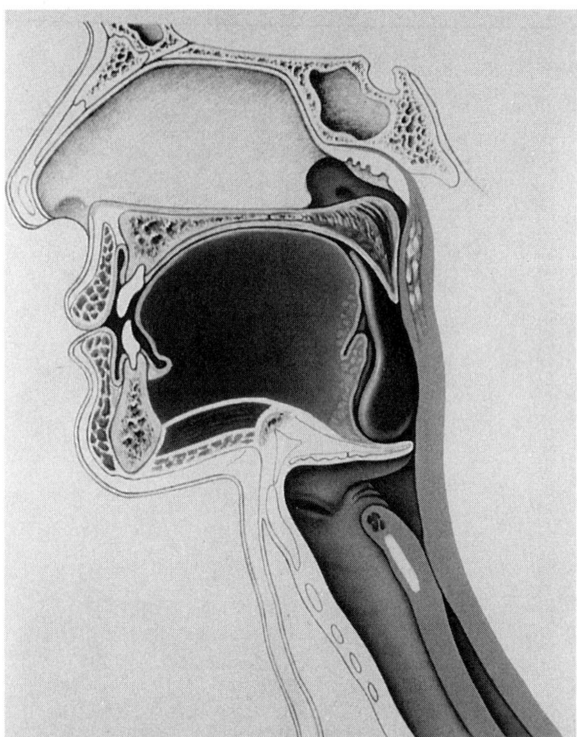

Figure 2.
Passage of the bolus into the pharynx, commencing the *pharyngeal phase* of deglutition. Note the extreme dorsal position of the tongue and the elevation of the soft palate. Of utmost importance is the contraction of the geniohyoid muscle, which results in anterior and superior movement of the larynx and posterior displacement of the epiglottis. *(From Schechter GL. When your patient complains "Doctor, I can't swallow." J Respir Dis 1985; 6:45–48; with permission.)*

■ DIFFERENTIAL DIAGNOSIS

History

The patient who has dysphagia is often concerned about the possibility of cancer. It is essential that from the outset the examining physician, and his or her staff, demonstrate serious interest in the patient's complaints and make it obvious that everything reasonable is being done to rule out a malignant or central nervous system process. Stating up-front that this will be your goal, and that you appreciate the patient's concern over the problem, is helpful. This kind of face-to-face confrontation with the patient's concerns creates a receptive atmosphere for patients in which their complaints may be heard, and it allows the patient and physician to be more comfortable with the exchange of information, which is necessary for obtaining a reliable history.

Establishing a differential diagnosis should be the first goal, and this begins with a detailed history. The single most important question is whether the difficulty in swallowing occurs while eating food or just between meals. A normal adult swallows unconsciously 600 times in a 24 hour period. Normally, between-meal swallowing involves an effortless passage of salivary secretions and the nasal mucous blanket through the pharynx into the esophagus. Obstructing disorders usually affect between-meal swallowing late in the course of the disease, whereas neurologic disorders affect between-meal swallowing in the early stages.

Nonfood-related dysphagia, traditionally termed *globus hystericus,* is the most common complaint heard in relation to the swallowing mechanism. Patients often introduce their complaint by stating that they are having a problem when they swallow. During some part of the day, they feel pressure, fullness, or a lump in the throat or neck. This complaint worsens with time, is not related to meals, and in fact, is often temporarily alleviated by eating food.

The classic teaching that nonfood-related dysphagia, or globus hystericus, is almost exclusively found in overweight, depressed, or obsessive, menopausal females is not only incorrect but also a dangerous idea to foster. This concept has introduced prejudice into the physician-patient relationship that may result in failure to diagnose significant pathology or, at the least, poor communications with patients who desperately need counseling from a concerned physician. It would be best if the term *globus hystericus* were eliminated. In fact, complaints relative to the nonfood-related swallowing cycle are not limited to any one sex or patients who have psychological problems, but are often associated with real

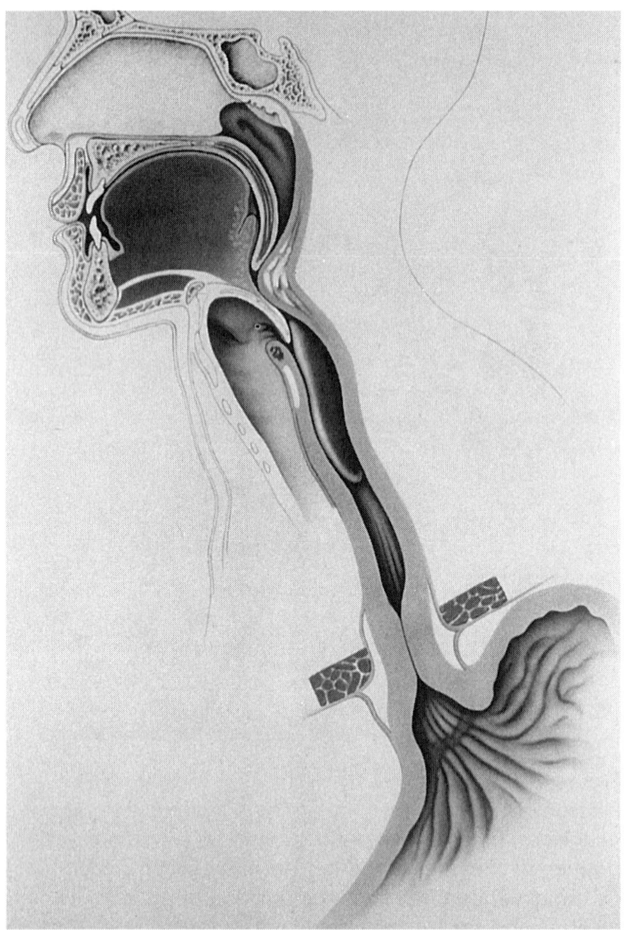

Figure 3.
During the final stage of the *pharyngeal phase* of deglutition, the bolus passes through the cricopharyngeal region into the cervical esophagus. Note the extreme anterior and superior position of the larynx, posterior displacement of the epiglottis, and the dilatation of the food passage posterior to the larynx, which represents relaxation of the cricopharyngeus muscle. *(From Schechter GL. When your patient complains "Doctor, I can't swallow." J Respir Dis 1985; 6:45–48; with permission.)*

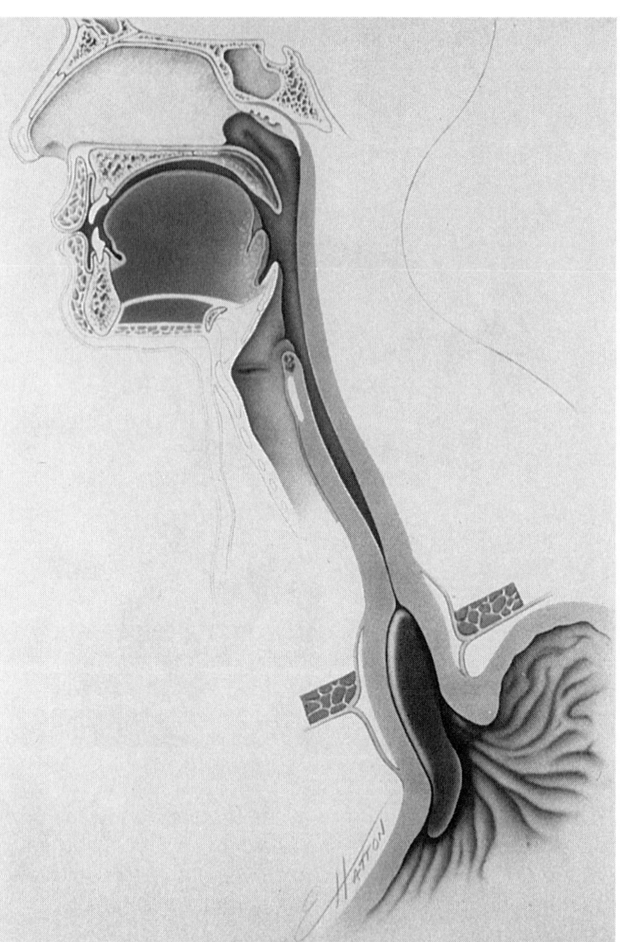

Figure 4.
The food bolus passing through the lower esophageal sphincter in the final stage of the *esophageal phase* of deglutition. *(From Schechter GL. When your patient complains "Doctor, I can't swallow." J Respir Dis 1985; 6:45–48; with permission.)*

pharyngoesophageal disorders such as gastroesophageal reflux disease (GERD).

Difficulty swallowing solid foods or liquids, with or without discomfort, or odynophagia, is a serious complaint usually caused by an obstructive or neuromuscular disease. The problem may be as mild as esophagitis or as serious as amyotrophic lateral sclerosis or cancer. The association of weight loss with food-related dysphagia increases the likelihood of a significant organic process. The corollary is nonfood-related dysphagia and the absence of weight loss usually indicate that there are no serious organic problems.

The history may help localize the site of the problem. Problems that occur in the initial 3 or 4 seconds after the initiation of swallowing can usually be localized to the oral cavity, pharynx, or cricopharyngeal regions. Problems occurring after 4 seconds are most often due to pathology in the esophagus.

Characteristics of the offending food, such as consistency and temperature, may be helpful. Liquids are the last to be affected by obstructing lesions, and the temperature of the food has no effect on the problem. Neuromuscular disorders, however, often present with aspiration of liquids first. In the latter circumstances, room temperature liquids, particularly plain water, cause aspiration, whereas those of extreme temperatures are easier to swallow.

Nasal regurgitation is an important indicator of significant neuromuscular dysfunction. It rarely occurs in association with obstructing lesions if the palate is intact. Escape of liquids through the nose is the most severe form of this problem, whereas symptoms of recurrent nasal and/or sinus infection may indicate that there is chronic nasal regurgitation.

Voice change may occur in patients who have reflux disorders, with either spillage of acid contents into the posterior laryngeal introitus or reflex cough and throat clearing from lower esophageal irritation. The voice may also change as a result of tumors or vocal cord paralysis. Elderly patients very commonly experience voice change as elasticity of the vocal ligaments diminishes and sensory function of the superior laryngeal nerves is lost. The latter not only results in voice change but also leads to a mild form of dysphagia for liquids, pills, and specific foods.

Close attention to medication history is important. Drug-induced dysphagia is a real entity. Common medications may affect smooth muscle function, produce xerostomia, and cause esophageal injury.

The patient's psychosocial history is extremely important, but avoid asking questions in this category too early in the encounter. Many patients have been seen by one or more other physicians before referral to your specialty, and have had negative experiences by being labeled as anxious or hysterical.

A considerable amount may be learned about the patient from the basic information sheet that is filled out for the physician's business office. Facts about age, marital status, number of children, type of employment, and location of the patient's home in the community often lead into conversation about the patient's background. Above all, make the patient feel as much at ease as possible under the circumstances of a new physician encounter. The major factor in achieving this is to demonstrate concern and interest in the patient's complaints and, as mentioned previously, to assure the patient that you are there to rule out the possibility of serious pathology.

Physical Examination

Examination of the patient begins while you are taking the history. Signs of chronic illness or recent weight loss may be detected from the patient's general appearance, skin color, fit of clothes, and general demeanor. Begin the traditional head and neck examination only after you have checked for signs of systemic nutritional difficulty, such as loss of skin turgor, character of the skin surface, condition of the nails and hair, color of nailbeds and conjunctivae, and the condition of the dorsum of the tongue.

The head and neck examination must be complete and include examination of the nasopharynx and laryngopharynx with the indirect mirror and the flexible fiberoptic endoscope. Topical anesthetics, such as Cetacaine or 10 percent lidocaine spray, are used to help with both the indirect and the direct examinations. The use of these drugs may also differentiate between the discomfort of organic and functional problems. The latter are usually unaffected by the anesthetic.

Flexible fiberoptic nasopharyngeal and laryngopharyngeal examinations with video documentation are essential when evaluating patients who have swallowing disorders. Video documentation allows the examiner to review the findings without examining the patient repeatedly. Subtle abnormalities are often noted when the videotape is played back several times. These tapes are also used to demonstrate positive and negative findings to the patient, his or her relatives, colleagues such as swallowing therapists and radiologists, and referring physicians.

Fiberoptic endoscopic evaluation of swallowing (FEES) disorders has become an important component of the dysphagia workup. Direct viewing of the liquid or food bolus through the flexible endoscope positioned high in the oropharynx allows observation of the vocal and arytenoid movements, elevation of the larynx and tongue base, and the patient's management of residual material after the initial swallow. Pooling of secretions and aspiration may be noted. Although there are strong arguments in the literature for and against FEES versus the modified barium swallow, I suggest that these two modalities are complementary and are both important parts of the dysphagia workup.

If any of the history or physical findings suggest a neurologic or lower gastrointestinal disorder, the patient must have a general physical examination. This should include examination of the chest and abdomen and a general neurologic examination.

Radiographic Studies

The modified barium swallow is the definitive study for evaluation of the swallowing mechanism. The standard barium swallow is performed using thin barium, and a quick view of the swallowing mechanism is carried out by the radiologist. This is not satisfactory for the evaluation of most swallowing disorders. In the modified barium swallow, all structures from the lips to the stomach are examined. It is helpful to have a speech pathologist who is trained and interested in swallowing disorders present during this examination. The studies should include both dynamic recordings with videofluoroscopy and double-contrast examination for evaluation of the mucosa. The spot film camera ideally should be high-speed, enabling 24 to 30 frames per second. Both the upright and recumbent positions are used to demonstrate the dynamics of the lower esophageal sphincter. A barium-impregnated bread sphere, bagel, or marshmallow is used to evaluate the system with a bolus similar to the food the patient will swallow when eating a regular meal. Some radiologists believe that acid barium is helpful in establishing the diagnosis of hiatal hernia with reflux esophagitis.

Videofluoroscopy is essential because it allows review by the radiologist, the physician, and the swallowing therapist, which enhances understanding of the problem and helps in the development of treatment plans.

Computed tomographic scans are necessary only to evaluate mass lesions in the neck. When neurologic disorders are suspected, the magnetic resonance image is useful in delineating mass lesions in the brain as well as degenerative processes in the brain and spinal cord. Dynamic ultrasound studies may help with the evaluation of tongue and pharyngeal muscles.

The radiographic studies should be completed and reviewed by the radiologist and the patient's physician, and then discussed with the patient via a prearranged telephone conversation. Serious findings require diplomacy on the telephone and an immediate office visit for personal contact with the patient. In most circumstances, endoscopy is indicated at this time. In some patients, it is appropriate to carry out special tests before endoscopy.

Special Tests

Manometric, pH monitoring, esophageal motility, nuclear scanning, and acid infusion tests may be required in some patients. These tests require careful interpretation and critical quality assurance relative to the equipment and technicians in the gastroenterology laboratory in which they are performed.

The pH study is carried out over a 24 hour period, but accuracy in diagnosis is not forfeited if the study is conducted during a 4 hour postprandial period followed by an 8 hour sleep period. A positive finding from a pH monitoring study suggests a diagnosis of GERD and laryngopharyngitis. Patients who have nonfood-related dysphagia with no significant reflux on barium swallow examination should have a pH study.

Manometry and motility studies are essential when the barium swallow examination demonstrates dysfunction of the cricopharyngeus, esophageal motility, or the lower esophageal sphincter. These studies must be carried out in a quality laboratory setting and interpreted by an experienced gastroenterologist. The gastroenterologist will be required for treatment of most motility disorders. Monitoring motility over 24 hours and even combined motility and pH monitoring are now considered in problematic cases.

Other tests may be helpful when those already mentioned fail to give definitive results. Nuclear esophageal or gastric scans may be used to evaluate gastric emptying, esophageal reflux, and the presence or absence of gastric contents in the hypopharynx and lungs. The Bernstein infusion test, which is conducted by infusing a dilute hydrochloric acid solution into the esophagus, is useful in determining if acid in the esophagus replicates the patient's symptoms.

Endoscopy

In most patients who have dysphagia, endoscopy may be carried out under local anesthesia. The only exceptions to this are patients who complain of persistent neck pain, pain on swallowing, or those who have obvious tumors demonstrated in the preliminary workup. Patients who have pain on swallowing, or odynophagia, must have a careful examination by rigid laryngoscopy of the piriform fossae, postcricoid region, and cervical esophagus, including microlaryngoscopy, if necessary, as well as cervical esophagoscopy, to rule out small tumors or areas of ectopic gastric mucosa with ulceration. Likewise, patients who have obvious hypopharyngeal or cervical esophageal tumors must have precise mapping of their lesions for treatment planning. In both situations, the endoscopy is best performed under general anesthesia with complete paralysis. This can be accomplished as outpatient surgery.

The best method for esophagoscopy must include the use of the flexible fiberoptic esophagoscope. Traditional rigid esophagoscopy, although sometimes essential, is not as useful in these circumstances. The rigid esophagoscope is uncomfortable for the patient who is under local anesthesia, places the examiner's eye a considerable distance from the mucosa, and does not provide the opportunity to use air for expansion of the mucosa ahead of the esophagoscope. The air under various pressure equates to visual palpation just as the Bruening otoscope allows for observation of tympanic membrane movement. The flexible esophagoscope also allows for easier video documentation, observation of the procedure by the operating room staff, and simultaneous teaching. For the examiner, the flexible fiberoptic esophagoscope provides excellent visualization because of its optical system and light source. The examiner has a sense of being down in the esophagus and pushing the walls apart as the esophagoscope is advanced.

The esophagus should be biopsied in all patients suspected of having esophagitis, a neuromuscular disorder, or collagen vascular disease. In patients who are found to have small (less than 5 mm) areas of ulcerated ectopic gastric mucosa in the cervical esophagus or postcricoid region, complete removal of the lesion with the biopsy forceps or an appropriate laser is therapeutic.

■ MEDICAL THERAPY

I have limited this section to general therapeutic concepts applied to the most common entities causing dysphagia. Detailed management regimens and techniques must be obtained elsewhere.

Nonsurgical problems that cause dysphagia are usually caused by disorders of the esophagus and its upper and lower sphincters. The most common of these problems is GERD with or without hiatal hernia. This disorder may demonstrate nonfood-related dysphagia in its mildest form or odynophagia when acute esophagitis is present. There may be associated symptoms related to spillage into the larynx, such as cough or hoarseness. The problem is suspected when there is a history of sour taste in the mouth shortly after eating or upon waking in the morning, chronic cough, or repeated throat clearing. Few patients complain initially of chest or abdominal dyspepsia. Further suspicion is aroused by the presence of acute inflammation involving the hypopharynx and arytenoids. Many patients complaining of dysphagia have already had a diagnosis of hiatal hernia established previously but do not relate their new symptoms to this old problem.

An aggressive antireflux regimen should be started as soon as the diagnosis of gastroesophageal reflux with esophageal or laryngopharyngeal complications is confirmed by barium swallow and endoscopy. Rapid relief of symptoms helps to confirm the diagnosis and is reassuring to both the patient and the referring physician. Of course, continued therapy must be under the direction of the gastroenterologist or the primary care physician. The antireflux regimen should consist of the following components:

1. Elevation of the head of the bed at a 20 degree to 30 degree angle. This is accomplished by elevating the head of the bed 6 to 8 inches on blocks, a plywood wedge under the mattress, or a foam rubber wedge pillow. The most luxurious manner in which to achieve the proper angle is by replacing the mattress and box spring with a hospital bed mechanism. Some insurance carriers will consider a hospital bed assembly as essential for the treatment of esophageal reflux if it is ordered by prescription.
2. No solid or liquid foods should be taken during the 3 hour period before bedtime. It is essential to allow complete emptying of the stomach before the patient assumes the recumbent position, whether it be at bedtime or before a daytime nap. This restriction will also assist the patient in any weight reduction or weight control program that may be prescribed as part of the long-term management of their GERD.

3. There must be a reduction of gastric acid during the hours of sleep. This is accomplished through the use of H_2-receptor blockers or proton pump inhibitors. The use of antacids before bedtime is controversial, but many patients find that these agents provide quick relief when other measures do not work.
4. The lower esophageal sphincter tone and esophageal contractions must be enhanced to promote esophageal emptying. This and promotion of gastric emptying may be accomplished with a variety of medications. The use of medications for reduction of acid production along with those that promote gastric emptying for the treatment of GERD remains controversial.
5. Alteration of the diet. Patients who have gastroesophageal reflux will benefit from avoiding hot and spicy foods. The traditional bland diet heavy in milk products is not thought to be beneficial. The diet recommended by the American Heart Association for prevention of cardiovascular disease appears to also be beneficial for patients who have gastroesophageal reflux. It is high in complex carbohydrates and roughage and low in cholesterol-containing products such as red meat and dairy products.

The diagnosis of pharyngeal and/or esophageal infections, for example, *Candida,* herpesvirus, and cytomegalic inclusion disease, may be established via endoscopy. In these cases, the presence of such predisposing factors as prolonged antibiotic therapy, diabetes, immune-suppressing cancers, and acquired immunodeficiency syndrome must be determined. *Candida* infections are treated with oral nystatin solutions at a dose of 500,000 U every 6 hours. Resistant cases may be treated with 200 mg of ketoconazole daily for 7 to 10 days. Antiviral therapy requires assistance from an infectious disease specialist.

The swallowing therapist is an extremely important part of medical and perioperative regimens for patients who have dysphagia. Swallowing therapy has been developed as a subspecialty of speech pathology. The swallowing therapist should be involved in the complete evaluation of the patient, including obtaining a history, performing swallowing evaluations, assisting with the observations of swallowing with flexible fiberoptic laryngoscopy, and interpreting the modified barium swallow. In clinical situations involving the need for alterations of swallowing technique, such as when there are neuromuscular disorders or postoperative defects, the swallowing therapist is indispensable. Further assistance may also be obtained from a nutritionist.

Dysmotility problems may be caused by surgical manipulations, degenerative disorders, autoimmune disease, thyroid myopathy, and diabetes, or they may occur spontaneously without evidence of serious systemic disease. Their diagnosis and management are usually in the hands of the gastroenterologist, but surgical therapy may be indicated in specific situations. Medical treatment includes reversal or management of any primary disorders, and medication to enhance esophageal and gastric emptying while preventing reflux. Alterations of diet and swallowing technique are often necessary.

■ SURGICAL THERAPY

In most patients who require surgical management of dysphagia, there is an identifiable lesion to treat. The following discussion includes the more common surgical solutions to dysphagia problems.

Dilation

The etiology of any stenosis noted on barium swallow must be determined immediately. Endoscopy is essential, and the endoscopist should be ready to perform dilation, if warranted. Stenoses vary and must be distinguished from disorders that cause obstruction through dysfunctional neuromuscular activity in isolated segments of the esophagus. Congenital rings or webs are usually covered with normal mucosa and are thin. Acquired stenoses from infection, trauma, burns, or esophagitis are usually irregular, covered by atrophic mucosa, and thick.

Dilation is very effective treatment for congenital and most acquired stenoses. It will also benefit some patients who have cricopharyngeal spasm. The initial dilation is often carried out at the time of diagnostic endoscopy. In situations in which the narrowed segment is too small to allow passage of the smallest esophagoscope, and the barium swallow has demonstrated a clear distal segment, the dilation is started with Fogarty or vascular dilating catheters. These come in very small sizes and are firm enough to pass through most tight stenoses. They are also capable of perforating the esophagus and developing false passages, a complication that can usually be avoided by using gentle technique and passing the bougie only where there is a visible lumen. The usual stenoses are dilated with mercury-weighted rubber or synthetic flexible dilators. These may be used under general anesthesia. However, they work best in the patient who is awake and in a sitting position.

Dilation regimens vary considerably. When the stenosis is thin and easily dilated, the patient may not require repeat dilation for many months or years. In the case of thick stenoses, however, multiple dilations may be required to achieve a lumen large enough for passage of a reasonable diet. Once the maximum lumen size has been achieved, and it is known that the patient requires frequent dilations, it is of great benefit to involve the patient or family in the dilation process. This is accomplished by having the patient purchase a flexible dilator one size smaller than the largest one used at the time of serial dilations, and then training the patient and family in the use of the dilator at home. Topical anesthetic spray and anesthetic jelly may be necessary to help with the process. Through trial and error, the patient learns the frequency of dilations necessary to keep the stenosis open.

Balloon dilators are helpful when there is narrowing in the distal esophagus, at the lower esophageal sphincter, and at the cricopharyngeal sphincter. These are used under manometric control and are designed to expand to a point that results in stretching of underlying sphincter muscles, such as in cricopharyngeal spasm.

Cricopharyngeal Myotomy

The cricopharyngeus muscle may require a relaxing procedure to treat cricopharyngeal spasm in association with suspension or resection of a Zenker's diverticulum, or when there is a more generalized neurologic problem. This operation should be performed in patients who have cricopharyngeal spasm only after more conservative measures have been tried.

The surgical approach to the cricopharyngeus muscle requires careful avoidance of the great vessels and laryngeal nerves. Because it is necessary to keep a dilator in place during the myotomy, it is preferable to perform the surgery under general anesthesia. A mercury-weighted rubber dilator is placed into the esophagus and taped to the patient's cheek before the preparation and draping of the neck. An oblique incision similar to the one used for carotid artery surgery is made opposite the thyroid cartilage along the medial border of the sternomastoid muscle. Dissection is then carried down to the carotid sheath and proceeds medially to enter the groove between the great vessels and the larynx. In some cases, it is necessary to ligate the superior thyroid artery in order to gain exposure to the entire cricopharyngeus muscle.

The dissection should be carried posteriorly to the fascia of the longus colli muscle and then medially to the posterior and lateral aspect of the pharyngoesophageal junction. This approach helps prevent damage to the superior and recurrent laryngeal nerves as they enter the larynx. The larynx is then rotated medially, and the cricopharyngeus muscle fibers are cut longitudinally down to the mucosa. The incision must be carried inferiorly into the muscle of the esophagus and superiorly into the muscle of the inferior constrictor in order to incise all fibers of the cricopharyngeus muscle. The wound is drained and closed in a standard fashion. It is preferable to wait several days before feeding these patients in order to allow resolution of the postoperative edema. Newer transoral approaches for cricopharyngeal myotomy using stapling devices or the laser have recently been described as well.

Feeding Tubes

In patients who have severe malfunction of their swallowing mechanism that will not respond to the spectrum of treatments previously discussed, it is necessary to provide access for tube feedings. In most cases, a nasogastric tube is not only uncomfortable and socially limiting, but also associated with postcricoid complications. Therefore, patients who have dysphagia that is expected to prevent adequate nutrition for more than 10 days should be considered for placement of a gastrostomy, usually by percutaneous endoscopic gastrostomy or a cervical esophagostomy.

The cervical esophagostomy has been maligned and associated with significant complications. However, in most cases in which problems occur, the procedure has not been carried out properly, and therefore a true cervical esophagostomy has not been performed. Entry into the piriform fossae or the cervical esophagus at the level of the cricopharyngeus has instead occurred, and these sites are associated with significant salivary leak, cricoiditis, and recurrent laryngeal nerve dysfunction.

Cervical esophagostomy may be performed under local or general anesthesia. A No. 18 nasogastric feeding tube is placed at the beginning of the procedure. It is preferable to place the esophagostomy in the patient's left neck because the cervical esophagus is more accessible on that side. The incision is made over the medial third of the sternomastoid muscle at the level of the thyroid gland in order to gain maximum exposure at the level of the middle thyroid vein. Dissection is then carried down to the prevertebral muscle fascia, as described for the approach to the cricopharyngeus, which allows entry into the cervical esophagus at its posterior and lateral border. This avoids injury to the recurrent laryngeal nerve.

The esophagotomy is performed after grasping the esophageal wall and the contained feeding tube with a Babcock clamp. A 5 to 7 mm vertical incision is then made into the esophagus down to the feeding tube, and the mucosal edges are grasped with small hemostats. The Babcock clamp is then released, and a fresh No. 18 feeding tube is inserted into the esophagus down to the stomach. A purse-string absorbable suture is then placed around the esophagotomy opening and the feeding tube. The medial border of the sternomastoid muscle is then sutured down to the prevertebral muscles, with avoidance of the cervical sympathetic chain, in order to protect the carotid artery. The tube is then led out through the skin and secured with a temporary silk suture and an umbilical tape. Feedings may begin within 48 to 72 hours.

Although the percutaneous gastrostomy technique has made placement of gastrostomy tubes much easier, cervical esophagostomy does have the following advantages: (1) it may be performed by the same surgeon at the time of other neck procedures, such as at staging endoscopy, primary tumor resection, tracheotomy, or cricopharyngeal myotomy; (2) the patient can perform self-feeding in the sitting position; (3) there is no problem with gastric juice leakage on the skin around the tube; and (4) the stomach is not violated and can be used for reconstruction at a later time.

Correction of Specific Defects

Some patients have dysphagia because of specific defects that arise from surgical procedures. This may be helped if defects demonstrated by the swallowing workup can be corrected. Tongue immobility after resection of tumors may improve with tongue release procedures. Velopharyngeal insufficiency is corrected with a pharyngeal flap. Epiglottoplasty may be useful in preventing aspiration in some patients who have immobile or ptotic larynges. Teflon injections are beneficial in correcting glottic insufficiency in patients who have vocal cord paralysis. Arytenoid and vocal cord medialization procedures are now considered the initial treatment of choice.

Tracheotomy in Patients Who Have Dysphagia

Tracheotomy may help or hinder patients who have dysphagia. In severe cases of dysphagia with aspiration, tracheotomy may be necessary for prevention of aspiration and to assist with pulmonary toilet. However, in these cases, and in patients who have tracheotomy for other reasons, the tracheotomy may be the cause of dysphagia and make aspiration worse. This results from binding of the trachea to the skin at the tracheotomy site and the presence of the tracheotomy tube preventing upward movement of the larynx during deglutition. These factors combine to prevent the epiglottis from moving over the laryngeal introitus for protection.

The tracheotomy may also prevent the development of subglottic pressure during the passage of the food bolus into the hypopharynx, a phenomenon that is thought to be helpful in preventing leakage of liquids through the vocal cords after they move to an abducted position for postdeglutition respiration. The tracheotomy tube cuff may also place pressure on the esophagus through the membranous tracheal wall and cause obstruction.

In patients who are made worse by tracheotomy, and who must have the tracheotomy for maintenance of their airway, it may be necessary to divert the trachea above the tracheotomy site or suture the larynx or cricoid closed in order to prevent aspiration. These patients usually have severe neurologic disorders and are the most extreme problems with dysphagia to manage.

Suggested Reading

Bastian RW. Videoendoscopic evaluation of patients with dysphagia: An adjunct to the modified barium swallow. Otolaryngol Head Neck Surg 1991; 104:339-350.

Brin MF, Younger D. Neurologic disorders and aspiration. Otolaryngol Clin North Am 1988; 21:691.

Hendrix TR. pH monitoring: Is it the gold standard for the detection of gastroesophageal reflux disease? Dysphagia 1993; 8:122-124.

Hendrix T, Ravich W, Bucholz D, et al. The multidisciplinary approach to dysphagia. Gastrointest Radiol 1985; 10:193.

Jones B, Donner MW. Examination of the patient with dysphagia. Radiology 1988; 167:319.

Jones B, Ravich WJ, Donner M. Dysphagia in systemic disease. Dysphagia 1993; 8:368-383.

Kennedy J, Kent R. Anatomy and physiology of deglutition and related functions. In Logemann J, ed. Relationship between speech and swallowing. New York: Thieme Stratton, 1985.

Kidder TM, Langmore SE, Martin BJW. Indications and techniques of endoscopy in evaluation of cervical dysphagia. Comparison with radiographic techniques. Dysphagia 1994; 9:256-261.

Krespi YP, Pelzer HJ, Sisson GA. Management of chronic aspiration by subtotal and submucosal cricoid resection. Ann Otol Rhinol Laryngol 1985; 94:580.

Logemann J. Manual for the videofluorographic study of swallowing. 2nd ed. Austin, Texas: Pro-Ed, 1993.

Logemann J. The role of the speech language pathologist in the management of dysphagia. Otolaryngol Clin North Am 1988; 21:783.

Lorenz R, Jory G, Classen M. The value of endoscopy and endosonography in the diagnosis of the dysphagia patient. Dysphagia 1993; 8:91-97.

McConnel FMS. Analysis of pressure generation and bolus transit during pharyngeal swallowing. Laryngoscope 1988; 98:71.

Miller A. A neurophysiologic basis of swallowing. Dysphagia 1986; 1:91.

Stuchell RN, Mandel ID. Salivary gland dysfunction and swallowing disorders. Otolaryngol Clin North Am 1988; 21:649.

SNORING

The method of
Eric F. Pinczower

Snoring, or upper respiratory noise while sleeping, is one of the most common afflictions of the United States adult population. As many as one-half of U.S. males and one-quarter of U.S. females may snore to varying degrees. However, snoring is only a medical problem if it is (1) part of a sleep apnea syndrome, or (2) socially disruptive, that is, interferes with the quality of life of the patient, or his or her bed partner, roommates, housemates, or neighbors. I discuss in this chapter the evaluation and treatment of the loud snorer as well as criteria for obtaining sleep studies and selecting patients suitable for snoring surgery. Once a patient has been deemed a candidate for snoring surgery, the various considerations that define the need for either nasoseptal, turbinate, or pharyngeal surgery are presented. In addition, the techniques that I use for laser turbinoplasty and laser-assisted uvulopalatoplasty are described. Figure 1 provides a general schematic of the diagnosis and treatment of the snorer. I also discuss common side effects and minor complications of the surgery and their management.

With careful patient selection and workup, more than 90 percent of patients who have a severe snoring disorder can be expected to obtain satisfactory results by following these methods.

■ SLEEP APNEA

Obstructive sleep apnea is a disease state characterized by pathologic obstruction of the upper airway in the deeper stages of sleep. Different authors have established different laboratory criteria for this diagnosis. The diagnosis is most frequently made with the assistance of the polysomnograph. Sleep apnea runs the gamut from the upper airway resistance syndrome, which is the disease's most mild form, to the pickwickian syndrome, which is the most severe. It is important to consider that the snoring patient may indeed have a component of obstructive sleep apnea. How does one decide whether to obtain polysomnography on each snoring pa-

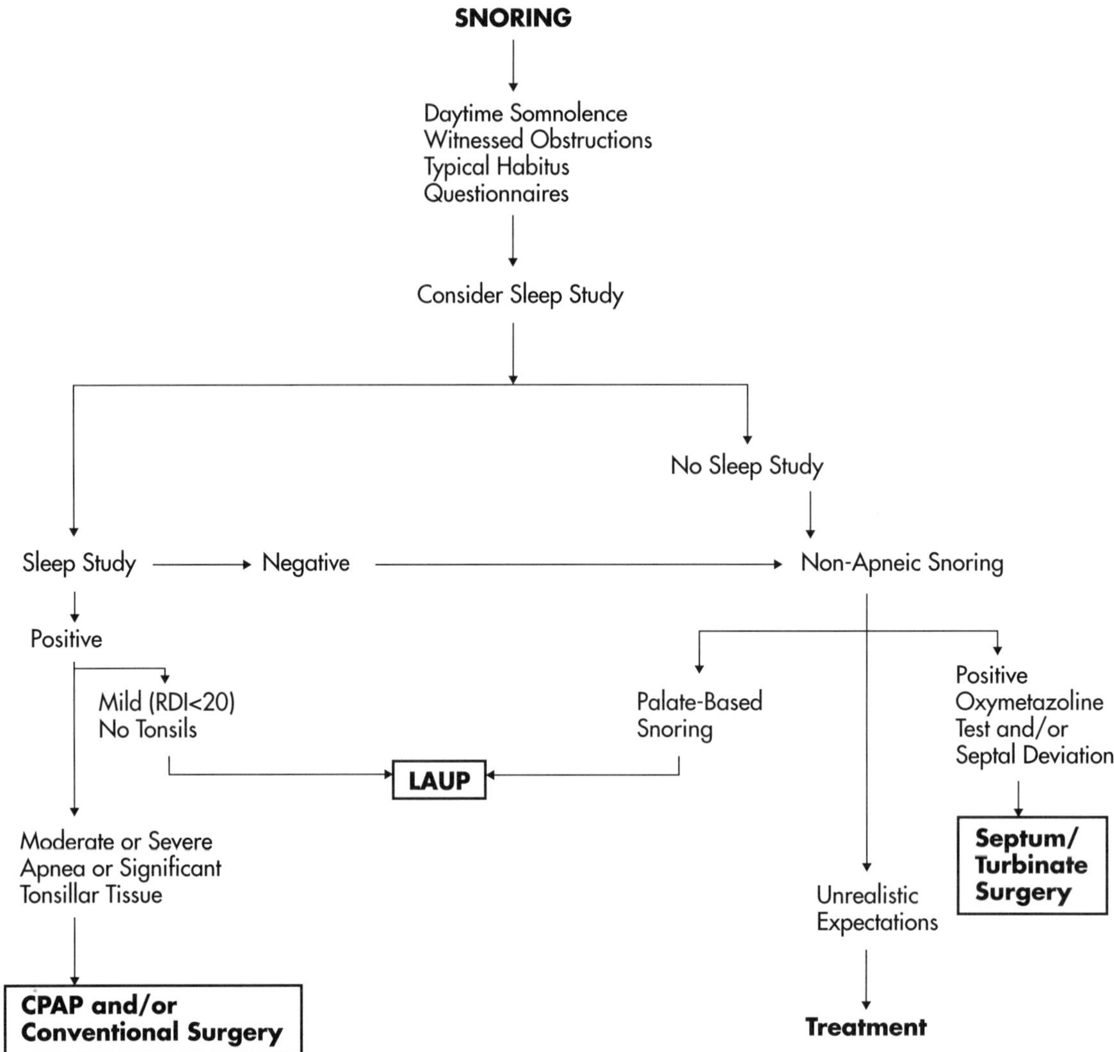

Figure 1.
Schematic diagram of snoring diagnosis and management. RDI, respiratory disturbance index; CPAP, continuous positive airway pressure; LAUP, laser-assisted uvulopalatoplasty.

tient? The Standards of Practice Committee of the American Sleep Disorder Association recommends polysomnography for every patient being considered for a surgical procedure to treat snoring. With the extremely high incidence of snoring in this country and the relatively smaller incidence of sleep apnea, clearly this recommendation is not always practical.

The cardinal feature of sleep apnea, be it the mild upper airway resistance syndrome or the severe pickwickian syndrome, is daytime somnolence. Other features characteristic of sleep apnea that need to be investigated are witnessed obstructions and morning headache. On physical examination, obesity, micrognathia, a very crowded pharynx, and a large posterior one-third of the tongue should alert the examiner to an increased likelihood of sleep apnea syndrome. The Epworth Sleepiness Scale, which was developed in Australia, is a reliable and accurate questionnaire for identifying daytime somnolence. It is a useful screening tool to help identify patients who may need polysomnography. In addition, the multiple sleep latency test, which is offered at sleep laboratories, provides a valid measure of daytime tiredness and is often combined with polysomnography. A patient of thin or moderate build with relatively normal pharyngeal and mandibular dimensions, who does not have excessive daytime sleepiness, morning, headache, or witnessed obstructions, is highly unlikely to have significant sleep apnea that requires intervention. A useful test is to allow the patient to sit quietly in a darkened examining room for 15 to 20 minutes before the physician visit. Virtually all patients who have significant daytime somnolence will fall asleep in the examining room. I recommend polysomnography for all of these patients. Once a decision has been made that the patient does not have significant sleep apnea or a sleep study has been obtained with either negative findings or findings showing only the mildest features of sleep apnea, the patient may be considered a candidate for snoring therapy.

■ PATIENT SELECTION

Patient selection for snoring surgery is crucial. The physician should carefully consider patients for snoring surgery in the same manner as patients are evaluated for cosmetic rhinoplasty surgery. It is in both the physician's and the patient's best interests to intervene surgically only on patients who have realistic expectations. Patients who have unrealistic expectations will not obtain satisfactory results. Whenever possible, I like to have the patient's bed partner, significant other, or roommate present during the initial interview. This is useful in providing an accurate appraisal of the nighttime noises. In addition, it is very useful in allowing one to better understand the dynamics of the patient's relationship and the true influence the snoring may have on these dynamics.

I consider the ideal candidate for snoring surgery to be part of a happily married or similarly stable couple who have recently begun sleeping either intermittently or constantly in separate rooms because of the nighttime noise. Their expectation would be to lower the level of snoring noise to enable them to sleep together in the same room.

A much less ideal situation would be a couple with marital problems who attribute a degree of their marital instability to nighttime noises. In my experience, snoring alone does not lead to dissolution of long-term relationships. If, however, the patient appears to be levelheaded, emotionally stable, and concerned that the nighttime noises have contributed to the inability to maintain a long-term relationship, I will consider the snoring surgery. I do, however, consider these patients to be less than ideal candidates.

On occasion, the physician is faced with patients who believe that they have never been able to maintain a long-term relationship or even establish a short-term relationship because of their snoring. Much like the rhinoplasty patient who believes that a rhinoplasty will change his or her entire social success level, these patients have unrealistic expectations regarding their snoring surgery, and one should avoid operating on them.

Other considerations regarding the suitability of snoring surgery include concurrent medical problems, professional voice usage, (i.e., singers), and patients unwilling to accept the possible pain and complications. As with any other surgical procedure, the risk-benefit ratio must be discussed with the patient.

■ EVALUATION FOR TREATMENT

Medical Versus Surgical Therapy

Upon determining that a patient does not have significant sleep apnea and is a suitable candidate for intervention, the physician should first attempt to rule out common medical causes of upper airway obstruction. Rhinitis, either allergic, vasomotor, or medicamentosus, should be identified and treated appropriately. Overweight patients should be encouraged to lose weight. Alcohol consumption before bedtime will increase pharyngeal relaxation and increase the degree of snoring. Position manipulation with pillows to elevate the head or a tennis ball in the back of the pajama top or nightshirt may help. I have found noise-reducing ear plugs for the bed partner particularly useful in elderly snoring patients. If the patient does not respond to either these suggestions or medical management of the common nasal complaints, I then consider surgical therapy for the snoring.

Nasal Versus Pharyngeal Surgical Therapy

Many patients who complain of snoring also have other complaints related to nasal obstruction. Patients who have nasal daytime obstruction due to a deviated nasal septum are obvious candidates for septoplasty. Patients with no septal deviation who have turbinate hypertrophy may be candidates for a turbinate reduction procedure. Generally, to determine whether a nasal procedure will help alleviate the nighttime noise, the patient and bed partner perform an oxymetazoline test. The patient uses oxymetazoline in both nostrils before going to sleep. The bed partner serves as an observer. If the oxymetazoline has a significant effect on the patient's snoring, one should consider improving the nasal airway before considering pharyngeal surgery. It is important that the patient try the vasoconstrictor test on at least 3 consecutive days in order to get an accurate assessment of whether the nighttime noise is improved.

If the patient has a deviated septum, daytime obstruction, and snoring, a septoplasty is indicated and performed using standard techniques. If the patient does not have a deviated septum but has daytime obstruction and/or a positive oxymetazoline test result, the physician may consider turbinate reduction surgery. This is performed using the CO_2 laser, which I describe later in this chapter. If the patient has no improvement with oxymetazoline, a straight septum, and no daytime obstruction, he or she is considered for pharyngeal surgery, usually a laser-assisted uvulopalatoplasty (LAUP).

Evaluation for Laser-Assisted Uvulopalatoplasty

LAUP is a relatively new operation that has gained popularity in the United States. It has been rapidly accepted by numerous otolaryngologists as well as a number of physicians from other medical fields. It is intended for the treatment of *palate-based* snoring. Hence, before using this technique, it is important to establish that the soft palate is indeed the source of the patient's snoring. This can be done in a number of ways. If the patient brings in a tape recording of the snoring, the characteristic sound of palate-based snoring can be identified. In addition, by having the patient perform a snorting type maneuver, getting the palate to vibrate, the physician can confirm with the bed partner that this is indeed the offending noise. While this maneuver is being done, the palate can either be examined directly in those patients who sleep with an open mouth, or via a flexible nasopharyngoscope in those patients who sleep with the mouth closed. This will confirm that the palate is indeed vibrating with each respiration. The LAUP treatment of pharyngeal snoring is more effective for inspiratory-phase than for expiratory-phase snoring.

It is crucial that the patient and the bed partner or roommate understand that LAUP is designed to reduce or eliminate the palate-based snoring noise. It will not eliminate every possible noise a patient may make throughout the night. One problem with the medical or surgical intervention of snoring is that patients and their bed partners become acutely aware of every sleeping noise. Before undergoing

LAUP procedure, they must understand that the procedure is designed only to remove the characteristic beating noise of a floppy soft palate.

Informed Consent

Before a LAUP is performed, the patient is presented with extensive information regarding the procedure. It is important for LAUP patients to understand that this is a relatively new procedure whose long-term benefits for both snoring and sleep apnea have not yet been ascertained. The procedure is painful; most patients call it the most severe sore throat of their lives. It frequently requires repetition; my patients require an average of 1.7 procedures each. It does not eliminate all nighttime noise, as mentioned previously. In addition, approximately 20 percent of the patients develop a transient globus sensation that lasts anywhere from 2 to 6 months. Bleeding, infection, and failure of the procedure are also rare risks. If the patient understands all of this and is willing to proceed, LAUP is performed using the following method.

Laser-Assisted Uvulopalatoplasty

The procedure is performed with the patient sitting upright in the otolaryngologic examining chair. The palate is prepped by a short spray of topical lidocaine, followed by an injection of a mixture of 1 percent lidocaine with epinephrine and 0.25 percent bupivacaine. Injections are as diagrammed in Figure 2; the physician should try to use the minimal amount of injection necessary to provide anesthesia for the area of the planned vaporizations. The anesthetic is allowed to work for a full 15 minutes before the laser procedure. Using a CO_2 laser at 15 W of continuous power and a handpiece with a backstop, 1 cm to 1.5 cm vertical trenches are created full thickness and slightly outward on either side of the uvula. This effectively doubles or triples the length of the uvula. Then with gentle traction downward on the uvula, a neouvula is sculpted at approximately the level of the old soft palate margin (Fig. 3). The small lateral pointed portions of the soft palate are further vaporized with the CO_2 laser. It is important that the vertical trenches are long enough to visibly identify relaxation of the soft palate. Patients are instructed throughout the procedure not to inhale, not to attempt to talk, and not to grab the surgeon. Should they need you to stop, they simply raise their hand, in which case all instrumentation is immediately withdrawn. Gagging is kept to a minimum using the usual psychological diversions employed in the indirect laryngoscopy examination.

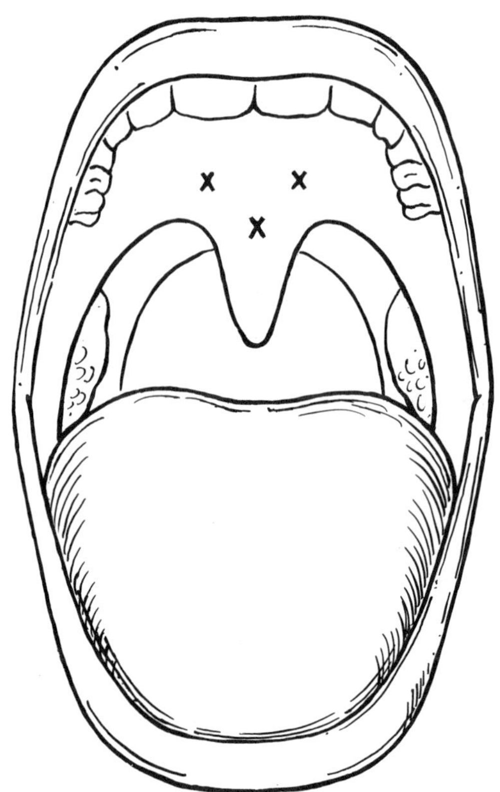

Figure 2.
Local anesthesia injection points.

After completion of the procedure, patients are discharged home with a 5 day supply of a broad-spectrum antibiotic (e.g., ampicillin, erythromycin), a nonsteroidal anti-inflammatory agent such as ibuprofen or naproxen to be first taken before the wearing off of the anesthetic agent, and a narcotic painkiller for breakthrough pain. The patient is instructed to use the nonsteroidal anti-inflammatory agent unless otherwise contraindicated for 7 to 10 days after the procedure. This greatly decreases reliance on postoperative narcotics. The patient returns in 6 to 8 weeks, with time scheduled for a possible repeat laser treatment. Upon return to the office, it is preferable to have both the patient and the bed partner available. Often, the patient and bed partner are satisfied, having succeeded in their goal to return to the same room at night. A small amount of snoring may persist, but if they are satisfied and have accomplished their primary goal, one can generally defer further treatment.

On occasion, a second, sometimes a third, and rarely a fourth or fifth procedure may be necessary for the patient to achieve the desired level of snoring reduction. One special situation that you may encounter is what I refer to as triangulation of the palate (Fig. 4). In this situation, the vertical trenches have healed straight across, tightening the posterior pharynx. Patients generally complain that the snoring has increased in pitch. In these patients, repeat trenches should be created in a more horizontal orientation. If the patient still complains of snoring after two, three, or four procedures, I carefully reinterview the patient about expectations and discuss whether these can realistically ever be achieved.

Postoperative Complications

I have seen no postoperative hemorrhage of consequence in over 100 consecutive patients. One patient developed an intraoperative hemorrhage that required transportation to the operating room for control. This was due to laser violation of an abnormally large uvular artery. In most patients, it would be a simple matter to control this condition in the office, but this was not possible in this particular patient. As mentioned earlier, approximately 20 percent of patients develop postoperative globus sensation. This appears to be due to denervation of the central palate from the vertical trenches. Patients may be reassured that this symptom will

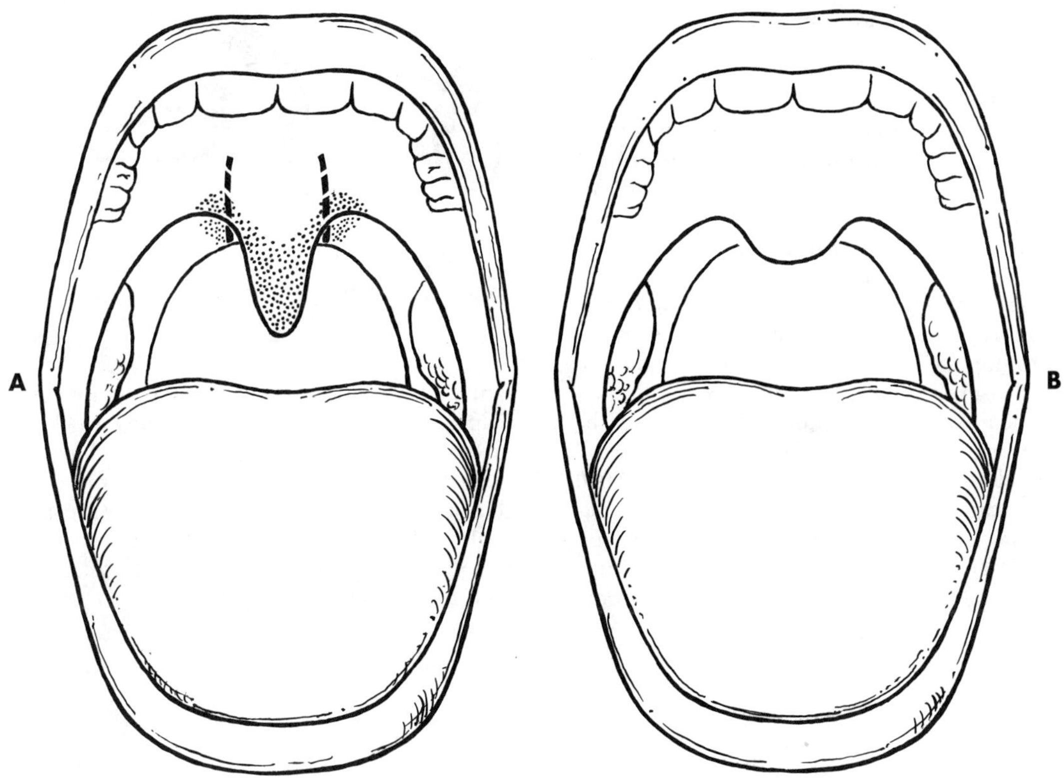

Figure 3.
A and *B*, Laser-assisted uvulopalatoplasty vertical trenches (dashed lines) and vaporization areas (stippled) should lead to a higher, stiffer palate with a short uvula.

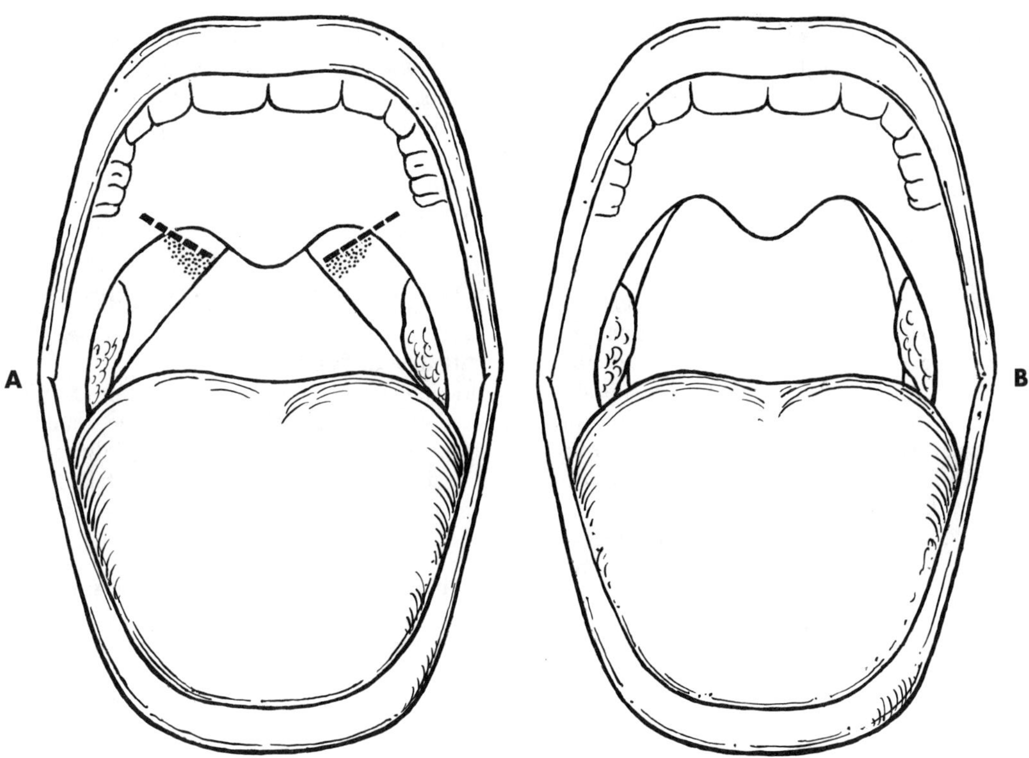

Figure 4.
A and *B*, Correction of palate triangulation.

disappear with time due to neurotization, that is, new nerve growth.

Laser Turbinoplasty

In patients who have both turbinate hypertrophy that is not responsive to nasal steroids or other allergy management and a positive vasoconstrictor test result, a laser turbinoplasty may be considered to improve nasal airflow. This procedure is very simple to perform in the otolaryngology clinic using a CO_2 laser. In addition, a similar result may be achieved by the judicious intraturbinate injection of steroids or other more formal turbinate reduction surgery.

For laser turbinoplasty, a topical anesthetic is applied to the patient's nose using 4 percent lidocaine mixed with oxymetazoline on neurosurgical cottonoids. The tip and the root of the inferior turbinate is then injected with as small amount as possible of 1 percent lidocaine with 1:100,000 epinephrine to achieve anesthesia of the anterior one-quarter of the inferior turbinate. Using the CO_2 laser at a power of approximately 8 W, multiple small islands of mucosal and submucosal vaporization are created. It is important to leave mucosal bridges to allow for rapid re-epithelialization of the anterior turbinate, which decreases the extensive crusting that often follows turbinate surgery (Fig. 5). Patients are instructed to use mupirocin ointment in their nose on a daily basis until the mucosa is completely healed. I have found this technique to be surprisingly effective as a treatment of chronic nasal obstruction, especially with regard to the snoring patient.

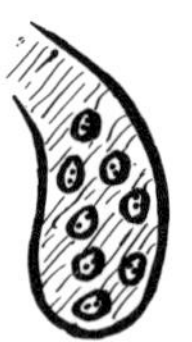
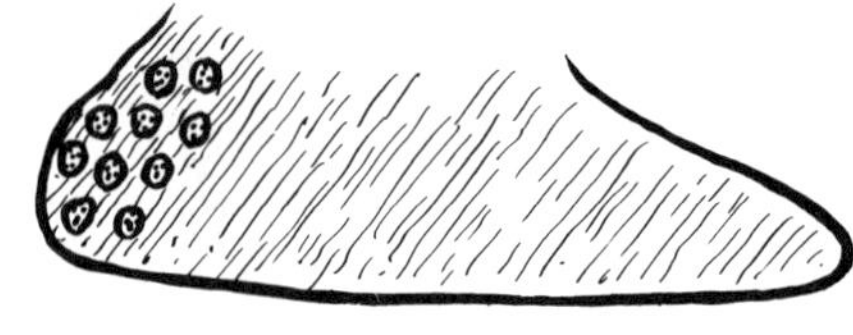

Figure 5.
Typical vaporization pattern of the anterior inferior turbinate; mucosal bridges left intact.

LARGE FACIAL WOUNDS

The method of
Lawrence P. Burgess*

Patients who have large facial wounds should be managed with a systematic approach. The most important aspect of care is to focus on the patient first, with care of the wound being secondary. The ABC's of advanced trauma life support should be used initially to manage the patient when appropriate. After the patient is stabilized and associated injuries are subject to diagnosis, treatment, and triage, attention is directed to the wound. Immediate primary closure is the goal, but delayed primary closure may be appropriate for infected or contaminated wounds. For patients who have significant soft-tissue or bony loss, early definitive repair within 7 to 10 days of injury is recommended.

The mechanism of injury provides important clues to potential associated injuries. Motor vehicle accidents are prone to cause associated cervical spine (C-spine) and central nervous system (CNS) injuries. A history of brief loss of consciousness may be the only indication of intracranial trauma. Gunshot wounds usually have deeper injuries than that which is readily apparent, with severe comminution of bony fragments. Bite injuries are prone to avulsion and infection.

INITIAL TREATMENT AND EVALUATION

Primary Survey

Patients are assessed, and treatment decisions are made based on the types of injuries and the stability of vital signs. The primary survey is conducted rapidly and efficiently, with resuscitation of vital functions undertaken in sequence. The primary survey is repeated frequently, because the patient's condition changes over time. The initial survey consists of:

- Airway maintenance with cervical spine control
- Breathing and ventilation
- Circulation with hemorrhage control
- Disability: Neurologic status
- Exposure/Environmental Control: Undress the patient, but prevent hypothermia.

The first priority is to open, clear, and stabilize the airway. Motor vehicle accidents that cause severe midfacial fractures and wounds extending into the tongue or pharynx usually

* The opinions or assertions contained in this chapter are the private views of the author and should not be considered as official or as reflecting the views of the Department of the Army or Department of Defense.

require a tracheostomy for eventual airway stabilization. In-line immobilization of the C-spine by an assistant should be maintained if intubation is required. C-spine extension, flexion, or rotation could turn a stable C-spine fracture into an unstable fracture with potential paralysis when establishing or maintaining the airway. Patients with maxillofacial or head trauma should be presumed to have a C-spine fracture, and the neck should be immobilized.

Once the airway is secured, breathing is assisted mechanically, if necessary, and supplemental oxygen is provided. Circulation is then closely assessed for signs of shock in multiple trauma patients. Large-bore intravenous lines are initiated, with central venous lines and Foley catheters for patients who have moderate to severe volume depletion. Pulse and level of consciousness are two elements that quickly provide key information. Decreased cerebral perfusion may result in altered levels of consciousness. Normal peripheral pulses usually indicate a relatively normovolemic patient, whereas a rapid, thready pulse is an early sign of hypovolemia. Both tension pneumothorax and cardiac tamponade should be considered as possible causes of poor ventilation and circulation in patients who have associated thoracic trauma.

External, severe hemorrhage is identified and controlled. Active bleeding from the majority of wounds in the head and neck can be controlled and stabilized with digital pressure until the vessel can be ligated or repaired under controlled circumstances. Blindly placing hemostats in an actively bleeding wound in an uncontrolled environment is discouraged. This action is usually ineffective, aggravates blood loss, and may damage surrounding vital structures.

The patient's neurologic status is then assessed. Level of consciousness and pupillary size and reaction should be determined. Level of consciousness can be simply described by the AVPU method: **A**lert, responds to **V**ocal stimuli, responds to **P**ainful stimuli, and **U**nresponsive. The Glasgow Coma Scale, a more detailed neurologic evaluation that can be substituted for AVPU, should be included in the secondary survey. A change in the level of consciousness may be due to either decreased cerebral perfusion or intracranial trauma. Alcohol or other drugs may also influence the level of consciousness in a patient. However, a combative or uncooperative patient might be dismissed as being intoxicated, when the real cause may be hypoxia, hypovolemia, or intracranial trauma.

The last step is to undress the patient to examine for other injuries. The patient should be appropriately covered after undressing to protect against hypothermia, and when possible intravenous fluids or blood should be warmed before administration. If not already done, appropriate radiographs of the C-spine, chest, or extremities should be ordered at this time. Early consultation with neurosurgery, general surgery, ophthalmology, and orthopedics should be obtained as appropriate.

Secondary Survey

The secondary survey is only initiated after the primary survey is completed, resuscitation is initiated, and the ABC's are reassessed. In this head-to-toe evaluation including vital sign assessment, each region of the body is thoroughly examined. Special procedures such as peritoneal lavage or radiologic evaluation are obtained at this time. The secondary survey also provides for the necessary time to obtain a more thorough history regarding the patient and mechanism of injury. The secondary survey is initiated with examination of the head and neck. The scalp should be thoroughly examined for lacerations, contusions, or underlying fractures. Scalp lacerations can be the cause of significant blood loss, which could lead to shock. The eyes should be examined for visual acuity; pupillary size and reactivity; hemorrhages in the conjunctivae, fundi, or anterior chambers; penetrating injury; lens dislocation; and contact lenses (remove).

Eardrums should be evaluated for hemotympanum or ruptured drums, which could indicate a temporal bone fracture. Battle's sign (ecchymosis over the mastoid tip) indicates a basilar skull fracture. Blood-tinged, free-flowing ear or nasal drainage could indicate a cerebrospinal fluid leak.

The bony skeleton should be examined for fractures. Dental occlusion is assessed for maxillary-mandibular fractures, and all teeth are accounted for. If a tooth is missing, a chest radiograph is necessary to evaluate for possible aspiration. Bilateral angle fractures should be considered and palpated for, because this could lead to airway compromise as the tongue displaces posteriorly. Like bilateral angle fractures, severe midfacial trauma will probably require tracheostomy for eventual airway stabilization. The neck should be palpated for crepitus, which could indicate airway penetration. The C-spine should also be palpated for tenderness if the patient is responsive.

Facial function is assessed for lacerations through the parotid region or for temporal bone trauma. These findings are often overlooked in the early stages of care. Clear fluid coming from a wound in the parotid region represents laceration of Stensen's duct or damage to glandular tissue. The otolaryngologist should use fiberoptic evaluation of the airway when possible to evaluate the upper airway and larynx.

■ THE WOUND

General Considerations

After completion of the secondary survey, the ABC's are reassessed. If the patient remains stable and there are no other more urgent injuries, the wound is assessed. During wound evaluation and treatment, the patient should be frequently reassessed for developing problems.

Before wound evaluation and treatment, photography is mandatory. Sequential steps in the closure should also be photographed. Because some of these cases will be the subject of either personal injury or medicolegal lawsuits, thorough chart documentation is also important. The patient and family members should be thoroughly counseled as to the potential for poor functional and cosmetic results. The need for revision surgery should also be emphasized.

Most isolated soft-tissue wounds can be closed under local anesthesia in a clinic or emergency room setting. Larger wounds often require general anesthesia, especially when airway stabilization is necessary with tracheostomy. Facial wounds in multiple trauma patients are usually closed under general anesthesia in the operating room, because other surgical services require general anesthesia for open reduction of extremity fractures or to explore the abdomen. Wounds with significant bone and soft-tissue loss can be closed as completely as possible, with early definitive repair to follow within 7 to 10 days.

Tetanus prophylaxis is indicated for clean wounds when the last booster has been given more than 10 years previously. For grossly contaminated wounds, tetanus prophylaxis is indicated for boosters given more than 5 years previously.

Wounds are thoroughly cleansed of debris, and conservative debridement is practiced. When necessary, a computed tomographic scan should be obtained in the subacute setting to evaluate the underlying bony architecture, and as a byproduct the scan is useful for detecting foreign bodies within the wound. A broad-spectrum antibiotic is used to cover staphylococci and streptococci in the postoperative period, and intravenous antibiotics should be used during initial treatment for contaminated wounds.

After the wound is healed, silicone gel sheeting helps reduce hypertrophic scarring. This material is also available in a liquid-gel form (Kelocote) that hardens to a less visible covering over which cosmetics can be applied.

Wound Types

Soft-tissue wounds may be broadly classified as abrasions, contusions, lacerations, and avulsions. Large wounds are likely to be a combination of all these types. Abrasions must be thoroughly cleansed to remove embedded foreign bodies. Brisk scrubbing with a surgical prep brush may be necessary. Solvents such as acetone or alcohol can be used to remove grease or tar. Antibiotic ointment or a synthetic biologic dressing should be used for wound coverage.

Contusions from blunt trauma or crash injuries have resultant ecchymoses and hematomas. Needle aspiration on one or more occasions may be necessary for treating hematomas. Cheek contusions and hematomas may have prominent swelling, but the amount of blood present is usually scant. Surrounding edema accounts for the majority of the swelling. Conservative treatment with ice and needle aspiration is recommended. If incision and drainage is believed to be necessary, it can usually be done in the gingivobuccal sulcus.

Lacerations require the careful examination of the wound's depths and closure in layers. For lacerations with ragged edges as seen with chain saw injuries, it is usually best to excise the ragged edges and close the wound with a linear scar when possible. Curvilinear lacerations combined with a flap of tissue can result in trapdoor deformities. The concave scar contracture, combined with venous and lymphatic obstruction, pushes the flap upward. The epithelial edges of the wound are usually beveled. If the beveling is excessive, it should be trimmed to create vertical skin edges for better wound approximation. During closure of the wound edge, the tendency is to have wound edges that are not level as the suture is passed full thickness on the flap side and partial thickness on the other. Attention to depth of suture placement as the wound is closed in layers helps prevent this.

Facial nerve function may be difficult to evaluate in combined laceration-contusions. Is the paralysis in one muscle group due to a lacerated or contused nerve branch? Electrical stimulation with a Hilger nerve stimulator proximal to the lesion will help show integrity of the nerve before the onset of swelling, when stimulation may be lost. Later in the subacute setting, evoked electromyography is another more sensitive alternative for testing. Without stimulation, nerve endings should be searched for under magnification in the region of the parotid.

A Stensen's duct laceration is suspected with clear fluid coming from the wound. The duct passes over the masseter muscle, in the middle of a line drawn from the tragus to the upper lip vermilion at Cupid's bow. The distal end of the laceration is found by passing a catheter from the duct intraorally into the wound. Long catheters or sheaths used for intravenous access serve this purpose well. The proximal end is found under magnification by manually compressing the parotid gland laterally and watching for salivary flow. Sialogogues might also be used. Using microvascular techniques, the duct is reanastomosed over the catheter. The tube is secured intraorally and remains in place for 3 weeks.

Avulsions usually result in some degree of tissue loss. These defects can be closed primarily (if small), skin grafted, or allowed to heal secondarily. The latter might be most appropriate if the wound is contaminated. Partial avulsions have a much higher success of healing with reattachment. For complete avulsions, attempting reattachment is generally thought to be a "nothing to lose" situation, but it may be risky on occasion, because infection may spread to surrounding structures. This is especially applicable in the ear, where infection can spread to and jeopardize the adjacent normal ear cartilage. Without microvascular reanastomosis, the rule of 2's applies: less than 2 cm in size and 2 hours since injury. Beyond these limits, success is less likely. Steroids, subcutaneous heparin, and aspirin may be used in an outpatient setting to improve vascularity. In addition, multiple stab incisions are useful for mechanically improving venous outflow, which takes longer to restore. Large defects with tissue loss might initially be dressed and debrided, as necessary, followed by microvascular free transfer, with the radial forearm free flap used most often. Likewise, avulsions of large segments of functional areas, for example, the eyelids or oral commissure, may require early definitive repair with a local flap or free tissue transfer.

Puncture wounds from humans or animals are a combination laceration-contusion, with infection being a significant problem because bacteria are buried deep within the wound. Amoxicillin-clavulanate potassium is the drug of choice for both human and animal bites.

Open fractures combine soft-tissue trauma with bony fractures or loss. Usually, the soft tissue is closed immediately under local anesthesia in the emergency room, with fracture repair following within 7 to 10 days. Mini- and microplating systems have revolutionized fracture repair and allow for piecemeal reconstruction of smaller fragments.

Gunshot wounds are a special example of open fractures that often represent significant reconstructive challenges. The mass of the bullet and the square of the velocity determine the energy of the projectile. Therefore, as the projectile's velocity increases, the energy and potential trauma increase exponentially. Low-velocity injuries from civilian handguns do not usually provide major problems, because there is not significant tissue loss. Intermediate-velocity (shotgun) and high-velocity (military) weapons can result in moderate to severe tissue loss, especially for close-range injuries.

Initially, the wound should be cleansed and debrided and primary closure accomplished, if possible. If soft-tissue loss is present, a second debridement may be necessary, followed by early definitive repair with a local or regional flap or free tissue transfer. Bony loss and fractures complicate the problem. Early definitive repair has emerged as the treatment of choice for these larger defects, because delayed reconstruction is prone to soft-tissue contraction without an underlying bony framework for support. During debridement, only small pieces of bone lying free within the wound are removed. Potential grafts that can be used are split calvarial for nose, orbital rim, and midface. For more extensive defects, contoured split rib grafts may be necessary. When significant soft-tissue loss is present, Gruss has described the use of free omentum to cover these fractures and grafts for vascularity. As a secondary benefit, the omentum also helps fill in dead space. Any omentum that is left exposed is skin grafted or covered with a second flap.

Open mandibular fractures with bony loss frequently communicate with the oral cavity. Unlike midface fractures, these wounds should be stabilized with plates or a biphase appliance, and the wound should be allowed to heal before placement of bone grafts. Grafts do poorly in the face of contamination with saliva. The space and overlying soft-tissue contour is maintained by the plate or appliance, so there is no urgent need for early definitive bony repair as exists in the midface.

Suggested Reading

American College of Surgeons Committee on Trauma. Advanced trauma life support instructor manual. Chicago: American College of Surgeons, 1993.

Goodman A. Soft tissue injuries to the face. In: Papel ID, Nachlas NE, eds. Facial plastic and reconstructive surgery. St. Louis: Mosby–Year Book, 1992:449.

Gruss JS, Antonyshyn O, Phillips JH. Early definitive bone and soft tissue reconstruction of major gunshot wounds of the face. Plast Reconstr Surg 1991; 87:436-450.

Pratt LW. Chain saw injuries of the head and neck. Ear Nose Throat J 1985; 64:15-22.

Schultz RC. Basic principles in management of facial injuries. In: Georgiade NG, Georgiade GS, Riefkohl R, Barwick WJ, eds. Essentials of plastic, maxillofacial, and reconstructive surgery. Baltimore: Williams & Wilkins, 1987:341.

Thorne CH. Gunshot wounds to the face. Clin Plast Surg 1992; 19:233-244.

HEAD AND NECK NEOPLASMS IN CHILDREN

The method of

Charles M. Myer III

In order to discuss head and neck neoplasms in children, one must have a clear understanding of all head and neck masses, including congenital, traumatic, and inflammatory lesions, in addition to true neoplasms. Certain generalities are present that allow a clinician to begin to classify lesions appropriately. Head and neck masses that are present from birth are most often congenital. When associated with infection, a lesion is more likely to be congenital or inflammatory. Implicit in this understanding is the fact that congenital lesions may not be present at birth but, rather, may be first seen later in childhood or adolescence, often following an upper respiratory infection. When a mass is inflammatory, it is usually painful and of rapid onset. When this type of lesion is associated with eating, one must strongly consider the affected structure to be one of the major salivary glands. If a hematoma is encountered, the usual etiology is trauma. However, bleeding into a congenital abnormality is an alternative explanation, especially if the hematoma develops slowly.

■ EVALUATION

History

Historical features that must be elicited include the presence of fevers, night sweats, cough, tuberculosis exposure, illness in the family, cat or other animal scratches, and a history of foreign travel. These symptoms all reflect the presence of an inflammatory process. The clinician should consider a possible mass lesion when symptoms such as prolonged nasal obstruction, recurrent epistaxis, or persistent unilateral middle ear effusion are detected. A mass lesion causing pressure on the upper aerodigestive tract may lead to dysphagia or dyspnea. Persistent or recurrent facial nerve paralysis may indicate the presence of a mass lesion in the posterior fossa, temporal bone, or parotid gland. A cervical mass associated with Horner's syndrome usually indicates cervical or upper medastinal neuroblastoma and is not indicative of inflammatory disease. Engorgement of the neck veins associated with facial plethora often indicates obstruction of the superior vena cava, which may be seen with lymphoma.

Physical Examination

A complete physical examination is mandatory when evaluating a patient who has a head and neck mass. As with any mass lesion, the physician must document its size, specific location, degree of firmness, tenderness, and fluctuance. With inflammatory lesions, there may be changes in the overlying skin that will aid in diagnosis. Additionally, there may be breaks in the mucosa of the oral cavity that aid in the diagnosis of such lesions. Face, scalp, and conjunctival lesions also may be seen with inflammatory disease. In dealing with pediatric patients, the physician must remember that skin lesions may be the first sign of Langerhans' cell histiocytosis (LCH). Patients typically demonstrate a scaly, erythematous, seborrhea-like rash that is especially prominent behind the ears. Superficial ulceration may occur, and the patient may present with areas similar to eczema.

Laboratory Studies and Imaging

Before performing a biopsy of a head and neck mass in a child, the physician should always obtain a complete blood count with differential, a chest radiograph, and determination of purified protein derivative reactivity. If changes in the smear indicate bone marrow involvement, including teardrop red blood cells, nucleated red blood cells, young myeloid cells, or young platelets, a bone marrow aspiration and biopsy is indicated. Older adolescents should be managed in a similar manner to adults who have neck masses and undergo panendoscopy before any biopsy procedures. This should include nasopharyngoscopy because of the relatively high incidence of nasopharyngeal carcinoma in patients who are in the second decade of life.

Plain radiographs have a relatively limited role in the assessment of head and neck masses in children. In the first month of life, ultrasonography can be used to localize a neck mass to the sternocleidomastoid muscle and thus assist the clinician in confirming the diagnosis of fibromatosis colli. Although computed tomography (CT) and magnetic resonance imaging (MRI) also can be used to make this diagnosis, ultrasound can be done much more inexpensively and without sedation. If the clinician believes that the mass is more likely not fibromatosis colli, an advanced imaging study would be appropriate initially. Outside of this age group, ultrasonography is generally used to differentiate a solid mass from a cystic one. Specifically, depending on the history and specific clinical circumstances, ultrasonography will be of most benefit in helping the clinician differentiate between a congenital cyst, an abscess, or a solid mass such as an inflammatory node or a neoplasm.

Depending on the ability of the patient to cooperate, needle aspiration may also be used to differentiate a solid from a cystic lesion. If the mass encountered is solid, the material aspirated can be sent for cytologic examination. This technique is not as well accepted in the pediatric population as in the adult population because of the types of pathology encountered. In adults, aspiration cytology is most effective in determining salivary gland pathology, thyroid abnormalities, and squamous cell carcinoma. Because these pathologic conditions are less common in children, many cytopathologists do not have experience with the lesions commonly encountered in pediatric patients. Thus, the technique is not as reliable in neoplasm determination in children as in adults and is used by many practitioners simply to differentiate cystic from solid masses. Liquid material should be sent for culture and sensitivity studies.

As previously mentioned, advanced imaging studies are indicated in many situations and include both a CT and an MRI. Depending on the location of the mass and the resources available, the physician should discuss the merits of both CT and MRI with the radiologist before obtaining a specific study. When midline lesions are present, the physician should consider performing thyroid function tests, thyroid scan, or both.

After obtaining a complete history, physical examination, and laboratory and imaging studies, the clinician should be able to differentiate neoplastic disease from non-neoplastic disease. Malignant neoplasms in children are typically first seen as solid, nontender masses that enlarge rapidly. Following trauma, cancer is the second leading cause of death in children in the United States. Approximately 5 percent of primary malignant neoplasms in children occur in the head and neck region. Reticuloendothelial, central nervous system, and connective tissue malignancies are more common than the epithelial malignancies usually seen in adults. Specifically, malignant lymphomas and soft-tissue sarcomas are the tumors seen most commonly. Approximately 70 percent of all pediatric head and neck malignancies occur as neck masses. However, the physician does not usually encounter thyroid carcinoma, nasopharyngeal carcinoma, and salivary neoplasms in children; these conditions, when seen, occur primarily during adolescence.

Biopsy

If a suspected inflammatory neck mass has not resolved or decreased substantially in size approximately 6 weeks following at least several weeks of administration of an appropriate antimicrobial agent, biopsy should be considered; an excisional biopsy should be attempted, if possible. Other factors that may prompt an earlier biopsy include palpable nodes in other parts of the body, an abnormal blood count or smear, a palpable liver or spleen, or a widened mediastinum on chest radiograph.

■ DIFFERENTIAL DIAGNOSIS

Depending on patient age, certain neoplasms should be considered more strongly in the differential diagnosis. Rhabdomyosarcoma in the head and neck region is seen most often in two specific age groups, between 4 and 6 years of age, and between 14 and 16 years of age. In contrast, neuroblastoma is seen most often within the first several years of life. Although Hodgkin's disease is seen more often in adolescents and adults, non-Hodgkin's lymphoma is identified more commonly in children under 12 years of age. Under the age of 2 years, LCH is the most commonly diagnosed malignancy. It is seen in an acute disseminated form (Letterer-Siwe disease) and is almost universally fatal. In children who are slightly older, the chronic disseminated form (Hand-Schüller-Christian disease) is seen and carries a better prognosis when treated with chemotherapy. Adolescent patients typically have the chronic unifocal form of LCH (eosinophilic granuloma), and treatment usually consists of limited surgical resection or curettage and, in some individuals, radiotherapy.

As patients live longer after treatment of primary malignancies of the head and neck region, clinicians more frequently will encounter mass lesions that represent second primary malignancies of the head and neck. Although the risk of having a second malignancy is increased substantially in a child who has a primary malignant neoplasm, both chemotherapy and radiotherapy further increase the chances of developing a second neoplasm. The most frequently reported radiation-associated malignancies are bone sarcomas, soft-tissue sarcomas, leukemia and/or lymphoma, and thyroid cancer. Patients undergoing organ transplantation and bone marrow transplantation may also be at increased risk because of the use of chemotherapy and, in some individuals, radiotherapy, which are requisite parts of their treatment protocols. The use of growth hormone also may be associated with an increased risk of developing second primary neoplasms.

■ THERAPY

It is difficult to generalize the role of the otolaryngologist in the treatment of head and neck neoplasms in children because of the diverse pathologic conditions encountered and the various sites from which the lesions arise. Regardless of the lesion encountered, an excisional biopsy should be performed whenever possible. If a biopsy procedure cannot be performed without injuring vital structures, an incisional biopsy should be performed in order to obtain a pathologic diagnosis before definitive therapy. With a benign neoplasm, the excisional biopsy will be curative. If a lesion is malignant, an excisional biopsy is indicative of a favorable staging in the development of a treatment protocol. If a malignancy cannot be removed totally, a less favorable staging results, which carries a poorer prognosis.

■ RHABDOMYOSARCOMA

Although the clinical grouping system has been the mainstay for staging with rhabdomyosarcoma, a new, nonsurgically based staging system (tumor, nodes, and metastases) is being evaluated to assist in the management of such patients. Because patients who have rhabdomyosarcoma are presumed to have, at a minimum, microscopic metastatic disease, therapy is focused on achieving local control and eradicating metastatic disease. The current multimodality therapy uses a combination of surgery, chemotherapy, and radiotherapy. Treatment decisions are based on the initial extent of the disease in addition to the site of origin of the primary tumor. This aggressive approach has resulted in an improvement in prognosis for patients who have rhabdomyosarcoma, especially those with locally extensive, unresectable, nonmetastatic disease. Similar advances are taking place in the staging and treatment of non-rhabdomyosarcoma soft-tissue sarcomas.

■ HODGKIN'S DISEASE

In the evaluation and management of patients who have Hodgkin's disease, the Ann Arbor system is used for staging, and CT is used for evaluation of spread. This has allowed clinicians to avoid laparotomy and splenectomy in their staging of these patients. In the treatment of this condition, low-dose irradiation and chemotherapy have been shown to be efficacious in some patients; these modalities have minimized growth impairment. This is especially useful in young patients who are still growing, because high-dose irradiation in large fields produces long-term growth effects. However, in adolescents and young adults who have attained full growth, the traditional treatment protocol has been maintained. Although nearly all Hodgkin's disease patients will achieve remission initially, prolonged remission is seen in only approximately one-half of patients who have advanced-stage disease.

■ NON-HODGKIN'S LYMPHOMA

In contradistinction to Hodgkin's disease, non-Hodgkin's lymphoma has been seen more frequently in pediatric patients who have acquired immunodeficiency syndrome, for whom there is an increased incidence of extranodal metastasis in comparison to children who have Hodgkin's disease. Recent changes in the classification system use immunologic subtyping based on identification of immunologic markers for lymphocyte subtypes, thus allowing for categorization into B cell, T cell, and true histiocytic origins. Similar to the treatment of Hodgkin's disease, the Ann Arbor staging system is used for determining therapy.

■ OTHER NEOPLASMS

Changes have occurred recently in the treatment of less common lesions as well. In nasopharyngeal carcinoma, Epstein-Barr virus titers have been used to evaluate markers of tumor burden and response to therapy. In addition to improved imaging and staging, advances in craniofacial surgery have allowed for surgical resection in some cases that was not possible previously. With neuroblastoma, new chemotherapy protocols have been developed for patients who have incomplete resection of tumor. When complete resection occurs, no adjuvant therapy may be indicated for some patients.

■ INTERDISCIPLINARY APPROACH

The treatment of head and neck tumors in children mandates an interdisciplinary approach between many medical subspecialties. Although the otolaryngologist often plays a relatively minor role in the overall management of such patients, this individual frequently performs the initial procedure that confirms the diagnosis of a malignancy. In this light, it is imperative for the otolaryngologist to guide the patient and family through the initial phase of diagnosis and treatment. However, when radical surgical excision is the appropriate form of treatment for a head and neck neoplasm in a child, it is essential for the otolaryngologist to possess that capability while maintaining the involvement of the other specialists who are so necessary for the care of such a child.

Suggested Reading

Angeli SI, Hoffman HT, Alcalde J, et al. Langerhans' cell histiocytosis of the head and neck in children. Ann Otol Rhinol Laryngol 1995; 104: 173-180.

Millman B, Pellitteri PK. Thyroid carcinoma in children and adolescents. Arch Otolaryngol Head Neck Surg 1995; 121:1261-1264.

Myer CM III. Second primary malignancies of the head and neck in children. Am J Otolaryngol 1995; 16:415-417.

Nasiri S, Mark RJ, Sercarz JA, et al. Pediatric sarcomas of the head and neck other than rhabdomyosarcoma. Am J Otolaryngol 1995; 16:165-171.

Tunkel DE, Baroody FM, Sherman ME. Fine-needle aspiration biopsy of cervicofacial masses in children. Arch Otolaryngol Head Neck Surg 1995; 121:533-536.

Wexler LH, Helman LJ. Pediatric soft tissue sarcomas. Ca Cancer J Clin 1994; 44:211-247.

VASOPROLIFERATIVE TUMORS IN CHILDREN

The method of
Carol J. MacArthur

Hemangioma is the most common hamartomatous lesion that occurs during infancy. Approximately 1 percent to 3 percent of all infants are born with hemangiomas. Of all hemangiomas, 35 percent to 60 percent are located in the head and neck region. Hemangiomas are made up of thin-walled, immature vessels of capillary size, lined by one layer of endothelial cells. Although most hemangiomas begin with a macular spot in the first few days of life, the proliferative phase (approximately the first year of life) causes a rapid growth in size, thickness, and density of the redness of the lesion. During the proliferative phase, hemangiomas have large numbers of mast cells and high mitotic activity. Hemangiomas must be differentiated from vascular malformations because both the treatment and the clinical course are different for these two entities. Figure 1 outlines the diagnostic pathway for vascular birthmarks. Hemangiomas involute over time, under the influence of hormones and angiogenesis factors. Involution begins with a change in the color of the hemangioma to a gray or fleshy color. With time, the hemangioma is replaced by fibrofatty tissue, usually leaving some residual mass effect in the area. Approximately 50 percent of hemangiomas have involuted by age 5 years and 70 percent have done so by age 7 years. Vascular malformations, on the other hand, are composed of mature blood vessels (capillary, venous, arteriovenous, or lymphatic) and do not involute over time. Clinically, hemangiomas usually appear within the first few days to weeks of life, whereas vascular malformations are present at birth.

Complications from large hemangiomas occur approximately 5 percent of the time and require intervention with medical or surgical therapy. Rapidly growing hemangiomas may ulcerate, bleed, or become infected. Hemangiomas may obstruct vision, if located in the periorbital area, and require urgent removal to prevent deprivational amblyopia. Hemangiomas may obstruct the airway anywhere from the nose to the trachea and cause breathing and feeding problems. Consumptive coagulopathy, thc Kasabach-Merritt syndrome, occurs from platelet trapping in large hemangiomas. This is a life-threatening complication with a 20 percent mortality rate that requires urgent treatment. High-output heart failure can occur as a result of multiple hemangiomas or hemangiomas with visceral involvement.

Therapeutic Alternatives

Treatment of small hemangiomas is usually expectant. For large hemangiomas causing complications, many treatment modalities have been tried. Medical therapy is the mainstay of treatment for complicated hemangiomas, although laser therapy, and even surgical excision, have been added to the armamentarium.

Steroids

The use of systemic steroids was begun in the 1960s for treating rapidly enlarging hemangiomas or hemangiomas in sensitive areas. High-dose prednisone (4 to 5 milligrams per kilogram daily) is used for short periods of time and tapered to 2 to 3 milligrams per kilogram daily. Steroids should be started as soon as it is determined that the hemangioma is growing rapidly and is likely to cause complications. After approximately 6 weeks' time (or after a good response has been obtained), alternate-day dosing is tried. Most infants who have hemangiomas in the proliferative phase respond well to systemic steroids. Most infants who respond to systemic steroids will need to be treated until approximately age 8 to 12 months, with periods of time off steroids approximately every 6 weeks. Steroids may need to be reinstated when there is obvious regrowth of the hemangioma off steroids. The reported response rate to systemic steroid use is

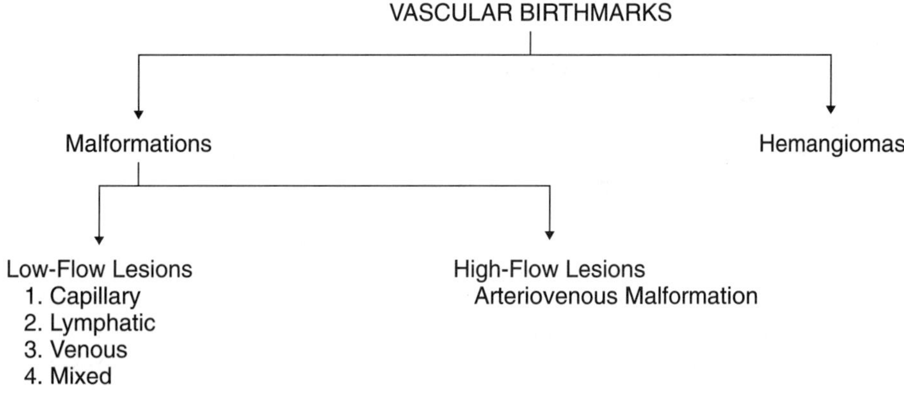

Figure 1.
Pathway for diagnosis of vascular birthmarks.

30 percent excellent response, 40 percent mixed response, and 30 percent no response. Those children who do not respond tend to be patients who have large hemangiomas, or older children whose hemangiomas are no longer in the proliferative growth phase. Complications of steroid use include growth retardation, cushingoid appearance, electrolyte imbalance, glucose metabolism disturbance, myopathy, behavioral disturbance, and peptic ulcer disease. Most of these problems are very infrequent in infants, especially with dosing every other day. Management of the small infant with systemic steroids should be coordinated with a pediatrician or pediatric endocrinologist who is familiar with long-term steroid use in infants.

Intralesional steroid injections can be very successful for small, localized hemangiomas that may require treatment due to their position in anatomically sensitive areas. Triamcinolone diacetate alone or as a mixture with betamethasone acetate can be injected directly into the lesion in small quantities (usually 1 to 5 cc per injection). Repeat injections can be performed every 6 weeks as needed, with careful watching for skin atrophy between injections. Usually no more than approximately a total of three injections is needed. Steroids injected into vascular lesions may cause adrenal suppression if large amounts are used. Steroid injections do not work well for high-flow or large hemangiomas, because it is impossible to get high concentrations of steroids into these types of hemangiomas.

Laser Therapy

Laser therapy has become more widely accepted as a form of treatment for hemangiomas, because lasers have been developed with more specificity for absorption in the wavelength spectrum of the hemoglobin pigment. Lasers used for the treatment of hemangiomas include CO_2, argon, neodymium (Nd):YAG (yttrium aluminum garnet), flashlamp pulsed-dye (585 nm), and copper vapor. The flashlamp pulsed-dye laser is useful for superficial or early hemangiomas and has the advantage of leaving virtually no cutaneous scarring after treatment. Hemangiomas can be re-treated as often as every 2 weeks with the flashlamp pulsed-dye laser. Another use for the flashlamp pulsed-dye laser is for "touch-up" obliteration of residual cutaneous markings from an involuted hemangioma. The copper vapor laser is used for thicker hemangiomas. The Nd:YAG laser is used for mucosal hemangiomas or is used by intralesional administration into thick hemangiomas because of its capacity for scarring. Of course, the CO_2 laser is very useful for airway hemangiomas due to its precision. Any hemangioma accessible via a suspension laryngoscope can be addressed by the CO_2 laser (supraglottic, glottic, subglottic). Care must be taken in treating circumferential subglottic hemangiomas, because they are more prone to result in subglottic stenosis. Avoiding stenosis can be accomplished by treating subglottic hemangiomas in stages, doing one side at a time, or by placing a tracheotomy and awaiting involution. Another alternative is open excision of subglottic hemangiomas. The Nd:YAG laser can also be used for airway hemangiomas in the trachea or bronchi, because it can be passed down the suction port of the ventilating bronchoscope. The use of the argon laser has virtually been replaced by the flashlamp pulsed-dye laser because of the specificity in targeting hemoglobin-containing tissues without damaging melanin-containing tissues.

Embolization

Angiographic embolization of large hemangiomas causing high-output heart failure also plays a role in the management of massive hemangiomas. Superselective angiographic embolization of feeding branches of large hemangiomas can induce early involution and decreased blood flow to huge lesions. This approach is not without morbidity in the young infant and must be considered after other, less invasive measures have failed.

Interferon Alfa-2a

Interferon alfa-2a (IFN alfa-2a) was first noted to modulate cutaneous vascular disease in a clinical trial for Kaposi's sarcoma. It was subsequently noted to cause regression of Kasabach-Merritt syndrome in two cases in 1989. In 1992, Ezekowitz and co-workers reported the first use of IFN alfa-2a for the treatment of life-threatening hemangiomas in infancy. These authors reported an excellent response rate in 18 of 20 patients. Ohlms and co-workers have reported the use of IFN alfa-2a for airway hemangiomas, with a response rate of 73 percent. MacArthur and co-workers have reported success (significant response in patients who were nonresponders to systemic steroids) in four of five patients treated with IFN alfa-2a for massive head and neck hemangiomas. The indications for use of IFN alfa-2a are large, complicated, steroid–nonresponsive hemangiomas, complex airway hemangiomas, and Kasabach-Merritt syndrome. Some clinicians have begun using IFN alfa-2a as primary therapy for large hemangiomas in young infants before trying steroids.

The treatment regimen is daily subcutaneous injections of 3 million units per square meter of body surface area, beginning with 1 million units per square meter, and advancing daily up to the goal of 3 million units per square meter as tolerated. Complete blood count and liver function tests should be monitored regularly during the treatment period. Most patients will experience some fevers and myalgias initially, but most pediatric patients tolerate IFN alfa-2a therapy well. There are anecdotal reports of spastic diplegia from the use of interferon; therefore, its use must be carefully contemplated. The expected length of treatment should be 12 to 18 months in order to obtain optimal involution before stopping therapy. IFN alfa-2a works best when instituted during the proliferative growth phase of the hemangioma.

Surgical Excision

Surgical excision can be very useful in selected cases: when the hemangioma is discrete, located in an anatomically sensitive area, and/or when rapid resolution is desired. Such areas include periorbital, nasal, and airway sites. In particular, subglottic hemangiomas that are not amenable to CO_2 laser excision (bilateral, airway reduction greater than 50 percent, extralaryngeal extension) may be best treated by surgical excision in order to avoid either a tracheotomy or subglottic stenosis from repeated laser excisions. An open approach can be used to excise the subglottic hemangioma, followed by cartilage augmentation, similar to a one-stage laryngotracheal tracheoplasty. This approach must precede laser airway surgery, or the submucosal dissection will be difficult and may risk the development of subglottic stenosis postoperatively.

Long-Term Sequelae

Although most hemangiomas do involute gradually over time, almost all leave behind residual changes in the skin and subcutaneous tissues. If these changes are small, no treatment is needed. However, for larger hemangiomas, a significant residual deformity may be present that will need addressing as the child matures. These residual changes include cutaneous telangiectasias, skin atrophy, scarring, hypo- or hyperpigmented areas, incomplete involution, subcutaneous fibrofatty tissue, and excess skin. Facial plastic surgery techniques may be necessary to remove bulky fibrofatty tissue and to reduce excess skin. The flashlamp pulsed-dye laser may be helpful in removing the remaining cutaneous telangiectasias and hemoglobin-containing areas in the area of the previous hemangioma.

■ LYMPHATIC MALFORMATIONS

A brief discussion of terminology is necessary in order to clarify the confusion between the terms *cystic hygroma*, *lymphangioma*, and *lymphatic malformation*. The preferred term is *lymphatic malformation*, because these lesions are a congenital malformation of lymphatic vessel development, not a tumor, which the suffix *-oma* would imply. These lesions do not have the capacity for cellular mitosis and invasion, as would a tumor. They also do not strictly have the capacity to "recur," as would a tumor; however, the multicystic variety are very difficult to completely eradicate, and incomplete excision often leads to some degree of persistent disease. There are basically three types of lymphatic malformations: lymphedema, solitary or multiple cystic lesions, and disorders of circulation of chyle. In this chapter, I discuss only the second entity, cystic lesions encountered in the head and neck, most commonly known as cystic hygromas. The anatomic location of these lesions dictates to some degree the clinical presentation. Lesions occurring in the neck, axilla, and mediastinum (areas with distinct tissue planes and loose areolar tissue) are able to expand, with multilocular or unilocular cysts insinuating along nerves and vessels. In other areas with restrictive tissue architecture such as the lips, cheeks, and tongue, lymphangiomatosis may occur without cystic changes.

Clinical Findings

Most lymphatic malformations are present at birth (65 percent), and 90 percent occur during the first 2 years of life. The cervicofacial region is the most common area of presentation. In the cervicofacial region, there are two main types of lymphatic malformations. The first and easiest to treat are the unilocular cystic lymphatic malformations, usually located in the anterior or posterior cervical triangle, below the mylohyoid muscle. The second type, and much more challenging to treat, is the suprahyoid mutiloculated lymphatic malformation. This second type tends to infiltrate into muscles and cross tissue planes, which makes complete excision impossible. I principally address the suprahyoid multiloculated type in this chapter, because its management is much more challenging and controversial.

Lymphatic malformations grow commensurately with the growth of the child. Rapid expansion can occur during times of upper respiratory infections or with bleeding into the lesion after trauma to the area (i.e., a fall). After the infection subsides, the lesion will slowly return to approximately its original size. Infections and cellulitis are common occurrences in lymphatic malformations, and are usually associated with upper respiratory infections; early administration of antibiotics, and sometimes steroids, is necessary. Rapid expansion of lesions in the tongue, pharynx, or neck can cause rapid respiratory embarrassment. Families of these children must be made aware of this potential complication. In many lesions with extensive and diffuse involvement near the airway (neck, tongue, pharynx, trachea), a tracheotomy will be necessary shortly after birth to control the airway until the lesion can be treated. Other complications of lymphatic malformations include feeding difficulty and soft-tissue and skeletal hypertrophy, which causes cosmetic disfigurement. Many of the patients who have suprahyoid extensive lesions will also require a feeding gastrostomy in infancy.

Skeletal hypertrophy and distortion occur in approximately 80 percent of large cervicofacial lymphatic malformations by age 10 years. It is most common that there is maxillary and/or mandibular overgrowth, causing prognathism, open bite, or other complex malocclusions. This probably occurs from primary bony mandibular involvement with the lymphatic malformation from birth, and not only from increased blood flow to the bony skeleton overlying the lymphatic malformation. Orthognathic surgical correction of the malocclusion and facial disharmony is often necessary when the child reaches an appropriate age for this intervention (i.e., teen years).

All patients who have lymphatic malformations should be evaluated with magnetic resonance imaging (MRI) to assess the extent of the lesion, because the lesion is often far more extensive than is appreciated from physical examination. Computerized tomography (CT) may also be helpful if bony detail is needed, depending on the anatomic area involved. Photographs should be taken at timely intervals, especially before and after surgical intervention, to objectively evaluate response to therapy.

Therapeutic Alternatives

The first tenet in the management of these challenging lesions is to remember that outcome depends most on anatomic location, and not as much on overall size, with the suprahyoid multicystic variety having a distinctly poorer prognosis for complete removal. Many approaches have been tried over time with these lesions, including surgical excision, sclerosing injections, aspiration, incision and drainage, radiotherapy, or chemotherapy, most of which are not recommended, except for careful, meticulous surgical excision.

Sclerosing Injections

Injections of boiling water, morrhuate sodium, hypertonic saline, iodized oil, and bleomycin into lymphatic malformations after aspirating the cyst contents have been used for the management of lymphatic malformations in the past. Most of these approaches have been discarded because of the poor results and complications such as scarring, systemic toxicity, and subsequent negative impact on success of surgical intervention. Orford and co-workers have reported complete clinical resolution after bleomycin injection in 44 percent of patients, a good response in 44 percent, and poor response in 12 percent. Those patients who had an excellent or good response had unilocular lymphatic malformations; those patients with poor outcomes had multicystic lymphatic malformations.

OK-432 has received renewed interest around the world in sclerosing therapy for treating lymphatic malformations. OK-432 is a lyophilized incubation mixture of group A *Streptococcus pyogenes* of human origin treated with penicillin G potassium. Injection of OK-432 causes an inflammatory response, followed by shrinkage of the cystic lymphatic spaces. By report, there is no significant surrounding fibrosis produced by OK-432. Ogita and colleagues have reported a 92 percent success rate in treating the unilocular variety of lymphatic malformations, but only a 44 percent response rate in treating the multicystic variety. The failure to produce a better response in the multicystic variety is thought to be related to the failure of intercommunication between the hundreds to thousands of cysts in the multicystic type. Although trials are under way with OK-432 in this country, this mode of therapy is not approved by the Food and Drug Administration at this time.

Cyclophosphamide

Turner and Gross, as well as other researchers, have reported on the use of intravenous cyclophosphamide for treating recurrent, unresectable lymphatic malformations. Cyclophosphamide was administered every 4 weeks, for approximately five cycles. In Turner's series, three of four patients responded, with a 50 percent to 75 percent reduction in overall tumor size. Little toxicity was reported. This approach has merit for unresectable, recurrent lymphatic malformations after surgical intervention has failed.

Laser

CO_2 laser therapy is very useful for airway involvement with lymphatic malformations. The CO_2 laser can be used to remove lymphatic malformations in areas such as the supraglottic larynx, tongue base, or pharynx. The Nd:YAG laser is very useful in ablating the vesicles that so often arise on the surface of the tongue and floor of the mouth in patients who have lingual lesions or extensive lesions that involve the neck, floor of the mouth, and tongue. Repeated Nd:YAG laser ablation of the tongue surface vesicles is often necessary to control local bleeding and for cosmesis of the tongue.

Surgical Excision

For most lymphatic malformations, well-planned and properly timed surgical excision is the mainstay of therapy. After careful physical examination and preoperative workup, including MRI and/or CT to image the extent of the lesion and possible airway compromise, surgery should be planned. Extensive preoperative counseling will be necessary with most families; the difficulty in total surgical extirpation of the extensive lesions must be explained. Timing is the first decision. Most of these lesions should not be resected immediately after birth. The baby often needs to gain weight and become strong enough for a lengthy surgery. Occasionally, a lesion will be amenable to complete removal during one procedure, or early removal may be necessary to alleviate airway obstruction. However, most of the complex lesions need to be addressed later, usually around 1 year of age. If an infant needs airway stabilization, or has feeding problems early on from the lymphatic malformation, a tracheotomy and feeding gastrostomy can be performed, and the surgical excision is then deferred until the child is older. Often, early surgery is fraught with more cranial nerve damage, because nerve dissection is much more difficult in infancy than in larger children of 1 to 2 years of age.

It is important to allow enough time for a careful, meticulous dissection, because these lesions are usually much more difficult to surgically remove than would be expected from physical examination. Usually, these dissections are prolonged and tedious and involve careful cranial nerve dissection. This is especially true with the multicystic lesions that are often insinuated into the surrounding muscles and nerves. There can also be surrounding fibrosis, depending on the number of preoperative infections. The basic surgical principles are to excise as much of the lesion as is possible, while preserving form and function. In other words, lymphatic malformations are not tumors and, therefore, radical resections are not indicated. Surgery must allow preservation of cranial nerve function and preserve form or cosmesis as much as possible. Therefore, the large, infiltrative lesions are by definition impossible to completely excise if the physician is to preserve normal structures invaded by the malformation. Staged excision is the best approach to the large cervicofacial lesions, with confinement of excision to one anatomic area at a time.

For lesions involving the tongue and floor of the mouth, surgical reduction of the tongue is often necessary. Macroglossia can be quite massive, with the tongue protruding from the mouth, becoming dry, and bleeding intermittently. Surgical reduction by wedge excision of the anterior tongue can restore the child's appearance to almost normal, and can help with returning the speech to near-normal function. Surgical tongue reduction should be done fairly early in life in order to try to avoid the mandibular prognathism and occlusal problems caused by the macroglossia.

Orthognathic correction of maxillomandibular discrepancy caused by the lymphatic malformation may be necessary in the young adult affected by large cervicofacial lymphatic malformations. Because cervicofacial lymphatic malformations involving the floor of the mouth and tongue may involve the mandibular bone at the outset, early surgical intervention for the large malformations may not completely prevent mandibular prognathism or open-bite deformity, but may lessen the overall severity of the occlusal problems.

Complications of surgery for these lesions are principally nerve damage (especially facial, hypoglossal, spinal accessory); postoperative fluid collections; infections; persistent edema; delayed healing; cosmetic disfigurement; and "recurrences." Parents need to be counseled about these possibilities. Nerve dissections should be carried out meticulously and with magnification, if necessary. Postoperative drains need to be placed, and these drains may need to be in place for a long time if prolonged serous drainage if present. Vesicular blebs may form in the incision lines, and these may require revision. "Recurrences" may occur in the months to years following surgical resection of lymphatic malformations. Recurrent lesions after surgical intervention for the multicystic and/or suprahyoid type occur as often as 80 percent of the time. Recurrences may occur by dilation of persistent lymphatic channels following postoperative scarring and fibrosis. Often, areas that were previously not involved clinically may dilate and become a "new" area of involvement that requires further surgery. It must be emphasized to the parents that for extensive lesions, complete excision is impossible, and that some disfigurement must be expected in the long run. The long-term psychological impact of these complex lesions on the patient and the family is complex and must not be underestimated.

Suggested Reading

Hemangiomas

Edgerton MT. The treatment of hemangiomas. Ann Surg 1976; 183:517-532.

Enjolras O, Riche MC, Merland JJ, Escande JP. Management of alarming hemangiomas in infancy: A review of 25 cases. Pediatrics 1990; 85:491-498.

Ezekowitz RAB, Mulliken JB, Folkman J. Interferon alfa-2a therapy for life-threatening hemangiomas of infancy. N Engl J Med 1992; 326: 1456-1463.

Folkman J. Toward a new understanding of vascular proliferative disease in children. Pediatrics 1984; 74:850-856.

Froehlich P, Seid AB, Morgon A. Contrasting strategic approaches to the management of subglottic hemangiomas. Int J Pediatr Otorhinolaryngol 1996; 36:137-146.

MacArthur CJ, Senders CW, Katz J. The use of interferon alfa-2a for life-threatening hemangiomas. Arch Otolaryngol Head Neck Surg 1995; 121:690-693.

Mulliken JB. Classification of vascular birthmarks. In: Mulliken JB, Young AE, eds. Vascular birthmarks: Hemangiomas and malformations. Philadelphia: WB Saunders, 1988:24.

Ohlms LA, Jones DT, McGill TJI, Healy GB. Interferon alfa-2a therapy for airway hemangiomas. Ann Otol Rhinol Laryngol 1994; 103:1-8.

Sloan GM, Reinisch JF, Nichter LS, et al. Intralesional corticosteroid therapy for infantile hemangiomas. Plast Reconstr Surg 1989; 83:459-467.

Wiatrak BJ, Reilly JS, Seid AB, et al. Open surgical excision of subglottic hemangioma in children. Int J Pediatr Otorhinolaryngol 1996; 34:191-206.

Lymphatic Malformations

April MM, Rebeiz EE, Friedman EM, et al. Laser therapy for lymphatic malformations of the upper aerodigestive tract. Arch Otolaryngol Head Neck Surg 1992; 118:205-208.

Ogita S, Tsuto T, Nakamura K, et al. OK-432 therapy in 64 patients with lymphangioma. J Pediatr Surg 1994; 29:784-785.

Orford J, Barker A, Thonell S, et al. Bleomycin therapy for cystic hygroma. J Pediatr Surg 1995; 30:1282-1287.

Padwa BL, Hayward PG, Ferraro NF, et al. Cervicofacial lymphatic malformation: Clinical course, surgical intervention, and pathogenesis of skeletal hypertrophy. Plast Reconstr Surg 1995; 95:951-960.

Ricciardelli EJ, Richardson MA. Cervicofacial cystic hygroma: Patterns of recurrence and management of the difficult case. Arch Otolaryngol Head Neck Surg 1992; 117:546-553.

Smith RJH, Burke DK, Sato Y, et al. OK-432 therapy for lymphangiomas. Arch Otolaryngol Head Neck Surg 1996; 122:1195-1199.

Turner C, Gross S. Treatment of recurrent suprahyoid cervicofacial lymphangioma with intravenous cyclophosphamide. Am J Pediatr Hematol/Oncol 1994; 16:325-328.

Young AE, Stewart G. Lymphatic malformations. In: Mulliken JB, Young AE, eds. Vascular birthmarks: Hemangiomas and malformations. Philadelphia: WB Saunders, 1988:215.

LACRIMAL OBSTRUCTION

The method of
Ralph B. Metson

Otolaryngologists who have developed expertise with endoscopic instrumentation for the treatment of chronic sinusitis can use similar skills to treat patients who have lacrimal obstruction. In the past, intranasal approaches to the lacrimal sac were rarely used because of poor exposure and visibility. The advent of nasal endoscopes has afforded the surgeon excellent visualization within the depths of the nasal cavity and allowed for a safe and effective method to open an obstructed lacrimal sac without the need for an external incision.

PREOPERATIVE EVALUATION

Most patients with obstruction of the lacrimal drainage system have epiphora, or excessive tearing, of the affected eye. Continued blockage of the sac can lead to chronic dacryocystitis, with drainage of purulent material from the canaliculi. Patients who have these symptoms should undergo nasal endoscopy to look for anatomic abnormalities that could contribute to such obstruction. The inferior meatus is inspected for any masses that could block the orifice of the nasolacrimal duct. The middle meatus is examined for polyps or mucopurulent drainage, which would be indicative of sinus inflammation adjacent to the lacrimal sac. The presence of a septal deviation or enlarged middle turbinate that may need to be addressed at the time of dacryocystorhinostomy (DCR) is also noted.

Ophthalmologic consultation is often obtained for patients who have idiopathic epiphora. Eye examination will serve to document any pre-existing ocular abnormality. In addition, probing and irrigation of the canaliculi can sometimes be helpful in identifying canalicular stenosis, which is a cause of epiphora that is not adequately treated with conventional DCR. The patency of the canaliculi can also be verified with a dacryocystogram, in which radiopaque contrast media is injected into the canaliculi while a radiograph is taken. Normally, the media should flow freely into the inferior meatus. When obstruction is present, dye will flow only to the site of obstruction and will not reach the nasal cavity. The most common site of obstruction is the distal region of the lacrimal sac, which appears as a dilated sac on the dacryocystogram.

ENDOSCOPIC PRIMARY DCR

Endoscopic DCR may be performed under either local or general anesthesia, depending on the condition of the patient and the preference of the surgeon. The operation is performed with a video camera attached to the endoscope so that the assistant surgeon can observe the entire procedure on a video monitor. The patient is placed in a supine position with the head slightly elevated to decrease venous pressure at the operative site. The nasal cavity is sprayed with oxymetazoline topical decongestant to initiate vasoconstriction. The nose and affected eye are draped in the operative field. A 4 mm diameter 0 degree nasal endoscope is used for visualization, while submucosal injections of 1 percent lidocaine with epinephrine 1 : 100,000 are placed in the middle turbinate and lateral nasal wall just anterior to the attachment of the turbinate. Nasal packing soaked in a 4 percent cocaine solution is then placed to maximize mucosal decongestion.

Surgical dissection begins with removing an approximately 1 cm diameter circle of mucosa and underlying bone along the lateral nasal wall. The maxillary line, a bony eminence that originates at the middle turbinate attachment and continues as a curvilinear eminence along the lateral nasal wall to the root of the inferior turbinate, serves as a critical landmark (Fig. 1). This line corresponds to the suture line that runs vertically through the lacrimal fossa between the lacrimal and maxillary bones. Although bone to the anterior of the maxillary line is generally thick and more difficult to remove, it is important that the portion of lacrimal sac anterior to this line be exposed during endoscopic DCR.

The upper half of the uncinate process, which attaches just posterior to the maxillary line, is removed early in the dissection (Fig. 2). The infundibulum is entered, and any agger nasi cells overlying the lacrimal sac are also opened.

Next, the maxillary bone, which forms the anterior aspect of the lacrimal fossa, is removed (Fig. 3). Resection of this thick bone is most easily accomplished with a drill that has a medium cutting bur; however, a curet, backbiting forceps, or rongeur can also be used for bone removal in this region.

After the medial sac wall has been exposed, it is entered with a sickle knife and an angled Blakesley forceps (Fig. 4). A lacrimal probe within the sac is used to tent up the medial sac wall as it is opened. This maneuver isolates the medial wall and prevents inadvertent injury to underlying structures. Once the sac interior has been entered, the probe will be visible. The medial sac wall is removed with a Blakesley forceps and sent as a separate specimen to ensure that an occult neoplasm is not the cause of the lacrimal obstruction. The sac opening is enlarged to a diameter of approximately 10 mm. It should extend inferiorly to the sac-duct junction and superiorly to above the level of the internal common punctum. No attempt is made to create mucosal flaps.

The location of the common punctum is verified by passing stents threaded to a Silastic catheter through the superior and inferior canaliculi. If these two probes can be seen entering the lateral sac wall with a 30 degree nasal endoscope (Fig. 5), the surgeon can be assured that enough bone and medial sac wall have been removed to ensure a high likelihood of surgical success. The stents are then grasped with a Blakesley forceps, withdrawn from the nasal cavity, and cut from the tubing. The ends of the tubing are then tied and trimmed within the nasal cavity to form a continuous

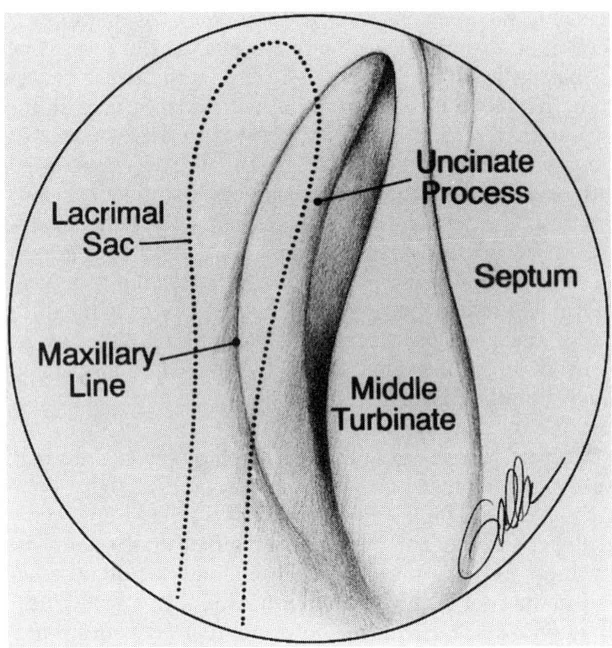

Figure 1.
Endoscopic view of right nasal cavity demonstrates location of the lacrimal sac (dotted outline) underlying the lateral nasal wall. The maxillary line, a bony eminence that originates at the middle turbinate attachment, is a reliable anatomic landmark for sac location.

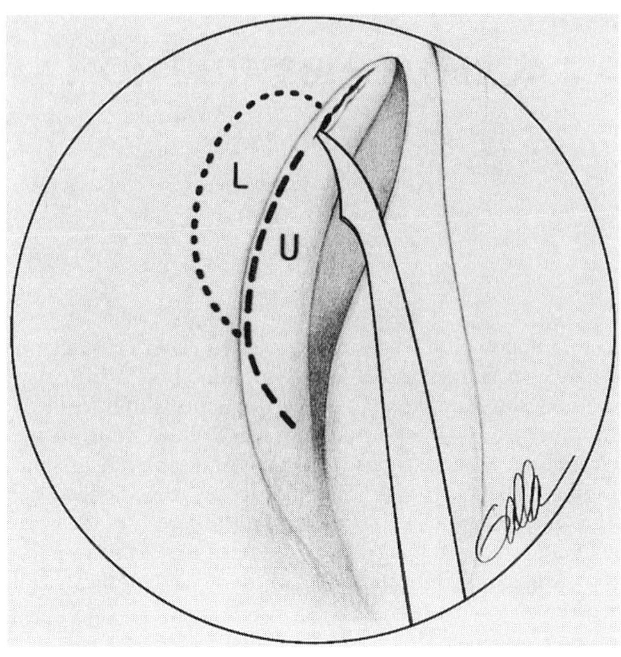

Figure 2.
After submucosal injections to promote hemostasis, the uncinate process (U) is incised just posterior to the maxillary line. An area of mucosa along the lateral nasal wall (L) is similarly incised and removed to expose bone that overlies the anterior portion of the lacrimal sac.

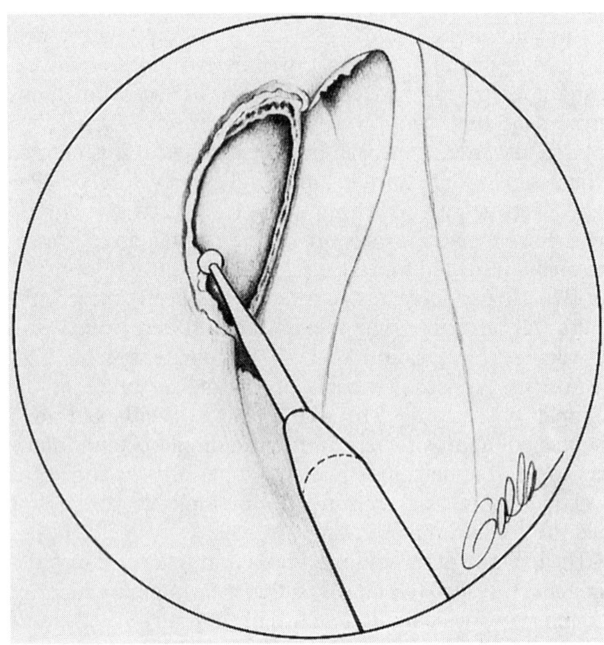

Figure 3.
The use of a drill with a medium-sized cutting bur facilitates removal of thick bone overlying the lacrimal sac. Rongeurs, curets, and bone-removal forceps can also be used.

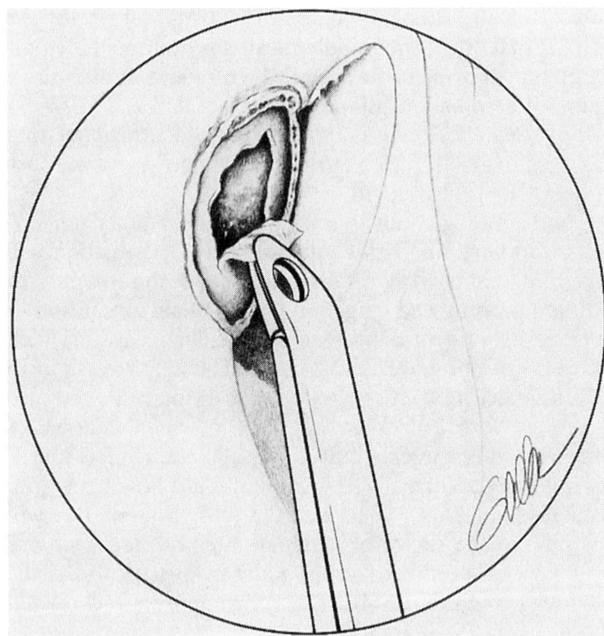

Figure 4.
The lacrimal sac is opened with a sickle knife, and the medial wall is removed with an angled Blakesley forceps. No attempt is made to create mucosal flaps.

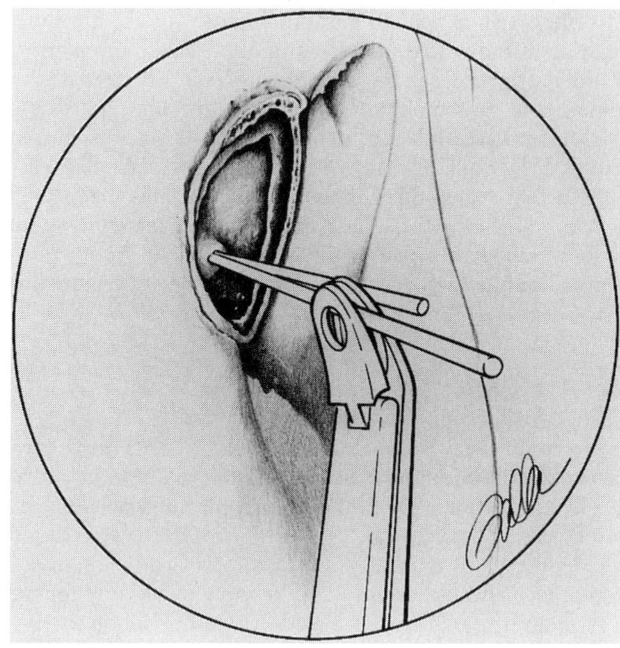

Figure 5.
Lacrimal probes threaded with a Silastic catheter are passed through the canaliculi and grasped with forceps. This catheter serves to stent the surgical opening during the healing period. Note the internal common punctum, which is visible where the probes enter the sac interior.

loop around the canaliculi. This tubing stents the surgical ostium during the postoperative healing period.

■ ENDOSCOPIC REVISION DCR

Because bone along the lateral nasal wall has already been removed during prior surgery, endoscopic revision DCR is technically easier than is primary endoscopic DCR and is more suitable for the surgeon who is learning the technique of endoscopic DCR.

Once the patient has been anesthetized and the nasal cavity prepared in the same manner as for primary DCR, the assistant surgeon passes a lacrimal probe through the canaliculi into the obstructed lacrimal sac. The tip of the probe can be observed with the endoscope as it tents the mucosa of the lateral nasal wall. The endoscopist then uses a sickle knife to make a curvilinear incision in the nasal mucosa approximately 1 cm anterior to the underlying probe tip. If extensive submucosal fibrosis exists from prior surgery, the mucosa posterior to this incision may have to be elevated sharply with a sickle knife. The posterior mucosal flap is then grasped with a straight Blakesley forceps and removed with a twisting motion. Similar bites of adjacent mucosa may be necessary in order to enlarge this intranasal opening to a diameter of at least 10 mm.

Once the lacrimal sac has been entered, the tip of the probe will be exposed. Frequently, however, additional scar tissue needs to be removed to enter the sac interior. The intranasal opening is deepened with an angled Blakesley forceps directed laterally toward the sac. Because scarring from previous surgery may obscure sac anatomy, the probe that lies within the sac is used as a guide for tissue removal. Care must be taken to remove only tissue directly surrounding the probe to avoid inadvertent exposure of periorbital fat. The assistant who is directing the lacrimal probe can alert the endoscopist if the section is getting too close to the medial canthus, which could injure the canaliculi. Once the intranasal opening has been sufficiently enlarged, the sac interior and internal common punctum are usually visible with a 30 degree endoscope. Lacrimal probes should pass freely into the nose from both the superior and the inferior canaliculi.

The lacrimal probe is then replaced by Silastic tubing that has its ends threaded over a rigid wire, as previously described for primary DCR. Unless bleeding is a problem or a concurrent septoplasty has been performed, no nasal packing is used.

■ POSTOPERATIVE CARE

If nasal packing is placed at the conclusion of surgery, it is removed the following morning. Patients are discharged with instructions to begin twice-a-day nasal saline irrigations with a bulb syringe. Any remaining intranasal debris is removed from the operative site under endoscopic guidance at the first postoperative visit 1 week following surgery.

The Silastic tubing used to stent the surgical ostium is typically removed 2 months after surgery by cutting the exposed tubing at the medial canthus and withdrawing it through the nose. It may be removed sooner if excessive granulation tissue formation occurs around the tube at the ostium. In revision cases in which postoperative scarring has been a problem, stents may be left in place for 6 months or longer. Patency of the lacrimal drainage system is verified by endoscopic observation of fluorescein dye flowing from the eye through the surgical ostium into the nose.

■ COMPLICATIONS

If excessive bleeding occurs during endoscopic DCR, the procedure should be terminated or converted to an external DCR. Occasionally, orbital fat is exposed while removing bone to uncover the lacrimal sac. Care must be taken not to disturb this fat so as to prevent injury to underlying orbital structures. Damage to the adjacent medial rectus and superior oblique muscles can lead to diplopia. Blindness can result from laceration of intraorbital vessels with subsequent hemorrhage or by direct injury to the optic nerve itself.

Postoperative adhesions are one of the most common causes of surgical failure for both external and endoscopic DCR. These adhesions usually span the lateral nasal wall and middle turbinate or septum, causing obstruction of the surgically created ostium. The incidence of this complication can be reduced by either avoiding surgical trauma to the turbinate mucosa or resecting the anterior half of the turbinate, so that it is not in the proximity of the ostium. Correction of a deviated septum also reduces the likelihood of postoperative adhesion formation, as does meticulous cleaning of debris from the intranasal operative site during the postoperative healing period.

Postoperative epistaxis severe enough to require nasal packing occurs in less than 3 percent of patients. Bleeding usually occurs within 1 week of surgery and is caused by a branch of the sphenopalatine artery supplying the remnant of a partially resected middle turbinate. Postoperative infection involving the nose or orbit after DCR is rare. Perioperative antibiotics are administered in an attempt to avoid this complication.

■ RESULTS

In my experience of more than 100 endoscopic procedures performed for lacrimal obstruction, a success rate higher than 90 percent has been achieved for primary endoscopic DCR surgery. Successful outcome of this procedure is technique-dependent and requires attention to the details that have been described previously. The surgeon must ensure that a sufficiently large intranasal opening is created into the lacrimal sac by removal of thick maxillary bone overlying the anterior sac. Reports in the literature of lower success rates for endoscopic DCR reflect techniques that involve limited bone removal and small sac openings. If the entire medial sac wall is removed and the internal common punctum is clearly visible at the end of the procedure, there is a high likelihood of successful surgical outcome.

Revision endoscopic DCR is a worthwhile surgical endeavor for those patients who have failed primary external DCR. I have a 75 percent success rate for revision surgery when patients present with recurrent epiphora or dacryocystitis after primary DCR. Common causes of DCR failure, such as intranasal adhesions, ethmoiditis, and an enlarged middle turbinate, can be easily identified and corrected with endoscopic instrumentation. When revision endoscopic DCR is unsuccessful, consideration must be given to missed causes of lacrimal obstruction, particularly canalicular scarring and stenosis. Such diagnoses are usually made with probing and attempted irrigation of the canaliculi by an ophthalmologist. These patients may benefit from endoscopic conjunctivodacryocystorhinostomy with Jones tube placement.

■ DISCUSSION

Endoscopic DCR allows for the opening of an obstructed lacrimal sac without the need for an external incision. Compared with external DCR, the endoscopic approach appears to offer an equivalent rate of success with decreased patient morbidity. In my opinion, these factors will lead to increased acceptance and utilization of endoscopic techniques for the treatment of patients who have lacrimal obstruction.

Suggested Reading

Mannor GE, Millman Al. The prognostic value of preoperative dacryocystography in endoscopic intranasal dacryocystorhinostomy. Am J Ophthalmol 1992; 113:134-137.

Metson R. Endoscopic dacryocystorhinostomy—an update on techniques. Otolaryngol Head Neck Surg 1995; 6:217-220.

Metson R. Endoscopic surgery for lacrimal obstruction. Otolaryngol Head Neck Surg 1991; 104:473-479.

Metson R. The endoscopic approach for revision dacryocystorhinostomy. Laryngoscope 1990; 100:1344-1347.

Metson R, Woog JJ, Puliafito CA. Endoscopic laser dacryocystorhinostomy. Laryngoscope 1994; 104:269-274.

VASOMOTOR RHINITIS

The method of
Robert M. Naclerio
by
Philip W. Rouadi
Robert M. Naclerio

Vasomotor rhinitis (VMR) is a poor term that clinicians use to describe a relatively common form of rhinitis characterized by symptoms of nasal obstruction, postnasal drainage, anterior rhinorrhea, or sneezing of unknown etiology. Although patients frequently associate their disease with a host of environmental irritants, there is no obvious cause of their symptoms. Symptoms are often exacerbated by fumes, tobacco smoke, spicy foods, alcohol, emotional factors, and weather changes. Traditionally, when a thorough clinical evaluation of such patients fails to identify an etiologic basis for the symptoms (e.g., allergic or infectious), many physicians use the term *vasomotor rhinitis* for this idiopathic disorder. This erroneously applied terminology implies a specific pathophysiology, when none is known. Currently, the term *VMR* is being replaced by *nonallergic* and *nonallergic, non-eosinophilic* rhinitis in Europe and America, respectively. Perhaps a better term would be *perennial, nonallergic, non-eosinophilic rhinitis,* or simply *idiopathic rhinitis.* The clinician should exhaust every effort in searching for all potential causes before labeling the patient's condition VMR or idiopathic rhinitis.

■ PATHOGENESIS

Investigations into the pathogenesis of VMR are limited. Most nasal irritants are believed to affect sensory neurons that send inputs to the central nervous system (CNS). In normal individuals, the nasal mucosal response to an irritant results in increased secretion and vascular changes that go unnoticed by the subject. The efferent limb of this nasal reflex is mediated by the parasympathetic fibers from the superior salivatory nucleus. In patients who have VMR, the same stimulus results in an exaggerated parasympathetic response manifested as hypersecretion. The net result is a wet, runny, and stuffy nose. Because the relationship between the magnitude of nasal symptoms and the physiologic magnitude of changes is limited, it is not known whether the symptoms expressed by the patients actually exceed normal variations of the physiologic nasal response. There is, unfortunately, little evidence for the existence of increased parasympathetic neuronal activity in patients who have vasomotor rhinitis. Added to this is the fact that the section of the vidian nerve that deprives the nasal mucosa of parasympathetic and sympathetic stimulation provides only temporary relief from rhinorrhea associated with this disease.

Positional rhinomanometry is a physiologic method that assesses quantitatively the changes in nasal resistance induced by different body positions. Altissimi and co-workers have demonstrated that alterations in nasal resistance on positional rhinomanometry are more marked in patients who have VMR than in healthy individuals. In testing of subjects in the supine and recumbent positions and comparison of the results to basal values in the seated position, positional rhinomanometry has indicated an 80 percent increase in nasal resistance in patients who have VMR compared with the nasal resistance seen in healthy subjects. These data indicate an abnormal response of the cavernous tissues in the turbinates to changes in body position that is quantitatively more marked in persons who have VMR than in normal individuals. In addition, the diving reflex, which is simulated by application of a cold stimulus to the face that produces bradycardia and peripheral vasoconstriction, resulted in significantly higher nasal airway resistance in VMR patients than in controls. This seems to reflect an abnormal autonomic control of the nasal vasculature in patients who have VMR.

For a better understanding of the pathogenesis of the disease and for delineating its potential cellular constituents, Blom and associates have performed immunohistochemical staining nasal biopsy sections obtained from patients who have VMR and compared the results to a group of normal subjects. There was no significant difference in the number of eosinophils, mast cells, and immunoglobulin E (IgE)–positive cells between the two groups. Whether this implies that these cells do not play a major role in the pathogenesis of VMR, or whether VMR is simply a variant of normal, could not be determined.

Patients who have VMR probably represent a heterogeneous group characterized by an exaggerated nasal response to environmental stimuli. The reason for this responsiveness is not known.

■ CLINICAL EVALUATION

History

The diagnosis of VMR should be made only after all other causes of perennial, nonallergic, noninfectious types of rhinitis are excluded (Table 1). This step is of primary importance before institution of any form of therapy. The workup of a patient who has VMR begins with obtaining a careful history defining the patient's own conception of the symptoms. The history obtained at the patient's initial visit serves as a baseline to which therapeutic interventions are directed. Some have suggested using a validated instrument like the Rhinitis Quality of Life Questionnaire for following up patients. The symptoms in VMR patients should be fully characterized in terms of temporal pattern, type, age of onset, and precipitating factors. Emphasis should be placed on the characteristics of secretions (clear versus purulent), the presence of postnasal drip, presence or absence of facial pain, and the characteristics of airflow obstruction. Severe nasal obstruction is often associated with a decrease in the sense of smell, which is frequently perceived as a loss of taste. Oral or topical prescribed medications consumed by the patient, in addition to over-the-counter medicines, should be identi-

Table 1. Causes of Nonallergic, Noninfectious Rhinitis

Drug-induced
Antihypertensives
Nasal decongestants
Oral contraceptive pills
Ophthalmic β-adrenergic blockers
Aspirin/NSAIDs
Systemic autoimmune diseases
SLE
Sjögren's syndrome
Granulomatous disease
Sarcoidosis
Wegener's granulomatosis
Metabolic conditions
Pregnancy
Hypothyroidism
Anatomic abnormalities
Septal deviations/spurs
Nasal polyps
Tumors
Atrophic rhinitis
Surgery
Ozena
Nonallergic rhinitis with eosinophilia syndrome
Conditions related to physical and chemical exposures
Gustatory rhinitis
Cold dry air–induced rhinitis
Occupational rhinitis
Pollutant-induced rhinitis

NSAIDs, nonsteroidal anti-inflammatory drugs; SLE, systemic lupus erythematosus.

fied. Antidepressants, antihypertensives, contraceptive pills, nonsteroidal anti-inflammatory drugs, and topical ophthalmic β-adrenergic blockers can cause nasal congestion. Also, tolerance to topically applied nasal decongestants can develop after their prolonged use and can cause rebound nasal obstruction (rhinitis medicamentosus). A variety of systemic and metabolic conditions can mimic the symptoms of VMR, and it is therefore important to recognize them in the process of history taking. Pregnancy, diabetes, hypothyroidism, and some granulomatous and autoimmune diseases can directly affect the function of the nose, leading to chronic nasal obstruction and rhinorrhea. The patient's occupation might give a clue to exposure to potentially harmful physical or chemical agents. The lack of symptoms during vacations and other off-work times should be evaluated. The chronicity of symptoms in VMR at times allows exclusion of acute, self-limited causes of rhinitis, such as viral infections. Chronic or recurrent acute disease states such as chronic sinusitis, immunodeficiency disorders, cystic fibrosis, and immotile cilia syndrome affect the nose in a protracted way. Virtually all patients who have chronic rhinitis, regardless of etiology, complain of symptoms related to abrupt changes in atmospheric conditions; the mechanism of this phenomenon is not understood.

The symptoms of VMR, unfortunately, overlap with those of many other types of rhinitis. Perennial allergic rhinitis (AR) is the disorder most frequently confused with VMR. A good history, including the age of onset of nasal complaints and the type of symptoms the patient manifests often allows differentiation (Table 2). In a retrospective study at the Johns Hopkins Allergy Clinic, the majority (70 percent) of patients diagnosed with nonallergic rhinitis developed their condition in adult life, whereas only 26.7 percent of patients with seasonal allergic rhinitis did so. Moreover, compared with patients who had perennial AR, those who had nonallergic disease reported significantly more sinus-related complaints, and less sneezing and conjunctival symptoms. On the other hand, patients who had perennial AR had a significantly higher association of their disease with asthma than did the nonallergic group. Also, a family history of atopy is common in patients who have allergy and uncommon in patients who have VMR. In contrast to patients who have AR, most of whom exhibit seasonal symptoms, those with VMR follow a perennial pattern of symptoms, but may also have seasonal variations. Another important clue is that patients who have AR can usually relate their attacks to exposure to a specific allergen. Allergic subjects have a hyperirritable mucosa, such that their symptoms can be triggered by irritants in the same manner as in patients who have VMR. Similarly, infective rhinitis and sinusitis frequently complicate both VMR and AR and can usually be diagnosed based on history and the presence of a purulent nasal discharge.

Physical Examination

During physical examination, the ear, nose, mouth, and throat areas should be thoroughly inspected. Inspection of the conjunctivae for injection, the chest for wheezing, and the skin for urticaria is also necessary. Gross examination of the nasal contour may show asymmetry which, in the presence of nasal obstruction, should alert the physician to the potential presence of an expanding mass, or a history of previous trauma. Also, gross examination of the nasal valve area, which is the major area of nasal airflow resistance between the external environment and the alveolus, might demonstrate loss of cartilaginous support. The nasal valve can be compromised by an edentulous upper alveolus, which causes the upper lip to hang, or sagging of the lower lateral cartilage associated with aging.

Nasal examination should focus on structural deformities that may impede nasal airflow, namely, those involving the septum, turbinates, and nasal mucosa. Considering the fact that most of the air entering the nose flows over the anterior edge of the inferior turbinates, passes up over the middle turbinate, and then descends into the nasopharynx, nasal septal deviations along this path have the greatest impact on airflow. Unless they are traumatic, septal deviations are unlikely to be the cause of a new-onset nasal obstruction. The color and consistency of the turbinates should also be noted. An edematous, boggy, pale turbinate, once considered diagnostic of AR, can also be encountered in patients who have VMR and hypothyroidism. Pooled secretions under the inferior turbinates should prompt the physician to investigate for the immotile cilia syndrome or total nasal obstruction. Thin crusts associated with a foul odor (ozena) are characteristic of atrophic rhinitis.

The contribution of the nasal mucosa to nasal obstruction can be determined by application of a topical nasal decongestant spray. A diseased, hyperplastic mucosa reacts poorly to such treatment. Turbinate hypertrophy that is sig-

Table 2. Patient History Used for Distinguishing Vasomotor Rhinitis (VMR) From Allergic Rhinitis (AR)

HISTORY	VMR	AR
Temporal pattern of symptoms	Perennial	Seasonal or perennial with seasonal exacerbation
Type of symptoms	Congestion, rhinorrhea, postnasal drip	Sneezing, pruritus, congestion, rhinorrhea, postnasal drip
Age of onset	Adulthood	Childhood
Precipitating factor		
Allergen	No	Yes
Nonspecific irritants	Yes	Yes
Family history of atopy	Not frequent	Frequent
Other atopic disease	Not present	Present
Asthma	Rare	Frequent

Table 3. Laboratory Tests Used for Differentiating Vasomotor Rhinitis From Other Types of Rhinitis

TEST	ALLERGIC RHINITIS	VASOMOTOR RHINITIS	EOSINOPHILIC NONALLERGIC RHINITIS	INFECTIOUS RHINITIS
Allergy testing	Positive	Negative	Negative	Negative
Nasal cytology	Marked eosinophilia	Few, if any, eosinophils	Marked eosinophilia	Neutrophils

nificant enough to cause nasal obstruction and is unresponsive to topical vasoconstrictive agents may require surgical intervention. Biopsy of the turbinates can also be performed for confirmation of a suspected diagnosis of systemic granulomatous disease, such as sarcoidosis. Decongestion allows better visualization of the anterior tip of the middle turbinate. This area, which is the region of greatest nasal airflow and greatest particle impaction, may be the first affected by environmental factors.

A complete workup of nasal obstruction should include flexible or rigid endoscopic evaluation of the nasal cavity. By fiberoptic endoscopy the physician detects abnormalities of the middle meatal region, septal spurs, obstruction of the sphenoid sinuses, adenoid hypertrophy, and other causes of nasal obstruction not seen by anterior rhinoscopy. The findings can be recorded on videotape and provide a permanent record that can be shared by the patient.

■ LABORATORY EVALUATION

Diagnostic tests are useful in excluding nasal conditions that mimic the symptomatology of VMR, namely, AR and nonallergic rhinitis with eosinophilia syndrome (Table 3).

In Vivo and In Vitro Testing

Skin testing and in vitro determination of specific IgE can be performed for differentiating between allergic and nonallergic rhinitis. Patients who have allergic rhinitis show a positive reaction to specific allergens. The measurement of total serum IgE in atopic diseases has only limited clinical significance: 50 percent of patients who have clinical evidence of allergy and detectable allergen-specific IgE have total IgE levels within normal limits. Patients who have elevated total IgE can have negative results from testing for a specific allergen. A variety of conditions unrelated to allergy, such as parasitic infections and hyperimmunoglobulinemia E with recurrent pyodermas (Job-Buckley syndrome), manifest high levels of total serum IgE. In VMR, the results of skin and radioallergosorbent testing for inhalant allergens are negative, and serum IgE levels are within normal limits.

Nasal Cytology

This diagnostic modality is the most useful in differentiating an acute infection from an allergic reaction. The presence of eosinophilia in nasal secretions or scrapings, regardless of the allergic status, is a positive prognostic factor for the efficacy of topical steroids (i.e., patients with eosinophils respond to steroids).

Various techniques have been described for obtaining nasal cytology specimens, including blowing secretions into wax paper; taking smears by using cotton wool swabs, imprints, or brushes; or performing nasal scraping, lavage, and biopsy. The selection of a sampling method depends on factors such as the age of the patient, the need for repeated sampling, or the requirement for simultaneous biochemical analysis. Nasal scraping with a Rhinoprobe is the best-studied technique. The wet contents of the sample are spread over a glass slide, fixed, stained, and evaluated by light microscopy. The nasal cytogram viewed at high power is graded semiquantitatively.

Increased numbers of eosinophils are found in the nasal mucosa of patients who have active AR. The degree of eosinophilia appears to correlate with the extent of allergen exposure, the magnitude of symptom, presence of positive allergy skin tests, and serum IgE levels. Patients who have VMR are characterized by the absence of eosinophils on nasal smear, whereas those who have negative findings from skin tests to common aeroallergens and marked eosinophilia on nasal cytology are referred to as having nonallergic rhinitis with eosinophilia syndrome (NARES). These latter patients have an increased incidence of sinusitis and polyp formation.

Nasal cytology can also be useful in differentiating infectious from other types of rhinitis. With bacterial infections such as rhinosinusitis, several histopathologic abnormalities are described: fewer ciliated cells, causing impaired mucociliary transport, and increased neutrophils, lymphocytes, and plasma cells. The presence of intracellular bacteria on a nasal cytogram is considered diagnostic for sinusitis. Another factor related to nasal cytology is that nasal eosinophilia is inconstant, and therefore one should perform the procedure several times to determine whether the condition is characterized by eosinophilia. We have not incorporated cytology into our practice because we rarely see patients who have acute nasal problems, and we find a therapeutic trial of intranasal steroids combined with allergy testing to be a more satisfactory approach.

Imaging

Imaging of the paranasal sinuses is ordered whenever sinusitis may be complicating the clinical picture. When the history and physical examination are completed, the paranasal sinuses are the only areas not fully evaluated. Plain radiographs do not provide good visualization of the ethmoid region and cannot detect subtle obstruction in the area of the osteomeatal complex. The clinical significance of plain radiographs resides in delineating the air-fluid level within the sinuses during acute infections. Computed tomographic (CT) scans visualize the sinuses better than do plain radiographs. Magnetic resonance (MR) imaging delineates clearly the extent of mucosal swelling, especially on T2-weighted images. However, air and bony interfaces, which are important for the diagnosis of sinus disease, are not visible on MR images.

Acoustic Rhinometry and Rhinomanometry

Acoustic rhinometry is a diagnostic modality that displays cross-sectional areas of the nasal cavity by distance from the nostrils. Its clinical importance stems from its ability to assess objectively hypertrophy of the inferior turbinates in patients who have VMR and in patients who have occult nasal obstruction in general. It also can distinguish deviations of the nasal structures from normal structures, such as valve stenosis and septal deviation. Its best use, however, is for showing a normal nasal volume in individuals who have abnormal symptoms and normal physical findings.

The minimal cross-sectional area, located at the isthmus nasi in normal individuals, becomes sited at the head of the inferior turbinates in patients who have inferior turbinate hypertrophy due to allergic or vasomotor rhinitis. After anterior turbinoplasty, improved nasal breathing is sometimes associated with an enlargement of the cross-sectional areas at the head of the anterior inferior turbinate.

Rhinomanometry is another diagnostic modality that evaluates airflow. Patients who have chronic rhinitis and obstruction to airflow, such as VMR, may exhibit increased nasal airway resistance on rhinomanometric studies. For all of these studies, limited normative data are available, and they may be subject to a number of errors.

■ MANAGEMENT

The history and physical examination, supported by diagnostic tests, will enable the physician to classify the patient who has nasal obstruction and rhinorrhea into one or several categories of chronic rhinitis (Table 1). In patients who have well-documented etiologies, management should be tailored according to the underlying problem. This includes allergy management, which is discussed in another chapter. This section focuses on the management of patients who have VMR.

Treatment of VMR is frustrating. Advocating multiple forms of therapy for its control reflects the variable, and often unpredictable, response to medical and surgical treatment. Avoidance of the offending irritant(s) and symptomatic control with pharmacotherapy constitute the fundamental strategy. Surgery is used as an adjunct to medical therapy.

Environmental Therapy

Treatment begins with avoidance of potential irritants. Organic dust, fumes, odors, powders, sprays, and tobacco smoke should be avoided at home and in the workplace. The normal nose can tolerate a wide range of temperature and humidity; the abnormal nose may not. Therefore, avoiding low room humidity, which may lead to nasal drying and a sensation of congestion, is prudent.

Venous congestion of the turbinates is maximal when the patient assumes the supine position because of decreased venous outflow. Instructing the patient to sleep on two pillows and/or to elevate the head of the bed a few inches may decrease congestion.

Pharmacotherapy

A practical approach to the management of VMR patients with pharmacotherapy is to categorize them as "runners," "blockers," and "sneezers." This approach helps the physician target therapy toward the predominant symptom. To date, therapy has included the following agents: anticholinergic drugs, antihistamines, alpha-adrenoreceptor agonists, and glucocorticoids. Other modalities described for the treatment of allergic diseases, such as immunotherapy, are not useful in treating VMR because their efficacy is dependent on an IgE-mediated pathophysiology. Treatment targeted at specific cellular mediators implicated in allergic diseases, such as leukotrienes and prostaglandins, has not been studied in VMR, to our knowledge.

Ipratropium Bromide

Anticholinergic agents are effective in the treatment of watery rhinorrhea regardless of the cause. Stimulation of parasympathetic nerve fibers to the nasal mucosa leads to watery nasal secretions. In contrast to normal individuals, patients with VMR have an abnormal hyper-responsiveness of the nasal mucosa to cholinergic stimulation, which is manifested as a significant increase in the volume of secretions in response to intranasal metacholine, a synthetic cholinergic agonist. The clear watery fluid, which is devoid of inflammatory cells but rich in proteins (lysozyme, secretory immunoglobulin A, lactoferrin), originates from the submucous glands of the nasal mucosa. The immediate and profuse rhinorrhea that follows nasal administration of metacholine is blocked by the topical application of anticholinergic agents, such as ipratropium bromide (IB) or atropine sulfate. The antirhinorrhea effect of atropine seems comparable to that of IB, although atropine has a shorter duration of action. IB is safer than atropine, because the topical application of the latter is associated with adverse reactions secondary to systemic absorption of the drug involving the ocular, cutaneous, gastrointestinal, cardiovascular, and central nervous systems.

Topical IB, or Atrovent, has its main application in patients with VMR in whom profuse watery rhinorrhea is the main symptom. Several studies have shown the efficacy of Atrovent in the control of rhinorrhea of perennial nonallergic rhinitis, in addition to the reduction of rhinorrhea associated with the common cold. In patients who have chronic clear watery nasal discharge for more than 1 hour per day, absent or mild nasal obstruction, no known allergies, and no satisfactory response to previous alternative medications, Atrovent produced a major reduction in the severity and duration of rhinorrhea. The dosage used, two sprays in each nostril (20 μg per spray) four times daily for 3 weeks, resulted in minimal side effects.

Nasal challenge studies with various chemical and physical stimuli have characterized the pharmacologic effects of IB. After nasal challenge with metacholine, histamine, allergens, and exercise, nasal secretions were reduced significantly in subjects premedicated with IB as compared to subjects who received placebo. On the other hand, IB had no effect on histamine- and allergen-induced itching, sneezing, or blockage. IB treatment also proved beneficial in subjects who had rhinorrhea after exposure to cold dry air, after ingested hot spicy food, had the common cold, and who aged.

IB can be delivered in two forms: as an aerosol from a metered-dose, pressurized canister, or as an aqueous solution in a pump spray. This latter is available in two concentrations, 0.03 percent and 0.06 percent. For perennial rhinitis, the recommended dosage is two puffs of 0.03 percent per nostril two to three times daily, whereas that for the common cold is two puffs of 0.06 percent per nostril three to four times daily. The total daily dose of the pressurized aerosol is 320 μg given as two puffs of 20 μg per nostril four times daily. This formulation is currently not available in the United States

Atrovent, which has a quaternary amine structure, is poorly absorbed after topical application to mucosal surfaces, and it is relatively slow to cross the blood-brain barrier. In clinical trials, no systemic side effects were reported. Local side effects, generally considered to be insignificant, are dose-dependent, and consist of nasal irritation; stuffiness; dryness of the nose, mouth, and throat; and bloody nasal secretions. Some reports have suggested that more dryness and irritation occur in elderly than in younger persons. Other variables, such as pulse rate and blood pressure, sneezing, nasal congestion, sense-of-smell threshold, nasal cytology, or appearance of the mucosa at rhinoscopy, were not affected by Atrovent treatment. Large intranasal doses (400 μg) applied topically to the nasal mucosa can be tolerated without systemic side effects. On the other hand, increasing the daily dose from 320 to 1,600 μg marginally increases the efficacy, but also markedly increases the local side effects.

In long-term follow-ups of patients who responded to Atrovent in clinical trials, the subjects were allowed to select their dose after the trial. The dose chosen was invariably lower than that used in the respective controlled trial. Also, it appears that patient-initiated doses elicit fewer side effects. This observation suggests that, after an initial response, patients should be permitted to titrate their dose.

Contraindications to the use of Atrovent by patients are hypersensitivity to the drug or to atropine, and a history of hypersensitivity to soya lecithin or related food products such as soybeans and peanuts. The drug should be used cautiously in patients who suffer from diseases that could potentially be aggravated by anticholinergic therapy, such as angle-closure glaucoma, prostatic hypertrophy, bladder-neck obstruction, and arrhythmias.

Antihistamines

Antihistamines compete with histamine at the H_1 receptors. In allergic rhinitis, symptoms of sneezing, itching, and rhinorrhea are treated most effectively with antihistamines, but with no effect on nasal congestion. Although rare among patients who have VMR, "sneezers" may also benefit from antihistamine treatment. The mechanism of histamine release that causes sneezing in these patients is still unclear. The older, more sedating class of antihistamines can be used in treating VMR because of their anticholinergic properties. On the other hand, second-generation H_1-receptor antagonists, which have much less affinity for cholinergic receptors than do their predecessors, have no clinical use in VMR. Antihistamines of the ethanolamine class, such as diphenhydramine, which have the greatest anticholinergic activity, might be more suitable for use in a patient who has VMR and rhinorrhea.

Dexchlorpheniramine maleate, available as tablets (2 mg) and in syrup form (2 mg per 5 milliliters), can be given for VMR at a dosage of 2 mg every 4 to 6 hours. Timed-release tablets, available in 4 and 6 mg, are prescribed three and two times daily, respectively. Dryness of the mucosa and sedation are common side effects. Other adverse CNS reactions include dizziness and stimulation. Sedation can frequently be avoided by administration of the drug at bedtime. Also, antihistamines can be associated with urinary retention in men who have enlarged prostates, and these drugs can interact with monoamine oxidase inhibitors and other CNS depressants, resulting in increased anticholinergic effects and sedation, respectively. Because small amounts of the drug are excreted in breast milk, antihistamine use is not recommended for breast-feeding women.

Decongestants

Sympathomimetic agents cause constriction of both resistance and capacitance vessels. The capacitance vessels are responsible for nasal congestion. Most topical vasoconstrictors, such as epinephrine and oxymetazoline, act directly on alpha-adrenergic receptors on blood vessels. Others, such as pseudoephedrine and phenylpropanolamine, act both directly on the vessels and indirectly by inhibiting the release of norepinephrine from sympathetic nerve fibers. The resultant effects are decongestion and an increase in nasal patency, regardless of the cause for the capacitance vessels' dilation. In a patient who has VMR, vasoconstrictors alleviate the symptom of nasal congestion, with no effect in reducing sneezing or nasal secretion; in some animal models, vasoconstrictors actually increased nasal secretion.

Nasal decongestants can be administered orally or topically (Table 4). For chronic nasal obstruction, such as occurs in VMR, oral vasoconstrictors should be prescribed first. Pseudoephedrine hydrochloride is available as 30 mg, 60 mg, and (extended-release) 120 mg, 160 mg, and 240 mg tablets; syrup preparations are available as 15 mg per 5 milliliters and 30 mg per 5 milliliters. Adults are prescribed 60 mg tablets orally every 6 hours, or 120 mg extended-release tablets twice per day, or 240 mg extended-release tablet once per day, with a maximum daily allowance of 240 mg. Prolonged therapeutic trials are unnecessary because systemically effective decongestants work within hours. Side effects include anxiety, nervousness, insomnia, palpitations, arrhythmias, and difficulty in urination in elderly persons. It is prudent to avoid these agents in the following conditions: coronary artery disease, hyperthyroidism, diabetes mellitus, narrow-angle glaucoma, and in patients receiving monoamine oxidase inhibitors. In oral doses necessary for decongestion of the nasal mucosa, these drugs seem to have no significant side effects in hypertensive patients whose blood pressure is adequately controlled.

Oral antihistamines and decongestants are often prescribed in combination. Initially, the stimulant effect of the decongestant was believed to counteract the sedative side effect of the antihistamine, but this has never been proved. Although these preparations are beneficial in reducing clinical symptoms of AR, clinical trials in VMR have not generated convincing evidence in terms of reduction of nasal airway resistance.

Vasoconstrictors administered as nasal drops or sprays are more effective in reducing nasal decongestion than are their oral counterparts. Oxymetazoline hydrochloride, an imidazole derivative, is available in 0.025 percent and 0.05 percent nasal solutions. It acts within minutes of administration and has a 10 to 12 hour duration of action. In adults, it is given as two to three drops or two sprays of 0.05 percent solution in each nostril twice daily. The same dosage of the 0.025 percent solution is used in children. Patients who have VMR and nasal obstruction that is unresponsive to other therapy might benefit from a single dose at bedtime.

Continued topical use of local decongestants for more than 10 consecutive days poses a significant risk for development of rhinitis medicamentosus. This condition, which is likely to occur in patients who have VMR because of chronicity of symptoms, manifests itself as nasal stuffiness that is no longer responsive to topical decongestant therapy. After prolonged use, when the vasoconstrictive effect of the drug has disappeared, nasal stuffiness occurs because of rebound swelling. Sustained use of oxymetazoline nasal spray, for example, induced a significant increase in nasal mucosal swelling, as measured optically by a microscope (rhinostereometry), as well as in nasal reactivity, as determined by the response to histamine challenge. These studies also suggest that the preservative used in these preparations, benzalkonium chloride, aggravates the symptoms by inducing a significant increase in nasal mucosal swelling, as shown by subjects sprayed only with the preservative as compared to subjects who received placebo. This swelling is treated by abstinence from the decongestant for 2 weeks. A patient who does not respond to simple withdrawal of the offending agent may benefit from a short course of topical intranasal steroids or systemic steroids.

Steroids

The major therapeutic impact that topical steroids have in the treatment of allergic rhinitis has generated enthusiasm for their use in treating VMR. Several studies have shown the efficacy of glucocorticoids in the symptomatic treatment of nonallergic perennial rhinitis. Fluticasone propionate, for example, significantly decreased the expiratory nasal airway resistance, as a response to a simulated diving reflex, in patients with nonallergic, non-eosinophilic rhinitis as compared to controls. This seems to reflect the efficacy of steroids in normalizing the nasal hyper-reflexia present in these patients. However, data describing the use of steroids in treating VMR according to strict inclusion criteria are still limited. As mentioned previously, in perennial nonallergic rhinitis, the presence of eosinophils on a nasal smear seems to indicate a high degree of symptomatic relief. However, the absence of these cells should not preclude a therapeutic trial in patients suffering from VMR.

A potential mechanism of action for these drugs in treating VMR is still under investigation. In dermal applications, glucocorticoids induce vasoconstriction of blood vessels. However, in the nasal mucosa, there seems to be no steroid-induced vasoconstriction. Treatment with budesonide in

Table 4. Different Types of Vasoconstrictors

DECONGESTANT DRUG	ATTRIBUTES	ROUTE OF ADMINISTRATION
β-PHENYLETHYLAMINE DERIVATIVES		
Ephedrine sulfate	Significant CNS stimulation	Oral and topical
Pseudoephedrine hydrochloride	Less CNS stimulation than ephedrine; less potent vasoconstrictor	Oral
Phenylephrine hydrochloride	Less CNS stimulation than ephedrine	Topical
Phenylpropanolamine hydrochloride	Rapid GI tract metabolism	Oral
IMIDAZOLINE DERIVATIVES		
Oxymetazoline hydrochloride	Long-acting	Topical
Xylometazoline hydrochloride	Long-acting	Topical
Naphazoline hydrochloride	Significant CNS depression in excess; mucosal irritation	Topical

CNS, central nervous system; GI, gastrointestinal.

Adapted from Malm L, Anggard A. Vasoconstrictors. In: Mygind M, Naclerio R, eds. Allergic and non-allergic rhinitis. Copenhagen: Munksgaard, 1993:95.

normal persons had no effect either on the capacitance vessels, as determined by measurement of nasal airway resistance, or on the resistance vessels, as determined by the xenon washout technique.

The steroid molecules that are widely used today for intranasal treatment are listed in Table 5. Although several studies have indicated a higher potency of some agents over others, all appear to be equally effective when used in recommended doses. The usual recommended dose is 200 to 400 μg daily in adults and half the dose in children. The dosage schedule varies with different preparations. In the lower airways, a clear dose-response curve has been demonstrated for these agents; in the nose, however, the results are less clear. In rhinitis, unlike asthma, high-dose therapy is not generally recommended, but a higher than normal dose can be tried for a short time in selected patients. At the initial visit, the drug is prescribed for a 2 week trial period. In subsequent follow-ups, the physician should assess the efficacy in alleviating the symptoms and evaluate any irritant effect of the drug. If no response occurs, the drug should be discontinued. The dose might be increased if slight, but insufficient improvement is noted. Should local irritation become bothersome to the patient, the physician might consider switching the patient to a different preparation or reducing the dose. If the patient reports symptomatic improvement, the dose should be tapered to the lowest level that provides efficacy. This should be done at weekly intervals because these agents can have a prolonged clinical effect. Once-a-day dosing is often possible; this is a major advantage for compliance. These agents have excellent clinical safety with long-term topical use. Biopsies of the nasal mucosa obtained from perennial rhinitis sufferers who received beclomethasone continuously for 5 years showed no signs of atrophy.

The major side effect of intranasal steroids is local irritation. Approximately 10 percent of patients will experience some sensation of irritation, burning, or sneezing after administration. Approximately 2 percent will note a bloody discharge, and rare septal perforations have been reported.

It is important to recognize some practical aspects of drug use in patients who receive topical steroid therapy. Frequently, severe nasal blockage and congestion preclude effective and even distribution of the drug in the nose. Therefore, when necessary, the patient should start by blowing the nose before spraying. Also, topical application of a nasal decongestant before steroid use might prove useful in "opening" the nasal airway. The physician might find that a patient who has a severely blocked nose must be started on a short course of systemic steroids.

It is necessary to teach the patient how to spray correctly. The delivery device should be directed toward the lateral nasal wall. Patients should also be instructed to use the drug regularly and not on an as-needed basis, because it will take several days before the beneficial results of the drug are maximum. In general, pump sprays provide a better distribution of drug compared with aerosols, but the choice of the preparation probably depends mostly on patient preference.

Surgical Therapy

The majority of patients who have VMR can be managed with the judicious use of pharmacotherapy. However, a small group of patients are resistant to all available forms of medical therapy, and in this group surgical treatment may be considered. The results of surgery are not uniform, and the long-term efficacy is not clear. Nonetheless, surgery can often complement the medical management of VMR by improving the airway and providing better access for topical therapy. The surgical procedures should be very conservative and should be aimed toward relief of nasal obstruction. The surgical interventions for correcting septal nasal valve deformities or inferior turbinate hypertrophy, or for modifying the autonomic innervation to the nasal mucosa, are described next. However, it should be emphasized to the patient that the goal of surgery is to provide symptomatic relief by improving the airway, and that surgery in itself will not provide a cure of the mucosal disease.

Surgery of the Nasal Septum and Nasal Valve

Patients with VMR in whom a moderately deviated septum is noted on physical examination should be initially started on a therapeutic trial of medical therapy. If pharmacotherapy improves the patient's symptoms, surgical correction of the septal deformity should be delayed. However, if no improvement with medical therapy is noted, or if the patient improves but still complains of symptoms that warrant further treatment, surgical intervention is indicated. A deviated septum requires surgical correction only if it is considered to be contributing to nasal obstruction or recurrent sinus infections. Occasionally, nasal obstruction can originate from abnormalities in the nasal valve area located at the anterior naris. This area, particularly in the elderly, can be compromised by sagging of the lower lateral cartilages, loss of cartilaginous support, or hypertrophy of the anterior portions of the middle or inferior turbinates. The surgical approach to these patients is individualized and depends on the underlying anatomic abnormality.

Surgery of the Turbinates

This can be accomplished in several ways, ranging from local application of silver nitrate to total turbinectomy. It is im-

Table 5. Topical Corticosteroids Used in Treating Rhinitis

PREPARATION	MODE OF DELIVERY	DOSAGE
Beclomethasone dipropionate	Aerosol or spray: 42 μg/puff; 50 μg/puff	1 puff/nostril 2 to 4 times daily
Flunisolide	Spray: 25 μg/puff (solution: 0.25 mg/mL)	2 puffs/nostril 2 to 3 times daily
Budesonide	Spray: 32 μg/puff	2 puffs/nostril 2 times daily
Triamcinolone acetonide	Aerosol: 55 μg/puff	2 puffs/nostril 1 to 4 times daily
Fluticasone propionate	Spray: 50 μg/puff	2 sprays/nostril once daily

portant to ascertain that the symptoms are due entirely or in part to turbinate dysfunction before any surgical intervention.

Silver Nitrate Application

This form of chemical cautery consists of topical silver nitrate application to the anterior portions of both inferior turbinates and to the corresponding anterior part of the nasal septum. Although some studies yielded good results and minimal side effects, reports on studies advocating such therapy have been poorly designed, and the studies lack objective outcome parameters and long-term follow-up data.

Corticosteroid Injection

In this method, 0.5 to 1 cc of depot corticosteroid preparations is injected, at multiple sites, throughout the length of each inferior turbinate. Because of their anti-inflammatory action and the induction of atrophy of the turbinate stroma, these agents may provide symptomatic improvement. Drawbacks include a short-term clinical effect (lasting for a period of weeks), which implies multiple therapeutic sessions; cumulative systemic effects; and rare instances of temporary and even permanent visual loss secondary to inadvertent intravascular injection of the steroids, with resultant retinal vasospasm or embolization.

Sclerosing Solutions

Sclerosing agents, such as 5 percent morrhuate sodium, can be injected into the inferior turbinates to sclerose vascular channels. Major disadvantages include prolonged crusting, edema, and rhinorrhea. Repeat injections may also be necessary.

Electrocautery

This appears to benefit mainly "nose blockers." Unipolar cautery can be performed either on the surface of the mucosa or submucosally. In the latter technique, where coagulation occurs in a linear submucosal fashion, less tissue damage ensues than with surface cautery. The bipolar submucosal technique also improves nasal obstruction by shrinking a hyperplastic mucosa. However, it does not relieve rhinorrhea or sneezing in a predictable fashion; it can result in considerable destruction of mucosa, with unpleasant crusting, and the results usually last only for several months.

Submucous Diathermy

Traditionally indicated for nose blocking secondary to mucosal turbinate hypertrophy, this procedure has much less effect on nasal hypersecretion than it does on blockage. Also, postnasal drainage and rhinorrhea frequently persist after the operation.

"Outfracturing" of Inferior Turbinates

Initially described as improving rhinorrhea in patients who have VMR, this technique consists simply of displacing the inferior turbinate first medially toward the nasal septum and then laterally into the inferior meatus. The fractured turbinate results in a greenstick fracture and can drift back to its original position after healing is complete, thus providing only temporary relief.

Cryosurgery

Cryosurgery with liquid nitrogen or nitrous oxide cryoprobes may benefit predominantly VMR patients who have nasal obstruction and, to a lesser extent, those who have rhinorrhea. Freeze times depend on the extent of mucosal disease. The longer the freeze time, the greater the sloughing of tissues, the more prolonged the healing period, and the greater the thaw pain. Some reports seem to suggest that tissue destruction does not extend beyond the grossly visible margin of the frozen area, which implies good control over the depth of freezing during the procedure. Regeneration of normal columnar epithelium with full ciliary activity is a consistent feature and occurs within 4 weeks of the operation. Biopsy studies of the regenerated epithelium show a reduction of nasal mucosal thickness, diminished glandular activity, and less vascularization. As with other procedures, initial success is followed by recurrence of symptoms; difficulty in avoiding the adjacent nasal septum, which results in formation of adhesions; and rather significant postoperative nasal congestion.

Turbinectomy

This procedure and its many variants aim at the conservation of the nasal mucosa with adequate excision of soft tissue and bone. Anterior turbinoplasty was initially advocated based on rhinomanometric studies that suggested a significant contribution of the anterior end of the inferior turbinate to nasal resistance. However, because nasal obstruction can be caused by a hyperplastic posterior segment, this procedure has limited usefulness. Submucosal resection of the inferior turbinate, which consists of elevating a submucosal flap off the anterior turbinate bone, followed by resection of the bone, is indicated in cases of bony rather than mucosal hypertrophy. Occasionally, it may result in significant bleeding or in a floppy residual mucosal flap that worsens obstruction. Total turbinectomy can result in chronic nasal crusting, adhesions, or a paradoxical situation in which the absence of objective evidence of airflow obstruction is associated with the subjective feeling of obstruction

Vidian Neurectomy

Originally described by Golding-Wood in 1961 and currently indicated for intractable VMR, this procedure seems to benefit "drippers" rather than "blockers." It involves interruption of both sympathetic and parasympathetic fibers in the vidian nerve through a transantral, septal, or direct transnasal approach. Laser ablation and/or electrocoagulation of the vidian nerve have also been reported. Regardless of the approach used, or modifications of the procedure itself, long-term follow-up of these patients has demonstrated recurrence of symptoms in the majority of cases, probably caused by reinnervation. Dryness of the eyes is a consistent postoperative finding in successfully operated patients, which occurs secondary to reduced lacrimal secretion. The development of IB has probably eliminated the need for this procedure.

Suggested Reading

Balle VH, Pedersen U, Engby B. Allergic perennial and nonallergic vasomotor rhinitis treated with budesonide nasal spray. Rhinology 1980; 18:135-142.

Blom HM, Godthelp T, Fokkens WJ, et al. Mast cells, eosinophils and IgE-positive cells in the nasal mucosa of patients with vasomotor rhinitis. An immunohistochemical study. Eur Arch Oto-Rhino-Laryngol 1995 (Suppl); 1:S33-S39.

Dolovich J, Kennedy L, Vickerson F, et al. Control of the hypersecretion of vasomotor rhinitis by topical ipratropium bromide. J Allergy Clin Immunol 1987; 80:274-278.

Graf P, Hallen H. Effect on the nasal mucosa of long-term treatment with oxymetazoline, benzalkonium chloride, and placebo nasal sprays. Laryngoscope 1996; 106:605-609.

Lenders H, Pirsig W. Diagnostic value of acoustic rhinometry: Patients with allergic and vasomotor rhinitis compared with normal controls. Rhinology 1990; 28:5-16.

Lindquist N, Balle V, Karma P, et al. Long term safety and efficacy of budesonide nasal aerosol in perennial rhinitis—A 12 month multicenter study. Allergy 1986; 41:179-186.

Meltzer EO, Orgel HA, Jalowayski A. Cytology. In: Mygind N, Naclerio R, eds. Allergic and non-allergic rhinitis. Copenhagen: Munksgaard, 1993:66.

Mygind N. Glucocorticoids and rhinitis. Allergy 1993; 48:476-490.

Mygind N, Borum P, Baroody FM, Naclerio RM. Anticholinergic medication. In: Mygind N, Naclerio RM, Durham SR eds. Allergic and non-allergic rhinitis. Copenhagen: Munksgaard, 1997 (in press).

Simons FER. Antihistamines. In: Mygind N, Naclerio R, eds. Allergic and non-allergic rhinitis. Copenhagen: Munksgaard, 1993:123.

ALLERGIC FUNGAL SINUSITIS

The method of
Jacquelynne P. Corey
by
Vincent P. Nalbone
Jacquelynne P. Corey

Allergic fungal sinusitis (AFS) is one of four types of fungal sinus infections. AFS and fungus ball are both chronic, noninvasive forms, whereas the two other types are invasive (acute-fulminant and chronic-invasive). Previous terms for AFS include *allergic aspergillus sinusitis,* but it has since been shown that dematiaceous fungi, not *Aspergillus,* are the most prevalent fungi. Although categorized as a fungal infection, AFS implicates an allergic process more than a true infection. AFS occurs in immunocompetent hosts and usually involves more than one of the paranasal sinuses.

AFS is the most common form of fungal sinusitis. It occurs in adolescents and young adults who have nasal polyposis. There is no gender or racial predilection. AFS is believed to occur more frequently in warm, humid climates (such as in the southwestern United States) due to airborne transmission and proliferation of fungi in such conditions. AFS accounts for approximately 5 percent to 10 percent of patients with sinusitis who undergo functional endoscopic sinus surgery (FESS).

■ EVALUATION

Clinical Presentation

Patients usually present initially with symptoms typical of sinusitis, such as nasal obstruction, local pain, rhinorrhea, and postnasal discharge. AFS is usually treated at first as routine chronic sinusitis, and patients have usually undergone several antecedent medical and surgical attempts at cure without success. Signs and symptoms that differentiate AFS from nonfungal sinusitis include discharge of thick nasal crusts and a history of atopy (75 percent) and asthma (50 percent). There is infrequently a history of sensitivity to aspirin. Most patients who have AFS harbor nasal polyps. If the polyps are extensive, there may be associated severe nasal obstruction, anosmia, excessive tearing, or orbital involvement with proptosis, cranial nerve involvement, and facial deformity.

Intranasal examination reveals extremely viscous mucus that is brown, yellow, or green. Nasal polyps or polypoid mucosal changes are usually evident. Concretions may be contained within polyps.

Plain radiographs or computed tomographic (CT) scans of the paranasal sinuses usually reveal soft-tissue opacification and areas of high attenuation that are due to calcium, magnesium, manganese, and iron released from the fungi. Frequently, there is expansion of sinonasal walls, and there may be bone destruction in long-standing cases. It is unclear whether bone is remodeled as a result of pressure or from the enzymatic action of inflammatory mediators. Unilateral sinus disease is present much more frequently than in nonfungal cases of sinusitis or polyposis. Areas of high attenuation on CT scans that have been imaged by magnetic resonance imaging (MRI) have decreased T1 signal intensity flanked by mucosal inflammation. On T2 images, there is a less intense signal than on T1. Chest radiographs are usually normal, but should be requested to rule out concomitant pulmonary involvement. There have been reported cases of simultaneous sinus and lung involvement.

Pathology

Histologically, there is a predominance of eosinophils in an edematous, chronically inflamed stroma. Thick, tenacious, rubbery mucin, termed *allergic mucin,* is characteristic of AFS. The mucin contains hexagonal or prism-appearing Charcot-Leyden crystals, which are degradation products of eosinophils. These crystals are diagnostic of AFS. Fungal hyphae are present, but do not invade the mucosa. This is an important pathologic distinction. The mucin also contains eosinophils, epithelial cells, and cellular debris. There is usually a laminar layering of cells and debris in the mucin.

Microbiology

Fungal stains and cultures should be requested if AFS is suspected, with the yield being higher for the former. Routine hematoxylin and eosin (H & E) stains may not detect fungi, so in suspected cases, potassium hydroxide or silver stains (Gomori's methenamine silver stain or Grocott's silver stain) should be performed. Culture of mucus or intranasal debris identifies the responsible organism. The most frequent fungi include members of the Dematiaceae family *(Curvularia, Bipolaris, Exserohilum,* and *Alternaria).* Aspergillus is the next most frequent organism. Other fungi reported in AFS include *Rhizopus, Chrysosporium, Cladosporium, Fusarium,* and *Nodulisporium.* In the past, *Helminthosporium* included dematiaceous fungi that were classified as *Bipolaris, Exserohilum,* and *Drechslera.* Species of *Drechslera* have now been recategorized as *Bipolaris.* Commercially available fungal antigens for in vitro and skin testing are listed in Table 1. The specific fungal organism isolated does not appear to influence treatment or prognosis. AFS is not believed to be contagious.

Pathogenesis

It is not clear how fungi in the nasal cavity progress to the clinical syndrome of AFS. Involved in the pathogenesis may be the tenacity of the mucus, multiple previous courses of broad-spectrum antibiotics allowing fungal proliferation, the allergenic load or amount of fungus present, a defective ciliary system, and entrapment of fungi in sinuses after ostiomeatal unit obstruction and/or tissue hypoxia.

Presumably, prolonged contact of the fungus with sinonasal mucosa in an individual who has an immunologic predisposition leads to an immune reaction that worsens the condition. One-half of patients with AFS have an elevated absolute eosinophil count and a raised level of total immunoglobulin E (IgE). One-third to one-half of patients have positive skin test results to multiple allergens. Fungal-specific IgE is detectable by radioallergosorbent testing (Gell and Coombs type I hypersensitivity reaction). Fungal-specific IgG can also be detected in the serum of AFS patients (Table 2). Type III (immune complex–mediated) reactions are also involved. AFS may derive from a fungus ball that progresses through an allergic process in an atopic host.

Diagnosis

A high index of suspicion is necessary to diagnose AFS. Suspicion is usually elevated during FESS, when viscid mucus is discovered. There are no universally agreed upon criteria

Table 1. Commercially Available Fungal Antigens

		IN VITRO TESTS FOR SPECIFIC IgE			
GENUS	SPECIES*	IMMUNOCAP (ELISA)	DISC METHOD (ELISA)	HYCOR (ELISA)	SKIN TEST ANTIGENS
Aspergillus	*Fumigatus*	Pharmacia	Sanofi	Hytec	Bayer
	Flavus	—	—	Hytec	—
	Niger	—	—	Hytec	Bayer
	Amstelodami	—	—	Hytec	—
	Versicolor	—	—	Hytec	—
	Clavatus	—	—	Hytec	Bayer
	Glaucus	—	—	—	Bayer
	Nidulans	—	—	Hytec	Bayer
	Restictus	—	—	—	Bayer
	Sydowi	—	—	—	Bayer
	Terreus	—	—	Hytec	Bayer
	Oryzae	—	—	Hytec	—
	Retens	—	—	Hytec	—
Curvularia	*Lunata*	Pharmacia	—	—	—
	Spicifera	—	—	Hytec	Bayer
Alternaria	*Alternata*	Pharmacia	—	—	—
	Tenius	—	Sanofi	Hytec	Bayer
Helminthosporium	*Halodes*	Pharmacia	—	Hytec	Bayer
	Interseminat	—	—	Hytec	Bayer
	Maydis	—	—	—	Bayer
Bipolaris		—	—	—	—
Exserohilum		—	—	—	—

ELISA, enzyme-linked immunosorbent assay; IgE, immunoglobulin E.

Company information is as follows: Pharmacia, Uppsala, Sweden; Sanofi Diagnostics, Chaska, Minn; Hytec, Hycor Biomedical, Irvine, Calif; Bayer Corporation, Spokane, Wash.

* AFS has not been reported with all species in this table. However, all species may be useful because cross-reactivity exists among species within the same genus.

Modified and updated from Corey JP, Delsupehe KG, Ferguson BJ. Allergic fungal sinusitis: Allergic, infectious, or both? Otolaryngol Head Neck Surg 1995;113:110–119.

Table 2. Immunologic Parameters of Allergic Fungal Sinusitis

MECHANISM	CLINICAL PRESENTATION	SKIN TEST IMMEDIATE/ LATE	TOTAL IgE	TOTAL EOSINOPHILS	IgE FUNGAL ANTIGEN	IgG FUNGAL ANTIGEN	PRECIPITATING ANTIBODIES
Types I and III (probable)	Recurrent sinusitis, refractory to conventional therapy	+/?	Elevated in some patients	Elevated	Elevated	Frequently elevated	?

IgE, immunoglobulin E; IgG, immunoglobulin G.
Modified from Corey JP, Bumstead RM, Panje WR, et al. Allergy and fungal screens in chronic sinusitis. Am J Rhinol 1990; 4:25–28.

Table 3. Suggested Diagnostic Criteria for Allergic Fungal Sinusitis

CRITERIA	COREY (1997)	BENT (1996)	CODY (1994)	SCHWEITZE (1992)	DE SHAZO (1992)
Allergic mucin present	+++	+++	+++	+++	+++
No mucosal invasion	+++	+++	+++	NI	+++
Fungus (stain or culture)	+++	+++	+++	+++	+++
Type I hypersensitivity	+++	+++	NI	NI	NI
Characteristic CT scan	+	+++	NI	NI	+++
Nasal polyps	+	+++	NI	NI	+
Eosinophilia	+	+	NI	+++	NI
Skin test reactivity	+	NI	NI	+++	NI
Elevated IgE	+	NI	+	+++	+
Elevated specific IgE	+	NI	+	+++	NI
Precipitating antibodies	+	NI	NI	+++	+
No diabetes mellitus or immunosuppression	+	NI	NI	NI	+++

IgE, immunoglobulin E; +++, major criteria for the diagnosis of AFS; +, minor criteria; NI, no information in this author's criteria.

to diagnose AFS. Central to most criteria is the presence of allergic mucin and detectable noninvasive fungus. Table 3 illustrates some recently suggested criteria for the diagnosis of AFS.

■ THERAPY

There have been no prospective published treatment trials to date, due to the relative rarity of this condition. Integral to what is believed to be appropriate treatment of AFS are eradication of fungal organisms and re-establishment of normal sinus ventilation and drainage through FESS. Larger fungal concretions or excessively thick mucus may require open procedures, such as the Caldwell-Luc operation, for adequate eradication. A conservative approach is indicated for this benign disease, in that uninvolved tissue is preserved. Much too frequently, even optimal surgical treatment is followed by recurrence, which indicates that AFS cannot be treated exclusively by surgery.

Also believed to be important in treatment are oral steroids (0.5 to 1.0 milligrams per kilogram daily) administered postoperatively to suppress immune hypersensitivity for several weeks. The duration of oral steroid use has not been established definitively; some authors discontinue steroids a few months postoperatively, whereas others maintain them indefinitely. Children should have steroids weaned at a faster rate than adults to prevent steroid-induced growth retardation. However, there are many reports of recurrence as steroids are weaned.

Waxman reported that different prognostic groups experienced recurrences at different rates. Unfortunately, no preoperative identifying features separated the prognostic groups. The role of topical steroids is unproved, but most physicians recommend their use.

Systemic or oral antifungals do not offer clinical benefit, but are recommended for intracranial or intraorbital involvement. Because the organism is extramucosal, topical antifungals may play a role in therapy, but this is unproved and has attracted considerable interest in anecdotal reports. In vitro testing of fungi against commonly used antifungal agents noted ketoconazole and amphotericin B to be the most active, which supports their theoretic use in nasal irrigations. Most clinicians recommend immunotherapy for nonfungal antigens if patients are sensitized. However, the use of immunotherapy for fungal antigens is controversial. There is some evidence that immunotherapy for fungal antigens may be helpful. Theoretically, immunotherapy may be counterproductive by elevating IgG, which is implicated in the pathophysiology of AFS (type III reaction). However, preliminary reports as well as the senior author's personal experience with AFS patients suggests the opposite—that patients do better with immunotherapy. The pathophysiology behind improvement could include a reduction in the "allergic load" presented to the patient.

FESS also reduces the allergic load; environmental measures to reduce fungal exposure are also indicated. The fungi that cause AFS are primarily soil organisms. Fungi proliferate in moist, dark sites such as basements, bathrooms, and areas with many houseplants.

Follow-up

Follow-up should involve close clinical, endoscopic, and radiographic evaluations. Recurrence is initially signaled by the resurgence of nasal symptoms, with crusting and polyps or polypoid mucosal change. Reculture and/or biopsy should be performed to identify fungal presence. Eosinophilia and elevated total serum IgE are present in most (but not all) patients who have AFS, and these markers have been anecdotally used to monitor disease activity. Reported recurrence rates range from 32 percent to 100 percent. Bent and Kuhn have had no long-term cures among their more than 50 patients who have AFS. Reasons for poor long-term outcome may be related to an incompletely treated surgical approach, repeat presentation and recolonization of fungi, or an "out of control" allergic diathesis.

Complications

Extension into the orbit or anterior cranial fossa may develop from bony dissolution by inflammatory mediators or pressure-induced bone necrosis. Visual loss and frontal lobe involvement have been reported. A theoretic progression of AFS to invasive fungal sinusitis with an increased morbidity and mortality is possible.

Suggested Reading

Allphin AL, Strauss M, Abdul-Karim FW. Allergic fungal sinusitis: Problems in diagnosis and treatment. Laryngoscope 1991; 101:815-820.

Bent JP, Kuhn FA. Allergic fungal sinusitis/polyposis. Allergy Asthma Proc 1996; 17:259-268.

Bent JP, Kuhn FA. Antifungal activity against allergic fungal sinusitis organisms. Laryngoscope 1996; 106:1331-1334.

Bent JP, Kuhn FA. Diagnosis of allergic fungal sinusitis. Otolaryngol Head Neck Surg 1994; 111:580-588.

Cody DT, Neel HB, Ferreiro JA, Roberts GD. Allergic fungal sinusitis: The Mayo Clinic experience. Laryngoscope 1994: 104:1074-1079.

Corey JP. Allergic fungal sinusitis. Otolaryngol Clin North Am 1992; 25: 225-230.

Corey JP, Bumstead RM, Panje WR, et al. Allergy and fungal screens in chronic sinusitis. Am J Rhinol 1990; 4:25-28.

Corey JP, Delsupehe KG, Ferguson BJ. Allergic fungal sinusitis: Allergic, infectious, or both. Otolaryngol Head Neck Surg 1995; 113:110-119.

Friedman GC, Hartwick WJ, Ro JY, et al. Allergic fungal sinusitis—Report of three cases associated with dematiaceous fungi. Am J Clin Pathol 1991; 96:368-372.

Goldstein MF. Allergic fungal sinusitis: An underdiagnosed problem. Hosp Pract 1992; 27:73-92.

Hartwick RW, Batsakis JG. Pathology consultation: Sinus *aspergillosis* and allergic fungal sinusitis. Ann Otol Rhinol Laryngol 1991; 100:427-430.

Katzenstein ALA, Sale SR, Greenberger PA. Allergic *Aspergillus* sinusitis: A newly recognized form of sinusitis. J Allergy Clin Immunol 1983; 72:89-93.

Kupferberg SB, Bent, JB. Allergic fungal sinusitis in the pediatric population. Arch Otolaryngol Head Neck Surg 1996; 122:1381-1384.

Mabry RL, Manning S. Radioallergosorbent microscreen and total immunoglobulin E in allergic fungal sinusitis. Otolaryngol Head Neck Surg 1995; 113:721-723.

Manning SC, Mabry RL, Schaefer SD, Close LG. Evidence of IgE-mediated hypersensitivity in allergic fungal sinusitis. Laryngoscope 103: 717-721.

Morpeth JF, Rupp NT, Dolen WK, et al. Fungal sinusitis: An update. Ann Allergy Asthma Immunol 1996; 76:128-140.

Schwartz HJ. Allergic fungal sinusitis: Experience in an ambulatory allergy practice. Ann Allergy Asthma Immunol 1996; 77:500-502.

Schweitze LA, Gourley DS. Allergic fungal sinusitis. Allergy Proc 1992; 13:3-6.

de Shazo RD, Swain RE. Diagnostic criteria for allergic fungal sinusitis. J Allergy Clin Immunol 1995; 96:24-35.

Travis WD, Kwon-Chung KJ, Kleiner DE, et al. Unusual aspects of allergic bronchopulmonary fungal disease: Report of two cases due to *Curvularia* organisms associated with allergic fungal sinusitis. Hum Pathol 1991; 22:1240-1248.

Waxman JE, Spector JG, Sale SR, Katzenstein AL. Allergic *Aspergillus* sinusitis: Concepts in diagnosis and treatment of a new entity. Laryngoscope 1987; 97:261-266.

Index

Page numbers followed by *f* indicate figures; page numbers followed by *t* indicate tables.

D

E

G

H

Q

R

U

V

W

X

Y

Z